E. N. T

THEATRES

Scott-Brown's Otolaryngology
Fifth edition

Basic Sciences

Scott-Brown's Otolaryngology

Fifth edition

General Editor

Alan G. Kerr FRCS

Consultant Otolaryngologist, Royal Victoria Hospital, Belfast and Belfast City Hospital;
Formerly Professor of Otorhinolaryngology, The Queen's University, Belfast

Advisory Editor

John Groves FRCS

Consultant Otolaryngologist, Royal Free Hospital, London

Other volumes

2 **Adult Audiology** *edited by* Dafydd Stephens

3 **Otology** *edited by* John B. Booth

4 **Rhinology** *edited by* Ian S. Mackay and T. R. Bull

5 **Laryngology** *edited by* P. M. Stell

6 **Paediatric Otolaryngology** *edited by* John N. G. Evans

Basic Sciences

Editor

David Wright MA, BChir, FRCS

Consultant Otolaryngologist, The Royal Surrey County Hospital, Guildford;
Honorary Consultant Otolaryngologist, The Cambridge Military Hospital

Butterworths

London Boston Durban Singapore Sydney Toronto Wellington

First edition, 1952
Second edition, 1965
  Reprinted, 1967, 1968
Third edition, 1971
  Reprinted, 1977
Fourth edition, 1979
  Reprinted 1984
Fifth edition, 1987

Butterworth International Edition, 1987
ISBN-0-407-00518-8   ISBN-0-407-00521-8
ISBN-0-407-00522-6   ISBN-0-407-00523-4
ISBN-0-407-00524-2   ISBN-0-407-00525-0
ISBN-0-407-00517-X (set of six volumes)

© **Butterworth & Co. (Publishers) Ltd, 1987**

British Library Cataloguing in Publication Data

Scott-Brown, Walter Graham
    Scott-Brown's otolaryngology.—5th ed.
    1. Otolaryngology
    I. Title   II. Kerr, A. G.   III. Groves, John,
    1925-   IV. Scott-Brown, Walter Graham.
    Scott-Brown's diseases of the ear, nose and throat
    617'.57   RF46

    ISBN 0-407-00511-0   ISBN 0-407-00512-9
    ISBN 0-407-00513-7   ISBN 0-407-00514-5
    ISBN 0-407-00515-3   ISBN 0-407-00516-1
    ISBN 0-407-00510-2 (set of six volumes)

Library of Congress Cataloging-in-Publication Data
Basic sciences.

    (Scott-Brown's otolaryngology; v. 1)
    Includes Bibliographies and indexes
    1. Otolaryngology.   I. Wright, David (David Arthur)
    II. Series.   [DNLM: 1. Otolaryngology. WV 100 S4313 v.1]
    RF46.B36   1987   617'.51   87-14624
    ISBN 0-407-00511-0

Photoset by Butterworths Litho Preparation Department
Printed and bound in Great Britain by Butler and Tanner, Frome, Somerset

Historical introduction

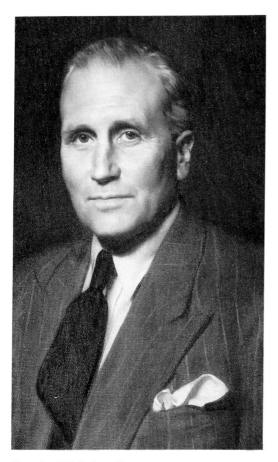

Portrait of W. G. Scott-Brown, CVO, MD, FRCS (1897–1987)

About 36 years ago Bill Scott-Brown suffered a major coronary infarct and being strictly ordered to 'rest' for six months set himself to create, as Editor (not author, because that would have been too strenuous, he thought) this work of his own inspiration. In 1952 I was among the first generation of FRCS candidates for whom it was the Bible. We all revered 'Negus' for the nose and throat (some of us still do) but Scott-Brown, in two volumes as it then was, provided the first post-war text for otolaryngology across the board. SB (as he was known) was probably the only person to be at all surprised by the success of his achievement, and to find himself in due course under notice from Butterworth's to prepare a second edition. It was at this stage that he recruited John Ballantyne and myself and the second, third and fourth editions were produced by the two of us under his friendly eye. For the third edition we succumbed to the inevitable by expanding two fat volumes into four (slightly) thinner ones, only to find that the fourth edition in its turn required four fat ones.

Throughout this 20 year period John Ballantyne and I derived constant satisfaction and pleasure from the ongoing association with so many willing friends and contributors past and present. We thank them warmly.

We know that the ENT fraternity world-wide has pleasure in the knowledge that SB continued in his retirement still to take satisfaction from the perpetuation of his work. The sad news of his death came just as this new edition went to press. Those who knew him will perhaps see in this Fifth Edition, and the 35th year of his book, a memorial to his achievement.

John Groves
Advisory Editor

Introduction

When I was first invited to edit the Fifth Edition of *Scott-Brown's Otolaryngology*, I thought I was aware of the enormity of the task and my own limitations. As time progressed, I realized that I had misjudged both.

This work has represented the mainstream of British otolaryngological thinking for over thirty years. However, the increase in the breadth and depth of our specialty is such that only a gifted few can be conversant with all aspects of it. Hence, I realized that I could not undertake the task without help. I have been most fortunate in having such a distinguished group of volume editors, all of whom are already well-known in British otolaryngology, and all of whom have beeen delightful and stimulating colleagues in this work. It has been a joy to work with them.

Modern otolaryngology has widened in recent decades, and procedures are now being performed that are no longer covered by the term 'ear, nose and throat surgery'. This work attempts to embrace all the areas that so-called ear, nose and throat surgeons are covering at the present time, and hence the change of the title to *Scott-Brown's Otolaryngology*.

For the new edition *Scott-Brown* has grown from four to six volumes. An entirely new volume has been introduced in recognition of the subspecialty of paediatric otolaryngology and the amount of material in audiological medicine is now great enough to justify its separation from the Ear volume. Although these are now specialties in their own rights, they are also, and will continue to be beyond the lifetime of this edition, part of the routine practice of most British otolaryngologists. To enable these new volumes to stand alone, a certain amount of overlap with other volumes has been necessary.

In any multi-author and multi-volume production, overlap is always necessary if each chapter is to be developed freely, and if there is to be easy reference to subjects dealt with in more than one volume. Consequently, I ask for the reader's indulgence in those sections where overlap has been planned and deliberate. Where it has occurred as a result of my ineptitude, I apologize.

The editorial team have been very pleased at the response of those invited to contribute, although, unfortunately, a few leading members of our specialty were unable to accept the invitation. However, by and large, those asked were both cooperative and energetic in their responses, and have given freely of themselves in their contributions. I have been most impressed by the spirit of goodwill among the otolaryngologists in this country, and I am grateful to them.

In the production of this edition, I have seen myself as custodian of a great British institution. I have always been aware of the privilege and responsibility of my position, and am grateful for the advice I have received from many senior and not so senior members of our specialty. I am particularly indebted to the Advisory Editor, John Groves, and to his former editorial colleague, John Ballantyne. My respect and admiration for these colleagues has risen, not simply because of the invaluable help they have given so freely in this edition, but because I now realise the enormity of their accomplishment and their contribution to British otolaryngology in editing the last three editions.

I also wish to express my thanks to those in Belfast who have helped with, or suffered because of, the Fifth Edition. Some have done both, and without their backing and encouragement this work would not have been possible. It would be invidious to try to name everyone. Various secretaries have been of enormous help, and without this I could not have produced this edition. My consultant colleagues have advised and encouraged me, and my junior colleagues have given very practical advice in their down-to-earth comments and invaluable help with proof-reading. My family have been both encouraging and remarkably tolerant of the long hours required to edit such a work as this.

The staff at Butterworths were helpful and encouraging throughout. Initially, Peter Richardson set the wheels in motion. He was followed as publisher by Charles Fry, who was assisted by Anne Smith and Jane Bryant. The sub-editors have been Anne Powell and Jane Sugarman. The general spirit of pleasant cooperation and tolerance has been delightful.

I am sufficiently optimistic to believe that there will be a Sixth Edition. I do not know who will be editing it. However, if the reader has any constructive comments or criticisms, I should be pleased to have them ... in writing! I can not guarantee to acknowledge these, but I promise that, if I am the editor, I shall give them due consideration, and, if not, I shall make them available to my successor.

Alan G. Kerr

Preface

Basic Sciences was a large and comprehensive volume in the earlier editions of *Scott-Brown* and to make it even larger for the Fifth Edition could have presented difficulties. However, an opportunity to update the information in a new scientific textbook should always be taken, and this has been done by combining and refining some of the chapters from the Fourth Edition and introducing seven new areas of study.

The chapter, 'The anatomy of the ear' has been expanded to include the ultrastructures of the ear and the chapter, 'Physiology of the ear' has been divided to give a completely new chapter–'The auditory perception of sound'. I am particularly pleased to include Mr Proops' chapter for I have always considered that most young ENT trainees have little opportunity to acquire knowledge about the mouth and maxillofacial structures as most present training programmes stand. Dr Patten has produced some remarkable drawings of the nervous system which I hope will clarify the presentation of the differential diagnosis of diseases affecting neuro-otolaryngological function.

Possibly there have been more new technical developments in radiography and imaging than any other, and the author Mr Peter Phelps has explained the basis for these new techniques and also contributed chapters to four of the other volumes of this edition. The chapter on laser surgery is new and includes clinical aspects of laser treatment. Each specialty now takes a greater interest in, and more responsibility for, its own plastic work and I am grateful to Dr Panje for writing a comprehensive chapter covering the basic principles of the subject. Intensive care units are now highly specialized and managed by anaesthetists, but every surgeon remains responsible for the immediate resuscitation of his or her patient, so I value the inclusion of Dr Leigh's contribution.

Finally, there is a totally new chapter on Biomaterials, a subject which may, in the future, have a significant place in reconsructive procedures in both the ear and nose.

Editing this volume has been a stimulating and rewarding experience for me. I am deeply aware of the significant contribution made by Mr W. G. Scott-Brown, CVO, MD, FRCS, in bringing out the First Edition of this widely accepted textbook, and to expansion of subsequent editions, by Mr John Ballantyne, CBE, FRCS and Mr John Groves, FRCS. It has been a privilege to follow them as I served my clinical apprenticeship with all three surgeons. I will have long-lasting gratitude to all thirty-two authors who have contributed from their experience on a wide range of subjects and to the Chief Editor, Alan Kerr, who, at all times, was available to offer advice. I am particularly grateful to Surgeon Captain Head for allowing the figures of his chapter in the previous edition to be included in the combined chapter on Pathophysiology of the ears and nasal sinuses in flying and diving. I would like to thank Linda Schabedly for assisting me with the proof reading, the editorial staff at Butterworths for their assistance, and finally to my family for their encouragement and indulgence.

David Wright
Guildford 1987

Contributors to this volume

Michael Apps, MA, MD, MRCP
Consultant Physician, Harold Wood Hospital, Essex

C. M. Bailey, BSc, FRCS
Consultant Otolaryngologist, The Hospitals for Sick Children, Great Ormond Street and The Royal National Throat, Nose and Ear Hospital, London

Patrick Beasley, MB, BS, FRCS, DLO
Consultant Otolaryngologist, The Department of Otolaryngology, The Royal Devon and Exeter Hospital, Exeter

Alan J. Benson, MSc, MB, ChB, FRACS
Senior Medical Officer (Research), Royal Air Force Institute of Aviation Medicine, Farnborough

J. A. S. Carruth, MA, MB, BChir, FRCS
Senior Lecturer in Otolaryngology at Southampton University and Consultant Otolaryngologist at the University Hospitals, Southampton

R. Y. Cartwright, MB, FRCPath
Consultant Microbiologist; Director Guildford Public Health Laboratory; Honorary Visiting Professor in Clinical Microbiology, University of Surrey

S. J. Challacombe, PhD, BDS, MRCPath
Consultant in Diagnostic Microbiology, Immunology and Oral Medicine; Head of Department of Oral Medicine and Pathology, United Medical and Dental Schools of Guy's and St Thomas's Hosptials, London

Henry J. L. Craig, MD, DA, FFARCS, FFARCSI
Consultant Anaesthetist, Royal Victoria Hospital, Belfast

Adrian Brendan Drake-Lee, MB, ChB, FRCS
Consultant ENT Surgeon, Royal United Hospital, Bath; Honorary Senior Lecturer, The Institute of Laryngology and Otology, London

Adrian Fourcin, PhD
Professor of Experimental Phonetics, University of London

Michael Gleeson, FRCS
Senior Lecturer and Consultant, Guy's and Lewisham Hospitals, London

J. J. Groté,
Clinical Professor, University of Leiden, The Netherlands

Bridget T. Hill, PhD, FRSC, FIBiol
Head, Laboratory of Cellular Chemotherapy, Imperial Cancer Research Fund, London; and Honorary Senior Lecturer, Institute of Urology, London

Guy Kenyon, BSc, FRCS
Consultant ENT Surgeon, The London Hospital

Air Vice-Marshal P. F. King, OBE, QMS, FRCS (Ed), DLO
The Senior Consultant RAF, and Consultant in Otolaryngology; Lately Whittingham Professor of Aviation Medicine, Royal College of Physicians, London

Julian M. Leigh, MD, FFARCS
Director, Intensive Care Unit, Royal Surrey
County Hospital, Guildford

W. S. Lund, MS, FRCS
Consultant Ear, Nose and Throat Surgeon, The
Radcliffe Infirmary, Oxford

Linda M. Luxon, BSc, MBBS (Hons), FRCP (UK)
Department of Neuro-otology, The National
Hospital for Nervous Diseases, London

Brian C. J. Moore, MA, PhD
University Lecturer in Experimental Psychology,
University of Cambridge

William R. Panje, BS, MS, MD, MS (Otol.), FACS
Professor and Chairman, Otolaryngology – Head
and Neck Surgery, The Pritzker School of
Medicine, The University of Chicago

John Philip Patten, BSc, MB, FRCP
Consultant Neurologist (South West Thames
Regional Health Authority), Guildford

Peter D. Phelps, MD (Lond.), FRCS, FRCR, DMRD
Consultant Radiologist, Walsgrove Hospital,
Coventry; Honorary Consultant, Royal National
Throat, Nose and Ear Hospital, London

L. A. Price, MD (Lond.), MRCP (UK)
United Kingdom Representative, Scientific
Advisory Council, New York Chemotherapy
Foundation

James O. Pickles, MA, MSc, PhD
Lecturer in Physiology, University of Birmingham

William J. Primrose, FRCS
Consultant ENT Surgeon, Royal Victoria Hospital,
Belfast

David W. Proops, BDS, MB, FRCS
Consultant ENT Surgeon, Queen Elizabeth
Hospital, and The Children's Hospital,
Birmingham

Lee S. Rayfield, BSc, PhD
Lecturer in Immunology, United Medical and
Dental Schools of Guy's and St Thomas's
Hospitals, London

P. H. Rhys Evans, MB, DCC, FRCS
The Head and Neck Unit, The Royal Marsden
Hospital, London

O. H. Shaheen, MS, FRCS
Consultant ENT Surgeon, Guy's Hospital, and
The Royal National Throat, Nose and Ear
Hospital, London

Neil Weir, MB, BS, FRCS
Consultant Ear, Nose and Throat Surgeon, Royal
Surrey County Hospital Guildford; Honorary
Consultant Neuro-otologist, St. George's
Hospital, London

Anthony Wright, DM, FRCS (Ed.) Tech RMS
Senior Lecturer in Otology, Institute of
Laryngology and Otology, London

W. F. White, MB, BS, MRCS, LRCP, DMRT, FRCR
Consultant Radiotherapist and Oncologist, St
Luke's Hospital, Guildford, and King Edward VII
Hospital, Midhurst

Contents

Colour plates in this volume

1

Anatomy and ultrastructure of the human ear

Anthony Wright

Development of the human ear

In accordance with longstanding convention, the adult ear is here described in terms of its three portions, namely the outer, the middle and the inner ear. The inner ear, comprising the bony and membranous labyrinth with its central connections, arises from a set of structures quite distinct from those which give rise to the outer and middle ears. The development of the inner ear, which is the first organ of the special senses to become fully formed in man, is considered first, following a short, general description of the growth of the nervous system.

Prenatal development is divided into a number of separate periods. The first period extends from the time of implantation of the developing blastocyst into the uterine wall until an intra-embryonic circulation has started to develop. During this short period of about 21 days, the three layers of ectoderm, mesoderm and endoderm develop to form a flat, elongated plate containing the notochord. This rod-like structure is derived from the ectodermal layer, and extends along the length of the embryonic disc from the buccopharyngeal membrane to the cloacal membrane, where ectoderm and endoderm are in direct contact (*Figure 1.1*). The second brief period of about 35 days, that is until the end of the eighth week, is termed the embryonic period. During this time there is rapid growth and cellular differentiation, so that by the fifty-sixth day all the major systems and organs are formed and the embryo has an external shape that is recognizably human. The remaining 7 months of gestation form the fetal period, during which there is rapid growth characterized by changes of shape, and by alterations in the position of one structure to another, rather than by the differentiation of new cell types.

During the embryonic period, the thickened mesoderm on each side of the notochord separates into paired cubical blocks called somites. The first occipital somite lies just behind the head end of the notochord, and no other somites develop further forward from this for the reason that here the mesoderm gives rise to, among other structures, the branchial (or pharyngeal) arches. Forty-one to forty-three more pairs of somites develop in a tailward direction during the first 9 days of the embryonic period.

The ectoderm not only assumes the shape of the underlying, developing mass of mesoderm but

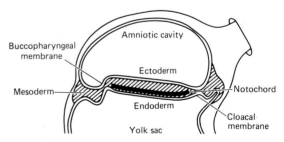

Figure 1.1 Highly diagrammatic representation of a longitudinal section of the developing embryonic disc. The structure never looks like this at any one time since development is progressing at different rates. Nevertheless, mesoderm lies between ectoderm and endoderm except at the buccopharyngeal and cloacal membranes where the two layers are in contact. The notochord, a derivative of the ectodermal layer, lies within the mass of mesoderm. A connecting stalk attaches the developing disc with its amniotic cavity and yolk sac to the uterine wall, and these structures lie within the extra-embryonic coelom at this stage of development

also thickens in the region of the notochord to form the midline neural plate. On each side of this plate, a longitudinal band of ectoderm called the neural crest develops. The neural plate subsequently sinks in to form the neural groove, the walls of which eventually close over to produce the neural tube surrounding the neural canal (*Figure 1.2*). While the neural groove is closing, the

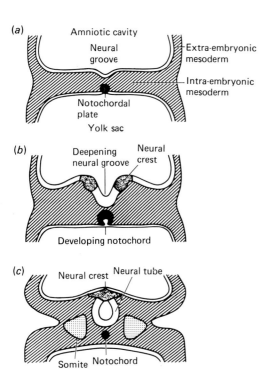

Figure 1.2 Transverse section of the developing embryonic disc at various stages of development. In the early presomite stage (*a*) a midline neural groove is present above the notochordal plate which is fused with the endodermal layer. The neural groove deepens (*b*) and specialized neural crest cells develop on the lips of the groove. The notochord separates from the endodermal layer. By the somite stage (*c*) the neural tube has formed and the neural crest cells are about to migrate to form cell clusters which at the head end of the embryo become the cranial sensory nerve ganglia. Cells from the neural crest also form the posterior root ganglion of the spinal cord and the cells of the sympathetic ganglia

neural crest cells sink in from the surface to lie alongside the completed neural tube. At the head end, the neural tube undergoes rapid enlargement and dilatation to form the hindbrain, the midbrain and the forebrain. These last two extend forward past the notochord and buccopharyngeal membrane, which by now has broken down to allow the formation of the buccal cavity.

The neural crest cells, lying alongside the developing brain and spinal cord, develop into a chain of cell clusters which, at the head end of the embryo, form three groups: trigeminal; facial and auditory; and glossopharyngeal and vagal. These clusters contain uni- or bipolar nerve cells and form the cranial sensory nerve ganglia. They link the peripheral sensory receptors with the afferent nuclei in the hindbrain. Motor nerve fibres arise directly from the cell bodies in the three efferent columns in the hindbrain and pass directly to striated muscles or, by way of a synapse, to non-striated muscle and glandular tissue.

The membranous labyrinth

When the embryo has reached the seventh somite stage (about 22 days), a thickening of the ectoderm forms just in front of the first occipital somite on each side of the still open neural groove. This thickening is the otic placode. The mesoderm surrounding this region proliferates and elevates the ectoderm around the placode, which subsequently sinks below the surface to become the otic pit. The ectoderm of the pit undergoes rapid growth, the mouth of the pit narrows and eventually closes, so that by the thirtieth somite (30 day) stage, an enlarging otocyst separated from the surface has been formed and lies anterior and medial to the combined facial and auditory cluster of neural crest cells. The geniculate ganglion migrates from this cluster leaving the auditory (vestibulocochlear) ganglion in close proximity to the otocyst (*Figure 1.3*).

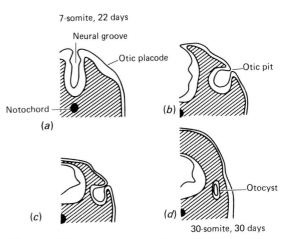

Figure 1.3 Diagram to represent the development of the otocyst from the otic placode which in turn is derived from the ectoderm cranial to the first occipital somite. During the seven days of its development the neural groove has also become converted into the future brainstem

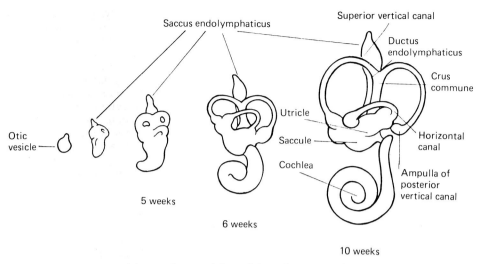

Figure 1.4 Development of the membranous labyrinth from the otocyst. This rapid and complex change occurs over a six-week period

Within 1 or 2 days, the otocyst has lengthened and an apparent infolding of the wall marks off a medial compartment, the endolymphatic duct, from a more lateral compartment, the utriculo-saccular chamber. This period is a time of rapid change, and complex alterations in the shape of different parts of the otocyst occur synchronously. The walls of the chamber grow inwards so that a number of constructions and folds appear, separating the utricle from the saccule. The major change is an ingrowth of the lateral wall assisted by a further enlargement of the initial fold (now called the utricular fold) that together separate the utricular chamber from the endolymphatic duct, and thus form the utricular duct. A lesser change is a separate ingrowth from the medial wall that divides the saccular chamber from the endolymphatic duct and thereby forms the saccular duct (*Figure 1.4*).

Meanwhile, the endolymphatic system is elongating in a medial direction towards the hindbrain; a proximal dilatation, the endolymphatic sinus, a middle, narrow endolymphatic duct and a widened distal endolymphatic sac are formed.

At the same time, other changes are occurring in the utricular chamber. At 35 days, three flattened hollow pouches push out approximately at right angles to each other, to form superior, posterior and lateral ridges. At the centre of each curved ridge, the opposing epithelial walls meet, fuse and break down to be replaced by the surrounding mesoderm. In this way, the superior ridge, at about 6 weeks, is transformed into the superior semicircular duct, with the transformation of the other two, the posterior before the lateral, taking place soon afterwards.

While the semicircular ducts are developing, and before the complete formation of the utricular and saccular duct has taken place, the saccule is putting out a single medially directed pouch which is the beginning of the cochlear duct. This grows medially and starts to coil, with the result that at the beginning of fetal life one coil is present, and by 25 weeks the adult form of two-and-one-half coils has been achieved. As the cochlear duct develops, it becomes isolated from the saccule by a construction called the ductus reuniens.

During this period of complex growth, other changes occur within the otocyst. Thickened epithelial areas develop in certain portions of its walls in relationship to the ingrowth of nerve fibres from the bipolar cells of the vestibulocochlear ganglion. The specialized areas of neuroepithelium are the maculae, the cristae and the organ of Corti.

The maculae

The maculae develop from the epithelium that overlies the areas where nerves enter the walls of the saccule and utricle. Two cell types differentiate: the sensory cells, with a single kinocilium and many stereocilia, projecting into the cavity of the otocyst; and the supporting cells. These latter cells appear to be responsible for the formation of the otoconia, although the early stages are not well understood. It seems likely that very small calcium-containing primitive otoconia are produced by the supporting cells and it is these that provide the nucleus for the multi-layered deposition of the calcite form of calcium carbonate to

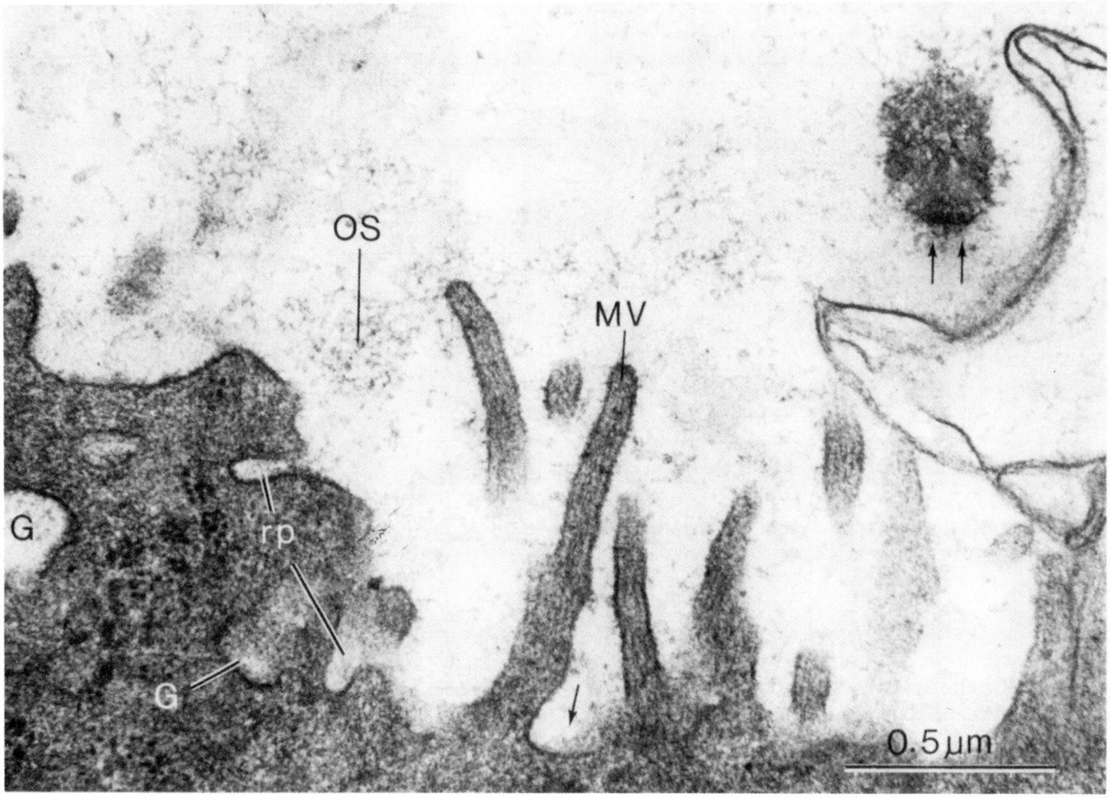

Figure 1.5 A small primitive otoconial crystal with recognizable shape (double arrows) is being formed near the long microvilli (MV) of the supporting cells of a 16.5-day mouse embryo. The specific granules that go to form the core of the crystal seem to come from pinocytic vesicles (G) that eventually fuse with the cytoplasmic membrane to release the granules (single arrow). Various organic substances (OS) which possibly form the gelatinous layer of the otoconial membrane seem to be secreted by reverse pinocytosis from the supporting cells. (Photograph courtesy of David Lim)

produce the mature otoconia with their characteristic shape (*see* section on adult anatomy) (*Figure 1.5*). The supporting cells also produce a gelatinous matrix that subsequently forms the gelatinous layer of the definitive otoconial membrane. In the very early stages of otoconial formation in man this matrix is not present. However, by 14–16 weeks, the individual parts of the maculae have assumed an adult form with the sensory and supporting cells being overlaid by the mature otoconial membrane (*see* Lim, 1984, for an excellent review).

The cristae of the semicircular ducts

At one end of each semicircular duct, a portion of the epithelial lining proliferates and heaps up to form the ridge-like cristae. Differentiation into sensory and supporting cells occurs and this takes place on what will eventually become the convex side of the definitive semicircular canal. The membranous duct in this region enlarges to form the ampulla and, subsequently, a fibrogelatinous structure – the cupula – develops with the lumen. It probably originates from the supporting cells and is present in the 24-week old fetus. Both the cupula and the otoconial membrane (as well as the tectorial membrane) are extremely sensitive to distortion and shrinkage during routine histological preparation; therefore, the shape seen in such preparations does not represent that found in life. Especial care has to be taken to preserve the real shape and form of these structures.

As the ampulla enlarges, the crista grows with it, so that by the time it has reached its adult size, at about 23 weeks, it has become a curved ridge covering the floor and extending part way up the side walls of the ampulla (*Figure 1.6*).

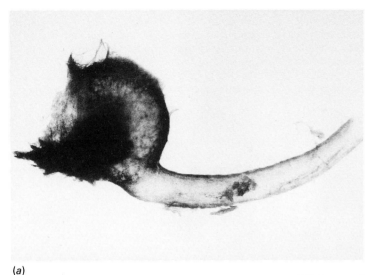

(a)

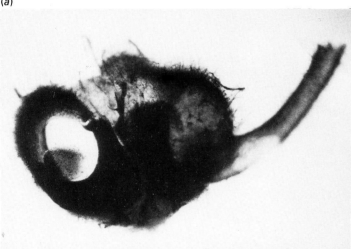

(b)

Figure 1.6 (*a*) Light micrograph of part of an osmium-stained semicircular duct and attached ampulla. This specimen comes from a young adult human. Within the ampulla the darkened crista can be seen. (*b*) View of the ampullae of the lateral and superior semicircular ducts. The crista is now seen more clearly as a saddle-shaped ridge in the open ampulla. Lying in the ampulla is the wedge-shaped cupula. With this method of preparation the cupula has shrunken considerably, but *in vivo* it extends to reach the walls of the ampulla

The organ of Corti

The coils of the cochlear duct are initially circular in cross-section, but with the growth of the surrounding mesoderm, they are converted into a triangular form with a floor and an outer wall at right angles to each other, and a sloping roof completing the triangle. The epithelium lining this duct is originally stratified; however, in the roof, it undergoes regression through columnar, then cuboidal stages, changing finally into a simple squamous epithelium that remains as the lining of the future Reissner's membrane. The epithelium of the outer wall develops into the stria vascularis, a three-layered structure which rests on, and is supplied by, a highly vascular strip developed in the surrounding mesoderm. The epithelium of the floor undergoes a series of spectacular changes to form the highly ordered organ of Corti. The structure of this is described in detail in the section on adult anatomy. During development, however, the stratified epithelium, under the influence of nerve terminals arriving from the cochlear ganglion, heaps up to form a ridge-like structure. This starts at about 11 weeks and the process is more rapid in the basal than the apical regions.

The future tectorial membrane, which is an ill-defined gelatinous membrane, develops and extends over the surface of the neuroepithelium. By 16 weeks, the ridge in the basal coil is more pronounced, so that an inner and outer sulcus are apparent. The inner sulcus is roofed in by the tectorial membrane, while in the outer sulcus the epithelial cells regress to a flattened low cuboidal form. Within the organ of Corti, sensory and supporting cells are developing. A space – the tunnel of Corti – appears within this mass of cells and separates the inner from the outer sensory cells. A cluster of stereocilia and a more laterally placed single kinocilium develop from the surface of each sensory cell, although the kinocilium subsequently degenerates and is not present in man at birth. The presence of the clusters of stereocilia has resulted in the sensory cells being called hair cells. The supporting cells become highly differentiated. Inner and outer pillar cells, on each side of the tunnel of Corti, give mechanical rigidity to the structure. Deiters' cells surround the base of the outer hair cells and send their processes up to the surface of the organ of Corti, which then expand to form the phalangeal processes which separate the upper surface of the outer hair cells. Hensen's and Claudius' cells form the lateral bulk of the organ of Corti, and it is to these that the tectorial membrane is attached laterally. The cells around the outer hair cells separate, so that definite spaces – the spaces of Nuel – develop and communicate with the tunnel of Corti.

As mentioned earlier, differentiation is occurring in a basal to apical direction, so that at any one time most stages of development can be seen in different parts of the cochlea as the duct is elongating. As the cochlear duct grows and coils, the cochlear ganglion also changes shape to complement the new form, to become known as the spiral ganglion. By 25 weeks, the organ of Corti and the spiral ganglion are complete, resembling those in the adult.

The bony labyrinth

Mesoderm surrounds the membranous labyrinth, and it is this which undergoes a series of changes that result in the formation of both the bony otic capsule and the perilymph spaces of the inner ear. The relatively unspecialized mesoderm of the presomite embryo becomes known as the mesenchyme in subsequent embryonic development as it undergoes differentiation into more specialized tissue. The mesenchyme surrounding the derivatives of the otocyst is initially quite dense and becomes chondrified to form the otic capsule. As the membranous labyrinth increases in size, the adjacent cartilage de-differentiates to form a loose periotic tissue. This subsequently regresses to form fluid-filled spaces adjacent to to most of the membranous structures. These are the perilymphatic spaces and they arise first in the region destined to become the vestibule. Subsequently, spaces develop around the cochlear duct, the scala tympani preceding the scala vestibuli. While this latter space is developing, other spaces form around the semicircular ducts so that the completed canals are formed. The perilymph space does not develop where vestibular and cochlear nerve fibres enter the sensory cell regions, and so these remain in close proximity to the cartilaginous otic capsule. Elsewhere, the developing perilymphatic spaces finally become continuous with the result that a tortuous but uninterrupted perilymph-filled space is formed.

The ossification of the remaining cartilaginous otic capsule takes place from 14 centres and begins in the fifteenth or sixteenth week. The last centre to begin ossification does so at 21 weeks, an indication that the otic capsule has, by this time, attained its maximum size. Each ossification centre develops as a three-layered structure comprising an inner periosteal layer, a central layer where mixed ossification of cartilage occurs and an outer periosteal layer. In the central layer, the cartilage cells enlarge, the matrix becomes calcified and the cells then shrink, atrophy and disappear leaving lacunae. Vascular invasion of the calcified cartilage occurs and osteogenic buds enter the lacunae and deposit an osseous lamina on the walls of the space. This is endochondral bone and its formation results in the development of a series of islands of bone enclosed in cartilage. Other osteoblasts derived from the vascular buds lay down endochondral bone on the surface of the remaining cartilage so that, with progressive growth, the vascular spaces are obliterated and the middle layer of the otic capsule will consist of one type of bone (intrachondral) embedded in another (endochondral), with remnants of calcified cartilage. Unlike all other cartilage-derived bones, no remodelling occurs, and the fetal architecture is maintained throughout life. The inner periosteal layer ossifies but remains thin, while the outer layer becomes greatly thickened by the laying down of interconnected plates of bone that form a dense hard petrous structure.

The 14 separate ossification centres fuse to form a single bony box (*Figure 1.7*), without the presence of a single suture line. (For a complete review, *see* Anson and Donaldson, 1981.) The interior of the bony labyrinth 'communicates' with the outside through seven or eight channels, and the facial nerve passing across and around it in a sulcus eventually becomes enclosed by a bony sheath on the lateral, tympanic aspect (*Table 1.1*).

The blood supply of the developing otic capsule comes mainly from the arteries of the tympanic plexus, which are supplied in turn predominantly by the stylomastoid arteries and its branches. The developing membranous labyrinth, however, is supplied almost entirely by branches of the internal auditory artery, and this pattern persists throughout life.

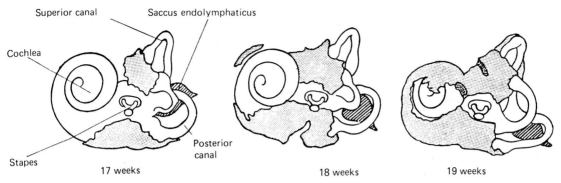

Figure 1.7 Diagram illustrating the progression of ossification of the cartilaginous labyrinth from 14 separate centres, not all of which are shown here. (Derived from Anson and Donaldson, 1981)

Table 1.1 Development of communication channels passing through the bony labyrinth

Internal auditory meatus	Persisting channel in cartilage model around VII and VIII nerves
Subarcuate fossa	Persisting vascular channel
Vestibular aqueduct	Fifth and sixth ossification centres fuse around the endolymphatic duct
Cochlear aqueduct	Resorption of precartilage
Fissula ante fenestram	Resorption of precartilage
Fossula post fenestram (inconstant)	Resorption of precartilage
Oval window	Otic capsule becomes footplate of stapes and annular ligament
Round window	Persisting cartilage becomes round window niche and membrane

The outer and middle ears

The mesenchyme surrounding the primitive pharynx differentiates into paired maxillary and mandibular processes above and below the level of the buccopharyngeal membrane. Shortly after the appearance of these processes, the membrane breaks down and the buccopharyngeal cavity is formed. Behind the level of the membrane, the mesenchyme which surrounds the pharyngeal tube separates on each side into five or six bars running around the pharynx; these are the pharyngeal arches. In each arch, a bar of cartilage, together with its associated muscles, differentiates from the mesenchyme. The muscle is supplied by a nerve (one of the special visceral efferents) and the endoderm which covers the arch internally is supplied not only by the nerve of the arch (pre-trematic) but also by a branch from the arch behind (post-trematic). Each arch also has an artery associated with it, at least for a short while during embryonic development. Between successive arches, the endoderm of the pharynx forms pouches which come into contact with the covering ectoderm which has sunk between the arches as the pharyngeal grooves (or clefts). In land-living vertebrates, a thin layer of mesoderm intervenes between the pouch and the cleft which does not break down, so that true gill clefts are never formed.

The first and second arches and their associated structures give rise to the middle and outer ears. *Table 1.2* outlines the details of the derivatives of these arches.

The auricle

The development of the auricle begins with the appearance of six hillocks around the first pharyngeal groove between the first and second arches. Three hillocks develop on each side of the groove; but as growth proceeds they tend to become obscured, and of those of the first (mandibular) arch, only that which later forms the tragus can be obviously identified throughout the process (*Figure 1.8*). It seems that the bulk of the auricle is derived from the mesenchyme of the second (hyoid) arch, which extends around the top of the groove to form a flattened extension that subsequently becomes the helix (Streeter, 1922). The cartilage of the auricle extends inwards partially to surround the future external meatus. The rudimentary pinna has formed by 60 days and in the fourth month the convolutions have attained

Table 1.2 Derivaties of 1st and 2nd branchial arches

	Cartilage	Pre-trematic nerve	Post-trematic nerve	Artery
1st arch Derivatives	Meckel's Malleus Incus 'Mandible' Anterior malleolar ligament Sphenomandibular ligament	Mandibular V	Chorda tympani VII	
2nd arch Derivatives	Reichert's Stapes superstructure Styloid process Lesser cornu of hyoid Stylohyoid ligament	Facial VII	Tympanic branch IX	Stapedial

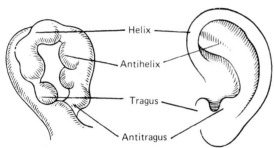

Helix

Antihelix

Tragus

Antitragus

Figure 1.8 Early stages in the development of the auricle. Six cartilaginous hillocks are visible around the first pharyngeal groove. During subsequent development these become the cartilage of the auricle although the bulk of the auricle appears to be derived from the cartilage of the second arch

their adult form, although further generalized enlargement continues during the remaining months of gestation and in the postnatal period.

The external canal

The external canal develops from the upper portion of the first pharyngeal groove. This extends inwards as a funnel-shaped tube and the meatus deepens by proliferation of its ectoderm which forms an epithelial plug. The ectoderm at the depths of this plug is in contact with the endoderm of the first pharyngeal pouch for a short while before the mesenchyme intervenes to become the middle fibrous layer of the future tympanic membrane.

The ectodermal plug breaks down and a narrow slit forms between the future walls of the external meatus and the tympanic membrane which lies in an almost 'horizontal' plane during fetal development (*Figure 1.9*).

Within the mesenchyme around the external meatus, four small centres of ossification arise in the ninth week. These are destined to fuse and to become the tympanic ring (not an accurate name as it is never a complete ring) and, subsequently, the tympanic bone. The ring develops a groove on its inner concave face, and this becomes the tympanic sulcus. The bony ring grows in diameter and extends laterally and inferiorly throughout fetal life to occupy the space between the mandibular fossa and the anterior surface of the developing mastoid bone, where it provides a sheath for the developing styloid process. By later

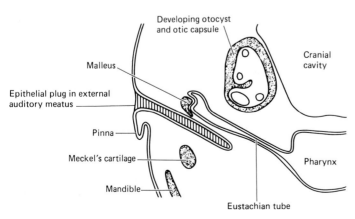

Developing otocyst and otic capsule

Cranial cavity

Malleus

Epithelial plug in external auditory meatus

Pinna

Meckel's cartilage

Pharynx

Mandible

Eustachian tube

Figure 1.9 Diagrammatic representation of the development of the external auditory canal and middle ear cleft. The endoderm of the first pouch is destined to become the lining of the eustachian tube and of the middle ear space. It is separated from the ectoderm of the ear canal by a thin layer of mesoderm in which develops the handle of the malleus

fetal life, the tympanic plate is widely open and the definitive bony canal unformed. After birth, anterior and posterior bony prominences, which have developed on the inner aspect of the ring, grow inwards and eventually fuse to form the floor of the canal. As the tips of the processes fuse, a space surrounded by bone is created; this is the foramen of Huschke which is usually obliterated by adolescence. The completed tympanic bone, therefore, makes contact with the mastoid process and part of the squamous bone posteriorly, and with another portion of the squamous and part of the petrous bone anteriorly. The petrotympanic fissure between the more medial aspect of the tympanic bone and the mandibular fossa allows the passage of the chorda tympani nerve, the post-trematic nerve of the first arch. The tympanic ring is deficient superiorly in the external meatus and this is the tympanic incisura.

The middle ear

The cavity and lining of the middle ear cleft and eustachian tube arise from the expanding first pharyngeal pouch with probably some contribution at the medial end from the second. By the 4-week stage, the distal end lies against the ectoderm of the first pharyngeal groove and expands to form a flattened sac, the precursor of the tympanic cavity. Mesenchyme grows between the ectoderm and the endoderm to form the third layer of the future tympanic membrane. The slit-like space within the sac expands and, as it reaches the developing ossicles and otic capsule, the epithelium lining the sac is draped over the lateral (tympanic) portion of the labyrinth, the bodies of the ossicles, and their developing ligaments and muscular tendons, so that a complex and variable network of mucosal folds is formed. 'Pneumatization' of the meso- and hypotympanum is complete at 8 months, while the epitympanum and mastoid antrum have developed by birth. The spaces are not filled with air but with amniotic fluid, and this is replaced shortly after birth. The mastoid antrum, which is an extension of the epitympanum, has started to develop in mid-fetal life. A few mastoid 'air-cells' are present late in fetal life, but the bulk of their development occurs in infancy and childhood.

The ossicles

The outer lateral ends of the first (Meckel's) and second (Reichert's) arch cartilages lie, respectively, above and below the developing first pharyngeal pouch. Before these arch cartilages are fully defined, condensations in the mesenchyme occur in this region at about 4–5 weeks. As development proceeds, the condensations form cartilage models

which, by 6.5 weeks, are well-defined as malleus, incus and stapes. By 5 weeks, the stapes can first be recognized as a circular mass at the end of the precursor of Reichert's (second arch) cartilage. Approximately 1.5 weeks later, this becomes annular as it is pierced by the first arch (stapedial) artery, and is now attached to the developing Reichert's cartilage by a membranous bar, the interhyale. At this time, the malleus and incus are developing from cartilage at the end of the precursor of Meckel's (first arch) cartilage. A groove represents the site of the future incudomalleolar joint, and the handle of the malleus and long process of incus are already apparent. By 7.5 weeks, the handle of the malleus lies between the layers of the developing tympanic membrane.

The stapes continues to grow and its ring-like shape is converted into the definitive arch-like stapedial form. It seems likely that the footplate of the stapes is formed primarily from the otic capsule, and that part of the stapedial ring which fuses with the otic capsule during ossification usually regresses. In the adult, therefore, the stapedial arches are derived from second arch cartilage, while the footplate is part of the labyrinthine capsule. Frequently, however, regression of the base of the stapedial ring is incomplete so that a dual origin for the mature footplate is possible. Ossification in the stapedial cartilage starts from a single centre at 4.5 months and is followed by a complex pattern of resorption, with the result that the base, the crura and the adjoining head are eventually hollowed out.

The malleus and incus start ossifying at the 4-month stage and progress is so rapid that, in the 25-week fetus, they are already of adult size and form.

The muscles of the tympanic cavity develop from the first and second arch mesenchyme to become the tensor tympani, which is supplied by a branch of the nerve of the first arch (mandibular), and the stapedius, which is supplied by the nerve of the second arch (facial). The pre-trematic nerve of the first arch is the chorda tympani and, with expansion of the tympanic cavity and resorption of the mesenchyme, its final course is within the layers of the tympanic membrane as it passes from the facial nerve to its destination in the floor of the mouth.

The temporal bone

The temporal bone is derived from four separate morphological elements that fuse with one another. The elements are the tympanic bone, already described previously, the squamous portion, the petromastoid complex, and the styloid process.

The squamous portion of the temporal bone, like the tympanic ring, develops in mesenchyme rather than in a preformed cartilage model. It is ossified from one centre that, as early as 8 weeks, appears close to the root of the zygomatic arch, and extends radially and also into the arch itself. The posteroinferior portion grows down behind the tympanic ring to form the lateral wall of the fetal mastoid antrum.

The petromastoid is morphologically a single element, although it is conveniently described in the adult in two separate units, the petrous and mastoid bones. The development of the cartilaginous otic capsule of embryonic and fetal life has already been described. The rapid progression of ossification completes the formation of the bony labyrinth. However, changes in the outer periosteal layer continue. A cartilaginous flange grows downwards and outwards from the lateral part of the petrosal cartilages, above the tubotympanic cavity, to form the roof of the middle ear and of the lateral bony wall of the eustachian tube. A separate flange grows outwards below the developing middle ear cavity to form the jugular plate. The facial nerve, which lies in a sulcus on the lateral, tympanic, aspect of the otic capsule, is also enclosed by growth from the capsule. Other changes gradually occur in the outer layers of the capsule. The subarcuate fossa, which carried a leash of blood vessels and was as large as the internal meatus, becomes progressively smaller. Anteriorly, the outer periosteal layer enlarges to form the petrous apex.

The styloid process develops from two centres at the cranial end of Reichert's (second arch) cartilage. That part closest to the tympanic bone is the tympanohyal and its ossification centre appears before birth. It fuses with the petromastoid during the first year of life and is surrounded at its root by a portion of the tympanic bone. The ossification centre for the distal part – the stylohyal – does not appear until after birth and fusion with the tympanohyal does not occur, if at all, until after puberty.

The tympanic ring unites with the squamous portion shortly before birth, while the petromastoid fuses during the first year of life, so that tympanosquamous (anterior) and tympanomastoid suture lines are present in the bony external meatus. At birth, the tympanic annulus lies beneath the skull in an almost horizontal plane. By the third month, as a result of the upward and lateral rotation of the petrous bone, caused by rapid enlargement of the forebrain, the annulus appears on the inferolateral aspect of the skull, and it is not until some months later that its accessible oblique position is attained.

The mastoid portion of the petromastoid is at first flat, and the stylomastoid foramen with the facial nerve lies on the lateral surface behind the tympanic bone. With the development of air cells in the mastoid, its lateral portion grows downwards and forwards so that the stylomastoid foramen is carried on to the undersurface of the bone and the facial nerve canal elongates. During the second year of life, the portion of the squamous bone adjoining the petromastoid enlarges and grows downwards, thereby concealing some of the petrous portion which also enlarges downwards to form the mastoid tip. A squamopetrous suture line is usually visible on the outer surface of the mastoid process. Within this process, a variable extension of the antral air cells occurs and a septum may be left between deep and superficial air cells. This is Korner's septum and is a remnant of the petrosquamous suture line. As the tympanic bone and the mastoid process develop, the lateral surface of the temporal bone takes up its vertical adult position.

Anatomy of the human ear

For the purpose of anatomical description, the ear is divided into four separate portions. These are: the auricle (or pinna), the external auditory canal, the middle ear and its derivatives and, finally, the inner ear.

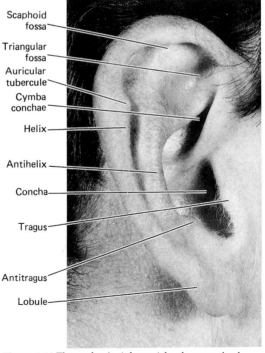

Figure 1.10 The author's right auricle, the growth of tragal hairs indicating the passing of youth

The auricle

The auricle (or pinna) projects to a greater or lesser angle from the side of the head and has some function in collecting sound (*see* Chapter 2). The lateral surface of the auricle has several prominences and depressions (*Figure 1.10*). The curved rim is the helix. At its posterosuperior aspect, a small auricular tubercle (Darwin's tubercle) is often present. Anterior to and parallel with the helix is another prominence, the antihelix. Superiorly, this divides into two crura between which is the triangular fossa; the scaphoid fossa lies above the superior of the two crura. In front of the antihelix, and partly encircled by it, is the concha. The anterior superior portion of the concha is usually covered by the descending limb of the anterior superior portion of the helix (the crus of the helix). This region is the cymba conchae. It is the direct lateral relation to the suprameatal triangle of the temporal bone. Below the crus of the helix and opposite the concha, across the external auditory meatus, is the tragus, which is a small blunt triangular prominence. This points posteriorly and overlaps the orifice of the external canal. Opposite the tragus, at the inferior limit of the antihelix, is the antitragus. The tragus and antitragus are separated by the intertragic notch. The lobule lies below the antitragus and is soft, being composed of fibrous and adipose tissue. The medial (cranial) surface of the auricle has elevations corresponding to the depressions on the lateral surface, and possesses corresponding names – for example, the eminentia conchae.

The body of the auricle is composed of a thin plate of cartilage covered with skin, and it is connected to surrounding parts by ligaments and muscles. It is continuous with the cartilage of the external meatus.

The skin of the auricle is thin and closely adherent to the perichondrium on the lateral surface. There is a definite but thin layer of subdermal adipose tissue on the medial (cranial) surface. The skin is covered with fine hairs which have sebaceous glands opening into their root canals. The glands are most numerous in the concha and scaphoid fossa. On the tragus and intertragic notch coarse, thick hairs may develop in the middle-aged and older male.

The cartilaginous skeleton comprises a single piece of elastic fibrocartilage which is absent in the lobule and deficient between the crus of the helix and the tragus, that is in the anterior superior portion, where it is replaced by dense fibrous tissue. The cartilage, in the same way as cartilage elsewhere, is dependent on its perichondrium for supply of nutrients and removal of by-products. The cartilage is connected to the temporal bone by two extrinsic ligaments. The anterior ligament runs from the tragus and from a cartilaginous spine on the anterior rim of the crus of the helix to the root of the zygomatic arch. A separate posterior ligament runs from the medial surface of the concha to the lateral surface of the mastoid prominence. Intrinsic ligaments connect various parts of the cartilaginous auricle; that between helix and tragus has already been described and another runs from the antihelix to the postero-inferior portion of the helix.

Extrinsic and intrinsic muscles are, in the same way as ligaments, attached to the perichondrium of the cartilage. The extrinsic muscles are supplied by temporal and posterior auricular branches of the facial nerve and, while being functionally unimportant, they do give rise to the postauricular myogenic response following appropriate auditory stimulation (Gibson, 1978). There are three extrinsic muscles: auricularis anterior, superior and posterior, the last being supplied by the posterior auricular branch of the facial nerve. All three radiate out from the auricle to insert into the epicranial aponeurosis. The intrinsic muscles – six in number – are small, inconsistent and without useful function, other than that of entertaining children in those who possess the ability to alter the shape of the pinna.

Three arterial branches of the external carotid supply the auricle. The posterior auricular provides twigs that supply the medial (cranial) surface and, by extension around the helix, the extremities of the lateral surface. The anterior auricular branches of the superficial temporal supply the bulk of the lateral surfaces, and a small auricular branch from the occipital artery assists the posterior auricular in supplying the medial surface.

Many nerves make up the sensory supply of the auricle. Their distribution is variable and the overlap may be extensive. The essential features are described in *Table 1.3*.

The lymphatic drainage from the posterior surface is to the lymph nodes at the mastoid tip, from the tragus and from the upper part of the anterior surface to the preauricular nodes, and from the rest of the auricle to the upper deep cervical nodes.

The external auditory canal

The external auditory canal extends from the concha of the auricle to the tympanic membrane. The distance from the bottom of the concha to the tympanic membrane is approximately 2.5 cm, although the length of the anterior canal wall is 1–1.5 cm more because of the length of the tragus, the obliquity of the tympanic membrane and the curvature of the canal wall. The supporting

Table 1.3 Sensory innervation of the auricle

Nerve	Derivation	Region supplied
Greater auricular	Cervical plexus C2,3	Medial surface and posterior portion of lateral surface
Lesser occipital	Cervical plexus C2	Superior portion of medial surface
Auricular	Vagus X	Concha and antihelix Some supply medial surface (eminentia concha)
Auriculotemporal	Vc mandibular	Tragus, crus of helix and adjacent helix
Facial VII		Probably supplies small region in the root of concha

framework of the canal wall is cartilage in the lateral one-third and bone in the medial two-thirds. In adults, the cartilaginous portion runs inwards slightly upwards and backwards, while the bony portion runs inwards slightly downwards and forwards. The canal is straightened, therefore, by gently moving the auricle upwards and backwards to counteract the direction of the cartilaginous portion. In the neonate, there is virtually no bony external meatus as the tympanic bone is not yet developed, and the tympanic membrane is more horizontally placed so that the auricle must be gently drawn downwards and backwards for the best view of the tympanic membrane.

In the adult, the lateral cartilaginous portion is about 8 mm long. It is continuous with the auricular cartilage and is deficient superiorly, this space being occupied by the intrinsic ligament between the helix and tragus. The medial border of the meatal cartilage is attached to the rim of the bony canal by fibrous bands.

The bony canal wall, about 1.6 mm long, is narrower than the cartilaginous portion and itself becomes smaller closer to the tympanic membrane. The anterior wall is longer by about 4 mm than the posterior wall because of the obliquity of the tympanic membrane. The medial end of the bony canal is marked by a groove, the tympanic sulcus, which is absent superiorly. Although the tympanic bone makes up the greater part of the canal, and also carries the sulcus, the squamous bone forms the roof. Therefore, there are two suture lines in the canal wall with the tympano-squamous anteriorly and the tympanomastoid posteriorly. Both these suture lines may be more or less developed; they project into the canal and the overlying skin is closely adherent. The tympanomastoid suture is a complex suture line between the anterior wall of the mastoid process, a portion of the squamous bone and the tympanic bone.

Apart from these intrusions into the canal, there are two constrictions: one at the junction of the cartilaginous and bony portions and the other, the isthmus, 5 mm from the tympanic membrane where a prominence of the anterior canal wall reduces the diameter. Deep to the isthmus, the anteroinferior portion of the canal dips forward so that a wedge-shaped anterior recess is formed between the tympanic membrane and the canal.

The skin of the external canal is continuous with that of the auricle and extends over the outer surface of the tympanic membrane. There is a definite subdermal layer in the cartilaginous portion, but in most of the bony segment this is very thin and the skin is adherent to the periosteum of the tympanic bone. In the superior portion of the deep meatus between the two suture lines, the subdermal layers are thickened and carry a leash of blood vessels. This is the vascular strip.

The skin itself has some properties not found in skin elsewhere. Instead of maturation occurring directly towards the surface there is lateral growth of the epidermis, with the consequence that layers of keratin are shed towards the surface opening of the external meatus (Johnson and Hawke, 1985). This is also true of the epidermal layers of the tympanic membrane, and Alberti (1964) has shown that migration occurs at the rate of about 0.05 mm/day, which is about the same rate of growth as that of fingernails.

The skin overlying the cartilaginous portion contains hairs and glands. The hairs are narrow and short and project towards the external opening of the meatus. The external surface of individual hairs has a series of overlapping 'scales' which are also directed externally (*Figure 1.11*).

The glands are of two types, ceruminous and sebaceous. The sebaceous glands are typical of sebaceous glands elsewhere and consist of a single wide duct from which arise a cluster of pear-shaped alveoli. Each alveolus consists of a basement membrane enclosing a mass of epithelial cells. The central cells, which contain fat, break down to form the sebaceous material (sebum), and are in turn replaced by a proliferation of epithelial

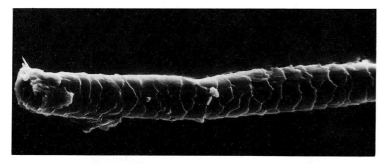

Figure 1.11 Scanning electron micrograph of a single short hair from an adult human external ear canal. A series of overlapping scales is present on the surface of the hair and directed to the external opening of the ear canal.

cells at the edge of the mass. The sebum passes along the ducts which nearly always open into hair follicles (*Figure 1.12*).

The ceruminous glands lie slightly deeper in the dermis and are simple coiled tubular structures lined with cuboidal secretory cells and surrounded by a myoepithelium. This contains smooth muscle, and its contraction compresses the duct which thus empties its contents into the root canal of the hair follicle from which these cells nearly always originate. The secretion is initially white and watery, but as it dries and is oxidized, it becomes sticky and semisolid, and thereafter slowly darkens in colour. The ceruminous glands are modified apocrine sweat glands and both react to the same stimuli. Adrenergic drugs, emotion resulting in an intrinsic release of adrenaline and noradrenaline, and mechanical manipulation, all result in a small increase in secretion.

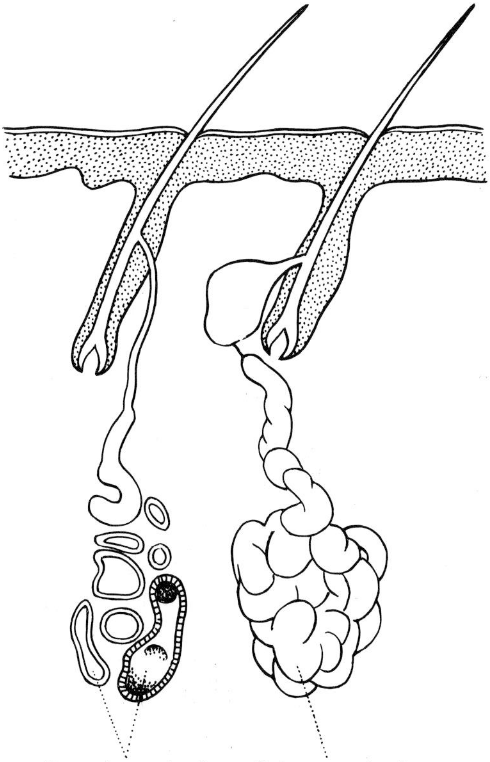

Wax (cerumen)

The mixture of the products of the sebaceous and ceruminous glands results in the formation of wax, of which there are two distinct forms – dry and wet. Dry wax is yellowish or grey, and is dry and brittle, while wet wax is yellowish brown, and is wet and sticky. The type of wax possessed by an individual is probably monofactorially inherited with the wet phenotype dominant over the recessive dry type. The Japanese, other mongoloid populations and the American Indians tend to carry the recessive gene and, in general, to have dry wax, whereas in white and black populations, the wet gene predominates.

Wax contains various amino acids, fatty acids, lysozymes and immunoglobulins and is to some extent bactericidal, being especially potent at killing dividing bacteria (Stone and Fulghum, 1984).

Blood supply and lymphatic drainage

The arterial supply of the external meatus is derived from branches of the external carotid. The auricular branches of the superficial temporal artery supply the roof and anterior portion of the canal. The deep auricular branch of the first part of the maxillary artery arises in the parotid gland behind the temporomandibular joint, pierces the cartilage or bone of the external meatus, and supplies the anterior meatal wall skin and the epithelium of the outer surface of the tympanic membrane. Finally, auricular branches of the posterior auricular artery pierce the cartilage of the auricle and supply the posterior portions of the canal. The veins drain into the external jugular vein, the maxillary veins and the pterygoid plexus.

Ceruminous gland   Sebaceous gland

Figure 1.12 Diagram of section of skin of external auditory canal showing ceruminous and sebaceous glands arising from hair follicles. (Courtesy of David Lim)

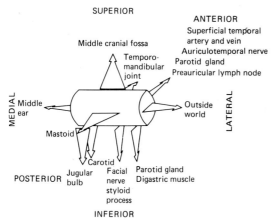

Figure 1.13 Relationships of the right external auditory canal

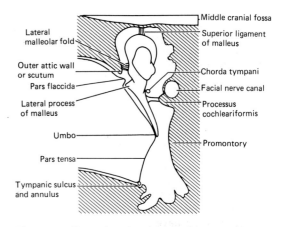

Figure 1.14 Coronal section through the external ear canal and middle ear at the level of the malleus handle

The lymphatic drainage follows that of the auricle.

The relationships of the external canal are depicted in *Figure 1.13*.

The middle ear cleft

The middle ear cleft consists of the tympanic cavity (tympanum), the eustachian tube and the mastoid air cell system. Included in this section are the extensions of the air cell system into the anterior and posterior petrous apex.

The tympanic cavity

The tympanic cavity is an irregular, air-filled space within the temporal bone and contains the auditory ossicles and their attached muscles. Other structures run along its walls to pass through the cavity. For descriptive purposes, the tympanic cavity may be thought of as a box with four walls, a roof and a floor. The corners are not sharp and, therefore, the precise localization of features lying at the edge of one wall may not be possible with this model.

The lateral wall of the tympanic cavity

The lateral wall of the tympanic cavity is part bony and part membranous. The tympanic membrane forms the central portion of the lateral wall, while above and below there is bone, forming the outer lateral walls of the epitympanum and hypotympanum respectively. The lateral wall of the epitympanum also includes that part of the tympanic membrane lying above the anterior and posterior malleolar folds – the pars flaccida (*see below*). This lateral epitympanic wall is wedge-

shaped in section and its lower bony portion is also called the outer attic wall or scutum (Latin = shield). It is thin and its lateral surface forms the superior portion of the deep part of the external meatus (*Figure 1.14*).

Three holes are present in the bone of the medial surface of the lateral wall of the tympanic cavity. The opening of the posterior canaliculus for the chorda tympani nerve is situated in the angle between the junction of the lateral and posterior walls of the tympanic cavity. It is often at the level of the upper end of the handle of the malleus, but a lower situation is very common. The opening leads into a small bony canal which descends through the posterior wall of the tympanic cavity. Near the tympanic opening, the chorda tympani lies anterior and lateral to the facial nerve; it descends obliquely to join the nerve, often at some point within the bone, but occasionally the channel remains separate and the two nerves join outside the skull. A branch of the stylomastoid artery accompanies the chorda tympani into the tympanic cavity.

The petrotympanic (Glaserian) fissure opens anteriorly just above the attachment of the tympanic membrane. It is a slit about 2 mm long which receives the anterior malleolar ligament and transmits the anterior tympanic branch of the maxillary artery to the tympanic cavity. The chorda tympani enters the medial surface of the fissure through a separate anterior canaliculus (canal of Huguier) which is short and is sometimes confluent with the fissure.

The tympanic membrane, forming the lateral wall of the mesotympanum and a small part of the epitympanum, separates the tympanic cavity from the external meatus. It is a thin, nearly oval disc, slightly broader above than below, forming an angle of about 55° with the floor of the meatus. Its longest diameter from posterosuperior to antero-inferior is 9–10 mm, while perpendicular to this the shortest diameter is 8–9 mm. Most of the circumference is thickened to form a fibrocartilaginous ring, the tympanic annulus, which sits in a groove in the tympanic bone, the tympanic sulcus. The sulcus does not extend to the roof of the canal which is formed by part of the squamous bone. From the superior limits of the sulcus, the annulus becomes a fibrous band which runs centrally as anterior and posterior malleolar folds to the lateral process of the malleus, the handle of which lies within the tympanic membrane. This leaves a small, rather squat, triangular region of tympanic membrane above the malleolar folds. It does not have a tympanic annulus at its margins, is lax and is called the pars flaccida. The pars tensa forms the rest of the tympanic membrane. It is taut and, when seen from the ear canal, is concave, with the maximal depression occurring at the inferior tip of the malleus handle (the umbo). However, each portion of the membrane, as the latter passes from the annulus to the umbo, is not flat but is gently curved, being slightly convex when seen from the external meatus (*Figure 1.15*).

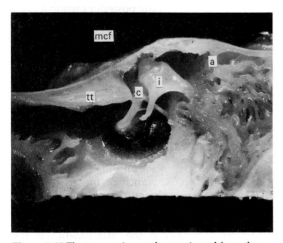

Figure 1.15 The tympanic membrane viewed from the middle ear. The corda tympani runs superior to the tensor tympani in its passage across the tympanic membrane. The aditus to the mastoid antrum lies posterosuperior to the short process of the incus which lies in the fossa incudis. a: aditus to mastoid antrum; c: chorda tympani; i: incus; mcf: middle cranial fossa; tt: tensor tympani

The tympanic membrane has three layers: an outer epithelial layer, the epidermis, which is continuous with the skin of the external meatus; a middle, mainly fibrous layer, the lamina propria; and an inner mucosal layer continuous with the lining of the tympanic cavity.

The epidermis is divided into the stratum corneum, the stratum granulosum, the stratum spinosum and stratum basale. In man (Hentzer, 1969), the stratum corneum, which is the outermost layer, consists of between one and six compressed layers of almost acellular structures, without organelles but with recognizable membranes and intercellular junctions (desmosomes). The stratum granulosum contains one to three layers of cells with smooth borders, and interconnecting desmosomes. Keratohyaline granules and lamellar granules are present among occasional tonofilaments, but other cell constituents are lacking. The cells of the stratum spinosum, which are two or three layers deep, have prominent interdigitations with neighbouring cells to which they are bound by desmosomes. These cells contain bundles of tonofilaments, with mitochondria and ribosomes also present, but have a high nucleus to cytoplasm ratio. The stratum basale, which is the deepest layer, consists of a single layer of cells separated from the lamina propria by a basement membrane. These cells have a polyhedral shape, or are elongated in a line parallel to the basement membrane. Occasionally, prolongations of the deep surface of the cell extend down into the lamina propria. Nerve endings and melanin granules have not been seen in any of the cell layers of the epidermis.

The predominant feature of the lamina propria, in both the pars tensa and the pars flaccida, is the presence of collagen fibrils. In the pars tensa, the fibrils closest to the epithelial layer are usually in direct contact with the basement membrane of the epidermal layer, although in places a thin layer of loose connective tissue intervenes. These lateral fibres are radial in orientation, while the deeper ones are circular, parabolic and transverse. A loose connective tissue layer, containing fibroblasts, macrophages, nerve fibres (mainly unmyelinated) and many capillaries, lies between the deep layers of the lamina propria and the inner mucosal layer. Neither the capillaries nor the nerves appear to penetrate the basement membrane or enter the mucosal layer.

In the pars flaccida, the lamina propria is less marked, but it still contains collagen fibres although they appear to lie in an almost random orientation.

The mucosal epithelium of the pars tensa varies in height from a low simple squamous or cuboidal type to a pseudostratified columnar epithelium. The adjoining cell borders have marked interdigitations with tight junctions between the apices of the cells facing the tympanic cavity. The free surface of the cells – that is the surface facing the middle ear – possess numerous microvilli and, where the epithelium is cuboidal or columnar, cilia with the typical 'nine plus two' internal ultrastructure are found. These true cilia are patchy in their distribution and a continuous sheet, such as that which covers the respiratory mucosa of, say, the eustachian tube, is not found. No goblet cells have been found in this layer, but in cells without cilia, secretory granules are present. The cytoplasm and nuclei of the cells are otherwise unremarkable. The mucosal layer is separated from the lamina propria by a basement membrane. In the pars flaccida, the overall picture is the same except that taller ciliated cells are not found.

Blood supply of the tympanic membrane

The arterial supply of the tympanic membrane is complex and arises from branches supplying both the external auditory meatus and the middle ear. These two sources interconnect through extensive anastamoses, but the vessels are found only in the connective tissue layers of the lamina propria. Within this layer there appears to be a peripheral ring of arteries connected by radial anastomoses, with one or two arteries that run down each side and around the tip of the malleus handle. The arteries involved include the deep auricular branch of the maxillary artery coming from the external auditory meatus; and, from the middle ear, the anterior tympanic branches of the maxillary artery, twigs from the stylomastoid branch of the posterior auricular and probably several twigs from the middle meningeal.

The venous drainage returns to the external jugular vein, the transverse sinus and dural veins and the venous plexus around the eustachian tube.

Nerve supply of the tympanic membrane

The nerves, in the same way as the blood vessels, run in the lamina propria and arise from the auriculotemporal nerve (Vc) supplying the anterior portion, from the auricular branch of the vagus (X), the posterior portion, and from the tympanic branch of the glossopharyngeal nerve (IX). The variations and overlap are considerable, but both the vascular supply and innervation are relatively sparse in the middle part of the posterior half of the tympanic membrane.

The roof of the tympanic cavity

The tegmen tympani is the bony roof of the tympanic cavity, and separates it from the dura of the middle cranial fossa. It is formed in part by the petrous and part by the squamous bone; and the petrosquamous suture line, unossified in the young, does not close until adult life. Veins from the tympanic cavity running to the superior petrosal sinus pass through this suture line.

The floor of the tympanic cavity

The floor of the tympanic cavity is much narrower than the roof and consists of a thin plate of bone which separates the tympanic cavity from the dome of the jugular bulb. Occasionally, the floor is deficient and the jugular bulb is then covered only by fibrous tissue and a mucous membrane. At the junction of the floor and the medial wall of the cavity there is a small opening that allows the entry of the tympanic branch of the glossopharyngeal nerve into the middle ear from its origin below the base of the skull (*see* Chapter 15).

The anterior wall of the tympanic cavity

The anterior wall of the tympanic cavity is rather narrow as the medial and lateral walls converge. The lower portion of the anterior wall is larger than the upper and consists of a thin plate of bone covering the carotid artery as it enters the skull and before it turns anteriorly. This plate is perforated by the superior and inferior caroticotympanic nerves carrying sympathetic fibres to the tympanic plexus, and by one or more tympanic branches of the internal carotid artery. The upper, smaller part of the anterior wall has two parallel tunnels placed one above the other. The lower opening is flared and leads into the bony portion of the eustachian tube which will be described in more detail later on in this chapter. The upper tunnel is separated from the eustachian tube by a thin plate of bone, and contains the tensor tympani muscle which subsequently runs along the medial wall of the tympanic cavity enclosed in a thin bony sheath. This muscle will also be further described in the section on the auditory ossicles.

The medial wall of the tympanic cavity

The medial wall separates the tympanic cavity from the inner ear. Its surface possesses several prominent features and two openings (*Figure 1.16*). The promontory is a rounded elevation occupying much of the central portion of the medial wall. It usually has small grooves on its surface and these contain the nerves which form the tympanic plexus. Sometimes the grooves, especially the groove containing the tympanic branch of the glossopharyngeal nerve, are covered by bone, with the consequence that small canals are present instead. The promontory covers part of the basal coil of the cochlea and in front merges with the anterior wall of the tympanic cavity.

Behind and above the promontory is the fenestra vestibuli (oval window), a nearly kidney-shaped opening that connects the tympanic cavity with the vestibule, but which in life is closed by the base of the stapes and its surrounding annular

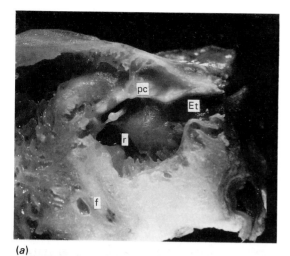

(a)

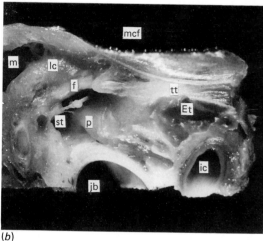

(b)

Figure 1.16 Two separate specimens cut at slightly different levels to show the medial wall of the tympanic cavity and the associated structures. (*a*) Section cut through a block of temporal bone just medial to the inferior part of the annulus; (*b*) section cut deeper, that is slightly more medial in a different temporal bone so as to expose the jugular bulb; Et: eustachian tube orifice; f: facial nerve in descending and intratympanic segments; jb: jugular bulb; lc: dome of lateral semicircular canal; m: mastoid antrum; mcf: middle cranial fossa; p: promontory; pc: processus cochleariformis; r: round window niche; st: sinus tympani; tt: tensor tympani. Other structures, that is subiculum and ponticulus can be seen clearly but are not labelled, to avoid confusion. They are described in the text

ligament. The long axis of the fenestra vestibuli is horizontal, and the slightly concave border is inferior. The size of the fenestra vestibuli naturally varies with the size of the base of the stapes, but on average it is 3.25 mm long and 1.75 mm wide. Above the fenestra vestibuli is the facial nerve and

below is the promontory. The fenestra, therefore, lies at the bottom of a depression or fossula that can be of varying width depending on the position of the facial nerve and the prominence of the promontory.

The fenestra cochleae (round window), which is closed by the secondary tympanic membrane (round window membrane), lies below and a little behind the fenestra vestibuli from which it is separated by a posterior extension of the promontory, called the subiculum. Occasionally, a spicule of bone leaves the promontory above the subiculum and runs to the pyramid on the posterior wall of the cavity. This spicule is called the ponticulus. The fenestra cochleae, which faces inferiorly and a little posteriorly, lies completely under cover of the overhanging edge of the promontory in a deep niche and is, therefore, usually out of sight. The niche is most commonly triangular in shape, with anterior, posterosuperior and posteroinferior walls. The latter two meet posteriorly and lead to the sinus tympani. The average length of the walls of the niche are: anterior – 1.5 mm; superior – 1.3 mm; and posterior – 1.6 mm (Nomura, 1984). There is great variation in the depth of the niche and, to enable the secondary tympanic membrane to be seen, bone frequently has to be removed from the anterior wall of the niche. Within the niche are mucosal folds or even complete membranes that partly or completely exclude the secondary tympanic membrane from view and may even be mistaken for it during surgery. In the adult, the secondary tympanic membrane lies almost horizontally in the roof of the niche. This membrane is not flat but curves towards the scala tympani of the basal coil of the cochlea, so that it is concave when viewed from the middle ear. It appears to be divided into an anterior and posterior portion by a transverse thickening within the membrane. The shape of the membrane varies, in different temporal bones, from round through oval and kidney-shaped to spatulate, with average longest and shortest diameters of 2.30 mm and 1.87 mm respectively.

The membrane consists of three layers: an outer mucosal, a middle fibrous and an inner mesothelial layer. The mucosal layer is rather like the mucosal layer of the primary tympanic membrane with flattened or cuboidal cells possessing microvilli and, occasionally, clusters of cilia on their surface. This layer is separated from the basement membrane by a single layer of loose connective tissue that often contains melanocytes. It is this layer that contains the capillaries and nerves. The rest of the middle layer, which forms the bulk of the membrane, contains fibroblasts and collections of collagen and elastic fibres. The fibres are not, however, ordered in the same way as in the pars tensa and do not form discrete bundles. The inner layer is a continuation of the cell layer lining the scala tympani. There are two or three layers of overlapping, flat mesothelial cells with wide intercellular spaces, but no tight junctions nor any connective tissue layer between this and the middle layer.

The membrane of the fenestra cochleae does not lie at the end of the scala tympani but forms part of its floor. The scala tympani terminates posterior and medial to the membrane. The ampulla of the posterior semicircular canal is the closest vestibular structure to the membrane and its nerve (the singular nerve) runs almost parallel to, and 1 mm away from, the medial attachment of the deep portion of the posterior part of the membrane. The membrane is therefore a surgical landmark for the singular nerve (Gacek, 1983).

The facial nerve canal runs above the promontory and fenestra vestibuli in an anteroposterior direction. It has a smooth rounded lateral surface that is occasionally deficient, and is marked anteriorly by the processus cochleariformis. This is a curved projection of bone, concave anteriorly, which houses the tendon of the tensor tympani muscle as it turns laterally to the handle of the malleus. Behind the fenestra vestibuli, the facial canal starts to turn inferiorly as it begins its descent in the posterior wall of the tympanic cavity.

The region above the level of the facial nerve canal forms the medial wall of the epitympanum.

The dome of the lateral semicircular canal extends a little lateral to the facial canal and is the major feature of the posterior portion of the epitympanum. In well-aerated mastoid bones, the labyrinthine bone over the superior semicircular canal may be prominent, running at right angles to the lateral canal and joining it anteriorly at a swelling which houses the ampullae of the two canals. In front and a little below this, above the processus cochleariformis, may be a slight swelling corresponding to the geniculate ganglion, with the bony canal of the greater superficial petrosal nerve running for a short distance anteriorly.

The posterior wall of the tympanic cavity

The posterior wall is wider above than below and has in its upper part the opening (aditus) into the mastoid antrum. This is a large irregular hole that leads back from the posterior epitympanum. Below the aditus is a small depression, the fossa incudis, which houses the short process of the incus and a ligament connecting the two. Below the fossa incudis and medial to the opening of the chorda tympani nerve is the pyramid, a small hollow conical projection with its apex pointing anteriorly. It contains the stapedius muscle, the tendon of which passes forward to insert into the stapes. The canal within the promontory curves downwards and backwards to join the descending portion of the facial nerve canal. Between the

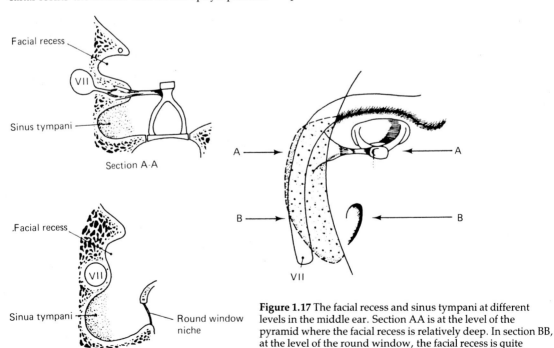

Figure 1.17 The facial recess and sinus tympani at different levels in the middle ear. Section AA is at the level of the pyramid where the facial recess is relatively deep. In section BB, at the level of the round window, the facial recess is quite shallow. The extent of the sinus tympani, deep and posterior to the facial nerve, is variable

promontory and the tympanic annulus is the facial recess (*Figure 1.17*). This is less marked lower down where the facial nerve canal forms only a slight prominence on the posterior wall. The facial recess is, therefore, bounded medially by the facial nerve and laterally by the tympanic annulus, but running through the wall between the two, with a varying degree of obliquity, is the chorda tympani nerve. This always runs medial to the tympanic membrane, which means that the angle between the facial nerve and the chorda allows access to the middle ear from the mastoid without disruption to the tympanic membrane. This angle can be small or large depending on the site of origin of the chorda from the facial nerve.

Deep to both the promontory and the facial nerve is a posterior extension of the mesotympanum – the sinus tympani. This extension of air cells into the posterior wall can be extensive, and Anson and Donaldson (1981) report that, when measured from the tip of the pyramid, the sinus can extend as far as 9 mm into the mastoid bone. The medial wall of the sinus tympani becomes continuous with the posterior portion of the medial wall of the tympanic cavity where it is related to the two fenestrae and the subiculum of the promontory.

The relationships of the middle ear space are shown diagrammatically in *Figure 1.18*.

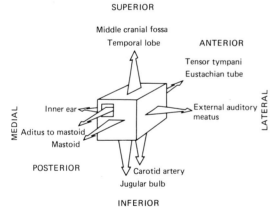

Figure 1.18 The relationships of the right middle ear

The contents of the tympanic cavity

The tympanic cavity contains a chain of three small movable bones – the malleus, incus and stapes – two muscles, the chorda tympani nerve and the tympanic plexus of nerves.

The malleus

The malleus (hammer), the largest of the three ossicles, comprises a head, neck and three processes arising from below the neck. The overall

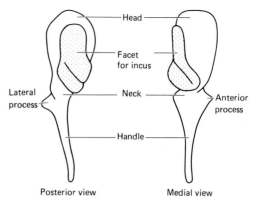

Figure 1.19 The left malleus. The stippling represents the cartilage of the synovial joint that articulates with the incus. *Figures 1.20* and *1.21* are on the same scale

length of the malleus ranges from 7.5 to 9.0 mm (*Figure 1.19*). The head lies in the epitympanum and has on its posteromedial surface an elongated saddle-shaped, cartilage-covered facet for articulation with the incus. This surface is constricted near its middle and the smaller inferior portion of the joint surface lies nearly at right angles to the superior portion. This projecting lower part is the cog, or spur, of the malleus. Below the neck of the malleus, the bone broadens and gives rise to the following: the anterior process from which a slender anterior ligament arises to insert into the petrotympanic fissure; the lateral process which receives the anterior and posterior malleolar folds from the tympanic annulus; and the handle. The handle runs downwards, medially and slightly backwards between the mucosal and fibrous layers of the tympanic membrane. On the deep, medial surface of the handle, near its upper end, is a small projection into which the tendon of the tensor tympani muscle inserts. Additional support for the malleus comes from the superior ligament which runs from the head to the tegmen tympani.

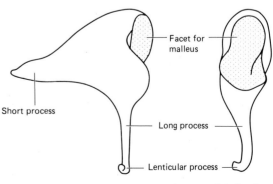

Figure 1.20 Left incus

The incus

The incus (*Figure 1.20*) articulates with the malleus and has a body and two processes. The body lies in the epitympanum and has a cartilage-covered facet corresponding to that on the malleus. The short process projects backwards from the body to lie in the fossa incudis to which it is attached by a short ligament. The long process descends into the mesotympanum behind and medial to the handle of the malleus, and at its tip is a small medially directed lenticular process which articulates with the stapes.

The stapes

The stapes consists of a head, neck, two crura (limbs) and a base or footplate (*Figure 1.21*). The head points laterally and has a small cartilage-covered depression for articulation with the lenticular process of the incus. The stapedius

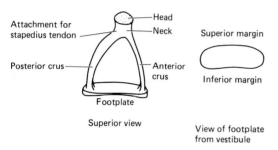

Figure 1.21 Left stapes

tendon inserts into the posterior part of neck and upper portion of the posterior crus. The two crura arise from the broader lower part of the neck and the anterior crus is thinner and less curved than the posterior one. Both are hollowed out on their concave surfaces. The two crura join the footplate which usually has a convex superior margin, an almost straight inferior margin and curved anterior and posterior ends. The average dimensions of the footplate are 3 mm long and 1.4 mm wide, and it lies in the fenestra vestibuli where it is attached to the bony margins of the labyrinthine capsule by the annular ligament. The long axis of the footplate is almost horizontal, with the posterior end being slightly lower than the anterior.

The stapedius muscle

The stapedius arises from the walls of the conical cavity within the pyramid and from the downward curved continuation of this canal in front of the descending portion of the facial nerve. A slender tendon emerges from the apex of the pyramid and inserts into the stapes. The muscle is supplied by a small branch of the facial nerve.

The tensor tympani muscle

This is a long slender muscle arising from the walls of the bony canal lying above the eustachian tube. Parts of the muscle also arise from the cartilaginous portion of the eustachian tube and the greater wing of the sphenoid. From its origins, the muscle passes backwards into the tympanic cavity where it lies on the medial wall, a little below the level of the facial nerve. The bony covering of the canal is often deficient in its tympanic segment where the muscle is replaced by a slender tendon. This enters the spoon-shaped processus cochleariformis where it is held down by a transverse tendon as it turns through a right angle to pass laterally and insert into the medial aspect of the upper end of the malleus handle. The muscle is supplied from the mandibular nerve by way of a branch, from the medial pterygoid nerve, which passes through the otic ganglion without synapse.

The chorda tympani nerve

This branch of the facial nerve enters the tympanic cavity from the posterior canaliculus at the junction of the lateral and posterior walls. It runs across the medial surface of the tympanic membrane between the mucosal and fibrous layers and passes medial to the upper portion of the handle of the malleus above the tendon of tensor tympani to continue forwards and leave by way of the anterior canaliculus, which subsequently joins the petrotympanic fissure.

The tympanic plexus

The tympanic plexus is formed by the tympanic branch of the glossopharyngeal nerve and by caroticotympanic nerves which arise from the sympathetic plexus around the internal carotid artery. The nerves form a plexus on the promontory and provide the following:

(1) Branches to the mucous membrane lining the tympanic cavity, eustachian tube and mastoid antrum and air cells.
(2) A branch joining the greater superficial petrosal nerve.
(3) The lesser superficial petrosal nerve, which contains all the parasympathetic fibres of IX. This nerve leaves the middle ear through a small canal below the tensor tympani muscle where it receives parasympathetic fibres from VII by way of a branch from the geniculate ganglion. The completed nerve passes through the temporal bone to emerge, lateral to the greater superficial petrosal nerve, on the floor of the middle cranial fossa, outside the dura. It then passes through the foramen ovale with the mandibular nerve and accessory meningeal artery to the otic ganglion. Occasionally,

the nerve runs not in the foramen ovale but through a separate small foramen next to the foramen spinosum. Postganglionic fibres from the otic ganglion supply secretomotor fibres to the parotid gland by way of the auriculo-temporal nerve.

The mucosa of the tympanic cavity

The middle ear mucosa is to some degree a respiratory mucosa carrying cilia on its surface and being able to secrete mucus (Sade, 1966). The extent of the mucociliary epithelium varies in normal middle ears, being more widespread in the young and ending at the line of the facial nerve in all ages. Above the facial nerve, that is in the epitympanum and mastoid, a flat non-ciliated epithelium, with only a very occasional mucus-producing cell, is found. The mucus comes from goblet cells and from mucous glands which are collections of mucus-producing cells linked to the surface by a short duct. In the middle ear, the glands are sometimes absent; however, in those ears where they are present, they tend to be clustered around the orifice of the eustachian tube, although they are never present in large numbers. Goblet cells eject mucus directly into the middle ear space (*Figure 1.22*) and are in highest concentration close to the eustachian tube opening (Tos and Bak-Pedersen, 1976). Again, large numbers of goblet cells do not occur, but their presence is indicative of the potential ability of the middle ear mucosa to undergo changes typical of respiratory epithelium.

The mucous membrane lines the bony walls of the tympanic cavity, and it extends to cover the ossicles and their supporting ligaments in much the same way as the peritoneum covers the viscera

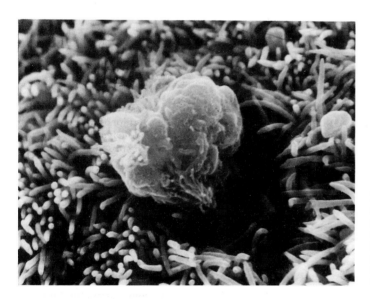

Figure 1.22 High magnification scanning electron micrograph of the surface of the respiratory mucosa from the nasopharyngeal end of the eustachian tube. A small volume of mucus is being secreted from a goblet cell. The cilia of the surrounding cells are clearly seen. Picture width 10 μm

Table 1.4 Blood supply to the middle ear

Branch	Parent artery	Region supplied
Anterior tympanic	Maxillary artery	Tympanic membrane, malleus and incus, anterior part of tympanic cavity
Stylomastoid	Posterior auricular	Posterior part of tympanic cavity, stapedius muscle
Mastoid	Stylomastoid	Mastoid air cells
Petrosal	Middle meningeal	Roof of mastoid, roof of epitympanum
Superior tympanic	Middle meningeal	Malleus and incus, tensor tympani
Inferior tympanic	Ascending pharyngeal	Mesotympanum
Branch from artery	Artery of pterygoid canal	Meso- and hypotympanum
Tympanic branches	Internal carotid	Meso- and hypotympanum

22

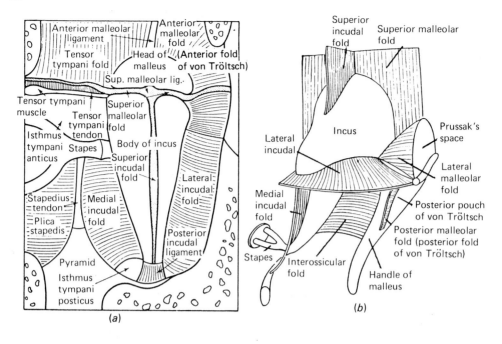

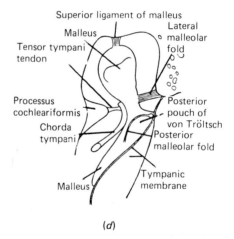

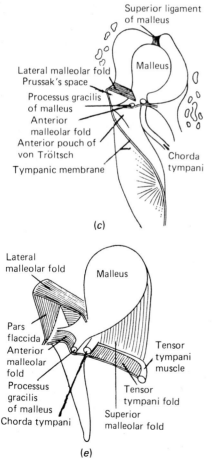

Figure 1.23 The compartments and folds of the middle ear (after Proctor 1964). (*a*) The attic folds. (*b*) Posterosuperior and lateral view of the right middle ear. (*c*) The anterior pouch of von Tröltsch viewed from an anterior aspect. (*d*) The posterior pouch of von Tröltsch viewed from a posterior aspect. (*e*) Prussak's spaces showing the posterior two-thirds of the space, seen from in front

in the abdomen. The mucosal folds also cover the tendons of the two intratympanic muscles and carry the blood supply to and from the contents of the tympanic cavity. These folds separate the middle ear space into compartments and the epitympanic space is only connected to the mesotympanum and is, therefore, ventilated only by way of two small openings between the various mucosal folds – the anterior and posterior isthmus tympani (*Figure 1.23*). The mucosal folds have been described in detail by Proctor (1964) and are depicted in *Figure 1.23*.

The blood supply of the tympanic cavity

Arteries supplying the walls and contents of the tympanic cavity arise from both the internal and external carotid system. The overlap between branches is extensive and there is great variability in the supply between individuals. *Table 1.4* outlines the general distribution of the arterial supply although the anterior tympanic and stylomastoid arteries are the biggest. Because of the great variability of the blood supply, and the difficulty of interpretation of injected specimens, an 'average' view of the blood supply has been presented. Different authors give different names to what appear to be the same vessels, and attach varying importance to the contribution made by each. However, most authors believe that a major contribution to the supply of the stapes and incudostapedial joint comes from a plexus of vessels derived from the stylomastoid artery and which surrounds the facial nerve to enter the tympanic cavity by way of the pyramid or directly through its posterior wall. Additional vessels reach the stapes from the meshwork of arterioles on the promontory, and probably derive mainly from the anterior and inferior tympanic arteries.

The eustachian tube (auditory or pharyngotympanic tube)

The eustachian tube is a channel connecting the tympanic cavity with the nasopharynx. In the adult, it is about 36 mm long and runs downwards, forwards and medially from the middle ear. There are two elements to the tube: a lateral bony portion arising from the anterior wall of the tympanic cavity, and a medial fibrocartilaginous part entering the nasopharynx. The tube is lined with respiratory mucosa containing goblet cells and mucous glands and having a carpet of ciliated epithelium (*Figure 1.24*). At its nasopharyngeal end, the mucosa is truly respiratory; but in passing along the tube towards the middle ear, the number of goblet cells and glands decreases, and the ciliary carpet becomes less profuse.

The bony portion is about 12 mm long and is widest at its outer tympanic end. It runs through the squamous and petrous portions of the temporal bone and gradually narrows to the isthmus which is the narrowest part of the whole tube, having a diameter of only 2 mm or less. The roof of the tube is formed by a thin plate of bone, above which is the tensor tympani muscle. The carotid artery, also separated by a plate of bone, lies medial to the tube. In cross-section, the tube is triangular or rectangular with the horizontal diameter being the greater.

The cartilaginous part of the tube is about 24 mm long and has a plate of cartilage forming its back (posteromedial) wall. At the upper border, the cartilage is bent forwards to form a short flange

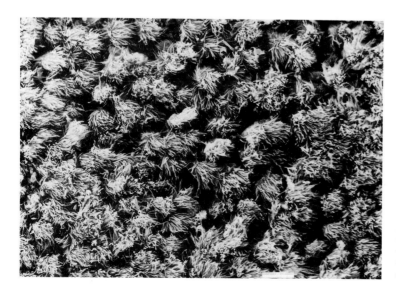

Figure 1.24 Scanning electron micrograph of surface of respiratory epithelium from nasopharyngeal end of human eustachian tube. A dense carpet of cilia is present on the surface. Marker 10 μm

that makes up part of the front (anterolateral) wall. The rest of the front wall comprises fibrous tissue (*Figure 1.25*). The apex of the cartilage is attached to the isthmus of the bony portion, while the wider medial end lies directly under the mucosa of the nasopharynx and forms the tubal elevation.

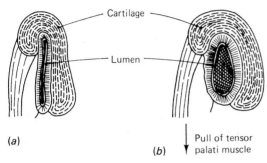

(a)

(b)   ↓ Pull of tensor palati muscle

Figure 1.25 Schematic diagram of the cartilaginous portion of the right eustachian tube. (*a*) Tube closed. (*b*) Tube open demonstrating the pull of the tensor palati muscle

The cartilage is fixed to the base of the skull in a groove between the petrous part of the temporal bone and the greater wing of the sphenoid. The groove terminates near the root of the medial pterygoid plate. In the nasopharynx, the tube opens 1–1.25 cm behind and a little below the posterior end of the interior turbinate. The opening is almost triangular in shape and is surrounded above and behind by the tubal elevation. The salpingopharyngeal fold stretches from the lower part of the tubal elevation downwards to the wall of the pharynx. The levator palati, as it enters the soft palate, results in a small swelling immediately below the opening of the tube. Behind the tubal elevation is the pharyngeal recess or fossa of Rosenmüller. Lymphoid tissue is present around the tubal orifice and in the fossa of Rosenmüller, and may be prominent in childhood.

Muscles attached to the eustachian tube

The tensor palati muscle arises from the bony wall of the scaphoid fossa, the spine of the sphenoid and from along the whole length of the short cartilaginous flange that forms the upper portion of the front wall of the cartilaginous tube. From these origins, the muscle descends, converges to a short tendon that turns medially around the pterygoid hamulus and then spreads out within the soft palate to meet fibres from the other side in a midline raphe. The tensor palati separates the tube from the otic ganglion, the mandibular nerve and its branches, the chorda tympani nerve and the middle meningeal artery. It is supplied by the mandibular nerve.

The salpingopharyngeus is a slender muscle attached to the inferior part of the cartilage of the tube near its pharyngeal opening, and it descends to blend with palatopharyngeus.

The levator palati contains a few fibres that arise from the lower surface of the cartilaginous tube. This muscle, which also originates from the lower surface of the petrous bone, just in front of the opening for the entrance of the carotid, and from fascia forming the upper part of the carotid sheath, first lies inferior to the tube, then crosses to the medial side and spreads out into the soft palate. Both the salpingopharyngeus and the levator palati are supplied from the pharyngeal plexus.

The mechanism of tubal opening during swallowing and yawning is not well understood. The tensor palati probably plays a major role, assisted by the levator palati and possibly by the salpingopharyngeus which is too slender to have much effect in raising the pharynx and larynx.

The tube is supplied by the ascending pharyngeal and middle meningeal arteries. The veins drain into the pharyngeal plexus and the lymphatics pass to the retropharyngeal nodes. The nerve supply arises from the pharyngeal branch of the sphenopalatine ganglion (Vb) for the ostium, the nervus spinosus (Vc) for the cartilaginous portion and from the tympanic plexus (IX) for the bony part.

The aditus to the mastoid antrum

This is a large irregular opening leading from the posterior epitympanum into the air-filled spaces of the mastoid antrum, often referred to as the aditus ad antrum. On the medial wall is the prominence of the lateral semicircular canal. Below and slightly medial to this is the bony canal of the facial nerve.

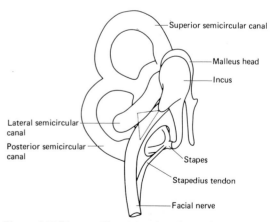

Figure 1.26 Diagram illustrating the relationship between the short process of the incus, the seventh nerve and the semicircular canal (lateral). The average dimensions are given in the text. This is the right ear with the structures viewed from behind and laterally

The short process of the incus is closely related to these two structures, and the average distances between them are: seventh nerve to semicircular canal – 1.77 mm; seventh nerve to short process incus – 2.36 mm; and short process incus to semicircular canal – 1.25 mm (Anson and Donaldson, 1981) (*Figure 1.26*).

The mastoid antrum

The mastoid antrum is an air-filled sinus within the petrous part of the temporal bone. It communicates with the middle ear by way of the aditus and has mastoid air cells arising from its walls. The antrum, but not the air cells, is well developed at birth and by adult life has a volume of about 1 ml – being 14 mm from front to back, 9 mm from top to bottom and 7 mm from side to side. The medial wall of the antrum is related to the posterior semicircular canal and more deeply and inferiorly is the endolymphatic sac and the dura of the posterior cranial fossa. The roof forms part of the floor of the middle cranial fossa and separates the antrum from the temporal lobe of the brain. The posterior wall is formed mainly by the bony covering of the sigmoid sinus. The lateral wall is part of the squamous portion of the temporal bone and increases in thickness during life from about 2 mm at birth to 12–15 mm in the adult. The lateral wall in the adult corresponds to the suprameatal (Macewen's) triangle on the outer surface of the skull. This region can be felt through the cymba conchae of the auricle and is defined by the supramastoid crest – which is the posterior prolongation of the upper border of the root of the zygoma – by a vertical tangent through the posterior margin of the external meatus and,

finally, by the posterosuperior margin of the external meatus itself.

The floor of the mastoid antrum is related to the digastric muscle laterally and the sigmoid sinus medially, although in a poorly aerated mastoid bone these structures may be 1 cm away from the inferior antral wall. The anterior wall of the antrum has the aditus in its upper part, while lower down, the facial nerve passes in its descent to the stylomastoid foramen. The relationships of the mastoid antrum are shown in *Figure 1.27*.

The mastoid air cell system

In the majority of the adult population, a more or less extensive system of interconnecting air-filled cavities arises from the walls of the mastoid antrum, and sometimes even from the walls of the epi- and mesotympanum. These air cells can extend throughout the mastoid process and may be separated from the sigmoid sinus and posterior and middle cranial fossae by thin bone, which is occasionally deficient. Cells often extend medial to the descending portion of the facial nerve as the retrofacial cells, down to the digastric muscle as the tip cells, and around the sigmoid sinus as the perisinus cells. They can reach the angle between the sigmoid sinus and the middle fossa dura (the sinodural angle), and may even extend out of the mastoid bone into the root of the zygoma and into the floor of the tympanic cavity underneath the basal turn of the cochlea. Occasionally, the apex of the petrous bone is pneumatized (*see* following subsection).

These air cells, like the mastoid itself, are lined with a flattened non-ciliated squamous epithelium. Pneumatization can be very extensive, as described previously, when the mastoid process is referred to in terms such as cellular, well-aerated, or by some similar name. Alternatively, the mastoid antrum may be the only air-filled space in the mastoid process when the name acellular or sclerotic is applied. This condition occurs in perhaps 20% of adult temporal bones. In between these two forms are the so-called diploeic or mixed types where air cells are present but are interspersed with marrow-containing spaces that have persisted from late fetal life.

The petrous apex

The petrous apex is, surgically, the most inaccessible portion of the temporal bone, and has the shape of a truncated pyramid with a base and three sides making up the medial part of the bone (*Figure 1.28*). The base of this pyramid is formed, from front to back, by the canal for the tensor

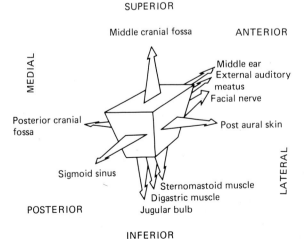

SUPERIOR

Middle cranial fossa   ANTERIOR

MEDIAL

Middle ear
External auditory meatus
Facial nerve

Posterior cranial fossa

Post aural skin

LATERAL

Sigmoid sinus

Sternomastoid muscle
Digastric muscle
Jugular bulb

POSTERIOR

INFERIOR

Figure 1.27 Relationships of the right mastoid antrum

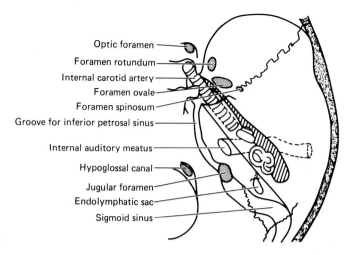

Optic foramen
Foramen rotundum
Internal carotid artery
Foramen ovale
Foramen spinosum
Groove for inferior petrosal sinus
Internal auditory meatus
Hypoglossal canal
Jugular foramen
Endolymphatic sac
Sigmoid sinus

Figure 1.28 Diagram showing the floor of the middle and posterior cranial fossae of the right side of the skull. The eustachian tube, middle ear and mastoid air spaces are represented by the dark cross-hatching while the paths of the internal and external auditory auditory canals are shown by interrupted lines. The text contains the description of the boundaries of the petrous apex

tympani and the carotid artery, by the cochlea, the vestibule and the semicircular canals. The superior surface is the floor of the middle cranial fossa extending forwards from the line of the superior semicircular canal (indicated by the arcuate eminence) to the foramen lacerum and the impression for the ganglion of the trigeminal nerve (V). The posterior surface forms the bony wall of the posterior cranial fossa and extends, again from back to front, from the endolymphatic sac and the line of the posterior semicircular canal to the pointed anterior tip of the petrous bone, from which arises the petroclinoid ligament. The junction between the superior and posterior surfaces is marked by the superior petrosal sinus, and the lower limit of the posterior surface is the suture line with the occipital bone. The third face of the pyramid has the jugular bulb and inferior petrosal sinus at its margins and the external opening of the carotid canal in the middle.

Two structures run through the petrous apex – the carotid artery and internal auditory meatus. The latter structure, on entering the posterior surface, divides the petrous apex into anterior and posterior parts. Chole (1985), from whom this description of the petrous apex is derived, reports that about 10% of normal human temporal bones have air cells within the anterior part, while perhaps 30% have a pneumatized posterior segment.

It is also of interest that the carotid artery loses its thick muscular medial layer as it enters the temporal bone from the neck, with the result that the mean thickness of the wall is only 0.15 mm. Sometimes, also, the medial bony wall of the eustachian tube is deficient or extremely thin, so that the carotid is separated from the mucosal lining of the tube by just a thin layer of fibrous connective tissue.

The internal auditory meatus

This is a short canal, nearly 1 cm in length and lined with dura, which passes into the petrous bone in a lateral direction from the cerebellopontine angle. It is closed at its outer lateral end, or fundus, by a plate of bone which is perforated for the passage of nerves and blood vessels to and from the cranial cavity. The meatus transmits the facial, cochlear and vestibular nerves and the internal auditory artery and vein.

Although various authors, having used different techniques for measurement, report dissimilar dimensions, on average the vertical diameter of the meatus in 90% of normal subjects lies between 2 mm and 8 mm, with an average of about 4.5 mm, and the difference between the two sides in an individual does not exceed 1 mm. The average length of the posterior wall is 8 mm, and the difference between the two sides does not exceed 2 mm (Valvassori and Pierce, 1964; Papangelou, 1972).

The bony plate separating the fundus from the middle and inner ears has a transverse crest on its inner medial surface. This is the crista falciformis and it separates a small upper region from a larger lower area (*Figure 1.29*). Above the crest and anteriorly is the opening of the facial canal carrying the facial nerve (VII). This is separated, by a small vertical ridge (Bill's bar), from the posterior region which transmits the superior vestibular nerve through several small foramina to the superior and lateral semicircular canals, to the utricle and a part of the saccule. Below the transverse crest, the cochlear nerve lies anteriorly and leaves the meatus through the cochlear area which comprises a spiral of small foramina and a central canal. The inferior vestibular nerve passes through one or two foramina behind the cochlear

SUPERIOR

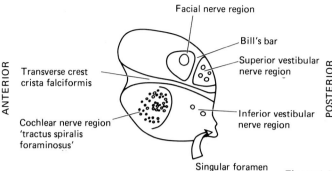

Facial nerve region

Bill's bar

Superior vestibular nerve region

Transverse crest crista falciformis

Inferior vestibular nerve region

Cochlear nerve region 'tractus spiralis foraminosus'

ANTERIOR

POSTERIOR

Singular foramen

INFERIOR

Figure 1.29 The right internal auditory meatus, viewed along its axis and from the posterior cranial fossa

opening to supply the saccule. Just behind and below the inferior vestibular foramen is the foramen singulare which contains the singular nerve. This runs obliquely through the petrous bone close to the fenestra cochleae (round window) to supply the sensory epithelium in the ampulla of the posterior semicircular canal.

The inner ear

The inner ear, or labyrinth, lies in the temporal bone, and for descriptive purposes it is divided into a bony and membranous portion. The membranous labyrinth containing the sensory epithelium of the cochlea and vestibular structures lies within cavities surrounded by the bony labyrinth.

The bony labyrinth

This is derived from the inner periosteal layer of the otic capsule, and in adult life consists of a thin,

but dense, bony shell surrounding the vestibule, the semicircular canals and the cochlea.

The vestibule

The vestibule is the central portion of the bony labyrinth and is a small flattened ovoid chamber lying between the middle ear and the fundus of the internal auditory meatus. It is about 5 mm long, 5 mm high, but only 3 mm deep. On its lateral wall is the opening of the fenestra vestibuli closed in life by the footplate of the stapes and its annular ligament. On the medial wall anteriorly is the spherical recess which houses the macule of the saccule and which is perforated by small holes that carry fibres from the inferior vestibular nerve (*Figure 1.30*). Behind the spherical recess is a ridge named the vestibular crest. At its lower end, the ridge divides to encompass the cochlear recess which carries cochlear nerve fibres to the very base of the cochlea. Above and behind the crest is an elliptical recess which contains the macule of the utricle. Nerve fibres, destined for the utricle and

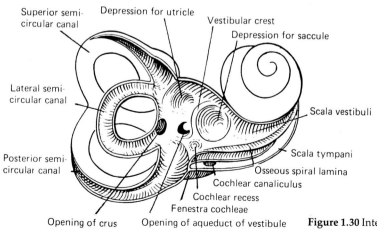

Superior semi-circular canal

Depression for utricle

Vestibular crest

Depression for saccule

Lateral semi-circular canal

Scala vestibuli

Scala tympani

Posterior semi-circular canal

Osseous spiral lamina

Cochlear canaliculus

Cochlear recess

Fenestra cochleae

Opening of crus commune

Opening of aqueduct of vestibule

Figure 1.30 Interior aspect of the right bony labyrinth viewed from the lateral aspect

superior and lateral semicircular canals, perforate the bony wall in an area close by which corresponds to the superior vestibular nerve region at the fundus of the internal auditory meatus. The opening of the vestibular aqueduct lies below the elliptical recess, and the aqueduct itself passes through the temporal bone to open in the posterior cranial fossa but outside of the dura. It carries the endolymphatic duct and several small blood vessels. The posterior wall of the vestibule contains five openings that lead into the semicircular canals. The anterior wall of the vestibule contains an elliptical opening into the scala vestibuli of the cochlea.

The semicircular canals

There are three semicircular canals – superior, posterior and lateral – situated above and behind the vestibule. Each occupies about two-thirds of a circle and the canals are unequal in length, although the lumen of each has a diameter of about 0.8 mm. At one end of each canal is a dilatation called the ampulla which contains the vestibular sensory epithelium and opens into the vestibule. For the superior and lateral canals, the ampullae are next to each other at their antero-lateral ends, while the ampulla of the posterior canal lies inferiorly near the floor of the vestibule. The non-ampullated ends of the superior and posterior canals meet and join to form the crus commune which enters the vestibule in the middle of its posterior wall. The non-ampullated end of the lateral canal opens into the vestibule just below the crus commune.

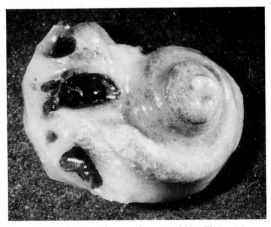

Figure 1.31 The right human bony cochlea. The petrous temporal bone has been drilled down until only a thin bony capsule enclosing the membranous labyrinth remains. The stapes has been removed from the oval window, and the bone overhanging the round window membrane partly removed. In this cochlea there are slightly more than two-and-one-half turns

In the two ears, the lateral canals lie nearly in the same plane which slopes downwards and backwards at an angle of about 30° to the horizontal when the individual is standing. The other canals are at right angles to this, so that the superior canal of one ear lies nearly parallel with the posterior canal of the other.

The lateral canal bulges the medial wall of the epitympanum, while the apex of the superior canal lies very close to the floor of the middle cranial fossa. The arcuate eminence of this portion of the petrous bone often, but not always, overlies this part of the superior canal.

The cochlea

The bony cochlea lies in front of the vestibule and has an external appearance rather like the shell of a snail (*Figure 1.31*). It is, however, a coiled tube, with the inside of one coil being separated from the lumen of an adjacent coil by a dense, but thin, bony wall. The shell has approximately two-and-one-half turns and its height is about 5 mm, while the greatest distance across the base is about 9 mm. The coils of the cochlea turn about a central cone or modiolus which arises from the cochlear nerve portion of the fundus of the internal auditory meatus, and points laterally and forwards, tapering from a wide base to a narrow apex. The apex of the cochlea, therefore, faces laterally and forwards towards the upper part of the medial wall of the tympanic cavity, while the basal coil forms the bulge of the promontory below this. Arising from the modiolus is a thin shelf of bone that spirals upwards within the lumen of the cochlea as the bony spiral lamina. A membrane – the membranous spiral lamina – extends from the edge of the bony spiral lamina to the outer wall of the cochlea, thereby dividing each coil into two major portions – the scala vestibuli and scala tympani.

Conventional anatomical nomenclature becomes very difficult within the cochlea because of its coiled shape and orientation, so that a separate system has arisen which defines the position of structures relative to the modiolus which is thought of as rising vertically from base to apex (*Figure 1.32*). Structures close to the modiolus are inner or medial, while other more distant structures are outer or lateral. A coil at the apex is above or apical to a coil at the base, while within one coil a structure on the apical side of the spiral lamina is above one below it. The scala vestibuli, therefore, lies above the scala tympani. This has greatly simplified relating one structure to another, and the terminology will be continued in this chapter.

At the apex, the spiral lamina continues for a short distance as a spur or crescent that is not

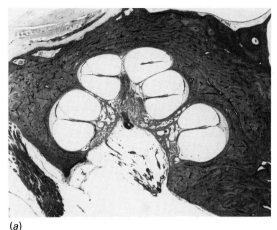

(a)

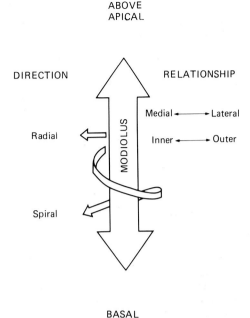

(b)

Figure 1.32 (a) Standard mid-modiolar section of the human cochlea. The spiral lamina is attached to the modiolus and separates the scala tympani below from the scala vestibuli above. The triangular scala media, or cochlear duct lies on the lateral or outer portions of the spiral lamina. (Courtesy of Professor L. Michaels, Institute of Laryngology and Otology.) (b) Diagram representing the nomenclature of the spatial relationships within the cochlea

attached to the modiolus (*Figure 1.33*). There is, therefore, communication between the perilymph spaces each side of the spiral lamina, and this channel is called the helicotrema.

At the base of the cochlea, the scala vestibuli opens into the vestibule with the fenestra vestibuli and stapes footplate close by on the lateral wall of the vestibule. The scale tympani is a blind-ended tube, but has in its floor the fenestra cochleae (round window) closed by the secondary tympanic membrane (round window membrane). A small opening into the cochlear aqueduct also

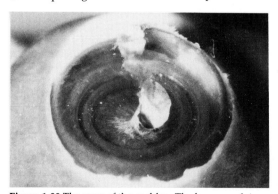

Figure 1.33 The apex of the cochlea. The bone overlying the apex of the cochlea has been removed to show the spiral lamina within. At the apex the spiral lamina continues on for a short distance as a spur or crescent not attached to the modiolus. The scala vestibuli and scala tympani are therefore in communication, and this channel is termed the helicotreme

arises from the basal end of the scala tympani. This aqueduct runs through the petrous bone and into the posterior cranial fossa well below the internal auditory meatus, establishing a communication between the subarachnoid space and the scala tympani.

The modiolus contains many small canals that spread out to enter the bony spiral lamina. The most central canals carry fibres to and from the apical regions, while the outermost canals carry fibres from more basal parts of the cochlea. Close to the origin of the bony spiral lamina, these canals dilate to accommodate the bipolar ganglion cells of the spiral (cochlear) ganglion, and the confluence of the dilated spaces has given rise to the name of the spiral canal of the modiolus. The name is slightly misleading as only a few unmyelinated efferent nerve fibres run along this apparent canal, with the vast majority of acoustic nerve fibres running across it from the organ of Corti, by way of the spiral ganglion, to form the cochlear nerve in the modiolus.

Perilymph

As well as containing the membranous labyrinth, the bony labyrinth is filled with perilymph. The exact origin of this fluid is not known, although it resembles plasma, interstitial fluid and cerebrospinal fluid in its make-up with major differences occurring in the concentration and type of proteins present (*see* Chapter 2 for further details).

The membranous labyrinth

The membranous labyrinth is a series of communicating sacs and ducts derived from ectoderm and filled with endolymph. Within the walls of the membranous labyrinth, the epithelium has become specialized to form the sensory receptors of the cochlear and vestibular labyrinth.

The cochlear duct (scala media)

The duct of the cochlea consists of a spirally arranged tube lying on the upper surface of the spiral lamina against the outer wall of the bony canal of the cochlea. The length of the cochlea, as measured by the length of the organ of Corti, varies enormously between individuals and much more than in experimental animals. The average length is around 34 mm (standard deviation about 2 mm) while the range is from 29 to 40 mm, which has interesting implications when the physiology of the cochlear function is considered (*see* Chapter 2). The length measurements are derived from the works of Retzius (1884), Bredberg (1968), Walby (1985) and Ulehlova, Voldrich and Janisch (1986).

The cochlear duct is triangular in section with a floor formed by the outer part of the bony spiral lamina and all of the membranous spiral lamina; with an outer wall lying against a fibrous thickening of the bony cochlear wall – the spiral ligament; and with a thin sloping roof – Reissner's membrane – that runs from the bony spiral lamina to the upper part of the outer wall. The scala vestibuli lies above the cochlear duct, the scala tympani below (*Figure 1.34*).

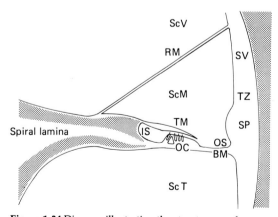

Figure 1.34 Diagram illustrating the structures and relationship of the cochlear duct. ScV = scala vestibuli; ScM = scala media; ScT = scala tympani; RM = Reissner's membrane; TM = tectorial membrane; OC = organ of Corti; BM = basilar membrane; IS = inner sulcus; OS = outer sulcus; SV = stria vascularis; TZ = transitional zone; SP = spiral prominence. ▓▓ = Bone

The floor of the cochlear duct

The inner part of the floor is formed by the bony spiral lamina which separates into two ridges one above the other. The upper ridge is the spiral limbus from which the tectorial membrane originates, while the lower ridge gives rise to the membranous spiral lamina and has acoustic nerve fibres running through it to the organ of Corti. The membranous spiral lamina has the flattened epithelium of the scala tympani on its underside, a fibrous middle layer and the organ of Corti on its upper surface. This is separated from the spiral limbus by the inner sulcus, and from the lateral wall by the outer sulcus. The organ of Corti is a ridge-like structure containing the auditory sensory cells and a complex arrangement of supporting cells. The sensory cells are arranged in two distinct groups as inner and outer 'hair cells' (*Figure 1.35*). They are called hair cells because a cluster of fine filaments, resembling hairs, projects from the upper surface of each sensory cell. There is a single row of inner hair cells, although occasionally extra hair cells may be apparent, and also three, four or five irregular rows of outer hair cells, with frequent gaps where individual hair cells are absent. The distribution of hair cells is markedly different from that seen in rodents (guinea-pigs, rats etc.) where there is nearly always a highly regular arrangement.

Each hair cell consists of a body, which lies within the organ of Corti, and a thickened upper surface called the cuticular plate, from which projects a cluster of stereocilia or 'hairs'. The stereocilia are not true cilia in that they do not have a central 'nine plus two' core of microtubules, but are more like large microvilli comprising a core of actin molecules packed in a paracrystalline array and covered with a cell membrane (Tilney, Derosier and Mulroy, 1980). The name 'cilia' is, therefore, inappropriate, but its use, like that of the term 'hair cell', has become entrenched in the literature and is unlikely to be replaced by a more convenient and correct term. The inner hair cells are separated from the outer ones by the tunnel of Corti. The bodies of the inner hair cells are flask-shaped, with a small apex and large cell body. The long axis of the cell is inclined towards the tunnel of Corti, and nerve fibres and nerve endings are located around the lower half of the body (*Figure 1.36*). The stereocilia projecting from the thickened cuticular plate are arranged in two or three rows parallel to the axis of the cochlear duct. The shortest row of stereocilia is innermost, while the longest row is outermost (*Figure 1.37*). Along the length of the cochlear duct, the height of the longest stereocilia increases linearly with distance from the base, although the variation from base to apex is not great.

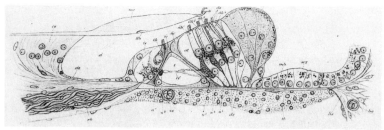

(a)

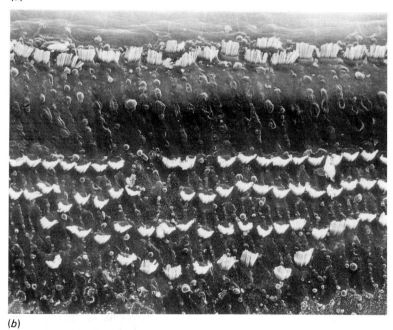

(b)

Figure 1.35 (*a*) Conventional light microscopic section of the human organ of Corti and tectorial membrane (from Retzius, 1884). (*b*) Scanning electron micrograph of a portion of the human organ of Corti. There is a single irregular row of inner hair cells with occasional extra inner hair cells. The outer hair cells lie in several irregular rows with gaps where the hair cells have been replaced by phalangeal scars. The rodent cochlea is by comparison remarkably regular. Picture width 200 μm

The body of the outer hair cell is cylindrical, with the nucleus lying close to the lower pole where afferent and efferent nerve endings are attached. The stereocilia that project from this have a different arrangement from those of the inner hair cells. There are several rows of stereocilia but the configuration varies from a W-shape at the base, through a V-shape in the middle coil, to an almost linear array at the apex. The number of stereocilia also decreases in the passage from base to apex, whereas the length increases although not in linear fashion (Wright, 1984) (*Figure 1.38*). Within a single cluster of stereocilia, individual members are linked by short transverse fibrils, and the tips of shorter stereocilia have fine fibrillar extensions running laterally to

adjoining longer stereocilia (Furness and Hackney, 1985). These linkages are also found between the stereocilia of both the inner hair cells and vestibular sensory cells (*Figure 1.39*). The role of these structures in cochlear mechanics is described in Chapter 2.

In the fetus and the newborn there are about 3500 inner hair cells and 13 000 outer hair cells (Bredberg, 1968), although the number of hair cells varies with the length of the cochlea, shorter cochleae having far fewer inner and outer hair cells. The distribution of hair cells, in terms of hair cell density related to place in the cochlea, can be plotted as a cytocochleogram, and it is found that with age there is a generalized reduction in the number of hair cells and an additional loss both at

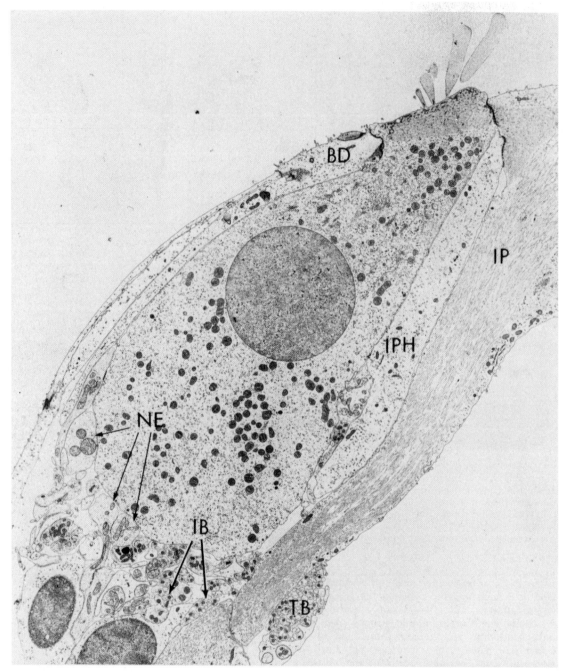

Figure 1.36 Transmission electron micrograph of an ultrathin section of a monkey's inner hair cell. The cell body is flask-shaped with a small apex, a large cell body and a central nucleus. Nerve fibres and nerve endings (NE) are located at the lower half of the cell body. Mitochondria are particularly plentiful in the lower half of the cell cytoplasm. The cell body makes contact with the inner phalangeal cell (IPH) laterally and with the border cell (BD) medially. IP = inner pillar cell; TB = tunnel spiral nerve bundle; IB = inner spiral nerve bundle. Picture width 13.5 μm (courtesy Robert Kimura)

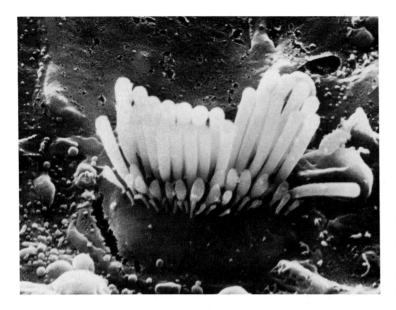

Figure 1.37 Scanning electron micrograph of a human inner hair cell. The stereocilia arise from a smooth cuticular plate and are arranged in an almost linear array. The short stereocilia are closer to the modiolus. Picture width 8 μm

the base and, to a lesser extent, at the apex. These changes are most marked in the outer hair cells but are also found in the inner hair cell population.

The hair cells are supported within the organ of Corti by several types of specialized, highly differentiated cells. These are the pillar cells, Deiters' cells and Hensen's cells.

The tectorial membrane arises from the spiral limbus and extends over the organ of Corti to attach close to the Hensen cell region (Kronester-Frei, 1979). The membrane is an acellular gel-like matrix containing fibrillar strands, and is extremely sensitive to distortion and shrinkage during most preparation techniques. The tips of the longest stereocilia of the outer hair cells are attached to, or embedded in, the undersurface of the tectorial membrane and leave an impression on this surface. In adults, however, no impression or attachment of the inner hair cells has ever been noted.

The lateral wall of the cochlear duct

The lateral wall of the cochlear duct has three distinct zones: the stria vascularis above, the spiral prominence below and a transitional zone between the two. The stria vascularis forms the bulk of the lateral wall and consists of three cell layers. The marginal cells face the endolymph and are separated by the intermediate cells from a basal cell layer which is rich in capillaries. The marginal cells have a carpet of microvilli on their endolymphatic surface and tight junctions between neighbouring cells, so that the stria vascularis is effectively isolated from the endolymph. These cells are also rich in mitochondria, have an extensive Golgi apparatus and endoplasmic reticulum, and complex foldings of their basal membranes, which interdigitate with the intermediate and basal cells. The stria is a metabolically active tissue and is thought to play an active role in the maintenance of the ionic composition and electrical potential of the endolymph.

The roof of the cochlear duct (Reissner's membrane)

Reissner's membrane is a thin membrane stretching from the bony spiral lamina to the upper part of the lateral wall of the cochlear duct. The endolymphatic surface consists of typical squamous epithelial cells with microvilli on their surface and joined together by tight junctions. A thin basement membrane separates these cells from those of the upper – scala vestibuli – side of the partition. These perilymphatic cells are thicker but have a dense cytoplasm only around the nucleus.

All of the cells lining the scala media are joined by tight junctions which effectively separate the endolymph from the outside and help in maintaining the unusual ionic content of this fluid (*see* Chapter 2 for details of the ionic constituents of endolymph).

The vestibular labyrinth

The vestibular labyrinth consists of a complex series of interconnecting membranous ducts and sacs which contain the vestibular sensory epithelium. Unlike the cochlea, the sensory epithelium is

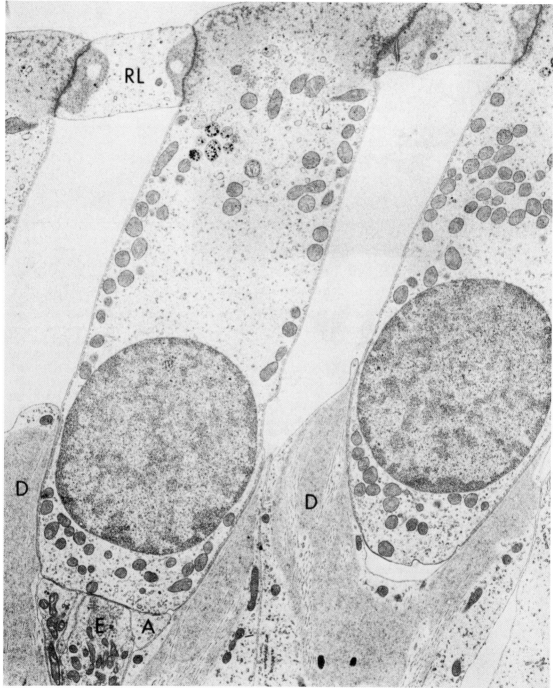

Figure 1.38 (*a*) Transmission electron micrograph of an ultrathin section of a monkey's outer hair cell. The cell body is cylindrical with the nucleus located in the lower pole. Mitochondria are present throughout the cell body but tend to be localized to the lateral cell membranes where, unlike the inner hair cell, there is a well-developed cisternal system. The apex of the cell is thickened to form the cuticular plate from which the stereocilia arise. The cell is supported at the apex by the phalangeal processes of Dieter's cells which form the reticular lamina (RL). At the base of the inner hair cell, the bodies of Dieter's cells (D) provide support. Afferent (A) and efferent (E) nerve endings synapse at the lower pole. The body of the hair cell is not supported but lies surrounded by perilymph in the spaces of Nuel. Picture width 13 μm (courtesy Robert Kimura).

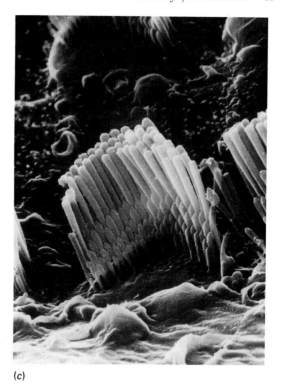

(b)

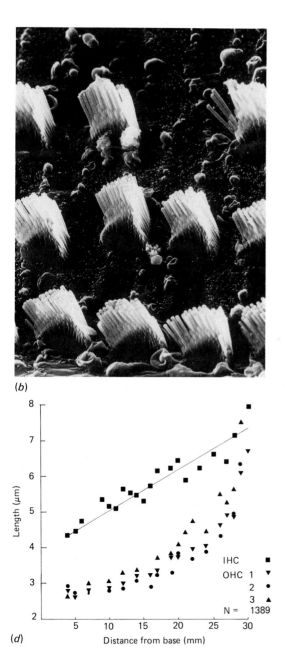

(c)

(d)

Figure 1.38 (*b*) Scanning electron micrograph of the outer hair cell region of the human organ of Corti. Three rows of outer hair cells are shown with a gap in the third row. Picture width 30 μm. (*c*) A single human outer hair cell. The stereocilia are arranged with the shortest ones being closest to the modiolus. Unlike the outer hair cells of rodents there are several rows of tall stereocilia. Picture width 9 μm. (*d*) Graphic representation of the length of the longest stereocilia of inner and outer hair cells related to position in the cochlea in terms of distance from the base in millimetres. There is a linear increase in the length of the stereocilia of the outer hair cells, but a more complex relationship for the stereocilia of the outer hair cells

found in localized collections in the three ampullae of the semicircular ducts and in the maculae of the saccule and utricle. The saccule lies in the spherical recess near the opening of the scala vestibuli of the cochlea. It is almost globular in shape but is prolonged posteriorly where it makes contact with the utricle. In the anterior wall there is an oval thickening – the macula. The saccule is connected anteriorly to the cochlea by a narrow duct, the ductus reuniens. From the posterior part arises the endolymphatic duct. This is joined by the utriculosaccular duct at an acute angle, and continues medially through the vestibular aqueduct to end as a blind pouch, the endolymphatic sac. The junction between the endolymphatic and utriculosaccular ducts has a Y-configuration with the lower limb continuing to the sac.

The utricle is the larger of the two vestibular sacs and is irregularly oblong in shape, occupying the posterosuperior part of the bony vestibule. The lower part of the lateral wall of the pouch contains the comma-shaped macula, the plane of which lies

36

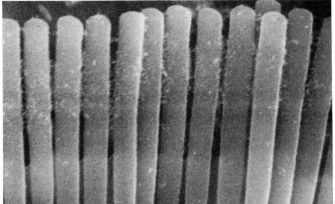

(a)

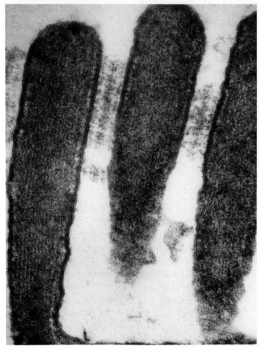

Figure 1.39 (a) Scanning electron micrograph of the inner hair cell stereocilia from a guinea-pig. The fine transverse cross links can be seen near to the tips. Picture width 6.5 µm. (b) Transmission electron micrograph of an ultrathin section of guinea-pig stereocilia showing not only the ordered structure of the actin molecules that form the core of these structures but also the nature of the crosslinks. Picture width 1.5 µm. (c) Transmission electron micrograph of the stereocilia showing the very fine apical crosslink which connects the tip of one stereocilia with the body of an adjacent one. (*Figures (a),* (b) and (c) courtesy of Dr A. Forge, EM Unit, Institute of Laryngology and Otology)

(b)

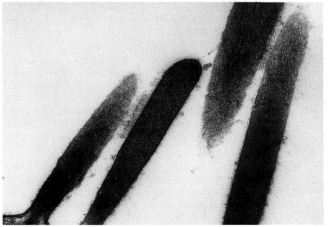

(c)

at right angles to that of the macule of the saccule. Apart from the utriculosaccular duct, there are five openings into the utricle which correspond to the utricular ends of the semicircular ducts.

The three semicircular ducts are about 0.2 mm in diameter and resemble the bony canals. Each duct has an ampulla at one end, and within this the sensory cells are collected on a saddle-shaped ridge – the crista – that runs across the lumen.

The vestibular sensory epithelium

The sensory cells of the ampullae and maculae have the same structure and comprise type I and type II cells. Type I cells are flask-shaped with a rounded base and a short neck. The body is surrounded by a large goblet-shaped nerve terminal, or chalice, which often extends to enclose more than one type I cell. The upper surface of the cell is thickened in the form of a cuticular plate and has a single kinocilium and between 20 and 100 stereocilia projecting from its surface. The kinocilium is slightly thicker than the stereocilia and has the internal structure of a true cilium with a 'nine plus two' arrangement of microtubules and an associated basal body and centriole. The stereocilia have the same internal structure as those of the cochlear sensory cells (*Figure 1.40*).

Type II cells are cylindrical in shape with the same collection of kino- and stereocilia as the type I cells. The cell body, however, is not surrounded by a nerve chalice but has many button-like nerve terminals associated with it. These button terminals are either granulated and thought to be efferent in origin, or non-granulated and presumed, conversely, to be afferent. The fibres arising from the type I cells are larger in diameter than those of the type II cells, and they are afferent. Efferent fibres to the type I cells appear to terminate on the nerve chalice itself rather than on the cell body (*Figure 1.41*).

The location of the kinocilium gives the sensory cells polarity and this is related to the changes that occur in the neural output when the ciliary bundle is deflected. Deviation in the direction of the kinocilium results in an increase in the resting output of nerve impulses of the afferent neurons, while deflection away from the kinocilium inhibits the resting discharge (*Figure 1.42*). The sensory

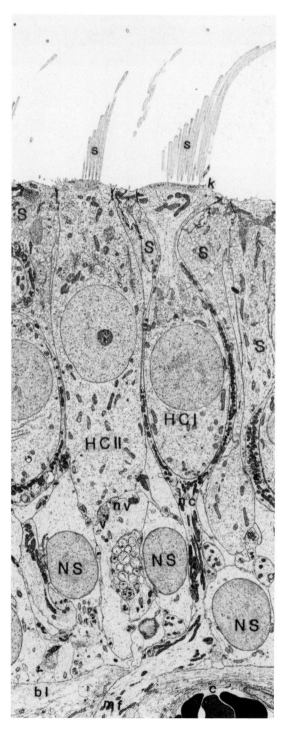

Figure 1.40 A portion of the macule of the utricle of the cat showing type I (HCI) and type II (HCII) sensory cells separated by supporting cells. Type I cells are partially surrounded by a nerve chalice (nc) which is the unmyelinated ending of a large myelinated nerve fibre (mf) seen crossing the basal lamina (bl). Vesiculated (v) and non-vesiculated (nv) nerve endings make synaptic contact with the infranuclear portion of type II cells. The nuclei of the supporting cells (NS) are located at the base of the epithelium. Each sensory cell has a single kinocilium (k) and many stereocilia (s) projecting from its free, endolymphatic surface. c = capillary containing red blood cells. Picture width 26 μm (courtesy Ivan Hunter-Duvar and Raul Hinojosa)

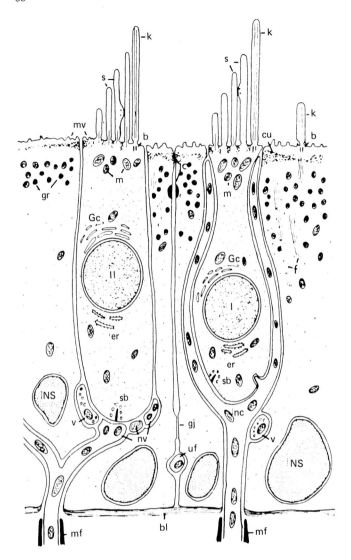

Figure 1.41 Diagram illustrating the general structure of vestibular sensory epithelium. The type I cell (I) is flask-shaped and is almost completely surrounded by a nerve chalice (nc). The type II cell (II) is cylindrical and innervated by vesiculated (v), and non-vesiculated (nv) button-like nerve terminals. b = basal body; j = junctional complex; cu = cuticular plate; m = mitochondria; Gc = Golgi complex; er = endoplasmic reticulum; sb = synaptic bar; f = tono filaments; gr = cytoplasmic vesicles in supporting cells; gj = gap junctions between supporting cells; uf = unmyelinated fibres; mf = myelinated fibres; NS = nucleus of supporting cell; bl = basal lamina. (Courtesy Ivan Hunter-Duvar and Raul Hinojosa)

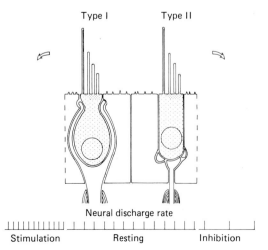

Figure 1.42 Diagram illustrating neural discharge pattern of vestibular sensory epithelium. As the ciliary bundle is deflected towards the kinocilium the resting discharge increases as the cell is stimulated. Inhibition and a decreased firing rate occurs when the opposite deflection occurs. The cells therefore have 'polarity'

cells are arranged in the cristae and maculae, so that there are strict patterns of orientation in the polarity of the cells (*see* Chapter 4 for further details and physiological relevance).

The sensory cells are surrounded by supporting cells. The apical surface of the supporting cells are covered with microvilli and it would appear that these cells have a secretory function. Close to the edges of the sensory cell regions of the cristae and maculae, and separated by a transitional zone in much the same way that the stria vascularis is separated from the organ of Corti, is a region occupied by 'dark cells'. These have an irregular surface, and resemble the marginal cells of the stria vascularis. Objects resembling degenerating otoconia are often found on the surface of the dark cells whose function is unclear but may, like the stria vascularis, have some role to play in the maintenance of the composition of the endolymph and, in addition, in the resorption of otoconia.

Structures associated with the vestibular sensory cells

In each ampulla, a gelatinous, wedge-shaped cupula sits astride the crista (*Figure 1.43*). The cupula, like the tectorial membrane, is extremely sensitive to alterations in its ionic environment and shrinks when standard preparative techniques are employed. In life, the cupula extends to the roof and lateral walls of the ampulla, and is attached firmly to each end of the crista. The rest of the dome of the ampulla also contains a loose fibrillar meshwork but there does appear to be a space between the cupula and the surface of the crista. The 'cilia' of the sensory cells project into this and the longest 'cilia' appear to enter the cupula. It seems most likely that during angular acceleration the cupula remains fixed, and the angle of the junction of the semicircular duct and the ampulla, along with the loose matrix within the dome of the ampulla, serve to direct endolymph into the subcupular space where deflection of the ciliary bundles occurs, with resulting stimulation or inhibition of the neural output of the sensory cells (Dohlman, 1981).

In each macula, a gelatinous material overlies the sensory cells, the ciliary bundles of which appear to project into a honeycomb meshwork in its undersurface. Embedded in the upper surface of the gelatinous layer are the otoconia. These have a characteristic shape with a barrel-shaped

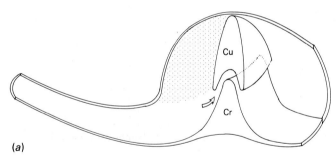

(a)

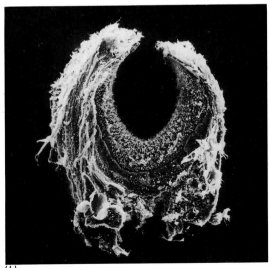

(b)

Figure 1.43 (*a*) Diagram of bisected semicircular duct and its associated ampulla (*see also Figure 1.6*). The arrow indicates that, during angular acceleration, the endolymph flows across the surface of the crista, beneath the cupula. Cu = cupula; Cr = crista.
(*b*) Scanning electron micrograph of the crista from the ampulla of the lateral semicircular canal of a young adult human. The dense carpet of stereocilia is apparent. Marker 100 µm

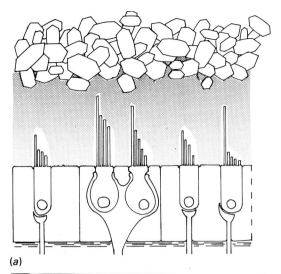

(a)

body and pointed ends (*Figure 1.44*). The size of the otoconia is not constant but varies across each macula. Small crystals are found near the central strip, or striola, and near to the margins, while the intervening zone has large, sometimes very large, crystals present in it. The term 'otoconial membrane' is used to describe the combination of the otoconia and the gelatinous membrane.

When the surface of the maculae is examined more closely, small globular bodies can be seen, apparently arising from the supporting cells (*Figure 1.44*). In experimental animals, these structures have a high calcium content and it has been suggested that the calcium of the otoconia is derived from this source (Harada, 1979). The otoconia are not static structures but appear to have a slow turnover with degenerating otoconia probably being resorbed by the dark cell regions (*see* Lim, 1984, for review).

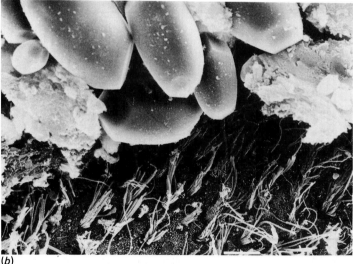

(b)

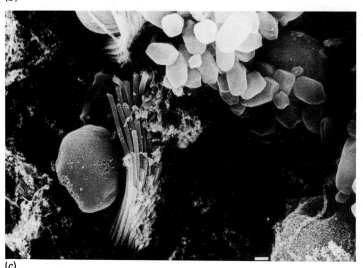

(c)

Figure 1.44 (*a*) Diagrammatic representation of the relationship of the sensory cells of the macula to the otoconial membrane. The ciliary bundles are embedded in the honeycomb-like meshwork of the gelatinous layer, which also contains the otoconia. (*b*) The surface of the human saccular macule. Some of the otoconia have been dislodged to reveal the amorphous gelatinous layer and the underlying sensory epithelium with the clusters of cilia. Picture width 100 μm. (*c*) A closer view of a single sensory cell and the otoconia from the striolar region. The wide range in the size of the otoconia can be appreciated from this and the preceding micrograph. A fine fibrillar meshwork, the remains of the gelatinous layer, clings to the surface of the cilia and the macula. A globular body is seen on the surface of the macula partly obscured by the bundle of stereocilia

The endolymphatic system

The endolymphatic system consists of a duct formed from the endolymphatic duct of the saccule and the utriculosaccular duct from the utricle, and a sac. The sac comprises three distinct portions. The proximal portion or isthmus is the first portion that is wider than the duct and lies within the bony vestibular aqueduct, as does the intermediate or rugose portion. The distal part of the sac is flattened and lies between the dura of the posterior fossa and the petrous bone. This arrangement is quite different from that found in most experimental animals where the rugose position, along with the distal position, is extra-dural.

The proximal part of the sac is lined with low cuboidal epithelium, whereas the intermediate, rugose, portion has a columnar epithelium that is extensively folded and, on cross-section, appears to consist of many small channels. The ultra-structural features suggest that the cells have an absorptive or secretory function. The distal part of the sac – that part which is surgically accessible – has a low cuboidal epithelium with no features suggestive of much metabolic activity, and an extremely narrow lumen as the opposing layers of the lining of the sac are frequently in contact (Lundquist *et al.*, 1984).

Innervation of the cochlea

The cochlea is connected with the brainstem by afferent and efferent nerves. The afferent nerves, carrying sensory information to the brainstem, have their cell bodies in the spiral ganglion and their terminal dendrites make contact with the hair cells. The efferent nerves pass directly through the spiral ganglion, their cell bodies being located within the brainstem.

There are major differences in the make-up of the cochlear nerve and spiral ganglion between the frequently studied small mammals and man, and because of the difficulty in obtaining suitable material much remains to be learnt about the anatomy in man. Nevertheless, each cochlear nerve in young, normal individuals contains about 30 000 myelinated nerve fibres. These are virtually all afferent, as the efferent fibres travel initially in the superior vestibular nerve (*see below*). The afferent fibres pass through the modiolus to the spiral canal where their cell bodies are found. Ninety-five per cent of the spiral ganglion cells are large type I cells, but unlike those found in other species the majority are unmyelinated as the afferent fibre loses its myelin sheath a short distance before entering the cell body. These type I cell bodies, both myelinated and unmyelinated, are bipolar and their terminal dendrites subse-

quently become myelinated for a short distance as they pass through the bony spiral lamina to reach the inner hair cells (Ota and Kimura, 1980). Each inner hair cells has about 10 dendrites synapsing around the lower part of the cell body.

The other 5% of spiral ganglion cells are small and may be myelinated or unmyelinated. The cell bodies can be unipolar or bipolar, and by analogy with animal work, it seems likely that the dendrites of these type II cells supply the outer hair cells. The fibres leave the spiral ganglion, run first across the floor of the tunnel of Corti and then descend the cochlea for up to 1 mm within an outer spiral bundle of nerve fibres before being distributed to 10 or more outer hair cells in various rows (*Figure 1.45*).

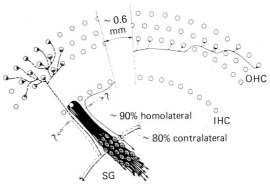

Figure 1.45 Horizontal innervation scheme of the organ of Corti in the cat. Although there are some differences between this animal and man the general pattern is much the same. The afferent nerve fibres are represented by solid lines, the efferent by interrupted lines. The efferent innervation of the outer hair cells (thick interrupted lines) originates (up to 80%) from the contralateral superior olivary complex while the efferents of the inner hair cell system (thin interrupted lines) originate (up to 90%) from the homolateral superior olivary complex. Virtually all of the afferent fibres (thick solid lines) arise from the inner hairs, only a few from the outer hair cells (thin solid lines). (Courtesy of Heinrich Spoendlin)

The efferent fibres are few in number and arise in both the homo- and contralateral superior olivary complex. They travel initially in the superior vestibular nerve which they leave in the internal auditory meatus to join the cochlear division by way of Oort's anastamosis. They enter the spiral canal within the modiolus and ascend or descend for a short distance. Some fibres subsequently supply the inner hair cells, while others run out across the tunnel of Corti as tunnel crossing fibres, to branch and terminate as large vesiculated nerve endings on several outer hair cells. The efferent innervation is most dense at the base of the cochlea but gradually diminishes towards the apex.

The other class of fibres entering the cochlea are adrenergic sympathetic fibres, some of which come from the superior cervical ganglion and are independent of the blood supply, whereas others originate in the stellate ganglion and arise from the plexus that surrounds the vertebral, basilar, anterior inferior cerebellar and labyrinthine arteries (*see* Spoendlin, 1984 for review).

The vestibular nerve

The vestibular nerve, like the cochlear nerve, contains afferent and efferent fibres as well as adrenergic sympathetic fibres. Unlike the cochlear nerve, however, there are a large number of efferent fibres and only 19 000 to 20 000 afferent fibres in the young adult. The calibre of the afferent fibres varies considerably between 2 and 15 μm (Spoendlin, 1972). The distribution of the various branches has already been described.

The vestibular ganglion (Scarpa's ganglion) contains the bipolar cell bodies of the afferent neurons as well as the efferent fibres that pass straight through. The ganglion lies at the lateral end of the internal auditory meatus partly covering the vestibular crest and being partially separated into a superior and inferior portion. Proximal to this, the vestibular nerve is a single bundle on its way to the brainstem by way of the cerebellopontine angle.

The central connections of the cochlear and vestibular nuclei are described in more detail in Chapter 2 (cochlear) and Chapter 4 (vestibular)

The blood supply of the labyrinth

The labyrinth is supplied principally from the labyrinthine artery which is usually a branch of the anterior inferior cerebellar artery, although it may arise directly from the basilar or even the vertebral arteries. The artery passes down the internal auditory meatus to divide into an anterior vestibular and a common cochlear artery, which subsequently divides into the cochlear artery and the vestibulocochlear artery.

The anterior vestibular artery supplies the vestibular nerve, much of the utricle and parts of the semicircular ducts.

The vestibulocochlear artery, on arrival at the modiolus, in the region of the basal turn of the cochlea, divides into its terminal vestibular and cochlear branches, which take opposite directions. The vestibular branch supplies the saccule, the greater part of the semicircular canals, and the basal end of the cochlea; the cochlear branch, running a spiral course around the modiolus, ends

by anastomosing with the cochlear artery. The vestibular and cochlear branches both supply capillary areas in the spiral ganglion, the osseous spiral lamina, the limbus, and the spiral ligament.

In the internal auditory canal, the cochlear artery runs a spiral course around the acoustic nerve. In the cochlea, it runs a serpentine course around the modiolus, as the spiral modiolar artery, which is an end artery. Arterioles leave this artery, to run either into the spiral lamina or across the roof of the scala vestibuli (*Figure 1.46*). Both

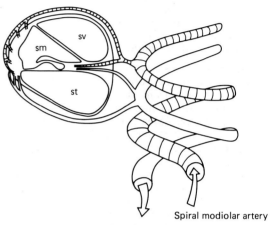

Spiral modiolar artery

Spiral modiolar vein

Figure 1.46 Diagram of the vascular supply to the organ of Corti and stria vascularis. sv = scala vestibuli; sm = scala media; st = scala tympani

sets of arteries end in capillary networks either in the spiral lamina or the stria vascularis on the lateral wall of the cochlear duct. The capillaries from the lateral wall drain into venules which run under the floor of the scala tympani to empty into modiolar veins which run spirally down the modiolus. The apical regions are drained by way of an anterior spiral vein, while the basal regions drain into the posterior spiral vein. These two branches of the spiral vein join with the anterior and posterior branches of the vestibular vein, in the region of the basal turn, to form the vein of the cochlear aqueduct – the principal vein of the cochlea – which empties into the jugular bulb.

The vestibular labyrinth is drained from the anterior part by the anterior vestibular vein, which becomes the labyrinthine vein and accompanies the artery of the same name, usually ending in the superior petrosal sinus; and also from the posterior part by the vein of the vestibular aqueduct which passes alongside the endolymphatic duct to the sigmoid sinus.

This description of the vascular supply of the cochlea is based on the work of Axelsson (1968).

The facial nerve

The seventh cranial nerve – the facial or intermediofacial – is a mixed nerve containing:

(1) motor fibres to the muscles of facial expression, the buccinator, stapedius, digastic and stylohyoid
(2) taste fibres from the palate and anterior two-thirds of the tongue
(3) secretomotor parasympathetic fibres to the lacrimal and nasal glands, and to the submandibular and sublingual salivary glands
(4) sensory fibres supplying part of the concha of the auricle and sometimes an area of skin behind the ear and part of the mucous membrane in the supratonsillar recess.

The motor fibres have their cell bodies in the facial nucleus in the pons. The nucleus receives pyramidal fibres from the contralateral motor cortex and a smaller number from the same side. The contralateral fibres reach all of the nucleus, while the ipsilateral fibres supply those parts of the motor nucleus involved with innervating the forehead and the muscles around the eyes (*Figure 1.47*). Other fibres also play on the facial motor nucleus and are involved in reflex movements. They come from the superior colliculus (an optic reflex centre), from the superior olive (acoustic reflex), as well as from sensory V nuclei and the nucleus of the solitary tract. The various inputs are involved in blinking and closing the eyes in response to strong light or touch on the cornea (corneal reflex), contraction and relaxation of the

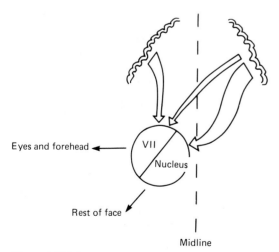

Eyes and forehead ← VII Nucleus

Rest of face

Midline

Figure 1.47 Schematic representation of innervation of nerve VII nucleus. The major supply is from the contralateral motor cortex but there is also a contribution from the ipsilateral side which supplies that part of the nucleus involved with innervating the muscles of the forehead and those around the eye

stapedius in response to sound, and sucking movements following the introduction of food into the mouth. Other fibres arrive from higher centres by way of the red nucleus, the mesencephalic reticular formation and probably the globus pallidus, and have been assumed to be involved with emotional facial movement.

The motor fibres leaving the facial nucleus do not pass directly out of the pons but first run medially and dorsally towards the floor of ventricle IV, turn around the nerve VI nucleus and then stream out laterally to leave the pons on the lateral aspect of the brainstem.

The sensory root of the facial nerve enters the brainstem as a separate nerve – the nervus intermedius. It carries the sensory fibres from the conchal skin and the supratonsillar recess, and the taste fibres from palate and tongue. The ganglion associated with these sensory fibres is the geniculate ganglion and the central processes of the unipolar ganglion cells leave the trunk of the facial nerve in the internal auditory meatus, as the nervus intermedius, to enter the brainstem at the lower border of the pons, and pass to the upper part of the nucleus of the solitary tract (tractus solitarius).

Secretomotor parasympathetic fibres also run in the nervus intermedius and have the superior salivatory nucleus as their origin.

At the fundus of the internal auditory meatus, the motor facial nerve – which, with the addition of the nervus intermedius, is now complete – enters the facial canal. In this canal, the nerve, surrounded by cerebrospinal fluid, runs between the cochlea anteriorly, the superior semicircular canal posteriorly and with the vestibule beneath it. This labyrinthine segment is the narrowest part of the facial canal with an average diameter of only 0.68 mm at the site of entry of the nerve (Fisch, 1979). As the nerve reaches the medial wall of the epitympanic recess, it turns sharply backwards to make an angle of about 60° with the subsequent tympanic segment. At this turn – the geniculum – lies the geniculate ganglion which is a reddish asymmetric swelling (*Figure 1.48*).

The tympanic portion of the nerve now begins as it runs posteriorly on the medial wall of the tympanic cavity. The nerve is surrounded by a bony shell and stands out clearly just above the promontory and oval window recess, but below the prominence of the lateral semicircular canal. The anterior end of the tympanic portion is marked by the processus cochleariformis which is a stable landmark rarely eroded by disease. From this level, the nerve slopes downwards and backwards at an angle of about 30° from the horizontal. Above the oval window recess the nerve starts to curve inferiorly, and at the level of the pyramid enters the descending or mastoid

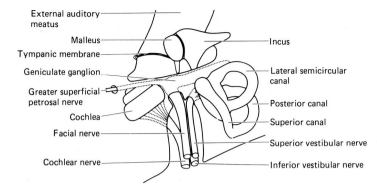

External auditory meatus
Malleus
Tympanic membrane
Geniculate ganglion
Greater superficial petrosal nerve
Cochlea
Facial nerve
Cochlear nerve
Incus
Lateral semicircular canal
Posterior canal
Superior canal
Superior vestibular nerve
Inferior vestibular nerve

Figure 1.48 Passage of the facial nerve through the right internal auditory meatus and middle ear, as seen from an approach through the middle cranial

portion of its intratemporal course. At this pyramidal turn, the short process of the incus always lies lateral to the nerve. In the descending portion, the nerve lies posterior and deep to both

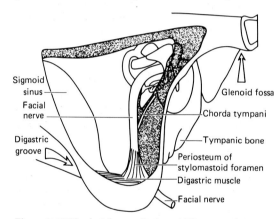

Sigmoid sinus
Facial nerve
Digastric groove
Glenoid fossa
Chorda tympani
Tympanic bone
Periosteum of stylomastoid foramen
Digastric muscle
Facial nerve

Figure 1.49 The facial nerve in the middle ear and mastoid segment as seen from a cortical mastoidectomy approach combined with a posterior tympanotomy. The stippling indicates the surface of bone that has been drilled during the cortical mastoidectomy

the tympanic annulus and the tympanomastoid suture line in the posterior wall of the external auditory meatus. This descending portion of the nerve lies deep within the mastoid portion of the temporal bone, rarely less than 1.8 cm from the outer surface of the bone in the adult (*Figure 1.49*).

The nerve emerges from the stylomastoid foramen to enter the neck. The posterior belly of digastric is attached to the digastric groove on the inferior surface of the mastoid process. This groove leads forwards to the stylomastoid foramen and the muscle provides a valuable landmark for the nerve. From the stylomastoid foramen, the nerve turns forward and passes laterally to the base of the styloid process and enters the parotid gland. Within the gland, the nerve separates into two primary divisions – an upper temporofacial and a lower cervicofacial. Each of these breaks up into several terminal branches which interconnect as the parotid plexus. From this plexus arise the terminal branches of the nerve.

During its course, the facial nerve makes communication with many other nerves, although the precise function of these is often unknown (*Table 1.5*).

Table 1.5 Branches of communication of the facial nerve

Location	Connection
Internal auditory meatus	Vestibulocochlear nerve
Geniculate ganglion	Greater petrosal nerve to pterygopalatine ganglion Via lesser petrosal nerve to otic ganglion Sympathetic plexus on middle meningeal artery
Facial canal	Auricular branch of vagus
At stylomastoid foramen	IX, X, greater auricular and auriculotemporal nerves
Behind the ear	Lesser occipital nerve
On the face	V nerve
In neck	Transverse cutaneous nerve of neck

Branches of the facial nerve

From the geniculate ganglion

(1) *Greater (superficial) petrosal nerve.* This leaves the geniculate ganglion anteriorly, runs forwards and receives a twig from the tympanic plexus. It enters the middle cranial fossa outside the dura, and runs in a groove in the bone to pass beneath the trigeminal ganglion where it is joined by the deep petrosal nerve from the sympathetic plexus on the internal carotid artery. The nerve is now called the nerve of the pterygoid canal and it runs through this canal to end in the pterygopalatine ganglion. Taste fibres pass on without interruption in the palatine branches of the ganglion. The secretomotor fibres in the nerve synapse within the ganglion and carry on by way of the zygomatic and lacrimal nerves to the lacrimal gland, and through the nasal and palatine nerves to the nasal and palatine glands.

Branches within the facial canal

(1) *Nerve to stapedius.* This arises from the facial nerve as the latter begins its descent, and reaches the muscle through a small canal in the base of the pyramid.
(2) *The chorda tympani.* This usually arises above the stylomastoid foramen but can occasionally leave the facial nerve outside the temporal bone and re-enter by way of a separate foramen. Its course in the middle ear has been described already and the nerve leaves the temporal bone by the petrotympanic fissure. It descends, sometimes grooving the medial surface of the spine of the sphenoid, and passes deep to the lateral pterygoid muscle to join the lingual nerve. The parasympathetic secretomotor fibres leave the lingual to enter the submandibular ganglion, which is suspended from the nerve by two fine neural filaments. The secretomotor fibres synapse within the ganglion and continue to supply the submandibular and sublingual salivary glands as well as other minor salivary glands in the floor of the mouth.

The majority of fibres in the chorda tympani are, however, taste fibres and these are derived from the mucous membrane of the presulcal part of the tongue but not from the vallate papillae which lie just in front of the sulcus.

Branches in the neck and face

(1) *The postauricular branch* arises close to the stylomastoid foramen and runs up between the external auditory canal and anterior surface of the mastoid. It has connections with other nerves as it continues on to supply the posterior auricular muscle, the intrinsic muscles of the posterior aspect of the pinna and the occipital muscle.
(2) *The diagastric branch* also arises close to the stylomastoid foramen and supplies the posterior belly of the digastric.
(3) *The stylohyoid branch* supplies the stylohyoid muscle and arises near or in conjunction with the digastric branch.

Branches from the parotid plexus

These are highly variable, as is the site of division of the facial nerve into temporofacial and cervicofacial divisions. Nevertheless, five major branches are nearly always found.

(1) *Temporal branches* cross the zygomatic arch and supply intrinsic muscles on the lateral surface of the auricle and the anterior and superior auricular muscles. Other branches supply the frontal belly of the occipitofrontalis, the orbicularis oculi and corrugator.
(2) *Zygomatic branches* run parallel to the zygomatic arch and also innervate orbicularis oculi. Some of the lower branches may join with the buccal branches to form an infraorbital plexus which innervates the muscles in the middle part of the face.
(3) *Buccal branches* pass horizontally forward to the muscles of the middle part of the face. These include the procerus, orbicularis oculi, zygomaticus, levator anguli oris, levator labii superioris, buccinator, orbicularis oris and the small muscles of the nose.
(4) *The mandibular branch* runs forward below the angle of the mandible under platysma and then turns upwards and forwards to cross the mandible under cover of depressor anguli oris which it supplies. It continues onwards and supplies the orbicularis oris and other muscles of the lips and chin.
(5) *The cervical branch* leaves the lower part of the parotid gland and runs down the neck under cover of platysma which it supplies.

Blood supply of the facial nerve

The facial nerve is supplied by the anterior inferior cerebellar artery in its intracranial course, by the superficial petrosal branch of the middle meningeal artery, and by the stylomastoid branch of the postauricular artery in its intratemporal course. Outside the skull, the stylomastoid artery, the posterior auricular or occipital, the superficial temporal and transverse facial artery are all involved.

The veins form a plexus around the nerve, and efferent veins run from this through the nerve sheath to lie on its outer surface. From the intratemporal portion, the venous drainage leaves the canal at the stylomastoid foramen and at the geniculum where it enters the venae comitantes of the stylomastoid and superficial petrosal arteries respectively.

References

ALBERTI, P. W. (1964) Epithelial migration over tympanic membrane and external canal. *Journal of Laryngology and Otology*, **78**, 808–830

ANSON, B. J. and DONALDSON, J. A. (1981) *Surgical Anatomy of the Temporal Bone*, 3rd edn. Philadelphia: W. B. Saunders

AXELSSON, A. (1968) The vascular anatomy of the cochlea in the guinea pig and in man. *Acta Oto-Laryngologica, Supplementum*, 243,6–134

BREDBERG, G. (1968) Cellular pattern and nerve supply of the human organ of Corti. *Acta Oto-Laryngologica Supplementum*, 236, 1–135

CHOLE, R. A. (1985) Petrous apicitis: surgical anatomy. *Annals of Otology, Rhinology and Laryngology*, **94**, 251–257

DOHLMAN, G. F. (1981) Critical review of the concept of cupula function. *Acta Oto-Laryngologica Supplementum*, 376, 1–30

FISCH, U. (1979) Facial paralysis. In *Clinical Otolaryngology*, edited by A. G. D. Moran and P. M. Stell, pp. 65–84. Oxford: Blackwell

FURNESS, D. N. and HACKNEY, C. M. (1985) Cross links between stereocilia in the guinea pig cochlea. *Hearing Research*, **18**, 177–188

GACEK, R. R. (1983) Cupulolithiasis and posterior ampullary nerve transection. *Annals of Otology, Rhinology and Laryngology*, Suppl. 112, 25–30

GIBSON, W. P. R. (1978) *Essentials of Clinical Electric Response Audiometry*, pp. 133–156. Edinburgh: Churchill Livingstone

HARADA, V. (1979) Formation area of statoconia. *Scanning Electron Microscopy*, III, 963–966

HENTZER, E. (1969) Ultrastructure of the human tympanic membrane. *Acta Oto-Laryngologica*, **63**, 376–390

JOHNSON, A. and HAWKE, M. (1985) Cell shape in the migratory epidermis of the external auditory canal. *Journal of Otolaryngology*, **14**, 273–281

KRONESTER-FREI, A. (1979) Localization of the marginal zone of the tectorial membrane *in situ* unfixed and with *in vivo* like ionic milieu. *Archives of Otorhinolaryngology*, **224**, 3–9

LIM, D. J. (1984) The development and structure of otoconia. In *Ultrastructural Atlas of the Inner Ear*, edited by I. Friedmann and J. Ballantyne, pp. 245–269. London: Butterworths

LUNDQUIST, P.-G. R., ANDERSEN, H., GALEY, F. R. and BAGGERSJOBACK, D. (1984) Ultrastructural morphology of endolymphatic duct and sac. In *Ultrastructural Atlas of the Inner Ear*, edited by I. Friedmann and J. Ballantyne, pp. 309–325. London: Butterworths

NOMURA, Y. (1984) Otological significance of the round window. *Advances in Oto-Rhinolaryngology*, No. 33, edited by C. R. Pfaltz, pp. 1–184. Basel: Kargel

OTA, C. Y. and KIMURA, R. S. (1980) Ultrastructural study of the human spiral ganglion. *Acta Oto-Laryngologica*, **89**, 53–62

PAPANGELOU, L. (1972) Study of the human internal auditory canal. *The Laryngoscope*, **82**, 617–624

PROCTOR, B. (1964) The development of the middle ear spaces and their surgical significance. *Journal of Laryngology and Otology*, **78**, 631–649

RETZIUS, G. (1884) *Das Gehororgan der Wilbeltiere*, Vol. II. Stockholm: Samson and Wallin

SADE, J. (1966) Middle ear mucosa. *Archives of Otolaryngology*, **84**, 137–143

SPOENDLIN, H. (1972) Innervation densities of the cochlea. *Acta Oto-Laryngologica*, **73**, 233–243

SPOENDLIN, H. (1984) Primary neurons and synapses. In *Ultrastructural Atlas of the Inner Ear*, edited by I. Friedmann and J. Ballantyne, pp. 133–164. London: Butterworths

STONE, M. and FULGHUM, R. S. (1984) Bactericidal activity of wet cerumen. *Annals of Otology, Rhinology and Laryngology*, **93**, 183–186

STREETER, G. L. (1922) Development of the auricle in the human embryo. *Contributions to Embryology*, **14**, 111–138

TILNEY, L. G., DEROSIER, D. J. and MULROY, M. J. (1980) The organization of actin filaments in the stereocilia of cochlear hair cells. *Journal of Cell Biology*, **86**, 244–258

TOS, M. and BAK-PEDERSEN, K. (1976) Goblet cell population in the normal middle ear and eustachian tube of children and adults. *Annals of Otology*, **85**, Suppl. 25, 44–50

ULEHLOVA, L., VOLDRICH, L. and JANISCH, R. (1986) Morphological aspects of cochlear tonotopy. *Hearing Research* (in press)

VALVASSORI, G. E. and PIERCE, R. H. (1964) The normal internal auditory canal. *American Journal of Roentgenology*, **92**, 1233–1242

WALBY, A. P. (1985) Scala tympani measurement. *Annals of Otology, Rhinology and Laryngology*, **94**, 393–397

WRIGHT, A. (1984) Dimensions of cochlear stereocilia in man and the guinea pig. *Hearing Research*, **13**, 89–98

2

Physiology of the ear

James O. Pickles

Sound and its analysis

An understanding of some of the basic physical properties of sound is a prerequisite for understanding the performance of the auditory system. The transmission of a sound wave from a loudspeaker can be seen in *Figure 2.1*. The wave shows variations in the pressure of the air, and the velocity and displacement of the molecules. This wave is traversing freely and, in such a case, when the pressure of the wave is at a maximum, the forward velocity of the air molecules is also at a maximum. However, the *displacement* of the molecules lags by one-quarter of a cycle. The displacement occurs around the mean position; the sound wave does not cause any *net* flow of air in the direction of motion, and the actual air pressure variations are only a small variation around the mean atmospheric pressure. A sound which is loud enough to be at the pain threshold – 130 dB sound pressure level (SPL) – is nevertheless only sufficient to produce pressure variations which are 0.2% of the resting atmospheric pressure.

A sound wave as shown in *Figure 2.1* has two basic properties: *intensity*, which has the subjective correlate of loudness; and *frequency*, which has the subjective correlate of pitch.

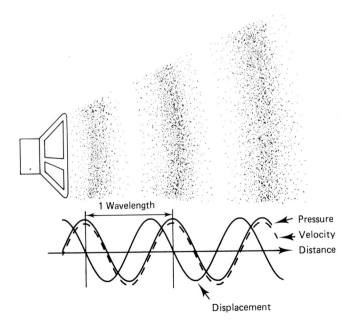

1 Wavelength

Pressure
Velocity
Distance

Displacement

Figure 2.1 The pressure, velocity, and displacement relations in a progressive sound wave

The pressure and intensity of sound waves

Basic relations

The peak pressure of the sound wave (P) can be related to peak velocity of the air molecules (V) by a constant of proportionality R:

$$P = RV \tag{1}$$

Here, R is called the impedance, and is a function of the medium in which the sound is travelling. From *Figure 2.1*, it can be seen that the pressure and velocity of the waveform vary together during the cycle. For such a wave, the same constant of proportionality holds over the whole cycle. This is the case if the wave is travelling freely and progressively in its medium. On the other hand, the situation becomes more complex if there are edges or other boundaries making reflections because, in such cases, the peak of pressure does not necessarily coincide with the peak of velocity. The ratio varies over the cycle and a simple number cannot be used to represent the ratio, and hence the impedance, of the air. Therefore, the impedance is a function not only of the medium alone, but also of its surroundings.

One basic property of the sound wave is that it involves the transfer of energy. The *intensity* is the *power* transmitted by the wave through a unit area. The intensity depends on both the pressure and the velocity, and is an average taken over a whole cycle. If the sound wave is sinusoidal (as in *Figure 2.1*), then there is a very simple relation between the power, the peak velocity and the peak pressure:

$$\text{Intensity} = \text{Peak pressure} \times \text{peak velocity}/2 \tag{2}$$

The factor of 2 is a function of the shape of the waveform. By using the dependence on R, it can also be expressed as a function only of P or V:

$$\begin{aligned}\text{Intensity} &= \text{Peak pressure}^2/2R \\ &= R \times \text{peak velocity}^2/2\end{aligned} \tag{2a}$$

This equation reveals the important parameters of the sound wave intensity. If the intensity of the sound wave is constant, the peak velocity and the peak pressure are also constant. The relation does not depend on the frequency of the sound wave. By contrast, the *displacements* produced by a sound wave do vary with frequency if the sound intensity is constant. The displacements vary in inverse proportion to the frequency, so that for a constant intensity, low frequency vibrations produce greater displacements.

The relation in equation (2) depends on the exact shape of the waveform. This dependency can be removed by measuring not the *peak* velocities and pressures but what is known as the root mean square (RMS). The RMS value is calculated by taking the value of the pressure or velocity at each moment in the waveform, squaring it, and then taking the average of all the squared values over the waveform. Finally, the square root is taken of the average. The RMS value is useful because the same relation between intensity, pressure and velocity holds over all shapes of waveform:

$$\begin{aligned}\text{Intensity} &= \text{RMS pressure}^2/R \\ &= \text{RMS velocity}^2 \times R\end{aligned} \tag{3}$$

The intensity of sound in air (that is in a medium with a constant and known value of R) can be measured by using the RMS pressure to specify the intensity of the wave. Pressure variations are also easily measurable by microphones. Therefore, the term 'sound pressure' is often used interchangeably with the term intensity. Caution is necessary, however, because in a medium of very different impedance, such as water, the intensity for a certain sound pressure will be very different (less in this case).

Decibels

A physicist would measure the RMS pressure in physical units, such as newtons/square metre (N/m^2 or pascals). Nevertheless, from the point of view of understanding the performance of the auditory system, it is easier to use a scale in which the vast range of sound pressures, from absolute threshold to pain threshold, is described by a convenient range of numbers. A wide range of numbers can be compressed into a smaller range by expressing these numbers as logarithms. The use of this method has other advantages, because the final scale corresponds in certain ways with the way in which sounds are heard. For instance, equal increments in sensation correspond approximately to equal increments in numbers on the logarithmic scale.

The scale is constructed by taking the logarithm of the sound intensity. However, the logarithm operation is best performed on quantities without dimensions – for example, ratios rather than, for instance, intensities. Therefore, the ratio of sound intensity to a reference intensity is used. If logarithms to the base 10 are used, the resulting units are called bels, after Alexander Graham Bell, the inventor of the telephone, since the scale was first used in telephony. The bel turns out to be rather too large to be convenient; therefore, the numbers are mulitplied by 10 to obtain units in terms of a smaller unit, one-tenth the size, known as the decibel. The formula for calculating decibels (abbreviated dB) is therefore as follows:

$$\text{Number of dB} = 10 \log_{10} \left[\frac{\text{sound intensity}}{\text{reference intensity}} \right] \tag{4}$$

Because it is usual to measure pressures rather than intensities, and because the intensity varies as the *square* of the pressure, decibels can be expressed in terms of pressure ratios, multiplying the logarithm by 20 instead of 10. Finally, a reference pressure has to be chosen. Any appropriate reference can be used. One scale in common use, the decibel sound pressure level (dB SPL) scale, uses a reference pressure of 2×10^{-5} N/m² RMS (20 μPa or 2×10^{-4} dyn/cm²). At standard temperature and pressure, air impedance is such that this corresponds to a power flow of approximately 10^{-12} W/m². In this scale, therefore,

$$\text{Intensity (dB SPL)} = 20\log_{10}\frac{(\text{RMS sound pressure})}{2 \times 10^{-5} \text{ N/m}^2} \quad (5)$$

Any other convenient reference pressure may be used. If the reference pressure is the subject's own absolute threshold at the frequency in question, the measure is known as decibels sensation level. Here, the subject's threshold is by definition 0 dB sensation level. The International Standards Organization (ISO) scale, uses as a reference the ISO standard human absolute threshold for the frequency being considered. Scales constructed in these ways are convenient for describing auditory performance. For instance, negative values of decibels sound pressure level (dB SPL; that is pressures below the reference) rarely have to be considered, since the reference is near the lowest absolute threshold. The range of numbers that has to be used is small, since 130 dB SPL is the human being's pain threshold. Similarly, step sizes less than 1 dB rarely have to be taken into consideration, since 1 dB is approximately the minimum intensity step detectable. Moreover, changes in intensity of equal numbers of decibels correspond to approximately equal steps in loudness.

The frequency of sound waves

Frequency, wavelength and velocity

The velocity of sound waves in free air is independent of the frequency, and at sea level has a value of 330 m/s. If the frequency of a wave is f cycles/s (or Hz), then f waves must pass any point in one second. The length of one wave is therefore $330/f$ metres. As an example, a 1-kHz wave has a wavelength of 0.33 m, and, as the equation shows, wavelengths become shorter with increasing sound frequency.

Relation between frequency and sensation

Frequency has the important subjective correlate of pitch. However, in complex sounds, the position is not necessarily clear. It is for instance important to specify what is meant by frequency in a complex sound. Sounds can be analysed mathematically into many separate frequency components, as will be discussed in detail below. This way of decomposing a complex sound is useful in discussing the physics and physiology of the system. While that approach is useful for some purposes, it does not necessarily mean that the individual frequency components in a complex sound can always be perceived, or that for certain stimuli the perceived pitch is always simply related to the frequency of the individual components in the complex.

The propagation of sound waves

Attenuation by distance

The way that sound waves progress through a medium depends on the nature of the medium, on the irregularities and inhomogeneities it contains, and on the boundaries of the medium. For the simplest source possible conceptually (although impossible to realize in practice), there is a point source of sound, situated in a completely even medium of infinite extent. The sound waves spread out evenly in all directions, so that the wavefronts make a series of expanding spheres centred on the source. In the idealized situation, the wavefront will not lose – or indeed gain – energy with time. Because the energy over the total area of the wavefront is constant, the energy in each *unit area* of wavefront decreases with distance. The total area increases as the square of the distance, and so the power passing through a unit area, which is the definition of sound intensity, falls as the inverse square of the distance. Thus the sound gets quieter with distance.

In many practical situations, however, obstructions will hinder the passage of the sound waves. Even where there is a clear path from the source to the receiver, objects may be present at the side, and often these serve to reflect the sound and prevent it spreading as rapidly as described above. Under these circumstances, the intensity will fall less rapidly than suggested by the square of the distance.

A further factor affects the attenuation of sound with distance. When the air is compressed, at the peak of the pressure wave, its temperature rises, and some of the energy of the sound wave is stored as heat. The reverse process takes place, and the energy is passed back into the wave, when the pressure is reduced in the trough of the wave. However, if heat is allowed to flow from the warmer to the cooler regions of the wave, some of the energy in the wave is irredeemably lost. This factor is particularly important for high frequency waves, where the short wavelength allows flow of heat between the peaks and the troughs of the wave.

Transmission between different media

If a medium, of which air is an example, is light and compressible, only small sound pressures will be needed to give a certain velocity of vibration, and hence displacement, of the air molecules. The pressures will be inadequate to give similar velocities of vibration in a denser, less compressible medium – in other words, in a medium with a higher impedance. If, therefore, a sound wave in air meets a medium of higher impedance, the sound pressures developed on the air side of the boundary will be inadequate to give the same amplitude of vibration of the medium on the other side of the boundary. The result is that much of the sound is reflected, with only a small proportion being transmitted. The pressure at the boundary stays high, but because the reflected wave travels in the reverse direction, it produces movements of the molecules in the reverse direction. Near the boundary, the movements arising from the incident and reflected waves substantially cancel one another, and the net velocity of the air molecules will be small. The resulting ratio of velocity to pressure in the air near the boundary is similar to that in the higher-impedance medium. Near the boundary, therefore, the impedance of the air is raised. This shows that the impedance of a medium is determined by its surroundings as well as by its intrinsic properties. It can be shown mathematically, that if the impedances of the two media are R_1 and R_2, the proportion of the incident power transmitted is $4R_1R_2/(R_1 + R_2)^2$.

This point is important physiologically when transmission of sound from the air into the cochlea is considered. The impedance of the cochlea is much higher than that of air. If the sound waves met the oval window directly, then, as can be calculated from the measured input impedance of the cochlea, only about 1% of the incident energy would enter the cochlea, with the rest being reflected. However, the following will show how the middle ear apparatus, by its action as an impedance transformer, improves this proportion considerably.

Fourier analysis

Figure 2.2 shows a portion of the waveform of a complex sound. The waveform has a regularly repeating pattern with two peaks per cycle. This pattern can be approximated by adding together the two sinusoids shown in the figure, one at 1 kHz, the other at 2 kHz. Such an analysis of a complex sound into its constituent sinusoids is known as Fourier analysis. The small irregularities in the waveform show that other frequency components, vibrating at higher frequencies, are present as well. If all the different sinusoids that have to be added together to give the waveform of *Figure 2.2a* are determined, and the required amplitude of each component is plotted as a function of the frequency of the component, a spectrum of the signal (*Figure 2.2b*) will result. The analysis of signals into spectra, that is Fourier analysis, is one of the essential tools for those trying to understand the workings of the auditory system.

There are several reasons why is it useful to analyse waveforms into sine waves (sinusoids) rather than into any other waveforms. A primary reason is mathematical, as any realistic waveform can be made out of sums of sinusoids. A second reason is that sinusoidal sound waves behave in a relatively simple way in many complex environments, such as a reflecting environment (for

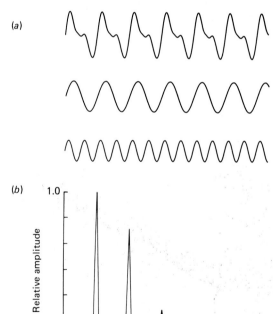

Figure 2.2 (*a*) A portion of a complex waveform. The waveform can be closely approximated by adding together the two waves shown. (*b*) A Fourier analysis of the waveform in part (*a*) shows the two main components, together with smaller ones of higher frequency

example the external auditory meatus), or one that has complex mechanical properties, such as the middle ear. In these cases, it is much easier to describe the way that sinusoidal waves would be affected by the system, and then, knowing how the complex sound can be described as the sum of sinusoids, to use this as a basis of working out how a complex wave would be transformed. A third reason, which is very important in understanding how the ear and the brain analyse sounds, is that the cochlea itself seems to perform a Fourier analysis. Therefore, if a complex sound has been analysed into sinusoids, it is often possible to understand how the auditory system itself would analyse it.

The principles of Fourier analysis can be illustrated most easily by the reverse process of Fourier synthesis – that is, the process of taking many sinusoids and adding them together to make a complex wave. *Figure 2.3* shows how, by adding sinusoids together, a good approximation to a square wave can be made. If this process were continued for more components, it would be possible to make a waveform indistinguishable from a square wave. Fourier analysis is simply the reverse of this – finding the elementary sinusoids which, when added together, will give the required waveform.

Periodic sounds

The sinusoids in *Figure 2.3* have 1, 3, 5, 7, 9 and so on, cycles respectively in the same time interval. Their frequencies are therefore multiples of the lowest, or fundamental, frequency. If the summed wave were repeated indefinitely, without any change of form in each period, then the higher frequencies would have to be *exact* multiples of the fundamental frequency. If the spectra of perfectly periodic sounds (*Figure 2.4a* and *b*) are drawn, it will be seen that the components are present only at certain discrete frequencies, as represented by the lines in the spectra, all of which are at exact multiples of the fundamental frequency. Such components at exact multiples of a frequency are called harmonics of the frequency.

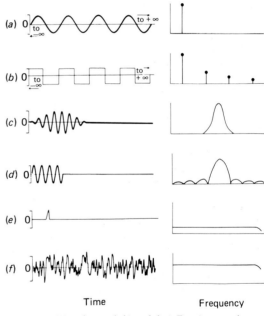

Figure 2.4 Waveforms (left) and their Fourier transforms (right). (*a*) Sine wave; (*b*) square wave; (*c*) and (*d*) Gated sine waves; (*e*) click; (*f*) white noise. (From Pickles, 1982)

In analysing complex sounds, not only do the frequency and amplitude of each frequency component have to be taken into consideration, but also the latter's timing, or phase. In *Figure 2.3*, each frequency component is in the same phase because, at the beginning of the fundamental cycle, each frequency component is moving upwards from its zero-crossing. However, the ear is relatively insensitive to the phase relations between components, so it is not always necessary to specify them.

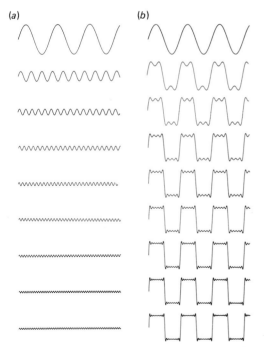

Figure 2.3 A square wave can be approximated by the addition of sinusoids of relative frequencies 1, 3, 5, 7, 9, 11, 13, 15 and 17. The column in (*b*) shows the effect of successively adding the sinusoids in (*a*)

Non-periodic sounds

Mathematically, a sinusoid repeats for an infinite time, and has a spectrum consisting of a line. The sounds encountered in everyday life do not continue for an infinite time. If the process of Fourier analysis is undertaken on a sound which is ramped on and off (for example *Figure 2.4c*), it will be found that the spectrum now contains not a certain discrete frequency or frequencies but rather a continuous range of frequencies. Moreover, what would be a single line in the spectrum (*Figure 2.4a*) is spread out into a band (*Figure 2.4c*). The fewer the number of cycles in the waveform, the wider is the band. In fact, the width of the band, in hertz, is inversely proportional to the time, in seconds, for which the sound is present.

The spectra of many everyday sounds can now be understood. For instance, spoken vowel sounds have a complex repeating waveform, which may continue steadily for half a second or so. In this case, there will be an approximation to a line spectrum, in which the components are harmonics of a fundamental. However, if the sound lasts for only 0.5 s, each component is spread into a band of closely adjacent frequencies, although in this case the frequency spread will be only about 2 Hz. The shorter the time for which the sound is present, the greater the frequency spread of each component.

As an extreme of a sound which is present for only a short time, a click should be considered. In this case, the spectrum has a very wide and uniform spread (*see Figure 2.4e*). Other transient sounds, which nevertheless give rise to some sort of a pitch sensation, such as the clash of a cymbal, will give rise to a wide frequency spectrum, with some frequency components present at greater intensities than others. Another sound with a wide spectrum is a continuous white noise, or hiss. Here, if the spectrum were averaged for a long period, a spectrum with a wide and uniform spread would be obtained. This differs from a click in the relative phases of the components, which are random in the case of white noise.

Linear systems

One concept which is useful in understanding hearing is that of a linear system. If a system – for instance the middle ear – is linear, it means that it transmits sounds without distortion. In this context, one particular kind of distortion, that of amplitude distortion, is meant. If a system is linear, it means that if the amplitude of the input signal is multiplied by a factor of, say, 10, the amplitude of the output also changes by a factor of 10 times. It also means that when two signals are presented at the same time, the response to both together is the same as the sum of the responses

that would be obtained if the signals were presented separately. In other words, linearity means that the presence of one signal does not change the responsiveness of the system to other signals. In the context of Fourier analysis, amplitude linearity has a simple implication. It means that the only frequencies (Fourier components) that are produced by the system are the ones that are put into it.

In some contexts, linearity is used differently: it is used to imply that the gain of a system is independent of frequency. Linearity will not be used in this sense in this chapter. It will be used only, as defined at the beginning of this section, in the sense of amplitude linearity, which is the way it is used in most of the physiological literature.

The outer ear

In man, the pinna forms a flat cartilaginous flange, with a raised rim and a dip in the centre called the concha. The external ear, which includes the pinna, concha, and external auditory meatus, is considered as having two main influences on the incoming sound. First, it increases the pressure at the tympanic membrane in a frequency-sensitive way, thus emphasizing certain frequencies in the input. Second, it increases the pressure in a way which depends on the direction of the sound source, and can therefore be used as an aid to sound localization. Although these two actions will be discussed separately, they are two aspects of the same phenomenon.

The gain in sound pressure at the tympanic membrane

In a free field, a portion of the incident sound is reflected off the head. This effect is at its maximum when the source is in the horizontal plane, and 90° to the side, being about 6 dB above 2 kHz, and becoming smaller at lower frequencies. If the sound source is on the opposite side of the head, there will be shadowing around the head, which can reduce the amplitude drastically. On top of this, the pinna–concha system itself can act like an ear trumpet, catching sound over a large area and concentrating it in the smaller area of the external meatus. Thus the total energy available to the tympanic membrane is increased.

A resonance in the external auditory meatus changes the sound pressure at the tympanic membrane in a frequency-selective way. If a tube is one-quarter of a wavelength long, and one end is open while the other is blocked with a hard termination, the pressure will be low at the open end and high at the closed end when the tube is

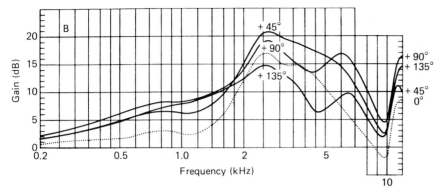

Figure 2.5 The pressure gain of the human external ear, for different frequencies of stimulation and different directions of the sound source. 0° is straight ahead. (From Shaw, 1974)

placed in a sound field. This phenomenon is seen in the human external meatus at a frequency of about 3 kHz. Here, the resonance adds 10–12 dB at the tympanic membrane, over the mid-concha position (Shaw, 1974).

Other resonances increase the sound pressure at other frequencies. The most important is a broad resonance, adding about 10 dB around 5 kHz, arising in the concha. The two main resonances are therefore complementary, and increase the sound pressure relatively uniformly over the range from 2 to 7 kHz. The total effect of reflections from the head and pinna, and the various external ear resonances, is to add 15–20 dB to the sound pressure, over the frequency range from 2 to 7 kHz (*Figure 2.5*) (Shaw, 1974).

The meatal quarter-wave resonance as described above can occur only if the meatus is terminated by a boundary with a higher impedance than the air in the canal. This implies that there is a mismatch of impedance between the ear canal and the tympanic membrane, with a loss of efficiency of transfer of energy. Such a mismatch can be measured in man from the standing wave pattern of sound reflected from the eardrum. The point made above is confirmed; although there is variation between the results of different investigators, the impedance of the tympanic membrane in man seems to be three or four times that of the air in the ear canal over a wide frequency range above 1 kHz. This leads to some 30% of the energy being reflected back into the meatus (Hudde, 1983). A function of the resonances is to reduce the loss of the incident energy around the resonant frequencies. An analysis of the performance of the whole system shows that in the range of the resonant frequencies (2 kHz and above), the external ear achieves a performance within 5 dB of the theoretically perfect value (Shaw and Stinson, 1983).

Sound localization and the outer ear

The most powerful cues for sound localization are provided by binaural interactions. However, the outer ear provides important cues which are useful in monaural localization and, where binaural hearing is concerned, in enabling us to distinguish in front from behind and up from down.

Figure 2.5 shows that as a sound source is moved around the head, starting in front and moving round to the side, the main change produced is an attenuation of up to 10 dB in the frequency range from 2 to 7 kHz. This arises from interference between the wave transmitted directly, and the wave scattered off the pinna. Changes in this frequency range could therefore indicate whether the source was in front of the subject or behind. In addition, the dip in the transfer function around 10 kHz gives information as to the elevation of the sound source. As a sound source is raised above the horizontal plane, the low-frequency edge of the dip moves to higher frequencies. The dip arises from cancellation between multiple out-of-phase reflections off the back wall of the pinna and concha. While, therefore, such transformations in the spectrum theoretically contain information as to the direction of the source, it would appear that judgement of direction of the source would require either previous familiarity with the spectrum of the sound, or the possibility of varying the transformation by making searching movements of the head.

At very high frequencies, where the wavelength is short compared with the dimensions of the pinna, it is possible for the pinna to become strongly directional and to produce a high gain on a narrow axis. This is taken advantage of in animals such as cats and bats. For instance,

Phillips *et al.* (1982) showed that at 16 kHz the cat pinna could provide 25 dB or more of amplification, but only for sound sources in a narrowly defined direction some 20° or less across. Combined with a mobile pinna, this would permit very accurate monaural localization of high-frequency sound sources.

The middle ear

The middle ear couples sound energy to the cochlea. As well as providing physical protection for the cochlea, the middle ear serves to match the impedance of the air to the much higher impedance of the cochlear fluids. The middle ear apparatus also serves to apply sound preferentially to only one window of the cochlea, thus producing a differential pressure between the windows, required for the movement of the cochlear fluids.

The mode of vibration of the middle ear structures

Calculation of the transformer action requires a detailed knowledge of the way that the middle ear structures move in response to sound. The measurements required are difficult to make, because the movements are complex ones in three dimensions, are submicroscopic and depend on the physiological state of the subject. For these reasons, the most reliable information available has come from experimental animals.

Von Békésy (1941, 1960), after measuring the vibration of the tympanic membrane in human cadavers, suggested that it moved like a stiff plate up to 2 kHz, hinging around an axis of rotation at one edge (*Figure 2.6a*). He found that the inferior edge of the membrane was flaccid and it was here that the movements were greatest. Khanna and Tonndorf (1972), working with live cats, did not confirm this pattern of movement at any frequency; rather, there were two maxima of vibration, one on either side of the manubrium (*Figure 2.6b*). Their results suggested that as the tympanic membrane moved to and fro, it buckled in the regions between the manubrium of the malleus and the anterior and posterior edges. The pattern of movement is shown in cross-section in *Figure 2.6c*. It suggests that the movement of the malleus is somewhat less than the mean movement of the tympanic membrane, and so of the air that drives it. Khanna and Tonndorf (1972) showed that for frequencies below 6 kHz the displacement of the malleus is some 0.5 times the mean displacement of the membrane. At frequencies above 6 kHz the pattern becomes much more complex: the vibra-

tion breaks up into many small zones with a reduction in the efficiency of the transfer of vibration to the malleus.

The axis of rotation of the ossicles and the axis of suspension by their ligaments nearly coincide with their centre of rotational inertia. Therefore, at high frequencies the bones are able to vibrate with very little loss through the suspending ligaments (*Figure 2.6d*). The relatively massive head of the malleus and incus in some species, including man, would therefore appear to aid determination of the appropriate centre of inertia. However, this factor is dominant at only mid and high frequencies. At low frequencies, where the mass effects are small, the ligaments play an important role in maintaining the position of the ossicles. Von Békésy (1941, 1960) showed this, by cutting the ligaments. Changing the suspension in this way affected transmission below, but not above, 200 Hz.

The actual mode of movement of the middle ear bones, like the mode of vibration of the tympanic membrane, has been a matter of controversy. It is not known whether the controversy has arisen as a consequence of species differences, or the better methods of measurement which have been used more recently, although of necessity in experimental animals rather than in human beings. For instance, von Békésy (1941, 1961), experimenting on human cadavers, suggested that the stapes rocked in the oval window as well as moving in and out. He ascribed this to an asymmetry in the annular ligament, which fits more tightly on its posterior edge. However, Guinan and Peake (1967) found that, in cats, the stapes simply moved in and out like a piston.

The impedance transformer action of the middle ear

Examination of the middle ear as an impedance transformer must begin with a consideration of the impedance of the structure to which it is connected, namely the cochlea.

Following the provisional and tentative conjecture made by Wever and Lawrence (1954), many authors have described the cochlea as having an impedance to sound equal to that of sea water (that is 1.5×10^6 N.s/m^3). While this comparison gains apparent precision by including the main solutes of the perilymph – although in concentrations four times too great – the basis of the comparison, as was indeed emphasized by Wever and Lawrence themselves, is in fact quite wrong. The above impedance is the specific impedance defined for progressive waves in an effectively infinite medium. However, the cochlea is many times smaller than the wavelength of sound in water, and it cannot develop such waves. Instead,

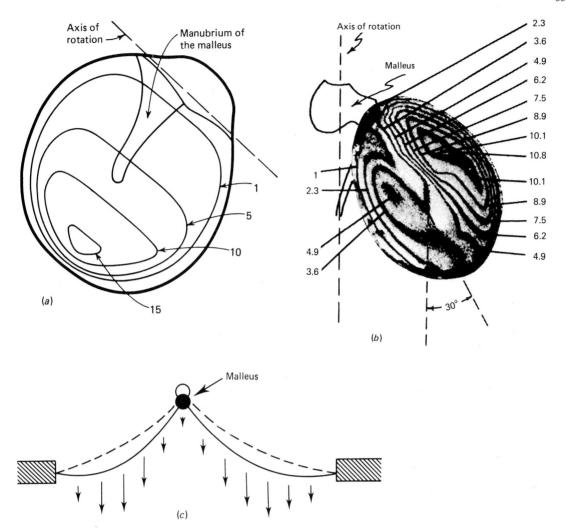

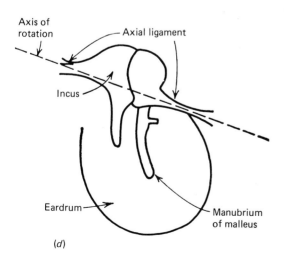

Figure 2.6 (*a*) The mode of vibration of the human tympanic membrane, according to von Békésy. The lines are contours of equal amplitudes of vibration. (From von Békésy, 1960; copyright McGraw-Hill, 1960).
(*b*) Vibration contours in the living cat's tympanic membrane, according to Khanna and Tonndorf (1972). The contours are produced by laser interference fringes. The corresponding amplitudes of vibration are shown by the numbers in units of 0.1 μm. (From Khanna and Tonndorf, 1972.) (*c*) The curved membrane principle.
(*d*) The axis of rotation of the ossicles. (From von Békésy, 1960; copyright McGraw-Hill, 1960)

the actual impedance of the cochlea is determined by factors such as the mass of the cochlear fluids, the stiffness of the round and oval windows and the other membranes, and by the pattern of motion of the cochlear fluids. Determination of the cochlear impedance is a complex matter, since it appears that the measurement must be made in a living specimen in good physiological condition. For this reason, the only reasonable measurements of cochlear input impedance that are available have been made on experimental animals. Probably the most reliable measurements to date are those of Lynch, Nedzelnitsky and Peake (1982), made on the cat. They showed that over a wide frequency range the input impedance of the cat cochlea had a value of $1.5 \times 10^5 \,\mathrm{N.s/m^3}$ (calculated here as a specific impedance), one-tenth that expected on Wever and Lawrence's approximation. Earlier authors had obtained much higher values than this, particularly at low frequencies. Lynch, Nedzelnitsky and Peake pointed out that these high values probably arose because the ligaments had dried out to some extent, thus increasing the stiffness of the system. Because air has a specific impedance of $415 \,\mathrm{N.s/m^3}$, the formula given above, where the transmission of sound between media of different impedances was considered (*see* Transmission between different media), would lead to the assumption that only 1% of the incident energy would be conveyed to the cochlea in the absence of a middle ear mechanism. This corresponds to an attenuation of the sound by 20 dB.

An efficient impedance transformer will change the low-pressure, high-displacement vibrations of the air into high-force, low-displacement vibrations suitable for driving the cochlear fluids. Three components have been identified in the mechanism by which this occurs.

(1) By far the most important factor depends on the large area of the tympanic membrane, in comparison with the area of the footplate of the stapes in the round window. The force collected over the tympanic membrane is expressed over the much smaller stapes footplate, with a corresponding increase in pressure. The pressure therefore increases in inverse proportion to the ratio of the areas.

(2) The ossicles act as a lever, with the malleus being longer than the incus. The displacement at the stapes is therefore decreased, while the force is increased.

(3) As described above, the tympanic membrane buckles as it moves to and fro (*see Figure 2.6c*). The reduction in the movement of the malleus means that the tympanic membrane acts as a mechanical lever, although of rather subtle shape. It therefore again increases the force and decreases the displacement at the stapes.

Measurements of the lever action of the ossicles suggest that the effective length of the manubrium of the malleus, taking into account the complex way that the vibration is connected to it, is some 1.15 times the length of the incus.

A value for the impedance transformer ratio can be calculated by multiplying these factors together. In the cat, the area of the tympanic membrane is $0.42 \,\mathrm{cm^2}$, and the area of the stapes footplate is $0.012 \,\mathrm{cm^2}$. The pressure is therefore increased $0.42/0.012 = 35$ times. The lever ratio increases the force 1.15 times, and decreases the displacement (and therefore velocity) 1.15 times. The impedance ratio, which is the pressure/velocity ratio, is therefore changed $1.15^2 = 1.32$ times. Finally, the buckling factor decreases the displacement 2.0 times, and increases the force 2.0 times, thus changing the impedance ratio 4.0 times. The overall transformer ratio, expressed as the pressure/velocity ratio is $35 \times 1.32 \times 4.0 \simeq 185$. The middle ear impedance transformer will therefore make the cochlear input impedance of $1.5 \times 10^5 \,\mathrm{N.s/m^3}$ appear as $1.5 \times 10^5/185 = 810 \,\mathrm{N.s/m^3}$ at the tympanic membrane. This is nearly twice the specific impedance of air which is $415 \,\mathrm{N.s/m^3}$. It agrees with the finding described above that the impedance of the tympanic membrane is rather higher than that of air, although it does not predict the exact value of the impedance, which, measurements suggest, is nearer three to four times the specific impedance of the air (Hudde, 1983).

The directly measured values of tympanic membrane impedance suggest that some 65% of the incident energy would be absorbed by the cochlea, as against the 1% expected in the absence of a middle ear transformer.

Transfer as a function of frequency

In order properly to describe the action of the middle ear, it is necessary to consider transmission over the whole audible frequency range, and not only at the mid-frequency (1 kHz) for which the calculations above are most nearly valid. Again, this is a measurement that is most easily made in experimental animals. The most direct way to measure the efficiency of transfer is to measure the sound pressure in the scala vestibuli, just behind the oval window, for a certain sound pressure at the tympanic membrane. Nedzelnitsky (1980) showed that in cats transmission reached a peak around 1 kHz; the transmission was less effective at lower and higher frequencies (*Figure 2.7*). Similar results were obtained with excised human temporal bones by Kringlebotn and Gundersen (1985); they also showed the bandpass transfer characteristic, with peak transmission occurring at

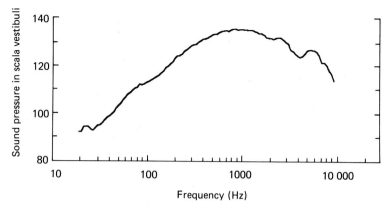

Figure 2.7 The transfer function of the middle ear in the cat, calculated from the pressure in the scala vestibuli, compared with that at the tympanic membrane. Sound pressure level at tympanic membrane = 105 dB. (From Nedzelnitsky, 1980)

around 1 kHz, when their data are used to plot the velocity of the inner ear input as a function of stimulus frequency.

The drop in transmission at low frequencies is probably due to the elastic stiffness of various components of the middle ear. One structure contributing considerable stiffness is the annular ligament fixing the circumference of the footplate of the stapes in the oval window. Lynch, Nedzelnitsky and Peake (1982), by comparing the movements produced by pressures applied to the stapes with the effect of pressures applied directly to the cochlear scalae, showed that this ligament contributed stiffness to the system below 500 Hz. Another factor is the air in the middle ear cavity. As the tympanic membrane moves in, the air is compressed, reducing the movement of the tympanic membrane. If the middle ear cavity is vented to the atmosphere, this effect disappears, and low-frequency transmission is improved (Guinan and Peake, 1967).

Stiffness is particularly important at low frequencies because, for constant sound pressure level, the *displacement* of the air, and so of auditory structures, increases in inverse proportion to frequency. The force on an elastic element is a function of its displacement, and so elasticity has most influence at low frequencies. The inverse relation between frequency and displacement is reflected in the curve shown in *Figure 2.7*, since at low frequencies transmission to the cochlea declines by almost exactly 20 dB/decade, that is in almost exact inverse proportion to stimulus frequency. The contention that elastic stiffness limits the movement at low frequencies is also supported by the phase data, which at these frequencies show that the tympanic membrane is displaced in phase with the sound pressure. This is the phase relation expected for a stiffness-

limited system, whereas a 90° phase lag would be expected if the energy were being coupled efficiently into the resistance of the cochlea.

The drop at high frequencies is affected by many factors. One important factor is the pattern of vibration of the tympanic membrane, which above 6 kHz breaks up into many independent zones, reducing the coupling to the malleus (Khanna and Tonndorf, 1972). A second factor, giving the dip around 4 kHz in the cat, depends on acoustic resonances within the middle ear cavity, with air resonating between the different compartments within the cavity. The mass of the middle ear system would also appear to have a significant effect at high frequencies. Mass is particularly important in limiting the movements at high frequencies because the forces on a mass are a function of the accelerations involved, which increase with frequency.

The data in *Figure 2.7* also allow the calculation of the transformer ratio to be checked in a different way, this time directly from the pressure ratio. In the mid-frequency range, the factors leading to transmission losses will be small, and the theoretical calculations detailed above will be most nearly accurate. The calculations lead to the assumption that the area ratio would increase the pressure 35 times, the lever ratio by 1.15 times, and the buckling factor by two. By multiplying these together, a total pressure increase of 80.5 times, corresponding to a 38 dB increase in pressure, is obtained. This is of the same order as, although rather greater than, the 30 dB maximum increase found by Nedzelnitsky (1980). The remaining discrepancy is probably mainly due to transmission losses in the middle ear, including friction in the tympanic membrane, ligaments, and ossicular joints, since they account for some 6 dB of transmission loss at the particular frequency under consideration. Shaw and Stinson (1983) described the different sites of loss in man.

If the total effect of outer and middle ear transmission on the power delivered to the cochlea at different frequencies is calculated, a curve is obtained that closely approximates the air-conduction audiogram for the absolute threshold between 200 Hz and 20 kHz (*see* for example Rosowski *et al.*, 1986). This suggests that the shape of the human audiogram is determined mainly by factors peripheral to the cochlea, at least until the sharp upper frequency cut-off of hearing is reached.

The role of the middle ear has been described so far as one of transferring sound from the ear canal to the cochlea. However, as in any matched system, transfer in the reverse direction is possible. The importance of this was recognized with the discovery of the *cochlear echo* (Kemp, 1978), a phenomenon in which sound is generated in the cochlea, either spontaneously or following an external stimulus, and transmitted to the external ear. The influence of middle ear transformer characteristics on the reverse transfer have been studied only superficially (for example Wilson, 1980). However, with a possible increase in the use of the echo as a diagnostic tool (*see below*), further information in this area will be required.

Influence of the middle ear muscles

The tensor tympani inserts on the top of the manubrium of the malleus, and contraction pulls the malleus medially and anteriorly, nearly at right angles to the normal direction of vibration. The second muscle, the stapedius muscle, inserts on the posterior aspect on the stapes. Contraction of the muscle, therefore, pulls the stapes posteriorly. Contraction of the tensor tympani can be detected as an inward movement of the tympanic membrane (Møller, 1964). On the other hand, different investigators have reported different effects for contraction of the stapedius muscle. Whereas Møller (1964) reported inward movements of the tympanic membrane in some experiments, and outward movements in others, Pang and Peake (1986) reported that stapedius contraction in cats was effective without *any* detectable movement of the incus, malleus, or tympanic membrane. Contraction of both muscles, however, influences transmission in the same way, by increasing the stiffness of the ossicular chain. The stapedius muscle achieves this by rocking the stapes in the oval window, so increasing the inward tension on the posterior edge of the annular ligament, and the outward tension on the anterior edge.

As pointed out above, when the factors limiting transmission through the middle ear at different frequencies were considered, stiffness has its greatest effects at low frequencies. Pang and Peake (1986) found that the strongest stapedius contractions could reduce transmission by up to 30 dB for frequencies less than 1–2 kHz. At higher frequencies, the effect was limited to 10 dB. However, the fact that any effects at all could be produced above the frequency range in which stiffness can be expected to limit the movement (that is above 1–2 kHz), suggests that contraction can do more than increase the stiffness. It may, for instance, change the direction of vibration of the ossicles so that the movement is less effectively coupled to the cochlea. Contraction of the muscles may also serve to damp out unwanted resonances in the middle ear system at these higher frequencies. In support of this, Simmons (1964) showed that in cats the middle ear muscles could remove a sharp dip in middle ear transmission which was seen around 4 kHz.

The middle ear muscles contract in response to sound. In man, only the stapedius can be driven acoustically, unless the sound is loud enough to give a startle reflex (Møller, 1974). However, in experimental animals such as cats and rabbits, both the stapedius muscle and tensor tympani contract in response to sound. The reflex arcs for such contractions contain only a few neurons (Borg, 1973). The arc to the stapedius muscle has three to four synapses, ending in the facial nerve, and that to the tensor tympani has four, ending in the trigeminal nerve. The few neurons lead to very fast reaction times; latencies as low as 6–7 ms in the responses to intense tones have been reported in cats, although under the more limited range of experimental conditions possible in man, the limit is nearer 25 ms (Metz, 1951). The latency is a function of the intensity of the stimulus, with longer latencies being found for low intensity stimuli. In man, the reflex threshold, below which no effects are found, has been reported to be some 80 dB above the subject's absolute threshold for stimuli in the frequency range from 250 Hz to 4 kHz (Møller, 1974). Both middle ear muscles can contract in response to stimuli other than external sound, including stimulation of the cornea by a puff of air, touching the skin around the eye or external ear, closing of the eyes, body movements, vocalization and, in some subjects, by voluntary effort (for review, *see* Møller, 1974).

The middle ear muscle reflex has various functions, which include the following. First, the reflex provides protection from noise damage. Although the reflex is too slow to protect the ear from sudden impulsive noise, it does seem to have an effect with longer lasting noises. Zakrisson and Borg (1974) showed that patients with Bell's palsy and paralysis of the stapedius muscle had greater temporary threshold shifts in response to intense low-frequency noises in the affected than in the unaffected ear. The reflex may, under some circumstances, also be useful with impulsive sounds; Hilding (1961) showed that if a sudden sound such as a gunshot is preceded by a 100 dB tone, the reflex contraction to the tone can provide protection from the gunshot. Second, the reflex may provide selective attenuation of low frequency stimulus components. Such stimuli are particularly effective at masking stimuli in the higher frequency range, and at high intensities they reduce the cues available concerning, for instance, the upper formants of speech sounds. Selective attenuation of the low frequency components by the middle ear muscle reflex could therefore be expected to improve the intelligibility of speech at high intensities. This received experimental support from Borg and Zakrisson (1973), whose patients with Bell's palsy showed deterioration in speech perception at stimulus intensities 25 dB lower than normal subjects. On the other hand, middle ear muscle contraction does not seem to reduce the masking produced by *internally* produced sounds (Irvine *et al.*, 1983), as has sometimes been suggested. Third, the reflex may also have a beneficial effect in reducing the influence of some of the resonances in the middle ear (Simmons, 1964). The reflex has been usefully reviewed by Silman (1984).

Transmission through damaged middle ears

If the middle ear is disordered, transmission can change by way of several mechanisms. The stimulus may be inadequately coupled to the tympanic membrane, the impedance transformer action may be lost, the ability of the ossicles to move may be reduced, and the differential application of sound pressure to the round and oval windows may be affected.

In the case of a total removal of the middle ear apparatus, the impedance transformer action and the differential application of pressure to the round and oval windows are lost. The loss of transformer action alone would be expected to lead to an increase of some 20 dB in auditory thresholds in the mid-range of frequencies. Von Békésy (1960) showed in excised human temporal bones that, under such circumstances, the pressures delivered to the round and oval windows were nearly equal. He argued that the scala vestibuli was more yielding than the scala tympani, because its blood vessels could be displaced out of the osseous labyrinth, so allowing equal pressures applied to the two windows to set up differential movements in the scalae of the

cochlea. This conjecture received support from the experiments of Tonndorf (1966), who showed that pressure release through structures such as the cochlear aqueduct was possible and could aid the detection of sound. As a second factor, the small compliance of the annular ligament of the stapes, in comparison with the much larger compliance of the round window membrane, will tend to enhance the differential movement. At the present time, it is not known whether the 40–60 dB loss observed clinically can be explained by known mechanisms. In the case of these severe losses, hearing by bone conduction may become significant.

If the middle ear apparatus is lost, but the round window is protected in some way from the incoming sound waves, then a differential pressure can be set up across the round and oval windows. Theoretically, the change in sensitivity is that resulting from the loss of the transformer mechanism alone.

If the tympanic membrane is intact and connected directly to the oval window, either by direct contact between the drumhead and the stapes or by means of a prosthesis, the major component of the impedance transformer, the area ratio, remains, although the lever action of the ossicles and possibly the buckling action of the tympanic membrane will be lost. As these two latter factors have a comparatively small influence on the impedance transformation, the transformation produced by the middle ear will be only a little affected, and good hearing is theoretically possible.

A hole in the tympanic membrane will reduce the effective area of the membrane in contact with the sound wave. Holes will also reduce the pressure differential across the tympanic membrane and, depending on their position, reduce the mechanical coupling between the remaining intact portions of the membrane and the malleus. The effects of different lesions were studied experimentally in the cat by Payne and Githler (1951). Averaging over all positions in which holes were made, small lesions (10% of the membrane) produced losses of 10–15 dB below 3 kHz, with smaller losses at higher frequencies. It would seem plausible that the pressure differential across the membrane would be maintained more at high frequencies, because the air has less time to flow through the perforation. However, large lesions produced severe losses over the whole range, particularly at the highest frequencies. With these lesions, the sound waves were acting directly on the round and oval windows. The size of the effects was highly dependent upon the site of the lesions. Small and moderate lesions (10–40% of area) had far more severe effects when placed on the posterior and superior margin of the membrane than when placed on the anterior and inferior margin.

Fixation of the stapes will cause decreased transmission of sound to the cochlea through decreased mobility. In severe cases, sound pressure changes arriving directly at the round window should still result in some differential movement of the cochlear fluid, because a release of pressure should be possible through the blood vessels and cochlear aqueduct. In this case, where the sound pressure has its effects directly at the round window, the impedance transformer action of the middle ear will also be lost.

Static pressure changes across the tympanic membrane, whether positive or negative, will increase the tension in the tympanic membrane and so increase its stiffness in response to applied sound. The increased stiffness will attenuate the transmission of sound in the frequency region in which it is stiffness limited, that is below about 1 kHz. The lowest stiffness occurs when the static pressure differential across the membrane is zero and, in the normal case, transmission decreases symmetrically for positive and negative changes in the pressure differential.

Mechanisms of bone conduction

Bone conduction is the normal route for hearing some of the components of one's own voice, is useful with severe conductive loss, and is used as a tool of considerable diagnostic power. The mechanisms of bone conduction have, however, been a matter of controversy over the years, and present knowledge of them owes much to the experiments of Tonndorf (1966). Tonndorf (1976) gives a useful recent review of these and other experiments.

By measuring cochlear microphonics in cats during bone stimulation, Tonndorf was able to measure the different factors leading to effective stimulation by bone conduction. He showed that it was determined by a multiplicity of factors, arising in the inner ear, the middle ear and the external ear.

Inner ear factors

In the most basic experiment, the skull was stimulated with a bone vibrator, and microphonics measured in a cochlea from which the middle ear apparatus had been entirely removed and the cochlear aqueduct blocked. If both the oval and round windows were sealed with rigid cement, bone conduction was substantial, although several decibels worse than in the normal animal. If, however, only the oval window was occluded, the microphonic responses of the cochlea were *better*

than normal by some 10 dB over the frequency range below 1 kHz.

The fact that substantial responses to bone conduction remained with the cochlear outlets sealed would suggest that differential flow of cochlear fluids between the windows, or to another opening such as the aqueduct, is not entirely necessary for the detection of bone vibrations. Tonndorf suggested that there was an intrinsic detection of distortional vibrations of the cochlear bone. Differential distortion of the bony walls of the cochlea, and of the walls of the other labyrinthine spaces closely connected to it, would produce a movement of the cochlear fluids. These would be coupled into the cochlear partition since the scala vestibuli is larger than the scala tympani. This is the *distortional vibration* factor.

Although detection is possible with the windows sealed, the windows will normally have some effect. As sealing the oval window while leaving the round window open actually improved bone conduction, it is apparent that a differential compliance can enhance the detection of bone vibration. Tonndorf suggested that leaving the round window open would release pressure and produce movements in phase with those resulting directly from the distortional vibration. On the other hand, increasing the mobility of the oval window would produce a shunt for the pressure changes, allowing them to bypass the cochlear partition and so reducing the response. This gives an explanation of the Weber test: an increased stiffness of the ossicular chain will reduce the shunting and so increase the detection of bone vibration.

The good response with one window sealed was seen, however, only when the vibrations were introduced into the bone. If the cochlea was stimulated by air vibrations led directly into the middle ear, it was necessary to have both windows open to obtain a response.

The experiment also suggested that release of pressure through the cochlear aqueduct, and hence also through the blood vessels, would influence the fluid flow resulting from bone vibration. Sealing the aqueduct reduced the response to vibration. This supports the notion of a 'third window' in the cochlea. Evidence was also presented for its role in the production of movements resulting from the inertia of the cochlear fluids, with a differential flow between the third window and the oval window.

Middle ear factors

The centre of inertia of the middle ear bones does not coincide exactly with their points of attachment. Translational vibrations of the skull will therefore produce a rotational vibration of the bones, which can be coupled to the inner ear. Obviously, this factor will be affected by any pathology in the mobility of the middle ear apparatus. It will also be affected by any natural resonances in the middle ear system. The middle ear acts as a broadly tuned bandpass filter with peak transmission around 1 kHz at its natural resonant frequency. If the degree of resonance of the system is reduced by damping the stapes, the main losses will be produced around the natural resonant frequency. This is the explanation given for the appearance of Carhart's notch with mild stapes fixation, although the notch usually appears at rather higher frequencies, namely 2 kHz.

Outer ear factors

Vibration of the bone is coupled to the walls of the ear canal and so to the air within it. These vibrations escape externally when the ear canal is open. When, however, the ear is occluded, the sound pressure changes in the canal are increased and are transmitted to the inner ear by the normal middle ear route (von Békésy, 1941; Tonndorf, 1976). Occlusion therefore increases bone conduction, but only if a significant area of the canal, or other part of the external ear which can radiate, is included behind the occlusion. Because the external radiation of sound normally occurs best for low frequencies, the change with occlusion occurs for those frequencies.

The cochlea

The fluid spaces of the cochlea

The principal divisions of the fluid spaces in the cochlea are the *perilymphatic space*, consisting of the scala vestibuli and scala tympani, and the *endolym-phatic space*, consisting of the scala media. The walls surrounding the endolymphatic space have occluding tight junctions between the cells, obstructing the movement of ions into and out of the endolymph (for example Smith, 1978). *Figure 2.8* shows the commonly accepted borders of the endolymphatic space in a cochlear cross-section. Between the scala media and the scala tympani, the border is drawn around the top edge of the organ of Corti, along the reticular lamina. Although that is the usually accepted position, the issue is in fact controversial, and will be discussed in more detail below.

The endolymphatic and perilymphatic spaces extend along the inner ear as shown diagrammatically in *Figure 2.9*. The perilymphatic space surrounds the membranous labyrinth and opens into the cerebrospinal fluid by way of the cochlear aqueduct. The endolymphatic space, as well as continuing throughout the membranous labyrinth, is joined to the endolymphatic sac by means of the endolymphatic duct.

Formation and absorption of the endolymph and perilymph

Endolymph

It is generally agreed that the endolymph of the cochlea is produced by the stria vascularis. The cells here have the morphological and biochemical properties of secretory cells. Under the light microscope, the cells of the stria vascularis can be divided into superficially located darkly staining cells, called the marginal cells, and more lightly staining basal cells (for example Fawcett, 1986). Under the electron microscope it can be seen that the marginal cells have long infoldings on their basal edge, that is on the edge furthest away from the endolymph. The infoldings contain many

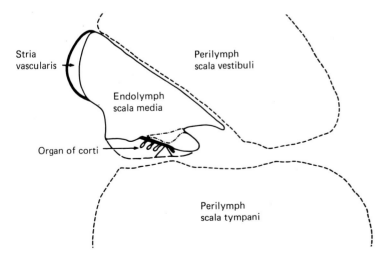

Stria vascularis

Perilymph scala vestibuli

Endolymph scala media

Organ of corti

Perilymph scala tympani

Figure 2.8 The compartments in the cochlea formed by occluding junctions. The thin continuous line surrounds the endolymphatic space, and the dotted line the perilymphatic space. (From Smith, 1978)

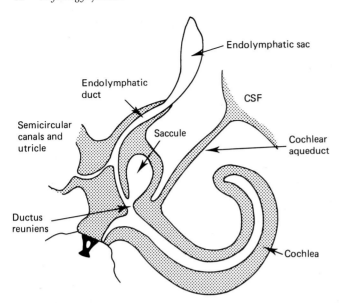

Figure 2.9 Schematic diagram of the perilymphatic space in the cochlea (stippled area) and the endolymphatic space (central clear area, running into the endolymphatic sac)

mitochondria. Presumably, this is the membrane across which most of the energy-consuming pumping of the stria vascularis occurs. There are also numerous capillaries coursing through the epithelium. The stria vascularis has a high concentration of Na^+/K^+ ATPase, adenylate cyclase and carbonic anhydrase, which are enzymes associated with the active pumping of ions and transport of fluid into the endolymph. The cells also contain high levels of the oxidative enzymes associated with glucose metabolism, as would be needed to provide fuel for a vigorous active transport system (reviewed in detail by Feldman, 1981).

Endolymph flows along the cochlear duct, through the ductus reuniens (which also communicates with the saccule), to the endolymphatic duct and thence to the endolymphatic sac (*see Figure 2.9*). Although there is a physical connection through to the endolymph of the utricle and semicircular canals, the connection is small and, in some cases, closed by obstructions. It is, for instance, thought unlikely that drugs in the cochlear and saccular division of the endolymph would enter the rest of the vestibular division (Brown, 1981). However, if the pressures are altered in disease states, as in Menière's disease, or by experimental perfusion, some communication may well occur.

Endolymph is absorbed in the endolymphatic sac. The cells here have a columnar shape and they appear specialized for absorption, containing long microvilli on the luminal surface, and many pinocytotic vesicles and vacuoles. It has also been suggested that free phagocytic cells cross the epithelium to remove cellular debris and foreign materials from the endolymph. Obliteration of the endolymphatic sac and duct in experimental animals causes endolymphatic hydrops, again confirming the view that it is the normal site of absorption of the endolymph (for example Kimura, 1967).

Perilymph

The perilymphatic space appears to be continuous between the vestibular and cochlear divisions. In contrast to endolymph, the site of production of the perilymph is controversial. It is undecided whether the perilymph originates from the cerebrospinal fluid, or is an ultrafiltrate of blood produced by the perilymphatic capillaries. The evidence for an origin in the cerebrospinal fluid comes from experiments in which substances appear in the perilymph after injection into the subarachnoid space. However, the position is by no means clear. It can be argued that the disruptions caused by the experiments change the patency of the cochlear aqueduct. In any case, the aqueduct in guinea-pigs, on which most of the experiments were performed, has a more open lumen than that in adult human beings. In one report, dye and radioactive proteins injected into the cerebrospinal fluid in patients did not appear in the perilymph (Ritter and Lawrence, 1965), although a lack of connection is contradicted in some individuals at least, by occasional reports of copious flows of perilymph or cerebrospinal fluid from the vestibule during stapedectomy.

Evidence in favour of the hypothesis that perilymph is an ultrafiltrate of blood comes from experiments in which the chemical composition of the perilymph has been analysed. The protein content of perilymph, while much lower than that of plasma, is nevertheless higher than that of the cerebrospinal fluid. In addition, if the composition of blood is changed experimentally, the changes are reflected more rapidly in the perilymph than in the cerebrospinal fluid (Schneider, 1974). It is obvious that if perilymph were derived indirectly by way of the cerebrospinal fluid rather than directly from the blood, the reverse would have been the case.

It is possible that there is a dual origin of perilymph, as proposed by Kellerhals (1979), with most of the perilymph being produced as an ultrafiltrate of blood, and the rest arising from the cerebrospinal fluid. The evidence is derived from experiments in which the relative speeds of dye tracer entry from the cerebrospinal fluid and the rate of production of perilymph were measured. The possibility of a dual origin for the perilymph is supported by analyses of the protein types in the perilymph, which showed it to be different from *both* blood plasma and the cerebrospinal fluid (Schiebe and Haupt, 1985).

The composition and electric potentials of the cochlear fluids

Endolymph

Endolymph is unique among the extracellular fluids of the body in that it has a high K^+ content, and a low Na^+ content, resembling intracellular fluid.

The K^+ content of endolymph can be measured by microsampling or by ion-specific electrodes, although the measurements are tricky because of the small volume of the endolymphatic space. Values obtained by different workers and a variety of techniques are in the range 144–171 mM, isotonic with intracellular K^+ (*see Table 2.1*). Na^+ concentrations are much more difficult to determine accurately because the Na^+ is present in low concentrations and the samples are susceptible to contamination from the higher levels of Na^+ in the surrounding perilymph. Thus, the earliest measurements of Smith, Lowry and Wu (1954), measured by means of microsampling, showed relatively high values, for example 38 mM. Much lower concentrations have been measured more recently with ion-selective electrodes, where the risk of contamination is lower (for example Johnstone and Sellick, 1972). The later measurements are in the range 1–6 mM. These values are also supported by some of the X-ray analyses of crystals of endolymph from the frozen cochlea (Ryan, Wickham and Bone, 1980). Because of the difficulties of making the measurements, the older tables of the ionic composition should be treated with suspicion so far as the endolymph is concerned. The more recent measurements are given in *Table 2.1*.

Although the endolymph has a high K^+ concentration similar to that found intracellularly, its electric potential, unlike that usually found inside cells, is strongly positive. Values obtained range from +50 to +120 mV with respect to the plasma, the higher values being found in the basal turn (von Békésy, 1952). The potentials are also higher near the stria vascularis (Tasaki, Davis and Eldredge, 1954).

The positive values suggest that the endocochlear potential is not a diffusion potential, such as is seen inside nerve cells. In other words, the potential is *not* produced by K^+ ions moving passively down their concentration gradient out of the endolymphatic space, taking positive charge with them, as this would leave the endolymph

Table 2.1 Endolymph electrolyte concentrations (mequiv./l unless stated otherwise)

Species	Cochlear duct			Utricle			Investigator
	Na^+	K^+	Cl^-	Na^+	K^+	Cl^-	
Guinea-pig	38‡			15.8	144		Smith, Lowry and Wu (1954)
	0.1–2.7			14.3			Sellick and Johnstone (1972)
	8	160.0		26	136.0		Silverstein, Takeda and Cox (1974)
	1.5*	152.3*	131.0±2.1				Konishi and Hamrick (1978)
		150	117		150	119	Morgenstern, Amano and Orsulakova (1982)
Rat	0.91	154					Bosher and Warren (1968)
	2.9±0.44	156.6±2.1	132.7±1.8				Sterkers *et al.* (1982)
Cat	6.1	171		14.8	155		Makimoto and Silverstein (1980)
Human	16.0±5.8	144.2±13.6	114				Rauch and Köstlin (1958)
	16	151†					Silverstein (1972)

*mM; †patients with Menière's disease; ‡now thought to be too high
Reproduced from Anniko and Wroblewski (1986), Table 1

with a negative potential. Instead, as is now recognized, the positive endocochlear potential is an electrogenic potential, directly dependent on ion-pumping in the stria vascularis. The potential arises because more K^+ ions are pumped into the endolymph than Na^+ ions out. Both ions are pumped against their concentration gradients, and therefore energy is required, this being supplied by ATP (Kuijpers and Bonting, 1969). There is evidence that the main component of the pumping occurs in the basal (that is non-endolymphatic or non-luminal) membrane of the marginal cells of the stria vascularis, and that the ions diffuse passively between the marginal cell cytoplasm and the endolymph (for example Johnstone and Sellick, 1972).

The most direct evidence that the potential is electrogenic comes from experiments in which the pump is poisoned or made anoxic. An electrogenic potential should disappear as soon as the pump stops. However, if the potential is a diffusion potential, it should be maintained as long as the ion gradients are present. Cyanide poisoning or anoxia causes the endocochlear potential to drop to zero within 1–2 minutes, too short a time for the ionic gradients to have disappeared (Johnstone and Sellick, 1972). The result is also supported by the effects of ouabain, which specifically affects electrogenic Na^+/K^+ ATPase, and which reduces the endocochlear potential in parallel with its effect on the ATPase (Kuijpers and Bonting, 1970).

In experiments in which the pump is poisoned or otherwise rendered inactive, the positive endocochlear potential is replaced within a few minutes by a negative potential of some $-40\,mV$, which can take several hours to disappear. This negative potential is thought to be a conventional diffusion potential, arising because K^+ diffuses across the boundaries of the endolymphatic space (mainly in this case through the organ of Corti),

taking positive charge with it, and so leaving the endolymph negative. The negative potential (called $-EP$) remains until the ionic concentrations decay. Because the membranes permit some diffusion even in the healthy cochlea, the negative potential will make a contribution in the normal state. The observed normal endocochlear potential of some $+80\,mV$ is therefore the sum of an electrogenic component of approximately $+120\,mV$, and the diffusion component of $-40\,mV$.

Perilymph

Measurement of perilymphatic ionic concentrations does not pose the same problems as that of endolymphatic concentrations, and the results are not controversial. *Table 2.2* shows that the results from different investigators are in close agreement. The values are in the range of normal extracellular concentrations, although they are interesting in suggesting that K^+ concentrations in the scala vestibuli are somewhat higher than in the scala tympani.

Johnstone and Sellick (1972) reported the electric potential of the scala tympani ($+7\,mV$) to be a little more positive than that of the scala vestibuli ($+5\,mV$). Voltages are given with respect to blood plasma. The small extra positivity may arise from leakage of K^+ through the organ of Corti, or may reflect small differences in ionic diffusion potentials because of the difference in the K^+ concentrations.

Organ of Corti and subtectorial space

The true border of the perilymphatic space in the organ of Corti is not the basilar membrane, but is likely to be situated more apically in the organ, for instance at the reticular lamina (*see Figure 2.8*). This

Table 2.2 Perilymph electrolyte concentrations (mM unless stated otherwise)

Species	Cochlear duct			Utricle			Investigator
	Na^+	K^+	Cl^-	Na^+	K^+	Cl^-	
Guinea-pig			127.8±2.0			128.6±1.9	Konishi and Hamrick (1978)
	154.5	7.3	123.2	124.3	3.5	155.4	Konishi, Salt and Hamrick (1979)
	133.5±2.7	7.4±0.57	120±5.8	138.6±2.6	3.7±0.33	107±4.2	Makimoto, Takedo and Silverstein (1980)
Cat	147±0.94	10.5±0.31	138.5±3.6	157.1±1.1	3.8±0.11	130.0±2.3	Makimoto, Takedo and Silverstein (1980)
Rat	137.5±1.2	4.0±0.15	127.1±0.9	137.0±0.96	3.1±0.15	127.7±0.71	Sterkers *et al.* (1982)
	129	5.9	119				Bosher and Warren (1968)
Human				142*	7*		Silverstein (1972)
				138.0±10.0	10.7±2.6	118.5*	Rauch and Köstlin (1958)

* mequiv./l
Reproduced from Anniko and Wroblewski (1986), Table 2

is supported by measurements of ionic concentrations in the spaces of the organ of Corti by X-ray microprobe analysis of quick-frozen tissue (Anniko, Lim and Wroblewski, 1984). These measurements show it to have the same ionic composition asa perilymph. The basilar membrane is readily permeable to macromolecular tracers, giving them access to the spaces in the organ of Corti. The same is therefore likely to be true for ions which are much smaller. However, Ryan, Wickham and Bone (1980) found that, with their freezing technique, fluid in the spaces of the organ of Corti did not give rise to crystals, suggesting that its protein content was relatively high. Fluid in this space has been named 'cortilymph'.

The fluid in the inner spiral sulcus and in the subtectorial space (between the tectorial membrane and the reticular lamina) has generally been thought to be continuous with the endolymph, and so would have a high positive potential. The chemical and electrical border between the endolymph and the perilymph would then be the reticular lamina, and would include the transducing surfaces of the hair cells. However, the position has been somewhat controversial, since Manley and Kronester-Frei (1980) found that fluid in the inner spiral sulcus had the same potential as the perilymph (near 0 mV), and the endocochlear potential was met only as the electrode entered the lower surface of the tectorial membrane. This suggests that the electrical, and hence chemical, border between the endolymph and the perilymph is the tectorial membrane and not the reticular lamina. Such a view is important because it would require revision of some of the existing ideas of hair cell transduction (*see below*). Studies of ion distribution with the X-ray microprobes have, however, not generally supported this view, although it must be said that it is difficult to ensure that the ions do not reorganize themselves during the freezing process. Ryan, Wickham and Bone (1980) and Anniko, Lim and Wroblewski (1984) both found that crystals from the subtectorial space had the high K^+ and low Na^+ concentrations characteristic of endolymph, not perilymph.

Cochlear mechanics

The mechanical travelling wave in the cochlea forms the basis of the frequency selectivity of the whole organism and, in addition, is the basis of our extreme sensitivity to sounds. A normal travelling wave is therefore fundamental to normal auditory function, and a pathological wave, as probably occurs in most cases of cochlear sensorineural hearing loss, can cause severe deficit.

The cochlear travelling wave was originally described by von Békésy (1943, 1960). Working in

excised human temporal bones, he opened a stretch of the cochlea, sprinkled reflecting particles on Reissner's membrane, and observed the movement of the membrane stroboscopically in response to applied sound stimuli. Intensities were in the range of 130–140 dB SPL. He showed the now classic travelling wave (*Figure 2.10*). He suggested that the pattern was similar to the pattern of movement of the other membrane, the basilar membrane, which carries the organ of Corti. The wave travels along the cochlea, comes to a peak, and dies away rapidly. *Figure 2.10* shows the

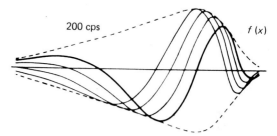

Figure 2.10 The travelling wave in the cochlea, according to von Békésy. The base of the cochlea is towards the left, and the apex towards the right. The solid lines show the displacements at four successive instants. The dotted lines show the envelope, which is static. Stimulus frequency: 200 Hz. (From von Békésy, 1960; copyright McGraw-Hill, 1960)

response, as a function of distance, for sinusoidal stimulation of a single frequency. Von Békésy made plots such as these for a variety of stimulus frequencies, and showed that high frequencies produced a travelling wave peaking near the base of the cochlea, whereas low frequencies produced a wave stretching further up to the apex.

Von Békésy (1943) also made plots in a different way. He opened the cochlea at single points, and measured the amplitude of vibration at the individual points as he varied the stimulus frequency. If the plots are recalculated for input stimuli of constant sound pressure, the basilar membrane is seen to have a purely low-pass filtering characteristic at each point. That is, the membrane vibrates with a constant amplitude for all low frequencies, until above a certain frequency the response drops abruptly. On the basis of von Békésy's results, the capacity of the basilar membrane for frequency filtering is therefore very poor indeed.

It is now known that single neurons of the auditory nerve have very sharp bandpass frequency filtering characteristics. That is, the response is large for only a very narrow range of sound frequencies and, if the sound frequency is changed either way, that is as if it is either increased or decreased, the response drops sharply (*see below*). This led to the suspicion that the sharp tuning might be derived from the mechanics, and that the basilar membrane was much more sharply tuned than von Békésy had shown. The most recent measurements, in which great care has been taken by the experimenters, and in which very sensitive methods have been used to make the measurements, have in fact shown that the mechanical response is very sharply tuned. The best, and probably definitive, measurements that are available were obtained from the guinea-pig by Sellick, Patuzzi and Johnstone (1982). Responses are plotted for one or more individual points on the basilar membrane, and the stimulus frequency is varied. However, instead of plotting the amplitude of response for a fixed input intensity, the converse is shown. That is, the stimulus intensity necessary to give a certain, criterion, amount of vibration is plotted, for different stimulus frequencies. The resulting curves are called 'tuning curves' or frequency threshold curves (FTCs). A tuning curve for the

mechanical response of one point on a basilar membrane of the guinea-pig is shown in *Figure 2.11*.

Two important points can be made from the response shown in *Figure 2.11*. First, the sharp dip around one frequency, 18 kHz, shows that only very low intensities of sound were necessary to give a response at that frequency. In the experiment illustrated in *Figure 2.11*, the criterion level of response (0.35 nm) was produced by a sound pressure level at the tympanic membrane of only 12 dB SPL. This is an indication that the mechanical system has a great responsiveness and sensitivity to sound. In fact, if the amplitude of the vibration of the membrane is calculated and this is compared with the vibration of the stapes at the input to the cochlea, it is found that the travelling wave amplifies the movement by about 40 dB. Second, the intensity necessary to give the criterion response rises sharply on either side of that frequency. The steep slopes of the function show that the system is very sharply tuned or, in other words, has great frequency selectivity. Sensitivity and frequency selectivity are two important properties of the normally functioning auditory system. The indications are that the sensitivity and frequency selectivity shown by the whole organism are derived from that of the basilar membrane.

Figure 2.11 also shows the tuning curves for the electrical response of a hair cell and an auditory nerve fibre, measured at nearly the same point along the basilar membrane. All three curves have similar, sharply tuned tips. This shows that they have the same degree of tuning.

Why was the sharply tuned response not seen by von Békésy? Two reasons have been suggested. First, the cochlea has to be in extremely good physiological condition to show a sharply tuned mechanical response. Any deterioration due to, for instance, anoxia, mixing of the endolymph or perilymph, interference with the blood supply, or bleeding into the scalae, will reduce the response. These factors set very stringent limits where it is necessary to open the cochlear scalae and place measuring instruments on the cochlear partition. In contrast, von Békésy performed his measurements on cadavers. Second, it is now known that the response becomes more broadly tuned at high intensities. It should be noted that the measurements of *Figure 2.11* are made down to 12 dB SPL. Von Békésy, because of the relative insensitivity of his measuring instruments, had to use far higher sound pressures, that is, 130–140 dB SPL.

Although the sharpness of tuning shown by von Békésy has to be revised, the tonotopicity of the cochlea does not. The modern evidence agrees with von Békésy in showing that high frequency tones produce their greatest effects near the base

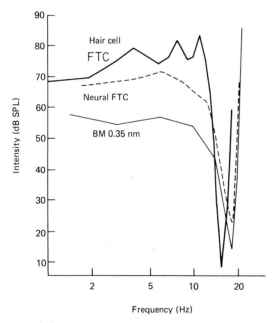

Figure 2.11 Tuning curve (frequency-threshold curve) for the mechanical vibration of the basilar membrane at 0.35 nm displacement criterion (——). The measurements were made at the 18 kHz place. Also shown is the tuning curve for an auditory nerve fibre (– – –) innervating the same place, and the tuning curve for an inner hair cell (——) situated a little more apically in the cochlea and so responding best to a lower frequency (14 kHz). (Basilar membrane and neural data from Sellick, Patuzzi and Johnstone, 1982, and hair cell data from Russell and Sellick, 1978. Reproduced from Pickles, 1985a)

of the cochlea, and low frequency tones at the apex, with a gradation in between for intermediate frequencies.

The fact that the basilar membrane tuning becomes less selective at high stimulus intensities is a reflection of the non-linearity of its response. That is, if the sound pressure is increased 10 times, the amplitude of the movement does not go up 10 times correspondingly, but by rather less. This is shown in the *amplitude functions* of *Figure 2.12*. If

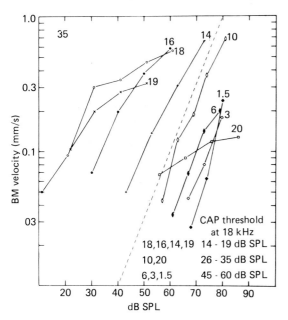

Figure 2.12 Amplitudes of basilar membrane vibration as a function of stimulus intensity, for different frequencies of stimulation (parameter on curves, in kHz). Responses were measured at the 18 kHz point on the basilar membrane. (From Sellick, Patuzzi and Johnstone, 1982, slightly modified)

the responses increased in proportion to stimulus pressure, the lines on the graph would all be parallel to the dotted line, which has been drawn for linear growth. However, the lines for stimuli of 18, 19 and 20 kHz (shown by the numbers on the curves) grow with a shallower slope – that is, non-linearly – for some of their range. If, for instance, the sound pressure at 18 kHz is increased from 30 to 50 dB SPL, the formula for calculation of decibels (*see* Decibels) will show that the sound pressure has gone up 10 times. However, the amplitude of response in the basilar membrane grew from 0.3 to 0.45 mm/s, an increase of only 1.5 times. The non-linearity makes the tuning less selective at high intensities because the responses in the sharply tuned tip of the tuning curve are influenced most by the non-linearity.

It has been questioned why the basilar membrane shows these very sharply tuned and non-linear responses, and why they are so vulnerable. The surprising answer suggested by many lines of evidence is that the basilar membrane contains an *active mechanical amplifier*, which uses biological energy to boost the mechanical vibration of the basilar membrane.

It is now believed that as a wave moves up the cochlea, towards its peak, it encounters a region in which the membrane is mechanically active. Triggered by the movement, the membrane starts putting energy into the wave. The amplitude of the movement then grows very sharply, but also dies away sharply because the wave soon reaches a region in which further wave motion for this frequency of stimulation is not possible. The travelling wave can therefore be considered as consisting of two components. There is a broadly tuned, relatively small component, which depends on the purely passive mechanical properties of the basilar membrane and cochlear fluids. In addition, there is a relatively large-amplitude active component, which gives sharp tuning and great frequency selectivity. The second component is produced by an input of biological energy from the cochlea. It is most prominent for low intensities of stimulation. It is less prominent with high intensity stimulation, and is reduced with cochlear pathology. Under these circumstances, the cochlea becomes more broadly tuned and relatively less sensitive. Because of this, von Békésy was able to see only the first component in his experiments.

The evidence for this process is still indirect, although all the individual elements of the sequence have been shown. For instance, mathematical models of cochlear mechanics have not been able to imitate the sharp tuning of *Figure 2.11* with purely passive mechanical systems. A feedback of mechanical energy has been required in the models, whereupon they have been successful in producing patterns as in *Figures 2.11* and *2.12*. It is known that the hair cells can move actively in response to stimulation. There is also strong evidence for active mechanical processes in the cochlea, because under some circumstances the cochlea can produce sound, either spontaneously or when triggered by acoustic stimulation (Kemp, 1978). Finally, the changes in tuning and sensitivity, observed with deteriorated cochleae in experimental animals, or psychophysically in human beings with sensorineural hearing loss of cochlear origin, are precisely the changes that would be expected with loss of the active process (*see below*). Pickles (1985b) reviewed current evidence in favour of the hypothesis. The details of the evidence require consideration of hair cell responses, the influence of the efferent nerve supply and pathological changes. These will be discussed in the following section, and points of relation to the active mechanical process pointed out.

Transduction by hair cells

The process of signal transduction in hair cells is becoming more clearly understood as a result of the advances that have been made in electrophysiological recordings from hair cells (for example Russell and Sellick, 1978; Holton and Hudspeth, 1986). There are anatomical suggestions as to the site of the transducer channels, and how the mechanical stimulus is coupled to them (Pickles, Comis and Osborne, 1984).

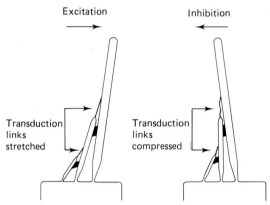

Figure 2.13 The role of tip links between stereocilia in transduction, according to Pickles, Comis and Osborne (1984). Three rows of stereocilia on a hair cell are shown in cross-section. (From Pickles, Comis and Osborne, 1984)

The individual stereocilia on the apical surface of the hair cell are mechanically rigid, and are braced together with cross-links so that they move as a stiff bundle. Therefore, as the bundle is deflected, the different rows of stereocilia could be expected to slide relative to one another (*Figure 2.13*). There are fine links running upwards from the tips of the shorter stereocilia on the hair cell, which join the adjacent taller stereocilia of the next row. When the stereocilia are deflected in the direction of the tallest stereocilia, the links are stretched, opening ion channels in the cell membrane. When the stereocilia are deflected in the opposite direction, the tension is taken off the links, and the channels close. This hypothesis is consistent with all the present electrophysiological evidence from hair cells (Hudspeth, 1985; Pickles, 1985b).

The tip links, which are likely to be responsible for coupling the movement to the transducer channels are shown for an outer hair cell, in *Figure 2.14.* Inner hair cells have similar links. The actual transducer channels are likely to be situated in the stereociliar membrane at one or both of the points of insertion of the tip link. The electrophysiological experiments of Hudspeth (1982) support the idea that these are the sites for the transducer channels, because if the extracellular environment is explored with an electrode while the stereocilia are being deflected, the currents resulting from transduction flow into the cell around the tips of the stereocilia.

The stimulus is coupled to the stereocilia by means of a shear or relative motion between the tectorial membrane and the reticular lamina. As the basilar membrane and organ of Corti are

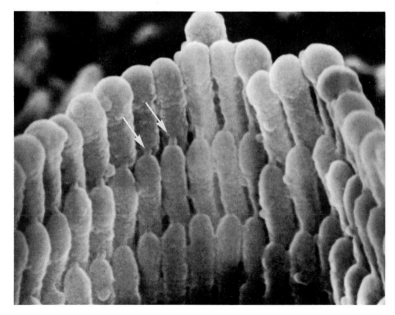

Figure 2.14 Guinea-pig: stereocilia at the apex of the V on an outer hair cell, showing tip links (arrows)

driven upwards and downwards by a sound stimulus, the stereocilia are moved away from and towards the modiolus (*Figure 2.15a* and *b*). Because the tallest stereocilia are situated on the side of the hair cell furthest away from the modiolus, an upwards movement of the basilar membrane is

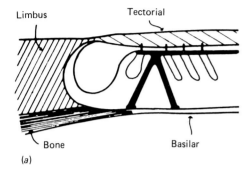

(a)

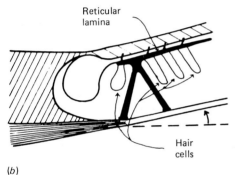

(b)

translated into a movement of the stereocilia in the direction of the tallest, as is shown in the left panel of *Figure 2.13*. This is the direction associated with opening of the ion channels. This is confirmed by recordings of the resistance variations of hair cells, which show that the resistance becomes low when the stereocilia are deflected in the direction of the tallest. The effective direction of shear between the tectorial membrane and the reticular lamina is therefore radial across the cochlear duct. It is no surprise that in both inner and outer hair cells the tip links are organized in such a way that they run in a direction most suited for picking up radial shear (Comis, Pickles and Osborne, 1985). In outer hair cells, where the stereocilia are closely packed in a hexagonal array, the rows of stereocilia need to be set diagonally across the cochlear duct if the tip links are to run radially (*see Figure 2.15c*). This is apparently the reason for the rows of stereocilia on outer hair cells having a V- or W-shaped arrangement. However, on inner hair cells the packing is looser, and these cells achieve a radial orientation of their tip links while the rows of stereocilia run in a straight line.

When the channels on the stereocilia are open, ions will enter or leave the cell depending on the electrical and chemical gradients across the apical cell surface. It appears that the ion channels are rather large and non-selective, so that, for instance, Na^+, K^+, and Ca^{2+} will enter with nearly the same efficacy (Corey and Hudspeth, 1979). Under the generally accepted position, the apical surface of hair cells is faced by endolymph with a

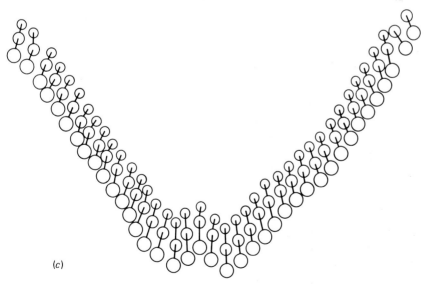

(c)

Figure 2.15 (*a,b*) Coupling of the movement of the basilar membrane to the stereocilia, by means of a shear between the tectorial membrane and the reticular lamina, in a direction radial across the cochlear duct. (From Davis, 1958.) (*c*) The direction of tip links on an outer hair cell, showing that they run nearly parallel to the cell's axis of bilateral symmetry, and so nearly radially across the cochlear duct. (From Comis, Pickles and Osborne, 1985)

high positive potential (+80 mV) and a high K⁺ concentration. Inside the cell, however, there is a negative intracellular potential, which is −45 mV for inner hair cells and −70 mV for outer hair cells. The potentials combine to give 125 mV (inner hair cells) or 150 mV (outer hair cells) of potential drop across the channel. When the channels are open, K⁺ from the endolymph will tend to be driven into the cell by this big potential gradient, thus making the cell become more positive inside (*Figure 2.16*). When the channels are completely shut, as during the opposite phase of the sound wave, even the resting current is shut off, and the cells will

become more negative. Most of the transducer current may be carried by K⁺, as this is the predominant ion in the endolymph. However, it is possible that some of the current is carried by other ions, such as Ca^{2+}. It is appropriate for K⁺ to be the main carrier of the transducer current. As K⁺ is automatically in equilibrium across the basal membrane of the hair cell, any excess K⁺ entering the cell through the transducer channel will flow out through the basal membrane without any pumping being necessary. The energy from the whole process comes from the stria vascularis, which, by ion pumping, stores energy in the 'battery' of the endolymph. This is the 'battery' or 'resistance modulation' theory of Davis (1965), as it appears in the light of modern evidence.

Because the stereocilia are driven by a radial shear between the tectorial membrane and the reticular lamina, and because this shear is produced by a vertical movement of the cochlear partition, the hair cells would be expected to have, to a first approximation at least, the same frequency tuning as the mechanical vibration of the basilar membrane. This is supported by the records available so far (*see* for example *Figure 2.11*), although it is still open as to whether there are differences of detail, particularly in the low-frequency part of the tuning curve.

The electrical responses of cochlear hair cells

Inner hair cells

The inner hair cells make a large number of synaptic contacts with the afferent fibres of the auditory nerve. In fact, some 95% of all afferent auditory nerve fibres make contact with the inner hair cells, and each inner hair cell has terminals from about 20 afferent fibres (Spoendlin, 1972). It must, therefore, be assumed that the role of inner hair cells is to detect the movement of the basilar membrane and transmit it to the auditory nerve.

It is one of the triumphs of recent cochlear physiology that intracellular records obtained from hair cells are now available. Those from inner hair cells have been obtained from several laboratories (for example Russell and Sellick, 1978, 1983). However, outer hair cells seem particularly difficult to record from and only a few reports are currently available.

If the electrical potential of an inner hair cell is measured during a low-frequency acoustic stimulus, approximately sinusoidal oscillations of the membrane potential are obtained, as the transducer channels open and close (*Figure 2.17a*, top traces). If such records are used to plot the instantaneous value of the input sound pressure against the intracellular voltage, the curves are

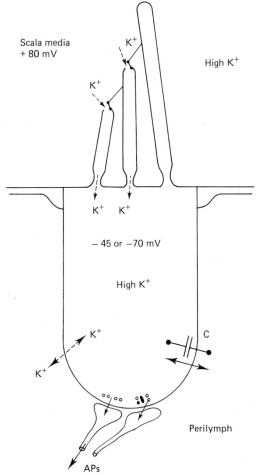

Figure 2.16 Suggested ion flows in a hair cell resulting from transduction. The transducer channels are shown on the ends of the shorter stereocilia, at the lower ends of the tip links, although their exact position is not known. After entering through the transducer channels, K⁺ can redistribute itself passively across the basal membrane of the hair cell. The capacitance (C) of the basal cell membranes provides a low-impedance path for high-frequency alternating currents. APs = action potentials

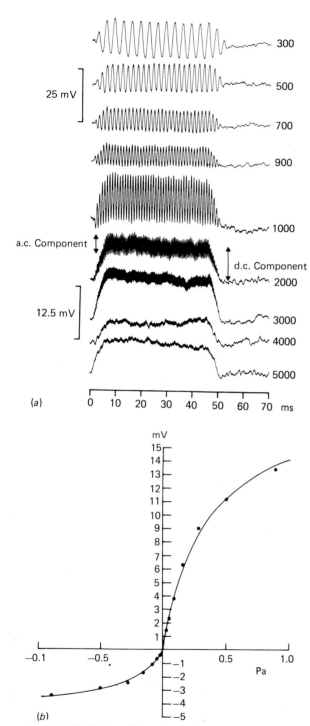

obtained as in *Figure 2.17b*. This record was obtained from an inner hair cell of the guinea-pig cochlea, driven by an acoustic stimulus. The values along the horizontal axis of *Figure 2.17b* are therefore plotted as sound pressure at the input, rather than as a direct deflection of the stereocilia. A few records have been made for mechanical displacements applied directly to the stereocilia, in cochlear hair cells in organ culture, where the tectorial membrane does not develop. These functions show a similar form (Russell, Richardson and Cody, 1986).

The function in *Figure 2.17b* is asymmetrical in two ways. First, the resting or zero point of the function shows that at rest only about 20% of the channels are open. Second, maximum channel opening is achieved much more gradually and for much more extreme deflections than is the case with channel closing. These asymmetries mean that, in response to sinusoidal stimulation, a distorted response will be obtained in the hair cell. The predominant distortion is that the positive excursions will be greater than the negative excursions and, as shown by some of the traces in *Figure 2.17a*, the whole record appears to shift upwards. Therefore, the responses of inner hair cells can be divided, to a first approximation, into an oscillating AC response, occurring at the stimulus frequency, and a DC depolarization.

The importance of these asymmetries is seen when the stimulus frequency is increased above about 1 kHz. Above this frequency, the electrical circuit properties of the hair cell walls begin to affect the response. The basal walls of the hair cell begin to act as a capacitor, and as the frequency is raised, more and more of the transducer current will flow out through the capacitance of the basal walls of the hair cells (*see Figure 2.16*). It therefore tends to short-circuit the AC component of the transducer current and, consequently, the AC voltage response in the cell drops (Russell and Sellick, 1983). This is why in *Figure 2.17a*, the AC changes become relatively smaller as the stimulus frequency is raised. However, the DC component is not affected by this process and remains large even at high frequencies of stimulation (*see Figure 2.17a*). The different roles of the AC and DC components of the response will be seen when the activity of auditory nerve fibres is discussed.

Consideration of inner hair cell responses is not complete without including the mode of coupling of the movement to the stereocilia. The tips of the inner hair cell stereocilia are not embedded in the tectorial membrane as are the tips of outer hair cell stereocilia. Rather, they are thought to fit loosely into a groove in Hensen's stripe. The stereocilia would therefore appear to be driven by viscous drag of the endolymph. Viscous forces increase with the velocity of the movements, and record-

Figure 2.17 (*a*) Intracellular voltage changes in an inner hair cell of the guinea-pig cochlea, for different frequencies of stimulation (number on left of traces, Hz). (From Palmer and Russell, 1986.) (*b*) Relation between instantaneous sound pressure (horizontal axis) and intracellular voltage change (vertical axis) for an inner hair cell. (From Russell and Sellick, 1983)

ings show that inner hair cells respond to the *velocity*, rather than just the displacement, of the basilar membrane (Russell and Sellick, 1983).

Outer hair cells

The great majority of the afferent auditory nerve fibres make their synaptic contact with inner rather than outer hair cells. Only a few make contact with outer hair cells. It does not, therefore, appear that outer hair cells form an essential step in transferring information about the basilar membrane vibration to the central nervous system. Rather, the outer hair cells are probably involved in generating the active mechanical amplification of basilar membrane vibration, which gives rise to the relatively large-amplitude and sharply tuned mechanical travelling wave. They also generate the cochlear microphonic, and this may be an essential step in the mechanical amplification.

The difficulty of recording from outer hair cells means that information about them is much more sketchy than for inner hair cells (*see* for example Dallos, 1985). In general, they would seem to respond rather like inner hair cells, although there is some evidence that the input–output functions (*see Figure 2.17b*) are more symmetrical than for inner hair cells, at least in the high frequency range (Russell and Sellick, 1983). Because the functions are relatively symmetrical, only small DC components will be generated in response to sinusoidal stimulation. As with inner hair cells, the AC currents resulting from high frequency stimulation will readily flow across the capacitance of the basal cell walls. The cells should therefore show only small AC and DC voltage responses to high-frequency stimuli. While this has undoubtedly contributed to the difficulty of recording from these cells, it also suggests that the cells contribute to cochlear function by way of some other route. One suggestion is that the heavy current flows through the outer hair cells, which give rise to the cochlear microphonic, are the critical elements in producing a mechanical amplification of the travelling wave (for example Pickles, 1985b).

Many attempts have recently been made to record movements generated by outer hair cells, which could be responsible for this mechanical feedback. As one example, Brownell *et al.* (1985) obtained movements from isolated outer hair cells which could be triggered either electrically or chemically. However, it is not yet known whether the effects have the right characteristics to be involved in the mechanical amplification of the travelling wave.

The gross electrical responses of the cochlea

If an electrode is placed within one of the cochlear scalae, or on the walls of the cochlea, or indeed anywhere in the vicinity of the cochlea, electric potentials can be recorded in response to acoustic stimuli. They can be divided into three components. First, there is the cochlear microphonic, which is an AC response that follows the waveform of the stimulus (*Figure 2.18*). Superimposed—

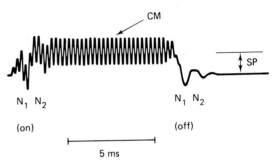

Figure 2.18 Diagram of the gross electrical responses to a tone burst, including the N_1 and N_2 neural potentials, the cochlear microphonic (CM) and the summating potential (SP). (From Pickles, 1982)

posed on that, a DC shift in the baseline of the microphonic is often seen. This is the summating potential. At the beginning of the stimulus, and sometimes at the end, a series of deflections in the negative direction can be seen, making the neural potentials. The first phase is called the N_1 potential and the second smaller phase, which is not always visible, the N_2 potential.

The cochlear microphonic is derived almost entirely from the outer hair cells, for if the cells are destroyed by the ototoxic antibiotic kanamycin, the response will drop drastically (Dallos, 1973). Electrode penetration through the organ of Corti shows the microphonic to be generated at the reticular lamina, which is the interface across which the transducing surface of the hair cell is situated (Tasaki, Davis and Eldredge, 1954). It is likely that the microphonic represents the massed effects of the transducer currents flowing through outer hair cells. Intracochlearly, the microphonic may be essential for the mechanical amplification of the travelling wave.

The summating potential can appear as either a positive or a negative shift, depending on the stimulus conditions. Unlike the cochlear microphonic, it can take some time to reach maximum amplitude after the onset of a stimulus. Evidence concerning the origin of the summating potential is still incomplete, but it is most likely generated as a distortion component of the outer hair cell response, with perhaps a small contribution from inner hair cells. At present there is insufficient information available about the responses of outer hair cells.

The neural potentials arise from the massed action potentials in the auditory nerve which are produced at the onset of a stimulus. They depend on the sum of a large number of synchronous action potentials. However, the delays involved in the travelling wave will affect the synchrony. Because the wave travels most rapidly in the base of the cochlea, high characteristic frequency fibres are the ones most likely to be activated together. Antoli-Candela and Kiang (1978) showed, in the normal cochlea at least, that fibres with characteristic frequencies of 4 kHz and above made the greatest contribution to N_1. The N_2 potential arose from the fibres firing a second time in response to the stimulus.

The responses of auditory nerve fibres

The activation of nerve fibres: phase-locking and frequency selectivity

Neurotransmitter is released in the synapses at the base of inner hair cells, and this gives rise to action potentials in the auditory nerve fibres. Single auditory stimuli are always excitatory, never inhibitory. Transmitter is released as a result of depolarization of the inner hair cells. For low-frequency stimuli, the transmitter will be released in packets concentrated during the depolarizing phases of the hair cell response (for example in the upward phases of the top five traces of *Figure 2.17a*). Because these occur in synchrony with the sound stimulus, transmitter release and action potential generation will also occur in synchrony with the individual cycles of the stimulus. This is known as *phase-locking*; an example from an experimental record is shown in *Figure 2.19*. Phase-locking is seen only at low frequencies, however, where the cyclic changes in inner hair cell intracellular potential are large. As explained earlier (*see* The electrical responses of cochlear hair cells), the AC component of the intracellular

response becomes smaller above about 1 kHz. The degree to which action potentials are phase-locked, therefore, declines above this frequency. By 3–5 kHz, the AC responses in the inner hair cells are so small that phase-locking of action potentials is negligible. Only the DC component of the intracellular change can play a part in the generation of action potentials, and then the action potentials are evoked equally in all phases of the sound stimulus (Palmer and Russell, 1986).

Phase-locking represents one way in which information about the sound stimulus is transmitted up the auditory nerve. For stimulus frequencies below some 5 kHz, therefore, the timing of the action potentials in the nerve is able to signal details of the temporal properties of the sound waveform. This is known as the *temporal coding* of stimuli.

A second important way that auditory nerve fibres code information is by means of their *frequency selectivity*. It should be recalled that inner hair cells detect the movement of the basilar membrane at one point along the cochlear duct, and that the mechanical response of the membrane is very sharply tuned (*see Figure 2.11*). Auditory nerve fibres, therefore, share the tuning characteristics of single points on the membrane and of the inner hair cells (for example Kiang *et al.*, 1965). If recordings are made from fibres at different points on the cochlear duct, the sharply tuned responses will be centred on different frequencies (*Figure 2.20*). *Figure 2.20* shows tuning

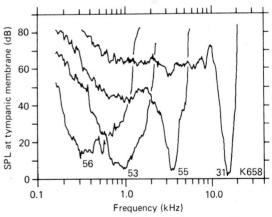

Figure 2.20 Tuning curves of four auditory nerve fibres. (From Kiang, 1980)

curves (frequency-threshold curves) in which the sound pressure level to give a certain criterion increase in firing has been measured automatically by computer for different frequencies of stimulation. Each fibre has a frequency of stimulation for which it is most sensitive, that is for which the sound pressure level was lowest for the criterion

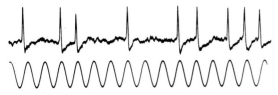

Figure 2.19 Phase-locked action potentials (upper trace), evoked by a 0.3 kHz tone (lower trace). In this record, the action potentials always occur just before the peak of the sound waveform. (From Evans, 1975a)

response. This is known as the best, or characteristic, frequency. As expected from the tonotopic organization of the mechanical travelling wave in the cochlea, fibres innervating the base have the highest best frequencies, and those innervating the apex the lowest.

Coding based on frequency selectivity is called *place coding*, for the reason that the fibres responding best to different frequencies arise from different places in the cochlea. It would therefore be possible to determine the frequency of a stimulus by telling which fibres were activated. It should be noted that the temporal code and the place code are not mutually exclusive. A low frequency stimulus will be frequency filtered, according to the place principle, before the fibre is stimulated. When stimulated, the pattern of firings will carry information about the frequency filtered waveform of the stimulus. The relative extent to which these two principles are actually *used* by the nervous system under different circumstances is at the moment a matter of debate. Pickles (1986) reviewed and analysed stimulus coding in auditory nerve fibres.

Figure 2.20 also shows that the auditory nerve fibres have their lowest thresholds at around 0 dB SPL. It is indeed a general finding that the most sensitive fibres have their lowest thresholds in an intensity range close to the behavioural absolute threshold. In fact, some 75% of fibres have their best thresholds within a 15-dB range of this (Liberman and Kiang, 1978). These low-threshold fibres have particularly high rates of spontaneous activity (that is random firing seen in

the absence of any stimulation). It is likely that the low thresholds arise because the fibres have very sensitive synapses on the hair cells. A second, minor population of fibres have much higher thresholds, in some cases 70 dB or more above the behavioural threshold. These fibres have particularly low rates of spontaneous activity (Liberman and Kiang, 1978).

The frequency selectivity of auditory nerve fibres can be characterized in a variety of ways. One way is to measure the bandwidth of the tuning curve at a set distance above the tip; bandwidths are often measured 10 dB above the tip. In that case, the bandwidth of cat auditory nerve fibres, in the range in which they are most frequency selective (around 10 kHz) is one-eighth of their characteristic frequency (for example Evans, 1975a). If the inverse of this is taken, and the 10-dB bandwidth divided by the characteristic frequency is measured, a number that increases with sharpness of tuning is obtained. This is called '$Q_{10\,dB}$', by analogy with the Q value of electrical filters. In the cat, it averages about 8 at 10 kHz.

Intensity responses of auditory nerve fibres

As the stimulus intensity is increased, the amplitude of basilar membrane vibration grows (*see Figure 2.12*). The activation of inner hair cells grows similarly and, as shown in *Figure 2.21*, so also does the firing rate of auditory nerve fibres. The functions for the different stages have many points of similarity. The slopes of the rate intensity functions, like the basilar membrane functions, are steeper for stimuli below the characteristic frequency than for those at and above it. Moreover, stimuli below the characteristic frequency can drive a fibre to greater firing rates than can stimuli of higher frequency. Above the characteristic frequency, the maximum firing rate that can be produced is lower still. It should also be noted that for stimuli at the characteristic frequency of the fibre, the maximum, or saturated rate has been reached by about 70 dB SPL. Therefore, it would seem that the intensity of an acoustic stimulus can be coded in the firing rates of the auditory nerve fibres, at least up to this intensity.

Non-linear interactions in auditory nerve fibres

Although single auditory stimuli are always excitatory, one stimulus can change the responsiveness of auditory nerve fibres to other stimuli. If one stimulus is already causing excitation in an auditory nerve fibre, a second stimulus can reduce

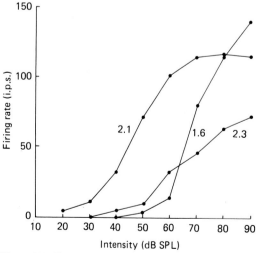

Figure 2.21 Firing rate plotted as a function of stimulus intensity for a guinea-pig auditory nerve fibre (characteristic frequency = 2.1 kHz), for different frequencies of stimulation, shown by parameter on each curve. (From Pickles, 1986)

the response. The reduction of activity is called *two-tone suppression*, because it is seen only during the interaction of two or more stimuli. It can, therefore, be distinguished from inhibition mediated by inhibitory synapses because spontaneous activity cannot be inhibited. Two-tone suppression is almost certainly related to the non-linearity of the basilar membrane, and two-tone suppression can be seen in the mechanical vibration of the basilar membrane (Robles, Ruggero and Rich, 1986) and in hair cell responses (Sellick and Russell, 1979), as well as in auditory nerve fibre responses. The actual mechanisms of two-tone suppression are a matter of debate. One suggested mechanism is that the suppressor, by driving the outer hair cells to the limits of their range of sensitivity, reduces the extent to which they can contribute to the active mechanical amplification of the travelling wave produced by the second stimulus (Johnstone, Patuzzi and Yates, 1986). Two-tone suppression may well be important functionally. In the firing of the auditory nerve fibre array, it aids in keeping separate the representation of the different elements of a complex stimulus.

Responses of auditory nerve fibres in pathological cochleae

As studied physiologically, it is apparent that most types of cochlear sensorineural hearing loss are related to loss of the sharply tuned portion of the travelling wave. This probably occurs because outer hair cells are among the most vulnerable elements in the organ of Corti. Moreover, it is likely that small deteriorations in the outer hair cell-travelling wave system are immediately noticeable. In the more severe cases, loss of inner hair cells and auditory nerve fibre responses will also reduce the detection of sounds. Here, it is possible that the great redundancy arising from the large number of auditory nerve fibres affords some protection from the effects of small losses.

The changes in the mechanical travelling wave resulting from the effects of cochlear damage are shown in *Figure 2.22a*. In this instance, as the experiment progressed, the tuning curve changed shape from a sharply tuned, low-threshold curve, to a higher-threshold and broadly tuned curve. This probably happened as a result of trauma from the acoustic stimuli used in making the measurements. After death, the curve had a still higher threshold and still broader tuning (*Figure 2.22a*). Here there would be complete loss of the active component of cochlear mechanics, and a resulting loss of the active mechanical amplification of the travelling wave. There would then be a return to a

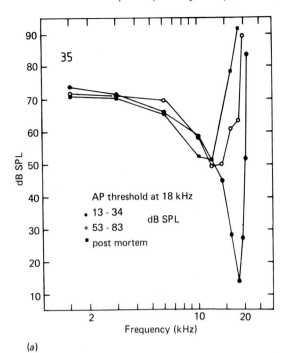

(a)

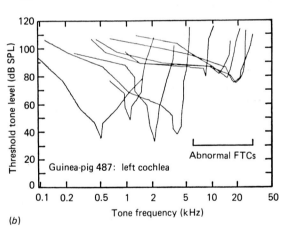

(b)

Figure 2.22 (*a*) Basilar membrane tuning measured when the cochlea was in good condition (●), poor condition (○), or after death (■). (From Sellick, Patuzzi and Johnstone, 1982.) (*b*) Auditory nerve fibre tuning curves in a guinea-pig treated with kanamycin. Fibres at the high-frequency end of the cochlea had high thresholds and broad tuning ('abnormal FTCs'). (From Evans and Harrison, 1976)

broadly tuned wave similar to the one shown originally in cadavers by von Békésy (1943, 1960).

Similar changes can be seen in the tuning curves of auditory nerve fibres in guinea-pigs that have been treated with kanamycin, an aminoglycoside antibiotic which preferentially destroys outer hair cells. *Figure 2.22b* shows that auditory nerve fibres recorded from the region of cochlear damage had high thresholds and broad tuning, comparable to the pathological basilar membrane responses of *Figure 2.22a.* Corresponding changes can be seen experimentally with a variety of manipulations, including anoxia, and the infusion of ototoxic loop diuretics, cyanide, and salicylates (for example Evans, 1975b; Evans, Wilson and Borerwe, 1981).

The changes initially produce a rise in the best thresholds of auditory nerve fibres, and then, with larger losses, a deterioration in the fibres' frequency resolving power. This is shown as an increase in the widths of the tuning curves. Such changes have an obvious correlate with the changes observed in man in many cases of sensorineural loss of cochlear origin, with an increase in absolute threshold and a loss of frequency resolution, apparent as a deterioration in the ability to understand complex sounds such as speech.

Recruitment is commonly seen with sensorineural hearing loss, and this too has its correlates in the activity of auditory nerve fibres. First, when the low-threshold tip of the tuning curve is lost, the rate–intensity functions steepen. It should be noted that, as in *Figure 2.21,* in a normal fibre the intensity function is relatively shallow for frequencies of stimulation at and above the fibre best frequency. This is a result of the active amplification of the cochlear travelling wave, which produces a shallow growth in the basilar membrane intensity functions at and above best frequency (*see Figure 2.12*). When the active component of the travelling wave is lost, the shallow growth disappears and the rate–intensity functions come to have a similar, steep, slope at all frequencies (Harrison, 1981). A second reason relates to the spread of activity along the array of nerve fibres. As pointed out by Evans (1975b), if the tuning curves are much broader than normal – say by a factor of 10 times – than for a certain level above fibre threshold, 10 times as many fibres will be activated as in the normal case. Increases in stimulus level will then produce changes in 10 times as many fibres as in the normal case, and loudness will grow correspondingly more quickly.

A different pattern of changes is seen with experimental endolymphatic hydrops. Harrison and Prijs (1984) showed that, in guinea-pigs with long-term experimental hydrops, low-frequency nerve fibres were affected most, with increases in their best thresholds, and a deterioration in sharpness of tuning. This can be contrasted with the pattern usually seen with cochlear damage, where the high frequency fibres seem most vulnerable. A specific effect on low frequency fibres can be expected if the *stiffness* of the cochlear partition has been increased by the hydrops, because this is the characteristic pattern of change with increases in stiffness in a mechanical system.

The centrifugal innervation of the cochlea

The cochlea receives a centrifugal, or efferent, nerve supply, arising in the superior olivary complex of the brainstem; it is called the olivocochlear bundle. One component of the bundle, which arises from the medial borders of the superior olivary complex and projects mainly contralaterally, innervates the outer hair cells directly. A smaller number of fibres arise laterally in the superior olivary complex, mainly on the ipsilateral side, and innervate the afferent dendrites below the inner hair cells (Guinan, Warr and Norris, 1983).

The functional importance of the olivocochlear bundle has long been a mystery. Dewson (1968) suggested that it aided the discrimination of complex sounds in noise. Speculations built on recent evidence suggest that, by affecting the state of the outer hair cells, the olivocochlear bundle can modify the active mechanical amplification of the travelling wave in the cochlea. Although effects on the basilar membrane vibration have not yet been measured directly, activation of the fibres can modify the extent to which the cochlea returns energy to the ear canal (*see* next section), suggesting an influence on the mechanics (Mountain, 1980). The changes that it can produce in inner hair cell and auditory nerve fibre tuning curves suggest an influence on mechanical tuning (Wiederhold, 1970; Brown, Nuttall and Masta, 1983). Rajan and Johnstone (1983) showed that stimulation of the bundle could protect the ear against moderate levels of noise damage, which is understandable if the olivocochlear bundle reduced the magnitude of the travelling wave. There is also the suggestion that its activity might normally help to keep the outer hair cells in the optimal mechanical state to participate in the active feedback process, and counter the effects of small static pressure changes in the scalae which might adversely affect this (Johnstone, Patuzzi and Yates, 1986).

Cochlear echoes

One of the most intriguing discoveries of recent years has been that the cochlea can emit sounds. It appears that the vibrations come from the hair cells themselves, or at least that the hair cells are an essential component of the process producing the sounds. It also seems likely that the production of sound by the cochlea is a by-product of the active mechanical amplification of the travelling wave. Cochlear echoes also open the possibility of a new objective tool for diagnosing cochlear abnormalities.

Cochlear echoes were discovered by Kemp (1978), who sealed a small microphone and speaker into the ear canals of human subjects. In response to a click applied to the speaker, there was a peak of pressure in the canal. However, there was also a later, and much smaller, peak. Amplification of the traces showed that the second peak was a complex wave, with a form different for each subject (*Figure 2.23*). If the wave had

would account for the relation between the predominant frequency in the response, and the time delay after the stimulus.

It can be shown that an active mechanical amplifier is involved in the echo, because for very low intensity stimuli more energy can be returned to the ear canal than was originally introduced (Kemp, 1978). In other cases, where the subject was hearing a tonal tinnitus, the tinnitus could be detected as a sound pressure fluctuation in the canal (Kemp, 1979), and in some cases an external stimulus of the right frequency could entrain the tinnitus. However, it is recognized that this is probably not the clinically important form of tinnitus, which is likely to arise by means of a different mechanism, perhaps centrally. Echoes seem to occur either in entirely healthy cochleae or on the borders of a region of sensorineural loss, while strong spontaneous emissions seem to be associated with localized hair cell pathology in the presence of normal hair cells (for example Clark *et al.*, 1984). The presence of emissions or echoes can therefore be used as an objective indication of the state of the cochlea.

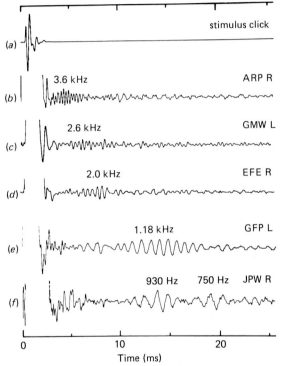

Figure 2.23 Cochlear echoes measured in five different subjects. (*a*) Sound pressure in canal produced by a click. (*b–f*) Sound pressures in canal, showed with a much magnified vertical scale. The input click has clipped (first 3 ms), but the waveform of the echo is visible (3–22 ms). The predominant frequency in each echo is marked on the trace. (From Wilson, 1980)

predominantly high frequency components, they appeared soon after the stimulus, and if it had predominantly low frequency components, they appeared later. It is suggested that, as the travelling wave progressed up the cochlea, it might meet impedance discontinuities, perhaps formed by irregularities in the active system feeding energy back into the travelling wave. The discontinuities would reflect a reverse pressure wave, which would emerge through the middle ear and be recorded in the canal. This model

References

ANNIKO, M., LIM, D. and WROBLEWSKI, R. (1984) Elemental composition of individual cells and tissues in the cochlea. *Acta Oto-Laryngologica*, **98**, 439–453

ANNIKO, M. and WROBLEWSKI, R. (1986) Ionic environment of cochlear hair cells. *Hearing Research*, **22**, 279–293

ANTOLI CANDELA, E. JR and KIANG, N. Y. S. (1978) Unit activity underlying the N_1 potential. In *Evoked Electrical Activity in the Auditory Nervous System*, edited by R. F. Naunton and C. Fernandez, pp. 165–189. New York: Academic Press

BORG, E. (1973) On the neuronal organization of the acoustic middle ear reflex. A physiological and anatomical study. *Brain Research*, **49**, 101–123

BORG, E. and ZAKRISSON, J. E. (1973) Stapedius reflex and speech features. *Journal of the Acoustical Society of America*, **54**, 525–527

BOSHER, S. K. and WARREN, R. L. (1968) Observations on the electrochemistry of the cochlear endolymph of the rat: a quantitative study of its electrical potential and ionic composition as determined by means of flame spectrophotometry. *Proceedings of the Royal Society, Series B*, **171**, 227–247

BROWN, R. D. (1981) Anatomy of the inner ear. In *Pharmacology of Hearing*, edited by R. D. Brown and E. A. Daigneault, pp. 3–18. New York: Wiley

BROWN, M. C., NUTTALL, A. L. and MASTA, R. I. (1983) Intracellular recordings from cochlear inner hair cells: effects of stimulation of the crossed olivocochlear efferents. *Science*, **222**, 69–72

BROWNELL, W. E., BADER, C. R., BERTRAND, D. and RIBAUPIERRE, Y. DE (1985) Evoked mechanical responses of isolated cochlear outer hair cells. *Science*, **227**, 194–196

CLARK, W. W., KIM, D. O., ZUREK, P. M. and BOHNE, B. A. (1984) Spontaneous otoacoustic emissions in chinchilla ear canals: correlation with histopathology and suppression by external tones. *Hearing Research,* **16,** 299–314

COMIS, S. D., PICKLES, J. O. and OSBORNE, M. P. (1985) Osmium tetroxide postfixation in relation to the cross linkage and spatial organization of stereocilia in the guinea-pig cochlea. *Journal of Neurocytology,* **14,** 113–130

COREY, D. P. and HUDSPETH, A. J. (1979) Ionic basis of the receptor potential in a vertebrate hair cell. *Nature,* **281,** 675–677

DALLOS, P. (1973) Cochlear potentials and cochlear mechanics. In *Basic Mechanisms in Hearing,* edited by A. R. Moller, pp. 335–372. New York: Academic Press

DALLOS, P. (1985) Response characteristics of mammalian cochlear hair cells. *Journal of Neuroscience,* **5,** 1591–1608

DAVIS, H. (1958) Transmission and transduction in the cochlea. *The Laryngoscope,* **68,** 359–382

DAVIS, H. (1965) A model for transducer action in the cochlea. *Cold Spring Harbor Symposia on Quantitative Biology,* **30,** 181–189

DEWSON, J. H. (1968) Efferent olivocochlear bundle: some relationships to stimulus discrimination in noise. *Journal of Neurophysiology,* **31,** 122–130

EVANS, E. F. (1975a) Cochlear nerve and cochlear nucleus. In *Handbook of Sensory Physiology Vol 5/2,* edited by W. D. Keidel and W. D. Neff, pp. 1–108. Berlin: Springer

EVANS, E. F. (1975b) Normal and abnormal functioning of the cochlear nerve. *Symposium of the Zoological Society of London,* **37,** 133–165

EVANS, E. F. and HARRISON, R. V. (1976) Correlation between cochlear outer hair cell damage and deterioration of cochlear nerve tuning properties in the guinea pig. *Journal of Physiology,* **256,** 43–44P

EVANS, E. F., WILSON, J. P. and BORERWE, T. A. (1981) Animal models of tinnitus. In *Tinnitus: CIBA Foundation Symposium no. 85,* edited by D. Evered and G. Lawrenson, pp. 108–129. London: Pitman

FAWCETT, D. W. (1986) *A Textbook of Histology.* Philadelphia: W. B. Saunders

FELDMAN, A. M. (1981) Cochlear biochemistry. In *Pharmacology of Hearing,* edited by R. D. Brown and E. A. Daigneault, pp. 52–80. New York: Wiley

GUINAN, J. J. and PEAKE, W. T. (1967) Middle-ear characteristics of anesthetized cats. *Journal of the Acoustical Society of America,* **41,** 1237–1261

GUINAN, J. J., WARR, W. B. and NORRIS, B. E. (1983) Differential olivocochlear projections from lateral versus medial zones of the superior olivary complex. *Journal of Comparative Neurology,* **221,** 358–370

HARRISON, R. V. (1981) Rate-versus-intensity functions and related AP responses in normal and pathological guinea pig and human cochleas. *Journal of the Acoustical Society of America,* **70,** 1036–1044

HARRISON, R. V. and PRIJS, V. F. (1984) Single cochlear fibre responses in guinea pigs with long-term endolymphatic hydrops. *Hearing Research,* **14,** 79–84

HILDING, D. A. (1961) The protective value of the stapedius reflex: an experimental study. *Transactions of the American Academy for Ophthalmology and Otolaryngology,* **65,** 297–307

HOLTON, T. and HUDSPETH, A. J. (1986) The transduction channel of hair cells from the bull-frog characterized by noise analysis. *Journal of Physiology,* **375,** 195–227

HUDDE, H. (1983) Measurement of the eardrum impedance of human ears. *Journal of the Acoustical Society of America,* **73,** 242–247

HUDSPETH, A. J. (1982) Extracellular current flow and the site of transduction by vertebrate hair cells. *Journal of Neuroscience,* **2,** 1–10

HUDSPETH, A. J. (1985) The cellular basis of hearing: the biophysics of hair cells. *Science,* **230,** 745–752

IRVINE, D. R. F., CLAREY, J. C., MORTON, R. E. and NEWMAN, R. G. (1983) Masking by internally generated noise and protection by middle ear muscle activity. *Hearing Research,* **10,** 371–374

JOHNSTONE, B. M. and SELLICK, P. M. (1972) The peripheral auditory apparatus. *Quarterly Reviews of Biophysics,* **5,** 1–57

JOHNSTONE, B. M., PATUZZI, R. and YATES, G. K. (1986) Basilar membrane measurements and the travelling wave. *Hearing Research,* **22,** 147–153

KELLERHALS, B. (1979) Perilymph production and cochlear blood flow. *Acta Oto-Laryngologica,* **87,** 370–374

KEMP, D. T. (1978) Stimulated acoustic emissions from within the human auditory system. *Journal of the Acoustical Society of America,* **64,** 1386–1391

KEMP, D. T. (1979) Evidence for mechanical nonlinearity and frequency selective wave amplification in the cochlea. *Archives of Oto-Rhino-Laryngology,* **224,** 37–45

KHANNA, S. M. and TONNDORF, J. (1972) Tympanic membrane vibration in cats studied by time-averaged holography. *Journal of the Acoustical Society of America,* **51,** 1904–1920

KIANG, N. Y. S. (1980) Processing of speech by the auditory nervous system. *Journal of the Acoustical Society of America,* **68,** 830–835

KIANG, N. Y. S., WATANABE, T., THOMAS, E. C. and CLARK, L. F. (1965) *Discharge Patterns of Single Fibers in the Cat's Auditory Nerve (Research Monographs no. 35).* Cambridge, Mass.: MIT Press

KIMURA, R. S. (1967) Experimental blockage of the endolymphatic duct and its effect on the inner ear of the guinea pig. *Annals of Otology, Rhinology, and Laryngology,* **76,** 664–687

KONISHI, T. and HAMRICK, P. E. (1978) Ion transport in the cochlea of guinea pig. II. Chloride transport. *Acta Oto-Laryngologica,* **86,** 176–184

KONISHI, T., SALT, A. N. and HAMRICK, P. E. (1979) Effects of exposure to noise on ion movement in guinea pig cochlea. *Hearing Research,* **1,** 325–342

KRINGLEBOTN, M. and GUNDERSEN, T. (1985) Frequency characteristics of the middle ear. *Journal of the Acoustical Society of America,* **77,** 159–164

KUIJPERS, W. and BONTING, S. L. (1969) Studies on the (Na^+-K^+)-activated ATPase. XXIV. Localization and properties of ATPase in the inner ear of the guinea pig. *Biochimica et Biophysica Acta,* **173,** 477–485

KUIJPERS, W. and BONTING, S. L. (1970) The cochlear potentials. I. The effect of ouabain on the cochlear potentials of the guinea pig. *Pflügers Archiv European Journal of Physiology,* **320,** 348–358

LIBERMAN, M. C. and KIANG, N. Y. S. (1978) Acoustic trauma in cats. *Acta Oto-Laryngologica Supplementum, 358,* 1–63

LYNCH, T. J., NEDZELNITSKY, V. and PEAKE, W. T. (1982) Input impedance of the cochlea in cat. *Journal of the Acoustical Society of America,* **72,** 108–130

MAKIMOTO, K. and SILVERSTEIN, H. (1974) Sodium and

potassium concentrations in the endolymph and perilymph of the cat. *Annals of Otology, Rhinology, and Laryngology*, **83**, 174–179

MAKIMOTO, K., TAKEDA, T. and SILVERSTEIN, H. (1980) Species differences in inner ear fluids. *Archives of Oto-Rhino-Laryngology*, **228**, 187–194

MANLEY, G. A. and KRONESTER-FREI, A. (1980) The electrophysiological profile of the organ of Corti. In *Psychophysical, Physiological and Behavioural Studies in Hearing*, edited by G. van den Brink and F. A. Bilsen, pp. 24–31. Delft: Delft University Press

METZ, O. (1951) Studies on the contraction of the tympanic muscles as indicated by changes in the impedance of the ear. *Acta Oto-Laryngologica*, **39**, 397–405

MØLLER, A. R. (1964) Effect of tympanic muscle activity on movement of the eardrum, acoustic impedance, and cochlear microphonics. *Acta Oto-Laryngologica*, **58**, 525–534

MØLLER, A. R. (1974) The acoustic middle ear muscle reflex. In *Handbook of Sensory Physiology Vol. 5/1*, edited by W. D. Keidel and W. D. Neff, pp. 519–548. Berlin: Springer

MORGENSTERN, C., AMANO, H. and ORSULAKOVA, A. (1982) Ion transport in the endolymphatic space. *American Journal of Otolaryngology*, **3**, 323–327

MOUNTAIN, D. C. (1980) Changes in endolymphatic potential and crossed olivocochlear bundle stimulation alter cochlear mechanics. *Science*, **210**, 71–72

NEDZELNITSKY, V. (1980) Sound pressures in the basal turn of the cat cochlea. *Journal of the Acoustical Society of America*, **68**, 1676–1689

PALMER, A. R. and RUSSELL, I. J. (1986) Phase-locking in the cochlear nerve of the guinea-pig and its relation to the receptor potential of inner hair-cells. *Hearing Research*, **24**, 1–15

PANG, X. D. and PEAKE, W. T. (1986) How do contractions of the stapedius muscle alter the acoustic properties of the ear? In *Peripheral Auditory Mechanisms*, edited by J. B. Allen, J. L. Hall, A. Hubbard, S. T. Neely and A. Tubis, pp. 36–43. Berlin: Springer

PAYNE, M. C. and GITHLER, F. J. (1951) Effects of perforations of the tympanic membrane on cochlear potentials. *Archives of Otolaryngology*, **54**, 666–674

PHILLIPS, D. P., CALFORD, M. B., PETTIGREW, J. D., AITKIN, L. M. and SEMPLE, M. N. (1982) Directionality of sound pressure transformation at the cat's pinna. *Hearing Research*, **8**, 13–28

PICKLES, J. O. (1982) *An Introduction to the Physiology of Hearing*. London: Academic Press

PICKLES, J. O. (1985a) Hearing and listening. In *Scientific Basis of Clinical Neurology*, edited by M. Swash and C. Kennard, pp. 188–200. Edinburgh: Churchill Livingstone

PICKLES, J. O. (1985b) Recent progress in cochlear physiology. *Progress in Neurobiology*, **24**, 1–42

PICKLES, J. O. (1986) The neurophysiological basis of frequency selectivity. In *Frequency Selectivity in Hearing*, edited by B. C. J. Moore, pp. 51–121. London: Academic Press

PICKLES, J. O., COMIS, S. D. and OSBORNE, M. P. (1984) Cross-links between stereocilia in the guinea pig organ of Corti, and their possible relation to sensory transduction. *Hearing Research*, **15**, 103–112

RAJAN, R. and JOHNSTONE, B. M. (1983) Crossed cochlear influences on monaural temporary threshold shifts. *Hearing Research*, **9**, 279–294

RAUCH, S. and KÖSTLIN, A. (1958) Aspects chimiques de l'endolymphe et de la périlymphe. *Practica Oto-Rhino-Laryngologica*, **20**, 287–291

RITTER, F. N. and LAWRENCE, M. (1965) A histological and experimental study of cochlear aqueduct patency in the adult human. *The Laryngoscope*, **75**, 1224–1233

ROBLES, L., RUGGERO, M. A. and RICH, N. C. (1986) Mössbauer measurements of the mechanical response to single-tone and two-tone stimuli at the base of the chinchilla cochlea. In *Peripheral Auditory Mechanisms*, edited by J. B. Allen, J. L. Hall, A. Hubbard, S. T. Neely and A. Tubis, pp. 121–128. Berlin: Springer

ROSOWSKI, J. J., CARNEY, L. H., LYNCH, T. J. and PEAKE, W. T. (1986) The effectiveness of external and middle ears in coupling acoustic power into the cochlea. In *Peripheral Auditory Mechanisms*, edited by J. B. Allen, J. L. Hall, A. Hubbard, S. T. Neely and A. Tubis, pp. 3–12. Berlin: Springer

RUSSELL, I. J. and SELLICK, P. M. (1978) Intracellular studies of hair cells in the mammalian cochlea. *Journal of Physiology*, **284**, 261–290

RUSSELL, I. J. and SELLICK, P. M. (1983) Low-frequency characteristics of intracellularly recorded receptor potentials in guinea-pig cochlear hair cells. *Journal of Physiology*, **338**, 179–206

RUSSELL, I. J., RICHARDSON, G. P. and CODY, A. R. (1986) Mechanosensitivity of mammalian auditory hair cells *in vitro*. *Nature*, **321**, 517–519

RYAN, A. F., WICKHAM, M. G. and BONE, R. C. (1980) Studies of ion distribution in the inner ear: scanning electron microscopy and x-ray microanalysis of freeze-dried cochlear specimens. *Hearing Research*, **2**, 1–20

SCHIEBE, F. and HAUPT, H. (1985) Biochemical differences between perilymph, cerebrospinal fluid and blood plasma in the guinea pig. *Hearing Research*, **17**, 61–66

SCHNEIDER, E. A. (1974) A contribution to the physiology of the perilymph. Part 1: the origins of the perilymph. *Annals of Otology, Rhinology, and Laryngology*, **83**, 76–83

SELLICK, P. M. and JOHNSTONE, B. M. (1972) Changes in cochlear endolymph Na^+ concentration measured with Na^+ specific microelectrodes. *Pflügers Archiv European Journal of Pathology*, **336**, 11–20

SELLICK, P. M. and RUSSELL, I. J. (1979) Two-tone suppression in cochlear hair cells. *Hearing Research*, **1**, 227–236

SELLICK, P. M., PATUZZI, R. and JOHNSTONE, B. M. (1982) Measurement of basilar membrane motion in the guinea pig using the Mössbauer technique. *Journal of the Acoustical Society of America*, **72**, 131–141

SHAW, E. A. G. (1974) The external ear. In *Handbook of Sensory Physiology Vol. 5/1*, edited by W. D. Keidel and W. D. Neff, pp. 455–490. Berlin: Springer

SHAW, E. A. G. and STINSON, M. R. (1983) The human external and middle ear: models and concepts. In *Mechanics of Hearing*, edited by E. de Boer and M. A. Viergever, pp. 3–18. The Hague: Martinus Nijhoff

SILMAN, S. (1984) *The Acoustic Reflex*. Orlando: Academic Press

SILVERSTEIN, H. (1972) A rapid protein test for inner ear fluid analysis. *Transactions of the American Academy for Ophthalmology and Otolaryngology*, **76**, 1030–1031

SILVERSTEIN, H., TAKEDA, T. and COX, M. (1974) Biochemistry of the inner ear following endolymph sac obstruction. *Bárány Society Proceedings* [*see* Anniko and Wroblewski (1986)]

SIMMONS, F. B. (1964) Perceptual theories of middle ear muscle function. *Annals of Otology, Rhinology and Laryngology,* **73,** 724–740

SMITH, C. A. (1978) Structure of the cochlear duct. In *Evoked Electrical Activity in the Auditory Nervous System,* edited by R. F. Naunton and C. Fernandez, pp. 3–19. New York: Academic Press

SMITH, C. A., LOWRY, O. H. and WU, M. L. (1954) The electrolytes of the labyrinthine fluids. *The Laryngoscope,* **64,** 141–153

SPOENDLIN, H. (1972) Innervation densities of the cochlea. *Acta Oto-Laryngologica,* **73,** 235–248

STERKERS, O., SAUMON, G., TRAN BA HUY, P. and AMIEL, C. (1982) Evidence for a perilymphatic origin of the endolymph. Application to the pathophysiology of Ménières disease. *American Journal of Otolaryngology,* **3,** 367–375

TASAKI, I., DAVIS, H. and ELDREDGE, D. H. (1954) Exploration of cochlear potentials in guinea pig with a microelectrode. *Journal of the Acoustical Society of America,* **26,** 765–773

TONNDORF, J. (1966) Bone conduction: studies in experimental animals. *Acta Oto-Laryngologica Supplementum,* 213, 1–132

TONNDORF, J. (1976) Bone conduction. In *Handbook of Sensory Physiology Vol. 5/3,* edited by W. D. Keidel and W. D. Neff, pp. 37–84. Berlin: Springer

VON BÉKÉSY, G. (1941) Über die Messung der Schwingungsamplitude der Gehörknöchelchen mittels einer kapazitiven Sonde. *Akustische Zeitschrift,* **6,** 1–16

VON BÉKÉSY, G. (1943) Über die Resonanzkurve und die Abklingzeit der verschiedenen Stellen der Schneckentrennwand. *Akustische Zeitschrift,* **8,** 66–76

VON BÉKÉSY, G. (1952) Resting potentials inside the cochlear partition of the guinea pig. *Nature,* **169,** 241–242

VON BÉKÉSY, G. (1960) *Experiments in Hearing,* edited by E. G. Wever. New York: McGraw Hill

WEVER, E. G. and LAWRENCE, M. (1954) *Physiological Acoustics.* Princeton: Princeton University Press

WIEDERHOLD, M. L. (1970) Variations in the effects of electric stimulation of the crossed olivocochlear bundle on cat single auditory nerve fiber responses to tone bursts. *Journal of the Acoustical Society of America,* **48,** 966–977

WILSON, J. P. (1980) Evidence for a cochlear origin for acoustic re-emissions, threshold fine structure and tonal tinnitus. *Hearing Research,* **2,** 233–252

ZAKRISSON, J. E. and BORG, E. (1974) Stapedius reflex and auditory fatigue. *Audiology,* **13,** 231–235

3

The perception of sound

Brian C. J. Moore

The commonest way of assessing hearing in the clinic is to measure the lowest intensity at which pure tones (sinusoids) can be detected, as a function of the frequency of the tones, giving what is called the pure-tone audiogram. The measurement is obtained separately for each ear using headphones. However, in everyday life we are rarely required to listen to pure tones at very low intensities through one ear only. Rather, the function of the auditory system is to analyse and discriminate sounds which typically contain many sinusoidal components, whose intensity may vary over a very wide range, and which may come from many different directions in space, creating complex time varying patterns of sound pressure which differ at the two ears. Thus the pure-tone audiogram tells us very little about how the auditory system normally functions.

This chapter is concerned primarily with how we perceive and discriminate sounds at intensities typical of those encountered in everyday life. A theme running through the whole chapter is the concept that the auditory system acts as a frequency analyser. When we listen to a complex sound containing a number of sinusoidal components, we are, to some extent, able to hear those components as separate tones. Thus when we strike two tuning forks simultaneously, we hear two different pitches. The action of the auditory system as a frequency analyser plays a role in many aspects of auditory perception, including the masking of one sound by another, the perception of loudness, the perception of pitch, and the perception of timbre.

The final part of the chapter is concerned with the perception of sound in the hearing impaired. It is shown that hearing impairment results not only

in an inability to detect faint sounds, but also in a loss of the ability to discriminate sounds which are well above the threshold for detection.

The action of the ear as a frequency analyser

Unlike the sinusoidal tones which are often used in the assessment of hearing, sounds encountered in everyday life are generally complex, containing a number of different sinusoidal frequency components. It is a central characteristic of the auditory system that it acts as a limited-resolution Fourier analyser; complex sounds are broken down into their sinusoidal frequency components. The initial basis of this frequency analysis almost certainly depends upon the tuning which is observed in the cochlea (*see* Chapter 2 for details). Indeed, it is possible that the tuning observed in the cochlea is sufficient to account for the analysing capacity of the entire auditory system (Moore, 1986; Pickles, 1986). It is largely as a consequence of this frequency analysis that we are able to hear one sound in the presence of another with a different frequency. This ability is known as *frequency selectivity* or *frequency resolution*.

The frequency analysis which takes place in the ear has consequences for many aspects of auditory perception, including the audibility of individual components in complex tones; the masking of one sound by another; musical consonance and dissonance; the perception of timbre (sound quality); and the perception of pitch. Hence, this chapter begins with a review of some of the ways in which the frequency selectivity of the ear has been measured.

Measurement of the frequency analysing capacity of the ear

Audibility of partials in complex sounds

When we are presented with a single sinusoid of a certain frequency, we perceive a single tone with a 'pure' sound. The pitch of the tone is related to its frequency, and the loudness mainly to its intensity. If we are presented with two sinusoids simultaneously, then what we perceive will depend upon their frequency separation. If the two components are widely spaced in frequency, for example 100 Hz and 10 000 Hz, we will perceive separate tones; thus the ear behaves as a frequency analyser, splitting the complex sound into its component sinusoids. If, on the other hand, the components are closely spaced in frequency, for example 1000 and 1030 Hz, then we will perceive a single sound corresponding to the mixture of the two. In this case, the ear's frequency resolution is insufficient to separate the components. Thus the limits of our ability to 'hear out' the components in a complex sound reflect the analysing capacity of the auditory system.

We can observe a continuum of effects as the frequency separation between two sinusoids is slowly increased from a very small value. When the two sinusoids are separated by a few hertz, they sound like a single tone fluctuating in loudness. The fluctuations, known as 'beats', have a physical basis, for the reason that the two sinusoids move alternately in and out of phase, producing first reinforcement and then cancellation. The number of beats per second is equal to the frequency separation between the two sinusoids; therefore, as the latter's frequency separation increases, the beats are perceived to occur more rapidly. For separations exceeding 20 Hz, we no longer perceive the amplitude fluctuations as such, but rather hear a harsh unpleasant sound, with a quality sometimes called 'roughness'. As the separation increases still further the roughness at first increases, and then decreases, and finally we start to hear two separate tones, each of which has a 'smooth' quality.

The minimum frequency separation at which the two tones can be heard separately varies depending on their mean frequency. At 500 Hz it is about 35 Hz, while at 5000 Hz it is about 700 Hz (Plomp, 1964a). This gives us a first indication of the characteristics of the ear's filtering mechanism; its resolution is not constant as a function of centre frequency, but decreases with increasing centre frequency.

When we listen to a complex tone containing many components, we are generally able to 'hear out' some of the individual frequency components or partials. Normally we do not listen in this way. For example, the complex tones produced by musical instruments or the human voice are usually heard as having a single pitch (*see below*). However, it is *possible* to 'hear out' individual partials provided that our attention is directed in an appropriate way, for example, by presenting a comparison sinusoidal tone whose frequency coincides with that of one of the partials.

For multi-tone complexes, it is generally slightly more difficult to hear the individual components than when only two are present; particularly for frequencies below 100 Hz, the frequency separation between adjacent components required to 'hear out' the components is greater than that required for a two-tone complex (Plomp, 1964a; Moore, 1973a). *Figure 3.1*, taken from Plomp (1976), summarizes results from Plomp (1964a), Plomp and Mimpen (1968) and Soderquist (1970). The figure shows the frequency separation between adjacent partials required for a given partial to be 'heard out' from a complex tone with either two equal-amplitude components (solid circles) or many equal-amplitude components (open symbols and crosses). In the latter case, for a centre frequency of 500 Hz the necessary separation is about 80 Hz, increasing to about 800 Hz at 5000 Hz.

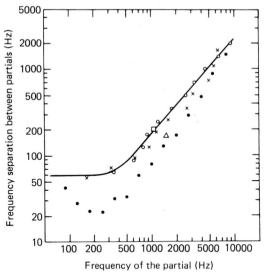

Figure 3.1 The frequency separation between adjacent partials required for a given partial to be 'heard out' from complex tones of various types plotted as a function of the frequency of the partial. The complexes were: a multicomponent harmonic complex (open circles fitted with the curve); a multicomponent inharmonic complex (crosses); and a two-tone complex (solid circles). The data are from Plomp (1964a) and Plomp and Mimpen (1968). The open square and triangle show results of Soderquist (1970) for inharmonic tone complexes for non-musicians and musicians, respectively. (From Plomp, 1976, *Aspects of Tone Sensation*, Academic Press, by courtesy of the author and publisher)

The difference between the results for two-tone and multi-tone complexes has been explained in terms of the use of information contained in the detailed timing of the firing patterns of neurons in the auditory nerve ('phase locking'; *see* Moore, 1982, and Chapter 2). When a two-tone complex is used, neurons with characteristic frequencies below the frequency of the lower partial, will phase lock primarily to that partial. Similarly, neurons with characteristic frequencies above the frequency of the upper partial will phase lock primarily to that partial. These patterns of phase locking might be used to extract the pitches of the individual partials (Moore, 1982; *see* also the discussion of pitch perception later in this chapter). When a partial is contained *within* a multi-tone complex, the patterns of phase locking in neurons with characteristic frequencies both above and below the frequency of the partial will be disrupted by the adjacent partials. Thus the partials have to be separated by a greater amount before the partial can be 'heard out'. It will be noticed that the results for the two-tone complex and the multi-tone complexes converge at about 5000 Hz. This is the highest frequency for which phase locking has been observed in the auditory nerve of mammals (*see* Chapter 2).

The results of Soderquist (1970), shown in *Figure 3.1*, indicate that the frequency separation of the partials required to 'hear out' a given partial in a complex tone is, on average, smaller for musicians than for non-musicians. It seems unlikely that there is any difference in the structure or function of the cochlea between musicians and non-musicians, which leads to the conclusion that factors other than peripheral filtering enter into this task.

Periodic complex tones, such as those produced by many musical instruments or the human voice (when the vocal cords are vibrating (*see* Chapter 14), consist of a fundamental component, whose frequency equals the repetition rate of the sound, and a series of harmonics, whose frequencies are integral multiples of the fundamental frequency. Hence, the harmonics are equally spaced on a linear frequency scale (*see* Chapter 2). The results shown in *Figure 3.1* indicate that, for a harmonic complex, the lower harmonics will be more easily 'heard out' or resolved than the higher harmonics. In fact, for a complex with equal-amplitude components, only about the first five to eight harmonics will be resolvable. It will be seen later that this plays an important role in modern theories of pitch perception for complex tones.

Masking and the critical band

We are all familiar with the fact that sounds we wish to hear are sometimes rendered inaudible by other sounds, a process known as 'masking'. The amount of masking is commonly defined as the number of decibels by which the threshold for the signal is raised above the absolute threshold (*see below* for a definition of absolute threshold). One conception of auditory masking, which has had both theoretical and practical success, assumes that the auditory system contains a bank of bandpass-filters, with continuously overlapping centre frequencies (Fletcher, 1940). In the simple case of a sinusoidal signal presented in a background noise, it is assumed that the observer will 'listen' to the filter whose output has the highest signal-to-masker ratio. The signal will be detected if that ratio exceeds a certain value. In most practical situations, the filter involved will have a centre frequency close to that of the signal.

A good deal of work has been directed towards determining the characteristics of the 'auditory filter'. Fletcher (1940) was one of the first people to apply the auditory-filter concept to the masking of sinusoidal tones by broad-band noise. He assumed that, to predict threshold, it would be reasonable to approximate the auditory filter as a simple rectangle, with a flat top and vertical edges. Thus all frequency components falling within the flat top or passband would be passed equally, whereas components outside the passband would be rejected. He called the width of this passband the *critical bandwidth* (CB). If the masker is a white noise, with a flat spectrum (equal amount of power per unit bandwidth), then the amount of noise passing through the auditory filter will be the product of the power per unit bandwidth (No) and the critical bandwidth. Therefore, if the power of the signal at threshold is P, then

$$P = K(CB)No \qquad (1)$$

where K is a constant of proportionality related to the efficiency of the detector mechanism following the auditory filter. Rearranging this formula, we get

$$CB = P/(K No) \qquad (2)$$

Fletcher pointed out that if K were independent of frequency, it would be possible to determine how the value of the critical bandwidth varied with frequency, by measuring the threshold of a sinusoidal signal as a function of frequency in a noise with a flat spectrum. However, recent measurements have suggested that K is not independent of frequency (Patterson *et al.*, 1982). Therefore, the measurement of tone thresholds in white noise does not give a reliable way of estimating the value of the critical bandwidth. The ratio P/No is often called the *critical ratio*. The term 'critical bandwidth' is reserved for more direct measures of the auditory filter bandwidth, such as those described below.

Although the approximation of the auditory filter as a simple rectangle works quite well for signals in broad-band noise, it does not work well for maskers which contain only a narrow range of frequencies. An example, taken from the results of Egan and Hake (1950), is given in *Figure 3.2*. The

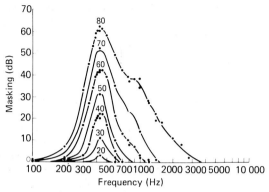

Figure 3.2 Masked audiograms for a narrow band noise masker centred at 410 Hz. Each curve shows the elevation in threshold of the sinusoidal signal as a function of frequency for a particular level of the masking noise. Masking stimulus: 90 Hz band of noise; parameter: overall sound pressure level. (From Moore, 1982. Original data from Egan and Hake, 1950; by courtesy of the publisher)

masker in this case was a narrow band of noise with a centre frequency of 410 Hz and a bandwidth of 90 Hz. The masker was set at a number of different overall levels, as indicated in the figure, and for each level the threshold of a sinusoidal signal was determined as a function of signal frequency. The masked audiograms obtained in this way have rounded tops and sloping edges, a fact which clearly indicates that the auditory filter is not a simple rectangle. It will be seen from *Figure 3.2* that at higher masker levels the slope of the masked audiogram tends to decrease on the high-frequency side. This means that at high sound levels, low frequencies become relatively more effective at masking high frequencies. This phenomenon is called the *upward spread of masking*. The masked audiograms obtained using sinusoidal maskers are basically similar to those shown in *Figure 3.2*, but the results are complicated by the occurrence of beats when the signal and masker are close in frequency (*see* the section on audibility of partials in complex sounds). The listener may not always detect the signal as such, but may detect the beats. The result is a local minimum in the masked audiogram when the signal frequency is close to that of the masker. This problem is avoided with narrow-band noise maskers, as such maskers have inherent amplitude fluctuations which preclude the use of beats as a cue.

Although masked audiograms of the type described above can give a rough idea of the shape of the auditory filter, they cannot be used to give a direct estimate of this shape. In principle, there is a different auditory filter for each centre frequency considered, and the shape may change with centre frequency. As the signal frequency changes, the auditory filter used to detect it will change. One method of reducing this problem is analogous to that used by neurophysiologists in determining a neural tuning curve (*see* Chapter 2). The resulting curves are often called psychophysical tuning curves. The signal used is a sinusoid which is presented at a very low level, for example 10 dB above the absolute threshold. It is assumed that this will excite only a small number of nerve fibres with characteristic frequencies close to that of the signal. Therefore, *to a first approximation*, only one auditory filter will be involved in detecting the signal. The masker is either a sinusoid or a narrow band of noise.

To determine a psychophysical tuning curve, the signal is fixed in frequency and level, and the level of the masker required to mask the signal is determined for various centre frequencies of the masker. If it is assumed that the signal will be masked when the masker produces a fixed amount of activity in the neurons which would otherwise respond to the signal, then the curve

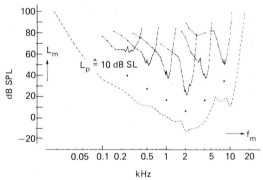

Figure 3.3 Psychophysical tuning curves (PTCs) determined in simultaneous masking using sinusoidal signals 10 dB above absolute threshold (called 10 dB sensation level). For each curve the solid diamond below it indicates the frequency and level of the signal. The masker was a sinusoid which had a fixed starting phase relationship to the 50-ms signal. The masker level required for threshold is plotted a a function of masker frequency. As the signal was brief, beats were not audible, but fluctuations in the waveform resulting from the interference of the signal and masker are probably responsible for the slight irregularities around the tips of the psychophysical tuning curves. The dashed line shows the absolute threshold for the signal. (From Vogten, 1974, in *Facts and Models in Hearing*, edited by E. Zwicker and E. Terhardt. Springer-Verlag, by courtesy of the author)

mapped out in this way is analogous to the neural tuning curve (Zwicker, 1974). Some examples are given in *Figure 3.3*. Returning to the concept of the auditory filter, the psychophysical tuning curve can be considered as representing the masker level required to produce a fixed output from the filter centred at the signal frequency. Normally, a filter characteristic is determined by plotting the output as a function of frequency for an input fixed in level. However, if the filter is linear the two methods are equivalent. Thus the filter characteristic can be obtained simply by turning the tuning curve upside-down.

The shapes of psychophysical tuning curves determined in humans are quite similar to neural tuning curves determined in the auditory nerve of other mammals, and this encourages the belief that the basic frequency selectivity of the auditory system is established at the level of the auditory nerve. However, it is important to remember that the assumptions which have been made in interpreting the psychophysical tuning curves may not be quite correct. For example, the detection of the signal will inevitably involve activity over an array of neurons, with a range of characteristic frequencies. It might be the case that, as the frequency of the masker changes, the neurons which are most effective in indicating the presence of the signal will change. An alternative way of expressing this idea is to say that the centre frequency of the filter used to detect the signal may change as the frequency of the masker is altered. When the signal is detected through a filter which is not centred at the signal frequency, this is called *off-frequency listening*.

Patterson (1976) has described an ingenious method of determining auditory filter shape which effectively prevents off-frequency listening. The method is illustrated in *Figure 3.4*. The signal is fixed in frequency, and the masker is a noise with a bandstop or notch centred at the signal

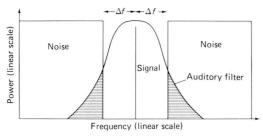

Figure 3.4 Schematic illustration of the method used by Patterson (1976) to determine auditory filter shape. The threshold of the sinusoidal signal is measured as a function of the width of a spectral notch in the noise masker. The amount of noise passing through the auditory filter centred at the signal frequency is proportional to the shaded areas. (From Moore, 1982, by courtesy of the publisher)

frequency. The deviation of each edge of the notch from the signal frequency is denoted by Δf. The threshold of the signal is determined as a function of notch width. Usually the notch is symmetrically placed around the signal frequency and the analysis assumes that the auditory filter is symmetric on a linear frequency scale. This assumption appears not unreasonable, at least for the top part of the filter and at moderate sound levels (Patterson and Nimmo-Smith, 1980). For a signal symmetrically placed in a notched noise, the highest signal-to-masker ratio at the output of the auditory filter will be achieved with a filter centred at the signal frequency, as shown in *Figure 3.4*. Shifting the filter upwards, for example, will reduce the amount of noise passing through the filter from the lower band, but this will be more than offset by the increase in noise from the upper band. Therefore, it seems reasonable to assume that for this task the subject uses only the filter centred at the signal frequency.

As the width of the spectral notch is increased, less and less noise will pass through the auditory filter; thus, the threshold of the signal will drop. The amount of noise passing through the auditory filter will be proportional to the area under the filter in the frequency range covered by the noise. This is shown as the shaded areas in *Figure 3.4*. Given the assumption that threshold corresponds to a constant signal-to-masker ratio at the output of the auditory filter, then the change in threshold with notch width indicates how the area under the filter varies with Δf. The area under a function between certain limits is obtained by integrating the value of the function over those limits. Hence, by differentiating the function relating threshold to Δf, the shape of the filter is obtained. In other words, the attenuation of the filter at given deviation, Δf, from the centre frequency is proportional to the slope of the function relating signal threshold to notch width at that value of Δf.

A typical set of results for such an experiment is shown in the left-hand panel of *Figure 3.5*, for three different signal frequencies. The notch width is plotted as a proportion of centre frequency, fc, so that the general form of the results is similar for all three frequencies; in the range $0.05 < \Delta f/fc < 0.3$ the data form a roughly straight line on these logarithmic-power against linear-frequency co-ordinates, but the curves tend to flatten at very narrow and very wide notch widths. Patterson and Nimmo-Smith (1980) pointed out that this form of threshold function implied that the auditory filter shape was like a pair of back-to-back exponential functions, but with a rounded rather than a sharp top, and with shallow skirts beyond $\Delta f/fc = 0.4$. They called this form of filter shape a rounded exponential. Although the auditory filter shapes can be estimated from the slopes of the

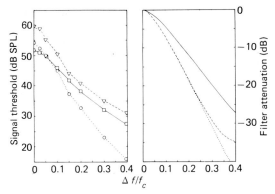

Figure 3.5 The left-hand panel shows the threshold of a sinusoidal signal plotted as a function of the relative width of a spectral notch in a noise masker ($\Delta f/fc$). The notch was always centred at the signal frequency which was either 0.4 (□), 1.0 (○) or 6.5 (▽) kHz. The right-hand panel shows the shapes of the auditory filters derived from the data on the left: 0.4 (–), 1.0 (· · · ·), 6.5 (--). (From Shailer and Moore, 1983, by courtesy of the publisher)

functions in the left panel of *Figure 3.5*, a better method is to assume a general form for the auditory filter – a rounded exponential – with a small number of free parameters. The assumed filter can then be used to predict the threshold data, and the parameters varied to find the values giving the smallest mean-squared deviation between the obtained and predicted thresholds. This procedure gives relatively robust estimates of auditory filter shape when the data are subject to errors, as is inevitably the case in psychophysical experiments.

Patterson *et al.* (1982) suggested that a good approximation to the auditory filter shape was given by the expression:

$$W(g) = (1 - r)(1 + pg)\exp(-pg) + r, \qquad (3)$$

where g is the normalized frequency deviation from the centre of the filter; $g = (f - fc)/fc$ where f is the frequency. The parameter p determines the sharpness of the passband of the auditory filter, and the parameter r approximates the shallower tail of the auditory filter. Details of how to use this expression to derive filter shapes from notched-noise data are given in Patterson *et al.* (1982). The filter shapes in the right-hand panel of *Figure 3.5* were derived in this way. Only half of each filter is shown as the filters are assumed to be symmetric on a linear frequency scale. For the values of r which are typically found, the equivalent rectangular bandwidth (ERB) of the auditory filter is equal to $4fc/p$. (The equivalent rectangular bandwidth is a measure of the 'effective' bandwidth of a filter. It is the bandwidth of an ideal rectangular filter which has the same peak transmission as the filter being studied, and which passes the same power of white noise. For the auditory filter, the equivalent rectangular bandwidth is about 10% greater than the 3-dB bandwidth.) The equivalent rectangular bandwidth of the auditory filter may be considered as a measure of the critical bandwidth.

Auditory filter shapes derived using notched-noise maskers have equivalent rectangular bandwidths which increase with increasing centre frequency. However, when expressed as a proportion of centre frequency, the bandwidth tends to be at its narrowest at middle to high frequencies. Over the range 100–6500 Hz, and at moderate sound levels, the equivalent rectangular bandwidth is well approximated by:

$$ERB = 6.23F^2 + 93.39F + 28.52 \qquad (4)$$

where F is frequency in kHz (Moore and Glasberg, 1983a). This expression is shown in *Figure 3.6*, together with estimates of equivalent rectangular bandwidth from several different experiments.

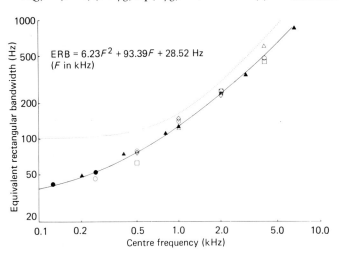

Figure 3.6 Estimates of the auditory filter bandwidth from a variety of experiments, plotted as a function of centre frequency. The solid line is a quadratic function, shown in the figure, which gives a good fit to the data. The dotted line shows the traditional critical bandwidth function. ● Fidell *et al.*, 1983; ▲ Shailer and Moore, 1983; ○ Houtgast, 1977; ◇ Patterson, 1976; □ Patterson *et al.*, 1982; △ Weber, 1977. (From Moore and Glasberg, 1983a)

The figure also shows the traditional 'critical bandwidth' function, as suggested by Zwicker and Terhardt (1980). It can be seen that the traditional critical bandwidth function flattens off below 500 Hz, whereas the estimates of auditory filter bandwidth continue to decrease. In fact, there have been a few estimates of critical bandwidth below 500 Hz, and some of the older measures do show a continuing decrease below 500 Hz (Zwicker, Flottorp and Stevens, 1957; Greenwood, 1961). Indirect estimates based on the critical ratio, which actually show an increase at very low frequencies, are almost certainly in error, as the efficiency of the detector mechanism following the auditory filter (given by the parameter K in equations **1** and **2**) appears to change with centre frequency (Patterson *et al.*, 1982).

The results given so far apply at moderate sound levels (noise spectrum levels up to 40 dB). There is now considerable evidence that the shape of the auditory filter changes somewhat with level, and that at high levels it can be markedly asymmetric. The asymmetry of the auditory filter can be investigated by using notched noise, with the notch placed both symmetrically and asymmetrically about the signal frequency. The auditory filter shape can be derived on the assumption that the subject always uses the filter giving the highest signal-to-masker ratio (Patterson and Nimmo-Smith, 1980). The results of such experiments indicate that the low-frequency side of the auditory filter becomes shallower with increasing level, whereas the high-frequency side may become slightly steeper (Patterson and Nimmo-Smith, 1980; Glasberg *et al.*, 1984; Lutfi and

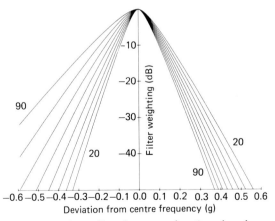

Figure 3.7 Auditory filter shapes as a function of masker level (20–90 dB sound pressure level) for a centre frequency of 1 kHz. The filter shapes are plotted as a function of the deviation from the centre frequency divided by the centre frequency. With increasing sound level the upper branch of the filter becomes slightly steeper and the lower branch becomes considerably less steep. (From Moore, 1987, by courtesy of the publisher)

Patterson, 1984; Moore, 1987). Thus the filter becomes increasingly asymmetric at high levels, and its equivalent rectangular bandwidth tends to increase (Weber, 1977). *Figure 3.7* shows auditory filter shapes as a function of level for a centre frequency of 1 kHz. The shapes were obtained by combining the data from a number of experiments, interpolating where necessary. The decrease in slope with increasing level of the low-frequency side of the auditory filter corresponds to the classical 'upward spread of masking'; at high levels, maskers well below the signal in frequency can have a pronounced masking effect (*see Figure 3.2*).

The excitation pattern

Measures of the auditory filter shape all use a fixed signal frequency, and they attempt to characterize frequency selectivity at that frequency. An alternative approach is to characterize the distribution of excitation across frequencies (or places within the cochlea) for a given masker: this distribution has been referred to as the excitation pattern of the masker. In terms of the filter bank analogy, the excitation pattern can be considered as the output of the auditory filters as a function of filter centre frequency. Many workers have attempted to derive the excitation pattern of a masker by measuring signal threshold as a function of signal frequency, on the assumption that the signal threshold is directly proportional to the masker excitation at the signal frequency/place (for example Zwicker and Feldtkeller, 1967). Thus the masked audiograms shown in *Figure 3.2* might be considered as giving a crude measure of the excitation pattern of the masker at each masker level. However, off-frequency listening and the detection of beats can markedly influence the form of the results.

It is instructive to consider in more detail the relationship that exists between filter shapes and excitation patterns. In order to do this, a simplified equation for the auditory filter shape will be used:

$$W(g) = (1 + pg)\exp(-pg) \qquad (5)$$

This simplified equation gives a good description of the main passband of the auditory filter. The equivalent rectangular bandwidth of the auditory filter will be assumed to vary with centre frequency according to equation **4**. The value of p at a given centre frequency can be derived from equation **4** by recalling that ERB = $4fc/p$. It is then a simple matter to calculate the filter output as a function of filter centre frequency for any given input stimulus. *Figure 3.8* illustrates this graphically for a 1-kHz sinusoid.

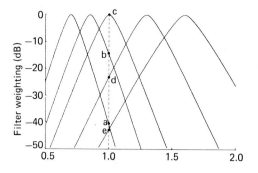

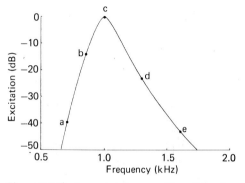

Figure 3.8 The top panel shows auditory filter shapes at several centre frequencies. The dotted line shows a 1-kHz sinusoidal tone which is applied to the filters. The bottom panel shows the output of the auditory filters as a function of filter centre frequency. This is the excitation pattern of the 1-kHz tone. (From Moore and Glasberg, 1983a, by courtesy of the publisher)

At the top of the figure are shown auditory filter shapes at several centre frequencies, with the form given by equation 5. The filters are assumed symmetric on the linear frequency scale, and the filter bandwidths increase with centre frequency in accordance with equation 4. For the filter with the lowest centre frequency shown, the relative output of the filter in response to the 1-kHz tone is about −40 dB, indicated by the point **a**. In the lower half of the figure this gives rise to point **a** on the excitation pattern; the point has an ordinate of −40 dB, and it is positioned on the abscissa at a frequency corresponding to the centre of the lowest filter illustrated. The relative outputs of the other filters shown are indicated, in order of increasing centre frequency, by the points **b** to **e**. These each give corresponding points on the excitation pattern. The entire excitation pattern was derived by calculating the filter output for filter centre frequencies spaced at 10-Hz intervals. Note that the derived excitation pattern is asymmetric; it has the same general form as the masked audiogram for a narrow-band noise maker (*see Figure 3.2*). This illustrates that the asymmetry

seen in masked audiograms is not incompatible with the idea that the auditory filter is roughly symmetric at moderate sound levels.

Non-simultaneous masking and suppression

It is now widely accepted that the normal peripheral auditory system is characterized by significant non-linearity. One manifestation of this non-linearity is' suppression, which may be crudely characterized as follows: strong excitation at one frequency/place will suppress weaker excitation at adjacent frequency/places. This results in the phenomenon of two-tone suppression (Sachs and Kiang, 1968; *see* Chapter 2). More generally, it will produce an enhancement in the sharpness of the excitation pattern produced by the initial filtering process; differences in level between peaks and dips in the excitation pattern will be increased by suppression, giving a greater 'contrast' in the pattern. Suppressive interactions between the different frequency components in a complex sound occur only when those components are presented simultaneously. The suppression produced by adding an extra component to a sound begins almost instantaneously, and also ceases very rapidly when the component is removed.

Although suppression is well established physiologically, it is only relatively recently that psychophysical evidence for suppression has been obtained. Suppression does not usually produce measurable effects in simultaneous masking. Houtgast (1972, 1974) has suggested that this is because suppression at a particular frequency/place does not change the signal-to-masker ratio at that place. Threshold in simultaneous masking appears to depend primarily on that ratio, as we have seen already, and so suppression has no effect on threshold. Houtgast presented evidence that non-simultaneous techniques, where the signal is presented out-of-time with the masker, could be used to demonstrate the effects of suppression. The signal can be viewed as a kind of 'probe' for estimating the excitation evoked by the masker in the frequency region of the signal. The signal itself will not be suppressed by the masker, as it is not presented simultaneously with the masker. However, if suppression alters the excitation evoked by the masker in the frequency region of the signal, then this will be revealed as a change in the threshold of the signal.

Two techniques have been widely used to study the influence of suppression, but both have drawbacks. Houtgast (1974) has made extensive use of the pulsation threshold technique, in which the signal and masker are alternated. When the signal is at a sufficiently low level, it may sound continuous even though it is actually being pulsed on and off. The subject is required to adjust the signal (usually its level) until it is on the borderline between sounding pulsatory and sounding continuous. Houtgast suggested that at the pulsation threshold, the excitation evoked by the signal was almost equal to the excitation evoked by the masker at the frequency/place of the signal. If this were correct, the pulsation threshold of the signal could be used to estimate the masker-evoked excitation, and to measure the effects of suppression. Unfortunately, it is not known whether Houtgast's suggestion is correct, and there is considerable uncertainty as to what criterion is actually adopted by the subject. The results are sometimes highly variable, and the method does not seem suitable for use with untrained subjects.

The other method which has been widely used to study suppression is forward masking. The

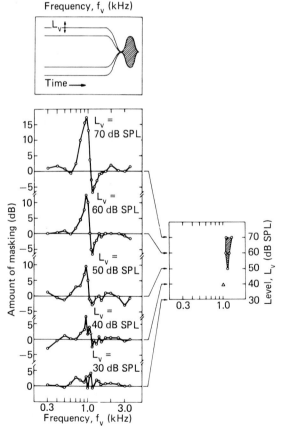

Figure 3.9 Results of an experiment demonstrating 'unmasking' in forward masking. The unmasking has been interpreted in terms of suppression. *See* text for details. (From Shannon, 1976, *Journal of the Acoustical Society of America*, **59**, 1460–1470, by courtesy of the author and publisher)

signal is presented just after the end of the masker. It is assumed that the threshold of the signal is determined by the amount of adaptation produced by the masker in the neurons tuned around the signal frequency. If the effective level of the masker is altered by suppression, that should change the amount of adaptation produced by the masker, which in turn should lead to a change in masked threshold.

An example of results obtained with this technique is given in *Figure 3.9*, taken from Shannon (1976). The time pattern of the masker and signal is shown at the top. The masker always contained a 1-kHz tone at 40 dB sound pressure level. The amount of masking produced by the 1-kHz tone is taken as a reference, and is called 0 dB in the five panels to the left of the figure. The effect of adding a second sinusoidal component to the masker is shown in the five panels by the points plotted as open circles. The frequency, f_V, of this extra component varied from 0.3 to 3.5 kHz, and its level, L_V, varied from 30 dB sound pressure level (bottom panel) to 70 dB sound pressure level (top panel). When f_V was very close to 1 kHz, the second component increased the amount of forward masking, as would be expected. However, when f_V was just above 1 kHz, the second component *reduced* the amount of forward masking, an effect called 'unmasking'. This effect has been attributed to suppression. It is assumed that the second component suppresses the response to the 1-kHz component when f_V is just above 1 kHz, which reduces the amount of forward masking produced by that component. The suppression increases as L_V is increased. The panel on the right shows values of f_V and L_V, for which more than 3 dB of unmasking was observed. The shaded area bounded by these values resembles the upper of the two-tone suppression areas observed neurophysiologically (*see* Chapter 2).

Forward masking, in the same way as the pulsation threshold, is not without problems of interpretation. It has been suggested that the unmasking produced by adding an extra component to a masker may be the result of changes in the cues available to the subjects, rather than being a result of the physiological process of suppression. Many demonstrations of unmasking seem to be confounded in this way (Moore, 1980; *see* Moore and O'Loughlin, 1986, for a review). Moore and O'Loughlin have suggested that this problem can be minimized by using sinusoidal signals and broad-band maskers (such as notched noise). The results which will be presented later in this chapter (in the section on frequency selectivity in impaired hearing) were obtained using such stimuli.

It is generally agreed that suppression can enhance contrast in the excitation pattern evoked by a given sound. While the effects of suppression can be revealed using either the pulsation threshold method or forward masking, the difficulties of interpretation discussed above make it difficult to quantify the size of the effect. Hence, the topic will not be pursued here. The interested reader is referred to Moore and Glasberg (1983b), Glasberg, Moore and Nimmo-Smith (1984) and Moore and O'Loughlin (1986).

Absolute thresholds and the perception of loudness

Absolute thresholds

The absolute threshold for a sound is defined as the minimum detectable level of the sound in the absence of any other sounds. The physical method of specifying the sound level is important, and two methods are in common use. In the first method, the sound pressure is measured at some point either close to or inside the entrance to the ear canal. This gives what is called the minimum audible pressure, and it is most commonly obtained using sounds delivered by earphone. In the second method, the sound is delivered by a loudspeaker. The sound level at the position of the centre of the listener's head is established after removing the listener from the sound field. This gives what is known as the minimum audible field. The two methods give slightly different results as the head, pinna and meatus do have an effect on the sound field. However, the general form of the results is similar.

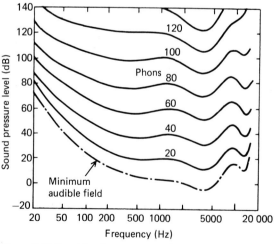

Figure 3.10 Equal-loudness contours for various loudness levels, as indicated on each curve. The dashed-dotted curve shows the absolute threshold (minimum audible field). (From Moore, 1982; original data from Robinson and Dadson, 1956, by courtesy of the publisher)

The lowest curve in *Figure 3.10* shows the average minimum audible field for healthy adult listeners. It should be noted that 'normal' listeners may have thresholds up to 20 dB above or below the average. Thresholds tend to increase with age, particularly at high frequencies (4 kHz and above). The range of frequencies to which we are most sensitive, 500–5000 Hz, is also the range most important for understanding speech; frequencies outside this range may be removed without any loss in intelligibility.

Equal-loudness contours

In describing the perception of sound, it is useful to have some kind of scale which allows the loudness of different sounds to be compared. A first step towards this is to construct equal-loudness contours for sinusoids of different frequencies. For example, a standard tone of 1 kHz, at a level of 40 dB sound pressure level, is presented and the listener is asked to adjust the level of a second tone (for example 2 kHz) so that it sounds equally loud. If this is repeated for many different frequencies of the second tone, then the sound level required, plotted as a function of frequency, maps out an equal-loudness contour. If this procedure is repeated for different levels of the 1-kHz standard tone, then a family of equal loudness contours will be mapped out. Such a family is shown in *Figure 3.10*.

When the standard tone is at 1 kHz, its loudness level is defined as being equal to its sound pressure level. Thus the loudness level of any sound is the level (in dB sound pressure level) of the 1-kHz tone to which it sounds equal in loudness. The unit of loudness level is the phon, and each equal-loudness contour in *Figure 3.10* is labelled with its phon value. It should be noted that the contours resemble the absolute threshold curve at low levels, but tend to become flatter at high levels. This finding has been taken into account in the design of sound-level meters, which weight the power at different frequencies according to the shapes of equal-loudness contours. At low sound levels, low-frequency components contribute little to the total loudness of complex sounds, and so an 'A' weighting is used, which reduces the contribution of low frequencies to the overall meter reading. At high levels, where the equal-loudness contours are flatter, a more nearly flat weighting characteristic, the 'C' weighting, is used.

It is important to understand two limitations of the readings obtained by means of sound level meters. The first is that readings in phons do not directly indicate the loudness of sounds, even for simple sinusoids. It is not true that a sound with a loudness level of 80 phons is twice as loud as one with a loudness level of 40 phons. The phon scale can be used only to indicate the order in which the loudness of sounds should be ranked. The second limitation is that the loudness of complex sounds, containing many frequency components, depends on how the energy is distributed over frequency (*see* the section on The role of frequency selectivity in determining loudness), and this is not taken into account in simple loudness level meters. In spite of these limitations (and others not mentioned here), 'loudness' meters have been widely used in the measurement of industrial and community noise.

Loudness scaling

Scaling methods have been used as a means of deriving the relationship between the physical intensity of sounds and their subjective loudness. There are many variations of the methods but they usually involve asking the listener to make a 'direct' estimate of the magnitude of the loudness sensation. In one method, called magnitude estimation, the listener might be presented with a standard sound, followed by a series of comparison sounds of different intensities (but the same frequency). The listener is asked to judge the loudness of each of the sounds, relative to the first sound, which might arbitrarily be called 100 units. Therefore, if a sound is judged twice as loud as the standard it is called 200 units of loudness, and if it is judged one-tenth as loud it is called 10 units. On the basis of results obtained with these methods, Stevens (1957) and others have suggested that loudness, L, is a power function of physical intensity, I:

$$L = kI^{0.3} \tag{6}$$

where k is a constant depending on the subject and the units used. In other words, the loudness of a given sound will be proportional to its intensity raised to the power 0.3. Roughly, this means that a two-fold change in loudness is produced by a 10 dB change in level.

Stevens proposed the sone as the unit of loudness. One sone is defined arbitrarily as the loudness of a 1-kHz tone at 40 dB sound pressure level. Thus a 1-kHz tone at 50 dB sound pressure level will have a loudness of 2 sones and a 1-kHz tone at 60 dB will have a loudness of 4 sones. The sone scale has been employed in models which allow the calculation of the loudness of complex sounds, and it has become quite widely used, being incorporated in a number of standard procedures for calculating loudness (for example Stevens, 1972). However, the interpretation of the scale, and the methods of deriving it, have been the subject of criticism. The results of loudness

scaling experiments can show great variability between listeners, and it is known that the exact way in which the experiments are conducted can have a large effect; biases of various kinds can be significant. Warren (1970) attempted to eliminate known biases and found that half-loudness corresponds to a 6 dB reduction in level, rather than the 10 dB suggested by Stevens.

Many researchers are unhappy with the whole concept of asking listeners to judge the magnitude of a sensation. What we do in everyday life is to judge the characteristics of sound sources, so that our estimate of loudness is affected by the apparent distance of the sound source, the context in which it is heard, the nature of the sound, and so on. In other words we are attempting to make some estimate of the properties of the source itself, and introspection as to the nature of the sensation evoked may be an unnatural and difficult process.

The role of frequency selectivity in determining loudness

It has been known for many years that if the total intensity of a complex sound is fixed, its loudness will depend on the frequency range over which the sound extends. The basic mechanism underlying this would seem to be the same critical band or auditory filter as is revealed in masking experiments (*see above*). Consider as an example a noise whose total intensity is held constant while the bandwidth is varied. The loudness of the noise can be estimated indirectly by asking the listener to adjust the intensity of a second sound, with a fixed bandwidth, so that it sounds equally loud. The two sounds are presented successively. When the bandwidth of the noise is less than a certain value, the loudness is roughly independent of bandwidth. However, as the bandwidth is increased beyond a certain point, the loudness starts to increase. This is illustrated in *Figure 3.11*, for several different overall levels of the noise. The bandwidth at which loudness starts to increase is known as the *critical bandwidth for loudness summation*. Its value is approximately the same as that of the equivalent rectangular bandwidth of the auditory filter.

The increase in loudness with increasing bandwidth can be understood if it is assumed that when the bandwidth of a sound is greater than one equivalent rectangular bandwidth, the loudness in adjacent, but non-overlapping, bands is summed to give the total loudness. Consider the effect of taking a band of noise whose width equals one equivalent rectangular bandwidth, and doubling the bandwidth, keeping the total intensity constant. The noise will now cover two bands of one equivalent rectangular bandwidth each, but the original intensity in each band will be half that

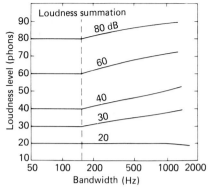

Figure 3.11 The loudness level in phons of a band of noise centred at 1 kHz, measured as a function of the width of the band. For each of the curves the overall level was held constant, and is indicated in the figure. The dashed line shows that the bandwidth at which loudness begins to increase is the same at all levels tested (except that no increase occurs at the lowest level). (Adapted from Feldtkeller and Zwicker, 1956, *Das Ohr als Nachrichtenempfänger*, S. Hirzel, by courtesy of the author and publisher)

in the original band. According to Steven's power law, $L = kI^{0.3}$, halving intensity is equivalent to a reduction in loudness to 0.81 of the original value. The total loudness in the two bands will be 2 × 0.81 = 1.62 times the original value. Therefore, increasing the bandwidth beyond the critical band results in an increase in loudness. At low sound levels, the power law appears to break down and loudness changes in proportion with sound intensity. As a result, the change in loudness with bandwidth is reduced or absent, as may be seen in the lowest curve of *Figure 3.11*.

The perception of pitch

The pitch of pure tones

Pitch is defined as that attribute of auditory sensation in terms of which sound may be ordered on a musical scale, that is that attribute in which variations constitute melody. For sinusoidal stimuli (pure tones), the pitch is closely related to the frequency; the higher the frequency the higher the pitch. One of the classic debates in hearing theory is concerned with the mechanisms underlying the perception of pitch. One theory, called the place theory, suggests that pitch is related to the distribution of activity across nerve fibres. A tone with a given frequency will produce maximum activity in nerve fibres with characteristic frequencies close to that frequency, and the 'position' of this maximum is assumed to determine pitch. Shifts in frequency will be detected as changes in the amount of activity at the place where the activity changes most. Such changes will usually

be maximal in neurons with characteristic frequencies below the stimulating frequencies; the frequencies will lie on the low-frequency side of the excitation pattern, where the slope is steep, and small changes in frequency will produce large changes in activity.

The alternative theory, which is called the temporal theory, suggests that pitch is determined by the time-pattern of neural spikes. For frequencies up to about 5 kHz, neural spikes are phase-locked to the stimulus, so that the time intervals between successive spikes carry information about the stimulus frequency (*see* Chapter 2).

One major fact which these theories have to account for is our remarkably fine acuity in detecting frequency changes. This ability is called frequency discrimination, and is not to be confused with frequency selectivity or frequency resolution. For two tones of 500 ms duration presented successively, a difference of about 3 Hz (or less in trained subjects) can be detected at a centre frequency of 1 kHz. It has been suggested that tuning curves (or auditory filters) are not sufficiently sharp to account for this fine acuity in terms of the place theory (*see* Moore and Glasberg, 1986a, for a detailed discussion of this issue). A further difficulty for the place theory comes from a consideration of the way frequency discrimination changes with centre frequency. *Figure 3.12* shows that discrimination worsens abruptly above 4–5 kHz (Moore, 1973b). This is difficult to explain in terms of a place theory, as neither neural measures of frequency selectivity (such as tuning curves) nor psychophysical measures of frequency selectivity

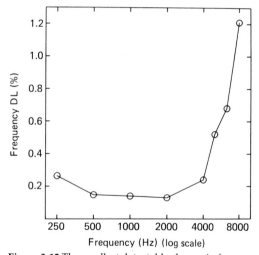

Figure 3.12 The smallest detectable change in frequency (called the frequency DL), expressed as a percentage of frequency, and plotted as a function of frequency. The stimuli were 200-ms sinusoidal tones. Note the worsening in performance above 4–5 kHz. (Data from Moore, 1973b)

(such as psychophysical tuning curves or auditory filter shapes) show any corresponding change.

These facts can be accommodated by the temporal theory. Changes in frequency discrimination with centre frequency (and with tone duration) can be predicted from the information available in inter-spike intervals (Goldstein and Srulovicz, 1977). The worsening performance at 4–5 kHz corresponds well with the frequency at which the temporal information ceases to be available (*see* Chapter 2). Studies of our perception of musical intervals also indicate a change in mechanism around 4–5 kHz. Below this, a sequence of pure tones with appropriate frequencies conveys a clear sense of melody. Above this, the sense of musical interval and of melody is lost, although the changes in frequency may still be heard.

The evidence, therefore, supports the idea that, for pure tones, pitch perception and discrimination are determined primarily by temporal information for frequencies below 4–5 kHz, and by place information for frequencies above this. The important frequencies for the perception of music and speech lie in the frequency range where temporal information is available.

The pitch perception of complex tones

In general, any sound which is periodic may have a pitch, provided that the repetition rate lies in the range 20–20 000 Hz. The pitch is related to the repetition rate, in the same way that it is related to frequency for pure tones. When a pitch value is assigned to a complex tone, this is generally understood to be the frequency of a sinusoid which has the same pitch. Theories concerned with the pitch perception of complex tones have changed considerably in recent years, and have become quite complex. Before introducing the theories, those physical properties of a complex sound which are important in determining its pitch will be considered.

Periodic sounds can be analysed into a series of sinusoids consisting of a fundamental component and a series of harmonics. For example, a brief impulse repeating 200 times/s has a fundamental component of 200 Hz, and harmonics at 400, 600, 800, ... Hz. The pitch of such a sound is close to that of a 200-Hz sinusoid; but what physical characteristics are essential for producing this pitch? The obvious answer, namely the presence of the fundamental component at 200 Hz, is not correct. The fundamental can be removed, or masked by low-frequency noise, and the pitch remains the same. This is called 'the phenomenon of the missing fundamental'. The pitch remains the same even when the sound is filtered so as to

contain only a few harmonics, say 1200, 1400, 1600 and 1800 Hz. The low pitch evoked by a group of harmonics (with a missing fundamental) has been given various names, including *residue pitch, virtual pitch* and *low pitch*.

Another possibility, that pitch is determined by the spacing between harmonics, is also incorrect. This can be shown by shifting all of the components upwards in frequency by an equal amount, say to 1219, 1419, 1619 and 1819 Hz. The spacing between components remains the same, but the pitch is heard to go up slightly.

The possibility that the pitch is related to some aspect of the time structure of the stimulus should now be considered. In so doing, it must be remembered that any sound entering the ear has to pass through the ear's filtering mechanism, so that the effective stimulus for each neuron resembles a bandpass-filtered version of the original waveform. A simulation of what the waveforms might look like at the outputs of the auditory filters for a typical periodic sound is shown in *Figure 3.13*. The sound in this case was the vowel /i/ as in 'weed'.

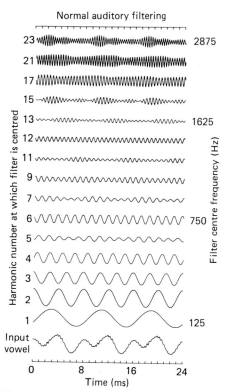

Figure 3.13 The waveforms at the outputs of simulated auditory filters in response to a complex periodic tone, the vowel /i/. *See* text for details. (From Rosen and Fourcin, 1986, in *Frequency Selectivity in Hearing*, edited by B. C. J. Moore, Academic Press, by courtesy of the publisher)

The auditory filter bandwidth increases with centre frequency, but the spacing between harmonics is constant. The lower harmonics of the sound are effectively resolved. Each produces activity in a different auditory filter, and the outputs of those filters are sinusoidal waveforms corresponding to the individual harmonics. The higher harmonics, on the other hand, are not completely resolved and interfere with one another. The waveform resulting from the interference of a group of harmonics has the same repetition rate as that of the waveform as a whole (shown at the bottom of the figure). Thus the repetition period of the waveforms at the outputs of auditory filters responding to higher harmonics could be the basis for pitch. However, this explanation is not entirely satisfactory. If a complex sound is filtered so as to contain only high unresolved harmonics (for example above the tenth), a pitch is still heard, but it is weak and ambiguous compared to that heard when lower harmonics are present (Moore and Rosen, 1979). It would appear that the lower, resolvable, harmonics are more important in determining pitch.

Most modern theories of pitch perception assume a two-stage process. In the first stage the lower harmonics are analysed. This analysis depends on the ear's filtering mechanism, but the time structure of the output from each filter, as represented in the temporal patterns of neural discharge, is probably also important (Moore, Glasberg and Shailer, 1984). In the second stage, some form of pattern recognizer determines a fundamental frequency whose harmonics match as closely as possible those of the stimulus (Goldstein, 1973). The perceived pitch corresponds to the frequency of this internally determined fundamental. In one model of this type, the pitch is determined by a mechanism which generates subharmonics of components which are present in the stimulus (Terhardt, 1974). These subharmonics coincide at certain frequencies. The frequency with the greatest number of coincidences corresponds to the perceived pitch of the sound. For the example shown in *Table 3.1*, the greatest number of coincidences in the subharmonics occurs at 200 Hz, which corresponds to the perceived pitch.

This model can explain the slight pitch shifts which occur when the frequencies of all components are shifted upwards by an equal amount. In this case, the subharmonics do not coincide perfectly, as the complex is no longer harmonic, but the frequency at which several subharmonics almost coincide matches the perceived pitch quite well.

In summary, modern theories assume that the pitch perception of complex tones is a kind of pattern-recognition process based on a preliminary analysis of the components present in the sound. The initial analysis may depend on both 'place' and temporal information. When only high harmonics are present, a pitch can still be heard but it is weaker. Presumably in this case, the harmonics cannot be resolved and the pitch is based purely on timing information. For a more comprehensive review of recent data and theories on pitch perception the reader is referred to Moore and Glasberg (1986a).

Table 3.1 An example illustrating Terhardt's model for the perception of the pitch of complex tones*

	Frequency of component (Hz)		
	800	*1000*	*1200*
Frequencies of subharmonics	400	500	600
	266.7	333.3	400
	200	250	300
	160	**200**	240
	133.3	166.7	**200**

*The complex in this case contains just three sinusoidal frequency components, 800, 1000 and 1200 Hz. A series of subharmonics of each component is generated. These subharmonics coincide at certain frequencies, the greatest number of coincidences occurring at 200 Hz. This corresponds to the perceived pitch.

The perception of timbre

Timbre may be defined as the characteristic quality of sound that distinguishes one voice or musical instrument from another. While pitch and loudness are one-dimensional, timbre is multidimensional; that is there is no single scale along which we can compare the timbres of various sounds. Timbre depends on several different physical properties of sound, including:

(1) Whether the sound is periodic, having a tonal quality for repetition rates from about 20 to 20 000 Hz, or irregular and having a noise-like quality.
(2) Whether the sound is continuous or interrupted. For sounds which have short durations, the exact way in which the sound is turned on and off can play an important role. For example, in the case of sounds produced by stringed instruments, a rapid onset (a fast rise time) is usually perceived as a struck or plucked string, whereas a gradual onset is heard as a bowed string.
(3) The distribution of energy over frequency (that is the spectrum), and changes in the spectrum with time. This is the correlate of timbre which has been studied most widely.

For steady-state periodic sounds, it is possible to use the more restricted definition of timbre given by the American Standards Association: 'that attribute of auditory sensation in terms of which a listener can judge that two steady-state complex tones having the same loudness and pitch, are dissimilar'. Timbre defined in this way depends primarily on the energy spectrum of the sound (Plomp, 1976). For example, sounds containing predominantly high frequencies have a 'sharp' timbre, whereas those containing mainly low frequencies sound 'dull' or 'mellow'. This is another example of the action of the ear as a frequency analyser. The components in a complex sound will be partially separated by the auditory filters, and the distribution of the excitation at the output of the filters, as a function of filter centre frequency (that is the excitation pattern), will determine timbre.

Plomp and his colleagues have conducted a series of experiments to investigate the perception of timbre for steady tones (for a review, *see* Plomp, 1976). Pols, Kamp and Plomp (1969) constructed a series of vowel sounds which all had the same fundamental frequency and loudness. The vowels may be considered as periodic complex sounds of the type discussed in the previous section. The differences between the vowels relate mainly to the differences in spectrum, that is to differences in the distribution of energy across harmonics. Groups of three vowels were presented to subjects. For each group, the subjects had to decide which pair was most similar and which pair was least similar; every possible combination of three was presented. They then used a technique known as multi-dimensional scaling (Shepard, 1962; Kruskal, 1964) to construct a perceptual space representing the similarities between the vowels. Each vowel is represented as a point in space, and the greater the distance between points, the more dissimilar the vowels are judged to be. The number of dimensions required to account for the judgements of similarity can be reduced at the expense of 'goodness of fit'. For the data of Pols *et al.*, six dimensions gave a very good fit, but the fit with three dimensions was not much worse.

Pols *et al.* also conducted physical analyses of their vowels using a bank of filters which were meant to simulate approximately the auditory filters. They used 18 filters, each one-third of an octave wide. Each vowel was applied to the filter bank and was characterized by a set of 18 numbers representing the levels at the outputs of the filters. This gave an 18-dimensional description of the set of vowels. However, the levels at the outputs of different filters are not independent, especially for filters with adjacent frequencies. Therefore, there is some redundancy or duplication of information

in the 18 dimensions. This redundancy can be eliminated by statistical procedures that yield the chief higher order dimensions underlying the physical differences between the vowels. Each higher order dimension is a weighted sum of the 18 original dimensions. In the same way as for the perceptual space, the number of dimensions can be reduced at the expense of a decrease in the accuracy with which the data are fitted. Pols *et al.* obtained a good fit with just three dimensions. Thus, physically, each vowel can be represented as a point in a three-dimensional space constructed from the results of the one-third octave analysis.

When Pols *et al.* compared the three-dimensional perceptual space with the three-dimensional physical space, they found a remarkably close correspondence between the two; the configurations of the two spaces were almost identical. They stated that, 'From this remarkable correspondence, it can be concluded that the subjects used for their perceptual judgements information comparable with that present in the physical representation of the sounds'. In view of the fact that the physical space was constructed using filters with bandwidths similar to those of the ear's auditory filters, it would seem that the frequency selectivity of the auditory system plays a key role in the perception of timbre for steady tones.

The temporal resolution of the ear

The auditory system is especially well adapted to detecting changes in sounds as a function of time. The limits of this ability can be determined by measuring the temporal resolution of the ear. A particularly straightforward method of doing this uses a gap-detection task. The subject is presented with two successive long-duration signals, one of which contains a temporal gap. The task of the subject is to identify whether the gap occurred in the first or second signal, and threshold is defined as the gap duration which is detectable on a given percentage of trials (for example 71%). The task is easy to explain to subjects, and gives stable results without the need for extended practice.

Many gap-detection experiments have used wideband noise as a stimulus, as introducing a temporal gap in such a noise does not change the spectrum of the noise. The results generally agree quite well, the threshold value being 2–3 ms (Plomp, 1964b; Penner, 1977). More recently, gap thresholds have been measured for band-limited noises, to determine whether gap threshold varies with centre frequency. Unfortunately, when a noise band is abruptly switched off and on, to produce the gap, a change in spectrum occurs. Energy is spread or 'splattered' to frequencies outside the nominal bandwidth of the noise. In order to prevent the detection of this 'spectral splatter', the noise bands have been presented with complementary band-reject noise, to mask off-frequency energy (Fitzgibbons and Wightman, 1982; Fitzgibbons, 1983; Shailer and Moore, 1983). Some results from Shailer and Moore (1983) are plotted in *Figure 3.14*.

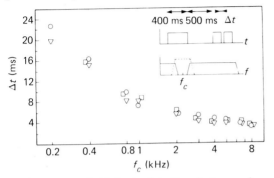

Figure 3.14 Thresholds for the detection of a temporal gap (Δt) in a bandpass noise stimulus, as a function of the centre frequency, fc, of the noise. Each symbol shows results for a different subject. The insets schematically illustrate the time course and frequency spectra of the stimuli. (From Shailer and Moore, 1983; by courtesy of the publisher)

The value of the gap threshold increases monotonically with decreasing centre frequency. At high frequencies, the gap threshold is similar to that found for wideband noise, suggesting that subjects listen primarily to high frequencies when detecting gaps in broadband noise. The increase in gap threshold at low frequencies may be connected with the temporal response of the auditory filter. When the input to a narrowband filter ceases abruptly, the filter continues to 'ring' for some time. Ringing in the auditory filters could partially fill in a brief gap in a signal, thus limiting gap-detection performance. In general, the narrower the bandwidth of a filter, the longer the time for which it rings. Therefore, the increase in gap threshold at low frequencies may be explained by the decrease in the bandwidth of the auditory filter at low frequencies.

Shailer and Moore (1983) measured auditory filter bandwidths in the same subjects that were used for the gap-detection task, using the notched-noise method described earlier. The results are shown in *Figure 3.15*, where the bandwidths of the auditory filters are plotted as a function of centre frequency. The figure also shows the reciprocals of the mean gap thresholds in *Figure 3.14*. For frequencies up to 1 kHz, the bandwidth of the auditory filter is highly correlated with the reciprocal of the gap threshold. This implies that ringing in the auditory filters does indeed limit

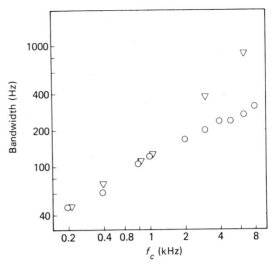

Figure 3.15 The circles show the reciprocals of the mean gap thresholds in *Figure 3.14*, plotted as a function of centre frequency, *fc*. The triangles show estimated equivalent rectangular bandwidths (ERBs) of the auditory filters of the same three subjects. Note the close correspondence between the two for frequencies up to 1 kHz. (Modified from Shailer and Moore, 1983)

gap detection. Above 3 kHz, the correspondence breaks down; gap thresholds are longer than would be the case if they were limited solely by ringing in the auditory filters. This suggests that, at high frequencies, other, presumably neural, processes limit gap detection. A decrease in gap threshold with increasing centre frequency has been found in all studies where centre frequency was varied (Fitzgibbons and Wightman, 1982; Tyler *et al.*, 1982; Fitzgibbons, 1983; Shailer and Moore, 1983).

At low sound levels, gap detection improves somewhat with increasing sound level. However, above a certain level (about 25–30 dB spectrum level for band-limited noise signals), performance changes only slightly with increasing level (Buus and Florentine, 1982; Fitzgibbons, 1983; Shailer and Moore, 1983).

The localization of sounds

Binaural cues

It has long been recognized that slight differences in the sounds reaching the two ears can be used as cues in sound localization. The two major cues are differences in the time of arrival and differences in intensity at the two ears. For example, a sound coming from the left will arrive first at the left ear and be more intense in this ear. For steady sinusoidal stimulation, a difference in time of arrival is equivalent to a phase difference between the sounds at the two ears. However, phase differences are not usable over the whole audible frequency range. Experiments using sounds delivered by headphones have shown that a phase difference at the two ears can be detected and used to judge location only at frequencies below about 1500 Hz. This is reasonable when we realize that, in order to convert a phase difference to a time difference, the listener must be able to determine which cycle of the sound in one ear corresponds to a given cycle in the other ear. At high frequencies, the wavelength of sound is small compared to the dimensions of the head, so the listener cannot determine which cycle in the left ear corresponds to a given cycle in the right; there may be many cycles of phase difference. Thus phase differences become ambiguous and unusable at high frequencies. On the other hand, at low frequencies our accuracy at detecting changes in relative time at the two ears is remarkably good; changes of 10–20 µs can be detected, which is equivalent to a movement of the sound source of 1–2° laterally.

Intensity differences between the two ears are useful primarily at high frequencies. This is because low frequencies bend or diffract around the head, which means that there is little difference in intensity at the two ears whatever the location of the sound source. At high frequencies, the head casts more of a 'shadow', and above 2–3 kHz the intensity differences are sufficient to provide useful cues. For complex sounds, containing a range of frequencies, the difference in spectral patterning at the two ears may also be important.

The idea that sound localization is based on interaural time differences at low frequencies and interaural intensity differences at high frequencies has been called the 'duplex theory' of sound localization, and it dates back to Lord Rayleigh (1907). However, it has been realized in recent years that this idea is not quite correct (for a review, *see* Hafter, 1984). *Complex* sounds, containing only high frequencies (above 1500 Hz), can be localized on the basis of interaural time delays, provided that they have an appropriate temporal structure. For example, a single click can be localized in this way no matter what its frequency content. Periodic sounds containing only high-frequency harmonics can also be localized on the basis of interaural time differences, provided that the *envelope* repetition rate (usually equal to the fundamental frequency) is below about 600 Hz (Neutzel and Hafter, 1981). As most of the sounds we encounter in everyday life are complex, and have repetition rates below 600 Hz, interaural time differences will be used for localization in most listening situations.

The role of the pinnae

Although binaural cues are traditionally considered as the most important in sound localization, it is clear that they are not sufficient to account for all of our abilities. For example, a simple difference in time or intensity will not tell us whether a sound is coming from in front or behind, or from above or below, but we are clearly able to make such judgements. Furthermore, under some conditions, localization with one ear can be as accurate as with two ears. About 20 years ago, Batteau (1967) showed that the pinnae play an important role in sound localization. They do so because the spectra of sounds entering the ear are modified by the pinnae in a way which depends upon the direction of the sound source (*see* Chapter 2). This direction-dependent filtering provides cues for sound source location. The pinnae are important not just in providing cues about the direction of sound sources, but also in enabling us to judge whether a sound comes from within the head or from the outside world. A sound is only judged as coming from outside if the spectral transformations characteristic of the pinnae are imposed on the sound. Thus sounds heard through headphones are normally judged as being inside the head; the pinnae do not have their normal effect on the sound when headphones are worn. Judgements of the position of a sound within the head are referred to as lateralization. However, sounds delivered by headphones can be made to appear to come from outside the head if the signals delivered to the headphones are synthetically processed (filtered) so as to mimic the normal action of the pinnae. Such processing can also create the impression of a sound coming from any desired direction in space.

The pinnae alter the sound spectrum primarily at high frequencies. Only when the wavelength of the sound is comparable with the dimensions of the pinnae is the spectrum significantly affected, which occurs mostly above about 6 kHz. This means that people with high-frequency hearing losses are generally unable to make use of the directional information provided by the pinnae. Hearing-aid users also suffer in this respect, because, even if the microphone is appropriately placed within the pinna, the response of most aids is limited to frequencies below 6 kHz.

The precedence effect

In everyday conditions, the sound from a given source reaches our ears by many different paths. Part of the sound will arrive by way of a direct path, but a great deal may reach our ears only after reflections from one or more surfaces. However, we are not normally aware of these reflections or echoes, and they do not appear to impair our ability to localize sound sources. The reason for this seems to lie in a phenomenon known as the precedence effect (Wallach, Newman and Rosenzweig, 1949). When several sounds reach our ears in close succession (that is the direct sound and its echoes), the sounds are perceptually fused into a single sound, and the location of the total sound is determined primarily by the location of the first (direct) sound. Thus the echoes have little influence on the perception of direction. Furthermore, we have little direct awareness of the echoes, although they may influence the timbre and loudness of the sound.

The precedence effect occurs only for sounds of a discontinuous or transient character, such as speech or music, and it can break down if the echoes are sufficiently intense compared to the direct sound. However, in normal conditions the precedence effect plays an important role in enabling us to locate and identify sounds in reverberant conditions.

The precedence effect seems to be primarily a binaural phenomenon. When one ear is blocked we become much more aware of room echoes. Sounds then generally appear 'boomy' or 'muddy' and localization is more difficult.

Perception of sound by the hearing impaired

Conductive hearing losses can be considered mainly as attenuating the sound reaching the inner ear. They do not have any marked effect on the ability to analyse or discriminate sound. Sensorineural losses, on the other hand, are commonly accompanied by reduced discrimination and/or distortion in the way sound is perceived. This section will concentrate on describing the changes in auditory perception associated with cochlear hearing losses, because most is known about them and because they constitute the largest category of the sensorineural hearing impaired.

Frequency selectivity in impaired hearing

There is now considerable evidence that in listeners with hearing impairments of cochlear origin there is a loss of frequency selectivity. This has been demonstrated using most of the masking techniques discussed earlier. In general, greater threshold elevations tend to be associated with broader auditory filters. However, the following cautions should be observed:

(1) There can be considerable variability among patients, even when the elevation in absolute threshold is similar. Although the bandwidth of the auditory filter is correlated with the threshold elevation (Pick, Evans and Wilson, 1977; Glasberg and Moore, 1986), some patients have broad filters and almost normal thresholds, while some have elevated thresholds but almost normal filters.

(2) The auditory filter tends to broaden with increasing age (Patterson *et al.*, 1982). As many hearing impaired patients are elderly, part of the broadening may be a 'normal' age effect. However, abnormally large filter bandwidths can be observed even in young hearing-impaired patients.

(3) The auditory filter becomes broader at high sound levels even in normal listeners (*see Figure 3.7*). As measurements with patients usually have to be made at high sound levels, part of the broadening may be attributed to a normal level effect.

One way around the first two problems is to use subjects with unilateral impairments. Each subject then acts as his/her own age-matched control. *Figure 3.16* shows a comparison of auditory filter shapes obtained separately from each of the ears of six patients with unilateral cochlear hearing losses. The left panel shows filter shapes for the normal ears and the right panel shows filter shapes for the impaired ears, which had threshold elevations at the test frequency (1 kHz) ranging from 40 to 60 dB. Losses were relatively flat as a function of frequency. A notched-noise masker was used, as described earlier, and the same noise spectrum level (50 dB) was used for testing all ears, so the results are not subject to the difficulty discussed in point (3) above.

It is clear that the auditory filters are considerably broader in the impaired ears. The most obvious feature is that the lower skirts of the filters are considerably and consistently less sharp in the impaired ears. This implies that these subjects are unusually susceptible to the upward spread of masking from low frequencies. This appears to be a common feature in cases of cochlear impairment, even in patients with relatively flat losses as a function of frequency. It may partially account for the fact that hearing aids are often most effective when their gain is greater at high frequencies than at low. A rising frequency-gain characteristic will help to alleviate the effects of the upward spread of masking.

There is also evidence that the suppression mechanism may be damaged, or even completely inoperative, in cases of cochlear impairment. The auditory filter shape measured in non-simultaneous masking is typically sharper than that

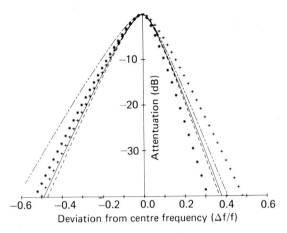

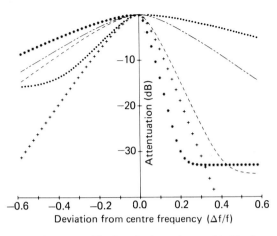

Figure 3.16 Auditory filter shapes for the normal ears (left) and the impaired ears (right) of six subjects with unilateral cochlear impairments. The centre frequency was 1 kHz. The filter shapes are plotted as a function of deviation from the centre frequency divided by the centre frequency. The impaired ear of one subject had too little frequency selectivity for a filter shape to be determined. (From Glasberg and Moore, 1986; by courtesy of the publisher)

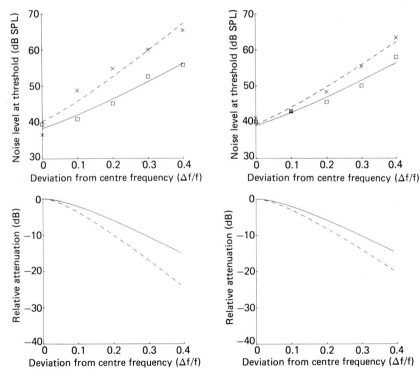

Figure 3.17 Results for a subject with a unilateral cochlear impairment. The top panels show the level of a notched-noise masker needed to mask a 1.5-kHz signal as a function of the width of the notch in the noise (expressed as the deviation of each edge of the notch from the signal frequency divided by the signal frequency). – and □ denote simultaneous masking and -- and × denote forward masking. Results for the normal ear are shown on the left, and those for the impaired ear on the right. The auditory filter shapes derived from the data are shown in the lower panels. The fact that the filters are sharper in forward masking has been interpreted as resulting from suppression. The results suggest that suppression is still operating in the impaired ear, but more weakly than normal. (From Moore and Glasberg, 1986b; by courtesy of the publisher)

measured in simultaneous masking, a difference which is commonly attributed to suppression (Houtgast, 1974, 1977; Moore and Glasberg, 1981; Glasberg, Moore and Nimmo-Smith, 1984). In patients with cochlear impairments, the differences are reduced or may even be zero (Festen and Plomp, 1983). However, in cases of moderate impairment (40–50 dB losses), the auditory filter shape measured with a notched-noise masker may still be slightly sharper in forward masking than in simultaneous masking. An example is given in *Figure 3.17*, which compares auditory filter shapes derived from simultaneous and forward masking, both for the normal and for the impaired ear of a patient with a unilateral cochlear loss (data from Moore and Glasberg, 1986b).

In the example shown, the signal level was fixed and the noise spectrum level was varied to determine threshold, as described in Moore and Glasberg (1981). The notched noise was always symmetrically placed around the signal frequency, and so it was not possible to determine the asymmetry of the auditory filter. Hence, only half of each filter shape is shown in the lower panel. For each ear, the noise level required for threshold was similar in simultaneous and forward masking for a notch width of zero. Thus the results are not confounded by differences in overall noise level between simultaneous and forward masking. The difference between the filter shapes for simultaneous and forward masking is smaller for the impaired ear than for the normal ear, but a difference nevertheless exists, indicating that suppression may be operating weakly in the impaired ear.

Consequences of impaired frequency selectivity

It is useful to consider briefly the perceptual consequences of a reduction in frequency selectivity. The first major consequence will be a greater susceptibility to masking by interfering sounds. When we are listening to everyday sounds, the frequency content (the spectrum) of sounds to which we wish to attend will usually differ from that of other sounds which may be present in the environment. By listening through the auditory filters tuned to the signal frequency or frequencies, the signal will be passed, but much of the background noise will be attenuated. When the auditory filters are broader than normal, the rejection of background noise will be much less effective. Thus background noise will severely disrupt the detection and discrimination of sounds, including speech. Indeed, difficulty in understanding speech in noise is one of the commonest complaints among people with hear-

ing impairments of cochlear origin. It has been shown that the intelligibility of speech in noise is related to frequency selectivity, worsening as frequency selectivity decreases (Dreschler and Plomp, 1980; Patterson *et al.*, 1982; Festen and Plomp, 1983).

A related difficulty arises in the perceptual analysis of complex sounds such as speech or music. The timbre of a musical note or a vowel sound depends strongly on the spectrum of the sound, and correspondingly on the shape of the excitation pattern evoked by the sound. When the ear's frequency selectivity is impaired, the excitation pattern of a sound becomes 'blurred'; the peaks and dips are less well represented. The situation may be made even worse if the suppression mechanism, which normally enchances the contrast between peaks and dips in the excitation pattern, is damaged. Thus it will be more difficult for the impaired listener to differentiate between different vowel sounds, or to distinguish musical instruments (for a review, *see* Rosen and Fourcin, 1986).

Loudness perception and recruitment in impaired ears

Damage to the inner ear, such as that produced by noise exposure, often results in an abnormality of loudness perception known as 'loudness recruitment'. Although the absolute threshold may be elevated, the rate of growth of loudness with intensity is more rapid than normal, so that at high intensities the sound appears as loud in the impaired ear as it would in a normal ear. The effect is most easily demonstrated when only one ear is affected, as then loudness matches can be made between the two ears, but it can also be detected in other ways. The presence of recruitment can limit the usefulness of conventional hearing aids, for if the gain of the aid is set so as to make sounds of low intensity clearly audible, sounds of high intensity will be uncomfortably loud. Hearing aids incorporating 'compression', especially multiband compression, can be useful in alleviating this effect (Laurence, Moore and Glasberg, 1983; Moore, Laurence and Wright, 1985).

It has been suggested (Evans, 1975) that recruitment may be a consequence of the impaired frequency selectivity which is commonly associated with it. If tuning curves (or auditory filters) are broader than normal, then, as the intensity of a tone is increased above threshold, the activity will spread across the nerve fibre array (or to adjacent auditory filters) more rapidly than it would in the normal ear. This rapid spread of activity could be the reason for the rapid growth of loudness with intensity.

Moore *et al.* (1985) tested this idea by measuring how the rate of growth of loudness of a tone in recruiting ears was affected by presenting that tone in a band-stop or notched noise. They argued that this noise should mask the excitation pattern of the tone at characteristic frequencies far removed from the tone frequency. Thus, if Evans' suggestions were correct, the noise should have reduced the rate of growth of loudness of the tone. They found instead that the noise had little effect on the loudness of the tone, and concluded that recruitment is probably not mediated by an abnormally rapid spread of excitation across the nerve fibre array. Therefore, the underlying cause of recruitment remains uncertain.

Pitch perception in impaired hearing

The data on this topic are sparse, and the results have been quite variable. Most people with cochlear hearing losses do have impaired frequency discrimination, but a few have almost normal discrimination. This applies to both pure and complex tones. The pattern-recognition theories of pitch perception would predict an impairment in pitch perception and discrimination of complex tones whenever frequency resolution is impaired, as the perception of pitch is assumed to depend upon the ability to resolve the lower harmonics. However, it may be the case that quite good discrimination is possible on the basis of temporal information alone. Only when temporal processing is also disrupted, will performance become very poor. Thus some subjects can show very broad psychophysical tuning curves, and almost normal pitch discrimination for complex tones (Hoekstra and Ritsma, 1977). For a review of this topic, *see* Rosen and Fourcin (1986).

Temporal resolution in impaired hearing

Measurements of temporal resolution in the hearing impaired show that considerable individual variability exists. Some listeners with cochlear impairments show almost normal temporal resolution, while others show marked impairments. Again, some caution is necessary in interpreting the results. We have seen that when wide-band stimuli are used, normal-hearing subjects listen primarily at high frequencies in order to perform the task. A subject with a loss primarily at higher frequencies will not be able to use high-frequency information effectively, and this alone could give rise to impaired performance; it is as if the impaired subject were listening to a low-pass filtered version of the stimulus (Bacon and Viemeister, 1985).

Several workers have measured gap detection for band-limited noise to determine whether listeners with cochlear impairments have reduced temporal resolution when compared with normal subjects at similar centre frequencies (Fitzgibbons and Wightman, 1982; Tyler *et al.*, 1982). On average, the impaired subjects did show reduced temporal resolution, and this impairment was observed whether the comparison with normal subjects was made at equal sound pressure level or at equal sensation level. Furthermore, gap thresholds decreased with increasing centre frequency for the impaired subjects, just as they do for normal-hearing subjects. Tyler *et al.* showed that increased gap thresholds were correlated significantly with a reduced ability to understand speech in noise.

Zwicker and Schorn (1982) have described a different method of measuring temporal resolution, which they recommend for use in clinical situations. The threshold is measured for a test tone which is pulsed on and off. The tone is presented first in quiet, then in continuous noise, and finally in noise which is square-wave amplitude modulated. In the latter case, the masker actually consists of brief bursts of noise with silent intervals between them. Listeners with good temporal resolution can take advantage of the brief interruptions in the noise to detect the tone, so that threshold in the modulated noise is lower than in the continuous noise. Zwicker and Schorn found that if the repetition period of the modulating square-wave was 72 ms, then the threshold in the modulated noise fell midway between the threshold in continuous noise and the threshold in quiet, for normal-hearing listeners. In the case of a patient, if the threshold in modulated noise is closer to the threshold in continuous noise than to that in quiet, this is taken to indicate a reduction in temporal resolution.

Zwicker and Schorn applied this method to several groups of listeners with different types of hearing loss. They used test tones and filtered masking noises at three frequencies: 500, 1500 and 4000 Hz. Patients with conductive hearing loss showed normal temporal resolution, and those with noise-induced, age-induced and sudden hearing loss showed normal resolution at the two lower frequencies and reduced resolution at 4000 Hz. Patients with retrocochlear losses, and those with Menières disease, showed a tendency for reduced resolution at all frequencies. Patients with ototoxic losses showed the greatest reduction in resolution at 1500 Hz.

It may be concluded that sensorineural hearing losses are commonly accompanied by reductions in temporal resolution. However, not all patients show impaired temporal resolution, and in some cases the impairments may occur only over a limited frequency range.

At first sight, it appears puzzling that temporal resolution is not better than normal in some patients. It was argued in the previous section that temporal resolution at low frequencies was limited in normal listeners by ringing in the auditory filters. As listeners with cochlear impairments typically have broader-than-normal auditory filters, the temporal response of their filters should be correspondingly more rapid than normal, and this in turn should lead to improved temporal resolution. As has been seen, the experimental results do not generally support this expectation. It may be the case that the reduced temporal resolution in hearing-impaired listeners is associated with a general impairment in neural functioning, possibly located more centrally than the cochlea, and that this impairment is sufficient to outweigh any improvement which might have resulted from a broadening of the auditory filter. It is still possible that improved resolution will be found in hearing-impaired patients at very low centre frequencies, as it is at these frequencies that ringing in the auditory filters has its greatest influence. However, there is little evidence at present to support or refute this idea.

General summary and conclusions

A central theme of this chapter has been the frequency-analysing capacity of the auditory system. This capacity plays a role in our ability to perceptually separate sounds presented simultaneously, to detect signals in masking noise, to identify the timbre of speech and musical sounds, and to perceive the pitch of complex tones. The basic properties of these abilities can be understood by conceiving of the peripheral auditory system as containing a bank of bandpass filters, whose centre frequencies cover the whole audible range. The bandwidths of the filters at different centre frequencies are characterized by the value of the auditory filter bandwidth or critical bandwidth. The value of the equivalent rectangular bandwidth increases in rough proportion with centre frequency above about 1 kHz (*see Figure 3.6*).

The basic frequency-analysing mechanisms seem to be well established at the level of the auditory nerve. Information about stimulus frequency, intensity and spectrum may be carried both in the distribution of activity across nerve fibres and in the temporal patterns of neural firing. Temporal patterns may be particularly important in the perception of pitch.

Damage to the inner ear results in an impairment in the frequency-analysing mechanisms. This has been shown both neurophysiologically, for single fibres in the auditory nerve, and

psychophysically, using masking techniques. Thus the ability to detect and discriminate signals in noise, to identify the timbre of sounds, and to perceive the pitch of complex sounds, may all be impaired. Temporal resolution may also be reduced in cases of cochlear hearing loss. In addition, changes in the loudness of sounds with changes in stimulus intensity and bandwidth may be abnormal. These disabilities are not corrected with a conventional hearing aid.

References

BACON, S. P. and VIEMEISTER, N. F. (1985) Temporal modulation transfer functions in normal-hearing and hearing-impaired listeners. *Audiology*, **24**, 117–134

BATTEAU, D. W. (1967) The role of the pinna in human localization. *Proceedings of the Royal Society B*, **168**, 158–180

BUUS, S. and FLORENTINE, M. (1982) Detection of a temporal gap as a function of frequency and level. *Journal of the Acoustical Society of America*, **72**, S89

DRESCHLER, W. A. and PLOMP, R. (1980) Relation between psychophysical data and speech perception for hearing-impaired subjects. *Journal of the Acoustical Society of America*, **68**, 1608–1615

EGAN, J. P. and HAKE, H. W. (1950) On the masking pattern of a simple auditory stimulus. *Journal of the Acoustical Society of America*, **22**, 622–630

EVANS, E. F. (1975) The sharpening of frequency selectivity in the normal and abnormal cochlea. *Audiology*, **14**, 419–442

FESTEN, J. M. and PLOMP, R. (1983) Relations between auditory functions in impaired hearing. *Journal of the Acoustical Society of America*, **76**, 652–662

FIDDELL, S., HORONJEFF, R., TEFFETELLER, S. and GREEN, D. M. (1983) Effective masking bandwidths at low frequencies. *Journal of the Acoustical Society of America*, **73**, 628–638

FITZGIBBONS, P. J. (1983) Temporal gap detection in noise as a function of frequency, bandwidth and level. *Journal of the Acoustical Society of America*, **74**, 67–72

FITZGIBBONS, P. J. and WIGHTMAN, F. L. (1982) Gap detection in normal and hearing-impaired listeners. *Journal of the Acoustical Society of America*, **72**, 761–765

FLETCHER, H. (1940) Auditory patterns. *Reviews of Modern Physics*, **12**, 47–65

GLASBERG, B. R. and MOORE, B. C. J. (1986) Auditory filter shapes in subjects with unilateral and bilateral cochlear impairments. *Journal of the Acoustical Society of America*, **79**, 1020–1033

GLASBERG, B. R., MOORE, B. C. J. and NIMMO-SMITH, I. (1984). Comparison of auditory filter shapes determined with three different maskers. *Journal of the Acoustical Society of America*, **75**, 536–544

GLASBERG, B. R., MOORE, B. C. J., PATTERSON, R. D. and NIMMO-SMITH, I. (1984) Dynamic range and asymmetry of the auditory filter. *Journal of the Acoustical Society of America*, **76**, 419–427

GOLDSTEIN, J. L. (1973) An optimum processor theory for the central formation of the pitch of complex tones. *Journal of the Acoustical Society of America*, **54**, 1496–1516

GOLDSTEIN, J. L. and SRULOVICZ, P. (1977) Auditory-nerve spike intervals as an adequate basis for aural frequency measurement. In *Psychophysics and Physiology of Hearing*, edited by E. F. Evans and J. P. Wilson, pp. 337–346. London: Academic Press

GREENWOOD, D. D. (1961) Critical bandwidth and the frequency coordinates of the basilar membrane. *Journal of the Acoustical Society of America*, **33**, 1344–1356

HAFTER, E. R. (1984) Spatial hearing and the duplex theory: How viable? In *Dynamic Aspects of Neocortical Function*, edited by G. M. Edelman, W. E. Gall and W. M. Cowan, pp. 425–448. New York: Wiley

HOEKSTRA, A. and RITSMA, R. J. (1977) Perceptive hearing loss and frequency selectivity. In *Psychophysics and Physiology of Hearing*, edited by E. F. Evans and J. P. Wilson, pp. 263–271. London: Academic Press

HOUTGAST, T. (1972) Psychophysical evidence for lateral suppression in hearing. *Journal of the Acoustical Society of America*, **51**, 1885–1894

HOUTGAST, T. (1974) Lateral suppression in hearing. *PhD Thesis*, Free University of Amsterdam, Amsterdam, The Netherlands

HOUTGAST, T. (1977) Auditory-filter characteristics derived from direct-masking data and pulsation-threshold data with a rippled-noise masker. *Journal of the Acoustical Society of America*, **62**, 409–415

KRUSKAL, J. B. (1964) Nonmetric multidimensional scaling: a numerical method. *Psychometrika*, **29**, 115–129

LAURENCE, R. F., MOORE, B. C. J. and GLASBERG, B. R. (1983) A comparison of behind-the-ear high-fidelity linear aids and two-channel compression aids, in the laboratory and in everyday life. *British Journal of Audiology*, **17**, 31–48

LUFTI, R. and PATTERSON, R. D. (1984) On the growth of masking asymmetry with stimulus intensity. *Journal of the Acoustical Society of America*, **76**, 739–745

MOORE, B. C. J. (1973a) Some experiments relating to the perception of complex tones. *Quarterly Journal of Experimental Psychology*, **25**, 451–475

MOORE, B. C. J. (1973b) Frequency difference limens for short-duration tones. *Journal of the Acoustical Society of America*, **54**, 610–619

MOORE, B. C. J. (1980) Detection cues in forward masking. In *Psychophysical, Physiological and Behavioural Studies in Hearing*, edited by G. van den Brink and F. A. Bilsen, pp. 222–229. Delft: Delft University Press

MOORE, B. C. J. (1982) *Introduction to the Psychology of Hearing*, 2nd edn. London: Academic Press

MOORE, B. C. J. (1986) Parallels between frequency selectivity measured psychophysically and in the auditory nerve. In *Cochlear Mechanics and Otoacoustic Emission*, edited by G. Gianfrone and F. Grandori, pp. 139–152. *Scandinavian Audiology*, Supplement 25

MOORE, B. C. J. (1987) Dynamic aspects of auditory masking. In *Functions of the Auditory System*, edited by G. M. Edelman, W. E. Gall and W. M. Cowan. New York: Wiley (in press)

MOORE, B. C. J. and GLASBERG, B. R. (1981) Auditory filter shapes derived in simultaneous and forward masking. *Journal of the Acoustical Society of America*, **70**, 1003–1014

MOORE, B. C. J. and GLASBERG, B. R. (1983a) Suggested formulae for calculating auditory-filter bandwidths and excitation patterns. *Journal of the Acoustical Society of America*, **74**, 750–753

MOORE, B. C. J. and GLASBERG, B. R. (1983b) Masking patterns for synthetic vowels in simultaneous and forward masking. *Journal of the Acoustical Society of America*, **73**, 906–917

MOORE, B. C. J. and GLASBERG, B. R. (1986a) The role of frequency selectivity in the perception of loudness, pitch and time. In *Frequency Selectivity in Hearing*, edited by B. C. J. Moore, pp. 251–308. London: Academic Press

MOORE, B. C. J. and GLASBERG, B. R. (1986b) Comparisons of frequency selectivity in simultaneous and forward masking for subjects with unilateral cochlear impairments. *Journal of the Acoustical Society of America*, **80**, 93–107

MOORE, B. C. J., GLASBERG, B. R., HESS, R. F. and BIRCHALL, J. P. (1985) Effects of flanking noise bands on the rate of growth of loudness of tones in normal and recruiting ears. *Journal of the Acoustical Society of America*, **77**, 1505–1513

MOORE, B. C. J., GLASBERG, B. R. and SHAILER, M. J. (1984) Frequency and intensity difference limens for harmonics within complex tones. *Journal of the Acoustical Society of America*, **75**, 550–561

MOORE, B. C. J., LAURENCE, R. F. and WRIGHT, D. (1985) Improvements in speech intelligibility in quiet and in noise produced by two-channel compression hearing aids. *British Journal of Audiology*, **19**, 175–187

MOORE, B. C. J. and O'LOUGHLIN, B. J. (1986) The use of non-simultaneous masking to measure frequency selectivity and suppression. In *Frequency Selectivity in Hearing*, edited by B. C. J. Moore, pp. 179–250. London: Academic Press

MOORE, B. C. J. and ROSEN, S. M. (1979) Tune recognition with reduced pitch and interval information. *Quarterly Journal of Experimental Psychology*, **31**, 229–240

NEUTZEL, J. M. and HAFTER, E. R. (1981) Lateralization of complex waveforms: spectral effects. *Journal of the Acoustical Society of America*, **69**, 1112–1118

PATTERSON, R. D. (1976) Auditory filter shapes derived with noise stimuli. *Journal of the Acoustical Society of America*, **59**, 640–654

PATTERSON, R. D. and NIMMO-SMITH, I. (1980) Off-frequency listening and auditory-filter asymmetry. *Journal of the Acoustical Society of America*, **67**, 229–245

PATTERSON, R. D., NIMMO-SMITH, I., WEBER, D. L. and MILROY, R. (1982) The deterioration of hearing with age: frequency selectivity, the critical ratio, the audiogram and speech threshold. *Journal of the Acoustical Society of America*, **72**, 1788–1803

PENNER, M. J. (1977) Detection of temporal gaps in noise as a measure of the decay of auditory sensation. *Journal of the Acoustical Society of America*, **61**, 552–557

PICK, G. F., EVANS, E. F. and WILSON, J. P. (1977) Frequency resolution in patients with hearing loss of cochlear origin. In *Psychophysics and Physiology of Hearing*, edited by E. F. Evans and J. P. Wilson, pp. 273–281. London: Academic Press

PICKLES, J. O. (1986) The neurophysiological basis of frequency selectivity. In *Frequency Selectivity in Hearing*, edited by B. C. J. Moore, pp. 51–121. London: Academic Press

PLOMP, R. (1964a) The ear as a frequency analyser. *Journal of the Acoustical Society of America*, **36**, 1628–1636

PLOMP, R. (1964b) Rate of decay of auditory sensation. *Journal of the Acoustical Society of America*, **36**, 277–282

PLOMP, R. (1976) *Aspects of Tone Sensation*. London: Academic Press

PLOMP, R. and MIMPEN, A. M. (1968) The ear as a frequency analyzer. II. *Journal of the Acoustical Society of America*, **43**, 764–767

POLS, L. C. W., KAMP, J. J. TH. VAN DER and PLOMP, R. (1969) Perceptual and physical space of vowel sounds. *Journal of the Acoustical Society of America*, **46**, 458–467

RAYLEIGH, LORD (1907) On our perception of sound direction. *Philosophical Magazine*, **13**, 214–232

ROBINSON, D. W. and DADSON, R. S. (1956) A redetermination of the equal-loudness relations for pure tones. *British Journal of Applied Physics*, **7**, 166–181

ROSEN, S. and FOURCIN, A. (1986) Frequency selectivity and the perception of speech. In *Frequency Selectivity in Hearing*, edited by B. C. J. Moore, pp. 373–487. London: Academic Press

SACHS, M. B. and KIANG, N. Y. S. (1968) Two-tone inhibition in auditory-nerve fibres. *Journal of the Acoustical Society of America*, **43**, 1120–1128

SHAILER, M. J. and MOORE, B. C. J. (1983) Gap detection as a function of frequency, bandwidth and level. *Journal of the Acoustical Society of America*, **74**, 467–473

SHANNON, R. V. (1976) Two-tone unmasking and suppression in a forward-masking situation. *Journal of the Acoustical Society of America*, **59**, 1460–1470

SHEPARD, R. N. (1962) The analysis of proximities: multidimensional scaling with an unknown distance function. *Psychometrika*, **27**, 125–140

SODERQUIST, D. R. (1970) Frequency analysis and the critical band. *Psychonomic Science*, **21**, 117–119

STEVENS, S. S. (1957) On the psychophysical law. *Psychological Review*, **64**, 153–181

STEVENS, S. S. (1972) Perceived level of noise by Mark VII and decibels (E). *Journal of the Acoustical Society of America*, **51**, 575–601

TERHARDT, E. (1974) Pitch, consonance and harmony. *Journal of the Acoustical Society of America*, **55**, 1061–1069

TYLER, R. S., SUMMERFIELD, Q., WOOD, E. J. and FERNANDES, M. A. (1982) Psychoacoustic and phonetic temporal processing in normal and hearing-impaired listeners. *Journal of the Acoustical Society of America*, **72**, 740–752

WALLACH, H., NEWMAN, E. B. and ROSENZWEIG, M. R. (1949) The precedence effect in sound localization. *Journal of Experimental Psychology*, **27**, 339–368

WARREN, R. M. (1970) Elimination of biases in loudness judgements for tones. *Journal of the Acoustical Society of America*, **48**, 1397–1403

WEBER, D. L. (1977) Growth of masking and the auditory filter. *Journal of the Acoustical Society of America*, **62**, 424–429

ZWICKER, E. (1974) On a psycho-acoustical equivalent of tuning curves. In *Facts and Models in Hearing*, edited by E. Zwicker and E. Terhardt, pp. 132–140. Berlin: Springer-Verlag

ZWICKER, E. and FELDTKELLER, R. (1967) *Das Ohr als Nachrichtenempfanger*. Stuttgart: Hirzel

ZWICKER, E., FLOTTORP, G. and STEVENS, S. S. (1957) Critical bandwidth in loudness summation. *Journal of the Acoustical Society of America*, **29**, 548–557

ZWICKER, E. and SCHORN, K. (1982) Temporal resolution in hard-of-hearing patients. *Audiology*, **21**, 474–492

ZWICKER, E. and TERHARDT. E. (1980) Analytical expressions for critical bandwidth and critical band rate as a function of frequency. *Journal of the Acoustical Society of America*, **68**, 1523–1525

4

Physiology of equilibrium and its application in the giddy patient

Linda M. Luxon

The statocyst, the most primitive gravity receptor organ, developed more than 600 million years ago and may be found today in the higher members of the phylum Coelenterata. With the evolution of the taxa, the balance receptor organ became more complex, attaining a more sophisticated form in modern fish some 100 million years ago, although little change has occurred since then (Gray, 1955). It is assumed that fish are more dependent on labyrinthine information than are higher animals – for example vertebrates – who possess well-developed systems of proprioception, vision and touch, which are intimately related to the vestibular system in the control of balance.

In humans, a highly sophisticated mechanism for maintaining balance has developed, which is dependent upon visual, vestibular, proprioceptive and superficial sensory information (*Figure 4.1*).

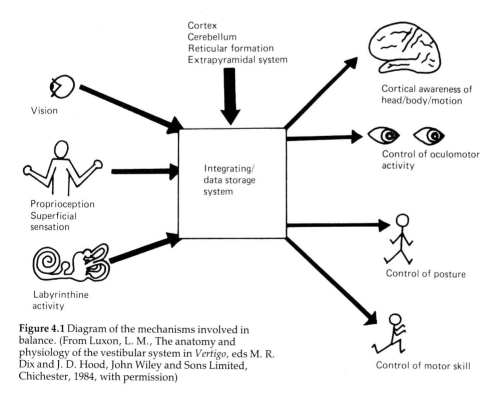

Figure 4.1 Diagram of the mechanisms involved in balance. (From Luxon, L. M., The anatomy and physiology of the vestibular system in *Vertigo*, eds M. R. Dix and J. D. Hood, John Wiley and Sons Limited, Chichester, 1984, with permission)

This is integrated in the central nervous system and is modulated by activity arising in the reticular formation, the extrapyramidal system, the cerebellum and the cortex.

Over 100 years ago, Mach (1875) identified the role of the vestibular apparatus in the perception of motion. He conducted a number of experiments, rotating a subject about a vertical axis inside a box, and oscillating a subject on a see-saw platform, which led him to the conclusion that the semicircular canals and the otolith organs were responsible for the perception of angular and linear acceleration, respectively. Physiologically, the vestibular labyrinth transduces mechanical energy (linear and angular acceleration) into electrical activity (nerve action potentials), which is interpreted by the brain to allow conscious awareness of the position of the head and body in space, and enables reflex control of eye movements, posture and body motion.

The ear is the first sensory organ to develop in the human embryo: by six weeks, the canal system is already clearly defined and between 6 and 14 weeks, the vestibular end organs are formed. It therefore becomes clear that vestibular function is not only a very primitive sense, in terms of the evolution of the species, but is also of paramount importance in the development and maintenance of balance. Furthermore, derangement of the vestibular apparatus itself, or of its multiple connections, may produce severely disabling and distressing symptoms.

Certain aspects of the vestibular system are undoubtedly unique. The sensory organs in man respond to stimuli external to the body, with the exception of the labyrinths which respond to changes within the body. Moreover, vestibular function is unique inasmuch as minor derangements frequently produce catastrophic vertigo as, for example, in early Menière's disease, while a gradual total loss of function, as may result from an acoustic neuroma, may produce no significant dysequilibrium. This fact merely reflects the complex and multiple connections of the vestibular system, which is not a feature of any other sensory system in the human body. As a consequence of these complex connections and the finely balanced nature of the vestibular system, balance is particularly susceptible to damage by insult or disease, and it is primarily for this reason that its study is of importance.

However, a number of additional reasons have focused interest on the vestibular apparatus during recent years. For practical purposes, it has become necessary to understand the role of the vestibular system in space sickness; and, on a more scientific level, the vestibular response lends itself to investigation by modern microelectrode

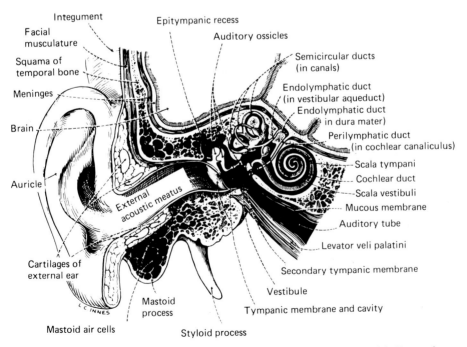

Figure 4.2 Anatomy of the ear. (From Anson and Donaldson, *Surgical Anatomy of the Temporal Bone and Ear*, W. B. Saunders Company, Philadelphia, 1973, with permission)

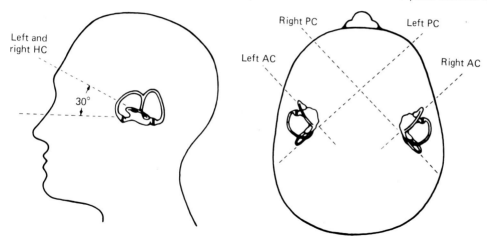

Figure 4.3 Planes of individual semicircular canals: HC = horizontal semicircular canal, AC = anterior semicircular canal and PC = posterior semicircular canal. (From Barber, H. O. and Stockwell, C. W., *Manual of Electronystagmography*, the C. V. Mosby Company, St Louis, 1976, p. 26, with permission)

techniques of studying subcortical reflex activity and the currently fashionable technique of mathematical modelling.

Peripheral vestibular apparatus

The ear may be divided into an external, middle and inner portion, which, with the exception of the auricle and soft tissue portion of the auditory canal, lie in the temporal bone of the skull (*Figure 4.2*). The temporal bone may be divided into four portions: the squamous, mastoid, petrous and tympanic segments. The *labyrinth* lies in the petrous portion, or pyramid, and consists of three chambers: the anterior bony cochlea; the vestibule, which is in a small oval chamber between the medial wall of the middle ear and the lateral part of the internal auditory canal; and a posterior vestibular chamber. Three bony semicircular canals open superiorly and posterolaterally into this latter chamber by means of five round apertures. The two vertical canals (the superior and posterior canals) join posteriorly to form a single crus commune. Clinically, it is of importance that the canals lie approximately at right angles to each other (Curthoys, Blanks and Markham, 1977), and that, in the erect position of the head, the horizontal canals slope downwards and backwards at an angle of 30° to the horizontal (*Figure 4.3*).

The *membranous labyrinth* is surrounded by perilymph and is suspended by fine connective tissue strands from the bony labyrinth. It consists of an anterior chamber, the cochlear duct, which subserves hearing, and which connects, by way of the round saccule, with the posterior vestibular

apparatus. This consists of the utricle and semi-circular canals (*Figure 4.4*). The three semicircular canals are small ring-like structures, each forming two-thirds of a circle, with a diameter of 6.5 mm and a cross-sectional diameter of 0.4 mm. One end of each canal is dilated and known as the ampulla, which completely fills the corresponding expansion of the bony canal. The membranous labyrinth forms a separate fluid compartment of *endolymph*, which is probably produced by the secretory cells of the stria vascularis of the cochlea and the dark cells of the vestibular labyrinth (Kimura, 1969). In common with all intracellular body fluids, endolymph has a high potassium and low sodium concentration, unlike perilymph which resembles extracellular fluid. The current hypothesis is that perilymph is a filtration product of the cerebro-spinal fluid or blood or possibly both (Silverstein,

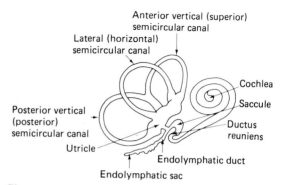

Figure 4.4 Diagram of membranous labyrinth. (From Ballantyne, J., Anatomy of the ear in *Scott-Brown's Diseases of the Ear, Nose and Throat*, Vol. 1, *Basic Sciences*, eds J. Ballantyne and J. Groves. Butterworths, London, 1979, p. 27, with permission)

1966; Kimura, Schuknecht and Ota, 1974). In spite of much research into the chemical composition of the inner ear fluids, the latter remain ill defined (O'Connor *et al.*, 1982).

Five *vestibular receptor organs* lie within the membranous labyrinth and may be divided into the two maculae of the otolith organs (utricle and saccule), which monitor linear acceleration, and the three cristae ampullares of the semicircular canals, which monitor angular acceleration (*Figure 4.5*).

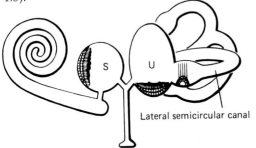

Lateral semicircular canal

Figure 4.5 Schematic drawing of the inner ear: S = saccule, U = utricle. (From Frenzel, H. In *Spontan-und Provokations-Nystagmus als Krankheitssymptom*, Springer Verlag, Berlin, 1955, with permission)

Each *macula* is a small area of sensory epithelium (less than 1 mm^2), which is found on the floor of the utricle in the horizontal plane, and on the medial wall of the saccule in the vertical plane. The macula supports a statoconial membrane (*Figure 4.6*), consisting of small calcium carbonate crystals (otoconia) embedded in a mucopolysaccharide gel

(Lindeman, 1969a). The position of the statoconial membrane, relative to the sensory epithelium, varies according to the magnitude and direction of the force acting upon it (De Vries, 1950); and the shearing force between the two structures results in the bending of the hairs of the hair cells embedded in the statoconial membrane (*Figure 4.7*). As early as 1874, Breuer postulated the mechanism by which the otolith organs sense linear acceleration. Recent studies (Fernandez and Goldberg, 1976) have confirmed the responsiveness of the maculae to static tilt and linear acceleration, and have estimated the sensitivity of the mammalian otolith organ to be 0.5 µm/g, thereby underlining the exquisite mechanical sensitivity of the otolith organs.

The receptor organ of the semicircular canals is the *crista ampullaris*, a crest of sensory epithelium supported on a mound of connective tissue and lying at right angles to the longitudinal axis of the canal (*see Figure 4.6*) (Wersall, 1956). The crista is surmounted by a bulbous gelatinous mass, the *cupula*, which extends from the surface of the crista to the ceiling of the ampulla, forming a watertight, swing-door seal (Igarishi, 1966). The specific gravity of the cupula is the same as that of the endolymph; therefore, unlike the statoconial membrane of the maculae, the cupula does not exert a resting force on the underlying sensory epithelium.

The semicircular canal system is sensitive to angular acceleration of the head. As the head is rotated, the endolymph within the duct tends to remain stationary in space because of its inherent

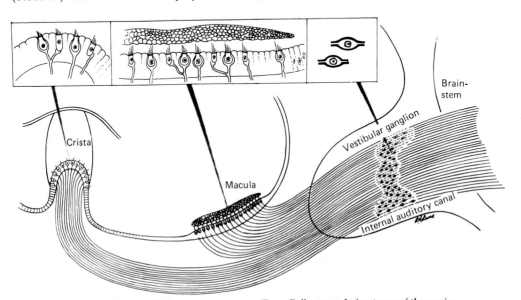

Crista

Macula

Vestibular ganglion

Internal auditory canal

Brain-stem

Figure 4.6 Diagram of the vestibular receptor organs. (From Ballantyne, J. Anatomy of the ear in *Scott-Brown's Diseases of the Ear, Nose and Throat*, Vol. 1 *Basic Sciences*, Eds J. Ballantyne and J. Groves, Butterworths, London, 1979, p. 29, with permission)

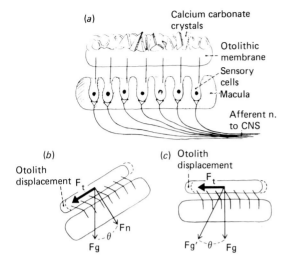

Figure 4.7 Illustration of the anatomy of the macula (*a*) and the distribution of forces associated with static head tilt (*b*) and linear acceleration tangential to the surface (*c*). (From Baloh, R. W. and Honrubia, V., *Clinical Neurophysiology of the Vestibular System*, F. A. Davis and Company, Philadelphia, 1979, p. 2, with permission)

inertia. The resultant flow of endolymph, with respect to the duct, is resisted by the elasticity of the gelatinous cupula, which becomes deflected, resulting in the bending of the hairs of the sensory hair cells (*Figure 4.8*). The function of the semicircular canal system was first established by Flourens in 1842, but it was Ewald's elegant experiments in 1892 that began to clarify vestibular

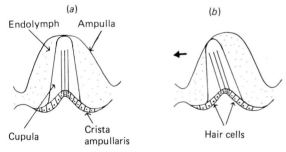

Figure 4.8 Diagram of cupula dynamics: (*a*) resting position and (*b*) swing door movement of cupula secondary to angular acceleration

physiology. Ewald attached a cannula to the lateral semicircular canal of the pigeon, thereupon producing head and eye movements in response to changes in pressure. Three major observations were made, which have become known as *Ewald's laws*:

(1) head and eye movements always occur in the plane of the canal being stimulated and in the direction of the endolymph flow

(2) in the horizontal canal, ampullopetal endolymph flow causes a greater response than ampullofugal flow
(3) in the vertical canals, ampullofugal endolymph flow causes a greater response than ampullopetal flow.

Recent work, which has more clearly delineated the anatomy and physiology of the vestibular sensory epithelium, has promoted an understanding of these three observations.

The vestibular sensory epithelium of the five receptor organs contains three basic components:

(1) sensory cells with hairs on their free surface
(2) supporting cells, which secrete a gelatinous substance

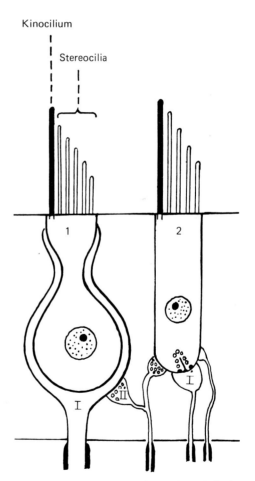

Figure 4.9 Diagram of type I and type II vestibular hair cells and their afferent and efferent connections. (From Wersall, J., Gleisner, L. and Lundquist, P. G. in *Symposium on Myotatic, Kinaesthetic and Vestibular Mechanisms*, J. A. Churchill, London, 1967, p. 110, with permission)

(3) the aforementioned substance, which is composed mainly of mucopolysaccharides, and into which the hairs of the hair cells are embedded.

The sensory cells themselves are of two types (*Figure 4.9*): *type I* are flask shaped and surrounded by a single, large challice-like nerve terminal, which is thought to be afferent in function; *type II* are cylindrical with multiple, button nerve terminals at their base, which are thought to subserve efferent function.

The hairs projecting from the free surface of the sensory cells are also of two types. Each cell has a single thick and long *kinocilium*, with 50–110 thin *stereocilia* (Spoendlin, 1964). The stereocilia are graded in height, with the shortest being at the most distant point to the kinocilium (*see Figure 4.9*). The kinocilium projects from the cell cytoplasm, through a segment of cell membrane, lacking the cuticular plate, and is anchored to the cell by the basal body, which closely resembles the centriole. The stereocilia of the cristae, projecting into the cupulae, are up to 36 μm in length, whereas the stereocilia of the maculae are shorter, being only a few micrometres in length.

As outlined previously, forces of acceleration cause the bending of the hairs of the receptor cells, and this bending, which is proportional to the force applied, results in the transduction of mechanical energy into neural activity. The maximal stimulus is a force parallel to the surface of the sensory epithelium, which bisects the bundle of stereocilia and passes directly through the kinocilium (von Békésy, 1966), while a force

perpendicular to the epithelial surface is ineffective in stimulating the hair cells (Fernandez and Goldberg, 1976). The exact mechanism of transduction has not been established although various hypotheses have been proposed (Malcolm, 1974; Goldberg and Fernandez, 1975). By extrapolation from cochlear mechanics (Honrubia, Strelioff and Sitko, 1976), it has been hypothesized that the bending of the hairs of the vestibular sensory cell results in the mechanical deformation of the hair-bearing surface of the hair cell, thereby altering the electrical conductance of the cell and allowing excitation. It has been documented that deflection of the hairs towards the kinocilium decreases the resting membrane potential of the sensory cells (depolarization), with an increase in the firing rate of action potentials in the vestibular nerve, while bending in the opposite direction, that is away from the kinocilium, produces the reverse effect (hyperpolarization) and a decrease in the resting activity in the primary afferent vestibular fibres (*Figure 4.10*) (Flock, Jorgenson and Russell, 1973).

In 1932, Hoagland made a fundamental discovery by identifying the continuous and spontaneous neural activity generated by lateral line organs. Although the mechanism of generation of this spontaneous activity remains unidentified, there is now a clear understanding of the modulation of this activity in response to movement. The recording of action potentials within the primary afferent fibres innervating the cupula has provided a direct method of measuring cupula endolymph dynamics and has enabled the effect

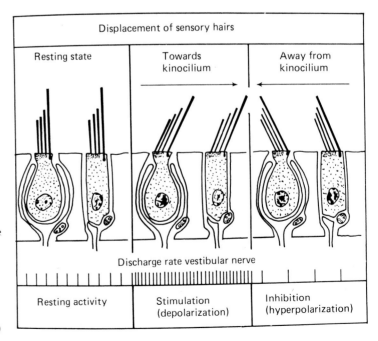

Figure 4.10 Schematic illustration of the relationship between hair cell orientation and the pattern of stimulation of the innervating fibres in the mammalian crista. (From Wersall, J., Gleisner, L. and Lundquist, P. G. in *Symposium on Myotatic, Kinaesthetic and Vestibular Mechanisms*, J. A. Churchill, London, 1967, p. 109, with permission)

of both static (Lowenstein and Roberts, 1950; Vidal *et al.*, 1971; Fernandez, Goldberg and Abend, 1972; Loe, Tomko and Werner, 1973) and dynamic stimuli (Lowenstein and Saunders, 1975; Fernandez and Goldberg, 1976) in the otolith organ to be investigated. In squirrel monkeys, the average resting discharge rate of both saccular and utricular units is approximately 65 spikes per second, while a higher rate of 70–90 spikes per second is recorded from the cristae. Studies of both the cristae (Fernandez and Goldberg, 1971) and the otolith organs (Fernandez and Goldberg, 1976) have demonstrated that some neurons have a regular spontaneous firing rate, while others have an irregular rate. The significance of this is not yet defined.

Anatomically, the polarization pattern for each of the sensory organs of the vestibular apparatus has been described (Lindeman, 1969b). The kinocilia of the sensory cells are orientated towards the utricle in the horizontal canal, whereas they are directed away from the utricle in the vertical canals (*Figure 4.11*). The magnitude of cupular deflection is precisely reflected by changes in the rate of discharge of neural impulses in the afferent fibres. A bidirectional response, with a slightly higher gain in the excitatory response, has

been documented in all vestibular sensory receptors. The different polarization patterns for the horizontal and vertical semicircular canals and the differential modulation of resting neural activity consequent upon utriculopetal or utriculofugal displacement of the hairs of the hair cells, provide an explanation of Ewald's second and third laws.

The maculae differ from the cristae in that the kinocilia within each organ are not uniformly orientated. A curved line, the *striola*, divides each macula into a medial and lateral zone, in each of which the kinocilia are orientated in opposite directions (*Figure 4.12*). In the macula utriculae, the kinocilia are orientated towards the striola, while on the macula sacculae the pattern is similar, although geometrically more complex, and the

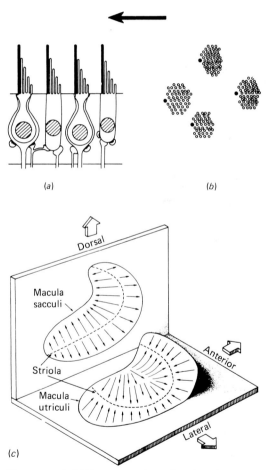

Figure 4.12 (*a,b*) Diagrams to show direction of orientation of kinocilia and (*c*) diagram to illustrate the position of the saccular and utricular macules; arrows indicate the directiton of hair cell polarization on each side of the striola. (From Barber, H. O. and Stockwell, C. W., *Manual of Electronystagmography*, the C. V. Mosby Company, St Louis, 1976, p. 31, with permission)

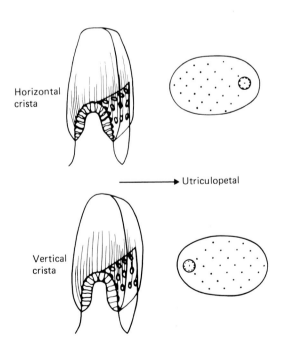

Figure 4.11 Diagram to show the orientation of the kinocilium and stereocilia of the sensory epithelium of the cristae of the semicircular canals. (From Spoendlin, H. H., Uber die Polarisation der Vestibularen Rezeptoren, *Practica Otorhinolaryngologica*, Vol. 26, pp. 418–432, 1964, with permission)

kinocilia are orientated away from the striola. Thus, displacement of either otolithic membrane in a particular direction produces an opposite physiological response from the hair cells on either side of the striola. It has been postulated (Benson and Barnes, 1973) that the signals from the hair cells are integrated spatially, so that information is provided with respect to both fore-and-aft and lateral acceleration of the head. This hypothesis is supported by the eye movements resulting from electrical stimulation of the otoliths (Fluur and Mellstrom, 1971). The combined polarization vectors of neurons over both maculae cover all possible positions of head in three-dimensional space.

A fine unmyelinated plexus of nerve fibres is found within the sensory epithelium. Type I fibres end in a nerve challice, each surrounding a type I hair cell, and are probably afferent in function, while type II fibres are richly granular, ending as button terminals on type II hair cells, and are probably efferent in function. From this plexus arise myelinated fibres, which pass to the large bipolar cells (the primary vestibular neurons) of *Scarpa's ganglion* in the internal auditory meatus. Scarpa's ganglion (*Figure 4.13*) may be divided into a superior portion, which innervates the cristae of the superior vertical and lateral semicircular

canals, the utricular macula and a small antero-superior portion of the saccular macula, and an inferior portion, which innervates the major part of the saccular macula and the posterior vertical canal (Gacek, 1968). The superior portion of the ganglion gives rise to large fibres, which occupy a central position within the ampullary nerves and terminate as the large challice endings of type I hair cells on the crest of cristae. The inferior portion gives rise to smaller fibres, which end in buttons on type II hair cells and are more numerous on the slopes of cristae (Sando, Black and Hemenway, 1972; O'Leary *et al.*, 1974).

The specific peripheral and central connections of the large and small nerve fibres suggest a different, but as yet unknown, functional role for each of the two types of vestibular hair cell.

The central processes of the primary vestibular neurons form an ascending branch, which synapses superiorly in the vestibular nuclei or cerebellum, and a descending branch, which synapses on the more inferior vestibular nuclei (Brodal, 1974).

An efferent supply to the vestibular sensory epithelium arises bilaterally from the area of the sixth nerve nucleus and adjacent to the ipsilateral, lateral and medial vestibular nuclei (Gacek and Lyon, 1974). The fibres emerge from the brain-

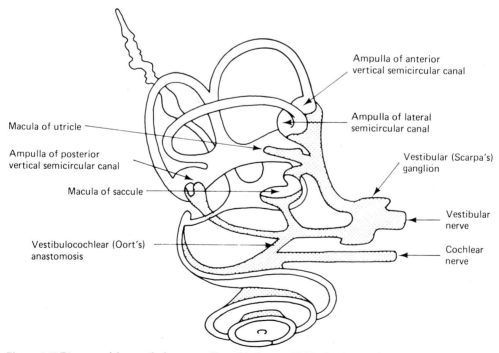

Figure 4.13 Diagram of the vestibular nerve. (From Lindeman, H. H., Studies on the morphology of the sensory regions of the vestibular apparatus, *Advances in Anatomy Embryology and Cell Biology*, Vol. 42, Springer Verlag, Berlin, 1969, with permission)

stem in the olivocochlear bundle and pass to the various components of the vestibular nerve, whereupon the cochlear division separates. Synapses are formed with both type I and type II hair cells.

Central vestibular connections

The vestibular nuclei lie on the floor of the fourth ventricle (Brodal, 1974). Four groups of cell bodies (the second order vestibular neurons) may be identified: the superior nucleus, the lateral nucleus of Dieter, the medial nucleus of Schwalbe, and the descending, or spinal, vestibular nucleus. There are a number of smaller groups of cells which are closely related anatomically to the major nuclei, but they have distinct morphological characteristics and anatomical connections. The majority of afferent fibres, from the receptor areas of the vestibular apparatus, terminate in the vestibular nuclei. A few neurons receive primary vestibular afferents alone but, with the exception of the neurons of the interstitial nucleus, the majority also receive afferents from the cerebellum, reticular formation, spinal cord and contralateral vestibular nuclei. Before neuronal impulses arriving in the vestibular nuclei are transmitted further, they pass at least one synapse and thus may be modified by impulses entering the nuclei from other sources. It is at the level of the vestibular nuclei that labyrinthine information is integrated with information from other somatosensory systems.

The activity of neurons within the vestibular nuclei, during vestibular stimulation, has been investigated for canal-dependent units (Shimazu and Precht, 1965; Fuchs and Kimm, 1975; Schneider and Anderson, 1976) and for otolith-dependent units (Milsum and Melvill-Jones, 1967; Peterson, 1970). Electrophysiological studies have identified two groups of neurons: one group which is monosynaptically innervated and a second group which is multisynaptically activated (Precht and Shimazu, 1965). Approximately 75% of the neurons of the vestibular nuclei receive innervation from the vestibular system, but only half of these are monosynaptically activated. Monosynaptic connections appear to be ipsilateral and excitatory, whereas neurons receiving multisynaptic input are frequently activated by contralateral vestibular nerve stimulation. It is worth noting that the largest afferent supply to the vestibular nuclei arises in the cerebellum (Brodal, 1974). The exact afferent connections to, and projections from, the vestibular nuclei have not been totally identified, but the following generalizations may be made.

Afferent input

See Figure 4.14a.

(1) Superior vestibular nucleus: cristae of the semicircular canal and cerebellum
(2) lateral vestibular nucleus: cerebellum and macula utriculae (a few spinal and commissural afferent fibres)
(3) medial vestibular nucleus: cristae and cerebellum (a few fibres from the reticular formation and the macula utriculae)
(4) descending vestibular nucleus: utricular and saccular maculae (a small supply from cristae and cerebellar afferent).

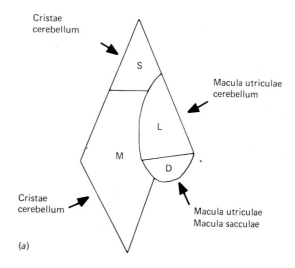

(a)

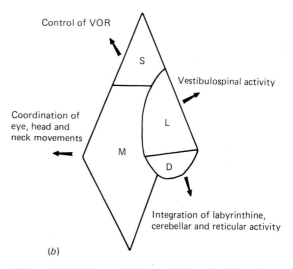

(b)

Figure 4.14 (*a*) Diagram to illustrate the main afferent inputs to each vestibular nucleus. (*b*) Diagram to illustrate the primary output of each vestibular nucleus

Efferent activity

The efferent activity of the vestibular nuclei reflects the integrated and modulated activity from a number of different afferent inputs (Brodal,

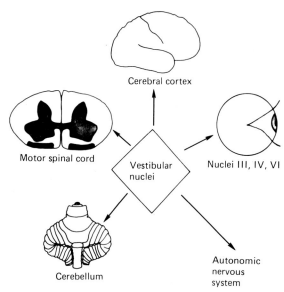

Figure 4.15 Diagram to illustrate the main efferent pathways of the vestibular nuclei

1974). The vestibular nuclei connect with five main systems (*Figure 4.15*):

(1) the oculomotor nuclei, by way of the median longitudinal fasciculus and multisynaptic connections in the reticular formation
(2) the motor part of the spinal cord, by way of the reticulospinal pathways and vestibulospinal pathways, and inferior part of the median longitudinal fasciculus
(3) the cerebellum
(4) the autonomic nervous system
(5) the cerebral cortex in the temporal lobe, by way of multisynaptic pathways.

It is now well established that, in addition to these five main efferent connections, there are important commissural connections between the vestibular nuclei on either side of the brainstem. No primary vestibular afferent crosses the midline, and all commissural connections, therefore, arise from second or higher order neurons. Shimazu and Precht (1966) initially documented the inhibitory effects, arising from the vestibular nuclei on one side of the brainstem, on the contralateral vestibular nuclei. Other commissural connections pass through the cerebellum (Furuya, Kawano and Shimazu, 1976). Physiologically, the existence of commissural, inhibitory connections

from one horizontal canal to another enhances the sensitivity of the vestibular system (Markham, Yagi and Curthoys, 1977). Such connections are also of clinical importance in certain forms of nystagmus, for example periodic alternating nystagmus, and, in a compensatory capacity, following a unilateral vestibular disturbance.

Apart from the anatomical considerations, each of the vestibular nuclei has a separate functional efferent role (*Figure 4.14b*). From the superior nucleus, fibres run predominantly to the median longitudinal fasciculus to innervate the motor nuclei of the extrinsic eye muscles, and this nucleus is, therefore, particularly important in the control of semicircular canal–ocular reflexes. The lateral nucleus is primarily involved in vestibulospinal activity; while the medial nucleus, as a result of projections in the median longitudinal bundle to both the oculomotor nuclei and the cervical cord, is of importance in coordinating eye, head and neck movements. Other efferents from this nucleus run to the vestibulocerebellum, the reticular formation and the contralateral vestibular nuclei. The descending vestibular nucleus sends fibres mainly to the cerebellum and the reticular formation. In addition, numerous commissural fibres supply the contalateral ascending medial and lateral nuclei.

The subjective awareness of motion is subserved by *vestibulocortical projections*, which were first identified electrophysiologically by Watzle and Mountcastle (1949), who identified monophasic potentials in the suprasylvian gyrus, following electrical stimulation of the contralateral vestibular nerve. In the human being, electrical stimulation of both the superior sylvian gyrus and the inferior intraparietal sulcus produces subjective sensations of rotation, or bodily displacement (Penfield, 1957). Studies in the cat and the squirrel monkey have demonstrated projections from the vestibular nuclei to the thalamus, and thence to the sensory motor cortex (Liedgren *et al.*, 1976; Liedgren and Rubin, 1976). Functionally, the vestibulothalamocortical projections allow some integration of labyrinthine and somatic proprioceptive signals, and thus facilitate conscious awareness of body orientation.

The threshold of subjective appreciation of angular acceleration is in the range of $0.1–0.5\,\text{deg/s}^2$ (Clark, 1967). Early tests of vestibular function attempted to correlate the threshold and magnitude of subjective sensation with the magnitude of angular acceleration. Van Egmond, Groen and Jongkees (1948) popularized the technique of cupulometry, in which a subject is rotated, at a constant velocity, and then suddenly stopped. The durations of 'after-turning sensation' and induced nystagmus are measured for impulses of different amplitude, usually 15–60 deg/s. The average sensation and nystagmus cupulogram for 15 or more subjects is shown in *Figure 4.16*. It is obvious that the average slope of the sensation cupulogram differs from that of the nystagmus cupulogram, although both are derived from a single cupular deflection from a given stimulus. This apparent discrepancy is almost certainly the result of the central nervous system altering in some way the stimulus–response relationship (Guedry, 1974). It is of importance that the central pathways which subserve subjective sensation and nystagmus are different, although they are both dependent upon the same input.

Otolith stimulation allows perception of linear movement in both the horizontal plane and tilt. Horizontal linear oscillation results in the perception of both types of motion. At low amplitudes of oscillation, the subject perceives motion, without specific direction. Increasing intensities of stimulation result in the perception of direction of linear movement and, at still higher intensities, a

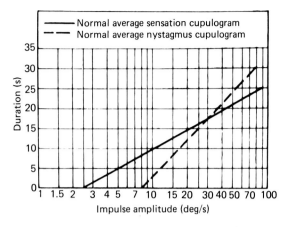

Figure 4.16 The average nystagmus and sensation cupulogram in 15 subjects. (From Van Egmond, A. A. J., Groen, J. J. and Jongkees, L. B. W., The turning test with small regulable stimuli, *Journal of Laryngology and Otology*, Vol. 62, pp. 63–69, 1948, with permission)

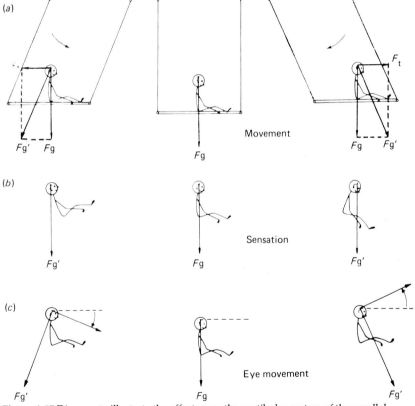

Figure 4.17 Diagram to illustrate the effect upon the vestibular system of the parallel swing. (*a*) Distribution of forces; (*b*) subjective sensation; (*c*) compensatory eye movements at different swing positions. Curved arrows indicate direction of acceleration. (From Baloh, R. W. and Honrubia, V., *Clinical Neurophysiology of the Vestibular System*, F. A. Davis, Philadelphia, 1979, p. 68; adapted from Jongkees, L. B. W., Pathology of vestibular sensation. In *Handbook of Sensory Physiology*, Ed. H. H. Kornhuber, Vol. VI, Part 2, Springer Verlag, New York, 1974, with permission)

perception of tilting. An explanation of this is given in *Figure 4.17*. When the swing is accelerating forwards (upper left), Ft/Fg interact to produce a resulting force Fg', which is perceived as the true earth vertical. The otolith organs respond by producing a compensatory eye movement, such that the nervous system perceives an angle of tilt proportional to Ft, whether or not the body is actually tilting.

Static tilt experiments (Clark, 1970; Graybiel, 1974), in which subjects are strapped to a tilt platform, in total darkness, and either estimate the deviation of the head from the earth's vertical or adjust a luminous line on a dark field to a vertical position, have shown that, up to 40°, normal subjects can perceive as little as 2–4° of tilt. The estimated angle of tilt is altered under different gravitational forces, and in experiments carried out in space, at 'zero g', subjects are unable to perceive tilt.

Having defined the basic vestibular pathways and function at each level of the vestibular system, it is now appropriate to consider the applied physiology of the vestibular system. For practical purposes, vestibular reflexes are most easily considered in terms of vestibulo-ocular activity and vestibulospinal activity (*Figure 4.18*).

Vestibulo-ocular reflex

Semicircular canal–ocular reflex

The vestibulo-ocular reflex represents one mechanism by means of which humans stabilize gaze, and the clinical measurement of the oculomotor response to precise vestibular stimuli, mediated through the semicircular canal–ocular reflex, enables quantification of labyrinthine function to be made.

The vestibulo-ocular reflex provides a simple example of a reflex arc, comprising the vestibular receptor, primary, secondary and tertiary neurons and the effector organ, the oculomotor muscle (Szentagothai, 1950). The connections between the individual semicircular canals and the extraocular muscles have been precisely defined by animal experiments, involving stimulation and ablation of individual semicircular canals (Lorente de No, 1933; Fluur, 1959; Cohen, Suzuki and Bender, 1964) (*Figure 4.19*). Under physiological circumstances, any angular acceleration produces an exact mirror image of events occurring simultaneously in opposite labyrinths. Each utriculopetal stimulus in one labyrinth is matched by an equal, but opposite, utriculofugal displacement in the functionally paired canal of the other ear. In this push–pull arrangement, the lateral canals

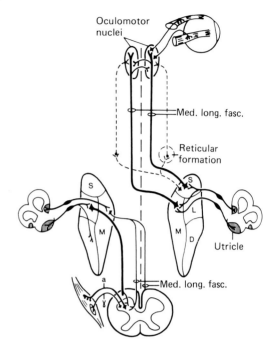

Figure 4.18 Simplified diagram of two reflex arcs involving the vestibular nuclei. S, D, L and M = superior, descending, lateral and medial vestibular nucleus, respectively. (From Brodal, A., *Neurological Anatomy in Relation to Clinical Medicine,* 3rd edn, Oxford University Press, New York, 1981, p. 482, with permission)

form one pair, while the posterior canal, because of its anatomical disposition, is parallel to, and therefore paired with, the opposite superior canal. The difference in input to the vestibular nuclei from the left and right labyrinths is the basis of the vestibular response and mediates all labyrinthine reflexes.

With regard to angular acceleration to the right in the plane of the horizontal canals (*Figure 4.20*), endolymph displacement occurs in the direction opposite to that of rotation, that is leftwards. Accordingly, utriculopetal deviation of the cupula of the right horizontal canal occurs with utriculofugal movement of the cupula of the left horizontal canal. This results in an increase in the firing rate of the right afferent ampullary nerve, with an equal, but opposite, response in the left vestibular nerve, that is a decrease in the neural activity. Thus the afferent information coming from the right ampullary nerve exerts an excitatory influence on the agonist muscles and an inhibitory influence on the antagonist muscles, while the response from the left ampullary nerve reduces the excitatory influence on the antagonist muscles and disinhibits the agonist muscles. As shown in

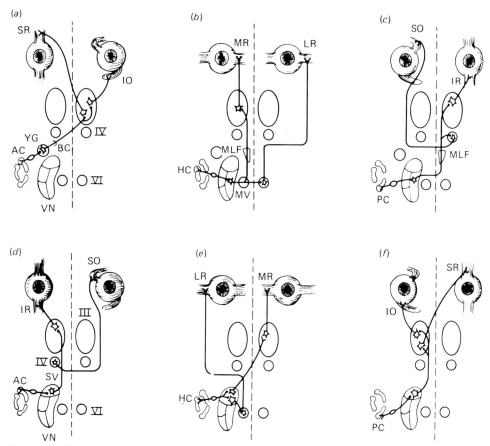

Figure 4.19 Exitatory (*a,b,c*) and inhibitory (*d,e,f*) pathways between the individual semicircular canals and eye muscles. SR, superior rectus; IO, inferior oblique; MR, medial rectus; LR, lateral rectus; SO, superior oblique; IR, inferior rectus; AC, anterior canal; HC, horizontal canal; PC, posterior canal; VN, vestibular nuclei; YG, satellite vestibular nucleus; SV, superior vestibular nucleus; MV, medial vestibular nucleus; BC, brachium conjunctivum; VI, abducens nucleus; IV, trochlear nucleus; III, oculomotor complex. (From Baloh, R. W. and Honrubia, V. (1979) *Clinical Neurophysiology of the Vestibular System,* p. 57; as adapted from Ito, M., The vestibulocerebellar relationships: vestibulo-ocular reflex arc and flocculus, In *The Vestibular System,* Ed. R. F. Naunton, Academic Press, New York, 1975, with permission)

Figure 4.21, this results in contraction of the left lateral rectus and the right medial rectus muscles, with relaxation of the left medial rectus and the right lateral rectus muscles, producing deviation of the eyes to the left.

If a small rotational head movement is made, a slow compensatory eye movement occurs in the opposite direction to the rotation. If a larger stimulus is applied, such that a compensatory eye movement cannot be contained within the confines of the orbit, the slow vestibular-induced eye deviation is interrupted by a fast eye movement, in the opposite direction. This combination of alternating slow and fast movements in opposite directions is called *nystagmus.*

The slow phase of the response is generated by the vestibular nuclei of the opposite side of the brainstem, as outlined previously, and the fast phase is an involuntary saccadic eye movement, which is generated as a result of the activity of neurons in the ipsilateral, parapontine reticular formation (Raphan and Cohen, 1978). The exact mechanism by means of which these saccades are generated is unclear, but it would appear that the nuclei of the parapontine reticular formation continuously 'monitor' vestibulo-ocular signals and intermittently discharge to produce corrective saccades. For clinical purposes, the direction of the nystagmus is defined by the direction of the fast phase.

Spontaneous nystagmus may be physiological or pathological in origin. *Physiological nystagmus* refers to end-point nystagmus, when the eyes are deviated more than 30° from the midposition of

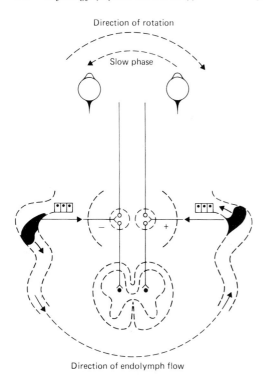

Figure 4.20 Diagram to illustrate the effect of angular acceleration in a clockwise direction. There is utriculopetal deviation of the cupula of the right horizontal ampulla and an increase in the activity of the corresponding ampullary nerve. In the left horizontal canal the cupula moves utriculofugally causing a decrease in the activity of the nerve. (From Henriksson, N. G., Pfaltz, C. R., Torok, N. and Rubin, W. in *A Synopsis of the Vestibular System*, The Barany Society, 1972, p. 12, by kind permission of Dr Nils Henriksson)

optic fixation (Hood, 1968), by other sensory stimuli, for example auditory, tactile or cervical information (Baloh and Honrubia, 1979), by age (Tibbling, 1969), and by drugs, for example anticonvulsants, (Nozue, Mizuno and Kaga, 1973). A prolonged constant stimulus to the semicircular canal system results in a slow decline in the firing rate of the afferent nerves, known as 'adaptation'. This phenomenon is transient, and should not be confused with 'habituation', which refers to a reduction in vestibular response following repeated stimulation (Collins, 1974b), as, for example, is observed in ice-skaters and dancers, who are subjected to repeated angular accelerations. The mechanism of habituation is unknown, but is undoubtedly related to visual suppression of the vestibular response (*Figure 4.22*), and the phenomenon may persist for a number of weeks.

Spontaneous vestibular nystagmus obeys Alexander's law, which states that nystagmus is maximal in the direction of the fast phase. Thus nystagmus to the right is most obvious with eyes to the right,

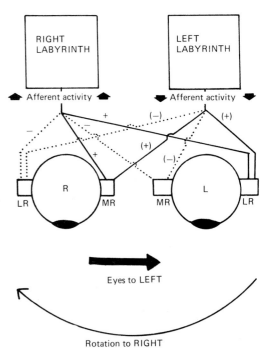

Figure 4.21 Diagram to illustrate the bilateral reciprocal arrangement of the semicircular canal–ocular reflex. Key: +, exitation; −, inhibition; (+), disinhibition; (−), disfacilitation; LR, lateral rectus muscle; MR, medial rectus muscle; R,L, right and left, respectively. (From Luxon, L. M., The anatomy and physiology of the vestibular system, in *Vertigo*, Eds. M. R. Dix and J. D. Hood, John Wiley and Sons, Chichester, 1984, p. 24, with permission)

gaze, induced (caloric or rotational) nystagmus and optokinetic nystagmus (*see below*). *Pathological nystagmus* implies an underlying abnormality and may be divided into congenital and acquired varieties. Acquired nystagmus may be further subdivided into spontaneous vestibular nystagmus, positional nystagmus, gaze paretic nystagmus, of which there are a number of varieties, and dissociated nystagmus. Spontaneous vestibular nystagmus results from an imbalance of afferent vestibular information, which may arise as a consequence of pathology at the level of the labyrinth, the vestibular nerve or the vestibular nuclei. If the lesion is small, or central compensation has occurred, spontaneous nystagmus may not be directly observed, but may be revealed as a directional preponderance upon inducing nystagmus, with caloric or rotational stimuli.

The nystagmic response may be modified by the degree of mental alertness (Collins, 1974a), by

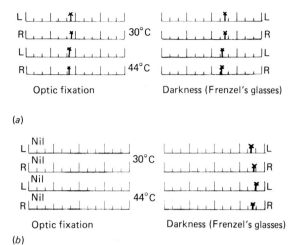

(a)

(b)

Figure 4.22 Diagram to illustrate the marked affect of optic fixation in a subject with vestibular habituation (*b*) compared with a normal subject (*a*), as demonstrated on caloric testing

less obvious with eyes in the primary position of gaze, and least obvious with eyes to the left. For the purposes of definition, nystagmus which is observable only in the direction of gaze of the fast component is defined as 'first degree nystagmus'; nystagmus which is observable with eyes in the primary position of gaze is defined as 'second degree nystagmus'; and nystagmus which is detectable with the eyes in the opposite direction to the fast component is defined as 'third degree nystagmus'. In general terms, second degree vestibular nystagmus is found only in the presence of first degree nystagmus, and third degree vestibular nystagmus is observed in the presence of first and second degree nystagmus. Furthermore, the amplitude and slow phase of first degree nystagmus is usually greater than second degree nystagmus and, similarly, second degree nystagmus is greater than third degree nystagmus. It should be emphasized, however, that these generalizations do not apply to nystagmus which is of central nervous system origin.

Spontaneous horizontal vestibular nystagmus may result from a labyrinthine, eighth nerve or vestibular nuclei lesion. Labyrinthine and eighth nerve pathology result in nystagmus with the fast component directed towards the affected side, while lesions of the vestibular nuclei may produce spontaneous nystagmus in either direction, depending on the involvement of inhibitory or excitatory pathways. The presence of brainstem signs may suggest a lesion at the level of the vestibular nuclei, but a more helpful point of differention is the effect upon the nystagmus of the removal of optic fixation. Nystagmus arising as

a result of pathology at the level of the labyrinth or eighth nerve is inhibited by optic fixation, whereas nystagmus of vestibular nuclei origin shows a reduction of the slow phase velocity but enhancement of the amplitude of the response (Dix and Hallpike, 1966; Korres, 1978). At the bedside, optic fixation may be abolished with Frenzel's glasses, or the eyes may be observed in total darkness with an infrared viewer.

Horizontal nystagmus of vestibular origin should be differentiated from *gaze paretic nystagmus*, although this differentiation may be difficult on clinical visual inspection alone. Characteristically, there is an exponential drift away from the intended position of gaze, followed by a corrective saccadic movement. Thus, the nystagmus is always observed in the direction of gaze and, as the angle of gaze increases, so the amplitude of nystagmus increases. Furthermore, in the absence of optic fixation, although the amplitude of gaze paretic nystagmus increases, the frequency and slow component velocity decrease. The underlying abnormality is a failure of gaze maintenance, which may be secondary to central nervous system or oculomotor pathology – for example, a brainstem glioma or the myasthenic involvement of the oculomotor muscles (*see below*).

Clinical measurement of the vestibulo-ocular reflex necessitates some consideration of the interaction of vestibularly induced eye movements with eye movements induced by visual and cervical information. The vestibulo-ocular reflex, stimulated by the perception of movement of the head in space, initiates compensatory conjugate ocular movements and provides one mechanism for stabilizing gaze. However, stability of gaze is a complex phenomenon and the relationship between the head and an object in the environment may change in a number of ways: either the head or the object may remain stationary while the other moves, or both may move simultaneously. The interaction between visual, vestibular and cervical information enables a more precise eye movement to be achieved, and thus better ocular stability than would be possible if only one system alone were functioning. Under certain circumstances vestibular and visual signals may conflict; for example, when the head and a visual target are moving at the same velocity, the vestibulo-ocular reflex is suppressed and gaze is maintained on the moving target. The vestibulocerebellum (flocculonodular lobe) is important in mediating visuovestibular interaction (Ito, 1975; Robinson, 1976). Electrophysiological studies have shown that the Purkinje cells of the flocculonodular lobes receive afferent visual and vestibular information, which is 'compared', and efferent information is related back to the vestibular nuclei (Baker, Precht and Llimas, 1973). It is at the level of the vestibular nuclei that the vestibular information is modulated and the 'required' oculomotor activity is generated (Miles, 1974).

There are three visually controlled oculomotor systems which are of clinical importance in terms of their interrelationships with the vestibulo-ocular reflex: the saccadic system, the smooth pursuit system and the optokinetic response.

The saccadic system

The saccadic system generates rapid eye movements (200–600 deg/s, depending on the size of the movement – Robinson, 1964) to both correct errors in the direction of gaze and bring the desired object of fixation to the fovea in the shortest possible time. Saccades may be produced voluntarily, or reflexly, as in the fast phase of nystagmus. Horizontal saccades are initiated by the activity of 'burst' cells in the parapontine reticular formation. This activity is transmitted by way of the median longitudinal bundle to the ipsilateral sixth nerve and the contralateral third nerve nuclei. The eye position is maintained by 'tonic' cells, which continue to fire after the saccadic movement is completed (Cohen and Henn, 1972). In mathematical jargon, the physiological mechanism which produces a saccadic eye movement is termed a 'pulse-step' of information (King, Lisberger and Fuchs, 1976) (*Figure 4.23*). Vertical saccades are generated and maintained in a similar manner by 'burst' and 'tonic' cells in the

pretectal region, through the third nerve complex (Hoyt and Daroff, 1971). Saccadic abnormalities are discussed later, but it may be readily appreciated that if the generation of normal saccades, that is fast phases of nystagmus, is not possible, a normal nystagmic response to vestibular stimulation cannot be obtained.

Smooth pursuit system

The smooth pursuit system subserves a low velocity, accurate, tracking eye movement, which enables a moving target to be stabilized on the fovea (Dodge, 1903). The stimulus is the presence of a moving target across the retina and, in the absence of such a target, pursuit cannot occur. Any attempt to move the eyes at a slow velocity, in the absence of a target, results in a saccade. In man, the smooth pursuit system is most efficient at low target velocities with a gain (eye velocity/target velocity) of approximately 0.95 (Baloh and Honrubia, 1979), but the gain rapidly falls off at target velocities greater than 60 deg/s and frequencies greater than 1 Hz (Young and Stark, 1963). A further point of interest is the comparison of the characteristics of the smooth pursuit system with those of the vestibulo-ocular reflex, which responds effectively to head movements with velocities greater than 100 deg/s and frequencies from 1 to 4 Hz (Baloh, Sills and Honrubia, 1979), but in man there is a gain of only 0.4 during sinusoidal oscillation in the dark at 0.05 Hz, and a maximum

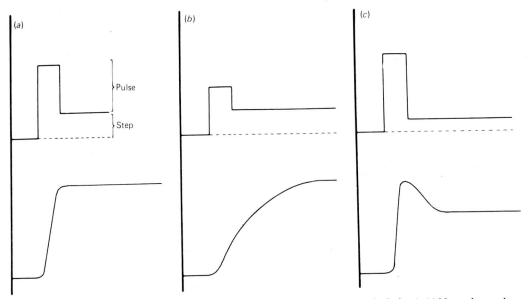

Figure 4.23 Diagram to illustrate the input (above) necessary for a normal saccade (below). (*a*) Normal saccade generation. Pulse and step input matched. (*b*) Type of saccade resulting from deficiency of pulse, that is slow but accurate. (*c*) Type of saccade resulting from deficiency of step, that is fast but not maintained. (From Rudge, P., *Clinical Neuro-otology*, Churchill Livingstone, Edinburgh, 1983, p. 32, with permission)

velocity of 30 deg/s. Thus the vestibulo-ocular reflex and smooth pursuit system are complementary in generating slow eye movements over a broad spectrum of target/head velocities and frequencies. The vestibular system makes possible the production of compensatory eye movements for head movement, and it provides a mechanism for stabilizing the retinal image at velocities or frequencies of head movement at which the visual pursuit system alone would not be capable of controlling eye movements (*Figure 4.24*). However, at the low frequencies of stimulation used in most clinical test procedures, the smooth pursuit system overrides the vestibulo-ocular reflex.

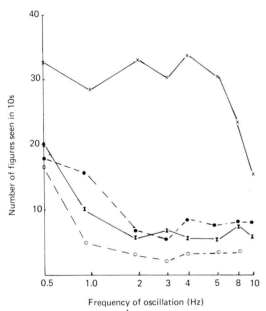

Figure 4.24 Diagram to illustrate leading performance during sinusoidal angular oscillation in yaw of the observer or of the target in eight normal subjects (mean) and a subject without labyrinthine function.
Key: normal – observer oscillation (×); normal – target oscillation (ⵏ); labyrinthine subject–observer oscillation (○); labyrinthine subject–target oscillation (●). (Adapted from Barnes, G. R., Vestibular mechanisms, in *Hearing and Balance in the Elderly*, Ed. R. Hinchcliffe, Churchill Livingstone, Edinburgh, 1983, p. 261, with permission)

The smooth pursuit system is also of particular clinical importance, as it is considered to be intimately related with the mechanism by means of which vestibular responses are suppressed by optic fixation (Lisberger and Fuchs, 1977). The clinical application of suppression of the vestibular responses is of the utmost importance in differentiating peripheral from central vestibular pathology (*see below*).

Optokinetic nystagmus

Optokinetic nystagmus is a reflex oscillation of the eyes, induced by movement of large areas in the visual field. The most common example of this phenomenon can be observed in the jerking eye movements of a train passenger as he views a landscape whose features traverse the field of vision with the motion of the train. In everyday life, the optokinetic response rarely acts independently, but interacts with the vestibulo-ocular reflex during the execution of spontaneous head movements, and with the smooth pursuit system during the visual following of a moving target, for example, a bird in flight. In these situations, the optokinetic stimulation results from the apparent displacement of the surroundings, which is attributable to eye movements induced by the primary response. Clinically, Bárány introduced tests of optokinetic nystagmus, as part of the neuro-otological examination, as early as 1922.

A qualitative assessment of the optokinetic response may be undertaken at the bedside, or in the out-patient department, by using either a hand-held rotating striped drum or a mechanically driven drum, or by moving a piece of striped cloth. For quantitative, diagnostic purposes, more precise and reproducible stimulus parameters are obtained by seating a patient inside a large, striped, rotating drum and stimulating the entire visual field. Alternatively, a moving field of parallel bars, projected on to a surface covering approximately 60° of visual angle, may be used.

Since Bárány's initial work, optokinetic nystagmus has been the subject of a wealth of literature, much of which is contradictory. Confusion has arisen as a result of inadequate consideration of patient and stimulus variables.

In ter Braak's (1936) outstanding work on optokinetic nystagmus, two types of response were identified: first, 'active' or 'look' nystagmus, elicited by attempting to follow, with the eye, a stripe on the surface of the drum as it traversed the visual field; secondly, 'stare' or 'passive' nystagmus, elicited by fixing the eyes on the surface of the drum. The characteristics of the 'active' response are large amplitude eye movements, with slow component velocities almost linearly related to the target velocity, with stimulus magnitude up to 60 deg/s. 'Passive' nystagmus has a much smaller amplitude, is of higher frequency and the slow component velocity falls behind the velocity of the target at speeds in excess of 30 deg/s (*Figure 4.25*).

An explanation of these two forms of response can be found in the consideration of certain experimental and clinical observations. While studying afoveate animals, for example the rabbit, ter Braak observed an optokinetic response to the

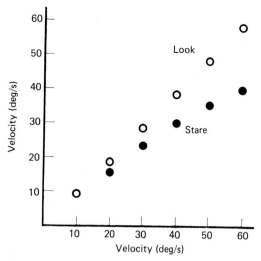

Figure 4.25 Diagram illustrating the velocity (deg/s) of the slow component of optokinetic nystagmus (ordinate) at the indicated velocities (deg/s) of the stimuli used in the test (abscissa) under two test conditions as indicated: look (○) and stare (●) (*see text*). (From Honrubia, V. and Luxon, L. M. in Optokinetic nystagmus with reference to the smooth pursuit function, in *Otoneurology*, Ed. W. J. Oosterveld, John Wiley and Sons Limited, Chichester, 1984, p. 197, with permission)

movement of large objects, such as vertical stripes, which were of no interest to the experimental animal. He further observed a gradual build-up of the slow component velocity of this response, in contrast to the response observed in humans, which reaches a maximum velocity of the slow component in one or two beats. In addition, he documented a marked difference in the optokinetic response between temporonasal and nasotemporal stimulation (the direction reflects the motion of the stimulus as seen by the experimental subject).

Further studies identified a second optokinetic response concerned with the tracking of small objects of interest to the experimental subject, such as pictures of rabbits in the case of a dog. This type of tracking is lost after the removal of the occipital lobes or cerebral hemispheres and would, therefore, appear to be subserved by cortical pathways. Nevertheless, ter Braak (1936) reported one patient who was completely blind from histologically proven infarcts of the occipital lobes, and who, although not able to track small, smoothly moving targets, did respond to stimulation by a full-field optokinetic drum.

On the basis of these observations, ter Braak hypothesized two anatomically separate smooth tracking systems: one subserved by subcortical pathways, which give rise to the 'passive' response observed in afoveate animals and in the

patient with infarcted occipital lobes, and the other subserved by cortical pathways, the 'active' response, which may be equated with smooth pursuit tracking. On the basis of further clinical observations in patients with congenital achromatopsia, glaucoma, cerebellar lesions and parietal lobe dysfunction, Yee and coworkers (1982) have lent support to this hypothesis of a dual system of visuo-ocular reflexes. They have suggested that the 'active' system involves the fovea and the calcarine cortex, while the 'passive' system originates in the peripheral retina and is subserved by the accessory optic tract and the vestibular nuclei, without cerebral cortical participation. It has been postulated that the cortical system is responsible for the production of the smooth pursuit reflex, while the subcortical system subserves the optokinetic response. In the normal course of events, optokinetic stimulation activates both systems and the resultant response is a combination of the reflex function of both pathways. The 'pure' optokinetic reflex is obtained only under special pathological circumstances, when the smooth

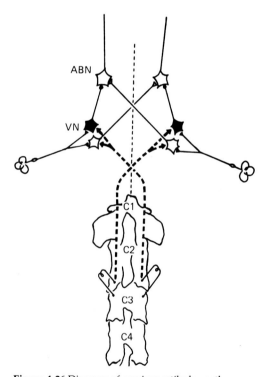

Figure 4.26 Diagram of cervicovestibular pathways. VN = vestibular nucleus; ABN = abducens nucleus; inhibitory interneurons in black. (From Hikosaka, O. and Maeda, M., Cervical effects on abducens motoneurons and their interaction with vestibulo-ocular reflex, *Experimental Brain Research*, Vol. 18, pp. 512–530, 1973, with permission)

pursuit system, which, in general, has precedence over the former, is deranged.

The clinical value of the optokinetic response lies in its ability to distinguish peripheral from central vestibular disorders (*see below*).

Having considered the role of visually induced eye movements and their interaction with vestibular induced eye movements, the role of cervical proprioception in ocular stability must not be overlooked (Bizzi, Kalil and Tagliasco, 1971). In humans, the observation and study of the cervico-ocular reflex has been hampered by the low gain of the system (a body torsion of 50–60°, in respect of the head, results in a compensatory eye deviation of only 4–5° – Takemori and Suzuki, 1971) and the difficulties in avoiding inadvertent vestibular stimulation. Recent work in patients with absent vestibular function has documented an increased gain of the cervico-ocular reflex, compared with normal controls (Bronstein and Hood, personal communication). This suggests that under normal circumstances, the vestibulo-ocular reflex overrides the cervico-ocular reflex, and it is only in the absence of vestibular function that the cervico-ocular reflex may be readily documented in man.

The cervico-ocular reflex is mediated by way of the medial and descending vestibular nuclei, although the pathways have not been fully elucidated (*Figure 4.26*). It is at the level of the vestibular nuclei that cervical proprioception and vestibular information is modulated (Hikosada and Maeda, 1973). The potent effect of the cervico-ocular reflex on the vestibulo-ocular reflex has been clearly demonstrated in rabbits by Baloh and Honrubia (1979) (*Figure 4.27*).

The otolith–ocular reflex

Stimulation of the utricular nerve induces eye movements (Suzuki, Tokumasu and Cohen, 1969), but the otolith control of extraocular muscles has proved more difficult to delineate than semicircular canal relationships. The sensory receptors of the otolith organs are orientated towards many different planes. Hence, any physiological stimulus results in a complex firing pattern of excitation and inhibition of many different units, which cannot be reproduced experimentally. Nevertheless, rotational and torsional compensatory eye movements, produced by static head tilt, are well documented. In humans, countertorsional movements are produced by lateral tilt (ocular counter-

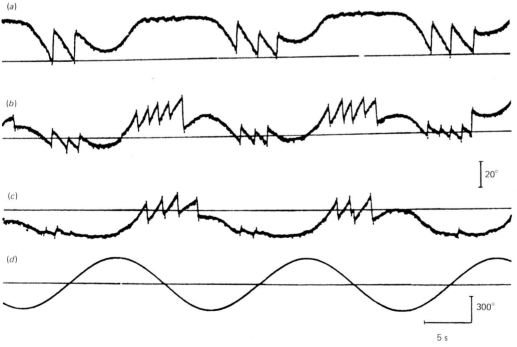

Figure 4.27 Nystagmus induced in a rabbit by sinusoidal angular rotation (*d*) with the head maintained at three orientations with respect to the torso. In (*a*), (*b*) and (*c*) the head is to the left, straight ahead and to the right, respectively. In (*a*) the mean eye position is displaced to the right, and left beating nystagmus is inhibited. The reverse occurs in (*c*). (From Baloh, R. W. and Honrubia, V., *Clinical Neurophysiology and the Vestibular System*, F. A. Davis and Company, 1979, p. 74, with permission)

rolling), while vertical rotation results in forward/backward tilt (Miller, 1962).

Vestibulospinal reflexes

The labyrinth influences posture and orientation through neck, axial and limb motoneurons. However, the influence of vestibular activity on postural muscles is more difficult to define and less clearly understood than the labyrinthine control of eye movements (Anderson, Soechting and Terzuolo, 1979). This can be explained partly by the fact that the vestibular system is only one of many afferent inputs to a complex multisensory orientation control system, and partly by the fact that vestibular activity produces postural change only after it has been 'processed and monitored' in the light of other learned responses. Furthermore, vestibular activity affects neck muscles in a different manner to that of the rest of the somatic musculature. Jones and Milsum (1965) have proposed that the vestibular–neck orientation system may be considered as a closed loop, negative feedback control system, in contrast to the vestibular–limb/torso system where changes in vestibular activity cannot be used directly to detect error or deviations in limb position. Similarly, afferent fibres from the extraocular muscles appear to exert little or no direct effect on the oculomotor response and have no direct representation within the vestibular nuclei. Thus the oculomotor reflex is also essentially an open loop system.

Vestibular information influences spinal anterior horn cell activity by means of three major pathways:

(1) the lateral vestibulospinal tract
(2) the medial vestibulospinal tract
(3) the reticulospinal tract.

The first two arise directly from neurons in the vestibular nuclei, while the reticulospinal tract arises from those neurons in the reticular formation that are influenced by vestibular activity as well as by other sensory inputs. In these three neural pathways, cerebellar activity is integrated with the activity of the vestibular apparatus and the reticular formation, in order to maintain equilibrium and coordinate locomotion (Pompeiano, 1974).

The lateral vestibulospinal tract

The lateral vestibulospinal tract originates primarily from neurons in the lateral vestibular nucleus and there is a clear topographic organization. The anterior/superior region of the nucleus supplies

the cervical cord, while the posterior/inferior region innervates the lumbosacral cord. Intermediate neurons supply the thoracic cord. Along the entire length of the tract, which runs ipsilaterally in the spinal cord, these fibres terminate on the anterior horn cells directly, or indirectly, by way of interneurons.

The lateral vestibulospinal tract fibres synapse with alpha- or gamma-motoneurons, as well as with interneurons in segmental reflex pathways. Direct disynpatic excitatory pathways exist to axial motoneurons, but limb pathways are polysynaptic.

The medial vestibulospinal tract

The medial vestibulospinal tract originates from neurons of the medial vestibular nucleus, and the fibres descend in the median longitudinal bundle. They synapse terminally with interneurons in the cervical cord, and do not appear to form direct connections with the cervical anterior horn cells. This tract is particularly important in cervicovestibulo-ocular reflexes, but is smaller than the lateral vestibulospinal trait or the reticulospinal tract.

The reticulospinal tract

The reticulospinal tract originates from neurons in the bulbar reticular formation, and both crossed and uncrossed fibres traverse the length of the spinal cord in the grey matter. Inhibitory and facilitatory stimuli are transmitted through this tract to the motoneurons throughout the spinal cord, but relatively little is known about the exact neural pathways.

It is well established that alterations in vestibular function may profoundly affect posture (Magnus, 1924); in animal experiments as early as 1892, Ewald was able to demonstrate such changes in posture. He did this by rotating animals on a turntable; when rotation ceased, the animal showed a tendency to fall in the direction of the slow phase of eye movement and head deviation. This tendency was counteracted by a reflex increase in extensor tone in the antigravity muscles of the limb on the side towards which the animal was falling, with a simultaneous reduction of extensor tone in the contralateral limbs. The animal, therefore, maintained its balance. These extremity muscle reflexes are mediated by the semicircular canals and are always appropriate to prevent falling, regardless of the direction of the acceleration force (Roberts, 1967). There is considerable species variation in the extent to which posture is influenced by the canal and otolith systems, with the postural alterations being less marked in the human being than in the cat.

It is of note that vestibulospinal reflexes are mediated in an exactly similar push–pull mechanism between the extensor and flexor muscles (*Figure 4.28*), as outlined previously for the extraocular muscles in the vestibulo-ocular reflex (*see Figure 4.21*).

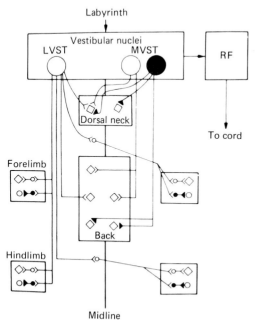

Figure 4.28 Diagram to illustrate connections between labyrinths and postural muscles. RF, reticular formation; ◇, extensor motoneurons; O, flexor motoneurons; O●, interneurons. Filled symbols, inhibitory neurons. (From Wilson, V. J. and Melvill Jones, G. in *Mammalian Vestibular Physiology*, Plenum Press, New York, 1979, p. 227, with permission)

The vestibular apparatus exerts an influence on the control of posture by way of the myotatic reflex (the deep tendon reflex), which is the elementary unit for the control of tone in the trunk and extremity skeletal muscles. Impulses are transmitted to the anterior horn cells of the spinal cord and body posture is maintained through the maculospinal reflex arc (Johanson, 1964). This reflex is under the influence not only of the vestibular system but also of the multiple supraspinal centres, including the basal ganglia, the cerebellum and the reticular formation. The vestibular influence may be demonstrated in animals by the ipsilateral reduction of muscular tone, following unilateral destruction of the labyrinth or the lateral vestibular nucleus (Fulton, Liddell and Rioch, 1930). The effect of tonic labyrinthine reflexes is observed when the brainstem is disconnected from higher neural centres as occurs, for example, when high brainstem tumours are present in man.

Alterations of head position then result in different postures, related to an increase in extensor tone in certain muscles (Magnus, 1924). These tonic labyrinthine reflexes, mediated by way of the otoliths, seldom occur in intact animals or human subjects, because of the inhibitory influence of the higher cortical and subcortical centres.

Much of the vestibular role in the control of posture and equilibrium has yet to be clarified. It is a gross oversimplification to assume that in humans the body acts as a rigid structure, such that tilt from the vertical is compensated only by activity in the limbs. Stabilization is a complex phenomenon and the corrective effects of vestibular function are probably of prime importance for the muscles of the neck. For practical purposes, Roberts (1978) has divided the reflexes which control posture into three categories: positional reflexes, which are 'static postural adjustments adopted when the animal's reference platform is displaced from its normal earth reference'; reflex effects of acceleration on the neck, body and limbs; and righting reflexes, which are considered to be specific combinations of vestibular, neck and limb reflex mechanisms. In man, such mechanisms, although they may be observed in infancy, tend to be overridden or dominated by a higher cerebral function such as vision.

Compensation

Sudden vestibular dysfunction produces a marked asymmetry in the neural activity passing from the labyrinth to the vestibular nuclei. This is perceived as movement and, in consequence, the patient develops a sense of disorientation and spontaneous vestibular nystagmus. Commonly, the patient complains that the world is spinning, in a contralateral direction to the disordered labyrinth, as the image of the environment sweeps across the retina during the slow phase of nystagmus. The patient feels nauseated, may vomit and prefers to lie with the unaffected ear lowermost. All symptoms are exacerbated by head movement.

Within approximately 10 days, the symptoms and signs decrease and eventually cease, as compensation occurs. The exact mechanisms of compensation are not fully understood. Precht, Shimazu and Markham (1966) have shown that in cats, labyrinthine destruction is followed by reactivation of activity in the ipsilateral vestibular nucleus, which is presumed to be consequent upon the release of inhibition of these neurons, by activity of commissural fibres, from the vestibular nuclei of the normal side. Thus a degree of vestibular symmetry is achieved. In addition, there is evidence to suggest that cerebellar activity inhibits vestibular activity on the normal side, again producing a degree of symmetry between the vestibular information within the two halves of the system (McCabe, Ryu and Sekitani, 1972; Schaefer and Meyer, 1973).

The importance of alternative sensory input in expediting vestibular compensation has been shown by several experiments. Lacour, Roll and Appaix (1976) demonstrated that if a baboon were restrained in a plaster cast, following vestibular neurectomy, recovery was delayed. When the animal was released from the restraining splint, it exhibited identical features to that which the unrestrained animal had exhibited immediately following the procedure. This implies that somatosensory input is important for recovery to occur. By the same token, Courjon *et al.* (1977) demonstrated the importance of vision in compensation. Following eighth nerve neurectomy, cats were either kept in the dark for a month or allowed to roam in the light. The animals which had been kept in the dark revealed nystagmus when brought into the light, whereas the animals that had been in the light constantly, following operation, had lost their nystagmus by this time. Finally, Schaefer and Meyer (1973) noted that in guinea-pigs subjected to cervical transection to remove spinal afferent information, the postural derangement of the head persisted after chemical labyrinthectomy, whereas in normal guinea-pigs the head position returned to normal.

Therefore, it would appear that multiple sensory inputs are important for compensation, and cerebellar function is particularly important in modulating long-term adaptation to a vestibular insult. The incidence of degenerative cerebellar disease and vascular involvement of the cerebellum with increasing age, may explain, in part, the observation that compensation occurs more slowly, if at all, following labyrinthine disease in the elderly.

The aforementioned observations in animal experiments provide a scientific basis for head and balance exercises originally documented by Cawthorne (1945) and Cooksey (1945). The exercises are of value in patients with peripheral vestibular disorders, and their purpose is that of providing maximal proprioceptive, somatosensory and visual input to expedite compensation. The foregoing discussion makes it clear that central vestibular disorders will not benefit from such an approach. From birth, the multiple information required for balance is integrated and stored in a 'data centre' (Roberts, 1967), which is thought to be in the reticular formation of the brainstem. New afferent information is constantly compared with these data and, under normal circumstances, 'immediate recognition' of sensory patterns enables vestibular activity to occur at a subconscious level. It would seem reasonable to hypothesize

that, by carrying out head and balance exercises, the dizzy patient 'repeatedly presents' the brain with the data necessary for new sensory patterns to be learned, following an alteration in the vestibular input. This learning process continues until a new pattern of information is developed in the storage mechanism which permits recognition of the unusual input, consequent upon labyrinthine pathology. For further details of vestibular rehabilitation, the reader is referred to Volume 2, Chapter 15.

Clinical applications

This review of the physiology of the vestibular system, and its connections, stresses the interrelationships of the many different systems necessary to achieve perfect balance. The clinical correlate of this fact is that the assessment of any disorder of equilibrium must be based on a multidisciplinary approach. A full and comprehensive history is essential, together with a complete general medical examination, with particular attention to the eyes, the ears, the central nervous system, the cardiovascular system and the locomotor system. Although the exclusion of otological pathology is essential in any balance disorder, many conditions will elude diagnosis if balance is equated purely with a disorder of vestibular function. Drachman and Hart (1972) have emphasized the importance of multisensory deficits, particularly in the elderly, and have postulated a syndrome, producing dizziness, when two or more of the following conditions are present: visual impairment (not correctable), neuropathy, vestibular deficits, cervical spondylosis and orthopaedic disorders which interfere with ambulation. An appreciation and understanding of the concept that dysequilibrium may be consequent upon multiple pathology are essential if appropriate investigation and interpretation of data are to be achieved.

Having established the need for a general medical approach to the problem of unsteadiness, it is essential to identify the presence or absence of a vestibular component. Clinically, vestibulo-ocular and vestibulospinal reflex functions must be assessed. Tests of vestibular function are fully discussed in Volume 2, Chapter 9, and the following discussion serves only to highlight the physiological aspects.

Vestibular examination

Stance and gait

Vestibulospinal function is assessed by the examination of stance and gait, which diagnostically are relatively non-specific and insensitive in comparison with the assessment of vestibulo-ocular function.

The Romberg test (Romberg, 1846) is widely used to assess a basic ability to stand, feet together, hands by the side, with eyes both open and closed. In the presence of an uncompensated, unilateral, peripheral vestibular lesion, or a unilateral cerebellar lesion, the patient tends to sway towards the affected side. In diseases of other areas of the central nervous system, the test may

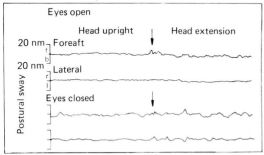

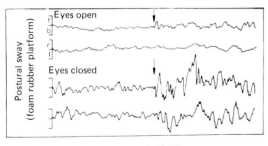

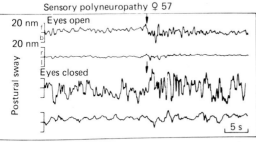

Figure 4.29 Diagram to illustrate the differential effects of head extension and normal head position upon forward–backward and lateral body sway (original recordings) with the eyes open or closed. Normal subjects standing on a firm balance platform (top); normal subjects standing on a slice of foam rubber (middle); and patient with sensory polyneuropathy standing on a firm platform (bottom). (From Brandt, T., Krafczyk, S. and Malsbenden, I., Postural imbalance with head extension: improvement by training as a model for ataxia therapy, in *Vestibular and Ocular Motophysiology:* International Meeting of the Barany Society. Ed. B. Cohen, *Annals of the New York Academy of Sciences*, Vol. 374, pp. 636–649, 1981, with permission)

provide evidence of instability, but is not helpful in terms of localization.

Quantitative assessment of body sway may be achieved by using a balance platform (Jansen, Larsen and Olsen, 1982; Trieson *et al.*, 1982), which monitors movement of the body about the centre of gravity by means of a plate mounted on four sensors, one at each corner. The data obtained have enabled the effect of various sensory modalities upon balance to be identified (*Figure 4.29*), and have allowed various pathological conditions, such as basal ganglia disorders, cerebellar dysfunction and incipient ataxia, to be differentiated (Dichgans, Diener and Müller, 1984).

Gait testing may be of particular value in providing information about the many systems which give rise to imbalance. Loss of proprioception, as seen in tabes dorsalis, and to a lesser extent in sensory neuropathy, results in a characteristic high-stepping, foot-slapping gait. A hemiplegic gait, with dragging of the leg and flexion of the affected arm, is instantly recognizable, as is the shuffling small-stepping gait of the parkinsonian patient, who walks with the head bowed and back bent, with little arm swing on the affected side. Midline cerebellar dysfunction tends to give rise to a broad-based, ataxic gait, while unilateral, cerebellar hemisphere pathology, like unilateral peripheral vestibular pathology, causes a tendency to veer to the affected side. The stiff painful gait of arthritis, or myopathy of the limb girdle muscles, resulting rotation of the pelvis from side to side with every step, may be noted. A hysterical gait is readily recognized by the bizarre features, which do not conform to any specific organic disease pattern. Thus, observation of gait may provide much information about derangement of sensory inputs required for balance, or may point to a disturbance of the integrating ability of the central nervous system which gives rise to unsteadiness – as, for example, in Parkinson's disease or in vascular disease associated with a stroke.

Although vestibular, visual and proprioceptive activity are all vital for the maintenance of perfect balance, spatial orientation can be controlled by any two of these mechanisms (Jongkees, 1953). However, man is unable to maintain his balance satisfactorily by using only one of the three systems. This physiological principle is admirably demonstrated on gait testing of a patient with bilateral vestibular failure. With eyes open and normal proprioception, it may be difficult to observe any gait disturbance, but if the patient is asked to walk in the dark, a marked difficulty and hesitancy of gait will be observed. If the patient is then deprived of all proprioception by being made to walk on a soft rubber mattress, with eyes closed or blindfolded, the patient will immediately fall to the ground, as all three of the main sensory modalities required for balance are removed.

Eye movements

The vestibulo-ocular reflex and its interrelationships, with the saccadic, pursuit and optokinetic systems, have already been discussed. From the clinical point of view, a thorough and careful examination of eye movements and nystagmus provides a wealth of information, in the siting of both peripheral and central vestibular disorders. Assessment at the bedside may provide much information, but quantitative data may be more accurately interpreted by using precise visual targets and recording the resultant eye movement, by, for example, electronystagmography.

Saccadic eye movements

Saccadic eye movements may be assessed by asking the patient to look back and forth, between two targets directly in front of him, for example at the examiner's index finger. Three variables of saccadic movements should be studied: latency, velocity and accuracy. Disease at various levels in the central nervous system results in abnormalities of different saccadic parameters (Henriksson *et al.*, 1981), whereas no such abnormalities are detected in peripheral labyrinthine disorders.

The latency of saccades is commonly prolonged in diseases which cause damage to the supranuclear control of the brainstem saccade-generating centres, for example basal ganglion disorders.

Impaired saccadic accuracy, with both undershooting and overshooting of the target, is characteristically seen in cerebellar pathology (Zee *et al.*, 1976). Disorders of the cortical saccade control centres may also affect the accuracy of saccades; for example, large frontoparietal lesions result in hypometria of horizontal saccades made in the contralateral direction (Baloh, Honrubia and Sills, 1977).

The slowing of saccadic eye movements may result from a lesion at any level from the pretectal and parapontine saccade-generating centres to the extraocular muscles. Both voluntary and involuntary saccades are involved.

Lesions of the median longitudinal bundle may result in the slowing of adducting saccades made by the medial rectus, on the side of the brainstem lesion, whereas abducting saccades by the lateral rectus muscle are normal. This is the commonest abnormality visible in an internuclear ophthalmoplegia (*see below*). Focal lesions may be identified as high or low in the brainstem, depending on involvement of vertical or horizontal saccades, respectively.

In terms of vestibular function, brainstem lesions which cause an abnormality of the saccadic eye movement will result in abnormal nystagmus, as the fast phase of the nystagmic response is impaired. Indeed, if the saccade-generating centre is destroyed, vestibular or optokinetic stimuli produce slow deviation of the eyes, with an absence of fast saccadic intrusions (Dix, Harrison and Lewis, 1971).

Smooth pursuit system

A smooth pursuit system may be examined clinically by moving a finger slowly backwards and forwards in front of the patient's eyes. Bilaterally impaired pursuit is a non-specific abnormality, which is observed when the patient is tired or inattentive, but, more importantly, is frequently seen as a consequence of psychotropic medication, such as tranquillizers, antidepressants or sedatives. Alcohol may produce a similar response. Unilateral derangement of pursuit, however, indicates organic disease of a cerebellar hemisphere, the brainstem or parieto-occipital dysfunction (Schalen, Henriksson and Pyykko, 1982).

Spontaneous nystagmus

Spontaneous nystagmus is an invaluable sign in siting vestibular and neurological disease (Rudge, 1983). If maximal diagnostic information is to be obtained, one must document alterations in the nystagmic response produced by: (1) change of eye position (30° right and left midposition of gaze); (2) presence and absence of optic fixation; or (3) various head positions.

Eye deviation greater than 30° to right and left may result in physiological end-point nystagmus in normal subjects. The generation of vestibular and gaze paretic nystagmus has been described previously. Experimental lesions at different levels of the vestibulo-ocular pathways in animals have allowed documentation of the resultant nystagmus. Bilateral labyrinthine destruction does not cause nystagmus, as there is no imbalance of vestibular information. Peripheral vestibular lesions of labyrinthine or eighth nerve origin result in spontaneous, vestibular nystagmus towards the side opposite to the lesion. Pathology at the level of the vestibular nuclei may produce spontaneous nystagmus either ipsilaterally or contralaterally, depending on the location and extent of the lesion and the imbalance produced between inhibitory and excitatory secondary vestibular neurons (Uemura and Cohen, 1973).

Lesions of the vestibulo-ocular pathways in the brainstem may affect either the slow vestibular component of the nystagmus (for example gaze paretic nystagmus), the fast saccadic component (as discussed previously) or both phases of nystagmus. Symmetrical gaze paretic nystagmus is commonly observed in association with deranged pursuit following the ingestion of psychotropic drugs and alcohol. Asymmetric horizontal gaze paretic nystagmus always indicates a structural brain lesion and, in the case of cerebellar or cerebellopontine angle disease, the nystagmus is of larger amplitude towards the side of the lesion (Brun's nystagmus).

Vertical nystagmus

Vertical nystagmus invariably implies central nervous system disease (Fisher *et al.*, 1983; Bogousslavsky, Regli and Hunberbuhler, 1980). Downbeat nystagmus is commonly associated with an intra-axial lesion, at the level of the foramen magnum and is well recognized in association with the Arnold–Chiari malformation (Cogan and Burrows, 1954). The patient complains of oscillopsia, and recognition of this malformation may enable surgical correction.

Neurological disease between the level of the vestibular nuclei and the oculomotor nerve may result in a variety of forms of nystagmus that are of diagnostic value.

Rebound nystagmus

Rebound nystagmus is characteristic of cerebellar dysfunction. It manifests itself as gaze paretic nystagmus, which disappears, or reverses, as the direction of gaze is held and, on recentring, a burst of nystagmus is initiated in the direction of the return saccade (Hood, Kayan and Leech, 1973; Baloh, Konrad and Honrubia, 1975).

Dysconjugate nystagmus

Dysconjugate nystagmus is commonly a correlate of central nervous system disease. Ataxic nystagmus, associated with an internuclear ophthalmoplegia, is the most well-recognized variety. It is the result of a lesion in the median longitudinal bundle (Cogan, Kubik and Smith, 1950) and most commonly occurs in multiple sclerosis. *Monocular nystagmus,* by definition, is dysconjugate, and has been reported in a number of ophthalmological and neurological conditions (Nathansan, Bergman and Berker, 1955; Donin, 1967). *See-saw nystagmus* is rare but is associated with lesions near the optic chiasm (Arnott and Miller, 1970; Williams *et al.*, 1982).

Periodic alternating nystagmus

Periodic alternating nystagmus changes direction without a change in head or eye position. The cycle length varies from 1 to 6 minutes, with null periods of 2–20 seconds. The precise site of the lesion which causes this nystagmus is unknown, but both the cerebellum (Baloh, Honrubia and Konrad, 1976; Rudge and Leach, 1976) and the caudal brainstem (Keane, 1974) have been implicated.

Optokinetic nystagmus

The physiology and pathways subserving optokinetic nystagmus have been outlined previously. Disorders affecting saccadic eye movements, or smooth eye movement, may result in derangements of optokinetic nystagmus. Neurological disease involving either the brainstem, cerebellum or third and sixth cranial nerves may result in derangement of the fast saccadic components. The slow component may be deranged by lesions of the afferent visual pathways, or lesions of the efferent motor pathways, within the central nervous system. Lesions at every level from the brainstem, basal ganglia, cerebellum and cortex have been shown to cause derangement of the slow component velocity of the optokinetic response. In contrast, peripheral vestibular abnormalities of the labyrinth or eighth nerve rarely give rise to optokinetic derangements (Abel and Barber, 1981; Yee *et al.*, 1982). Optokinetic nystagmus is, therefore, of great clinical value in distinguishing peripheral from central vestibular disorders.

It cannot be overemphasized that careful inspection of eye movements provides invaluable information in identifying the presence of a vestibular lesion and in defining whether it is of peripheral or central origin. It is notable that the pathophysiological mechanisms subserving positional nystagmus remain poorly understood, and for this reason alone, positional nystagmus is not discussed. It must be emphasized, however, that as a clinical sign in the diagnosis of vestibular pathology, positional nystagmus is of the utmost importance (*see* Volume 2, Chapter 9).

Vestibular tests

The physiological aspects of the caloric test and rotational tests will be briefly considered.

Caloric test

In the normal situation, a steady stream of electrical activity arises in each vestibular end

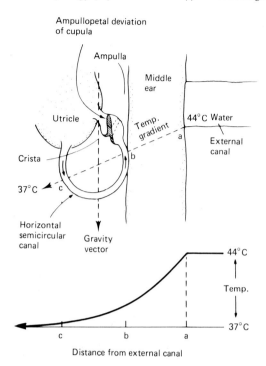

Figure 4.30 Diagram illustrating the mechanism of caloric stimulation of the horizontal semicircular canal. (From Baloh, R. W. and Honrubia, V. *Clinical Neurophysiology of the Vestibular System*, F. A. Davis and Company, 1979, p. 113, with permission)

organ and tends to drive the eyes towards the opposite side, by way of the vestibulo-ocular reflex. For practical purposes, the vestibular system may be considered in two halves, the activity of each being balanced in an equal and opposite manner, such that the eyes are maintained in a central position. The basis of the caloric test lies in the development of an asymmetry of information in the two halves of the vestibular system, as a result of the application of a thermal gradient across the horizontal canal of each labyrinth in turn (*Figure 4.30*). The patient lies in the supine position, with the head tilted 30° upwards, so that the horizontal semicircular canal is brought into the vertical plane, the position of maximal sensitivity to a thermal gradient. The thermal stimulus is standardized for each of four irrigations, · that is 7° below and above body temperature in the right and left ears. The induced nystagmus may be measured by using a number of parameters (duration, slow component velocity and/or amplitude) and reflects the integrity of the vestibulo-ocular reflex derived from each labyrinth independently.

Hot irrigations result in an ampullopetal flow of endolymph, with bending of the cupula and an increase in activity in the vestibular division of the eighth cranial nerve. There is a slow deviation of the eyes away from the irrigated ear, with fast saccadic phases directed towards the irrigated ear. Precisely the converse situation appertains for cold irrigations (*Figure 4.31*). The nystagmic response from the onset of irrigation to the end of observable nystagmus is documented, in both the presence and absence of optic fixation.

The caloric test, as described, was established on a quantitative basis in 1942 by Fitzgerald and Hallpike, and remains the best method of assessing the integrity of each labyrinth and its central nervous system connections. The results of the test are well documented in a large range of vestibular and neurological conditions. The localizing value in siding and siting vestibular pathology is high, and the value of the test in revealing an organic basis to symptoms of vestibular derangement remains unchallenged.

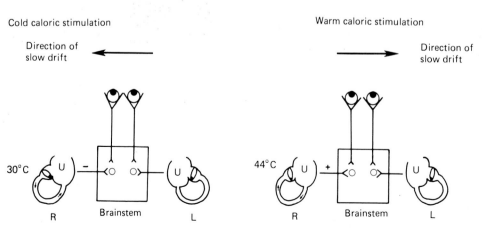

Figure 4.31 Diagram to illustrate the direction of nystagmus produced by cold and warm caloric irrigation. U = utricle; R = right and L = left

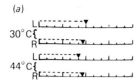

(a)

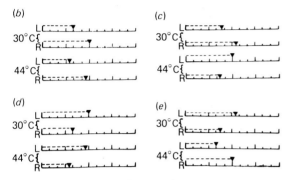

Figure 4.32 Diagram to illustrate the two main patterns of abnormal response observed upon caloric testing. (*a*) Normal; (*b*) left canal paresis; (*c*) directional preponderance to left; (*d*) right canal paresis; (*e*) directional preponderance to the right. L = left ear; R = right ear

Pathology may give rise to two distinct patterns of response, which may appear separately, or in combination (*Figure 4.32*). The first of these, named 'canal paresis' by Fitzgerald and Hallpike, is characterized by a reduced response to both hot and cold stimuli applied to one ear, and is a manifestation of depression of function of one labyrinth, the ipsilateral eighth nerve or the vestibular nuclei, within the brainstem. The second derangement, a 'directional preponderance', is defined as a preponderance of the responses to stimuli, which give rise to nystagmus in one direction, and is a sign of imbalance between the two halves of the vestibular system. As already outlined, the vestibular system may be considered as two halves, which are normally maintained in a state of equilibrium by tonic discharges from a number of sources. These may be modified by lesions of the labyrinth, the vestibular nerve, the vestibular nuclei, the cerebellum and/or the corticofugal fibres deep in the temporal lobe. A derangement of any of these centres may result in an imbalance between the vestibular inputs, and hence a tendency for the eyes to drift either to the right or to the left. A vestibular stimulus will, therefore, produce a nystagmus, which is more exaggerated when the slow component is in the direction of the tendency of eye drift. With more pronounced degrees of tonic imbalance, spontaneous nystagmus will appear.

An understanding of the pathophysiological mechanisms of canal paresis and directional preponderance make it clear that bithermal testing of both ears is necessary. If both ears are irrigated at one temperature only, it is impossible to be certain whether one is dealing with a canal paresis, a directional preponderance, a combined pattern or a normal response (*Figure 4.33*).

The effect of optic fixation upon vestibular nystagmus has already been discussed, and the application of this principle is of importance in the caloric test. Demanez and Ledoux, in 1970, were the first to demonstrate that a caloric-induced nystagmus is much enhanced by eye closure in normal subjects and in cases of peripheral vestibular lesions, but appreciably less so, or even inhibited, in the case of a central vestibular disturbance, as illustrated in *Figures 4.34a, b* and *c*, respectively. This phenomenon is readily explicable on the basis of vestibulo-ocular reflex suppression in the presence of a visual stimulus, and provided that the central nervous system and cerebellar pathways subserving this mechanism are intact, there will be excellent suppression of caloric-induced nystagmus in both normal subjects and in patients with peripheral disorders. If these central pathways are deranged, however, there will be little suppression, as was clearly visualized in the aforementioned responses.

In the caloric test, this phenomenon has been documented by calculation of a 'fixation index', which compares the magnitude of the nystagmus in the absence and presence of optic fixation (Hood and Korres, 1979).

It must be emphasized that, in the literature, there are many different methods of conducting the caloric test and the foregoing discussion merely underlines the relevant physiology and pathophysiological mechanisms of importance in this procedure. For full details of the various techniques, their advantages and disadvantages, and the clinical interpretation of the results, the reader is referred to Volume 2, Chapter 9.

Rotation testing

Rotation about the vertical axis (*Figure 4.35*) provides another method of modulating the resting activity in the vestibular system. *Figure 4.20* illustrates the effect of angular acceleration in a clockwise direction. The imbalance generated in the vestibular system by such a stimulus is 'sensed' by the central nervous system connections, and a compensatory slow eye deviation in the opposite direction to that of rotation is initiated. With increasing rotational stimulus, the slow phase is interrupted by a rapid corrective saccadic eye movement, giving rise to induced nystagmus.

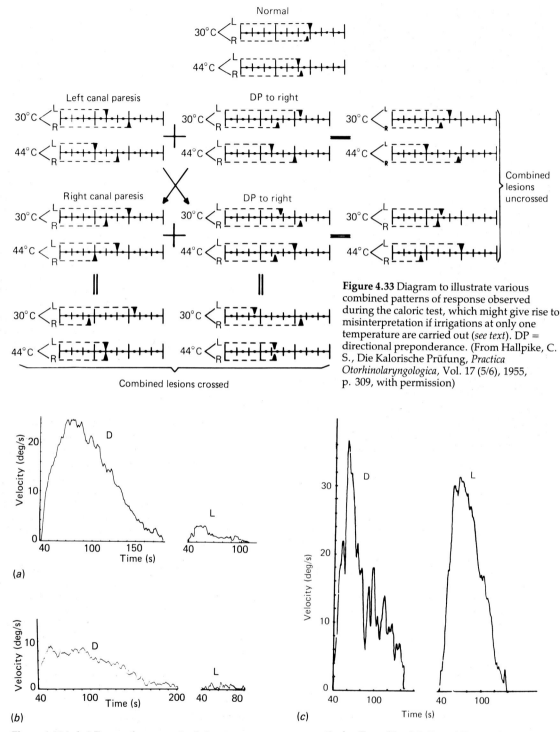

Figure 4.33 Diagram to illustrate various combined patterns of response observed during the caloric test, which might give rise to misinterpretation if irrigations at only one temperature are carried out (*see text*). DP = directional preponderance. (From Hallpike, C. S., Die Kalorische Prüfung, *Practica Otorhinolaryngologica*, Vol. 17 (5/6), 1955, p. 309, with permission)

Figure 4.34 (*a,b,c*) Traces of computerized slow component velocity of nystagmic response to irrigation carried out in the darkness (D) and in the light (L) in a normal subject, a patient with a peripheral vestibular lesion and a patient with a central vestibular lesion, respectively. (From Hood, J. D. and Korres, S., Vestibular suppression in peripheral and central vestibular disorders, *Brain*, Vol. 102, pp. 785–804, 1979, with permission)

unilateral vestibular dysfunction, an asymmetrical response to rotatory stimuli may be observed because of the difference in excitation and inhibition between ampullopetal and ampullofugal stimulation of the labyrinth. This asymmetry is most pronounced after high intensity stimuli, but is consistent only in identifying complete unilateral, peripheral, vestibular paralysis (Honrubia *et al.*, 1980). Furthermore, the results do not allow patients with eighth nerve lesions to be distinguished from those with peripheral labyrinthine lesions.

Rotation testing is of particular value in certain situations. If the caloric test reveals no observable response, high frequency oscillation or high intensity acceleration may provide evidence of some residual vestibular function. Vestibular thresholds may be identified by applying minimal angular accelerations; it may therefore be possible to identify ototoxic damage, for example, before total vestibular failure supervenes. Caloric testing is too crude a technique to allow identification of such minor dysfunction. Undoubtedly, the investigation of visuovestibular interactions, by using rotational stimuli, facilitates the investigation of dysfunction of the central nervous system connections of the vestibular apparatus (Baloh *et al.*, 1982).

Motion sickness

Consideration of the clinical applications of vestibular physiology must include the entity of motion sickness, which is a normal physiological response to certain types of real or apparent motion. Motion sickness is characterized by nausea, vomiting, pallor and cold sweating, and may occur during sea, air, car, space and camel travel. However, it is also commonly encountered in children on swings or at fun fairs, and in the more serious environment of space and aircraft simulators.

For many years, motion sickness has been ascribed to vestibular 'overstimulation', but this hypothesis is difficult to substantiate as certain observations cannot be explained on this basis. Strong, unfamiliar stimuli, such as the repeated stops of a rotating chair, do not tend to induce motion sickness, whereas combinations of linear and angular accelerations, such as voluntary or involuntary head movements during simultaneous rotation about the vertical axis, are highly provocative (Guedry, 1970). In addition, it is well established that the purely visual stimuli may also produce a 'motion sickness' syndrome (Dichgans and Brandt, 1973). The currently accepted explanation of motion sickness is based on a suspected mismatch between sensory information arising from the eyes, the labyrinth or other

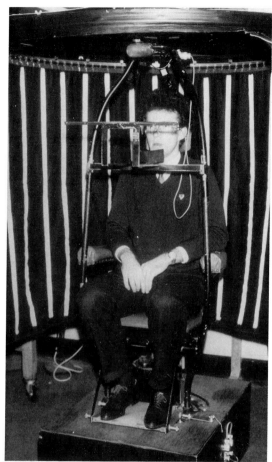

Figure 4.35 Illustration of subject seated in a rotating chair with attached chin rest and facility for electronystagmographic recordings of induced eye movements

Clinically, the caloric test is invaluable as a simple test which allows each vestibular system to be assessed independently. However, in certain situations, for example middle ear disease, it is not possible to carry out a caloric test, and rotational tests may therefore be of value. In general, these tests have not been widely used, partly because both labyrinths are stimulated simultaneously and partly because of the expense of the equipment required to generate precise rotatory stimuli. Nevertheless, as electronystagmographic techniques have become available for the recording of nystagmus during rotation; tests which make use of both constant and sinusoidal acceleration have become increasingly popular (Honrubia *et al.*, 1980; Rubin, 1981).

The patient is seated in a chair that rotates about its vertical axis, and the patient's head is tilted 30° forward so that the angular rotation occurs in the plane of the horizontal semicircular canals. In

receptors stimulated by motion forces, or between these signals of actual sensory input and those of the expected sensory input, as determined by the central nervous system in the light of previous experience (Reason, 1970; 1978).

The pathways subserving the neurophysiological mechanisms which result in motion sickness are poorly established. It is well recognized that the vestibular apparatus and the vestibular projections in the cerebellum are essential for the development of motion sickness. Convergence of vestibular, visual and somatosensory afferents can be identified at the level of the vestibular nuclei (Wilson and Melvill-Jones, 1979), and it is at this level, therefore, that matching of actual and expected motion cues may occur. Although supratentorial structures are involved in motion sickness, they are not essential, as the condition has been documented in both the decorticate dog and man (Reason and Brandt, 1975). It therefore seems likely that the vestibulocerebellum and the vestibular nuclei are prerequisites for the development of motion sickness. Although some people are sensitive to the development of motion sickness, others are highly resistant (Jongkees, 1974), and the reasons influencing susceptibility are not fully understood.

Conclusion

Man has developed an exceedingly complex mechanism for the purpose of maintaining equilibrium. A clear understanding of the vestibular system and its multiple connections is essential, if the correct cause(s) of dysequilibrium in any individual patient is (are) to be identified. The pathophysiology of many vestibular disorders remains poorly understood and it is only by further investigation and by careful interpretation of data that advances in the diagnosis and treatment of disorders of equilibrium will be made.

References

ABEL, S. and BARBER, H. O. (1981) Measurement of optokinetic nystagmus for otoneurological diagnosis. *Annals of Otorhinolaryngology*, **90**, 1–12

ANDERSON, J. H., SOECHTING, J. F. and TERZUOLO, C. A. (1979) Role of vestibular inputs in the organization of motor output to the forelimb extensors. *Progress in Brain Research*, **50**, 582–596

ARNOTT, F. J. and MILLER, S. J. H. (1970) Seesaw nystagmus. *Transactions of the Ophthalmological Society of the UK*, **84**, 251–257

BAKER, R. G., PRECHT, W. and LLIMAS, R. (1973) Cerebellar modullatory action on the vestibulo-trochlear pathway in the cat. *Experimental Brain Research*, **15**, 364–385

BALOH, R. W. and HONRUBIA, V. (1979) *Clinical Neurophysiology of the Vestibular System*. Philadelphia: F. A. Davis Company

BALOH, R. W., HONRUBIA, V. and KONRAD, H. R. (1976) Periodic alternating nystagmus. *Brain*, **99**, 11–26

BALOH, R. W., HONRUBIA, V. and SILLS, A. (1977) Eye tracking and optokinetic nystagmus: Results of quantitative testing in patients with well-defined nervous system lesions. *Annals of Otology, Rhinology and Laryngology*, **86**, 108–114

BALOH, R. W., KONRAD, J. R. and HONRUBIA, V. (1975) Vestibulo-ocular function in patients with cerebellar atrophy. *Neurology*, **25**, 160–168

BALOH, R. W., SILLS, A. W. and HONRUBIA, V. (1979) Impulsive and sinusoidal rotatory testing: a comparison with results of caloric testing. *The Laryngoscope*, **89**, 646–654

BALOH, R. W., YEE, R. D., JENKINS, H. A. and HONRUBIA, V. (1982) Quantitative assessment of visual-vestibular interaction using sinusoidal rotatory stimuli. In *Nystagmus and Vertigo: Clinical Approaches to the Patient with Dizziness*. Eds V. Honrubia and M. A. B. Brazier, pp. 231–239. New York: Academic Press

BÁRÁNY, R. (1922) Zur Klinik und Theorie des Eisenbahnnystagmus. *Acta Oto-Laryngologica*, **2**, 260–265

BENSON, A. J. and BARNES, G. R. (1973) Responses to rotating linear acceleration vectors considered in relation to a model of the otolith organs. *Fifth NASA Symposium on the Role of the Vestibular Organs in the Exploration of Space*, Pensacola Fla. SP-314, pp. 221–236. Washington DC: NASA

BIZZI, E., KALIL, R. E. and TAGLIASCO, V. (1971) Eye–head coordination in monkeys: evidence for centrally-patterned organisation. *Science*, **173**, 452–454

BOGOUSSLAVSKY, J., REGLI, F. and HUNBERBUHLER, J. P. (1980) Downbeat nystagmus. *Neuro-ophthalmology*, **1**, 137–143

BREUER, J. (1874) Uber die Funktion der Bogengange des Ohrlabyrinthes. *Weiner Medizinische Jahrgang*, **4**, 72–73

BRODAL, A. (1974) The anatomy of the vestibular nuclei and their connections. In *Handbook of Sensory Physiology: The Vestibular System.*, edited by H. H. Kornhuber, Vol. VI, Part 1. New York: Springer-Verlag

CAWTHORNE, T. E. (1945) Vestibular injuries. *Proceedings of the Royal Society of Medicine*, **39**, 270–273

CLARK, B. (1967) Thresholds for the perception of angular acceleration in man. *Aerospace Medicine*, **38**, 443–450

CLARK, B. (1970) The vestibular system. *Annual Review of Psychology*, **21**, 273–306

COHEN, B. and HENN, V. (1972) Unit activity of the pontine reticular formation associated with eye movements. *Brain Research*, **46**, 403–410

COHEN, B., SUZUKI, J. I. and BENDER, M. B. (1964) Eye movements from semicircular canal nerve stimulation in the cat. *Annals of Otology, Rhinology and Laryngology*, **73**, 153–169

COLLINS, W. E. (1974a) Arousal and vestibular habituation. In *Handbook of Sensory Physiology: The Vestibular System*, edited by H. H. Kornhuber. Vol. VI, pp. 361–368. New York: Springer-Verlag

COLLINS, W. E. (1974b) Habituation of vestibular responses with and without visual stimulation. In *Handbook of Sensory Physiology: The Vestibular System*, edited by H. H. Kornhuber. Vol. VI, pp. 369–388. New York: Springer-Verlag

COGAN, D. G. and BURROWS, L. J. (1954) Platybasia and the Arnold–Chiari malformation. *Archives of Ophthalmology*, **52**, 13–29

COGAN, D. G., KUBIK, C. S. and SMITH, W. L. (1950)

Unilateral internuclear ophthalmoplegia: report on 8 clinical cases with post-mortem study. *Archives of Ophthalmology,* **44,** 783–796

COOKSEY, F. S. (1945) Rehabilitation of vestibular injuries. *Proceedings of the Royal Society of Medicine,* **39,** 273–278

COURJON, J. H., JEANNEROD, M., OSSUZIO, I. and SCHMID, R. (1977) The role of vision in compensation of vestibulo-ocular reflex after hemilabyrinthectomy in the cat. *Experimental Brain Research,* **28,** 235–248

CURTHOYS, I. S., BLANKS, R. H. I. and MARKHAM, C. H. (1977) Semi-circular canal functional anatomy in cat, guinea pig and man. *Acta Oto-Laryngologica,* **83,** 258–265

DEMANEZ, J. P. and LEDOUX, A. (1970) Automatic fixation mechanisms and vestibular stimulation. *Advances in Oto-Rhino-Laryngology,* **17,** 90–98

DE VRIES, H. (1950) The mechanics of the labyrinth otoliths. *Acta Oto-Laryngologica,* **38,** 262–273

DICHGANS, J. and BRANDT, T. (1973) Optokinetic motion sickness and pseudo-Coriolis effects induced by moving stimuli. *Acta Oto-Laryngologica,* **76,** 339–348

DICHGANS, J., DIENER, J. C. and MÜLLER, A. (1984) Characteristics of increased postural and abnormal long loop responses in patients with cerebellar disease and parkinsonism. International EMG Conference, Munich

DIX, M. R. and HALLPIKE, C. S. (1966) Observations on the clinical features and neurological mechanisms of spontaneous nystagmus resulting from unilateral neurofibromata. *Acta Oto-Laryngologica,* **61,** 1–22

DIX, M. R., HARRISON, M. J. G. and LEWIS, P. D. (1971) Progressive supranuclear palsy (the Steele–Richardson–Olszewski syndrome): A report of 9 cases with particular reference to the mechanism of the oculomotor disorder. *Journal of the Neurological Sciences,* **13,** 237–256

DODGE, R. (1903) Five types of eye movements in the horizontal meridian plane of the field of regard. *American Journal of Physiology,* **8,** 307–329

DONIN, J. F. (1967) Acquired monocular nystagmus in children. *Canadian Journal of Ophthalmology,* **2,** 212–215

DRACHMAN, D. A. and HART, C. (1972) An approach to the dizzy patient. *Neurology,* **22,** 323–334

EWALD, J. R. (1892) *Physiologische Untersuchungen über das Endorgan des Nervus Octavus.* Wiesbaden: Bergmann

FERNANDEZ, C. and GOLDBERG, J. M. (1971) Physiology of peripheral neurons innervating semicircular canals of squirrel monkey. II. Response to sinusoidal stimulation and dynamics of peripheral vestibular system. *Journal of Neurophysiology,* **34,** 661–675

FERNANDEZ, C. and GOLDBERG, J. M. (1976) Physiology of peripheral neurons innervating otolith organs of the squirrel monkey. *Journal of Neurophysiology,* **39,** 970–1008

FERNANDEZ, C., GOLDBERG, J. M. and ABEND, W. K. (1972) Response to static tilts of peripheral neurons innervating otolith organs of the squirrel monkey. *Journal of Neurophysiology,* **35,** 978–997

FISHER, A., GRESTY, M. A., CHAMBERS, B. and RUDGE, P. (1983) Primary position upbeating nystagmus. *Brain,* **106,** 949–964

FITZGERALD, G. and HALLPIKE, C. S. (1942) Studies in human vestibular function: 1. Observations on the directional preponderance ('Nystagmusbereitschaft') of caloric nystagmus resulting from cerebral lesions. *Brain,* **65,** 115–137

FLOCK, A., JORGENSEN, M. and RUSSELL, I. (1973) The physiology of individual hair cells and their synapses. In *Basic Mechanisms in Hearing,* edited by A. Miller, pp. 273–307. New York: Academic Press

FLOURENS, P. (1842) *Recherches Expérimentales sur les Propriétes et les Fonctions du Système Nerveux dans Les Animaux Vertébrés.* Paris: Crevot

FLUUR, E. (1959) Influences of the semicircular canal ducts on extra-ocular muscles. *Acta Oto-Laryngologica Supplementum,* **149,** 5–46

FLUUR, E. and MELLSTROM, A. (1971) The otolith organs and their influence on oculomotor movements. *Experimental Neurology,* **30,** 139–147

FUCHS, A. F. and KIMM, J. (1975) Unit activity in vestibular nucleus of the alert monkey during horizontal angular acceleration and eye movement. *Journal of Neurophysiology,* **38,** 1140–1161

FULTON, J. F., LIDDELL, E. G. T. and RIOCH, D. M. (1930) The influence of unilateral destruction of the vestibular nuclei upon posture and the knee jerk. *Brain,* **53,** 327–343

FURUYA, N., KAWANO, K. and SHIMAZU, M. (1976) Transcerebellar inhibitory interaction between bilateral vestibular nuclei and its modulation by cerebello-cortical activity. *Experimental Brain Research,* **25,** 447–463

GACEK, R. R. (1968) The innervation of the vestibular labyrinth. *Annals of Otology, Rhinology and Laryngology,* **77,** 676–685

GACEK, R. R. and LYON, M. (1974) Localisation of vestibular efferent neurones in the kitten with horseradish peroxidase. *Acta Oto-Laryngologica,* **77,** 92–101

GOLDBERG, J. M. and FERNANDEZ, C. (1975) Vestibular mechanisms. *Annual Review of Physiology,* **37,** 129–162

GRAY, O. (1955) A brief survey of the phylogenesis of the labyrinth. *Journal of Laryngology and Otology,* **69,** 151–179

GRAYBIEL, A. (1974) Measurement of otolith function in man. In *Handbook of Sensory Physiology: The Vestibular System,* edited by H. H. Kornhuber, Vol. VI, Part 2, pp. 233–266. New York: Springer-Verlag

GUEDRY, F. E. (1970) Conflicting sensory cues as a factor in motion sickness. In *Fourth Symposium on the Role of the Vestibular Organs in Space Exploration.* Report SP-187, pp. 45–52, NASA, Washington, DC

GUEDRY, F. E. (1974) Psychophysics of vestibular sensation. In *Handbook of Sensory Physiology: The Vestibular System,* edited by H. H. Kornhuber, Vol. VI, Part 2, pp. 3–154. New York: Springer-Verlag

HENRIKSSON, N. G., HINDFELT, B., PYYKKO, I. and SCHALEN, L. (1981) Rapid eye movements reflecting neurological disorders. *Clinical Otolaryngology,* **6,** 111–119

HIKOSAKA, D. and MAEDA, M. (1973) Cervical effects on abducens motoneurons and their interactions with vestibulo-ocular reflex. *Experimental Brain Research,* **18,** 512–530

HOAGLAND, H. (1932) Impulses from sensory nerves of catfish. *Proceedings of the National Academy of Sciences of the USA,* **18,** 701–705

HOOD, J. D. (1968) Electronystagmography. *Journal of Laryngology and Otology,* **82,** 697–710

HOOD, J. D., KAYAN, A. and LEECH, J. (1973) Rebound nystagmus. *Brain,* **96,** 507–526

HOOD, J. D. and KORRES, S. (1979) Vestibular suppression in peripheral and central vestibular disorders of the brain. *Brain,* **102,** 785–804

HONRUBIA, V., BALOH, R. W., YEE, R. D. and JENKINS, H. A.

(1980) Identification of the location of vestibular lesions on the basis of vestibulo-ocular reflex measurements. *American Journal of Otolaryngology*, **1**, 291–301

HONRUBIA, V., STRELIOFF, D. and SITKO, S. T. (1976) Physiological basis of cochlear transduction and sensitivity. *Annals of Otology, Rhinology and Laryngology*, **85**, 697–710

HOYT, W. F. and DAROFF,F R. B. (1971) Supranuclear disorders of ocular control in man. In *The Control of Eye Movements*, edited by P. Bach-Y-Rita, C. C. Collins and J. E. Hyde, pp. 175–263. New York: Academic Press

IGARISHI, M. (1966) Dimensional study of the vestibular end organ apparatus. In *Second Symposium on the Role of the Vestibular Organs in Space Exploration*, US Government Printing Office, Washington DC

ITO, M. (1975) The vestibulo-cerebellar relationships: vestibulo-ocular reflex arc and flocculus. In *The Vestibular System*, edited by R. F. Naunton. New York: Academic Press

JANSEN, C., LARSEN, R. E. and OLESON, M. B. (1982) Quantitative Romberg's test. *Acta Neurologica Scandinavica*, **66**, 93–99

JOHANSON, W. H. (1964) The importance of the otoliths in disorientation. *Aerospace Medicine*, **35**, 874–877

JONES, G. M. and MILSUM, J. H. (1965) Spatial and dynamic aspects of visual fixation. *IEEE Transactions on Biomedical Engineering*, **12**, 54–62

JONGKEES, L. B. W. (1953) Über die Untersuchungsmethoden des Gleichgewichtsorgans. *Fortschritte der Hals-Nasen-Ohrenheilk*, **1**, 1–147. Basel: Kargen

JONGKEES, L. B. W. (1974) Motion sickness. II. Some sensory aspects. In *Handbook of Sensory Physiology*, edited by H. H. Kornhuber, Vol. VI, Part 2. New York: Springer-Verlag

KEANE, J. R. (1974) Periodic alternating nystagmus with downbeating nystagmus: a clinical anatomical case study of multiple sclerosis. *Archives of Neurology*, **30**, 399–402

KIMURA, R. S. (1969) Distribution, structure and function of dark cells in the vestibular labyrinth. *Annals of Otology, Rhinology and Laryngology*, **78**, 542–561

KIMURA, R., SCHUKNECHT, H. and OTA, C. (1974) Blockage of the cochlear aqueduct. *Acta Oto-Laryngologica*, **77**, 1–12

KING, W. M., LISBERGER, S. G. and FUCHS, A. F. (1976) Responses of fibres in medial longitudinal fasciculus (MLF) of alert monkey during horizontal and vertical conjugate eye movements evoked by vestibular or visual stimuli. *Journal of Neurophysiology*, **39**, 1135–1149

KORRES, S. (1978) Electronystagmographic criteria in neuro-otological diagnosis. 2: Central nervous system lesions. *Journal of Neurology, Neurosurgery and Psychiatry*, **41**, 254–264

LACOUR, M., ROLL, J. P. and APPAIX, M. (1976) Modifications and development of spinal reflexes in the adult baboon (Papio papio) following unilateral vestibular neurotomy. *Brain Research*, **113**, 255–269

LIEDGREN, S. R. C., MILNE, A. C., RUBIN, A. M., SCHWARZ, D. W. F. and TOMLINSON, R. D. (1976) Representation of vestibular afferents in somatosensory thalamic nuclei of the squirrel monkey (*Saimiri sciureus*). *Journal of Neurophysiology*, **39**, 601–612

LIEDGREN, S. R. C. and RUBIN, A. M. (1976) Vestibulo-thalamic projections studied with antidromic technique in the cat. *Acta Oto-Laryngolica*, **82**, 379

LINDEMAN, H. H. (1969a) Studies on the morphology of the sensory regions of the vestibular apparatus. In *Advances in Anatomy, Embryology and Cell Biology*, Vol. 42, pp. 1–113. Berlin: Springer

LINDEMAN, H. H. (1969b) Regional differences in structure of the vestibular sensory regions. *Journal of Laryngology and Otology*, **83**, 9–17

LISBERGER, G. G. and FUCHS, A. F. (1977) Role of the primate flocculus in smooth pursuit eye movements and rapid behavioural modification of the vestibulo-ocular reflex. In *Control of Gaze by Brainstem Neurons*, edited by R. Baker and A. Berthoz, pp. 381–389. Elsevier/North Holland: Amsterdam

LOE, P. R., TOMKO, D. L. and WERNER, G. (1973) The neural signal of angular head position in the primary afferent vestibular nerve axons. *Journal of Physiology*, **230**, 29–50

LORENTE DE NO, R. (1933) Anatomy of the eighth nerve. 1. The central projection of the nerve endings of the internal ear. *The Laryngoscope*, **43**, 1–38

LOWENSTEIN, O. and ROBERTS, T. D. M. (1950) The equilibrium function of the otolith organs of the Thornback Ray *Raja Clavata*. *Journal of Physiology*, **110**, 392–415

LOWENSTEIN, O. and SAUNDERS, R. D. (1975) Otolith-controlled responses from the first-order neurones of the labyrinth of the bullfrog (Rana Catesbeina) to changes in linear acceleration. *Proceedings of the Royal Society of London*, Series B, **191**, 475–505

MACH, E. (1875) *Grundlinien der Lehre von den Bewegungsempfindungen*. Engelman, Leipzig. Bonset, Amsterdam (translation) 1967

MAGNUS, R. (1924) *Köperstellung*. Berlin: Springer-Verlag

MALCOLM, R. (1974) A mechanism by which the hair cells of the inner ear transduce mechanical energy into a modulated train of action potentials. *Journal of General Physiology*, **63**, 757–772

MARKHAM, C. H., YAGI, T. and CURTHOYS, I. S. (1977) The contribution of the contra-lateral labyrinth to second order vestibular neuronal activity in the cat. *Brain Research*, **138**, 99–109

McCABE, B. F., RYU, J. H. and SEKITANI, T. (1972) Further experiments on vestibular compensation. *The Laryngoscope*, **82**, 381–396

MILES, F. A. (1974) Single unit firing patterns in the vestibular nuclei related to voluntary eye movements and passive body rotation in the conscious monkey. *Brain Research*, **71**, 215–224

MILLER, E. F. (1962) Counterrolling of the human eye produced by head tilt with respect to gravity. *Acta Oto-Laryngologica*, **54**, 479–501

MILSUM, J. H. and MELVILL-JONES, G. (1967) Trigonometric resolution of neural responses from the vestibular otolith organ. *Digest 7th International Conference of Medical Biology Engineering*, p. 203. Stockholm

NATHANSON, M., BERGMAN, T. S. and BERKER, M. B. (1955) Monocular nystagmus. *American Journal of Ophthalmology*, **40**, 685–692

NOZUE, N., MIZUNO, M. and KAGA, K. (1973) Neuro-otological findings in diphenylhydantoin intoxications. *Annals of Otology*, **82**, 389–394

O'CONNOR, A., LUXON, L. M., SHORTMAN, R. C., THOMPSON, E. J. and MORRISON, A. W. (1982) Electrophoretic separation and identification of perilymph proteins in cases of acoustic neuroma. *Acta Oto-Laryngologica*, **93**, 195–200

O'LEARY, D. P., DENNIS, P., DUNN, R. F. and HONRUBIA, V. (1974) Functional and anatomical correlation of afferent responses from the isolated semicircular canal. *Nature*, **251**, 225–227

PENFIELD, W. (1957) Vestibular-sensation and the cerebral cortex. *Annals of Otology*, **66**, 691–698

PETERSON, B. W. (1970) Distribution of neural responses to tilting within vestibular nuclei of the cat. *Journal of Neurophysiology*, **33**, 750–767

POMPEIANO, O. (1974) Cerebello-vestibular interrelations. In *Handbook of Sensory Physiology: The Vestibular System*, edited by H. H. Kornhuber, Vol. VI, Part 1, pp. 417–476. New York: Springer-Verlag

PRECHT, W. and SHIMAZU, H. (1965) Functional connections of tonic and kinetic vestibular neurons with primary vestibular afferents. *Journal of Neurophysiology*, **28**, 1014–1028

PRECHT, W., SHIMAZU, H. and MARKHAM, C. H. (1966) A mechanism of central compensation of vestibular function following hemilabyrinthectomy. *Journal of Neurophysiology*, **29**, 996–1010

RAPHAN, T. and COHEN, B. (1978) Brainstem mechanisms for rapid and slow eye movements. *Annual Review of Physiology*, **40**, 527–552

REASON, J. T. (1970) Motion sickness: a special case of sensory rearrangement. *Advances in Science*, **26**, 386–393

REASON, J. T. (1978) Motion sickness adaptation: a neural mismatch model. *Journal of the Royal Society of Medicine*, **71**, 819–829

REASON, J. T. and BRANDT, J. J. (1975) *Motion Sickness*. London: Academic Press

ROBERTS, T. D. M. (1967) *Neurophysiology of Postural Mechanisms*. New York: Plenum Press

ROBERTS, T. D. M. (1978) *Neurophysiology of Postural Mechanisms*, 2nd edn. London: Butterworths

ROBINSON, D. A. (1964) The mechanics of human saccadic eye movement. *Journal of Physiology*, **174**, 245–264

ROBINSON, D. A. (1976) Adaptive gain control of vestibulo-ocular reflex by the cerebellum. *Journal of Neurophysiology*, **39**, 954–969

ROMBERG, M. H. (1846) *Lehrbuch der Nerven Krankheiten des Menschen*. Berlin: A. Duncker

RUBIN, W. (1981) Sinusoidal harmonic acceleration test in clinical practice. *Annals of Otology, Rhinology and Laryngology*, **90**(3) (Suppl. 86), 18–25

RUDGE, P. (1983) *Clinical Neuro-otology*. Edinburgh: Churchill Livingstone

RUDGE, P. and LEECH, J. (1976) Analysis of a case of periodic alternating nystagmus. *Journal of Neurology, Neurosurgery and Psychiatry*, **39**, 314–319

SANDO, I., BLACK, F. O. and HEMENWAY, W. G. (1972) Spatial distribution of vestibular nerve in internal auditory canal. *Annals of Otology*, **81**, 305–314

SCHAEFER, K. P. and MEYER, D. L. (1973) Compensatory mechanisms following labyrinthine lesions in the guinea pig. A simple model of learning. In *Memory and Transfer of Information*, edited by H. P. Zippel, pp. 203–232. New York: Plenum

SCHALEN, L., HENRIKSSON, N. G. and PYYKKO, I. (1982) Quantification of tracking eye movements in patients with neurological disorders. *Acta Oto-Laryngologica*, **93**, 387–395

SCHNEIDER, L. W. and ANDERSON, D. J. (1976) Transfer characteristics of first and second order lateral canal and vestibular neurons in gerbil. *Brain Research*, **112**, 61–76

SHIMAZU, M. and PRECHT, W. (1965) Tonic and kinetic responses of cats vestibular neurons to horizontal angular accelerations. *Journal of Neurophysiology*, **28**, 989–1013

SHIMAZU, M. and PRECHT, W. (1966) Inhibition of central vestibular neurons from the contralateral labyrinth and its mediating pathway. *Journal of Neurophysiology*, **29**, 467–492

SILVERSTEIN, H. (1966) Biochemical studies of the inner ear fluids in the cat. *Annals of Otology, Rhinology and Laryngology*, **75**, 48–63

SPOENDLIN, H. (1964) Uber die Polarisation der Vestibularen Rezeptoren. *Pratica Otorhinolaryngologica*, **26**, 418–432

SUZUKI, J. I., TOKUMASU, K. and COHEN, B. (1969) Eye movements from single utricular nerve stimulation in the cat. *Acta Oto-Laryngologica*, **68**, 350–362

SZENTAGOTHAI, J. (1950) The elementary vestibulo-ocular reflex arc. *Journal of Neurophysiology*, **13**, 395–407

TAKEMORI, S. and SUZUKI, J. I. (1971) Eye deviations from neck torsion in humans. *Annals of Otology*, **80**, 439–444

TER BRAAK, J. W. G. (1936) Untersuchungen ueber optokinetischen Nystagmus. *Archives Neerl de Physiologie*, **21**, 309–376

TIBBLING, L. (1969) The rotatory nystagmus response in children. *Acta Oto-Laryngologica*, **68**, 459–467

TRIESON, H. H., BRINSCOMBE, J., JANSEN, E. and SWENSON, J. M. (1982) Normal ranges in the reproducibility for the quantitative Romberg's test. *Acta Neurologica*, **66**, 100–104

UEMURA, T. and COHEN, B. (1973) Effects of vestibular nuclei on vestibulo-ocular reflexes and posture in monkeys. *Acta Oto-Laryngologica Supplementum*, 315

VAN EGMOND, A. A. J., GROEN, J. J. and JONGKEES, L. B. W. (1948) The turning test with small regulable stimuli. *Journal of Laryngology and Otology*, **62**, 63–69

VIDAL, J., JEANNEROD, M., LIFSCHITZ, W., LEVITAN, H., ROSENBURG, J. and SEGUNDO, J. P. (1971) Static and dynamic properties of gravity-sensitive receptors in the cat vestibular system. *Kybernetik*, **9**, 205–215

VON BÉKÉSY, G. (1966) Pressure and shearing forces as stimuli of labyrinthine epithelium. *Archives of Otolaryngology*, **84**, 122–130

WATZL, E. and MOUNTCASTLE, V. (1949) Projection of vestibular nerve to cerebral cortex of the cat. *American Journal of Physiology*, **159**, 594

WERSALL, J. (1956) Studies on the structure and innervation of the sensory epithelium of the crista ampullaris in the guinea pig. *Acta Oto-Laryngologica Supplementum*, 126

WILLIAMS, I. M., DICKINSON, P., RAMSAY, R. J. and THOMAS, L. (1982) Seesaw nystagmus. *Australian Journal of Ophthalmology*, **10**, 19–25

WILSON, V. J. and MELVILL-JONES, G. (1979) *Mammalian Vestibular Physiology*. New York: Plenum Press

YEE, R. D., BALOH, R. W., HONRUBIA, V. and JENKINS, H. A. (1982) Pathophysiology of optokinetic nystagmus. In *Nystagmus and Vertigo. Clinical Approaches to the Patient with Dizziness*, edited by V. Honrubia and M. Brazier, pp. 251–296. New York: Academic Press

YOUNG, L. R. and STARK, L. (1963) Variable feedback experiments testing a sample data model for eye tracking movements. *IEEE Trans Human Factors in Electronics HFE-4*, 38–51

ZEE, D. S., YEE, R. D., COGAN, D. G., ROBINSON, D. A. and ENGLE, W. K. (1976) Oculomotor abnormalities in hereditary cerebellar ataxia. *Brain*, **99**, 207–234

5

Anatomy of the nose and paranasal sinuses

P. H. Rhys Evans

Embryology

The complex anatomy of the midfacial structures, including the nose, the paranasal sinuses, the mouth and the pharynx, can be fully understood only if it is considered in relation to the embryological development of those structures. In the original yolk sac vesicle, the fundamental structural change which initiates a number of other important developments is the rotation of the cephalic end of the embryonic disc with the formation of the embryo head.

In the early embryo, the pericardial cavity and heart tube lie cephalic to the notochordal plate, from which they are separated by the buccopharyngeal membrane (*Figure 5.1*). The ectodermal and endodermal layers of the embryonic disc are separated by a layer of mesoderm, which later differentiates laterally into the somites, the so-called 'paraxial' structures, which include the pharyngeal arches.

Rotation of the heart tube caudally around the axis of the buccopharyngeal membrane brings the cardiogenic region, the future septum transversum, and the cranial mesoderm from their original position to lie ventral to the foregut (*Figure 5.2*). The folding of the original ventral mesodermal layer, which lined the yolk sac cavity, results in the formation of an endodermal-lined diverticulum lying between the cardiogenic complex and the anterior end of the notochord. At the closed

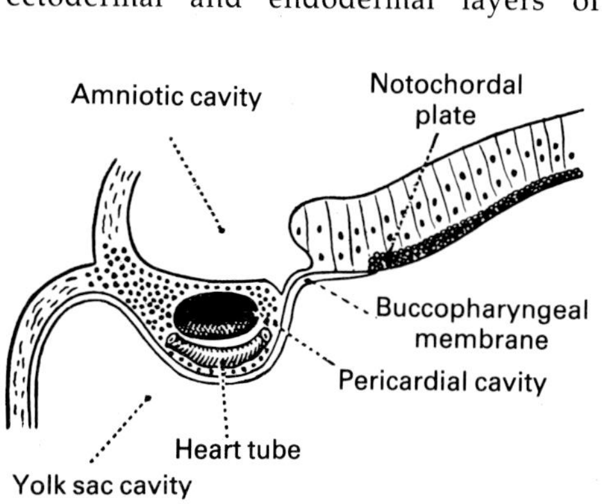

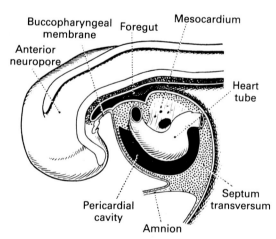

Figure 5.1 A diagrammatic longitudinal midline section through the cranial half of the embryonic disc in a presomite human embryo to show the relationships of the pericardial cavity and the buccopharyngeal membrane before the formation of the head fold. (Reproduced by courtesy of Professors W. J. Hamilton and R. J. Harrison)

Figure 5.2 A diagrammatic longitudinal midline section through the cranial half of the embryonic disc of a 14 somite embryo to show the rotation of the heart tube resulting from the formation of the head fold. (Reproduced by courtesy of Professors W. J. Hamilton and R. J. Harrison)

anterior end of this 'primitive foregut' is the buccopharyngeal membrane, which consists of an endodermal layer and the adjacent ectoderm.

The differentiation of the paraxial mesoderm on either side of the notochord, which results in the formation of somite ridges, occurs almost synchronously with the foregoing changes. Between the somites and lateral plate mesoderm lie the intermediate cell masses of mesoderm. The

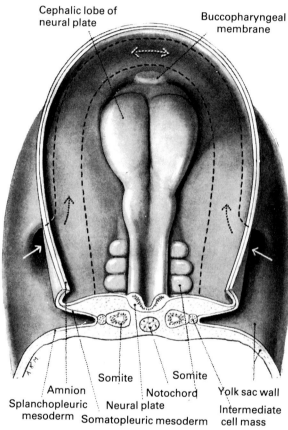

Cephalic lobe of neural plate

Buccopharyngeal membrane

Amnion

Splanchopleuric mesoderm

Somite

Neural plate

Somatopleuric mesoderm

Somite

Notochord

Yolk sac wall

Intermediate cell mass

Figure 5.3 A schematic representation of the cranial part of a somite embryo to show the relationships of the intraembryonic coelom, the development of the neural plate and the continuity between the intraembryonic and the extraembryonic coelom. (Reproduced by courtesy of Professors W. J. Hamilton and R. J. Harrison)

lateral plate mesoderm subsequently splits to enclose the intraembryonic coelom, and cranially this extends forwards to fuse in the midline, forming the coelomic ducts (*Figure 5.3*). It is the mesoderm at the cephalic end of the embryonic disc which condenses cranially, differentiating into the branchial arch structures surrounding the caudal derivatives of the foregut.

Development

The development of the nose and paranasal sinuses is a continuous process which commences in the third week of gestation, when the primordial structures first appear, and continues until completion in early adulthood, when sinus pneumatization and bony growth have ceased. Knowledge of the intrauterine developmental changes is essential for a basic understanding of the anatomical relation of these structures, but it is equally important for the clinician to appreciate the important anatomical changes which continue to take place throughout childhood.

The external nose

The nose develops from the cranial ectoderm above the stomatodaeum, where paired thickenings – the olfactory or nasal placodes – become apparent in the fourth intrauterine week when the embryo has a crown–rump length of 5.6 mm (Streeter, 1945). Proliferation of the surrounding mesoderm into the medial and lateral nasal folds results in the gradual depression of the placodes to form olfactory pits, which eventually deepen by the fifth week to form the nasal sacs (*Figure 5.4*)

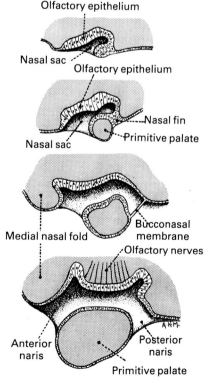

Olfactory epithelium

Nasal sac

Olfactory epithelium

Nasal sac

Nasal fin

Primitive palate

Medial nasal fold

Bucconasal membrane

Olfactory nerves

Anterior naris

Posterior naris

Primitive palate

Figure 5.4 The development of the nasal sac, nasal cavity and primitive palate (after Streeter). (Reproduced by courtesy of Professors W. J. Hamilton and R. J. Harrison)

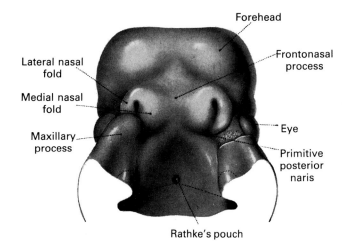

Forehead

Lateral nasal fold

Medial nasal fold

Maxillary process

Frontonasal process

Eye

Primitive posterior naris

Rathke's pouch

Figue 5.5 The roof of the stomatodaeum of a 12 mm human embryo to show the development of the primitive and posterior nares by approximation of the maxillary processes to the lateral and medial nasal folds. The previous site of attachment of the buccopharyngeal membrane is represented by the interrupted line. Part of the left maxillary process has been removed. (Reproduction by courtesy of Professors Hamilton, Boyd and Mossman)

(Streeter, 1948). Between these pits, the medial nasal folds fuse below the frontonasal process, and eventually develop into the central portion of the upper lip, the premaxilla and the primitive nasal septum (*Figure 5.5*).

The nasal cavity

In the 12.5 mm embryo, the maxillary process of the first branchial (mandibular) arch grows anteriorly and medially below the developing eye, across the inferior border of the nasal pits, to fuse anteriorly with the medial nasal folds and the frontonasal process. The nasal pits then become closed inferiorly and form the primitive nasal cavities (*Figures 5.6 and 5.7*). The nasolacrimal furrow is also obliterated by fusion of the outer aspect of the maxillary process and the lateral nasal process. At this junction, the adjacent layers of ectoderm fuse to form a solid cellular rod, producing a surface elevation of the nasolacrimal ridge, which later sinks into the mesenchyme. The solid rod later becomes canalized to form the nasolacrimal duct.

The primitive palate is formed at this stage by proliferation of mesoderm in the free lower border of the frontonasal process (*see Figures 5.4 and 5.7*). The blind ends of the nasal sacs continue to extend posteriorly with progressive thinning of the bucconasal membrane, so that by the thirty-eighth day this membrane is just a thin layer of nasal and oral epithelium. This eventually ruptures in embryos of crown–rump length 12–14 mm, with formation of the choanae, which are the posterior apertures of the nose (*see Figure 5.4*). The position of the bucconasal membrane (or primitive posterior naris) (*see Figure 5.7*) is more anterior to the eventual position of the definitive posterior naris, which does not become established until the third month because of the continued posterior growth of the palate (Warbrick, 1960). Choanal atresia, caused by failure of rupture of the bucconasal membrane, may therefore lie in a more anterior position in the nasal cavity. Membranous and bony atresia may also occur to a variable degree because of failure of recanalization of the nasal cavity, which temporarily becomes filled with proliferating epithelial cells between the sixth and eighth weeks.

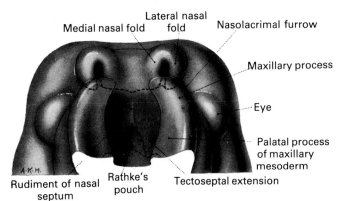

Medial nasal fold

Lateral nasal fold

Nasolacrimal furrow

Maxillary process

Eye

Palatal process of maxillary mesoderm

Tectoseptal extension

Rathke's pouch

Rudiment of nasal septum

Figure 5.6 The roof of the stomatodaeum of a 12.5 mm human embryo. The interrupted line indicates the extent of the lateral and medial nasal folds and the frontonasal process. (Reproduced by courtesy of Professors Hamilton, Boyd and Mossman)

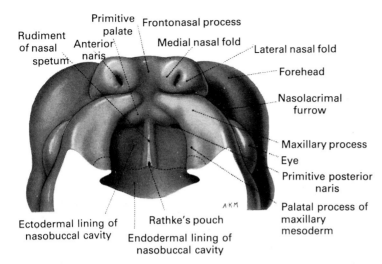

Rudiment of nasal septum

Primitive palate

Anterior naris

Frontonasal process

Medial nasal fold

Lateral nasal fold

Forehead

Nasolacrimal furrow

Maxillary process

Eye

Primitive posterior naris

Palatal process of maxillary mesoderm

Ectodermal lining of nasobuccal cavity

Rathke's pouch

Endodermal lining of nasobuccal cavity

A K M

Figure 5.7 The roof of the stomatodaeum of a 135 mm human embryo. (Reproduced by courtesy of Professors Hamilton, Boyd and Mossman)

At this stage, the cranial boundary of the oral opening consists of the fused premaxillary and maxillary regions, and only later does the upper lip separate from the deeper tissues which will ultimately form the maxillary alveolus. The eventual contribution made by the frontonasal process and the maxillary processes to the formation of the premaxilla, external nose and upper lip is in some doubt. Frontonasal process derivatives are supplied by the ophthalmic nerve, a branch of which – the anterior ethmoidal nerve – supplies the external nose. The upper lip, including the philtrum, is supplied by the maxillary nerve and is therefore considered to be derived from the maxillary processes. Others believe that the philtrum is derived entirely from premaxillary tissue (Keith, 1948; King, 1954; Warbrick, 1960; Wood, Wragy and Stuteville, 1967), and that the maxillary innervation extends into the frontonasal derivative in the upper lip.

The palate and nasal septum

By the time the embryo is 13.5 mm, the primitive palate is beginning to form by fusion of the maxillary processes with the caudal end of the frontonasal process (*see Figure 5.7*). Behind this are the openings of the primitive posterior nares, and in the midline the rudiment of the nasal septum (*see Figure 5.7*). At this stage, therefore, only the ventral (or anterior) part of the palate is formed. As the head increases in size, mesenchymal proliferation occurs between the forebrain and buccal cavity, and the nasal cavities deepen towards the forebrain. A midline ridge develops from the posterior edge of the frontonasal process in the roof of the buccal cavity, extending posteriorly to the opening of Rathke's pouch. This

becomes the nasal septum which is continuous anteriorly with the partition between the primitive nasal cavities. On either side of the elongating septum, the nasal cavities continue to deepen and extend dorsally from the primitive choanae to become two deep, narrow grooves in the roof of the oral cavity (*Figure 5.8*). At this stage, the tongue is almost in contact with the broad dorsocaudal (inferior) border of the developing septum, and there is free communication between the nasal cavities (behind the primitive palate) and the mouth (*Figure 5.8*).

As the nasal cavities enlarge, the palatal processes, derived from the lateral maxillary mesoderm, grow medially towards each other and the developing septum (*see Figure 5.8*). The free edges are at first directed vertically on either side of the tongue, but with further growth the latter structure and the mandibular region are drawn ventrally. This is followed by a rapid change in directional growth of the palatal processes, occurring at about the eighth week, so that these processes now approach each other horizontally and fuse. The mechanism of this directional change is of particular relevance to maldevelopment of the palate, and is the subject of much controversy (Kraus, Jordan and Pruzansky, 1966). The fusion initially occurs along the posterior margin of the primitive palate, except for a small dehiscence in the midline, where the nasopalatine canal remains patent for a time between the two cavities, later marking the site of the incisive foramen. The palatal processes then fuse progressively with each other and with the caudal border of the septum in an anteroposterior direction (*Figure 5.9*). The nasal and oral cavities are thus separated from each other, and the choanae are progressively moved in a posterior direction until they lie adjacent to the free dorsal margin of the

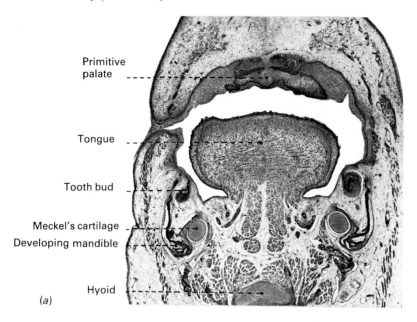

Primitive palate

Tongue

Tooth bud

Meckel's cartilage
Developing mandible

Hyoid

(a)

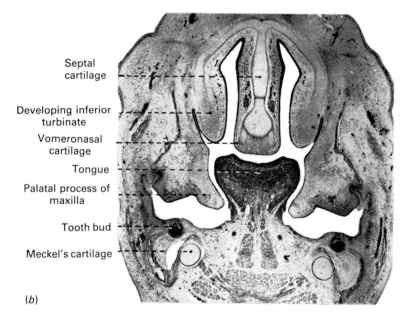

Septal cartilage

Developing inferior turbinate

Vomeronasal cartilage

Tongue

Palatal process of maxilla

Tooth bud

Meckel's cartilage

(b)

Figure 5.8 Two sections through the developing palate of a 20 mm human embryo. (Reproduced by courtesy of Professors W. J. Hamilton and R. J. Harrison)

nasal septum. The palatal processes continue to fuse posteriorly, forming the soft palate and uvula, thereby separating the nasopharynx from the oral cavity.

At the anterior (ventral) end of the nasal septum, above the primitive palate, are situated the paired vomeronasal organs of Jacobson. The ectoderm becomes invaginated on either side to form a diverticulum, which is directed dorsally adjacent to the developing septal cartilage (*see*

Figure 5.9). The vomeronasal organs become well developed auxiliary olfactory organs in many vertebrates, but they are vestigial in man. In some adults, a residual small slit or pit can be identified on each side of the anterior septum, just above the nasal floor (Johnson, Josephson and Hawke, 1985).

The paired vomeronasal cartilages (*see Figures 5.8* and *5.10*) are narrow longitudinal strips, 7–15 mm in length, which lie alongside the lower

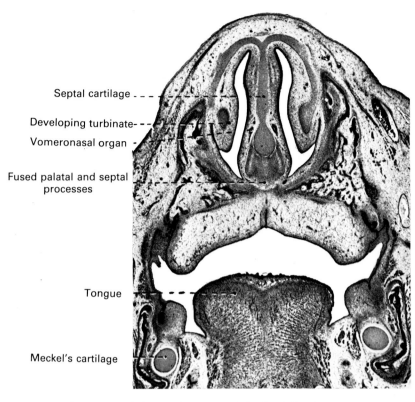

Septal cartilage

Developing turbinate

Vomeronasal organ

Fused palatal and septal processes

Tongue

Meckel's cartilage

Figure 5.9 Section through the palate of a 48 mm human embryo. (Reproduced by courtesy of Professors W. J. Hamilton and R. J. Harrison)

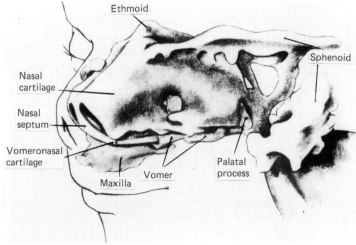

Ethmoid

Sphenoid

Nasal cartilage

Nasal septum

Vomeronasal cartilage

Vomer

Maxilla

Palatal process

Figure 5.10 The cartilaginous nasal capsule from a human fetus aged 4 months (after Schaeffer, 1920a). (From Schaeffer, J. P. (1920a) *The Nose, Paranasal Sinuses, Nasolacrimal Passageways and Olfactory Organ in Man. A Genetic Developmental and Anatomico-physiological Consideration*. Philadelphia: Blakiston Co, by courtesy of the publisher)

border of the septal cartilage. They are attached anteriorly to the maxillary crest and posteriorly to the vomer. In the adult, they may be identified as a cartilaginous bulge along either side of the lower border of the septum, or may remain as separate, discrete strips of cartilage.

The bony and cartilaginous structures of the midface develop from the primitive nasal capsule (*Figure 5.10*), which is formed by mesenchymal condensation during the third fetal month. This is the primary skeleton of the upper and midface, just as the Meckel's cartilage is for the lower face. In the sixth month, this capsule differentiates anteriorly into the alar, the upper lateral and septal cartilages, which are the only parts of the capsule to remain cartilaginous into adult life. The greater part of the capsule becomes ossified posteriorly into the ethmoid bones, the turbinates, part of the sphenoid bone and the vomer, and laterally into the maxillae and nasal bones.

The paranasal sinuses

Progressive changes in the lateral nasal walls with formation of the paranasal sinuses occur simultaneously with development of the palate. In the 40-day-old fetus, as the nasal cavity expands, so horizontal grooves appear on the lateral wall, which will later form the inferior and middle meatus. Between them, the maxilloturbinate mesenchyme proliferates, bulging into the lumen, and later becomes the inferior turbinate (*see Figures 5.8 and 5.9*). The upper turbinates develop from ethmoidturbinate folds which appear later, and by term as many as five may be present. The upper ones regress after birth and remain vestigial (Schaeffer, 1920a). Development of the sinuses occurs once the turbinate folds are established; this is a slow process which continues until cessation of bony growth in early adult life. Of the four named sinuses, only the maxillary and ethmoid sinuses have their origin in early fetal life.

Maxillary sinus

The maxillary sinus is the first to appear as an ectodermal depression just above the uncinate ridge on the inferior turbinate (*Figure 5.11*). This pit, which is the site of the eventual maxillary ostium in the central part of the middle meatus, deepens laterally and expands so that by term a cavity measuring $7 \times 4 \times 4$ mm is present (Ritter, 1973). The expansion continues after birth at an estimated growth rate of 2 mm vertically and 3 mm anteroposteriorly each year (Proetz, 1953). By the age of 12 years, the floor of the sinus has descended to the level of the nasal floor and further downgrowth is achieved by expansion of the lumen into spaces vacated by the erupting teeth.

Ethmoid sinus

During the fifth fetal month, small ectodermal evaginations develop on the lateral nasal wall and grow laterally into the ethmoid bone. By term, these diverticula are globular shaped and they continue to grow until late puberty, or until they abut against compact bone or against another sinus (Ritter, 1973).

Frontal sinus

At the anterosuperior part of the middle meatus, a small evagination, the frontal recess, develops during the third month. This gradually deepens and by term a small diverticulum is present. The formation of the frontal sinuses occurs with gradual upwards expansion of the diverticulum into the frontonasal region. At 6 years, this may just be recognizable in the frontal bone on X-ray. The sinus may, on rare occasions, develop as an extramural expansion of one of the anterior ethmoid cells (Schaeffer, 1920b). Medially, the two sinuses come to lie in close proximity, divided by a thin intersinus septum.

Sphenoid sinus

The primitive sphenoid sinus develops, during the fourth fetal month, as an ectodermal pit in the posterosuperior aspect of the nasal capsule. At birth, it measures $2 \times 2 \times 1.5$ mm and is still only rudimentary. In the fourth postnatal year, when the nasal capsule resorbs, sphenoid pneumatization begins at a rate of 0.25 mm growth each year in a posterior direction, although progress may well be irregular (Hinck and Hopkins, 1965). It is the first of the paranasal sinuses to reach full development.

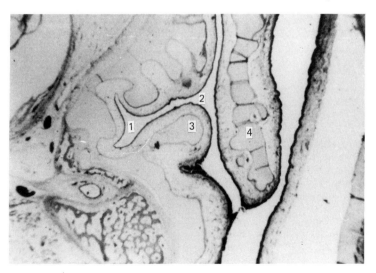

Figure 5.11 Coronal section at the site of the ostium of the future maxillary sinus showing evagination from the right nasal chamber. 1 Rudimentary maxillary sinus; 2 ostium; 3 uncinate ridge; 4 middle turbinate. (From Ritter, F. N. (1973) *The Paranasal Sinuses; Anatomy and Surgical Technique.* St Louis: C. V. Mosby Company, by courtesy of the author and publisher)

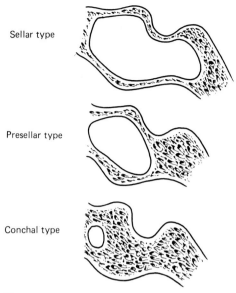

Sellar type

Presellar type

Conchal type

Figure 5.12 Sagittal section diagram of the sphenoid to show degrees of pneumatization of the sphenoid sinus

The degree of pneumatization of the sphenoid sinus varies considerably, and three main types are recognized (*Figure 5.12*):

(1) Sellar type. In 90% of individuals, pneumatization extends beyond the tuberculum sellae by early adulthood. In 20% of these, it extends underneath the sella turcica, or even beyond it towards the basiocciput.
(2) Presellar type. In under 10% of adults, pneumatization extends only as far posteriorly as the tuberculum sellae, although in childhood, as pneumatization is progressing, the proportion is much greater.
(3) Conchal type. In 2–3% of cases, pneumatization does not progress beyond the rudimentary infantile stage (Hammer and Radberg, 1961).

Anomalies and variations in development

The external nose

The shape of the nose is determined by genetic and racial factors and there is wide individual variation. Cleft-palate and cleft-lip deformities are always associated with nasal abnormality, as their development is intimately related. The nasal dermoid cyst is a common developmental midline abnormality on the dorsum of the nasal bridge, resulting from failure of fusion of the medial nasal folds. Failure of fusion more caudally may result in a bifid nasal tip.

The upper lip and palate

The commonest congenital anomaly in this region is the cleft palate, which is often associated with a cleft or hare lip. These deformities are a consequence of failure of fusion of the maxillary processes medially with the frontonasal process and the developing nasal septum. The condition may be unilateral or bilateral.

The septum and nasal cavities

Deviation or asymmetry of the nasal septum occurs in approximately 80% of individuals (Gray, 1978), often involving the junction of the ethmoid plate and the vomer. However, the posterior border of the septum, where it articulates with the rostrum of the sphenoid, is always in the midline, an important landmark in transethmoidal hypophysectomy.

Choanal atresia results from failure of recanalization of the nasal cavities and may be unilateral or bilateral. Simple membranous atresia may occur if the bucconasal membrane fails to rupture.

The external nose
Surface anatomy

The skin covering the nose is thicker towards the tip, and at this point contains a large number of sebaceous glands. It is also more tightly adherent to the underlying alar cartilages, whereas the skin over the upper part of the nose is more loosely attached to the underlying nasal bones and, to a lesser extent, to the upper lateral cartilages. Muscles also intervene between the skin and upper part of the nasal skeleton. The descriptive anatomical features are indicated in *Figure 5.13*.

Bony and cartilaginous structures

The supporting framework of the nose is derived from the nasal capsule, most of which becomes ossified. Anteriorly, the capsule remains cartilaginous, forming the paired alar (lower lateral) cartilages, the upper lateral cartilages and the septal cartilage in the midline. Small accessory alar cartilages are present laterally in the alar fold. The lateral crus of the alar cartilage forms the lateral boundary of the nasal vestibule (the external nasal valve), and is moved by the compressor and dilator naris muscles. The medial crus is attached to its counterpart forming the support of the columella. The alar cartilage is thin and consists of elastic cartilage, while the other cartilages, by contrast, are of the hyaline type. The upper lateral cartilage is overlapped by the cephalic edge of the alar cartilage, to which it is attached by dense connective tissue. This creates a

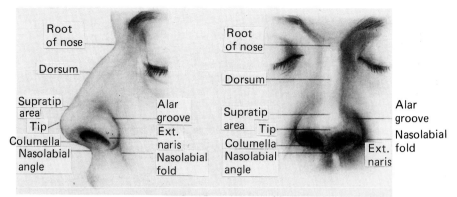

Figure 5.13 Surface anatomy of the external nose with its component parts. (From Converse, J. M. (1977) Plastic surgery of the nose. *Reconstructive Plastic Surgery Vol. 2,* Philadelphia: W. B. Saunders Co, by courtesy of the author and publisher)

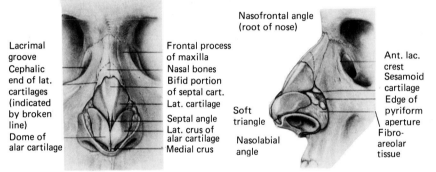

Figure 5.14 The skeletal framework of the external nose. (From Converse, J. M. (1977) Plastic surgery of the nose. *Reconstructive Plastic Surgery Vol. 2,* Philadelphia: W. B. Saunders Co, by courtesy of the author and publisher)

ridge across the roof of the nasal vestibule which forms the inner nasal valve. The outer aspect of the upper lateral cartilage is firmly attached to the frontal process of the maxilla, but the alar cartilage is separated by fibroareolar tissue containing the accessory and sesamoid cartilages, thereby allowing mobility.

Along its cephalic border, the upper lateral cartilage is also overlapped by the caudal margin of the nasal bone, to which it is closely adherent (*Figure 5.14*).

The medial aspects of the upper lateral cartilages are continuous with the cartilaginous part of the nasal septum. This is a quadrangular-shaped cartilage whose tapering posterior prolongation articulates with the perpendicular plate of the ethmoid and the vomer (*see Figure 5.21*). Caudally, the septal cartilage articulates with the nasal spine anteriorly, and with the vomer where it normally rests in a groove. On either side, the vomeronasal cartilage may be separate from, or fused with, the lower border of the septal cartilage (*see Figure 5.10*). The free anterior caudal margin of the

septum is separated from the medial crura of the alar cartilages by the membranous portion of the septum, which aids mobility of the tip of the nose. A short length of the dorsal margin of the septum can be identified between the alar and upper lateral cartilages, the so-called 'septal angle' (*see Figure 5.14*). Above this, the cartilage becomes bifid, forming a shallow median groove, and merges into the upper lateral cartilages on each side.

The bony nasal pyramid, to which the cartilaginous structures are attached, consists of the paired nasal bones above, and the frontal processes of the maxillae laterally (*see Figure 5.14*). The fusion inferiorly of the bodies of the maxillae complete the pear-shaped opening. Because of the recessed position of the anterior border of the bony septum, which divides the nasal cavity posteriorly, it is a single aperture, and in the centre of its inferior border is the elevated anterior nasal spine.

The nasal bones articulate with each other in the midline and with the medial part of the nasal notch of the frontal bone superiorly. Additional

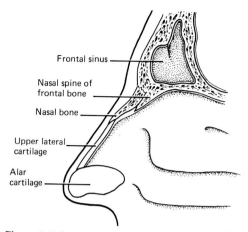

Figure 5.15 Sagittal section diagram to show relations of the nasal bone to the nasal spine and upper lateral cartilage

support is also obtained on the deep aspect from the nasal spine of the frontal bone (*Figure 5.15*). Laterally, the nasal bone articulates with the medial border of the frontal process of the maxilla. The nasal bones are quadrangular in shape and are flatter and wider at the bottom, but where they articulate with the frontal bone they are narrow and thick.

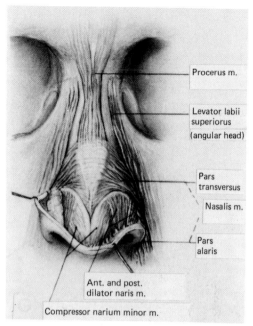

Figure 5.16 The muscles of the nose. (From Converse, J. M. (1977). *Reconstructive Plastic Surgery Vol. 2*, Philadelphia: W. B. Saunders Co, by courtesy of the author and publisher)

Musculature of the nose

Movements of the tip of the nose, including the alae and the lower part of the septum, are controlled by procerus nasalis, consisting of transverse fibres (compressor naris) and alar fibres (dilator naris), and depressor septi. Other smaller muscles are attached to the alar cartilage: the anterior and posterior dilator naris muscles and the compressor narium minor muscles (*Figure 5.16*). The muscle fibres are either attached to the cartilages or, as in the case of the compressor naris, pass across the upper lateral cartilages to be inserted into a median aponeurosis. Their actions are indicated by their names, but they are less well developed in humans than in other primates.

Nerves and vessels of the nose

The cutaneous sensation of the external nose is through the infratrochlear nerve above, and the external nasal nerve towards the tip, the latter being a continuation of the anterior ethmoidal nerve. Both are branches of the ophthalmic division of the trigeminal nerve. Laterally, branches of the infraorbital nerve encroach on to the side walls of the nasal skin. The nasal muscles are

all supplied through the buccal branches of the facial nerve, and paralysis of the nerve will cause collapse of the alae with nasal obstruction on that side.

There is a rich blood supply, partly from the facial artery to the alae and lower part of the septum, but also from the external nasal branch of the ophthalmic artery superiorly, and from branches of the infraorbital artery to the lateral surface and septum laterally. The marginal vein, which continues as the facial vein, is situated at the medial canthus on the side wall of the nose, and here it may be quite prominent.

Surgical anatomy of the nose

The nose is the most prominent feature of the face and, as such, is easily subject to traumatic injury. Fractures of the nose usually involve only the thinner, distal portions of the nasal bones. Injuries to the tip of the nose often cause fracture or dislocation of the cartilaginous septum, with the resulting deformity depending on the direction and force of the impact. Disruption of the external nasal artery by bony fractures may often cause severe bleeding, which may need to be controlled by ligation of the anterior ethmoid artery. In corrective surgery, dissection should be carried out close to the bony and cartilaginous framework to avoid unnecessary injury to the vessels in the soft tissues.

The nasal cavity

Functional anatomy

The anatomical structure of the nasal cavity is intimately related to its important functions of respiration and olfaction. As in other primates, the sense of smell in humans has become less well developed and the olfactory area is confined to a small area around the cribriform plate in the roof of the nasal cavity. In man, the main function of the nose is respiratory and, apart from providing an airway, the nasal cavity is also important for humidification and cleaning of the inspired air.

The nasal cavity is closed off from the mouth by the bony hard palate, so that mastication of food can take place without compromising breathing. During the initial phase of swallowing, the soft palate is elevated, closing off the nasopharynx and, momentarily, interrupting breathing. One other function of the nasal cavity, in conjunction with the paranasal sinuses, is to contribute to resonance of speech.

The importance of adequate patency of the nasal cavity is demonstrated by the effects of pathological obstruction which, apart from impairment of the above functions, may also lead to secondary sinus and eustachian tube problems. In spite of there being an apparently adequate alternative upper airway through the mouth, oxygen tension levels in the blood are significantly reduced in nasal obstruction.

Bony structure

The nasal cavity extends from the external nares (nostrils), anteriorly, to the posterior choanae where it becomes continuous with the nasopharynx. The nasal septum is a midline partition which divides the cavity into two halves. In the prepared skull, the anterior opening of the nasal cavity presents as a single pyriform aperture because of the deficiency of the bony septum anteriorly. The cavity is wide across its floor, but narrows to a maximum of 5 mm across the cribriform plate in its roof. The medial walls are formed by the nasal septum, and the lateral walls are characterized by the presence of horizontal, curved bony projections called nasal turbinates. The paired maxillary, frontal, ethmoid and sphenoid sinuses communicate with the nasal cavity of the same side.

The roof is concave in an anteroposterior direction, with the nasal bones and the supporting nasal septum forming the sloping anterior (frontonasal) portion (*Figure 5.17*). The central part is made up of the cribriform plate of the ethmoid bone, while the posterior, sloping part of the roof is formed by the floor of the sphenoid sinus. In the midline posteriorly, the vomerine portion of the bony septum flares out on either side as the alae of the vomer, which articulate laterally with the

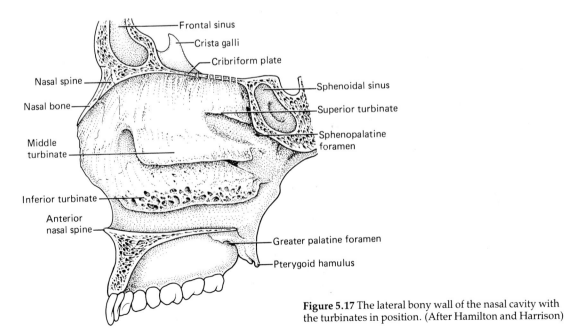

Figure 5.17 The lateral bony wall of the nasal cavity with the turbinates in position. (After Hamilton and Harrison)

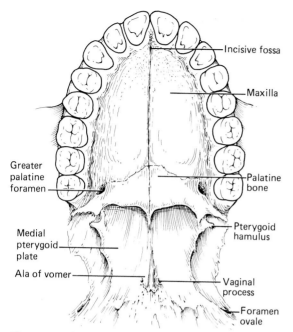

Figure 5.18 The palate and posterior nasal apertures seen from below. (After Hamilton and Harrison)

may be deviated, the rostrum itself is invariably in the midline and, as such, forms an important landmark in transethmoidal or trans-sphenoidal hypophysectomy. However, its posterior projection, which forms the intersphenoid sinus septum, is almost always deviated to one side or the other.

The posterior nasal apertures (choanae) are thus divided medially by the free posterior edge of the vomer. Their roof is formed by the body of the sphenoid with the overlapping, flared alae of the vomer and the vaginal process of the medial pterygoid plate. Their lateral walls are formed by the medial pterygoid plate, and the floor by the free posterior edge of the horizontal plate of the palatine bone (*see Figure 5.18*).

The floor of the nasal cavity is concave from side to side and slightly concave in an anteroposterior direction (*see Figures 5.17* and *5.19*). The anterior three-quarters is formed by the palatine processes of the two maxillae, and the posterior quarter by the horizontal plate of the palatine bones (*see Figure 5.18*). Anteriorly, close to the base of the septum, is the incisive fossa. In the upper part of the fossa are two lateral incisive canals and two median incisive foramina. The lateral incisive canals represent the site of the embryonic communication between the nasal and oral cavities, and thus define the line of union on the palate of the premaxilla with the maxillae. The incisive foramina transmit the nasopalatine (long sphenopalatine) nerve and the terminal branch of the greater palatine artery.

The lateral wall of the nasal cavity has a complex

medial (vaginal) process of the medial pterygoid plate and the sphenoidal process of the palatine bone (*Figure 5.18*). Higher up, the front of the body of the sphenoid projects as a prominent midline ridge called the rostrum, which articulates with the vertical plate of the ethmoid at the upper part of the septum. Although the bony septum

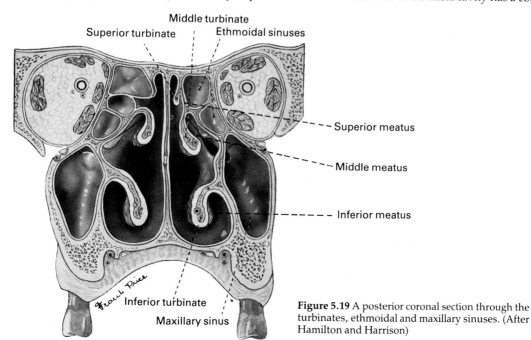

Figure 5.19 A posterior coronal section through the turbinates, ethmoidal and maxillary sinuses. (After Hamilton and Harrison)

anatomical contour as a result of the presence of three scroll-like projections, the superior, middle and inferior turbinate bones (*see Figure 5.17*). Anteriorly, the wall is formed by the inner aspect of the nasal bone, the frontal process and by the anterior part of the body of the maxilla, and is overlapped by the anterior end of the inferior turbinate. The medial wall of the ethmoidal labyrinth forms the upper middle part of the lateral wall, with its superior turbinate bone projecting from the posterosuperior part and the middle turbinate from the anterior and middle surfaces (*see Figures 5.17* and *5.19*).

The superior turbinate is the smallest of the turbinates and may be reduced to only a small ridge about 1.25 cm below the cribriform plate. The sphenoid sinus ostium opens above and behind the superior turbinate into a small depression, the sphenoethmoidal recess. Occasionally, a fourth rudimentary turbinate bone – the supreme turbinate – may lie above and behind this recess.

The middle turbinate bone is large and its anterior part extends forward to articulate with the ethmoidal crest on the frontal process of the maxilla. The posterior edge extends as far back as the medial surface of the perpendicular plate of the palatine bone. The line of attachment is like an inverted 'V', that is with a short, almost vertical anterior limb and a long, sloping posterior limb. The free edge is directed downwards and medially, and overhangs the middle meatus (*Figure 5.20*).

The inferior turbinate is a separate bone, unlike the superior and middle turbinates which are projections from the ethmoid labyrinth. It extends from the body of the maxilla to the ethmoidal crest on the perpendicular plate of the palatine bone. Its central portion is arched so that the inferior meatus, which it overhangs, is both wider and higher at this point; the anterior and posterior ends are narrowed.

The spaces overhung by the turbinates are called the meatus (*see Figure 5.19*), whose lateral walls can be studied on removal of the turbinate bones at their attachments (*see Figure 5.20*). The superior meatus has one opening from the posterior ethmoid sinus, and below and posterior to this is the sphenoethmoidal recess into which the sphenoid sinus drains (*see Figure 5.22*).

The middle meatus has a number of important landmarks and openings on its lateral wall. The highest point of the attachment of the middle turbinate at the angle of its anterior and posterior limbs lies above the frontal recess, into which the frontal sinus and some of the anterior ethmoidal cells may drain. Behind this, the sloping posterior ramus of the middle meatus overlies the uncinate process, the hiatus semilunaris and the bulla ethmoidalis (*see Figure 5.20*). The uncinate process is a sharp, curving ridge of bone projecting upwards from the anterior extremity of the ethmoidal labyrinth to articulate with the ethmoidal process of the inferior turbinate. The posterosuperior border of the uncinate process partially covers the opening of the maxillary sinus (antrum

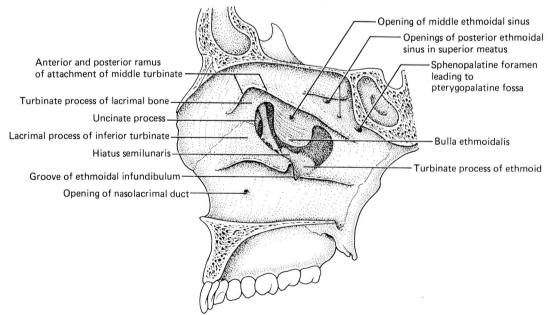

Figure 5.20 The lateral bony wall of the nasal cavity. The turbinates are trimmed to show the three meatus. (After Hamilton and Harrison)

of Highmore), and forms the lower boundary of a curved fissure, the hiatus semilunaris. The hiatus semilunaris leads into the ethmoidal infundibulum, which is the vertical groove between the lateral nasal wall and the uncinate process. Its average depth, depending on the height of the uncinate process, is about 5 mm. The anterior ethmoidal cells open into the infundibulum anteriorly, and behind these is the opening of the maxillary sinus. Posteriorly, the infundibulum becomes continuous with the middle meatus; anteriorly, it is directly continuous with the ostium of the frontal sinus. The lateral wall of the infundibulum and adjacent parts of the lateral nasal wall may be membranous and, in up to 40% of cases, there may be accessory ostia leading into the maxillary sinus (Hollinshead, 1982).

The upper border of the hiatus semilunaris is formed by the bulla ethmoidalis, which is a rounded projection immediately below the middle turbinate. This swelling is produced by the bulging of one or more middle ethmoidal cells which open on to or above the bulla. The anterior border of the uncinate process articulates with the lacrimal process of the inferior turbinate and the turbinate process of the lacrimal bone, which together from the medial bony wall of the nasolacrimal duct (*see Figure 5.20*). Behind the posterior end of the middle turbinate is the sphenopalatine foramen leading into the pterygopalatine fossa (*see Figure 5.20*).

The inferior meatus is the largest of the three meatus, and the only structure of importance to

open into it is the nasolacrimal duct. The ostium is usually situated quite high on the lateral wall in the anterior part of meatus, just below the attachment of the inferior turbinate bone. The shape of the ostium varies from a narrow oval slit to a rounded opening, and may tend to be larger when it is placed at a higher level in the meatus (Hollinshead, 1982). Narrow openings may be protected by a fold of mucous membrane, the plica lacrimalis or valve of Hanser.

The nasal septum is made up of a cartilaginous anterior portion and a larger, bony, posterior part consisting of the vertical plate of the ethmoid and the vomer below. The anterior, free caudal border of the septum or columella contains the paired medial crura of the alar cartilages, which are connected to the septal cartilage by the membranous septum. The perpendicular plate of the ethmoid articulates with the nasal spine of the frontal bones and with the nasal bones anterosuperiorly behind this. It is continuous with the cribriform plate and it articulates posteriorly with the crest of the sphenoid. Posteroinferiorly it articulates with the vomer and anteroinferiorly with the septal cartilage. Its size varies inversely with the size of the septal cartilage.

The vomer forms the posterior part of the nasal septum, articulating inferiorly with the nasal crest of the maxilla and palatine bone (*Figure 5.21*). Posterosuperiorly, it flares out to form two alae which spread out on to the undersurface of the sphenoid, lying between the vaginal processes of the medial pterygoid plates (*see Figure 5.18*). The

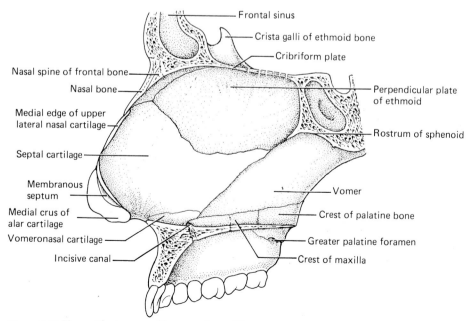

Figure 5.21 The cartilaginous and bony septum of the nose

rostrum of the sphenoid bone – a small anteriorly directed wedge of bone projecting from the body of the sphenoid bone – fits in between the posterior junction of the vomer and ethmoid bones. The anterior border of the vomer is grooved to support the posterior edge of the septal cartilage. Anatomical variation and deformities of the septovomerine junction and deviations of the septal cartilage are common in humans, but are unusual in lower primates and other vertebrates. Lateral ridges may also occur along the maxillary crest and vomeroethmoidal articulation, thereby contributing to nasal obstruction. The perichondrium of the septal cartilage and the periosteum fuse along the groove, but mobility of the cartilaginous septum is facilitated by looser connective tissue between the cartilage and the bone, in which there may be fat (Aymard, 1917).

Nasal cavity lining

Each half of the nasal cavity can be divided into four parts: the vestibule, the atrium, and the respiratory and olfactory regions (*Figure 5.22*). The vestibule is the anterior portion of the nasal cavity bounded laterally by the ala of the nose. It is lined with skin containing sebaceous and sweat glands, which are more abundant in the lower part. Strong hairs, or vibrissae, project into the vestibule from its medial wall and floor to trap coarse inhaled particles. The skin of the roof and lateral wall is

thinner, and the vibrissae here are much finer. The inner margin of hairs across the roof and lateral wall correspond to the cephalic margin of the alar cartilage. The vestibule is demarcated from the rest of the nasal cavity by a ridge across its roof – the limen nasi (limen vestibuli) – which is formed by the caudal margin of the upper lateral cartilage. The narrowed airway at this point is often referred to as the inner nasal valve and corresponds to the margin of transition from the skin of the vestibule to the mucous membrane of the remainder of the cavity. On the medial wall of the vestibule, the thicker skin changes more abruptly to mucous membrane at the level of the valve, and can be easily identified. Anterior to this line, the skin is tightly bound by connective tissue to the underlying cartilage, which makes surgical elevation more difficult. Incisions are best made at the mucocutaneous junction, as behind this line the mucous membrane is delicate and more easily torn.

Behind the posterior aspect of the limen nasi, the lateral wall of the nasal cavity forms a shallow depression corresponding to the atrium. This space is limited posteriorly by the anterior edge of the middle turbinate and superiorly by a ridge – the agger nasi – which runs from the upper end of the middle turbinate, above the atrium and then downwards towards the vestibule. The agger nasi is most marked in the newborn and represents the nasoturbinate bone which is found in many mammals. The groove above the agger nasi,

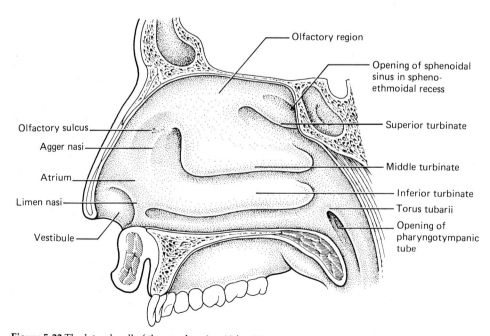

Figure 5.22 The lateral wall of the nasal cavity. (After Hamilton and Harrison)

leading up to the olfactory region, is called the olfactory sulcus.

The olfactory region corresponds to the upper third of the nasal cavity and is bounded by the superior turbinate, the upper part of the septum and the cribriform plate. The remaining portion of the nasal cavity forms the respiratory region.

The mucous membrane of the nasal cavity is tightly applied to the periosteum and perichondrium of its walls. Moreover, the mucosa is continuous through the sinus ostia and also lines the paranasal sinuses. It is thick and vascular and contains numerous goblet cells. Over the turbinates, the septum and the floor, the mucous membrane is especially vascular and thickened, but in the paranasal sinuses it is relatively thin. This respiratory mucosa (Schneiderian membrane) is covered by pseudostratified, columnar, ciliated epithelium, but its structure does vary in different parts of the nasal cavity. In the newborn, the epithelium is almost all of the columnar ciliated type. However, as a response to the drying effect of inspiration, the anterior third of the nasal cavity, to a point about 1 cm behind the anterior end of the inferior turbinate, gradually loses its cilia. The squamous epithelium of the vestibule progresses through transitional epithelium (stratified epithelium with cuboidal surface cells covered by microvilli) in the atrium area, through pseudostratified columnar epithelium (few ciliated cells), to the typical ciliated columnar type of epithelium

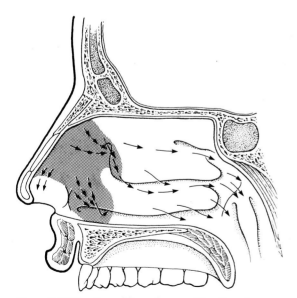

Figure 5.23 Direction of flow of mucus (direction of ciliary beat) on the lateral wall of the nose. The area of less active ciliary movement (corresponding to areas of transitional and pseudostratified epithelium) is stippled. (After Hilding, 1932)

(Mygind, 1978). This metaplastic change in the epithelium may be partially reversed when the nasal airway is obstructed.

Numerous goblet cells are present in the epithelium, beneath which is an almost continuous layer of mucous and serous glands (*Figure 5.23*). In addition, there are aggregations of lymphoid tissue, particularly prominent at the posterior edge of the nasal septum.

Over the medial surfaces of the inferior and middle turbinates, the lamina propria is very vascular and its deeper layer contains a rich plexus of large veins or cavernous sinusoids. This vascular network, similar to erectile tissue, is of great functional importance in controlling the patency of the nasal airways.

The olfactory region is covered by specialized olfactory epithelium, and has a yellowish appearance in man. It is covered by non-ciliated epithelium containing bipolar olfactory nerve cells and supporting cells with oval nuclei. Beneath the olfactory epithelium is a layer of serous, tubular, branched nasal glands. The mucous membrane lining the paranasal sinuses is thin, relatively avascular, and loosely applied to the underlying bone. It is covered with typical columnar ciliated respiratory epithelium.

Near the floor of the nose, on the lower part of the septum, a small depression or pit, which marks the site of the vomeronasal organ, may be found. An extensive study by Johnson, Josephson and Hawke (1985) has shown that in 39% of subjects, at least one vomeronasal pit was identified, and in 9% this was present bilaterally. The mean distance from the anterior naris to the pit was found to be 22 mm. Sectioning of the adult septum shows a much higher prevalence of a vomeronasal structure (70%), compared with clinical examination. The pit is lined with thin mucoperichondrium and extends posterosuperiorly for a variable distance to end as a blind diverticulum. The thin strip of vomeronasal cartilage is closely related to the organ at the lower border of the cartilaginous septum. Although the vomeronasal organ has a well-recognized chemoreceptor function as an accessory olfactory organ in many species, its function among primates is probably limited to the New World monkeys. Olfactory epithelium in this organ has not been identified in humans.

Mucus secreted by the glands in the respiratory mucosa is cleared efficiently from the sinuses and nasal cavity by ciliary activity. In the sinuses this is directed towards the ostia, and in the nasal cavity the direction of ciliary beat is backwards and downwards, carrying the mucus towards the nasopharynx (*see Figure 5.23*). Ciliary activity may be greatly reduced by changes in temperature and by various chemicals.

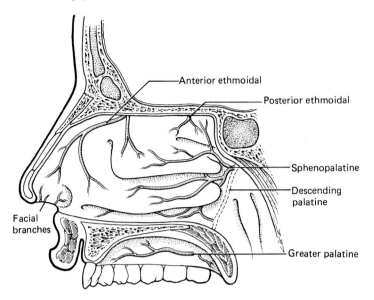

Figure 5.24 Arteries of the lateral nasal wall. (From Hollinshead, W. H. (1982) *Anatomy for Surgeons Vol. 1,* Philadelphia: Harper and Row, by courtesy of the author and publisher)

Blood vessels

The nasal cavity derives its blood supply from both the internal and external carotid arteries, through various branches. The anterior and superior quadrants of the lateral wall and septum receive branches of the anterior and posterior ethmoidal arteries from the ophthalmic artery, which comes from the internal carotid (*Figure 5.24*). The vestibular area is supplied laterally by twigs from the facial artery and medially by the septal branch of the superior labial artery. The posterior and inferior quadrants are supplied on

the lateral wall by branches of the sphenopalatine artery, through its large lateral nasal branches which run along the middle and inferior turbinates. A septal branch of the sphenopalatine artery passes across the anterior aspect of the sphenoid bone to descend diagonally down the septum towards Little's area (Kiesselbach's plexus), where it anastomoses with branches of the superior labial, greater palatine and anterior ethmoidal arteries (*Figure 5.25*). The sphenopalatine artery is given off the maxillary artery in the pterygopalatine fossa. Another branch is the greater palatine artery, which descends through the greater

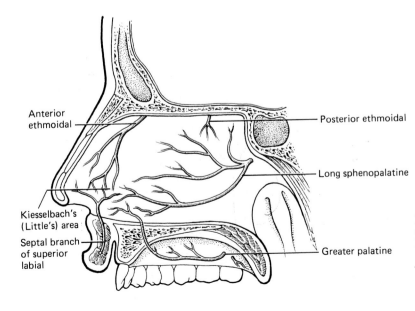

Figure 5.25 Arteries of the nasal septum. (From Hollinshead, W. H. (1982) *Anatomy for Surgeons Vol. 1,* Philadelphia: Harper and Row, by courtesy of the author and publisher)

palatine canal to emerge on the oral surface of the palate through the greater palatine foramen (*see Figure 5.18*). It runs forwards in a groove on the palatal surface of the maxilla to the incisive canal, and branches pass through this canal to anastomose over Little's area. In the greater palatine canal, a number of branches penetrate the perpendicular plate of the palatine bone, and anastomose on the lateral wall with the lateral nasal branches of the sphenopalatine artery.

The arrangement of blood vessels in the mucous membrane consists of a superficial venous plexus and a deeper arteriolar system, arranged parallel to the long axis of the nose (Swindle, 1935; 1937). The arterioles do not contain an internal elastic membrane, so that their endothelial basement membrane is continuous with that of the smooth muscle cells. Also, the increased porosity of the nasal blood vessels means that the subendothelial musculature of these vessels is influenced by agents, such as histamine, in the blood more readily than elsewhere (Mygind, 1978). The cavernous sinusoids are usually found in the contracted state, but can rapidly dilate. Other arteriovenous anastomoses are also found in the nasal mucosa so that blood can bypass the capillary bed.

Venous drainage is to the neighbouring sphenopalatine vein, the anterior facial vein, the anterior and posterior ethmoidal veins and to the cerebral veins through the cribriform plate. A communicating vein may pass through the foramen caecum, which lies between the crista galli and the frontal crest, and when this foramen is patent, the vein opens into the superior sagittal sinus.

Nerve supply

The olfactory mucous membrane contains the cells of origin of the olfactory nerve fibres and is lined with neuroepithelium. The basal parts of the cells are thin and pass upwards to form a dense plexus of non-myelinated nerve fibres, from which about 20 olfactory nerves are formed. These nerves pierce the cribriform plate and pass to the olfactory bulb on each side of the crista galli. The number of fibres in the olfactory nerve begins to decrease shortly after birth at a rate of about 1% a year (Smith, 1941; 1942). Smith found that over 60% of the fibres had been lost in 55% of adults, and no olfactory fibres could be identified in 13%. He concluded that the fibres had been lost partly in consequence of degenerative changes with age and partly in consequence of pathological changes in the mucosa.

General sensory fibres to the respiratory mucous membrane are derived from the ophthalmic and maxillary divisions of the trigeminal nerve. The anterior ethmoidal branch of the nasociliary nerve (ophthalmic division) supplies the anterosuperior lining of the nasal cavity on the lateral wall and septum. Branches of the infraorbital nerve innervate the lateral wall of the vestibule (*Figure 5.26*). The anterior superior alveolar branch, the nerve of the pterygoid canal, the long sphenopalatine (nasopalatine) nerve, the greater palatine nerve and nasal branches of the sphenopalatine ganglion complete the maxillary nerve innervation of the nasal cavity (*Figures 5.26* and *5.27*).

In addition to tactile and sensory fibres, these nerves also carry secretomotor fibres to the mucous and serous glands of the palate, nose and paranasal sinuses. The chief autonomic nerve supply of the nasal cavity is through the pterygopalatine (sphenopalatine) ganglion, which is a relay station between the superior salivatory nucleus in the pons and the nasal cavity mucous membrane. The autonomic root is through the nerve of the pterygoid canal (Vidian nerve) which is formed by the union between the greater superficial petrosal nerve, containing parasympathetic secretomotor fibres, and the deep petrosal nerve, containing sympathetic vasoconstrictor fibres from the carotid plexus. These two nerves join to form the nerve of the pterygoid canal, which runs forwards to the ganglion to be

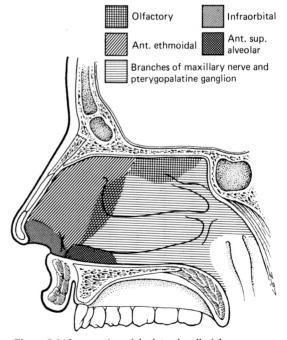

	Olfactory		Infraorbital
	Ant. ethmoidal		Ant. sup. alveolar
	Branches of maxillary nerve and pterygopalatine ganglion		

Figure 5.26 Innervation of the lateral wall of the nose. (From Hollinshead, W. H. (1982) *Anatomy for Surgeons Vol. 1*, Philadelphia: Harper and Row, by courtesy of the author and publisher)

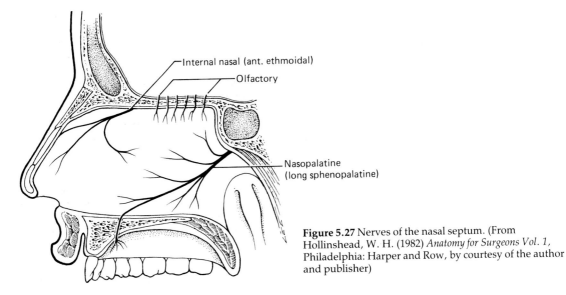

Internal nasal (ant. ethmoidal)

Olfactory

Nasopalatine
(long sphenopalatine)

Figure 5.27 Nerves of the nasal septum. (From Hollinshead, W. H. (1982) *Anatomy for Surgeons Vol. 1*, Philadelphia: Harper and Row, by courtesy of the author and publisher)

distributed through its various branches. Only the parasympathetic fibres relay in the ganglion and, therefore, each branch to the nasal cavity contains sensory, postganglionic, parasympathetic, secretomotor fibres and sympathetic fibres (*Figure 5.28*).

The paranasal sinuses

The paranasal sinuses are a group of air-containing spaces that surround the nasal cavity, extending superiorly to the skull base and laterally

to encompass the medial wall and floor of the orbit. At birth, they are mostly rudimentary and their development continues during childhood into early adult life. Because of their origin and growth as pneumatic diverticula from the primitive nasal cavity, their mucous membrane lining is continuous with and similar in structure to that of the nose. The pseudostratified, ciliated, columnar epithelium, however, is thinner, less vascular and contains fewer mucous glands than that of the nasal mucosa. The cilia direct the mucous blanket in a spiral fashion towards the ostium and, although gravity does not play a role in drainage of the normal sinus, negative air pressure during inspiration does assist ciliary clearance in the maxillary sinus.

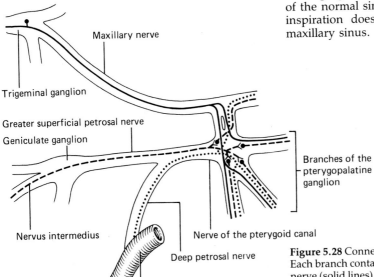

Maxillary nerve

Trigeminal ganglion

Greater superficial petrosal nerve

Geniculate ganglion

Branches of the
pterygopalatine
ganglion

Nervus intermedius

Nerve of the pterygoid canal

Deep petrosal nerve

Internal carotid artery

Figure 5.28 Connections of the pterygopalatine ganglion. Each branch contains sensory fibres from the maxillary nerve (solid lines), sympathetic postganglionic fibres which traverse the ganglion (dotted lines) and postganglionic parasympathetic fibres which relay in the ganglion (long broken lines)

The arterial blood supply of the paranasal sinuses comes from branches of the internal and external carotid arteries which supply the adjacent midfacial structures. The veins and the lymphatics, however, pass through the sinus ostia to drain into the venous and lymphatic plexuses in the nasal cavity. This may be of great significance in inflammatory and allergic conditions of the nasal cavity, where venous and lymphatic congestion may lead to congestion of the sinus openings, with secondary sinus pathology as well as impaired mucus drainage.

The function of the paranasal sinuses is not clear, and most suggestions are speculative rather than factual. They do improve resonance of the voice, but they are also well developed in many silent animals. One of their functions may be to allow warming of the inspired air in the nasal cavity, while they act as insulators to prevent cooling of the surrounding structures.

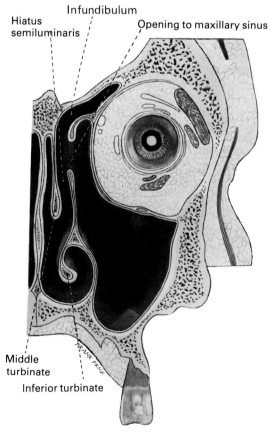

Figure 5.29 A coronal section through the maxillary sinus. (Reproduced by courtesy of Professors W. J. Hamilton and R. J. Harrison)

Maxillary sinus (antrum of Highmore)

The maxillary sinus is the largest of the paranasal sinuses and is contained within the body of each maxilla on either side of the nasal cavity. It is pyramidal in shape with its apex directed laterally, extending into the zygomatic process of the maxilla or into the zygomatic bone itself (*Figure 5.29*). Its base lies medially and forms the lateral wall of the nasal cavity. The bone of the medial wall is thin and is composed of the medial wall of the maxilla, the maxillary process of the inferior concha, the perpendicular plate of the palatine bone, the uncinate process of the ethmoid bone and the descending portion of the lacrimal bone. The roof slopes downwards from medial to lateral and is formed by the orbital surface of the maxilla. It is ridged in the sagittal plane by the canal of the infraorbital nerve. The anterior and posterior walls of the sinus are the corresponding surfaces of the maxilla, and are directly related to the facial surface of the cheek and the infratemporal fossa respectively.

The floor of the sinus consists of the alveolar and palatine processes of the maxilla. In the adult, it lies at a level 1.0–1.2 cm below that of the floor of the nasal cavity, but in the child and also in the edentulous skull, the level corresponds more with the floor of the nasal cavity. The size of the maxillary sinus varies considerably, but average dimensions in the adult skull are 33 mm in height, 23 mm in width and 34 mm in anteroposterior depth. The approximate volume is 14.75 ml but a large antrum may hold 30 ml. The sinuses are usually equal in size; on rare occasions, they may be virtually absent.

The relation of the maxillary sinus to the teeth depends not only on age and the state of dentition, but also on the degree of development of the sinus into the alveolar process. The canine tooth raises a ridge on the anterior surface of the maxilla but does not indent the sinus which lies behind it. The three molar teeth are most constantly directly related to the floor of the sinus and the premolars less frequently (Schaeffer, 1910). The floor of the sinus in relation to these teeth may be ridged or smooth, depending on the projection of the root. Normally the roots are covered with a layer of compact bone, but when this is absent the root lies in direct contact with the mucous membrane. Extraction of these teeth might easily result in oroantral fistulae, the majority of which close spontaneously.

The incidence of dental caries in relation to maxillary sinusitis has been studied by Berry (1930). He found that in 18% of 152 patients, the sinusitis could be directly traced to apical infection; in 30%, a dental abscess was present which was thought probably to be the aetiological cause;

and in 41%, a dead tooth was found in relation to the floor of the sinus, which might possibly have been the origin of the infection. In only 11%, were all the teeth seemingly healthy.

The ostium of the maxillary sinus is situated high up on its posteromedial wall and opens indirectly into the middle meatus of the nasal cavity through the narrow ethmoidal infundibulum (*Figure 5.30*). It is 3–4 mm in diameter, but in

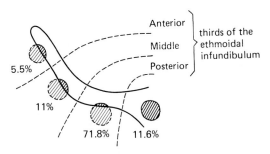

Figure 5.30 Location of sites of the maxillary sinus ostium in the ethmoidal infundibulum and the adjacent uncinate groove. Percentages according to Van Aylea (1936). (From Hollinshead, W. H. (1982) *Anatomy for Surgeons Vol. 1*, Philadelphia: Harper and Row, by courtesy of the author and publisher)

the prepared skull, the bony ostium is larger because the opening is normally partially covered by membrane. Van Aylea (1936) found that in the 163 specimens he examined, 83.4% of ostia were situated in the posterior third of the infundibulum or at the adjacent tip of the uncinate groove (*see Figure 5.30*); only a small proportion were found in the anterior or middle third of the infundibulum. Accessory ostia are present in about 30% of specimens in the adjacent, thin nasal wall (Schaeffer, 1920a; Myerson, 1932; Van Aylea, 1936).

The blood supply to the maxillary sinus is through small arteries that pierce its bony walls, mostly originating from the maxillary, facial, infraorbital and greater palatine arteries. Its largest artery is a branch of the superior artery on the inferior concha which enters the ostium of the sinus (Hollinshead, 1982). Veins accompany these vessels and drain mainly to the anterior facial vein and the pterygoid plexus. The lymphatic drainage of the sinus is mainly through the ostium into the nasal cavity or through the infraorbital foramen, but all lymphatics drain to the submandibular lymph nodes.

The mucous membrane of the sinus is innervated by the superior alveolar nerves (anterior, middle and posterior), the anterior palatine nerve and the infraorbital nerve. All are branches of the second (maxillary) division of the trigeminal nerve

and they supply sensation to the upper teeth and sinus, as well as secretomotor fibres to the mucous membrane through branches from the pterygopalatine ganglion.

Frontal sinus

The frontal sinus is the last of the paranasal sinuses to develop. There is dispute as to whether it is a separate sinus or merely one of the more extensive anterior ethmoidal outgrowths from the frontal recess, growing into the frontal bone. Normally there are two frontal sinuses which lie deep to the supraciliary ridges (*see Figures 5.15, 5.17* and *5.21*). They are of unequal size and are divided by a thin, intersinus bony septum which is seldom in the midline and may occasionally be deficient. Two or more frontal sinuses may be present on each side, but a more common finding is the presence of partial or incomplete septa which give the roof of the sinus a scalloped radiological appearance on the occipitofrontal projection. In the sagittal plane, the sinus has a pyramidal shape, based inferiorly, where there is usually prolongation of the sinus posteriorly over the orbital roof or even a separate accessory frontal (or anterior ethmoidal) sinus. Superiorly, the sinus extends to a variable degree between the inner and outer table of the frontal bone; it is usually larger in men than in women, but there is great individual variation. Occasionally, the sinuses may be absent.

The anterior wall of the sinus is composed of diploic bone and is fairly thick (1–5 mm), but the posterior wall which separates the sinus from the anterior cranial cavity is thinner and formed of compact bone. This thin bone may easily be eroded by mucocoele compression, infection or careless operative technique. The floor separates the sinus from the orbital cavity and slopes downwards and medially towards the opening of the frontonasal duct. The bone here is also thin and is the most frequent site of erosion secondary to mucocoele formation.

The frontonasal duct runs downwards through the front of the ethmoidal labyrinth to open into the middle meatus. In 100 dissections, Kaspar (1936) found that in 62% the duct opened into the frontal recess, and in the remaining 38% it drained directly, or indirectly by way of an anterior ethmoidal cell, into the ethmoidal infundibulum. The duct may, therefore, vary in length and diameter, depending on the distribution of the anterior ethmoidal cells which sometimes bulge into the floor of the frontal sinus. Van Aylea (1946) suggested that the presence of these cells adjacent to the ostium may compromise drainage of the frontal sinus.

The innervation of the frontal sinus is from branches of the supraorbital nerve which pierce the roof of the supraorbital foramen, and there are also branches direct from the nasociliary nerve. The main blood supply is from the supraorbital artery, by way of its diploic branch, and the anterior ethmoidal artery. The venous drainage follows the arterial pattern to the supraorbital veins of the nose. In addition, there are connections with the superior ophthalmic vein, and through the diploic veins to the veins of the scalp and dura. These connections probably account for the spread of osteomyelitis of the frontal bone from frontal sinus infection, and the occurrence of Pott's puffy tumour. Lymphatic drainage is to the submandibular lymph nodes.

Ethmoidal sinus

The ethmoidal sinuses lie within each lateral mass of the ethmoid bone, situated between the nasal cavity and the orbit. Each sinus consists of a variable number (3–18) of air-containing cavities – the ethmoid air cells – which together form a honeycomb network called the ethmoidal labyrinth. In the midline between the two labyrinths is the vertical portion of the ethmoid bone, consisting of the crista galli and the vertical plate of the bony septum which project above and below the cribriform plate respectively. A small part of the roof of each ethmoidal labyrinth is formed medially by lateral bony projections of the cribriform plate (fovea ethmoidalis), but the main part is formed by the frontal bone with which it articulates. The roof has an undulating contour, as a result of the bulging of the domes of the ethmoid air cells, and it slopes gradually downwards at an angle of 15° in an anteroposterior direction. Each ethmoidal sinus has a pyramidal shape based posteriorly, and is 4–5 cm in length. Its height is 2.5–3 cm and its width is 1.5 cm posteriorly, narrowing to 0.5 cm anteriorly (Mosher, 1929; Van Aylea, 1942, 1951).

The bony labyrinth is contained within a delicate but rigid framework. On its lateral aspect is the lamina papyracea which separates it from the orbit (*Figure 5.31*). This part of the ethmoid bone is deficient anteriorly where the ethmoid cells are bounded laterally by the lacrimal bone. The lamina papyracea articulates inferiorly with the maxilla, posteriorly with the lesser wing of the sphenoid and superiorly with the frontal bone. This latter suture line is an important landmark in external ethmoid surgery as it indicates the plane of the roof of the ethmoid air cells (*see Figure 5.31*). Medially, the sinus is bounded by the middle and superior turbinate bones, and posteriorly it is separated from the sphenoid sinus by a thin, bony septum. The middle turbinate bone is continuous superiorly with the fovea ethmoidalis at the lateral aspect of the cribriform plate.

The internal framework of the ethmoid sinus is composed of incomplete, irregular portions of thin bone – the basal lamellae – which traverse the sinus from the medial aspect of the lamina papyracea to the middle and superior turbinates. They divide the ethmoid cells into anterior and posterior air cells whose ostia drain into the middle and superior meatus respectively. Some of the anterior cells behind the hiatus semilunaris form a convex bulge on the lateral wall of the middle meatus, the bulla ethmoidalis. These bullar cells, which vary in number from one to four, are often referred to as the middle ethmoid cells (Van Aylea, 1939) (*see Figure 5.20*).

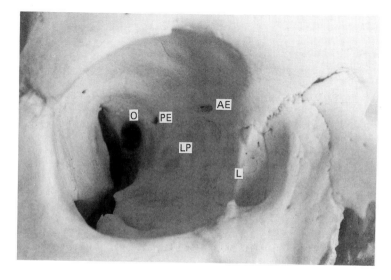

Figure 5.31 The medial wall of the orbit, showing the anterior (AE) and posterior (PE) ethmoid foramina, the lamina papyracea (LP), the lacrimal bone (L) and the optic foramen (O). (By courtesy of Alison Orchard)

The anterior ethmoid cells may otherwise be categorized according to their position and the site of their drainage into the middle meatus. The most anterior of the infundibular cells are the agger cells (one to four in number), which lie laterally to the agger nasi ridge and may invade the lacrimal bone and ascending ramus of the maxilla. Above these, the three to four frontal recess cells invade superiorly into the frontal bone, encroaching on the frontal sinus. As their name implies, they open into the frontal recess. The bullar cells are the most constant of the ethmoid cells and usually open from the medial or anterior surface of the bulla directly into the meatus (*see Figure 5.20*). The posterior ethmoid cells vary in number from two to six and tend to be larger than the anterior cells. Posteriorly, they may grow into the sphenoid bone and may even largely displace the sphenoid sinus. The close proximity of the optic nerve to the posterior ethmoid cells is a very important surgical relation in ethmoidectomy and also may account for possible retrobulbar neuritis in ethmoid infections. The ostia of the posterior cells are usually found in the upper anterior recess of the superior meatus; they vary in diameter from 1 to 2 mm, although they are usually larger than the anterior ethmoid cell openings.

The main arterial supply to the ethmoid sinus is from the anterior and posterior ethmoidal branches of the ophthalmic artery and from the sphenopalatine artery. The ethmoidal arteries pass medially across the roof of the ethmoid cells, often forming a ridge, but sometimes they lie in a bony canal suspended by a thin bony mesentery from the roof. As such, they should be distinguished from an incomplete bony septum at ethmoidectomy, as they may otherwise be accidentally divided.

The nerve supply is from the maxillary branch of the trigeminal nerve and nasociliary branches of the ophthalmic nerve which form the anterior and posterior ethmoidal nerves. Lymphatic drainage of the anterior and middle cells is to the submandibular lymph nodes, and from the posterior cells to the retropharyngeal node.

The sphenoid sinus

The sphenoid sinus is rudimentary at birth but begins to grow after the third year, expanding within the body of the sphenoid bones. Occasionally it invades laterally into the greater and lesser wings and the medial and lateral pterygoid plates of the sphenoid. Posterior extension may occur into the basilar part of the occipital bone. The two sinuses are separated by a bony septum which is rarely in the midline. Other partitions may be present which partially divide the sinus

into several large, intercommunicating cells as well as into lateral recesses. The overall size of the sinus varies enormously (*see Figure 5.12*) and its capacity may range from 0.5 to 30 ml, with an approximate average size of 7.5 ml. Van Aylea (1944) found that in 100 sinuses, the dimensions varied in length from 4 to 44 mm, in height from 5 to 33 mm and in width from 2.5 to 34 mm.

The ostium from each sinus drains into the sphenoethmoidal recess above the superior turbinate. The openings lie in the centre of the sphenoidal turbinates (bones of Bertin) which were originally associated with the primitive nasal capsule. These bones cover the anterior walls of the sinus and, although they are separate bones initially, they fuse with the rest of the body of the sphenoid after the tenth year.

The anatomical relations of the sphenoid sinus are of great surgical importance, especially as the sinus forms the most accessible approach to the pituitary gland. The gland lies in the sella turcica in the roof of the sinus posteriorly, and on either side of this the optic nerves are closely related and sometimes indent the roof more anteriorly. Laterally, the sinus is directly related to the cavernous sinus, the internal carotid artery and divisions of the trigeminal nerve. The posterior wall is usually thick, and separates the sinus from the pons and basilar artery. Inferiorly, the floor of the sinus is related to the roof of the nasopharynx. The close lateral relation of the sinus may become more evident in well pneumatized bones where they form ridges on the lateral wall. Van Aylea found that 65% of the sinuses he examined had a prominent ridge on the posterolateral wall caused by the internal carotid artery. In some cases, the bony wall may be absent at this site (Dixon, 1937). The optic canal may indent the sinus in up to 40% of cases (Van Aylea, 1941), sometimes presenting dehiscences. The maxillary nerve may ridge the sinus in most cases and, more inferiorly, the nerve of the pterygoid canal may also cause an indentation in 48% of cases (Val Aylea, 1941).

The blood supply to the sphenoid sinus is from the posterior ethmoid and the sphenopalatine artery, and its innervation is from branches of the pterygopalatine ganglion. Veins drain into the nasal cavity and accompany lymphatics through the ostium, the latter draining to the retropharyngeal lymph node.

References

AYMARD, J. L. (1917) Some new points in the anatomy of the nasal septum and their surgical significance. *Journal of Anatomy*, **51**, 293

BERRY, G. (1930) Further observations on dental caries as a contributing factor in maxillary sinusitis. *Archives of Otolaryngology*, **11**, 55

CONVERSE, J. M. (Ed.) (1977) Plastic surgery of the nose. In *Reconstructive Plastic Surgery,* Volume II. London: W. B. Saunders

DIXON, F. W. (1937) A comparative study of the sphenoid sinus; a study of 1600 skulls. *Annals of Otology, Rhinology and Laryngology,* **46,** 687

GRAY, L. P. (1978) Deviated nasal septum, incidence and aetiology. *Annals of Otology, Rhinology and Laryngology,* **87** (Suppl. 50), 3–20

HAMMER, G. and RADBERG, C. (1961) Sphenoidal sinus; anatomical and roentgenologic study with reference to transphenoid hypophysectomy. *Acta Radiologica; Diagnosis,* **56,** 401–422

HILDING, A. (1932) Experimental surgery of nose and sinuses: changes in morphology of epithelium following variations in ventilation. *Archives of Otolaryngology,* **16,** 9–18

HINCK, V. C. and HOPKINS, C. E. (1965) Concerning growth of the sphenoid sinus. *Archives of Otolaryngology,* **82,** 62–66

HOLLINSHEAD, W. H. (1982) *Anatomy for Surgeons: The Head and Neck,* 3rd edn. Philadelphia: Harper and Rowe

JOHNSON, A., JOSEPHSON, R. and HAWKE, M. (1985) Clinical and histological evidence for the presence of the vomeronasal (Jacobson's) organ in adult humans. *Journal of Otolaryngology,* **14,** 71–79

KASPAR, K. A. (1936) Nasofrontal connections: a study based on 100 consecutive dissections. *Archives of Otolaryngology,* **23,** 322

KEITH, A. (1948) *Human Embryology and Morphology,* 6th edn. London: Arnold

KING, T. S. (1954) The anatomy of hare lip in man. *Journal of Anatomy,* **88,** 1–12

KRAUS, B. S., JORDAN, R. E. and PRUZANSKY, S. (1966) Dental abnormalities in the deciduous and permanent dentitions of individuals with cleft lip and palate. *Journal of Dental Research,* **45,** 1736–1746

MOSHER, H. P. (1929) Symposium on the ethmoid: the surgical anatomy of the ethmoidal labyrinth. *Transactions of the American Ophthalmological Society,* 376

MYERSON, M. C. (1932) The natural orifice of the maxillary sinus. I. Anatomic studies. *Archives of Otolaryngology,* **15,** 80

MYGIND, N. (1978) *Nasal Allergy.* Oxford: Blackwell Scientific Publications

PROETZ, A. W. (1953) *Essays on the Applied Physiology of the Nose,* 2nd edn. St Louis: Annals Publishing Co

RITTER, F. N. (1973) The paranasal sinuses – anatomy and surgical technique. St Louis: C. V. Mosby Co

SCHAEFFER, J. P. (1910) The sinus maxillaris and its relations in the embryo, child and adult man. *American Journal of Anatomy,* **10,** 313

SCHAEFFER, J. P. (1920a) *The Embryology, Development and Anatomy of the Nose, Paranasal Sinuses, Nasolacrimal Passageways and Olfactory Organ in Man.* Philadelphia: P. Blakiston Co

SCHAEFFER, J. P. (1920b) *The Nose, Paranasal Sinuses, Nasolacrimal Passageways and Olfactory Organ in Man. A Genetic Developmental and Anatomico-pathological Consideration.* Philadelphia: Blakiston Co

SMITH, C. G. (1941) Incidence of atrophy of the olfactory nerves in man. *Archives of Otolaryngology,* **34,** 533

SMITH, C. G. (1942) Age incidence of atrophy of olfactory nerves in man. A contribution to the study of the process of ageing. *Journal of Comparative Neurology,* **77,** 589

STREETER, G. L. (1945) *Contributions to embryology at the Carnegie Institution.* **31,** 27

STREETER, G. I. (1948) *Contributions to embryology at the Carnegie Institution.* **32,** 133

SWINDLE, P. F. (1935) Architecture of blood vascular networks in erectile secretory lining of nasal passages. *Annals of Otology, Rhinology and Laryngology,* **44,** 913

SWINDLE, P. F. (1937) Nasal blood vessels which serve as arteries in some mammals and as veins in some others. *Annals of Otology, Rhinology and Laryngology,* **46,** 600

VAN AYLEA, O. E. (1936) The ostium maxillae; anatomic study of its surgical accessibility. *Archives of Otolaryngology,* **24,** 553

VAN AYLEA, O. E. (1939) Ethmoid labyrinth: an anatomic study. *Archives of Otolaryngology,* **29,** 881

VAN AYLEA, O. E. (1941) Sphenoid sinus: anatomic study with consideration of the clinical significance of the structural characteristics of the sphenoid sinus. *Archives of Otolaryngology,* **34,** 225

VAN AYLEA, O. E. (1942; 1951) *Nasal Sinuses: an Anatomic and Clinical Consideration.* Baltimore: The Williams and Wilkins Co.

VAN AYLEA, O. E. (1944) Sphenoid sinus drainage. *Annals of Otology, Rhinology and Laryngology,* **53,** 493

VAN AYLEA, O. E. (1946) Frontal sinus drainage. *Annals of Otology, Rhinology and Laryngology,* **55,** 267

WARBRICK, J. C. (1960) The early development of the nasal cavity and upper lip in the human embryo. *Journal of Anatomy,* **94,** 351–362

WOOD, N. K., WRAGG, L. E. and STUTEVILLE, O. H. (1967) The premaxilla: embryological evidence that it does not exist in man. *Anatomical Record,* **158,** 485–490

6

Physiology of the nose and paranasal sinuses

A. B. Drake-Lee

Physiology is the science of the normal function and phenomena of living things and their parts. Whereas most works on the physiology of the nose devote considerable attention to the pathophysiology, this chapter will concentrate on the normal nose and its homeostatic reactions. The development of medical sciences has led to considerable overlap between physiology, biochemistry, microanatomy and immunology, and so any work on the physiology of an organ will include some details of other subjects. For example, the humidification of the air is facilitated by the specialized endothelial cells of the nasal capillaries; the ultrastructure of these show that there are pores facing the surface epithelium.

The role of the otolaryngologist is to distinguish patients with a normal nose from those who have a pathological condition. This can be very difficult in some cases where factors in the environment modify the normal response. The variable blockage of the nasal cycle may be exaggerated by underfloor heating or irritant chemicals in the furniture or flooring, but no pathological process is present. An understanding of the physiology of the normal nasal functions will prevent unnecessary surgery to the septum and turbinates.

Although the nose is a paired structure, divided coronally into two chambers, it acts as a functional unit. The paranasal sinuses are mirror images of each other. The relative importance of the sinuses in the physiology appears to be small. When their function is questioned more deeply, no single use can be found. They seem to be like the appendix, although phylogenetically the latter was useful; they are both notable only when diseased.

The nose contains the organ of smell as well as that of respiration. The nose warms, cleans and humidifies the inspired air, and alters the expired air; it also adds quality to speech production. A brief summary of nasal physiology is given in *Table 6.1.*

Table 6.1 Physiological functions of the nose

Respiration
Heat exchange
   direction of blood flow
   latent heat of evaporation
   thermoregulation
Humidification
   anterior serous glands
   mixed serous and mucous glands
   capillary permeability
   other body fluids, e.g. tears
Filtration
   vibrisal
   air flow pattern: laminar/turbulent
Nasal resistance
   anatomical, fixed
   neurovascular, variable
Nasal fluids and ciliary function
   mucus, mucins
   proteins including immunoglobulins
   ciliary structure and function
Nasal neurovascular reflexes
Parasympathetic
   acetylcholine
   vasoactive intestinal polypeptide
Sympathetic
   noradrenaline
   neuropeptide Y
Sensory
   axon reflexes
   substance P
Axon reflexes
Sneezing
Central nasopulmonary reflexes
Nasal cycle
Reflexes initiated in the nose
Reflexes acting on the nose

Olfaction

Respiration

Respiration provides oxygen for metabolism and removes carbon dioxide from the body. Most of the transfer occurs in the alveoli of the lungs, and it is the function of the nose to modify air so that it is ideal for this purpose and so that exchange can occur without damaging the alveoli. The nose performs three functions: humidification, heat transfer and filtration. The nose can be bypassed during exercise because there is such a great reserve of function within the respiratory tract (Dretner, 1979). Becaue of its ability to transfer heat, the nose may be more important in temperature regulation than in respiration.

The humidity and temperature of the ambient air in the home is changed by central heating of various types and by air-conditioning. The inspired gases themselves are non-irritant but contain pollutants, such as oxides of nitrogen and sulphur, which are irritant, and carbon monoxide, which affects the oxygen carrying capacity of haemoglobins. The inspired air contains not only domestic dust particles and pollens but also industrial products, bacteria and viruses. Many people burden their respiratory tract further by smoking tobacco. As an adult will inspire over 10^4 litres of air a day, it is surprising that the nose is not diseased more frequently.

Heat exchange

The temperature of the inspired air can vary from $-50°C$ to $50°C$ and the nose has become modified to suit the local ambient temperatures. Most of the work on heat exchange has been performed on Europeans in temperate or Mediterranean climates.

Conduction, convection and radiation

Heat may be transferred by conduction, convection and radiation. When conduction occurs alone there must be no flow and heat is transferred by increased molecular movement. A temperature gradient in gases will lead to convection currents; this will affect air flow in the nose and cause turbulence. The gases in the nose are in motion, so forced convection will occur. Empirically, a formula to express this can be applied:

$$F_H = h\,(T_{wall} - T_f)$$

where F_H is the heat flux in J/m per s, T_f is the bulk temperature and h is the heat transfer coefficient in J/m per s per °C.

The effectiveness of the system's functioning can be expressed by the heat transfer coefficient (Prandtl number),

$$Pr = \frac{C_p\eta}{K_H}$$

where C_p is the heat capacity of the gas in J/g per °C, η is the viscosity and K_H is the thermal conductivity in J/m per °C.

The nose may be considered as a heat exchange system where two 'fluids' are in thermal but not direct contact. One of the fluids is the inspired air, the other is the blood supply of the nose. The main blood supply comes from the sphenopalatine artery, the branches of which run forward in the nose, particularly over the turbinates. During inspiration, the blood flow is opposite or countercurrent to air flow, and is thus more efficient in warming the inspired air. The efficiency of the system can be measured by comparing the temperature difference between the two 'fluids' (blood and air) at one end, ΔT_1, with that at the other end, ΔT_2. A log mean temperature difference is used to express the relationship

$$\Delta T_{LM} = \frac{\Delta T_1 - \Delta T_2}{\log \Delta T_1 - \log \Delta T_2}.$$

Radiation does not play a significant part in warming the inspired air, but the process is complicated by humidification. The surface membrane of the nose is cooled by vaporization. The energy required to vaporize water is 2.352×10^9 J/kg.

In temperate climates, the temperature in the nasopharynx varies by 2–3°C between inspiration and expiration, and the temperature of the expired air on expiration is the core temperature (Swift, 1982). Because humidification and temperature change in the respired gases are complementary, further changes of temperature will be considered in the next section.

Humidification

Inspiration

Saturation of the inspired air rapidly follows the temperature rise. Energy is required for two functions: raising the temperature of the inspired air and the latent heat of evaporation. These functions require about 2100 kJ every day in the adult, of which only one-fifth is used to raise the temperature (Cole, 1982). The amount of energy is dependent on the ambient temperature and the relative humidity of the inspired air. Because the process is inefficient, over 10% of the body heat loss occurs through the nose. In some animals, particularly dogs, which do not sweat, respiration forms the main source of heat loss. In spite of the variations in temperature of the inspired air, the air in the postnasal space is about 31 °C and is 95% saturated.

Expiration

The temperature of the expired air in the nose is slightly below body core temperature and is saturated; it drops during passage along the nose and this allows some water to condense into the mucosa. The temperature in the anterior nose at the end of expiration is 32° C, and approximately 30° C at the end of inspiration. About one-third of the water required to humidify the inspired air is recovered this way. People who breathe in through the nose and out through the mouth will dry the nasal mucosa.

Water production

It is generally assumed that the water from humidification comes directly from the capillaries through the surface epithelium. However, fluorescent studies have shown that, except during acute inflammation, little water comes directly through the surface epithelium (Ingelstedt and Ivskern, 1949), but originates in the serous glands which are extensive throughout the nose. Humidification is reduced by atropine, probably acting on the glands rather than the vasculature. During the nasal cycle, reduction of secretions occurs on the more obstructed side. Additional water comes from the expired air, the nasolacrimal duct and the oral cavity.

Air flow

The nasal air flow is very different between rest and exercise; most studies have been performed during quiet respiration.

For the purpose of explaining how air flow occurs, the nose may be considered as a tube: most of the work of heat and mass transport has been performed on simple structures with constant cross-sections. Mathematical formulae have been derived to describe behaviour (Swift, 1982).

Air flow: $\bar{V}A$ = constant

where $\bar{V}$ is the average velocity in m/s and A is the cross-sectional area in m^2.

It follows that if the cross-section is decreased then the velocity increases. Gases flow faster through the anterior and posterior nasal apertures. If the shape of the tube changes then the magnitude and direction of velocity also change. This can be seen most clearly when dye is photographed in fluid which has been applied to casts of the nasal passages.

The flow is maximal at the centre of the tube and drops towards the edge. Near the boundaries, flow is further retarded by viscosity of the medium, and at the edge it is zero. Pressure changes which result from viscous changes are irreversible – that is energy is used in overcoming viscosity.

If there is a change in velocity then the pressure will also alter. This process is reversible and is described by Bernouilli's equation:

$$P + \tfrac{1}{2}\rho V^2 = \text{constant}$$

where ρ is the density.

However, because some viscous forces are always active in the nose, the Bernouilli equation is not strictly applicable. The nose has a variable cross-section and therefore the pressure and velocity will alter continuously. The pressure also varies independently during respiration. The inspiratory phase lasts approximately 2 seconds and reaches a pressure of $-10\,\text{mmH}_2\text{O}$, whereas expiration last about 3 seconds and reaches a pressure of $8\,\text{mmH}_2\text{O}$. The respiratory rate is between 10–18 cycles a minute in adults at rest (*Figure 6.1*).

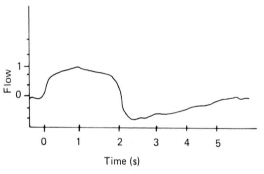

Figure 6.1 A diagram of a pneumotachogram which shows the flow characteristics against time for quiet respiration

Laminar and turbulent air flow

In circular tubes, the change between laminar and turbulent flow is denoted by changes in the Reynolds number (Re):

$$\text{Re} = \frac{dv\rho}{\eta}$$

where d is the diameter in m
v is the average velocity in m/s
ρ is the 'fluid' density in g/m^3
η is the viscosity in g/s per m.
When the Reynolds number varies between 2000 and 4000, the flow changes from laminar to turbulent.

Initial studies by Proetz (1953) were performed on models made from liquid latex, cast at postmortem. Although there is considerable variety of nasal shape, Swift and Proctor (1977) showed that the characteristics of air flow are similar in different noses. These studies used only one side of the nose, but more recently a technique using cast wax has been developed to study the flow in both sides of the nose together (Collins, 1985). Flow studies performed in this way do not take into account the variation in the nasal lumen produced by alterations of the blood flow within the nasal mucosa.

Inspiration

During inspiration, the air flow is directed upwards and backwards from the nasal valve mainly over the anterior part of the inferior turbinate, below and over the middle turbinate and then into the posterior choana. Air reaches the other parts of the nose to a lesser degree (*Figure 6.2*). The velocity at the anterior valve is 12–18 m/s during quiet respiration, and it is considered laminar for rhinomanometry, although, in practice, it is turbulent even in quiet respiration, producing eddies in the olfactory region.

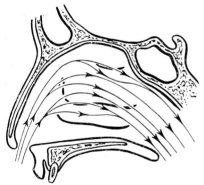

Figure 6.2 Diagram of inspiratory air currents

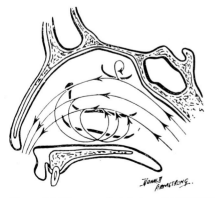

Figure 6.3 Diagram of expiratory air currents

Expiration

Expiration lasts longer than inspiration and flow is more turbulent (*Figure 6.3*). Extrapulmonary air flow is turbulent because the direction changes, the calibre of the airway varies markedly and the walls of the nasal cavity are not smooth. The surface area is enlarged by both the turbinates and the microanatomy of the epithelium. The Reynolds number is exceeded.

Protection of the lower airway: mechanical and chemical

One of the functions of the nose is to remove particles from the inspired air in order to protect the lower airway. The nose is able to filter out particles as small as 30 μm. This includes most pollen particles, which are among the smallest particles deposited, and it accounts for the fact that the nose is the commonest site of hay fever.

The nose is able to achieve this level of filtration because of its morphology. The inspired air travels through up to 180° and during this time not only the direction but also the velocity changes, dropping markedly just after the nasal valve. Turbulence encountered in the flow will increase the deposition of particles.

Particles in motion will tend to carry on in the same direction: the larger the mass, the greater the tendency. The resistance to change in velocity will be greater in irregular particles because of the larger surface area and the number of facets or surfaces.

The nasal hairs will stop only the largest particles and are therefore relevant only to other organisms, which try to crawl into the nose.

Nasal resistance

The nose accounts for up to half the airway resistance.

The nasal resistance is produced by two resistors in parallel, and each cavity has a variable value produced by the nasal cycle. The resistance is made up of two elements: the bone, cartilage and attached muscles; and the mucosa. The narrowest part of the nose is the nasal valve which, physiologically, is less well defined than the anatomical structures which constitute it. It comprises the lower edge of the upper lateral cartilages, the anterior end of the inferior turbinate and the adjacent nasal septum, together with the surrounding soft tissues. Electromyography shows contraction of the dilator naris alone during inspiration (van Dishoek, 1965). Loss of innervation can result in alar collapse even in quiet respiration. The anterior valve, being the narrowest part of the nose, is one of the main factors in promoting turbulent air flow as it is the largest resistor in the whole airway (Bridger and Proctor, 1970).

During quiet respiration, the flow is more laminar in quality so that the resistance may be calculated by dividing the pressure by the flow rate. When the flow is turbulent, because the nose is an irregular tube, the resistance is then inversely proportional to the square of the flow rate (Otis, Fenn and Ryhn, 1950).

The nasal resistance is high in infants who, initially, are obligatory nose breathers. Adults breathe preferentially through the nose at rest even though a significant resistance is present and work is required to overcome the resistance. The resistance is important during expiration because the positive pressure is transmitted to the alveolae and keeps them expanded. Removal of this resistance by tracheostomy is a mixed blessing because, although it reduces the dead space, it also allows a degree of alveolar collapse. Furthermore, it may result in reduced alveolar ventilation and a degree of right to left shunting of the pulmonary blood.

Nasal cycle

The air flow and nasal resistance are modified by mucosal changes. These changes are produced by vascular activity, in particular by the veins of the pseudoerectile tissue of the nose (capacitance vessels). The changes are cyclical and occur between every 4 and 12 hours; they are constant for each person. The cycle consists of alternate nasal blockage between passages, which passes unnoticed by the majority of people. The cycle has been known by yogis since antiquity, although Kayser (1895) gave it its first physiological description.

The nasal cycle can be demonstrated in over 80% of adults, but it is more difficult to demonstrate in children. It has been shown to be present in early childhood (Van Cauwenberge and Deleye, 1984). The cycle may be demonstrated both by rhinomanometry or, more recently, by thermography (Canter, 1986). The physiological significance has not been established but, in addition to a resistance and flow cycle, nasal secretions are also cyclical, with an increase in secretions from the side with the greatest air flow (Ingelstedt and Ivskern, 1949).

A number of factors may overcome or modify the nasal cycle; these include allergy, infection, exercise, hormones, pregnancy, fear, emotions generally and sexual activity. The nasal cycle is controlled by the autonomic nervous system and vagal overactivity may cause nasal congestion. Drugs which block the action of noradrenaline may cause nasal congestion in the same way as hypotensive agents. The anticholinergic effects of antihistamines can block the parasympathetic activity and produce an increase of sympathetic tone, hence an improved airway. Times of hormonal changes, such as puberty and pregnancy, will affect the nasal mucosa. The hormones act directly on the blood vessels.

Oestrogens are actively concentrated in nasal tissue, and levels up to a thousand times the serum levels have been demonstrated (Reynolds and Foster, 1940). They also inhibit the function of acetylcholinesterase and so may affect the autonomic sensitivity of the nose as well (Michael, Zumpe and Keverne, 1972).

Rhinometry

The nasal air flow is usually measured as a volume flow in litres/minute and plotted against pressure. Quiet respiration is studied and a sample point of the flow found at 150 pascals pressure is the standard reference (Clement, 1984). Flow is now measured in SI units (*Figure 6.4*). The details of rhinomanometry are considered in Volume 4.

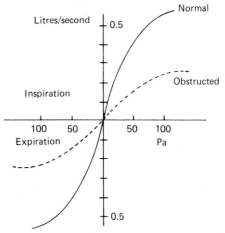

Figure 6.4 The pattern of quiet nasal breathing showing flow (litres per second) against pressure (pascals)

A number of newer techniques have been developed to try to measure nasal resistance practically, as up to one-third of subjects will not be able to perform rhinomanometry adequately. Thermography of the expired air has been used and the sounds of nasal respiration have been analysed, either directly or by the forced random noise technique (Fullton *et al.*, 1984).

Nasal secretions

Nasal secretions are composed of two elements, namely glycoproteins and water with its proteins and ions. Most information on the nature and action of mucus has been obtained from the lower respiratory tract. The glycoproteins are produced by the mucous glands, and the water and ions are produced mainly from the serous glands and indirectly from transudation from the capillary network. The nasal mucus film is divided into two layers: one upper more viscous layer; and a lower more watery layer in which the cilia can move freely, with the tips of the cilia entering the viscous layer to move it. There are also two secretory cell types in the mixed nasal glands, the mucous and serous cells. The glycoproteins found in mucus are produced in two cell types, the goblet cells within the epithelium and the glandular mucous cells.

Glandular mucous and goblet cells contain large secretory granules which can be seen as lucent areas on electron microscopy and which contain the acidic glycoproteins (Lamb and Reid, 1970) (*Figures 6.5* and *6.6*). Serous cells contain electron dense granules which are discrete; the granules may have material of two densities and the cores of these are of a greater density (*Figure 6.7*). The serous cells contain neutral glycoproteins, enzymes such as lysozymes, and lactoferrin, as well as immunoglobulins of the IgA type class. The IgA dimers are conjugated with a secretory piece which is produced in the serous cells. The submucosal glands may be mixed and are arranged around ducts. The anterior part of the nose contains serous glands only in the vestibular region. When stimulated, these glands produce a copious watery secretion. The sinuses have goblet cells and mixed glands although lower in density.

Composition of mucus (*Table 6.2*)

The water, ions and some enzymes may arise outside the nose, for example in tears, and the watery layer in mucus merges gradually into the more viscous upper layer. The two layers may be considered a sol layer and a gel layer. The gel layer contains more of the glycoproteins which contribute many of the properties of mucus. The

Table 6.2 Nasal secretions

Water and ions from transudation
Glycoproteins
    sialomucins, fucomucins, sulphomucins
Enzymes
    lysozymes, lactoferrin
Circulatory proteins, complement
    α_2-macroglobulin, C reactive protein
Immunoglobulins
    IgA, IgE, IgG, IgM, IgD
Cells
    surface epithelium, basophils, eosinophils, leucocytes

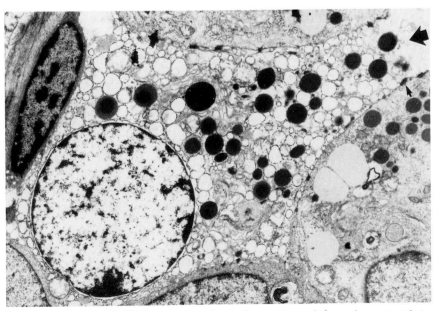

Figure 6.5 Holocrine cell. The large arrow points to the opening and shows the contents being discharged directly. The small arrow shows the tight junctions. (Magnification ×10 000, reduced to 65% in reproduction)

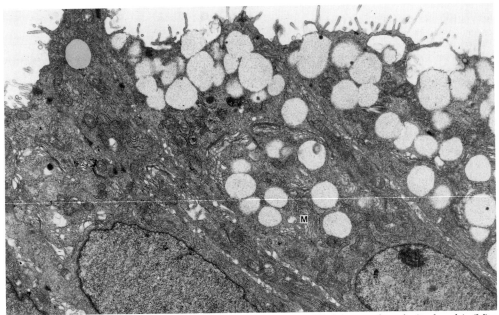

Figure 6.6 Goblet cells. The mucus is removed during preparation. The large number of mitochondria (M) should be noted. (Magnification ×10 900, reduced to 60% in reproduction)

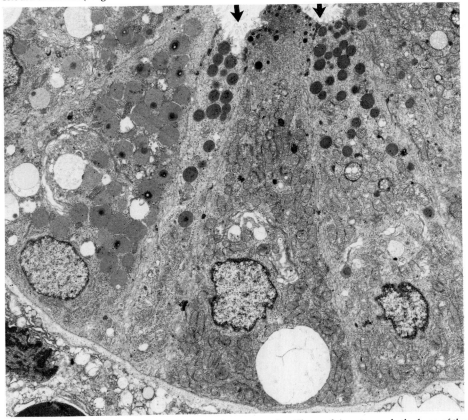

Figure 6.7 Serous cells. These contain electron dense granules. The nuclei are towards the base of the cells. The lumen is arrowed. Several cell types are found. (Magnification ×8545, reduced to 60% in reproduction)

glycoproteins form about 80% of the dry weight of mucus (Masson and Heremans, 1973). They consist of a single sugar side chain and a polypeptide chain which are linked covalently. These units are polymerized by disulphide linkages. Complexes in secretions may weigh up to 10^6 daltons. These polymers interact with water and ions to form a gel. Analysis results in dissolution, which alters the mechanical properties.

Hydroxyamino acids form up to 70% of the amino acids and the most common one in nasal mucus is serine (Boat *et al.*, 1974). The glycoproteins are classified as neutral or acidic. The acid is either sialic acid (sialomucins) or a sulphate group (sulphomucins), and the neutral glycoproteins contain fucose (fucomucins). Sialomucins can be subdivided into those that are digested by sialidases and those that are not. Cells contain a mixture of different mucins.

The glycoproteins give mucus its two most commonly measured properties, namely viscosity and elasticity. The role of mucus in covering the nasal mucosa, and the action of cilia upon it, are dependent on its elastic properties as the ciliary beat frequency is between 10 and 20 Hz (Widdicombe and Wells, 1982). The viscosity and elasticity may be easier to measure but within the nose, adhesiveness and fluidity may be more important.

The viscosity of mucus is lowered by reducing the ionic content. The temperature of the nasal cavity is fairly constant and therefore does not have much effect on flow characteristics. However, the temperature of the nasal cavity is lower than that of the tracheobronchial tree, although both the constituents and flow have yet to be compared. In conclusion, the rheology of nasal mucus requires further study.

The other compounds, such as immunoglobulins, albumin etc., do not add much to the flow characteristics. Most of the protein structures help to defend the host from the environment, whereas the water and ions have a role in the respiratory function.

Proteins in nasal secretion

The proteins in nasal secretion are derived from the circulation or are produced within the mucosa or the surface cells. Comparison of levels within the circulation with levels contained in fluids or nasal secretions will give an indication of local production. Some compounds, such as lactoferrin, are present only in nasal secretions.

Many of the proteins are involved in the immunological responses of the nose and will be considered briefly later.

Lactoferrin

This is present in nasal secretions and is not present in serum. Its action is to bind iron in a similar way to transferrin, although the latter is not found in secretions in any great quantity. They both bind two divalent metal ions, particularly iron, and have a molecular weight of 76 000–77 000 daltons. Lactoferrin is produced by the glandular epithelium, mainly by the serous cells. Its action of removing heavy metal ions prevents the growth of certain bacteria, in particular *Staphylococcus* and *Pseudomonas* spp.

Lysozymes

These are produced by secretion in the nose from the serous glands, but some originate from tears which gain entry by way of the nasolacrimal duct. They are also produced from leucocytes which are found in nasal secretions and mucosa. The action of lysozymes is non-specific and depends on the absence of bacterial capsules for effect.

Antiproteases

A number of different antiproteases have been demonstrated and they increase with infection; however, their role remains open. They include α-antitrypsin, α_1-antichymotrypsin, α_2-macroglobulin and other antiproteases produced by leucocytes.

Complement

All components have been identified and C3 is produced by the liver and, locally, by macrophages. Its activation is produced by nonspecific as well as specific immunological responses through the alternative and classic pathways. It has a variety of functions, acting both on microorganisms including lysis, and neutrophil function including leucotaxis.

A number of other proteins and macromolecules have been identified from plasma, and are probably present as a result of capillary leakage.

Lipids

Phospholipids and triglycerides are present; their exact function is unknown.

Ions and water

The evaporation of water may account for some of the hyperosmolar Na^+ and Cl^- in mucus, but active ion transport also exists (Widdicombe and Welsh, 1980). This occurs within the serous glands which also account for the major proportion of the water in nasal secretions.

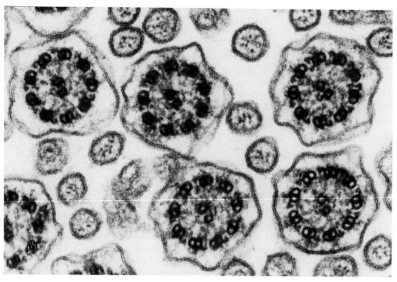

Figure 6.8 Ultrastructure of cilia. The nine plus two structure is clearly seen. The inner and outer dynein arms may be seen occasionally. The radial links may just be inferred. The smaller structures are microvillae

Immunoglobulins

Immunoglobulins are part of the immune system and all classes have been found in nasal secretions. Because the nose is a mucosal surface, the two immunoglobulins involved with mucosal defence, IgA and IgE, have been found to be present in greater quantities than in serum. IgA accounts for 70% of the total protein content. The immune system will be considered later.

Cilia

Ultrastructure

Cilia are found on the surface of the cells in the respiratory tract, and their function here is to propel mucus backwards in the nose towards the nasopharynx. All cilia have the same ultrastructure although nasal cilia are relatively short, measuring 5 µm, with over 200 per cell. The cilium comprises a surface membrane which encloses an organized ultrastructure of nine paired outer microtubules and a single inner pair of microtubules. The outer paired microtubules are linked together by nexin links and are linked to the inner pair by central spokes. The outer pairs also have inner and outer dynein arms which consist of an ATPase which is lost in Kartagener's syndrome. The microtubules become the basal body, the outer pairs become triplets, and the inner pair disappear. The three outer microtubules are similar to centrioles of mitotic cells and it has been suggested that centrioles migrate to the cell surface to form these structures (Sleigh, 1974) (*Figures 6.8* and *6.9*).

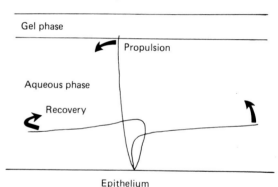

Figure 6.9 The beat pattern of a cilium; only the tip is in the gel layer

Ciliary action

The beat frequency is between 10 and 20 Hz at body temperature. The beat consists of a rapid propulsive stroke and a slow recovery phase. During the propulsive phase the cilium is straight and the tip points into the viscous layer of the mucous blanket, whereas in recovery the cilium is bent over into the aqueous layer. Energy is produced by the conversion of ATP to ADP by the ATPase of the dynein arms and the reaction is dependent on Mg^{2+} ions. Motion is initiated by the pair of outer microtubules sliding in relation to each other. ATP is generated by the mitochondria near the cell surface next to the basal bodies of the cilia.

The mucous blanket is propelled backwards by the metachronous movement of the cilia, which means that only those at right angles to the direction of flow are in phase. All those in the direction of flow are slightly out of phase until the cycle is complete. Initiation of ciliary movement is by mechanical action, a reversible domino effect. Mucus flows from the front of the nose posteriorly. Mucus from the sinuses joins that flowing on the lateral wall, with most going through the middle meatus. Most mucus passes around the eustachian orifice and is then swallowed.

The time taken for the cilia to transport mucus may be measured by the progress of saccharin, dye and radiolabelled particles. Saccharin is very inexpensive and is reliable clinically. The time taken is variable and lies between 5 and 20 minutes.

Factors affecting ciliary action

The nose is a remarkably constant environment and changes in it will affect ciliary function. Drying will stop the movement of the cilia but, if this is for only a short period, it is reversible. Temperature will also affect function, with cessation of movement below 10°C and above 45°C. *In vitro* ciliary beat frequency should be studied on a microscope with a warmed stage. Isotonic saline will preserve activity, but solutions above 5% and below 0.2% will cause paralysis. Similarly, cilia will beat above pH 6.4 and will function in slightly alkaline fluids of pH 8.5 for long periods. The commonest factor affecting ciliary function *in vivo* is an upper respiratory tract infection, which may damage the epithelium to such a degree that the surface cells slough away.

Drugs

The neurotransmitters will affect ciliary beat frequency. Acetylcholine increases the rate while adrenaline decreases the rate. The effects are reversible and dose dependent for adrenaline below a concentration of 1:1000. Topically active drugs such as ephedrine have not been shown to affect function, but cocaine hydrochloride, in solutions above 10%, causes immediate paralysis. Corticosteroids have been shown to reduce the rate of saccharin clearance following one week's therapy (Holmberg and Pipkorn, 1985).

Protection of the lower airways: immunological

The effect of altering the direction and velocity of the inspired air is to deposit particles on the surface epithelium. If the particles are not inert there are other factors which prevent damge to the host. Mucus is a barrier but the respiratory mucosa is not as effective as skin in protecting the internal environment from invasion. Mucus contains a number of different compounds which are able to neutralize antigenically active compounds. It may do this by the innate mechanisms or by the learned or adaptive immunological responses. The two main surface immunoglobulins are IgA and IgE. If the mucosa is breached then the IgM and IgG immunoglobulins are activated. These mechanisms cope with certain bacterial allergens. However, several bacteria and viruses require the activation of the cell-mediated immune response to protect the host.

Lymphocytes are conveniently subdivided into B and T types, and T lymphocytes are further subdivided by surface markers into suppressor, helper and killer cells, respectively. T and some B cells interact with macrophages. Macrophages, in turn, have both specific and non-specific immunological properties.

The lymphatic system can be divided into two types depending on the type of immunoglobulins produced. The first is the unencapsulated type of system, which includes the tonsils, adenoids, Peyer's patches and the aggregations within the respiratory and gastrointestinal tract. The plasma cells produce mainly IgA and IgE and are called either the gut or mucosal associated lymphoid tissue (GALT or MALT). If this system is overcome in the nose then the encapsulated system is activated; this is situated in the lymph nodes and the spleen and it produces IgG and IgM. Certain respiratory diseases can affect a lymphocyte cell type, and the virus causing glandular fever (infectious mononucleosis) replicates in B lymphocytes and may produce tonsillar hypertrophy, lymphadenopathy and splenomegaly (*Table 6.3*).

Table 6.3 Nasal immune system

Surface properties
  mechanical
  physical characteristics of mucus
Innate immunity
  bactericidal activity in mucus
  proteins
    lactoferrin, lysozymes, α_2-macroglobulin, C reactive protein, complement system
  cellular, polymorphs and macrophages
Acquired immunity
  surface IgA, IgM, IgE and IgG
  primed macrophages
  submucosa macrophages IgM, IgG, T and B lymphocytes
  mucosal associated lymphoid tissue
Distant sites
  adenoids, lymph nodes and spleen

Non-specific immunity

Lactoferrin, lysozymes, complement, antiproteases and other macromolecules interact with a number of bacteria, particularly those without capsules, to give an innate immunity. The actions of polymorph leucocytes and macrophages result in phagocytosis and destruction of foreign material. Many organisms and viruses are resistant and specific reactions are therefore required.

Acquired immunity

Acquired immunity may be produced by the immunoglobulins and interferon. IgG also activates complement which will result in cell lysis and phagocytosis. Viruses and mycobacteria initiate cell-mediated immunity. The nose has two types of acquired cell reaction as a first line defence: the production of IgA which produces insoluble complexes in mucus; and immunologically primed surface active cells which are capable of phagocytosis. IgA is found in considerable quantities in nasal secretions, and for this reason its production will be considered further. IgE produces allergic reactions and, as the nose is the commonest site of allergic reactions, a few comments about it will also be included here.

IgA

IgA is divided into two subgroups – IgA1 and IgA2. The former is more frequent in the serum and is a monomer, the latter is more common in nasal secretions and is a dimer. IgA accounts for up to 70% of the total protein in nasal secretions. The monomer has a molecular weight of 160 000 daltons, and two units are joined by a junctional chain (molecular weight 16 000 daltons). These units are produced in the same plasma cell so that antigenically similar IgAs are linked together. The IgA dimer is then transferred passively through the interstitial fluid and is actively taken up by the seromucin glands and the surface epithelium.

In the epithelium, a secretory piece is attached to the IgA dimer which makes it stable in mucus. When it reacts with an antigen it forms an insoluble complex which is swallowed and destroyed by the stomach acid. IgA does not activate complement.

IgE

IgE is the main immunoglobulin to cause allergic reactions and was first identified by Ishizaka and Ishizaka (1967). It is produced mainly in lymphoid aggregates, such as the tonsils and adenoids, and within the submucosa. IgE is firmly attached to mast cells and basophils, and two molecules of allergenic specific IgE have to sit on adjacent receptor sites on mast cells to cause degranulation. IgE has a molecular weight of 190 000 daltons and does not activate complement. It is usually directed against intestinal parasites.

Surface cells

In addition to its molecular components, mucus also contains cells. These consist of epithelial cells, leucocytes, basophils, eosinophils, mast cells and macrophages. Leucocytes and macrophages are important for phagocytosis on the surface and may help prevent bacterial or viral invasion. Cytology of the secretion may help in diagnosis. The surface cells migrate through the interstitium from the circulation.

Nasal vasculature and nerve supply

Nasal vasculature

Comparisons between the nose and the trachea and bronchial tree have limitations. The nose is a rigid box which is devoid of a constricting smooth muscle, thus the changes in its resistance are produced by alterations in the blood flow in resistance vessels and the amount of blood within capacitance vessels. The arrangement of the blood vessels is complex and varies at different sites within the nose (*Figure 6.10*). It is best developed where the air flow is maximum, which is over the turbinates and part of the nasal septum, and is less well developed in the sinuses and the floor of the nose. The vascular anatomy was described extensively by Burnham (1935), and the microanatomy has been further studied by Cauna (1970). The blood supply is derived from deep vessels traversing through the bone.

Figure 6.11 is a diagram of the blood vessels within the turbinate. In general, the arteries and arterioles produce the resistance, and the venules and sinusoids the capacitance. Shunting between the arteries and veins deep in the mucosa bypasses the surface vessels and reduces the amount of blood within the system. The anastomotic arteries spiral upwards through the cavernous plexus of veins where most of the shunting occurs. Towards the surface, the arteries ramify and give rise to arterioles which lack an elastic lamina, and end in capillaries which run parallel to and just below the surface epithelium. They also run around the mucous glands. The capillaries are fenestrated with more 'holes' towards the epithelium (Cauna, 1970); this allows transudation to occur, and the parallel course permits maximum heat exchange.

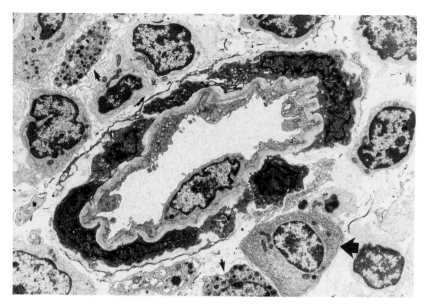

Figure 6.10 Arteriole. The endothelial cell is surrounded by darker smooth muscle cells. Next to the blood vessel is a plasma cell identified by the larger arrow. The two smaller arrows point to mast cells. (Magnification ×4000, reduced to 65% in reproduction)

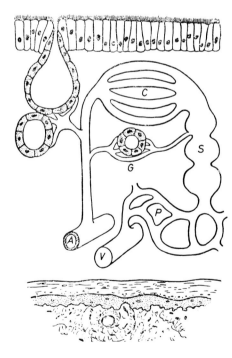

Figure 6.11 Schematic representation of the blood supply of the turbinates. It shows the arteriole (A) supplying the subepithelial capillaries (C), the glandular capillaries (G) which drain into the sinusoids (S) and the venous plexus (P)

The capillaries drain into a superficial venous system; the smooth muscle is best developed just before the superficial veins drain into the venous sinusoids.

The venous sinusoids are a cavernous plexus of large tortuous anastomotic veins without valves. The sinusoids receive both arterial and venous blood. The drainage of the sinusoids is regulated by cushion or throttle veins which have a circular muscle coat and an incomplete longitudinal crest. They do not close the lumen completely but are able to regulate the flow into the bone through the deep venous plexus. In cats, about 60% of the blood flow is shunted through arteriovenous anastomosis (Anggard, 1974), and the actual blood flow per cubic millimetre is greater than muscle, brain or liver (Drettner and Aust, 1974).

Although the arterial supply is from a number of different sources, the main supply is from the maxillary artery, and the arterial flow is forward through the nose against the incoming air. The vascular arrangement within the turbinates is often called pseudoerectile because of similarities to the blood supply of the penis.

Blood flow

Measurement of the nasal blood flow is difficult because material introduced into the nose will alter the nasal resistance. Blood flow may be inferred by

(1) direct changes in the colour
(2) photoelectric plethysmography
(3) alteration in the temperature which may be measured by thermocouples.

As the nasal resistance is related to blood flow, rhinometry may be used to assess blood flow indirectly. Capillary leakage may be gauged either by the appearance of labelled albumin in nasal secretion following intravenous injection or by the xenon wash-out method.

A number of combinations of blood flow may exist depending on the balance between arterial flow, arteriovenous shunting and venous pooling: hyperaemia with congestion of the cavernous sinuses, hyperaemia without venous congestion, ischaemia and reduced arterial perfusion with no shunting, giving rise to venous congestion. Control of vascular flow is by both the autonomic nervous system and the local inflammatory reactions, which may sometimes be independent of each other.

Autonomic nervous system

The autonomic nervous system controls the vascular reflexes in the nose and the distribution may be seen schematically (*Figure 6.12*). The reflexes may be initiated or modified by the sensory input which is by way of the trigeminal nerve. The ethmoid nerves are mainly sensory, whereas the sphenopalatine nerves are mixed.

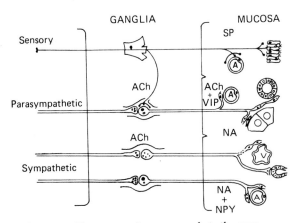

Figure 6.12 The autonomic nerve supply to the nose. Substance P (SP) of the sensory nerves act on arterioles. The action of acetylcholine (ACh) and vasoactive intestinal peptide (VIP) on the vessels and glands is shown. Noradrenaline (NA) and neuropeptide Y (NPY) act on the venules (V) in addition to the arterioles. (With kind permission of Dr A. Anggard)

Sympathetic nerve supply

The sympathetic nerve supply is derived from the lateral horn of the grey matter of the spinal cord at the level of the first and second thoracic vertebrae. Preganglionic axons run through the anterior nerve roots, anterior primary rami and white rami, and communicate with the sympathetic chain. They synapse in the superior cervical ganglion. Postganglionic fibres travel along the carotid artery to the deep petrosal and nerves of the pterygoid canal. They continue through the sphenopalatine ganglion and pass into the nerves of the nasal cavity.

Parasympathetic nerve supply

The pons contains the superior salivary nucleus in which preganglionic fibres have their cell bodies. They proceed by way of the intermediate branch of the facial nerve to the geniculate ganglion through which they pass. After continuing along the greater superficial petrosal nerve, and the nerve of the pterygoid canal, they synapse in the sphenopalatine ganglion. Postganglionic fibres then pass to the nasal mucosa.

Sensory nerves

The main sensory nerve supply is mediated by way of the trigeminal nerve. The ophthalmic and maxillary nerves which arise in the trigeminal ganglion supply the nose; sneezing is mediated through the vidian nerve (Malcolmson, 1959). It is uncertain precisely to which modalities the nose may be sensitive, but temperature, pain (or discomfort) and touch or irritation can be appreciated. Thermoreceptors are limited to the nasal vestibule. Proprioception does not appear to be present. It may be impossible to define nasal nerve endings in the same manner as the nerve endings in the skin and the locomotor system. There is some evidence that sensory nerve endings have H_1 receptors (Mygind and Lowenstein, 1982). Olfaction will be considered separately.

Neurotransmitters

Both parasympathetic and sympathetic nerve fibres supply the vasculature and glandular epithelium. Postganglionic fibres have been shown to have more than one neurotransmitter, which may account for the discrepancy in behaviour between expected experimental responses and actual reflexes. Classic cholinergic antagonists do not block parasympathetic vasodilation completely (Eccles and Wilson, 1973). (There is a similarity to mast cell reactions where antihistamines do not completely block reactions since there is more than one cellular mediator.)

In addition to acetylcholine and noradrenaline, neuropeptides are present in sympathetic, parasympathetic and sensory nerves (Uddman *et al.*, 1978; Anggard *et al.*, 1979; Lundberg *et al.*, 1982). Detection is by immunofluorescent techniques.

Parasympathetic

The main transmitter in the parasympathetic supply is acetylcholine, but vasoactive intestinal polypeptide (VIP) is present in postganglionic fibres. There are specific receptors for this on the blood vessels but not within the glandular epithelium. The transmitters probably act in combination. The action of acetylcholine is on both the blood vessels and the secretory tissue. Acetylcholine produces widespread vasodilation and increased glandular activity. If the rate of firing is low then acetylcholine probably acts alone on blood vessels. At higher rates, vasoactive intestinal polypeptide causes vasodilation which is atropine resistant, but acetylcholine may cause suppression of vasoactive intestinal polypeptide release by negative feedback (Uddman, Malm and Sundler, 1980). Acetylcholine is secretor motor for glandular tissue alone, but the effects of vasoactive intestinal polypeptide on neighbouring blood vessels may indirectly affect secretion.

Sympathetic

The transmitter to postganglionic fibres is acetylcholine, and the main postsynaptic transmitter is noradrenaline. Two neuropeptides may be found, namely neuropeptide Y and pancreatic polypeptide; neuropeptide Y is probably the more effective of the two. In contrast to noradrenaline, which causes both arterial, arteriolar and venous constriction, neuropeptide Y causes only arteriolar constriction (Lundberg and Tatemoto, 1982). Avian pancreatic polypeptide is similar morphologically to substance P and shares its action of vasodilation (Lundberg *et al.*, 1980).

Sensory

A number of nasal sensory neurons have been shown to contain the neuropeptide substance P. They are present in the sphenopalatine ganglion, near blood vessels and under the surface epithelium (Anggard *et al.*, 1979). Substance P causes vasodilation and is found in the C fibres.

Reflexes

Reflexes may be mediated through the brainstem, but axon reflexes may occur through the sensory nerves alone.

Axon reflexes

The neuropeptide substance P has been shown to transmit the reflex, and it may be initiated by mechanical irritation or by way of the mast cells which produce histamine. The reflex is antidromic. In addition to histamine's causing the reflex, substance P is also able to liberate histamine from mast cells. The concept of neurovascular reflexes and mast cell reactions being separate entities may need to be revised.

Reflexes from nasal stimulae

Chemical irritation, temperature change and physical stimuli of the nose may all cause widespread cardiovascular and respiratory responses. The degree of the response depends on the intensity of the stimulus, and ranges from sneezing to cardiorespiratory arrest. Sneezing is associated with facial movements, lacrimation, nasal secretions and vascular engorgement. More usually, a change in respiratory rate with closure of the larynx and a variable cardiovascular response occurs.

Animal studies have shown that sensory stimulation of the nose can result in intense vasoconstriction of skin, muscles and visceral arteries, and is accompanied by a lowered cardiac output. This is a modification of the submersion reflex which diverts blood away from the skin to the brain.

Nasopulmonary reflexes

Increasing the air flow through one side of the nose is associated with an increased ventilation of the homolateral lung. This follows the nasal cycle. Blowing air through the nose will cause the bronchial muscle to relax on the same side and increase its respiratory activity (Samzelius-Lejdstron, 1939).

Reflexes acting on the nose

The resistance of the nose may vary because of changes in the metabolic requirements of the individual. Exercise, emotion and stress may all cause vasoconstriction. These changes are mediated by increasing the sympathetic tone and are abolished by stellate ganglion block. An increase in arterial CO_2 mediated by the chemoreceptors will result in nasal vasoconstriction. Hypoxia has the same effect. Hyperventilation will cause nasal congestion.

Cutaneous stimulation

Heating the skin of parts of the body, such as that of the feet, arms or neck, will produce an increase

Table 6.4 Drugs acting on the nasal mucosa

Group	Examples
Sympathomimetics and their antagonists	Adrenaline and synthetic analogues
	Antihypertensives particularly β-blockers
Parasympathomimetics and their antagonists	Atropine, pilocarpine
	Antihistamines with this activity
Histamine and antihistamines	Mainly H_1 blockers
	Sedative and non-sedative
Local anaesthetics	Cocaine, lignocaine
Hormones	Sex hormones, thyroxine, corticosteroids

in nasal resistance. Cooling will result in vasoconstriction (Cole, 1954). Adaptation to both will occur and is followed by rebound. Pressure to the axilla on the dependent side will cause ipsilateral nasal blockage (Burrows and Eccles, 1985).

Central control

The hypothalamus is associated with cardiorespiratory responses and stimulation causes marked nasal vasoconstriction. Exercise, fight and flight reflexes and reflexes following emotional change are mediated by way of the hypothalamus. The relationship between the rhinencephalon and nasal function needs further evaluation.

Drugs acting on the vascular tissue of the nose *(Table 6.4)*

A brief review will be included of the drugs which affect the vasculature of the nasal mucosa. Drugs may be grouped into four sections: sympathomimetics and their antagonists; parasympathomimetics and their antagonists; histamine and antihistamines; and local anaesthetics. The mode of action in humans has not been fully evaluated and some of these drugs, particularly the antihistamines, rely on animal work in cats and dogs for evaluation of their behaviour.

Sympathomimetics and their antagonists

The two naturally occurring sympathomimetics, namely noradrenaline and adrenaline, act on the nose mainly through α_1-receptor sites, although it has been suggested that there may be some α_2-receptors which have a physiological role in the nose. It would appear that, opposed to the action of receptors which vasoconstrict, the agonists such as isoprenaline act on α_2-receptors and cause vasodilation. There are a number of sympathomimetics, related to ephedrine, that are used for

vasoconstriction; some, such as neosynephrine hydrochloride, are strong and cause a prolonged vasoconstriction. The main nasal complication is rebound hyperaemia which is associated with rhinorrhoea. Drugs such as cocaine block the uptake of noradrenaline and potentiate their own vasoconstriction. Drugs used in the treatment of hypertension may result in nasal obstruction by blocking sympathetic activity. Reserpine, which is no longer used, was the worst offender. Methyldopa and β-blockers may all give rise to nasal symptoms.

Parasympathomimetics and their antagonists

Intravenous pilocarpine and carbachol will cause nasal congestion, vasodilation and watery secretions. These actions are blocked by atropine and are a cholinergic effect. As mentioned earlier, atropine-resistant vasodilation does occur and is mediated by vasoactive intestinal polypeptide. Other mediators, such as histamine, are present in normal nasal secretions and may also cause vasodilation.

Histamine and antihistamines

The pharmacology of histamine is complex and both H_1 and H_2 receptors have been demonstrated in the nasal mucosa, with H_1 receptors predominating. Histamine acts both on the vasculature, giving vasodilation together with leakage from capillary walls, and on the sensory nerve endings where it is an irritant, resulting in the sensation of irritation and sneezing. Histamine has been shown to be present only in the mast cells and basophils. Histamine, although not as powerful as other inflammatory mediators from mast cells, is present in the greatest quantity. The actions of histamine, therefore, account for only some of the mast cell reactions.

Antihistamines are used widely in medicine and have a number of properties which include blockage of H_1 receptors, anticholinergic activity, local anaesthesia and sedation. Not all actions are present in each compound and the new antihistamines, such as terfenadine and astemizole, have no sedative effect, which makes them safer.

Although antihistamines work clinically, one study would suggest that they do not have any action against histamine in the nose (Bentley and Jackson, 1970), in spite of being shown to block the action of histamine on isolated guinea-pig ileum in other experiments.

Local anaesthetics

Local anaesthetics work by the action of an amide group which blocks conduction through the transmembrane channels and affects ion exchange. Two main groups are lignocaine and derivatives, and cocaine. Cocaine is a powerful vasoconstrictor, and it also potentiates the action of noradrenaline by blocking its recycle through re-uptake into the sympathetic nerve endings. Lignocaine has an effect on the precapillary sphincters which it dilates; thus it has, in fact, a slight vasodilatory activity. If lignocaine is used, it should have a vasoconstrictor added to the solution. All local anaesthetics, if given in high concentrations, have systemic effects on the heart and central nervous system.

Hormones

A close link exists between the anterior pituitary and the hypothalamus by way of the hypothalamohypophyseal tract. A complex interrelationship is present between emotional states, the autonomic nervous system and the hormones of the body. In all animals, olfaction is part of sexual behaviour and will be considered in more detail later.

Sex hormones

The nasal mucosa is susceptible to sex hormones, particularly oestrogens which it can concentrate. Conditions where oestrogen levels are high are associated with nasal obstruction and with rhinorrhoea. There are changes in nasal function during menstruation, pregnancy, and puberty in both sexes. Higher dose oestrogen contraceptives were associated with rhinitis in some women.

Thyroxine

Hyperthyroidism may give rise to rhinitis, although the exact mechanism is unclear, whereas hypothyroidism is associated with nasal obstruction resulting from the deposition of mucopolysaccharides in the extracellular spaces of the submucosa, which is similar to the condition found in the larynx and elsewhere.

Corticosteroids

Glucocorticosteroids affect nasal function indirectly and do so mainly during inflammatory reactions which involve mast cells. They affect the mast cell surface membrane and vascular endothelium, making them less permeable.

Adrenal medulla

The sympathomimetics have been considered elsewhere, but they produce a direct intense vasoconstriction on the nasal vasculature.

Emotional states

Three different responses may be categorized: fight or flight, which causes vasoconstriction; sexual behaviour, which produces a number of different responses; and stress. Vagal overactivity is found in patients with stress. This condition manifests itself in the abdomen by duodenal ulceration, whereas in the nose it results in prolonged congestion and may be the cause of some of the blocked noses encountered in patients in the clinic. Stress may result in migraine which, by way of the hypothalamus, gives rise to nasal symptoms, usually congestion and clear rhinorrhoea.

The nose and the voice

The voice is produced by modifying the vibrating column of air from the larynx. The larynx gives rise to the vowel sounds and the pitch voice and the main frequencies are under 1000 Hz (F_1 300–400 Hz, F_2 500–1900 Hz, F_3 1800–2600 Hz). High frequency sound which produces the consonants is added by the pharynx, tongue, lips and teeth. The nose adds quality by allowing some air to escape through it. The sound resonates within the nose and mouth; if too little air escapes from the nose then rhinolalia clausa occurs, if too much then rhinolalia aperta ensues. The nose is most effective when resonating at the laryngeal F_1

frequencies. It is doubtful whether the sinuses have any effect on modifying the voice, although they may help with auditory feedback. Transmission of sound through the facial skeleton helps monitor voice quality.

Olfaction

Olfaction initiates and modifies behaviour in many creatures. Humans minimize its importance, however, by concentrating on the audiovisual aspects of behaviour; and yet much money is spent annually on products which modify body odour and are supposed to make the wearer less offensive and more attractive to the opposite sex.

Odours are a complex mixture of different compounds, each one at a low concentration; however, studies in olfaction concentrate on single compounds or mixtures with two or three chemicals. Olfactory compounds have to come into contact with the nasal mucosa and, in order to produce a smell, need both a high water and lipid solubility. Man discriminates a large number of different smells, and the olfactory mucosa and pathway are rapidly fatigued, although they recover quickly.

Sniffing

The maximum exposure of the olfactory area to the smell is produced by sniffing which causes a turbulent air flow. Animal studies suggest that by increasing the velocity of air flow, the olfactory stimulus is increased (Ottoson, 1956).

Olfactory area

The olfactory area varies according to species, with dogs and rabbits having larger areas than human beings. The human being has $200-400\,mm^2$ with a density of about 5×10^4 cells/mm^2. The receptor cells carry modified cilia which increase the surface area and project like normal cilia into the mucus.

Stimulus

Odours are absorbed into the water of the mucus, and the lipid reacts with the lipid bilayer of the receptor cells at specific sites, which causes K^+ and Cl^- to flow out and thus to depolarize the cells (Tagaki *et al.*, 1968). After a latent period of up to 400 ms, a slow compound action potential may be recorded from the olfactory mucosa (Ottoson, 1956), and this is called the electro-olfactogram.

The speed of the rising phase varies with the intensity of the stimulus. The recovery phase or falling phase is an exponential decay with time constant of 0.9–1.45 ms.

Threshold

The olfactory response shows variation in both threshold and adaptation. The threshold concentration can vary by 10^{10} depending on the chemical nature of the stimulus. The threshold of perception is lower than identification: that is, a smell is sensed before it is recognized. Threshold values vary widely between studies and they reflect the nature of smell and the different methods of detection. Smell does not have an absolute threshold, but the threshold depends on the level of inhibitory activity which is generated by the higher centres. Some animals, particularly dogs, have a much lower threshold for detection.

Adaptation

The olfactory response shows marked adaptation: the threshold increases with exposure and recovery of the electro-olfactogram is rapid when the stimulus is withdrawn.

$$R = a + bc^t$$

where R is the perceived intensity, a is the asymptote, b is a constant and c is the rate of decline which is a function of time (t). Adaptation is both a peripheral and a central phenomenon. Cross-adaptation is present between odours at high concentrations, whereas cross-facilitation occurs near threshold values.

Other factors affecting threshold

Changes in the nasal mucus and its pH will alter olfactory perception. Threshold increases with age and is both decreased and altered by hormones, particularly the sex hormones. In man, some genetic variation occurs which is similar to colour blindness: there is a familial lack of perception of certain odours which is more common in males.

Discrimination

Man appears to be better at detecting the pleasantness of an odour than at recognizing it. The pleasantness is largely determined by cultural factors and is therefore learned. If two odours are mixed, the resulting intensity is always less than the sum of the two individually perceived intensities and is dominated by the stronger component.

Pathways

There is no interaction between the individual receptor cells, and receptor cells are connected to the olfactory bulb by non-myelinated nerve fibres. These fibres end on olfactory glomeruli; about 25 000 fibres end on each glomerulus, which then acts as an integrator. The conduction time between the receptor cells and the glomerulus is 50 ms for, even though the fibres are slow, they are short. The glomerulus fires with an all or none response into the mitral or tufted cells whose axons transport the signal through the lateral olfactory tract. Inhibition comes from feedback from the high cortical centres.

Higher centres

The anterior olfactory nucleus sends impulses to the opposite bulb and to the ipsilateral forebrain through the anterior commissure. The primary olfactory cortex lies rostral to the telencephalon and includes the olfactory tubercle, the prepyriform and preamygdaloid areas. There are projections into the thalamus where they are integrated with taste fibres, and there are also projections to the hypothalamus. Communication between the receptor cell and the brainstem occurs with only two synapses.

Perceived intensity

The perception of smell is a complex activity involving both the pathways and the higher centres which have learned to recognize the smell. It is possible to determine a mathematical relationship between the perceived intensity of the stimulus R and the stimulus concentration S:

$$R = CS^n$$

where C is a constant and the value of n is below one. As n is below one, the system attenuates particularly at high concentrations.

Trigeminal input

Most smell is independent of the trigeminal nerve, but at high concentrations irritation occurs which is a factor in detecting the intensity of certain compounds, such as butyl acetate, and may account for 30% of the odour intensity (Cain, 1974). Patients who are anosmic can distinguish only sweet, sour, salt and bitter and whether a compound is irritant. The irritant effect cannot be bypassed in normal people and does contribute to the nature of smell. It is important when testing olfaction to use compounds which are not irritant.

Classification of odours

There is no satisfactory classification of odours but Amoore (1969) has suggested that there are up to 30 primary odours for humans, basing his theory on the stereochemistry of compounds and the variations of anosmia to substances which are present in man. The human being has difficulty in detecting and recognizing variation in intensity of more than 17 odours. Furthermore, because the human being does not rely on conscious detection of odour, only its quality, training is necessary for scientific experiments and for occupations which require a 'good nose'. An obvious discriminatory mechanism has not been found in the nose at either the receptor site or in the olfactory bulb. Some cells in the olfactory bulb increase their discharge rate and some decrease their rate of discharge on stimulation.

Theories of smell

It is a general rule in medicine and science that if there is no single theory of function then no one really knows or has proven the mechanism involved. There are a number of hypotheses which have been advanced to explain the nature of smell.

Molecular structure

Moncrieff (1967) has suggested that molecular structure is important; however, no stereospecific olfactory receptors have been demonstrated.

Electrochemical reactions

Some cells contain carotenoids similar to those in the eye and these could be responsible for the occurrence of reactions similar to the photochemical reactions in the eye (Briggs and Duncan, 1962).

Stereospatial patterns

Certain receptors could have a stereospatial, lock and key form, and receptor cells fire when the surface membrane is altered (Mozell, 1970).

Molecular properties

A modification of the previous theory would hold that basic molecular properties account for receptor specificity and include molecular volume at boiling point, proton affinity and donation, and local polarization within the molecule (Laffort, Patte and Etcmeto, 1974). Theoretical thresholds correlate with experimental values.

Olfactory mucosa morphology

The pattern of the stimulus within the mucosal configuration of the receptor cells detects the nature of the smell. This theory of discrimination is based partly on specific receptor sites and partly on their position within the olfactory mucosa (Holley and Doving, 1977).

Olfaction may well be an analogue system. A number of different patterns from a few receptor sites would give rise to a large number of different smells.

Olfaction and behaviour

Olfaction is important in regulating behaviour in all animals, including man and insects. The degree of development depends on the species. Smell is used in four main areas of behaviour: the detection and consumption of food, recognition, territorial markings, and sexual behaviour. In humans, eating and sexual behaviour are highlighted.

Eating

Olfaction is related to two aspects of eating, namely the recognition of food types and the initiation of digestion. The initiation of digestion is mediated by way of the lateral and ventromedial hypothalamus, and it causes salivation and increases the output of gastric acid and enzymes.

Sexual behaviour

Pheromones were first described in relation to insects. The term was used to describe the chemicals which were produced by glands and were responsible for sexual attraction. They have since been encountered widely in all animals. Three types of pheromone have been described, which are releaser pheromones, primer pheromones and imprinting pheromones. Releaser pheromones produce an immediate and reversible response and act through the nervous systems, whereas primer pheromones require prolonged stimulation and act on the anterior pituitary where they cause hormones to be released. Imprinting pheromones, which are chemicals encountered during development, modify behaviour and may subsequently initiate a response.

The degree of involvement in human behaviour is uncertain but the influence of smell is probably underestimated as most activity occurs at the subconscious level.

The paranasal sinuses

The physiological role of the paranasal sinuses is uncertain. They are a continuation of the respiratory cavity and are covered by a respiratory mucosa. They share certain features with the nose but the responses are much less marked on account of the relatively poorly developed vasculature and nerve supply. In man, the sinuses' main interest is in disease, and this subject is outside the scope of this chapter.

The development of the paranasal sinuses takes up to 25 years: the ethmoids and maxillary sinuses are present rudimentarily at birth, while the frontal sinuses develop after the age of 6 years but may be completely absent; the sphenoid sinus differs considerably in the degree of development. It holds true that whatever physiological role the sinuses play, it is not essential and of only minor importance.

Mucosa

The mucosa runs in continuity from the nose and is respiratory in type; however, there are differences between the nose and the sinuses. In the sinus mucosa, goblet cells and cilia are less numerous in general but more frequent near the ostia; the blood supply is less well developed with no cavernous plexuses. The poorer blood supply results in a pale, semitranslucent mucosa. As the nerve supply is less well developed, the sinus mucosa is able to give only a basic vasomotor response and increase mucus production on parasympathetic stimulation.

Drainage

Mucociliary clearance in the maxillary sinus is spiral, and towards the natural ostium, and may be seen by means of dyes and carbon particles (Toremalm, Mercke and Reimor, 1975). Drainage of the frontal and sphenoidal sinuses is downwards and is aided by gravity; the blood supply is better developed in the frontal sinuses and the ostium is relatively large in the sphenoid sinus. The secretions join the nasal mucus in the middle meatus and may contribute to the total amount and effectiveness of the nasal mucus.

Oxygen tension

The P_{O_2} is lower in the maxillary sinuses than in the nose and it is lower still in the frontal sinuses. If the ostium becomes blocked, the oxygen tension drops further. Ciliary motion remains normal if the blood supply is adequate. If the blood supply is impaired then ciliary activity is reduced and stasis of secretions results.

Ostium size

Blockage of the natural sinus ostium results in a reduction of ventilation and stasis of secretions. If the ostium size is below 2.5 mm, it predisposes to the development of disease (Aust, Drettner and Hemmingsson, 1976).

Pressure changes

The pressure in the maxillary sinus varies with respiration but lags behind by 0.2 s. There is little fluctuation when the nose is patent, and the variation of pressure during quiet respiration is ± 4 mmH$_2$O which reaches 17–20 mmH$_2$O on exercise. If the nose is blocked then the pressure fluctuations are much more marked.

Barotrauma is five times less common than in the ear and is most frequently seen in the maxillary sinuses, particularly in divers.

Physiological functions of the sinuses

The possible functions of the sinuses are as follows:

air conditioning
pressure damping
reduction of skull weight
heat insulation
flotation of skull in water
increasing the olfactory area
mechanical rigidity
vocal resonance and diminution of auditory feedback.

On the other hand, the sinuses may have no function at all.

Comments

The volume of the largest sinus is under 50 ml and, therefore, the sinuses contribute little to air conditioning. Similarly, a damper has to have a large volume to be effective. The reduction of skull weight is small compared to the overall weight. Most of the cranial activity is away from the sinuses so they play little part in insulating the brain. Man has long ceased to be an amphibian.

It is probable that apart from mucus production and some strengthening of the facial bones, the paranasal sinuses have little or no physiological function.

References

AMOORE, J. (1969) A plan to identify most primary odors. *Olfaction and Taste*, edited by C. Pfaffman, pp. 158–171. New York: Rockefeller University Press

ANGGARD, A. (1974) Capillary and shunt blood flow in the nasal mucosa of the cat. *Acta Oto-Laryngologica*, **78**, 419

ANGGARD, A., LUNDBERG, J. M., HOKFELT, T., NILSSON, G., FAHRENKRUG, J. and SAID, S. (1979) Innervation of the cat nasal mucosa with special reference to relations between peptidergic and cholinergic neurones. *Acta Physiologica Scandinavia Supplementum*, 473, 50

AUST, R., DRETTNER, B. and HEMMINGSSON, A. (1976) Elimination of contrast medium from the maxillary sinus. *Acta Oto-Laryngologica*, **81**, 468–474

BENTLEY, A. and JACKSON, R. (1970) Changes in patency of the upper nasal passage induced by histamine and antihistamines. *The Laryngoscope*, **80**, 1859–1870

BOAT, T. F., KLEINERMAN, J. I., CARLSON, D. M., MALONEY, W. H. and MATTHEWS, L. W. (1974) Human respiratory tract secretions. 1 Mucous glycoproteins secreted by cultured nasal polyp epithelium from subjects with allergic rhinitis and with cystic fibrosis. *American Review of Respiratory Diseases*, **110**, 427–441

BRIDGER, G. P. and PROCTOR, D. P. (1970) Maximum nasal inspiratory flow and nasal resistance. *Annals of Otology*, **79**, 481–488

BRIGGS, M. and DUNCAN, B. (1962) Pigment and olfactory mechanism. *Nature*, **195**, 1313–1314

BURNHAM, A. H. (1935) An anatomical investigation of blood vessels of the lateral nasal walls and their relation to turbinates and sinuses. *Journal of Laryngology and Otology*, **50**, 569–593

BURROWS, A. and ECCLES, R. (1985) Reciprocal changes in nasal resistance to airflow caused by pressure applied to the axilla. *Acta Oto-Laryngologica*, **99**, 154–159

CAIN, W. S. (1974) Contribution of the trigeminal nerve to perceived odor magnitude. *Annals of the New York Academy of Science*, **237**, 28–34

CANTER, R. (1986) A non-invasive method of demonstrating the nasal cycle using flexible liquid crystal thermography. *Clinical Otolaryngology*, **11**, 329–336

CAUNA, N. (1970) Electron microscopy of the nasal vascular bed and its nerve supply. *Annals of Otorhinolaryngology*, **79**, 443–450

CLEMENT, P. (1984) Committee report on standardisation of rhinomanometry. *Rhinology*, **22**, 151–155

COLE, P. (1954) Respiratory mucosal vascular responses, air conditioning and thermoregulation. *Journal of Laryngology and Otology*, **68**, 613–622

COLE, P. (1982) Modification of inspired air. In *The Nose: Upper Airway Physiology and the Atmospheric Environment*, edited by D. Proctor and I. Anderson, pp. 351–375. Amsterdam: Elsevier

COLLINS, M. P. (1985) A practical guide to the construction of a 'cire perdue' model of the human nose. *Rhinology*, **23**, 71–78

DRETTNER, B. (1979) The role of the nose in the functional unity of the respiratory system. *Rhinology*, **17**, 3–11

DRETTNER, B. and AUST, R. (1974) Plethysmographic studies of the blood flow in the mucosa of the human maxillary sinus. *Acta Oto-Laryngologica*, **78**, 259

ECCLES, R. and WILSON, H. (1973) The parasympathetic nerve supply of the nose of the cat. *Journal of Physiology*, **230**, 213–223

FULLTON, J., FISCHER, N., DRAKE, A. and BROMBERG, P. (1984) Frequency dependence of effective nasal resistance. *Annals of Otology, Rhinology and Laryngology,* **93,** 140–145

HOLLEY, A. and DOVING, K. (1977) Receptor sensitivity, acceptor distribution, convergence and neural coding in the olfactory system. In *Olfaction and Taste VI,* edited by J. Le Magna and P. Macleod, pp. 113–123, London: Information Retrieval

HOLMBERG, K. and PIPKORN, U. (1985) Mucociliary transport in the human nose. The effect of topical glucocorticoid treatment. *Rhinology,* **23,** 181–186

INGLESTEDT, S. and IVSKERN, B. (1949) The source of nasal secretion in normal conditions. *Acta Oto-Laryngologica,* **37,** 446–450

ISHIKAZA, K. and ISHIZAKA, T. (1967) Identification of E antibodies as a carrier of reaginic activity. *Journal of Immunology,* **99,** 1187–1198

KAYSER, R. (1895) Die exakte Messung der Luftdurchgängigkeit der Nase. *Archives of Laryngology,* **3,** 101–210

LAFFORT, P., PATTE, F. and ETCMETO, O. (1974) Olfactory coding in the basis of physiochemical properties. *Annals of the New York Academy of Science,* **237,** 193–208

LAMB, D. and REID, L. (1970) Histochemical and autoradiographic investigation of the serous cells of the human bronchial glands. *Journal of Pathology,* **100,** 127–138

LUNDBERG, J., ANGGARD, A., FAHRENKRUG, T., HONFELT, T. and MUTT, V. (1980) Vasoactive intestinal polypeptide in cholinergic neurones of exocrine glands: functional significance of coexisting transmitters for vasodilation and secretion. *Proceedings of the National Academy of Science of the USA,* **77,** 1651–1655

LUNDBERG, J. and TATEMOTO, K. (1982) Pancreatic polypeptide family (APP, BPP, NPY and PYY) in relation to sympathetic vasoconstriction resistant to α-adrenoceptor antagonists. *Acta Physiologica Scandinavica,* **116,** 393–402

LUNDBERG, J. M., HOKFELT, T., ANGGARD, A., TERENIUS, L., ELDE, R., MARKEY, Y. *et al.* (1982) Organisational principles in the peripheral sympathetic nervous system. *Proceedings of the National Academy of Science of the USA,* **79,** 1303–1307

MALCOLMSON, K. G. (1959) The vasomotor activities of the nasal mucous membrane. *Journal of Laryngology and Otology,* **73,** 73–98

MASSON, P. L. and HEREMANS, J. F. (1973) Sputum proteins. In *Sputum: Fundamentals and Clinical Pathology,* edited by M. J. Dulfano, pp. 412–474. Springfield Illinois: Charles C. Thomas

MICHAEL, R. P., ZUMPE, D. and KEVERNE, D. B. (1972) Neuroendocrine factors in the control of primate behaviour. *Recent Progress in Hormonal Research,* **28,** 665

MONCRIEFF, R. (1967) *The Chemical Senses.* London: Leonard Hill

MOZELL, M. (1970) Evidence for a chromatographic model of olfaction. *General Physiology,* **56,** 46–53

MYGIND, N. and LOWENSTEIN, H. (1982) Allergy and other environmental factors. In *The Nose: Upper Airway Physiology and the Atmospheric Environment,* edited by D. F. Proctor and I. Anderson, pp. 377–397. Amsterdam: Elsevier

OTIS, A., FENN, W. and RYHN, H. (1950) The mechanics of breathing in man. *Journal of Applied Physiology,* **2,** 597–607

OTTOSON, D. (1956) Analysis of the electrical activity of the olfactory epithelium. *Acta Physiologica Scandinavica, Supplementum,* 122, 1–83

PROETZ, A. W. (1953) *Applied Physiology of the Nose,* 2nd edn. St Louis: Mosby

REYNOLDS, S. R. M. and FOSTER, F. (1940) Acetylcholine equivalent content of nasal mucosa in rabbits and cats, before and after administration of oestrogen. *American Journal of Physiology,* **131,** 422

SAMZELIUS-LEJDSTROM, I. (1939) Respiratory movements. *Acta Oto-Laryngologica Supplementum,* 35, 3–104

SLEIGH, M. (1974) *Cilia and Flagella.* London: Academic Press

SWIFT, D. L. (1982) Physical principles of airflow and transport phenomena influencing air modification. In *The Nose: Upper Airway Physiology and the Atmospheric Environment,* edited by D. F. Proctor and I. Anderson, pp. 337–349. Amsterdam: Elsevier

SWIFT, D. L. and PROCTOR, D. F. (1977) Access of air into the respiratory tract. In *Respiratory Defense Mechanisms,* edited by J. D. Brain, D. F. Proctor and L. M. Reid, Vol I, Chapter 3. New York: Dekker

TAKAGI, S., WYSE, F., KITAMURA, H. and ITO, K. (1968) The roles of sodium and potassium ions in the generation of the electro-olfactogram. *Journal of General Physiology,* **51,** 552

TOREMALM, N., MERCKE, U. and REIMOR, A. (1975) The mucociliary activity of the upper respiratory tract. *Rhinology,* **13,** 113–120

UDDMAN, R., ALUMETS, J., DENSERT, O., HAKANSSON, R. and SUNDER, P. (1978) Occurrence and distribution of VIP nerves in the nasal mucosa and tracheobronchial wall. *Acta Oto-Laryngologica,* **85,** 448–555

UDDMAN, R., MALM, L. and SUNDLER, F. (1980) VIP increases in nasal venous blood after stimulation of the vidian nerve. *Acta Oto-Laryngologica,* **87,** 304–308

VAN CAUWENBERGE, P. B. and DELEYE, L. (1984) Nasal cycle in children. *Archives of Otolaryngology,* **110,** 108–110

VAN DISHOEK, H. A. G. (1965) The part of the valve and turbinate in total nasal resistance. *International Rhinology,* **3,** 19–26

WIDDICOMBE, J. and WELSH, M. (1980) Ion transport by dog tracheal epithelium. *Federation Proceedings,* **39,** 3062–3066

WIDDICOMBE, J. G. and WELLS, U. K. (1982) Airway secretions. In *The Nose: Upper Airway Physiology and the Atmospheric Environment,* edited by D. F. Proctor and I. Anderson, pp. 215–244. Amsterdam: Elsevier

7

Pathophysiology of the ears and nasal sinuses in flying and diving

A. J. Benson and P. F. King

No study of otolaryngology is complete without a description of the physiological and pathological conditions which may affect the ears and nasal sinuses in aerospace and underwater. This is borne out by the importance of aviation, both civil and military, in the modern world and by the rapid development of the underwater industry. This view is consolidated by the millions of passengers who fly each year, and the thousands who fly and dive for a hobby.

Physical laws relating to aerospace and the underwater environment

The response of gases when subjected to pressure must be understood as this governs the behaviour of gas in the tympanic cavity, the middle ear, and the nasal sinuses. This is exemplified by Boyle's law, which states that the pressure and the volume of an enclosed fixed mass of gas are inversely proportional.

It is convenient for descriptive purposes to start at sea-level; during an *ascent* through the atmosphere there is a progressive reduction in pressure (*Figure 7.1*). In general terms, at 18 000 ft (5500 m) above sea-level the pressure is half that at sea-level, and is halved again at 34 000 ft (10 300 m); the change in differential pressure with altitude is greater at relatively low altitudes than at a greater height. In practice, during ascent through the atmosphere, a given mass of gas contained within an elastic structure will expand.

In the middle ear, this gaseous expansion will push the tympanic membrane to the natural limit of its excursion, to be followed by an easy and involuntary escape of air along the eustachian tube (*Figure 7.2a*) (Hartmann, 1879; Armstrong and

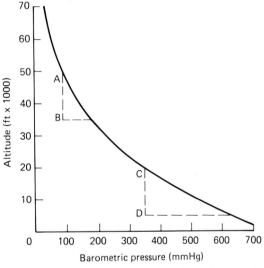

Figure 7.1 Relationship between altitude and barometric pressure in flight. For any given rate of descent, the rate of pressure change increases as the altitude is reduced. A descent of 15 000 ft (4570 m) is shown at AB and CD: in AB the pressure change is 91 mmHg (12.1 kPa) and in CD it is 283 mmHg (37.6 kPa)

Heim, 1937). Movement of the membrane may be restricted by scarring or by calcareous deposits, and this may give rise to aural pain during ascent.

During *descent* from altitude, with an increase in the atmospheric pressure, there is a decrease in volume of the middle-ear gas (*Figure 7.2b*). The eustachian tube must be opened by swallowing movements to adjust the volume. If this mechanism fails or if it is delayed, an increasing differential pressure will act on the soft

183

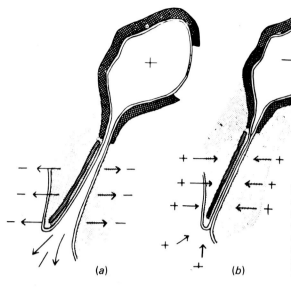

Figure 7.2 Diagrammatic representation of the middle ear during ascent (*a*) and descent (*b*). With reducing ambient pressure on ascent, the air in the middle ear expands, bulges the tympanic membrane and passively opens the eustachian tube. In descent, with increasing ambient pressure, the tympanic membrane is forced inwards, and the soft parts of the eustachian tube are held in apposition

nasopharyngeal end of the tube to close it. When this pressure is greater than can be generated by the tubal dilator muscles, the tube will stay closed and is said to be 'locked'. Thereafter, with continued descent the pathophysiological changes of barotrauma are inevitable. Armstrong and Heim (1937) showed that positive extratympanic

pressure of 90 mmHg (12 kPa) will lock the tube, but this figure depends on the intrinsic strength of the tubal dilator muscles, and so it is variable.

Boyle's law is still applicable underwater. At water surface, the ambient atmospheric pressure is 14.7 pounds per square inch (psi) or a pressure of 1 atmosphere (1 atm or 101 kPa). In descent from the water surface, the pressure increases rapidly in a linear fashion as a result of the density of the water, so that at 33 ft (10 m), the pressure is double that at the surface (2 atm or 202 kPa). Every 33 ft (10 m) of descent adds 1 atmosphere of pressure (101 kPa). Compare this with the aviator's situation, when descent from 18 000 ft (5500 m) to sea-level will encompass a change in pressure of only 0.5 atmosphere (50.5 kPa). In ascent to the surface from depth, a reverse state of affairs will apply (*Figure 7.3*).

The role of pressurization and the pressure cabin

The adverse physiological effects of flight at high altitude are almost entirely a consequence of the accompanying reduction of barometric pressure, so that the most logical way of securing satisfactory conditions for the occupants of high-flying aircraft is to provide within the aircraft an atmosphere that is at a pressure appropriate to bodily needs (*Figure 7.4*).

As the cabin pressure has to be greater than that of the surrounding atmosphere, the difference between the two pressures will be represented by a differential pressure tending to force the cabin wall outwards. It follows that the absolute pressure within the pressure cabin will be equal to

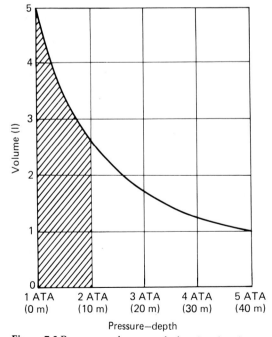

Figure 7.3 Pressure–volume graph showing that the maximum change occurs during the first 10 m (33 ft) of a dive. (Reproduced by permission of Surgeon Captain P. W. Head)

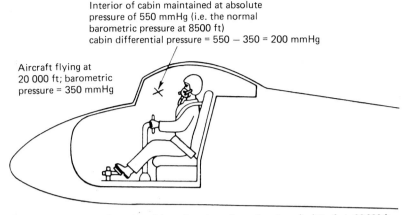

Interior of cabin maintained at absolute
pressure of 550 mmHg (i.e. the normal
barometric pressure at 8500 ft)
cabin differential pressure = 550 − 350 = 200 mmHg

Aircraft flying at
20 000 ft; barometric
pressure = 350 mmHg

Figure 7.4 Pressure cabin aircraft in a situation where the aircraft altitude is 20 000 ft
(6100 m) and the cabin altitude is 8500 ft (2600 m)

the barometric pressure existing at an altitude below that at which the aircraft is flying. It is convenient to consider conditions inside the aircraft in terms of the altitude that is being simulated by pressurization. In pressure cabin aircraft, the terms 'aircraft altitude' and 'cabin altitude' are appropriate.

The effect of employing a pressure cabin is to reduce the range over which barometric pressure is acting, but it should be remembered that below 15 000 ft (4500 m), the rate of pressure change will predispose to barotrauma, and this is an important factor in deciding the rate at which pressurization should diminish when an aircraft is descending.

The practicalities of the situation have resulted in the concept of both a high and a low differential cabin. The high differential cabin is employed in transport aircraft in which the conveyance of passengers makes it necessary to maintain a cabin altitude of 8000 ft (2440 m), even when the aircraft, like the supersonic transport, is flying at 60 000 ft (18 300 m). The maximum differential pressure involved is 430 mmHg (56.9 kPa). The low differential cabin is employed in military aircraft, when failure of the pressure cabin in combat must be accepted as an operational hazard. The risks of too great a pressure change occurring during sudden decompression are minimized by employing a relatively low cabin differential pressure. In spite of this, many military aircraft are commonly fitted with cabin pressure controllers, whose characteristics can be altered in flight. Although no variation can be made in the maximum permissible differential pressure, it is possible to select the altitude at which pressurization will start after take-off, and the rate of change of cabin pressure during ascent and descent.

In the example shown in *Figure 7.5* (Brown, 1965), the alternative pattern, if adopted, would reduce the risk of barotrauma when carrying out a rapid descent below 8000 ft (2400 m). For example, if the aircraft were descending at 1000 ft/minute (5 m/s) below 8000 feet, the rate of change of the cabin altitude would be 500 ft/minute (2.5 m/s) – an effective reduction.

Physiology of the eustachian tube

The function of the auditory tube is to maintain the equality of air pressure around the tympanic membrane, necessitated by the absorption of gas through the mucous membrane, and variations of ambient atmospheric pressure. This is achieved by opening the tube to permit the passage of air. In its natural state the tube is collapsed, so that its closure is a passive process, assisted by relaxation of the associated muscles. Other related factors, probably acting in combination, are the elasticity of the cartilaginous support, the venous pressure, and the presence of a blanket of mucus in the lumen of the tube (Farmer, 1985).

The auditory tube is opened by swallowing, yawning and gaping movements. The muscles involved in the control of patency of the tube can be divided into two groups:

(1) those muscles which by having an insertion into the walls of the tube exert direct action
(2) those muscles which by anatomical association assist and influence tubal opening.

The muscles in the first group comprise the tensor palati, the levator palati, the salpingopharyngeus and the tensor tympani muscles. The tensor palati muscle is the most important, and McMyn (1940) believed it to be the prime mover in opening the tube, a view supported by Rich (1920) and Macbeth (1960). It is likely that tensor palati

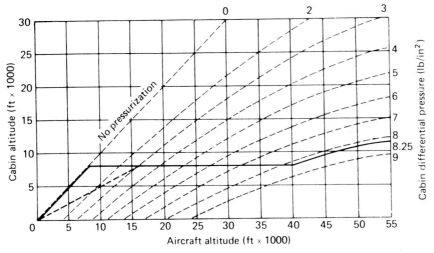

Figure 7.5 Graph illustrating, for a typical passenger aircraft, the relationship between aircraft altitude, cabin altitude and cabin differential pressure. (From Brown, 1965)

and tensor tympani muscles, with a common embryological origin, and with the same nerve supply, act synergistically. The levator palati muscle supports and holds the tubal cartilage (*Figure 7.6*) to permit the tensor palati to act on the curve of the tubal cartilage, and so open the lumen. The muscles in the second supporting group are the upper parts of the superior constrictor of the pharynx, and the spincter of the nasopharyngeal isthmus, of which the palato-pharyngeus is a major contributor.

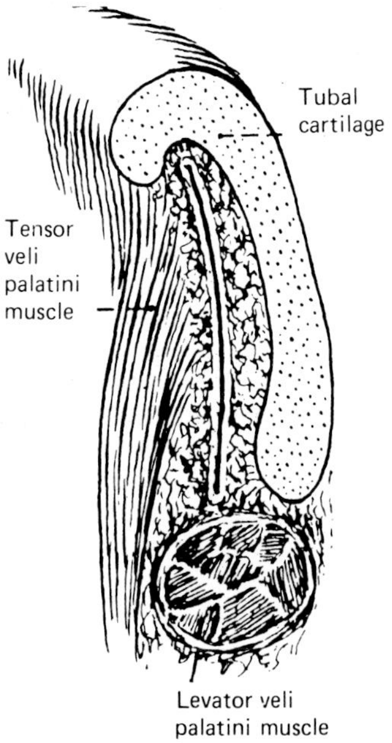

Otic barotrauma

Unobstructed ventilation of the middle ear will produce no changes and hence no symptoms. The term 'otic barotrauma' defines any damage to the ear which results from pressure, and it has been known as aerotitis media, aviation pressure deafness, and otitic barotrauma. This condition is likely to occur in any situation where a change of pressure acts on the middle ear and tubal system. However, concern here is with the occurrence of such a mechanism in flight, in diving, and in the simulation of these physical environments in decompression and compression chambers. In addition, patients treated in hyperbaric chambers may also suffer from otic barotrauma (Morrison, 1972).

Factors contributing to barotrauma

Any condition which narrows the tubal lumen by oedema or by increasing the amount or viscosity of the mucus coating the mucous membrane will, by impeding the flow of gas along the tube, or by impairing the ability of the tube to open, predispose to barotrauma. The commonest predisposing causes of acute barotrauma are acute and chronic infections in the nose, particularly coryza, nasal allergy and vasomotor rhinitis – and to these should be added malformation of the nasal skeleton.

Tubal cartilage

Tensor veli palatini muscle

Levator veli palatini muscle

Figure 7.6 A diagram of a cross-section of the cartilaginous portion of the auditory tube, showing the relative positions of the tensor palati and levator palati muscles. (After Holmquist, 1976)

The role of overpressure in the nasopharynx

It has been seen that the eustachian tube will open passively in ascent, from overpressure of gas in the middle ear. In descent, the tube will also open from overpressure of some degree applied at the end of the tube, as in the Valsalva manoeuvre. This technique is frequently used in flight and, in effecting tubal clearance, it is no less successful when used in diving. The subject attempts forcible expiration with the lips closed, and the nostrils occluded by digital compression of the nose. In doing so, the air pressure in the nasopharynx is raised to force air along the auditory tube to the middle ear. The manoeuvre has the disadvantage that it may cause syncope from the increase in central venous pressure and pooling of the venous blood resulting from the raised intrathoracic pressure. In addition, pulmonary stretch reflexes may induce cardiac arrhythmia (Duvoisin, Kruse and Saunders, 1962), so that there is a potential hazard with this method.

A procedure developed by Frenzel (1938, 1950) consists of closing the glottis, the mouth and nose, while at the same time contracting the muscles of the floor of the mouth and the superior pharyngeal constrictors. It is independent of intrathoracic pressure and can be performed in any phase of respiration. Chunn (1960) found that with this manoeuvre, the mean tubal opening pressure was 6 mmHg (0.8 kPa) compared with a mean opening pressure of 33 mmHg (4.4 kPa) with the Valsalva method.

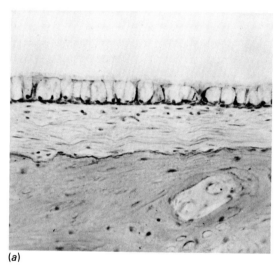

(a)

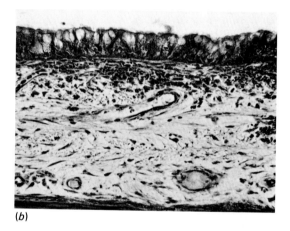

(b)

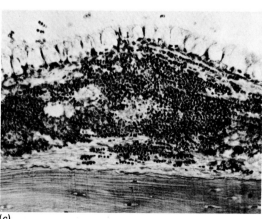

(c)

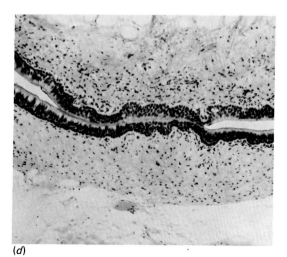

(d)

Figure 7.7 Histological preparations showing the tissue changes occurring in barotrauma induced experimentally in the ear of cats. (*a*) Normal mucosa of middle ear. (*b*) Oedema of middle-ear mucosa, with subepithelial cellular infiltration. (*c*) Haemorrhage in middle-ear mucosa. (*d*) Tubal obstruction

Pathophysiology of barotrauma

The pathophysiology of otic barotrauma was given a definitive description in the work of Dickson, McGibbon and Campbell (1947), in which cats were decompressed to a pressure corresponding to an altitude of 20 000 ft (6100 m) and then recompressed. The histological changes seen (shown in *Figure 7.7a–d*) were all vascular in nature, and included mucosal congestion, oedema, haemorrhage, effusion and polymorph infiltration. These are related to the subambient pressure in the middle ear, which will become clinically manifest by invagination of the drumhead, congestion, solitary or multiple haemorrhagic bullae, blood or fluid in the middle ear and, in some instances, rupture of the tympanic membrane. These features are shown in *Plate 1*.

In the situation of a descent without ventilation of the middle ear from, say, an altitude of 10 000 ft (3050 m) to sea-level, where the ambient pressure is 760 mmHg (101 kPa), the middle ear will contain air at a theoretical pressure of 523 mmHg (70 kPa) and the pressure difference across the tympanic membrane will be 237 mmHg (31 kPa). The absolute pressure within the blood vessels in the tympanic membrane is the sum of the ambient pressure (atmospheric pressure) plus the present blood pressure. If the capillary pressure is of the order of 20 mmHg (2.7 kPa), then the absolute blood pressure in the capillaries will be 780 (760 + 20) mmHg (103.7 kPa); and as the pressure of the tissue fluid surrounding the vessels is only 523 mmHg (70 kPa) the vessels will become passively engorged.

Rupture of the tympanic membrane

The anteroinferior portion of the tympanic membrane is the site where tears commonly occur, but previous scars are also a site of predilection. In flight, barotrauma associated with a fast rate of descent may cause avulsion of the drumhead from the tympanic ring. King (1976) reported rupture of the drumhead in 38 of 897 ears which had sustained barotrauma in flight. Underwater, rupture of the drumhead is likely with unrelieved tubal obstruction on descent to depths greater than 16 ft (4.8 m).

Rupture of the labyrinthine windows: inner ear barotrauma

Hughson and Crowe (1933) demonstrated that, during a rise in pressure of the cerebrospinal fluid, the round window membrane would bulge outwards into the tympanic cavity. In 1971, Goodhill reported spontaneous rupture of the round window membrane caused by a rise in intracranial pressure resulting from coughing, sneezing or straining, and he believed that a sudden change in the middle-ear pressure in flight might have the same effect. Work by Tingley and MacDougal (1977) suggested window rupture as the cause of symptoms of alternobaric vertigo (*see below*) in some instances.

The operation of stapedectomy may involve a special risk in flying and diving. The possible fate of the stapedectomized ear in flight has been investigated by Rayman (1972); sudden pressure change may involve the disruption of the artificial stapes from the oval window, or its impaction into the inner ear. Either of these situations will produce sudden severe sensorineural loss, and possibly incapacitating vertigo. This places a special responsibility on the surgeon when advising this operation and he should warn of the possible hazards to the ear. In this connection, a fat and wire assembly is considered the safest of the many different combinations of prosthesis and graft that are utilized in this procedure.

The concept of round window fistula is of particular relevance to the hyperbaric environment of the diver (Edmonds and Freeman, 1972; Edmonds, 1973b). Goodhill (1971) suggested that in some individuals an infantile type of cochlear aqueduct persisted, with the consequent loss of the protective effect of the long, narrow adult aqueduct in the reduction of fluctuations in pressure differential between the cerebrospinal fluid and the perilymph. Increased cerebrospinal fluid pressure could cause a sudden rise in perilymph pressure within the scala tympani, leading to rupture of the round window membrane. In diving, the physical exertion plus the hyperbaric environment will increase the cerebrospinal fluid pressure. A susceptible diver, if exposed to a sudden and rapid increase in depth, may thus suffer both from middle-ear barotrauma and round window fistula.

Delayed otic barotrauma

Otic barotrauma is normally associated with physiological changes at the time of the alteration in pressure. However, there are occasions when subjects may experience an incidence of deafness and discomfort in the ear several hours later. This delayed form of barotrauma occurs after long flights, when the breathing of 100% oxygen has resulted in a raised tension of that gas in the middle ear. With passive collapse of the tube, as happens in sleep, and with no active inflation of the middle ear, the absorption of oxygen through the middle-ear mucosa results in the development of a significant pressure differential. Comroe *et al.*

(1945) reported the condition originally, and Jones (1958, 1959) has also studied the significance of oxygen absorption in this context. The signs are minimal, consisting of invagination of the drumhead and, in some cases, a suspicion of fluid in the middle ear.

Chronic otic barotrauma

This is a clinical rather than a physiological entity in which one episode of barotrauma predisposes to another. Two factors are considered to be responsible:

(1) the original predisposing factor may itself be chronic
(2) oedema and interstitial bleeding in the tubal mucosa, resulting from the original barotrauma, may reduce the tubal lumen, so predisposing to further attacks; in practice, in both aviation and diving, sufficient time is not always given for the basic lesion to recover before the patient is again exposed to pressure change.

'Reversed ear' (reverse ear squeeze) – barotrauma of the external auditory meatus

This condition will occur on descent, both in water and in the air, if an obstruction at the meatal entrance prevents an increase in pressure in the external canal, in the presence of ambient atmospheric pressure in the middle ear through an open eustachian tube. The tympanic membrane bulges outwards leading to possible rupture, and blood blisters may form in the external canal which may also rupture. In flying, reverse ear squeeze is caused by the fitting of a tight earplug, whereas in diving, the most likely cause is the compression, by increasing water pressure, of the soft hood of a Scuba suit against the pinna (*Figure 7.8*) (Jarrett, 1961).

The management of otic barotrauma

The immediate aim of treatment is to relieve pain, and simple analgesics will usually suffice. Pain is greatest at the time of change of pressure, and eases once the situation has stabilized. Persistence or worsening of pain suggests that otitis media has supervened, although this is rare.

The second principle of treatment involves the ventilation of the middle-ear cleft. Decongestants in spray form for the nose, or antihistamines, are helpful both as a first-line treatment and as a continuing supportive measure. Early eustachian catheterization and inflation used to be the popular form of treatment, but they are considered unproductive in a severe otic barotrauma. Instant relief can be obtained by myringotomy, a method much in favour in the USA, and this was recommended over 40 years ago by Canfield and Bateman (1944).

Delay in recovery, the persistence of fluid in the middle ear, or recurrent barotrauma all call for myringotomy, suction, and the insertion of a ventilation tube. This method is of value to professional aviators as it permits the continuation of trouble-free flying while the aural condition resolves. This is not the case in divers, who, once a ventilation tube is fitted, are advised to stay out of water until resolution is complete. As a precipitating factor for otic barotrauma is commonly found in the nose or sinuses, a thorough search of this area must be made for any lesion or abnormality, which, if present, should be treated on its merits. It has been shown (Dickson and King, 1956) that, where surgical treatment is indicated and carried out, a high rate of functional recovery can be expected. The passage of time has not changed this view, which has been reaffirmed by McNicholl (1982). He found that 34 of 37 naval divers were able to equilibrate middle-ear pressure during descent only after undergoing nasal septal surgery.

If rupture of the tympanic membrane occurs it is best left undisturbed, apart from careful cleansing of the ear to remove blood or loose clot. Many of these ears will heal of their own accord. Of those that do not heal, some form of tympanoplasty may be required to produce a safe ear, although it should be stressed that there is no physiological reason why an individual with a clean dry central perforation should not fly.

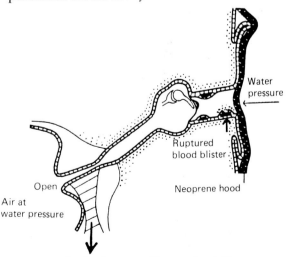

Figure 7.8 The development of 'reversed ear'. (From Roydhouse, reproduced by permission of the publisher)

Where flying personnel and divers are concerned, the surgical result from tympanoplasty must conform to the physiological requirements demanded by the individual's working environment. This means that the repaired tympanic membrane should look reasonably normal, move well during pressure change, and that the hearing should be within the practical limits required by the patient's occupation. These functional and practical criteria are not always easy to meet. In any event, and no matter what treatment is given for barotrauma, sufficient time should be allowed for the condition to resolve itself, and for the eustachian tube to open properly, before a return to flying or diving is permitted. Apart from visual inspection, pure-tone audiometry and tympanometry are useful and often assist in making an assessment.

Sinus barotrauma

The paranasal sinuses also contain air, with the consequence that barotrauma of these structures may occur in flying and diving. The syndrome encompassing the development of pain in the frontal area or the cheeks during or shortly after pressure change, and sometimes associated with rhinorrhoea and epistaxis, is called sinus barotrauma. Other descriptive terms are aerosinusitis, barotraumatic sinusitis and dysbarism.

The real frequency of the condition is not known, and estimates vary. Dickson and King (1954) reported a ratio of 5:2 when comparing otic with sinus barotrauma in a series of 328 patients suffering from barotrauma. In describing the distribution, King (1965) reported involvement of the frontal sinus(es) in 80% of cases of sinus barotrauma, with antral implication in 29%, with some 10% of cases having both the antra and the frontal sinuses affected.

The production of pathology as a result of a change of pressure will hinge on the degree of patency of the sinus ostium, and hence, to a large degree, on nasal function. Unlike the middle ear, with ventilation through the eustachian tube, there is no voluntary control over the diameter of the sinus ostium so that equalization of pressure may be difficult. The Valsalva manoeuvre may sometimes be effective, but it cannot be relied upon.

The sinus ostium may be reduced by a plug of mucus, mucosal oedema, or by some mechanical feature such as a polyp or neoplasm, although this latter occurrence is rare. The obstruction is often of a valvular nature, so that air passes easily in one direction only. Adequate ventilation of the nasal sinuses is related closely to nasal function, with the consequence that factors creating oedema of the nasal mucosa are commonly found as predisposing causes, for example coryza and its infective sequelae, vasomotor rhinits, seasonal allergy, and the effects of mechanical obstruction from nasal injury and deflection of the nasal septum.

During descent in air or water (the compression phase), sinus barotrauma may be caused by obstruction of the ostium from the nasal side (*Figure 7.9b*). With unrelieved obstruction, and continuing descent, the decreasing volume of air in the affected sinus exerts a suction effect on the lining mucosa and enhances the ostial block. On ascent, the ostium may be blocked from within the sinus cavity (*Figure 7.9a*), and the symptoms are caused by the unrelieved expansion of the gas contained in the sinus.

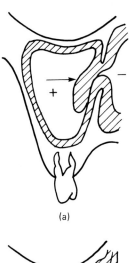

(a)

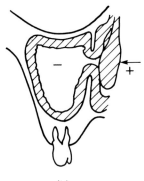

(b)

Figure 7.9 (*a*) Diagram to indicate how antral barotrauma is caused during ascent. The air in the sinus expands with decreasing ambient pressure and, in this instance, has forced a polyp into the ostium so blocking it. With continued ascent, an increasing differential pressure is built up between the sinus and the environment. (*b*) The mode of causation of antral barotrauma in descent. With increasing environmental pressure, a polyp in the nasal fossa has been forced into the sinus ostium, so blocking it. With continued descent, and unrelieved obstruction, antral barotraum will occur

During descent, either in air or in water, the absolute blood pressure increases steadily. If there has been ostial obstruction during this phase, the gas in the sinus will remain at a relatively low pressure. The pressure differential between the mucosa and the interior of the sinus will increase, and the mucosa will become engorged. This can lead to rupture of mucosal vessels, the formation of a subepithelial haematoma, and even frank haemorrhage (*Figure 7.10*). The degree of pathological change is proportional to the magnitude of the pressure differential and the period of time over which the pressure inequality is

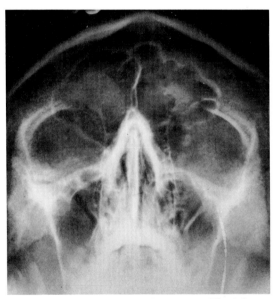

Figure 7.10 Right frontal sinus barotrauma. The right frontal sinus shows a pear-shaped swelling, the result of submucosal haemorrhage

unrelieved. Because of the greater pressure differential in diving, the mucosal changes can be expected, on average, to be greater than those experienced in flight.

Pain is the main symptom, which is frequently localized to the affected sinus. It often originates above the eyes, and spreads to the temples and the vertex; facial discomfort and pain in the upper teeth may also occur. The pain is of sudden onset, it is often severe, and may precipitate fainting. Nasal bleeding can be profuse and there is often a discharge of straw-coloured fluid from the nose. There may be a blood clot in the nasal fossae (*Figure 7.11*), and the affected sinus may be tender.

Radiological examination can help to determine the site and size of the lesion in as many as 75% of cases, and the use of radiology can be useful in assessing the progress of treatment. However, it should be remembered that this type of examination does not necessarily distinguish between lesions contributing to the production of barotrauma, and those which are the result of it (McGibbon, 1947).

Management

Treatment follows accepted principles which are aimed at relieving pain and achieving adequate ventilation of the affected sinus. This latter is accomplished by nasal decongestants and antihistamine preparations. Any predisposing factor should be dealt with in order to reduce the risk of recurrence, and simple surgical treatment, such as submucous resection of the septum, antrostomy, polypectomy, or enlargement of the frontonasal duct, may be required.

Delayed sinus barotrauma

The production of delayed sinus barotrauma is uncommon, and generally occurs after flights in which high concentrations of oxygen are inhaled,

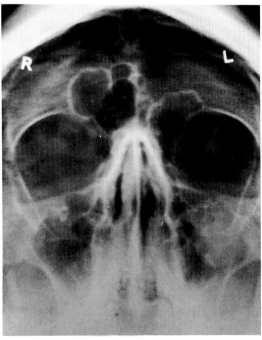

Figure 7.11 Left antral barotrauma. The left antrum shows a well-defined polypoid swelling, apparently arising from the upper outer angle of the antrum. Lavage yielded blood clot on this side

thus raising the tension of the gas in the sinuses. If an ostial block occurs, oxygen is absorbed through the mucosa; a pressure differential develops which may engender local sinus pain and may be followed by generalized headache.

Pneumocoele

Pneumocoele of the antrum is rare, and is aggravated by high altitude flying. Although few cases have been reported (Noyek and Zizmor, 1974; Zizmor *et al.*, 1975), the condition is included here for completeness. A structural anomaly at the ostium creates a valve that permits air easily to enter the antrum, but prevents it from escaping. Flight may induce a feeling of pressure in the cheek, worsened by sneezing. In one reported case, the Valsalva manoeuvre produced a fluctuant swelling through a dehiscence in the lateral wall of the antrum; radiology showed an expanded translucent antrum.

Dental barotrauma

Pain of dental origin may occur both in flying and diving. In view of the close proximity of the second premolar and the first two molars to the antral floor, it is important to differentiate dental barotrauma from maxillary sinus barotrauma. In the case of military air-crew, pain of this type is not uncommon. Ashely (1977) reported that one in five fighter pilots in the US Air Force suffered from such pain, while a French Air Force survey reported an incidence of 6% in flying personnel. In non-vital teeth, the pulp may become necrotic, probably in consequence of restoration or the use of instant fillings. Gas formation occurs in the autolysing pulp, and its expansion on ascent forces infected material into the periapical tissue, with the likely development of an abscess in the following day or two. In partially vital teeth, there may be gas bubbles in the pulp cornua under a deep cavity, although the source and composition of the gas is unknown. Severe pain in such teeth may be experienced in flight at altitudes up to 5000 ft (1500 m).

The commonest occurrence of dental pain in flight is in vital teeth with pulpitis and, in these cases, pain typically occurs on ascent at about 7000 ft (2000 m). Such teeth need treatment, and it is sensible to stop flying for 10–14 days after the completion of treatment of a suspect tooth. In diving, implosion of a tooth can occur in descent when a cavity with thin cementation is present (Edmonds, 1976), while in ascent, pain has resulted from lifting of enamel or crown (Leitch, 1985). In view of the poor critical localization of pain from the dental pulp, all suspect teeth should be checked and their response to cold stimulation determined.

Inner ear injuries in a hyperbaric environment

Injuries to the cochlea and the vestibular apparatus can occur after exposure to a stable, hyperbaric environment in diving, particularly during deep dives. According to Dalton's law, each gas in a mixture of gases exerts its own pressure independently of the other contained gases, and the total pressure of the gas mixture is the sum of the partial pressures. The solubility of a gas is proportional to its partial pressure. Of the inspired air, oxygen constitutes 21%, while nitrogen comprises 78%. Nitrogen is inert and, with increasing depth, more dissolves in body tissues and fluids. During decompression, nitrogen may be released as bubbles from the tissue, which will cause the 'bends'. To prevent or reduce the possibility of bends and nitrogen narcosis, an oxyhelium gas mixture is employed for deep and 'saturation' dives. In saturation diving, divers must stay at a pressure level for a sufficient time to enable their tissues to reach a state of equilibrium with the gases to which they are exposed. The usual method is for the divers to live in a complex of chambers, and to move to and from their working site in a pressurized bell (Leitch, 1985).

Lesions of the cochlea or vestibular apparatus are precipitated at the beginning of decompression when the oxyhelium gas mixture is changed to compressed air. It is unusual for both cochlea and vestibular mechanism to be damaged. The 'isobaric countercurrent diffusion theory', developed by Farmer (1977), attempts to explain the formation of bubbles in the peri- and endolymphatic fluids by the counterdiffusion of two inert gases across the round window membrane. This is not surprising in view of the fact that when the breathing mixtures are changed, the perilymph and endolymph are saturated with helium, while the middle ear rapidly fills with compressed air.

Decompression sickness

Decompression sickness is a condition which has been recognized in divers and caisson workers since the middle of the nineteenth century, yet only in the last 50 years has its effect on those exposed to subatmospheric pressures been clearly described (Fryer, 1969). Paralysis, fits and other neurological manifestations from this cause are rare in aviators, and disturbances of taste, smell and hearing have not been recorded in this group.

In otological terms, consideration must be given to the way this condition affects divers, for whom decompression sickness remains a limiting factor on ascent from deep or prolonged saturation dives. As a dive increases in depth, the respired gases in the diver are absorbed into the circulation. The quantity of gas absorbed will depend on its solubility and partial pressure; it will also depend on the vascularity of the tissue, and the rate of diffusion of the gas. During decompression a reversal of this process occurs; the dissolved gases come out of solution and appear in a gaseous state in the lungs, or as bubbles in the tissues or body fluids. In accordance with Boyle's law, bubbles increase in size as decompression proceeds. Bubbles may be present within the inner ear, as well as in the eighth nerve pathway and its central connections. Intravascular gas emboli can also occur. The pathological changes, including haemorrhage, and the diverse signs and symptoms of decompression sickness have been described by McCormick, Philbrick and Holland (1973) (*Figures 7.12* and *7.13*). This risk may be reduced by careful control of the depth and duration of the dive and the rate of ascent to the surface. Susceptibility to decompression sickness increases with age and obesity, while the effects of cold and dehydration, and the after-effects of alcohol, have been recognized.

The aural symptoms of decompression sickness, vertigo and hearing loss, either singly or together, are not common but are well recognized; the imbalance which can occur is referred to by divers as 'staggers'. Coles (1976) reported the incidence of these symptoms as 6 or 7% in some 100 cases of decompression sickness affecting experimental deep divers at the Royal Naval Physiological Laboratory (Alverstoke, Hants, UK). As long ago as 1909, Keays suggested that in 5% of all cases of decompression sickness, vertigo was the most characteristic symptom. It should be remembered that signs of sensorineural hearing loss in a diver may not be evidence of decompression sickness, but can be related to the high ambient noise in which the diver works, as well as to noise exposure unrelated to diving.

Other changes in hyperbaric states

In addition to bubbling, hyperbaric states are associated with a reduction in capillary flow and with stasis in the microcirculation. Combined with this is an elevation of the level of the serum lipid and serum cholesterol. Workers at the Institute of Naval Medicine (Alverstoke, Hants, UK) (Martin and Nichols, 1972) have found a significant reduction in the circulating platelet level after decompression. Platelet aggregates form around

developing gas bubbles, and have been shown to initiate clotting (Philip, Schacham and Gowdey, 1971). This contributes a potential hazard to the cochlea and vestibule, although no part is more at

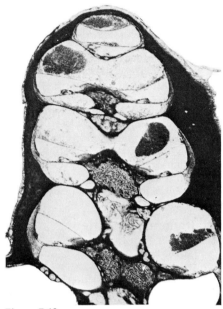

Figure 7.12

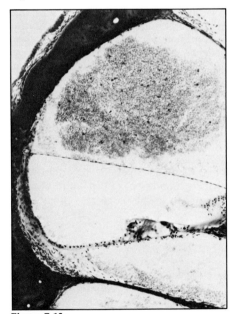

Figure 7.13

Figures 7.12 and **7.13** Haemorrhage into the cochlea of guinea-pig following simulated oxyhelium dive in a pressure chamber. (From McCormick, Philbrick and Holland, 1973; reproduced by permission of authors and publisher)

risk than another. Microemboli from lipid, platelets or gas bubbles will lead to degeneration of the affected sensorineural epithelium.

High pressure nervous syndrome

Compression, particularly rapid compression, in an oxyhelium atmosphere to depths greater than 500 ft (152 m) may produce symptoms of the high pressure nervous syndrome (Bennet and Towse, 1971). These symptoms are dizziness, nausea, intention tremor, and decrement in standing steadiness. The symptoms abate in a matter of hours. Electronystagmographic (ENG) studies during high pressure nervous syndrome (Farmer, 1977) have shown no evidence of vestibular end organ dysfunction and the mechanism of these symptoms remains unknown, although an alteration in cerebellar function has been postulated.

Pressure (alternobaric) vertigo

Attention so far has been directed to the traumatic effects of pressure change on the ear and sinuses, but it has long been recognized that changes in ambient pressure can also cause a transient disturbance of vestibular function in the absence of overt aural pathology. The occurrence of vertigo in aviators during ascent and descent was first described by van Wulfften Palthe (1922). However, the condition was not clearly recognized until Jones (1957) reported that 10% of the Royal Air Force pilots whom he had interviewed had experienced such symptoms. A later survey by Lundgren and Malm (1966) found an incidence of 17% in flying personnel of the Royal Swedish Air Force. The disability is even more common among divers who are exposed to greater and more rapid changes in pressure than air-crew. In a group of Swedish sports divers, no fewer than 33% reported that they had experienced vertigo when diving, which Lundgren (1973) attributed to pressure change in 26% of those responding to his questionnaire.

Clinical features

The characteristic features of the syndrome, termed 'pressure vertigo' by Jones (1957) and 'alternobaric vertigo' by Lundgren (1965), is the vertigo, of sudden onset, which coincides with the passive equalization of middle-ear pressure, either during a rapid ascent or on producing an overpressure in the middle ear by means of a Valsalva manoeuvre during descent or when on the ground. Typically, the vertigo is short lived, decaying within 5 seconds or less, although it can

be of such an intensity that the induced nystagmus impairs vision. Less commonly, the vertigo is weaker, with only a sensation of turning without impairment of vision, but the vertigo is more persistent, lasting for up to one minute or longer. There is considerable intersubject variability in the plane and direction of the vertigo, although it is usually of a consistent pattern in any one individual. Pressure vertigo is more likely to affect air-crew and divers when there is difficulty in equilibrating middle-ear pressure, usually from congestion and inflammation of the nasal mucosa resulting from a common cold or other infection of the upper respiratory tract; such an association is found in about 70% of cases. There are, however, a few individuals who suffer from pressure vertigo even in the absence of infection. Studies by Ingelstedt, Ivarsson and Tjernström (1974) suggest that these susceptible individuals require a higher pressure differential between the middle ear and ambient pressure than is the norm in order to open the eustachian tube and vent gas to the immediate surroundings.

Pathophysiology

The mechanism by which the sensory receptors of the vestibular apparatus are stimulated by changes in middle-ear pressure is still a matter for conjecture. The dominant symptom, vertigo, strongly suggests that it is the ampullary receptors of the semicircular canals, rather than the maculae, that are stimulated. Furthermore, the transient nature of the disturbance accords with the theory proposed by Jones (1957), namely that the cupula is deflected when the overpressure in the middle ear is suddenly relieved on passive venting, or when middle-ear pressure is raised momentarily above ambient pressure by a Valsalva manoeuvre. Overpressure in the middle ear may not be transmitted equally to the fluid systems of the inner ear by the round and oval windows, for the stapes footplate might move against the pressure gradient caused by the outward displacement of the tympanic membrane. It is conceivable that, with the sudden restoration of middle-ear pressure, there is a movement of endolymph and perilymph which causes a displacement of the cupula of one or more of the semicircular canals of the ear involved. Unfortunately, little is known about the transient response of the hydrodynamic systems of the inner ear to large amplitude pressure changes, even in the normal ear, so it is difficult to explain why some individuals show an altered pattern of end-organ activity with such a stimulus while others do not.

The work of Ingelstedt, Ivarsson and Tjernström (1974) and Tjernström (1974a) has shown that five out of 79 otologically healthy subjects exposed to simulated ascents with a pressure change of 66 mmHg (8.8 kPa) in 25 s (equivalent to an ascent from ground level at approximately 5000 ft (1500 m)/minute) developed vertigo when middle-ear volume was allowed to equilibrate passively. Indirect measurement of the middle-ear volume was used to identify the timing of tubal opening. It was found that vertigo and the concomitant nystagmus were not induced at the moment of tubal opening but, rather, that vestibular stimulation occurred when the relative overpressure in one ear was about 44 mmHg (5.9 kPa) or higher. However, not all subjects who had a high opening pressure developed vertigo. The additional requirement for the induction of symptoms was a definite asymmetry of the middle-ear pressures, caused by one ear equilibrating with low tubal opening pressures and the other needing a high opening pressure.

The demonstration that vertigo and nystagmus could be induced in susceptible subjects by an overpressure in the middle ear when there was free communication of air between the middle ear and the external canal led Tjernström (1977) to propose that pressure vertigo might be caused by a relative ischaemia of the sensory epithelium. He suggested that the overpressure in the middle ear is effectively transmitted to the fluid system of the inner ear because of poor patency of the cochlear aqueduct when there is a rapid pressure change. The estimated pressure in the capillaries of the inner ear is less than 40 mmHg (5 kPa) above ambient pressure, so if fluids of the inner ear were pressurized to more than 40 mmHg above ambient pressure, by an overpressure in the middle ear, then circulatory insufficiency affecting structures within the inner ear would be likely to ensue.

Although such a mechanism cannot be refuted, it must be pointed out that the vestibular reactions induced by the pressure change in the experimental studies of Ingelstedt and Tjernström were relatively weak. Vascular insufficiency could well be responsible for the low grade and sometimes sustained vertigo that is reported by a minority of flying personnel with 'pressure vertigo', but in the authors' opinion, it is unlikely to account for the severe, although brief, disturbance of vestibular function that can be precipitated by equilibration of middle-ear pressure during ascent or active over-inflation (Valsalva manoeuvre) during descent.

Management

The established association between the incidence of pressure vertigo and the impairment of middle-ear ventilation by upper respiratory tract infections implies that the most important prophylactic measure is the restriction of the duties of air-crew and divers when they are suffering from coryza or other conditions in which there is congestion of the mucous membrane of the nasopharynx. Unfortunately, in some cases, it is the occurrence of pressure vertigo that first tells the individual that he is developing a common cold.

On their return to flying or diving following an upper respiratory tract infection, susceptible individuals should be advised to equilibrate middle-ear pressure frequently so as to minimze the development of high pressure differentials. The use of nasal decongestants may also be beneficial.

The repeated occurrence of vertigo associated with changes of middle-ear pressure, in the same way as any other form of persistent vertigo, merits withdrawal from flying or diving duties, and a full investigation. If evidence of tubal dysfunction is not found, the integrity of the round window should be determined by tympanotomy. Tingley and MacDougal (1977) have described two air-crew with symptoms not dissimilar to those of pressure vertigo, who were found to have a small defect in the round window membrane when this structure was visualized.

Motion sickness

Motion sickness, or kinetosis, is a syndrome characterized primarily by nausea, vomiting, pallor and cold sweating, which is induced when an individual is exposed to certain types of real or apparent motion stimuli. Motion sickness is a generic term which embraces sea-sickness, air-sickness, car-sickness, space-sickness, swing-sickness, simulator-sickness and so on, the name identifying the provocative environment or vehicle. Yet despite this diversity of causal stimuli, the responses of the afflicted individual are essentially the same and have a common aetiology. Motion sickness is not a pathological condition but is the normal response of an individual, with an intact vestibular system, to motion stimuli with which he is unfamiliar and to which he is consequently unadapted; only those individuals without labyrinthine function are truly immune.

However, it should be pointed out that the signs and symptoms of the motion-sickness syndrome are a common feature of organic disease of the vestibular sensory system, in particular those conditions in which there is a sudden and asymmetrical modification of the activity of the sensory receptors of the vestibular apparatus. Although the primary cause of the malaise engendered by motion stimuli and by vestibular dysfunction may differ, the basic aetiology is the same, as is the process of adaptation to the altered sensory information and the therapeutic benefit of certain drugs.

Clinical features

The development of the motion-sickness syndrome typically follows an orderly sequence, the time-scale being determined by the intensity of the provocative motion and susceptibility of the individual. There are, however, considerable individual differences in susceptibility as there are in the incidence and order of occurrence of particular signs and symptoms. The earliest symptom is commonly a sensation of epigastric discomfort, best described as 'stomach awareness'. With continued exposure, nausea increases in intensity and the cardinal autonomic signs appear, namely pallor and sweating. Vasoconstriction is most noticeable in the face, particularly about the mouth, while sudomotor activity is usually confined to those areas of skin where thermal rather than emotive sweating occurs. There is frequently a feeling of bodily warmth and the afflicted individual seeks cool air to obtain symptomatic relief, although this is short-lived. Associated, but more variable, early signs and symptoms are increased salivation, eructation and flatulence, headache, and an ill-defined dizziness. There may be an alteration in the pattern of respiration, with sighing and yawning, which may lead to hyperventilation, particularly in those who are anxious about their disability or their safety in a hostile motion environment (for example, storm conditions at sea or severe turbulence when flying).

The aforementioned signs and symptoms develop relatively slowly, but with continued exposure to the provocative motion there is commonly a sudden intensification of malaise which culminates in vomiting or retching. This is usually followed by a temporary amelioration of symptoms before the subject's condition again deteriorates and emesis ensues. This cyclical pattern of recurrent vomiting, with waxing and waning symptoms, may continue for several days if there is no escape from the provocative motion environment. Those so afflicted can be severely anorexic, depressed and apathetic, incapable of carrying out allotted duties or even caring for their own safety. Their debility may be further compounded by dehydration and a disturbance of electrolyte balance brought about by repeated vomiting (*see* Money, 1970; Reason and Brand, 1975; or Benson, 1984, for a more detailed review of the clinical features of motion sickness).

In those situations where there is continued exposure to provocative motion, as aboard ship in storm conditions, most individuals exhibit a progressive reduction in the severity of symptoms as they adapt to the motion. The time course of this adaptation is variable, but typically it takes 2–4 days before a significant level of protective adaptation is achieved and the signs and symptoms of motion sickness are dispelled.

In conventional aircraft, prolonged exposure to provocative motion is, these days, relatively uncommon and flights are rarely longer than 10–12 hours. The situation is different in space-flight where the astronaut is in an abnormal force environment (that is null gravity or weightlessness) for many days or even months. The natural history of space-sickness is in most respects similar to that of terrestial motion sickness, as described previously (Benson, 1977; Homick *et al.*, 1983). The important difference is not in the signs and symptoms, but rather in the nature of the provocative stimulus. In conventional (terrestrial) motion sickness, it is the complex motion of the vehicle imposed on the person within that induces malaise, whereas in space-flight, it is the movement of the astronaut within the vehicle that is the provocative factor. The time-scale of adaptation to space-sickness is similar to that described for sea-sickness. Most astronauts who have suffered from space-sickness have been able to move about and make rapid head movements without discomfort after 3 days in weightlessness, and all but one have been symptom-free by the sixth day of space-flight.

Adaptation to an atypical motion environment involves a modification in the way sensory information is processed by the central nervous system and establishment of new motor patterns that are beneficial to the individual. However, on return to a normal (that is a stable 1 *g*) environment, these sensory and motor patterns are no longer appropriate and can cause perceptual and equilibratory disturbances until readaptation has taken place. The *mal de debarquement* that sailors experience on return to land after a voyage of sufficient duration for them to adapt to the motion of the vessel, is but one example of this phenomenon. Likewise, astronauts on their return to earth have reported vertiginous sensations on making head movements, and they have an impairment of postural equilibrium that is present for many days, or even weeks, after a long flight.

Aetiology

The vestibular system has a significant role in the genesis of motion sickness because the human being, like other susceptible animals, does not suffer from motion sickness unless possessing a functional labyrinth (James, 1882). The knowledge that the absence of vestibular function afforded protection against the disability led to the hypothesis that motion sickness was caused by *vestibular overstimulation*, but this concept is untenable. Quite strong and unfamiliar motion stimuli, such as repeated stops of a rotating chair or the cyclical oscillation experienced on horseback, do not readily induce sickness, whereas much weaker stimuli, such as the cross-coupled (Coriolis) stimulation of the semicircular canals (produced by head movement while rotating on a turntable) can be highly provocative. Furthermore, the vestibular overstimulation hypothesis does not account for the visually induced forms of motion sickness (for example simulator- or Cinerama-sickness), neither does it attempt to explain adaptation and readaptation (*mal de debarquement*) phenomena.

The alternative and more acceptable explanation is that the essential cause of motion sickness is the presence of sensory information about bodily motion which is at variance with inputs that, from past experience, the central nervous system would 'expect' to receive (Reason, 1970). Central to the *sensory conflict* or *neural mismatch* hypothesis is the existence, within the central nervous system, of a model of afferent and efferent activity associated with body movement that is derived through daily experience of the process of volitional control of body movement and maintenance of postural equilibrium. In normal locomotor activity, disturbances of body movement, such as when one accidently trips, are typically brief and the mismatch between actual and expected sensory inputs from the body's motion detectors is employed to initiate corrective motor responses. However, when there is a sustained change in the sensory input – as occurs, for example, in atypical

motion environments or when there is vestibular disease – then the presence of the mismatch, between actual and expected sensory inputs, indicates to the central nervous system that the internal model is no longer appropriate. The process of adaptation thus involves the modification or rearrangement of the internal model so that it corresponds more closely with the contemporary sensory afference, and the mismatch signal is reduced to an acceptable level.

An essential feature of the neural mismatch hypothesis is that the presence of a sustained mismatch signal has two effects: one, it causes a rearrangement of the internal model; and two, it evokes the sequence of neural responses that constitute the motion-sickness syndrome. There is clearly benefit to the organism to be derived from modifying sensory and motor responses, for this allows it to function more effectively in a novel environment. The question, however, of whether motion sickness has survival value, or whether it is just a design defect that has only recently (in an evolutionary time-scale) become apparent with the use of mechanical aids to transportation, is a matter for debate (Oman, 1980).

Figure 7.14 is a diagramatic representation of the functional components and processes embraced by the neural mismatch hypothesis. Motion of the body is detected principally by the eyes and the vestibular apparatus, although changes in the body's orientation to gravity and imposed linear accelerations are also transduced by mechanoreceptors in the skin, muscle, capsules of joints and supporting tissues, which may be considered to act synergistically with the otolith organs. It is postulated that within the central nervous system there is a neural centre that acts as a comparator of the signals from the receptors with those from the internal model that stores the signature of

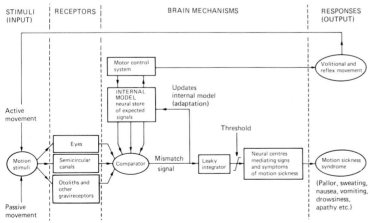

Figure 7.14 Heuristic model of motor control, motion detection and motion sickness based on the 'neural mismatch' hypothesis. (From Benson, 1984; reproduced by permission of the publisher)

'expected' signals. The output of this comparator is the mismatch signal that, on the one hand, is responsible for modifying the internal model and, on the other, for activating the neural structures mediating the signs and symptoms of motion sickness. How this activation is achieved, that is whether by purely neuronal or whether by neurohumoral mechanisms, has yet to be determined. However, in the heuristic model, the presence of a leaky integrator serves to explain the slow development of symptoms following exposure to provocative motion. In addition, it is necessary to postulate the existence of a threshold function in the system, in order to account for the development of protective adaptation without induction of motion sickness and for the large intersubject differences in susceptibility.

Features of provocative stimuli

Two categories of motion cue mismatch can be identified, according to the sensory systems involved: one is a visual–vestibular mismatch, the other a semicircular canal–otolith (or intravestibular) mismatch (Reason, 1970). Within each category, the nature of the mismatch may be further subdivided by identifying those situations in which both sensory systems simultaneously provide discordant cues (type 1 mismatch), and those in which one sensory system signals motion in the absence of the expected signal in the other modality (type 2 mismatch). Examples of the different types of mismatch causing motion sickness in aerospace and maritime environments are presented in *Table 7.1*.

Intravestibular mismatch of one type or another

is the most frequent cause of motion sickness. For example, when a head movement is made in an aircraft which is turning, both the semicircular canals and the otoliths can provide erroneous and incompatible signals which are likely to differ substantially from those generated by the same head movement in a normal, stable, $1g$ environment. Likewise, in the weightless environment of space flight, head movements, particularly in pitch and roll (that is in the sagittal and coronal planes) are provocative because the canals correctly signal the angular movement, but the otoliths fail to provide information about head orientation (as they do on earth) or are stimulated atypically by the linear accelerations produced by the head movement.

Another potent cause of motion sickness is the changing linear accelerations to which those aboard an aircraft flying through turbulent air or a ship in rough seas are exposed. Such motion is provocative because it is the otoliths (and other gravireceptors) that are stimulated in the absence of the expected signals from the semicircular canals. However, it is worthy of note that the incidence of sickness bears an inverse relationship to the frequency of the linear oscillatory motion (*Figure 7.15*); stimuli at frequencies above $0.5\,Hz$ rarely cause motion sickness but, as the frequency decreases, susceptibility rapidly increases to reach a peak at 0.1–$0.2\,Hz$ (O'Hanlon and McCauley, 1974).

Space-sickness may be attributed to a type 2a mismatch in which the canals are stimulated without the expected otolithic signals. This category of mismatch can be identified as the cause of the malaise, with all the signs and symptoms of the motion-sickness syndrome, but without a motion stimulus, that is commonly associated

Table 7.1. Identification of type of motion cue mismatch in aviation and marine environments where motion sickness is provoked

	Category of motion cue mismatch	
	Visual (A)–vestibular (B)	*Canal (A)–otolith (B)*
Type 1 A and B simultaneously signal contradictory information	(a) Looking from side or rear window of aircraft (b) Inspection through binoculars of ground or aerial targets from moving aircraft (c) Watching waves from side of ship	(a) Making head movement while rotating (cross-coupled or Coriolis stimulation) (b) Making head movement in abnormal force environment which may be stable (e.g. hyper- or hypogravity) or fluctuating
Type 2(a) A signals without expected B signal	(a) 'Simulator-sickness'. Piloting of fixed base simulator with moving external visual display (b) Cinerama-sickness	(a) Making head movement in weightless environment (space-sickness) (b) Pressure (alternobaric) vertigo (c) Caloric stimulation of semicircular canals
Type 2(b) B signals without expected A signal	(a) Looking inside aircraft or ship when exposed to motion	(a) Low frequency (<0.5 Hz) linear oscillation (b) Rotation about non-vertical axis

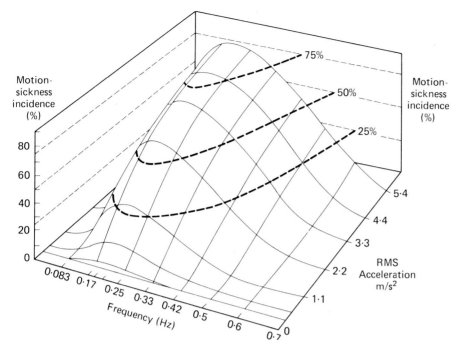

Figure 7.15 Motion sickness incidence as a function of wave frequency and acceleration for 2-hour exposures to vertical sinusoidal motion. (From McCauley *et al.*, 1976)

with the atypical stimulation of the semicircular canal receptors by physical agents or disease processes. Both aviators and divers may experience such symptoms in association with pressure (alternobaric) vertigo (*see above*). Sickness accompanying caloric stimulation is seen more frequently in the clinic than elsewhere, but asymmetrical thermal stimulation of the vestibular apparatus does occasionally occur in divers and may engender nausea as well as disorientation.

Motion sickness can be induced in the absence of vision, but in many provocative environments the visual stimulus contributes to the sensory conflict. Furthermore, there are circumstances, such as certain aircraft simulators or cinematic displays, in which the dynamic visual cues, in the absence of motion of the observer, cause sickness (that is a type 2a visual–vestibular mismatch); but more commonly, visual information is in conflict with information about whole-body motion provided by vestibular and other mechanoreceptors. A person who is within the cabin of an aircraft or boat has no visual information about his motion in space even though he may be receiving complex vestibular cues about the motion of the vehicle (type 2b mismatch). Conversely, when he is on deck or looking out of the aircraft, visual motion cues can be in accord with inertial cues if a stable reference, such as the horizon, is available, and this can be of benefit in reducing the incidence of sickness. However, if the object of regard has real or apparent motion, as, for example, when looking at waves close to the ship or when using binoculars to observe objects on the ground from a helicopter, then the visual motion cues contribute to sensory conflict (type 1 mismatch) and they increase the probability of the observer becoming motion sick.

Neural centres and pathways involved in motion sickness

Neural mismatch is a useful concept with which to collate aetiological factors of motion sickness, but it is now necessary to try to give neurophysiological and neuroanatomical substance to the theory. Regrettably, the picture is far from complete, although certain elements are reasonably well understood as a result of experimental work on animals (*Figure 7.16*). It is well established that the vestibular apparatus and the vestibular cerebellum (uvula and nodulus) are essential for the development of the motion-sickness syndrome and, by inference, the integrity of the vestibular nuclei is also mandatory (Money, 1970). The activity of the vestibular nuclei is influenced not only by the vestibular input but also by visual, somatosensory and cerebellar afferents, so the convergence necessary for the comparator to function can be

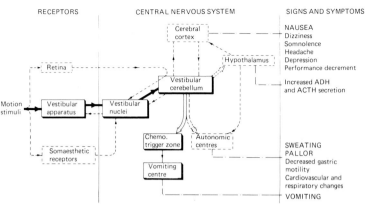

Figure 7.16 Structures involved in motion sickness. (From Benson, 1977; reproduced by permission of the publisher)

identified at this level. However, it is perhaps more likely that the vestibular cerebellum functions both as a comparator and as a neural store, and that it controls and mediates the process of adaptation.

The nature of the 'mismatch signal' and the means by which it initiates the sensory and autonomic responses of the motion-sickness syndrome are even more speculative. The signal acts, whether by neural or by humoral mechanisms, through centres in the area postrema of the medulla, close to the chemoreceptive trigger zone, and also through the vomiting centre, to initiate the integrated motor response of vomiting (Borison, 1985). Modification of the activity of hypothalamic nuclei is reflected by the increased secretion of anterior pituitary (antidiuretic) hormone, and there is also increased secretion of other pituitary hormones, notably prolactin, growth and adrenocorticotrophic hormones. The secretion of antidiuretic hormone parallels the development of the motion-sickness syndrome and is responsible for the oliguria that is a consistent finding in those suffering from motion sickness (Eversmann *et al.*, 1977). Yet, neither hypophysectomy nor partial destruction of the hypothalamus prevents the development of motion sickness in dogs. Indeed, decerebrate dogs and, anecdotally, decerebrate humans are not immune.

Incidence of motion sickness and factors influencing susceptibility

There are very considerable intersubject differences in susceptibility to motion sickness, but provided that the motion is of sufficient intensity and duration, only those without a functioning vestibular system will not develop symptoms. The incidence of sickness in a particular motion environment is determined by, on the one hand, the physical characteristic (for example, intensity, frequency, duration) of motion, and, on the other hand, by the intrinsic susceptibility of the person exposed to the motion stimulus and the nature of the task he or she has to perform.

In large civil transport aircraft, the incidence of air-sickness is a fraction of 1% of passengers, although in smaller aircraft of 'feeder' airlines, which fly at lower altitudes with greater exposure of the passengers to gusts and turbulence, the incidence can be of the order of 5–10%. In military aviation, and in particular in high performance training and combat aircraft, 50–60% of the student pilots and navigators experience sickness at some time during training and in about 5% it is of sufficient severity and frequency to lead to the withdrawal of the student from flying training. The severe turbulence to which the crew of 'hurricane penetration' flights are exposed causes symptoms in 90% of experienced flight personnel and all air-crew who have not previously flown in such conditions are affected (Benson 1984).

Space-motion sickness of varying severity affects approximately 50% of astronauts. Perhaps somewhat surprisingly, susceptibility to space-sickness does not appear to correlate with the individual's susceptibility to sickness induced by provocative motion on earth (Reschke *et al.*, 1984).

Sea-sickness, apart from its greater antiquity, can have a numerically higher incidence than that of air- or space-sickness, for, in general, the motion is more severe and more prolonged than in other modes of transportation. The severity of the motion stimulus is determined by the sea state and vessel size. Thus in an inflatable life raft in a rough sea, all but the very resistant succumb within a few hours, while aboard a Royal Navy frigate in a similar sea state, the incidence of sickness was of

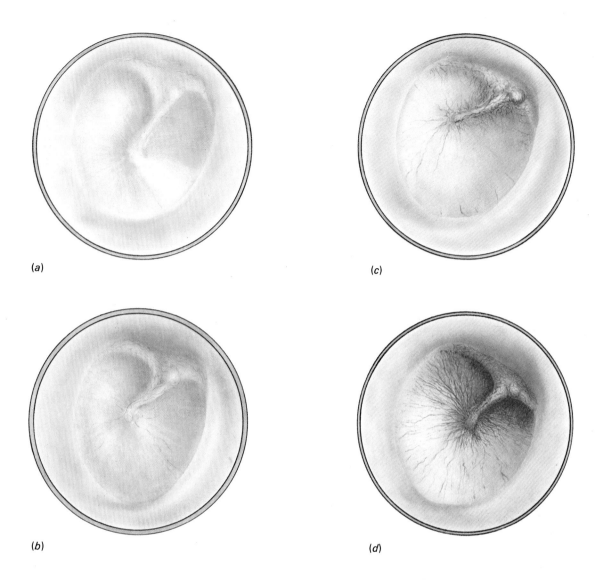

(a)

(c)

(b)

(d)

Plate 1 Appearance of the tympanic membrane in otic barotrauma: (*a*) normal right tympanic membrane; (*b*) tympanic membrane invaginated, with minimal congestion, during descent; (*c*) invagination of the tympanic membrane with congestion along the handle of the malleus; (*d*) attic congestion from a relatively mild otic barotrauma;

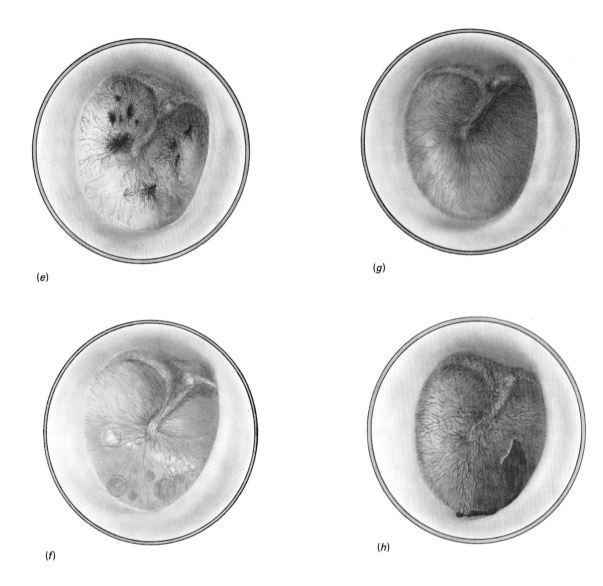

(e)

(g)

(f)

(h)

Plate 1 Contd. (*e*) scattered interstitial haemorrhages in tympanic membrane: these are usually residual in nature; (*f*) unresolved otic barotrauma with amber-coloured effusion in the middle ear: the bubbles indicate attempts to ventilate the ear via the eustachian tube; (*g*) marked congestion, with fresh haemorrhage into the middle ear; (*h*) rupture of the anterior portion of the tympanic membrane

the order of 25%. A survey of Royal Navy sailors (Pethybridge, Davies and Walters, 1978) revealed that 70% admitted to having suffered from sea-sickness during their service afloat and 49% had been sea-sick in the preceding year.

In a particular individual, motion sickness may be more readily evoked by one type of provocative motion than another. Nevertheless, there is a correlation, if not a highly significant one, between susceptibility in one motion environment and that in another, although, as noted previously, susceptibility to space-sickness would appear to be an exception to this relationship. The intensity, character and duration of the motion stimulus is the principal determinant of whether a person develops sickness, but a number of factors concerning the physical and mental constitution of the individual have been identified as influencing susceptibility (Reason and Brand, 1975). It is well established that susceptibility changes with age. Motion sickness is rare below the age of 2 years, but with maturation, tolerance decreases rapidly and susceptibility is at a peak between the ages of 3 and 12 years. Over the following decade, susceptibility decreases quite markedly and this decrease continues, if more slowly, with increasing age. The increase in tolerance has been documented for both air-sickness and sea-sickness, although the elderly are not immune. A recent survey of sickness aboard a Channel Islands ferry revealed that 22% of those suffering from sea-sickness were over the age of 59 years (Lawther and Griffin, 1981).

Females are more suceptible to motion sickness than males of the same age (Reason, 1967). The reason for this sex difference, which has long been recognized and which applies to both children and adults, is not understood. It is most likely to be a consequence of hormonal factors, as in women the incidence of motion sickness reaches a peak during menstruation and susceptibility increases during pregnancy.

Nausea and vomiting are not uncommon symptoms of fear and anxiety, hence it is commonly assumed that anxiety increases susceptibility to motion sickness. Positive but weak correlations have been established between psychometric measures of neuroticism and susceptibility, which show that extroverts have a higher tolerance and adapt more rapidly than introverts. Significant correlations have also been demonstrated between susceptibility and performance of the rod and frame test, with 'field dependent' subjects having a higher tolerance than those who were 'field independent' (Barrett and Thornton, 1968). However, these dimensions of personality are not sufficient to explain the large differences in susceptibility that exist in a group of men or women of similar age and exposure to motion.

Studies carried out by Reason (1970) suggest that these differences are attributable to other constitutional factors relating to the way the individual transduces sensory signals (receptivity), how he or she adapts to motion stimuli (adaptability) and to the ability to retain protective adaptation (retentivity). Thus a person who has low receptivity, high adaptability and good retentivity has a high tolerance to provocative motion, whereas the highly susceptible individual has high receptivity, adapts slowly and has poor retention of the little protective adaptation acquired.

Although fear and anxiety are considered to be of only secondary importance in the aetiology of true motion sickness, it must be acknowledged that the motion-sickness syndrome can be a conditioned response or the manifestation of a phobic neurotic reaction. The student pilot whose symptoms become progressively more severe on successive flights, or the passenger who is sick on stepping aboard a boat, are examples of those conditions in which the mind, rather than the motion, is the cause of the malaise.

Prevention and treatment

Behavioural measures

Motion sickness can be regarded as a self-inflicted condition, for it is effectively prevented by avoidance of exposure to provocative motion. If so wished, people need not travel in aircraft, ships, space vehicles etc., although few in the modern world could accept such a restriction on their mobility. For those who do find themselves exposed to motion stimuli that are likely to induce sickness, there are a number of simple measures that are of benefit in preventing, or at least delaying, the onset of symptoms. These may be summarized as follows:

(1) occupy a position aboard the ship or aircraft close to its centre of gravity in order to minimize the intensity of motion stimuli
(2) minimize unnecessary head movements; this is facilitated by the provision of head support and good body restraint, and may be further aided by a reclined or supine position
(3) take up a position in which there is a good view forward of a stable external visual reference, such as the horizon when aboard an aircraft or ship
(4) if deprived of an external visual reference, close the eyes to reduce visual–vestibular conflict
(5) be involved in a task which occupies the mind and minimizes introspection; optimally, be in control of the vehicle; pilots rarely suffer from air-sickness except when flying as passengers.

These measures can be of immediate value to those who find themselves exposed to provocative motion, but in the long term, it is adaptation which is the most powerful prophylactic. Adaptation is 'nature's own cure' and is the preferred method of preventing, or at least reducing susceptibility to, motion sickness. It is of special importance to air-crew who, in general, should not fly when under the influence of anti-motion-sickness drugs. The basic principle governing the acquisition and maintenance of protective adaptation is that air-crew should be introduced gradually to the provocative motions of the aircraft, and that adaptation, once achieved, should be maintained by regular and repeated exposures. Inter-subject differences in receptivity, adaptability and retentivity do, however, imply that adaptation schedules must be tailored to the individual, and must preclude definition of the interval between exposures. Some air-crew are troubled by air-sickness if 2–3 days elapse between flights; others, with better retentivity, can spend several weeks on the ground without any increase in susceptibility.

There is, unfortunately, a small percentage of air-crew who do not develop sufficient adaptation during the course of their normal flying duties and who continue to suffer from air-sickness. In a number of studies (Dobie, 1974; Cramer, Graybiel and Oosterveld, 1976; Stott and Bagshaw, 1984), it has been shown that the majority of those who fall into this category can be helped by ground-based training which, in general, involves graded incremental exposure to cross-coupled (Coriolis) and other provocative stimuli. This desensitization therapy may be coupled with biofeedback training aimed at teaching the subject how to control autonomic responses (Levy, Jones and Carlson, 1981), although this procedure does not appear to have yielded better results than were obtained by a more mechanistic approach to therapy. The procedure currently employed by the Royal Air Force has allowed 80% of the air-crew, referred because of intractable air-sickness, to return to normal flying duties without disability from air-sickness (Bagshaw and Stott, 1985).

Drugs

Many studies, both in the laboratory and in the field, have demonstrated that certain drugs can reduce the incidence of motion sickness in a given population at risk (Graybiel *et al.*, 1975). A large number of drugs have been studied, but none can afford complete protection. Of the relatively few drugs with proven prophylactic potency, all have side-effects, commonly that of sedation, which limit the usage of these drugs by those in whom the impairment of skilled performance would jeopardize safety. There is a place, however, for the administration of anti-motion-sickness drugs to student air-crew, particularly in the early stages of flying training, but under no circumstances should drugs be taken by a pilot when he flies solo. Such a restriction does not apply to the use of drugs by passengers to alleviate air- or sea-sickness. Nevertheless, where personnel are required to work at peak efficiency, the possible decrement in performance as a result of sickness must be balanced against that produced by medication.

The choice of drug is, in part, dependent upon the duration of exposure to provocative motion and, in part, upon individual differences in effectiveness, and upon the incidence of side-effects. The pharmacokinetics of drugs of proven efficacy differ considerably. A single oral dose of 0.3–0.6 mg hyoscine hydrobromide acts in 30–60 minutes and provides protection for about 4 hours, whereas promethazine hydrochloride (25 mg) and meclozine hydrochloride (50 mg) take 1–2 hours to act and are effective for 12 hours or longer. The other useful drugs, dimenhydrinate (50 mg), cyclizine hydrochloride (50 mg) and cinnarizine (30 mg), are absorbed at about the same rate as promethazine, but their duration of action is shorter (around 6 hours). Thus for short exposure, as in training flights, hyoscine is the drug of choice unless its side-effects – sedation, blurring of vision and dry mouth – are particularly troublesome. For more protracted exposure, one of the longer-acting drugs should be given, with repeated dosage if indicated. The repeated administration of oral hyoscine is not recommended because the side-effects are cumulative. However, with the advent of the Transdermal Therapeutic System (Ciba-Geigy), an adhesive 'patch', placed behind the ear can provide a loading dose of 200 µg of hyoscine and controlled release at 10 µg/h for up to 48 hours. Although a therapeutic efficacy comparable to oral drugs has been claimed (Graybiel, Cramer and Wood, 1981), more recent studies have indicated greater variability between subjects in the protection afforded (Homick *et al.*, 1983).

The prophylactic potency of hyoscine or one of the antihistamines has been shown to be enhanced when the drug is administered in conjunction with either 5 mg *d*-amphetamine sulphate or 25 mg ephedrine sulphate. The combination has the further advantage that sedation is less than when the anti-motion-sickness drug is given alone.

Most of the drugs, detailed above, may be given by intramuscular injection, promethazine hydrochloride (25 mg) being preferred when the accompanying and relatively long-lasting sedation is acceptable, or even, as in passengers aboard ship, desirable.

Spatial disorientation

Spatial disorientation is a term used to describe a variety of incidents in which the aviator or diver fails to sense correctly his position, motion or attitude with respect to a fixed reference, such as the gravitational vertical or the surface of the earth or sea. The erroneous or illusory perception that characterizes a disorientation incident may, on the one hand, be no more than a trivial and transient distraction, but, on the other, it can jeopardize safety and lead to loss of life. In aviation, spatial disorientation of the pilot has long been recognized as a cause of aircraft accidents, but despite the benefits afforded by modern flight instruments, accidents still occur. In military aviation, spatial disorientation is a primary or contributory cause of some 10% of accidents, whereas in private flying the incidence is even higher (25% in the USA). In diving, as in flying, it is the inexperienced divers who are most at risk, for they are the more likely to be alarmed by unexpected and bizarre sensations and, as a result, may fail to carry out those basic procedures, such as ascent to the surface, that would ensure their safety.

Aetiology

Man's ability to determine his spatial orientation is dependent upon information provided by the eyes, the vestibular apparatus and other mechanoreceptors stimulated by accelerations acting on his body. Although visual information is of primary importance, on the ground man can still maintain his postural equilibrium and spatial orientation during normal locomotor activities, even when deprived of vision. The non-visual receptors, and their associated central sensory processing, are functionally adapted to transduce and perceive the motion stimuli experienced in everyday life on the surface of the earth, where the sustained force of gravity (indistinguishable from linear acceleration) is a stable reference of verticality. However, in the aerial or subaquatic environments, the human being is subject to motion which has angular and linear accelerations which may differ substantially in direction, intensity or frequency from those normally experienced on the ground. Consequently, errors in the perception of spatial orientation occur in these atypical environments, primarily because of the functional limitations of the human's sensory mechanisms.

Many different kinds of erroneous sensations and perceptions, falling within the broad definition of spatial disorientation, have been described and there are many different causes (*see* Benson, 1978; Gillingham and Wolfe, 1985, for more detailed reviews of the topic), but in the context of this chapter discussion will be confined to perceptual errors attributable to vestibular mechanisms. Although spatial disorientation can be caused by misinterpretation of visual information, in general, most disorientation incidents and accidents occur when normal visual cues are either absent or deficient, as, for example, when flying in cloud or at night, or when diving in turbid water or an enclosed space.

Failure to perceive motion and changes in attitude

In the absence of vision, detection of angular and translational (linear) movements is governed by the transduction of the motion stimulus by the receptors of the semicircular canals and otolith organs. These sense organs are functionally adapted to respond to the motion stimuli that occur during normal locomotor activity, but both in flight, and underwater, the body can be exposed to linear and angular movements which are below the threshold of detection. Thresholds are dependent upon a number of variables, notably, the axis or plane of motion, its frequency spectrum and its duration. Transient movements (that is those taking less than 10 s) are unlikely to be detected if the change in angular velocity is less than about 2°/s or the linear acceleration is less than 0.05 m/s^2. With more prolonged stimuli (that is greater than 20 s) typical threshold values are 0.3°/s^2 for rotational movements and 0.1 m/s^2 for linear movements. It is worthy of note that for such sustained stimuli the critical factor is the acceleration of the movement, which, if below threshold, can engender large changes of attitude of which the aviator or diver may be completely unaware in the absence of visual cues for orientation.

False sensations of angular motion

In general, misleading sensations of angular motion are a consequence of the dynamic limitations of the semicircular canals. These end-organs correctly transduce the angular *velocity* of transient (that is less than 10 s) head movements, provided that the threshold is exceeded. However, once a steady rate of turn is achieved, there is no longer an adequate stimulus and the deflected cupulae in the plane of the motion slowly return to their neutral position and the associated sensation of turn dies away. Provided there is no appreciable change in angular velocity, the turn can continue without the aviator having any sensation that the aircraft is in fact turning (*Figure 7.17*).

Recovery from the turn is associated with an angular acceleration in the opposite direction to that on entering the turn. The cupulae are deflected from their rest position and will

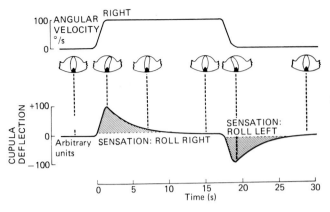

Figure 7.17 Response of semicircular canal and sensations of turning during and on recovery from sustained rotation. The upper graph shows the speed of rotation; the lower graph shows the deflection of the cupula of a semicircular canal stimulated by angular acceleration in the plane of the canal. (From Benson, 1978; reproduced by permission of the publisher)

erroneously signal rotation in the opposite direction, at a rate commensurate with the *change in velocity* that has occurred. This false sensation decays somewhat more quickly than the decay of the correct sensation during the initial phase of the turn, but the presence of inappropriate eye movements induced by the vestibular stimulus can degrade vision and impair the pilot's only reliable source of information. The intensity of these post-rotational effects is a function of the duration of the rotational manoeuvre and of the angular velocity achieved; accordingly, disorientation is most likely to be a problem on recovery from prolonged, high-rate, rolling or spinning manoeuvres.

Cross-coupled or Coriolis stimulation of the semicircular canals occurs whenever an angular movement of the head is made while rotating about another axis. However, disorientating sensations are evoked only when rotation is prolonged and the semicircular canals do not correctly signal the sustained turn. For example, if the pilot were to move his head in pitch at the beginning of a prolonged spin, his sensation of both head and aircraft motion would be correct, but if the same head movement were made some 15–20 s later, the head movement would elicit an entirely illusory sensation of rotation in roll. Head movements made during the recovery phase cause even stronger and more bizarre sensations. As a general rule: a head movement made in one axis, after rotating for some time about an orthogonal axis produces an illusory sensation in the third orthogonal axis.

The semicircular canals may also be stimulated other than by angular accelerations. The effect of pressure change is discussed earlier in this chapter and it will suffice to point out that, on occasion, the onset of vertigo can be quite intense and can be accompanied by nystagmus of sufficient severity to impair vision and degrade the pilot's or the diver's only reliable source of information about his spatial orientation.

Pressure vertigo is a potential cause of spatial disorientation in both aviators and divers, but it is only the latter who are likely to experience vertigo caused by thermal stimuli. As is well known from the caloric test, irrigation of the external canal with water at a temperature more than a few degrees above or below body temperature is an effective stimulus to the semicircular canals, although if both ears are at the same temperature, little nystagmus or vertigo will be evoked. However, problems arise when diving without a hood if there is inequality in the thermal stimulus to each ear. This most commonly occurs when there is wax in the external canal which impedes the heat transfer between the labyrinth and the water (Edmonds, 1973a).

False sensations of attitude

In the presence of the constant acceleration of earth's gravity, the otolith organs and the other gravireceptors provide information which allow the orientation of the head and body to be sensed with accuracy. Normally, one is able to distinguish changes of attitude from transient linear accelerations, but perceptual errors occur when the imposed linear acceleration or deceleration is sustained, as in an aircraft when power is applied or dive-brakes are operated (*Figure 7.18*). In such circumstances, the resultant of the imposed acceleration and gravity is accepted as the vertical reference and consequently there is an illusory sensation of a nose-up attitude during acceleration in the line of flight and of a nose-down change of attitude during deceleration. This somatogravic illusion may also be accompanied by a perceived movement of visual objects, particularly isolated lights, which appear to move upwards during acceleration and downwards during deceleration.

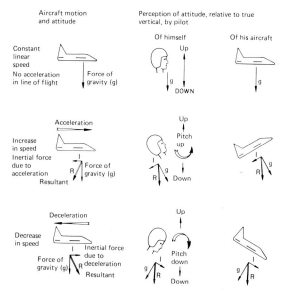

Aircraft motion and attitude | Perception of attitude, relative to true vertical, by pilot

Of himself — Of his aircraft

Constant linear speed — No acceleration in line of flight — Force of gravity (g)

Increase in speed — Inertial force due to acceleration — Force of gravity (g) — Resultant

Deceleration — Decrease in speed — Force of gravity (g) — Inertial force due to deceleration — Resultant

Figure 7.18 Somatogravic illusions during linear acceleration or deceleration in the line of flight are responsible for errors in the perception of pitch attitude. (From Benson, 1978; reproduced by permission of the publisher)

This visual or oculogravic illusion, in the same way as the somatogravic illusion, takes time to develop and does not reach maximum intensity until the imposed acceleration has been sustained for 40–60 seconds.

The failure to sense accurately the angle of bank during a turn is also attributable to the resultant of the radial and gravitational accelerations being accepted as vertical, for in a coordinated turn the resultant vector remains normal to the aircraft's longitudinal axis and aligned with the long (z) axis of the pilot's head and body.

A false sensation of roll attitude, 'the leans', is one of the commonest illusions experienced by air-crew. It usually occurs on recovery from a prolonged turn or from a previously undetected banked attitude to straight and level flight. In both of these conditions, the aviator feels that he is straight and level before he rolls out. The change in roll attitude is made within a few seconds and is a suprathreshold stimulus to the semicircular canals. This vestibular information is interpreted as roll from the wing-level attitude to one of bank in a direction opposite to that which existed before recovery was initiated. The curious feature of 'the leans' is that it may persist for many minutes even though instruments indicate level flight; yet, characteristically, the illusion disappears as soon as an unambiguous external visual reference is present.

The disorientating sensations produced when head movements are made in a turning aircraft are not solely due to a cross-coupled stimulation of the semicircular canals. The presence of a linear acceleration greater than $10 \, \text{m/s}^2$ $(1 \, g)$ means that the otoliths will also be stimulated in an atypical manner when the head is moved. The principal effect on moving the head in hypergravity is that of generating an otolithic signal which corresponds to a greater change in attitude, relative to the acceleration vector, than has actually occurred. The semicircular canals and receptors in the neck signal the angular movement of the head with little error, so there is a mismatch which is interpreted as a change of attitude of the aircraft in the plane and direction of the head movement. At higher accelerations (for example $50–60 \, \text{m/s}^2$), vertigo and sensations of tumbling, as well as an apparent change in attitude, can be evoked by a head movement.

Prevention

In general, spatial disorientation, whether in the air or underwater, is not caused by pathology, but is a normal psychophysiological response to abnormal motion stimuli in an environment deficient in reliable visual orientation cues. Thus the aviator's or diver's knowledge about the different causes and manifestations of spatial disorientation, and the conditions in which it is most likely to occur, is of principal importance in the prevention of orientation error accidents. On the one hand, this knowledge will allow him to avoid potentially provocative aerial or underwater environments or, when this is not practicable, to exercise special care in such situations. On the other hand, knowledge that when visual cues are inadequate (for example when flying in cloud or at night), control of the aircraft can be maintained only be reference to flight instruments, implies that proficiency at instrument flying is mandatory if the aviator is correctly to resolve conflicting sensory cues and maintain proper control of the aircraft.

It is generally agreed that aviators and divers should be advised not to fly or dive when they are suffering from an upper respiratory tract infection, in order to minimize the occurrence of pressure vertigo. In addition, they should be made aware that any impairment of higher mental function, consequent on intoxication by alcohol or other drugs, may not only increase their susceptibility to spatial disorientation but also degrade their ability to resolve perceptual conflict and to make the correct decision in the event of their experiencing any disorientating sensations.

References

ARMSTRONG, H. G. and HEIM, J. W. (1937) The effect of flight on the middle ear. *Journal of the American Medical Association*, **109**, 417–421

ASHLEY, K. F. (1977) Aerodontalgia – pain felt in the teeth during flight. *Medical and Dental Newsletter*, **26**, 15–17. London: Ministry of Defence, (RAF)

BAGSHAW, M. and STOTT, J. R. R. (1985) The desensitisation of chronically motion sick aircrew in the Royal Air Force. *Aviation Space and Environmental Medicine*, **46**, 1144–1151

BARRETT, G. V. and THORNTON, C. L. (1968) Relationship between perceptual style and simulator sickness. *Journal of Applied Psychology*, **52**, 304–308

BENNET, P. B. and TOWSE, E. J. (1971) The high pressure nervous syndrome during a simulated oxygen-helium dive to 1500 feet. *Electroencephalography and Clinical Neurophysiology*, **31**, 389–393

BENSON, A. J. (1977) Possible mechanisms of motion and space sickness. In *Life-Sciences Research in Space*, Report SP-130, pp. 101–108, Paris: ESA

BENSON, A. J. (1978) Spatial disorientation. In *Aviation Medicine: Vol 1 Physiology and Human Factors*, edited by G. Dhenin and J. Ernsting, pp. 405–467. London: Tri-med Books

BENSON, A. J. (1984) Motion sickness. In *Vertigo*, edited by M. R. Dix and J. D. Hood, pp. 391–426. Chichester: J. Wiley and Sons

BORISON, H. L. (1985) A misconception of motion sickness leads to false therapeutic expectations. *Aviation Space and Environmental Medicine*, **56**, 66–68

BROWN, H. H. S. (1965) The pressure cabin. In *A Textbook of Aviation Physiology*, edited by J. A. Gillies, pp. 152–186. London: Pergamon Press

CANFIELD, N. and BATEMAN, G. H. (1944) Myringopuncture for reduced intratympanic pressure, report of pressure chamber experiments. *Journal of Aviation Medicine*, **15**, 340–343

CHUNN, S. P. (1960) A comparison of the efficiency of the Valsalva manoeuvre and the pharyngeal pressure test and the feasibility of teaching both methods. *ACAM Thesis, Brooks AFB*, Texas: USAF School of Aerospace Medicine

COLES, R. R. A. (1976) Cochleo-vestibular disturbances in diving. *Audiology*, **15**, 273–278

COMROE, J. H., DRIPPS, R. D., DUMKE, R. R. and DEMING, M. (1945) Oxygen toxicity: effect of inhalation of high concentrations of oxygen for 24 hours on normal men at sea level and at simulated altitude of 18 000 feet. *Journal of the American Medical Association*, **128**, 710–717

CRAMER, D. B., GRAYBIEL, A. and OOSTERVELD, W. J. (1976) Successful transfer of adaptation acquired in a slow rotation room to motion environments in Navy flight training. In *Recent Advances in Space Medicine*, Conference Proceedings, **203**, C.2, 1–6, Neuilly sur Seine: AGARD/NATO

DICKSON, E. D. D. and KING, P. F. (1954) The incidence of barotrauma in present day Service flying. *Flying Personnel Research Committee Report* No. 881. London: Air Ministry

DICKSON, E. D. D. and KING, P. F. (1956) Results of treatment of otitic and sinus barotrauma. *Journal of Aviation Medicine*, **27**, 92–99

DICKSON, E. D. D., McGIBBON, J. E. G. and CAMPBELL, A. C. P. (1947) Acute otitic barotrauma – clinical findings, mechanism and relationship to the pathological changes produced experimentally in the middle ears of cats by variations of pressure. In *Contributions to Aviation Otolaryngology*, edited by E. D. D. Dickson, pp. 60–83. London: Headley Bros

DOBIE, T. G. (1974) *Airsickness in Aircrew.* Report AG-177; Neuilly sur Seine: AGARD/NATO

DUVOISIN, R. C., KRUSE, F. and SAUNDERS, D. (1962) Convulsive syncope induced by Valsalva manoeuvre in subjects exhibiting low G tolerance. *Aerospace Medicine*, **33**, 92–96

EDMONDS, C. (1973a). Vertigo and disorientation in diving. In *Otological Aspects of Diving*, edited by C. Edmonds, P. Freeman, R. Thomas *et al.*, pp. 55–62. Sidney: Australian Medical Publishing Co.

EDMONDS, C. (1973b) Round window rupture in diving. *Försvarsmedicin*, **9**, 404–405

EDMONDS, C. (1976) Barotrauma. In *Diving Medicine*, edited by R. H. Strauss, pp. 49–62. New York: Grune and Stratton

EDMONDS, C. and FREEMAN, P. (1972) Inner ear barotrauma. *Archives of Otolaryngology*, **95**, 551–563

EVERSMANN, T., GOTTSMANN, M., UHLICH, E., ULBRECHT, G., VON WERDER, K. and SCRIBA, P. C. (1977) Increased secretion of growth hormone, prolactin, antiduretic hormone and cortisol induced by the stress of motion sickness. *Aviation Space and Environmental Medicine*, **49**, 53–57

FARMER, J. C. (1977) Diving injuries to the inner ear. *Annals of Otology, Rhinology and Laryngology*, **86** (Suppl. 36), 1–20

FARMER, J. C. (1985) Eustachian tube function: physiology and role in otitis media. *Annals of Otology, Rhinology and Laryngology*, **94** (Suppl. 120), 1–6

FRENZEL, H. (1938) Nasen-Rachendruckversuch zur Sprengung des Tubenverschlusses. *Luftfahrtmedizin*, **2**, 203–205

FRENZEL, H. (1950) Otorhinolaryngology. In *German Aviation Medicine World War II*, **2**, 977–984. Washington: Government Printing Office

FRYER, D. I. (1969) *Subatmospheric Decompression Sickness in Man.* AGARDograph 125, Slough, England: Technivision Services, AGARD/NATO

GILLINGHAM, K. K. and WOLFE, J. W. (1985) Spatial orientation in flight. In *Fundamentals of Aerospace Medicine*, edited by R. L. DeHart, pp. 299–381. Philadelphia: Lea and Febiger

GOODHILL, V. (1971) Sudden deafness and round window rupture. *The Laryngoscope*, **81**, 1462–1474

GRAYBIEL, A., CRAMER, D. B. and WOOD, C. D. (1981) Experimental motion sickness: efficacy of transdermal scopolamine plus ephedrine. *Aviation Space and Environmental Medicine*, **52**, 337–339

GRAYBIEL, A., WOOD, C. D., KNEPTON, J., HOCHE, J. P. and PERKINS, G. F. (1975) Human assay of antimotion sickness drugs. *Aviation Space and Environmental Medicine*, **46**, 1107–1118

HARTMANN, A. (1879) *Experimentelle Studien uber die Funtion der Eustachishen Rohre.* Leipzig

HOLMQUIST, J. (1976) Auditory tubal function. In *Scientific Foundations of Otolaryngology*, edited by R. Hinchcliffe and D. F. N Harrison, pp. 252–257. London: Heinemann

HOMICK, T. L., KOHL, R. L., RESCHKE, M. F., DEGIOANNI, J. and CINTRON-TREVINO, N. M. (1983) Transdermal scopolamine in the prevention of motion sickness: evaluation of time course of efficacy. *Aviation Space and Environmental Medicine*, **54**, 994–1000

HUGHSON, W. and CROWE, S. J. (1933) Experimental investigations of physiology of the ear. *Acta Oto-Laryngologica*, **18**, 291–339

INGELSTEDT, S., IVARSSON, A. and TJERNSTRÖM, Ö. (1974) Vertigo due to relative overpressure in the middle ear. *Acta Oto-Laryngologica*, **78**, 1–14

JAMES, W. (1982). The sense of dizziness in deaf-mutes. *American Journal of Otolaryngology*, **4**, 239–254

JARRETT, A. (1961) Ear injuries in divers. *Journal of Royal Naval Medical Service*, **47**, 13–19

JONES, G. M. (1957) A study of current problems associated with disorientation in man-controlled flight. *Flying Personnel Research Committee Report*, No. 1006. London: Air Ministry

JONES, G. M. (1958) Pressure changes in the middle ear after flight. *Flying Personnel Research Committee, Report* No. 1059, London: Air Ministry

JONES, G. M. (1959) Pressure changes in the middle ear after simulated flights in a decompression chamber. *Journal of Physiology*, **147**, 43P

KEAYS, F. L. (1909) Compressed air illness, with a report of 3692 cases. In *Researches from the Department of Medicine*, **2**, Ithaca: Cornell University Medical School

KING, P. F. (1965) Sinus barotrauma. In *A Textbook of Aviation Physiology*, edited by J. A. Gillies, pp. 112–121. London: Pergamon Press

KING, P. F. (1976) Aural problems in the armed services: otitic barotrauma and related conditions. *Proceedings of the Royal Society of Medicin*, **68**, 817–818

LAWTHER, A. and GRIFFIN, M. J. (1981) Motion sickness incidence in sea-going passenger vessels: an interim report. *Human Factors Research Unit, ISVR*, Southampton University

LEITCH, D. R. (1985) Complications of saturation diving. *Journal of the Royal Society of Medicine*, **78**, 634–637

LEVY, R. A., JONES, D. R. and CARLSON, E. H. (1981) Biofeedback rehabilitation of airsick aircrew. *Aviation Space and Environmental Medicine*, **52**, 118–121

LUNDGREN, C. E. G. (1965) Alternobaric vertigo – a diving hazard. *British Medical Journal*, **2**, 511–513

LUNDGREN, C. E. G. (1973) On alternobaric vertigo – epidemiological aspects. *Försvarsmedicin*, **9**, 406–409

LUNDGREN, C. E. G. and MALM, L. U. (1966) Alternobaric vertigo among pilots. *Aerospace Medicine*, **37**, 178–180

MACBETH, R. (1960) Some thoughts on the Eustachian tube. *Proceedings of the Royal Society of Medicine*, **53**, 151

McCAULEY, M. E., ROYAL, J. W., WYLIE, C. D., O'HANLON, J. F. and MACKIE, R. R. (1976) Motion sickness incidence: exploratory studies of habituation, pitch and roll, and the refinement of a mathematical model. *Technical Report*, No. 1733-2, Goleta, California: Human Factors Research Inc.

McCORMICK, J. G., PHILBRICK, T. and HOLLAND, W. (1973) Diving induced sensorineural deafness: prophylactic use of heparin and preliminary histopathology results. *The Laryngoscope*, **83**, 1483–1501

McGIBBON, J. E. G. (1947) Nasal sinus pain caused by flying. In *Contributions to Aviation Otolaryngology*, edited by E. D. D. Dickson, pp. 134–155. London: Headley Brothers

McMYN, J. R. (1940) Anatomy of salpingo-pharyngeus muscle. *Journal of Laryngolgoy*, **55**, 1–22

McNICHOLL, W. D. (1982) Remediable eustachian tube dysfunction in diving recruits: assessment, investigation and management. *Undersea Biomedical Research*, **9**, 37–43

MARTIN, K. J. and NICHOLS, G. (1972) Platelet changes in man after simulated diving. *Aerospace Medicine*, **43**, 827–848

MONEY, K. E. (1970) Motion sickness. *Physiological Reviews*, **50**, 1–38

MORRISON, R. (1972) Radiotherapy of the larynx and laryngo-pharynx. In *Modern Trends in Diseases of the Ear, Nose and Throat*, edited by M. Ellis, Vol. 2, pp. 324–325. London: Butterworths

NOYEK, A. M. and ZIZMOR, J. (1974) Pneumocele of the maxillary sinus. *Archives of Otolaryngology*, **100**, 155–156

O'HANLON, J. F. and McCAULEY, M. E. (1974) Motion sickness incidence as a function of the frequency of vertical sinusoidal motion. *Aerospace Medicine*, **45**, 366–369

OMAN, C. M. (1980) A heuristic mathematical model for the dynamics of sensory conflict and motion sickness. *Report MVT-80-1*. Cambridge, Mass.: MIT Man Vehicle Laboratory

PETHYBRIDGE, R. J., DAVIES, J. W. and WALTERS, J. D. (1978) A pilot study on the incidence of sea-sickness in Royal Navy personnel on two ships. *Report INM 55/78*, Alverstoke, Hants: Institute of Naval Medicine

PHILIP, R. B., SCHACHAM, P. and GOWDEY, G. W. (1971) Platelets and microthrombi in decompression sickness. *Aerospace Medicine*, **42**, 494–502

RAYMAN, R. B. (1972) Stapedectomy: a threat to flying safety? *Aerospace Medicine*, **43**, 545–550

REASON, J. T. (1967) An investigation of some factors contributing to individual variation in motion sickness susceptibility. *Flying Personnel Research Committee Report No. 1277*, London: Ministry of Defence (Air)

REASON, J. T. (1970) Motion sickness: a special case of sensory rearrangement. *Advances in Science*, **26**, 386–393

REASON, J. T. and BRAND, J. J. (1975) *Motion sickness*. London: Academic Press

RESCHKE, M. F., HOMICK, J. L., RYAN, P. and MOSELEY, E. C. (1984) Prediction of space adaptation syndrome. In *Motion Sickness: Mechanisms, Prediction, Prevention and Treatment*, Conference Proceeding No. 372, 26, 1–11. Neuilly sur Seine: AGARD/NATO

RICH, A. R. (1920) A physiological study of the eustachian tube and its related muscles. *Bulletin of the Johns Hopkins Hospital*, **31**, 206–214

STOTT, J. R. R. and BAGSHAW, M. (1984) The current status of the RAF programme of desensitisation for motion sickness. In *Motion Sickness: Mechanisms, Prediction, Prevention and Treatment*, Conference Proceeding No. 372, 40, 1–9. Neuilly sur Seine: AGARD/NATO

TINGLEY, D. R. and MacDOUGAL, J. A. (1977) Round window tear in aviators. *Aviation Space and Environmental Medicine*, **48**, 971–975

TJERNSTRÖM, Ö. (1974) Middle ear mechanics and alternobaric vertigo. *Acta Oto-Laryngologica*, **78**, 376–384

TJERNSTRÖM, Ö. (1974b) Function of the eustachian tubes in divers with a history of alternobaric vertigo. *Undersea Biomedical Research*, **1**, 343–351

TJERNSTRÖM, Ö. (1977) Effects of middle ear pressure on the inner ear. *Acta Oto-Laryngologica*, **83**, 11–15

VAN WULFFTEN PALTHE, P. M. (1922) Function of the deeper sensibility and of the vestibular organs in flying. *Acta Oto-Laryngologica*, **4**, 415–448

ZIZMOR, J., BRYCE, M., SCHAFER, S. L. and NOYEK, A. M. (1975) Pneumocoele of the maxillary sinus. *Archives of Otolaryngology*, **101**, 387–388

8

The mouth and related faciomaxillary structures

David W. Proops

The mouth is not only the province of the sister speciality of dentistry, but has enormous social importance to man. All creatures eat to live, but humans have transformed this energy acquiring necessity into the focus of much of their social life.

The development of conceptual thought and the ability to express this through speech is what has most separated the human being from the rest of the animal kingdom. The physiological complexities of speech, as with eating, demand the attention of the speciality. Diseases of the mouth will interfere with these most vital activities.

To the otolaryngologist, therefore, the mouth is not only the route to the pharynx and beyond, but increasingly a meeting ground for the disciplines of oral and maxillofacial surgery, dental surgery and speech therapy. A thorough knowledge of this region, combined with an understanding of modern practices, is therefore essential.

The mouth or oral cavity extends from the lips and cheeks externally to the pillars of the fauces internally. Its boundaries are the lips anteriorly, the cheeks laterally, the hard and soft palate superiorly and the floor of the mouth inferiorly.

The mouth is divided into the vestibule outside the teeth, the alveolar arches, and the oral cavity proper within the dental arcades, which contains the tongue.

Developmental anatomy

The primitive oral cavity or *stomatodaeum* is first apparent in the four-week old embryo as a slit-like space, bounded by the brain above and the pericardial sac below. The *buccopharyngeal membrane* at the back of the cavity forms a thin septum

between the stomatodaeum and the foregut, which later breaks down so that the mouth cavity becomes continuous with the developing pharynx (*Figure 8.1*). The branchial arches originate from a

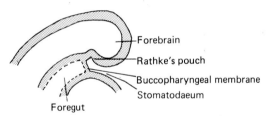

Forebrain

Rathke's pouch

Buccopharyngeal membrane

Stomatodaeum

Foregut

Figure 8.1 Sagittal section of human embryo showing early development of oral cavity

number of mesodermal condensations in the lateral wall and floor of the pharynx. Between the arches, successive clefts on the pharyngeal aspects are matched by corresponding clefts in the overlying ectodermal surface.

Within these mesodermal condensations, differentiation produces a cartilaginous bar and branchial musculature together with a branchial arch artery (Paten, 1953). Each arch receives an afferent and an efferent nerve to supply the skin, the musculature and the endodermal lining of the arch concerned. In addition, each arch receives a branch from the nerve of the succeeding arch. The branch from its own arch is known as the *post-trematic branch* and the second branch from the succeeding arch is called the *pre-trematic branch*. The mandibular division of the trigeminal nerve is the post-trematic nerve of the first branchial arch. The pre-trematic nerve to the first arch is represented by the chorda tympani branch of the facial nerve.

The facial nerve itself is the post-trematic branch of the second arch, while the pre-trematic branch of this arch is derived from the tympanic branch (Jacobson's nerve) of the glossopharyngeal nerve. The glossopharyngeal is the post-trematic nerve of the third arch. The nerves of the remaining arches (fourth and sixth) are derived from the vagus and accessory nerves by their superior and inferior (recurrent) laryngeal branches and from the pharyngeal branches.

By the sixth week of embryonic life, the two mandibular processes, which have arisen from the lateral aspect of the developing head, have met and fused in the midline, to form the tissue of the lower jaw. Meanwhile, the maxillary processes develop as buds from the mandibular process, and grow forward on each side of the face beneath the developing eyes to make contact with the lower ends of the descending nasal processes (*Figure 8.2*).

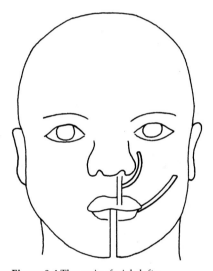

Figure 8.2 Development of the face in 7-week-old fetus

The fusion of the maxillary processes both creates the primary palate and separates the primitive nasal cavity from the primitive oral cavity. The inwardly directed extensions of each maxillary process produce tissues which later will form the nasal septum and secondary palate, and which will fuse following the descent of the developing tongue (*Figure 8.3*) (Kraus, Kitamura and Latham, 1966; Sperber, 1976).

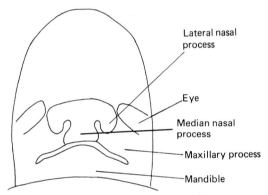

Figure 8.3 View from below of developing palate in 6-week-old embryo

Anomalies of development

Normal development depends upon the crucially timed convergence of tissue processes from different origins. Failures result in anomalies along the lines of normal fusion. The most common of the orofacial clefts is that of the secondary palate, followed by lip clefts and then clefts of the primary palate. The embryological basis for these is failure of fusion of the palatal shelves of the maxillary process, and the medial and lateral limbs of the frontonasal process, respectively. Failure of the tongue to descend in consequence of abnormal embryonic head flexion has been postulated as a cause, although genetic factors do play a part in some cases (Poswillo, 1975). Less common clefts are oblique facial clefts, midline clefts and congenital macrostomia or microstomia, which represent failures in the earlier stages of development (*Figure 8.4*).

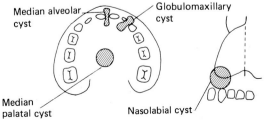

Figure 8.4 The major facial clefts

Other common abnormalities, such as developmental cysts and fistulae, result from the entrapment of epithelium along the lines of fusion, and these include nasolabial, nasoglobular, median alveolar and median palatal cysts which usually do not present until adult life (*Figure 8.5*).

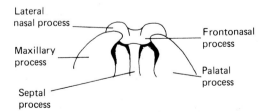

Figure 8.5 Developmental cysts of the maxilla

Development of the tongue

The tongue develops in two parts: the anterior part arises from the mandibular arches, in the form of paired eminences and, from a midline structure, the tuberculum impar in the floor of the mouth; the posterior part is derived from the *hypobranchial eminence* of the third visceral arch which grows forward over the second arches to become continuous with the anterior part of the tongue (*Figure 8.6*). The V-shaped *sulcus terminalis*

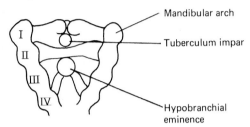

Figure 8.6 Development of the tongue. Floor of the mouth in 9-mm fetus

lies posterior to the site of union of the two parts. At the apex of this V, just behind the row of *circumvallate* papillae, there is a small median pit in the dorsum of the adult tongue, the *foramen caecum*. This is a vestige of invagination from the floor of the pharynx which gives rise to the thyroid gland. By using the foramen caecum as a landmark, it becomes apparent that the mucosal covering of the body of the tongue arises from the first arch tissue and thus its sensory innervation is by the lingual branch of the *trigeminal* nerve, which is the nerve to the first arch.

The sensory innervation to the part of the tongue posterior to the sulcus terminalis is derived from the third arch and hence its innervation is by the *glossopharyngeal* nerve.

Trapped between these two parts of the tongue is some tissue from the second arch, and this tissue is innervated by the nerve to the second arch, the seventh or facial nerve. In fact, the function of the nerve supply is gustatory and served by the *chorda tympani* branch of the facial nerve.

During the early part of its development, the tongue lies partly within the nasal cavity, and a delay in its descent may impede the uniting of the palatal folds, thereby producing clefts in the secondary palate.

Development of the mandible

The mandible is formed in the lower or deeper part of the first visceral arch. It is preceded there by *Meckel's cartilage* which represents the primitive

vertebrate mandible. The dorsal end of this unbroken rod of cartilage gives rise to the malleus of the middle ear, but Meckel's cartilage itself plays little direct part in the development of the bony mandible. A band of dense fibrocellular tissue on the lateral side of Meckel's cartilage undergoes ossification and traps the associated mandibular arch nerves (*Figure 8.7*). Thus the

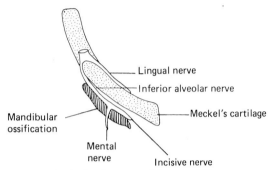

Figure 8.7 Early development of the mandible

inferior alveolar nerve comes to lie in the inferior dental canal after entering the mandible through the mandibular foramen, and the mental nerve to the lower lip and chin exits through the mental foramen. The two bony halves are united anteriorly by connective tissue, but bony union of this suture takes place before the end of the first year of life. All of Meckel's cartilage, except for the sphenomandibular ligament, the malleus and the malleolar ligament, disappears.

Surface anatomy

The lips

The lips are covered externally by skin and internally by mucous membrane. The vermillion border of the lips is a characteristic of the human species, and the red zone in the upper lip protrudes in the midline to form the *tubercle*. From the midline to the corners of the mouth the lips widen and then narrow. In the midline of the upper lip is the *philtrum* and the corners of the lips, known as the *commissures*, lie adjacent to the canine teeth. The skin surrounding the lips in the adult male is hirsute, a secondary sexual characteristic. At rest, the lips are lightly closed together when they are said to be *competent*.

The oral vestibule

The oral vestibule is a slit-like space between the lips and cheeks, and the teeth and alveolus. When the teeth are occluded, the vestibule is a closed space which communicates with the oral cavity proper only in the retromolar regions. The reflection of the mucosa from the alveolus to the lips and cheeks is the *fornix of the vestibule*. The upper and lower labial *frenula* are consistent folds of mucosa running from lip to the alveolus.

The cheeks

The cheeks extend from the labial commissures anteriorly to the ascending ramus posteriorly, and are bounded superiorly and inferiorly by the upper and lower vestibular *sulci*. Yellow granules on the mucosal surface are ectopic sebaceous glands known as *Fordyce granules*. The parotid salivary duct drains into the cheek opposite the maxillary second molar tooth. In front of the pillar of the fauces, a fold of mucosa containing the pterygomandibular raphe extends from the upper to the lower alveolus.

The palate

The palate is divided into the bony anterior hard palate and the mobile posterior soft palate. Immediately behind the anterior teeth, the mucosa of the hard palate shows the distinct prominence of the *incisive papilla*. Extending posteriorly to this is the midline raphe and the irregular folds of bound mucosa known as the palatal *rugae*. The junction of the hard and soft palate can be discerned, without palpation, by the change of colour from the pink of the hard palate to the yellow-red of the soft palate. In the middle of the free posterior edge of the soft palate is the *uvula*.

The floor of the mouth

The floor of the mouth is divided into two parts by the lingual frenulum which extends up to the base of the tongue. On either side of the frenulum are the sublingual papillae which mark the entry into the mouth of the ducts of the submandibular glands. On either side of this duct are the sublingual folds overlying the sublingual salivary glands.

The tongue

The tongue has both a dorsal and a ventral surface. The dorsal surface is divided by the V-shaped groove or the *sulcus terminalis* into the larger palatal and smaller posterior pharyngeal parts. Just anterior to these lie the large *circumvallate papillae*, while the remainder of the dorsum is covered with numerous white, conical elevations, the *filiform* papillae, between which are interspersed isolated reddish prominences, the *fungiform* papillae. On the posterolateral aspect of the tongue are the leaf-like *foliate* papillae, which can cause much anxiety when first discovered by the cancerophobic patient (*Figure 8.8*).

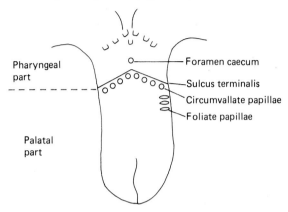

Figure 8.8 Dorsum of the tongue

The ventral surface of the tongue is covered by a smooth mucous membrane through which vessels are clearly visible. It is divided into two by the lingual frenulum, on either side of which are fringed folds of mucous membrane, the *fimbriated folds* (Liebgott, 1982).

Bony anatomy

Maxilla

The right and left maxillae are the principal bones of the facial skeleton and superior aspect of the mouth. Each maxilla consists of a body and four processes, the frontal, palatine, zygomatic and alveolar processes, the first three of which articulate with separate bones of the same name while the alveolar process supports the maxillary teeth. In the midline, the two maxillae meet at the intermaxillary suture which is continuous with the suture between the two palatal processes (*Figure 8.9*).

Each maxilla is hollowed by the paranasal sinuses and contains the following foramina: the posterior superior dental, incisive, palatine canal (with palatine bone), nasolacrimal canal (with lacrimal and inferior turbinate bones), infraorbital groove canal and foramen, and ostium to the maxillary antrum (Scott and Symons, 1977).

Growth of the maxilla

The maxilla develops in the fetal maxillary process as a membranous ossification. At birth, the infant

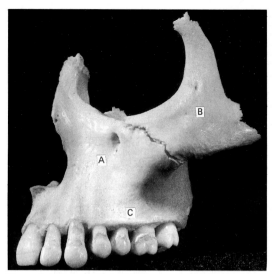

Figure 8.9 The maxilla and the zygoma. (*a*) Maxilla; (*b*) zygoma; (*c*) alveolar process

maxilla differs from the adult maxilla in having small alveolar processes and rudimentary maxillary sinuses. Growth is by bone apposition, but the forward and downward growth of the mid-third of the facial skeleton also depends on endochondral growth at the *spheno-occipital synchondrosis*.

The zygoma

The zygoma is an important element in the facial buttress system. It is a paired bone, triradiating into a maxillary, frontal and temporal process (*see Figure 8.9*). Clinically, this bone, the malus or malar bone, can undergo fracture dislocation following trauma. This may result in an inability to close the mouth because the coronoid process of the mandible impinges on the medially displaced zygoma. Reduction is achieved by passing an instrument under the zygoma from above using the fascia of the temporalis muscle as a guide.

The palatine bone

The horizontal plates of these paired bones articulate with each other and with the palatal process of the maxilla to form the posterior aspect of the bony palate (*Figure 8.10*).

The mandible

The mandible consists of a horizontal horseshoe-shaped component, the *body* of the mandible, and

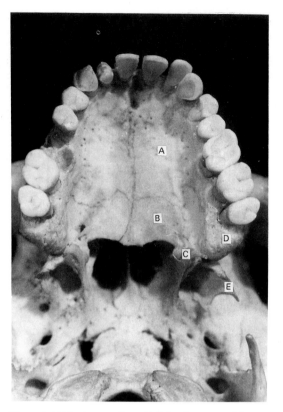

Figure 8.10 The bony palate. (*a*) Palatal process of the maxilla; (*b*) horizontal process of the palatine bone; (*c*) pterygoid hamulus; (*d*) tuberosity of maxilla; (*e*) lateral pterygoid plate

two vertical plates, the *rami*, which form the body at an obtuse angle. The two lateral halves of the mandible fuse in the midline soon after birth and the lower half of this forms the mental protuberance or chin. The upper border of the ramus carries two processes, the coronoid process anteriorly, and the condyloid process posteriorly, the latter of which articulates with the temporal bone at the *temporomandibular* joint.

The upper border of the mandible is the alveolar margin which contains the sockets for the roots of the mandibular teeth (*Figure 8.11*).

On the medial side of each ramus is the inferior dental foramen, opening into the inferior dental canal which runs through the body of the mandible to terminate laterally at the mental foramen.

On the medial aspect of the body of the mandible, the transverse mylohyoid ridge runs anteriorly almost to the genial tubercles at the midline (*Figure 8.12*). (Berkovitch, Holland and Moxham, 1977).

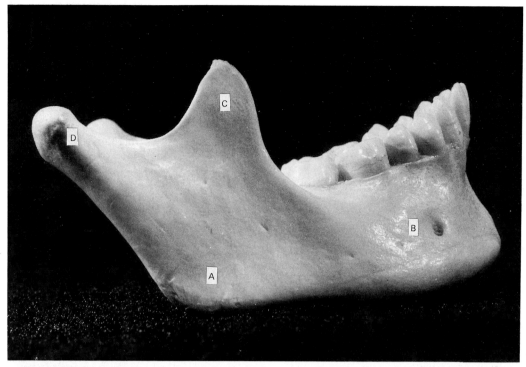

Figure 8.11 Lateral view of mandible. (*a*) Ramus; (*b*) body; (*c*) coronoid process; (*d*) condyloid process

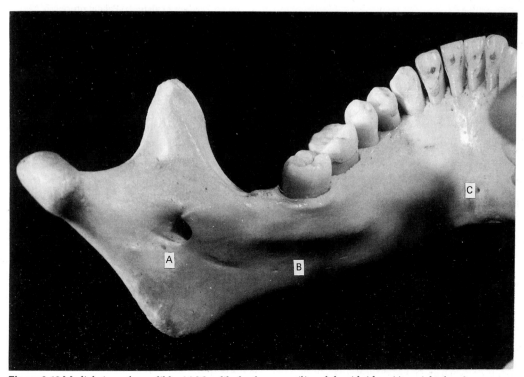

Figure 8.12 Medial view of mandible. (*a*) Mandibular foramen; (*b*) mylohyoid ridge; (*c*) genial tubercles

Growth of the mandible

The ramus of the mandible is composed largely of bone, with the exception of the condylar process which differentiates into a cone-shaped mass of cartilage. This zone of cartilage beneath, and separate from, the articular cartilage persists until the end of the second decade of life and, by its continued proliferation and endochondral ossification, is responsible for the growth in length of the mandible. Damage to this cartilage will result in failure in growth of the mandible.

Renewed activity by this centre after completion of growth accounts for the prognathism of acromegaly. The change in width and general architecture of the mandible is produced by the remodelling process of resorption and apposition to which all bones are subject. During life the mandible changes in shape. At birth, there is a wide mandibular angle, the ramus is small compared to the body and the chin is poorly developed. By the end of life, if all the teeth have been prematurely lost, the mandible once again approaches its fetal form (*Figure 8.13*) (Scott, 1967).

Clinical aspects of the facial skeleton

Trauma to the facial skeleton is common, and is usually the result of either a road traffic accident or violent assault. Many combinations of fracture of the mandible can occur but most fractures involve, either singly or in combination, the body, the ramus or the neck of the condyle of the mandible. Treatment of most fractures requires the application of intermaxillary fixation, although fractures distal to the tooth-bearing areas may require additional techniques. Injuries to the mandibular condyle should be mobilized early to prevent ankylosis of the temporomandibular joint (*Figure 8.14*).

Fractures of the maxilla and facial skeleton were classified by Le Fort at the turn of the century. Le Fort 1 fractures involve the maxilla alone, Le Fort 2 fractures involve the orbits, and Le Fort 3 fractures consist of a separation of the maxilla, nose and ethmoids from the base of the skull (*Figure 8.15*).

Severe disproportion between the mandible and the maxilla or between these and the face can be treated surgically by maxillary or mandibular

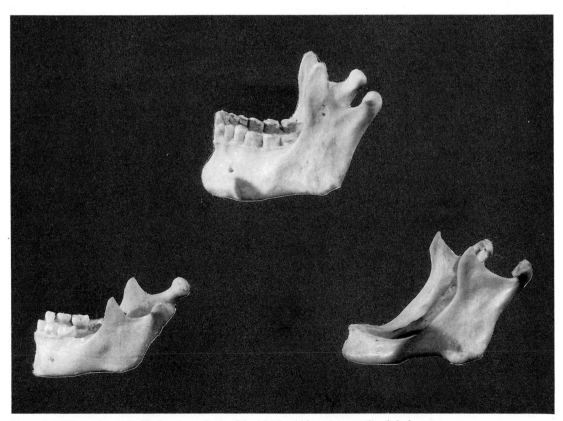

Figure 8.13 Changes in mandibular shape during life. (*a*) Mandible at 6 years; (*b*) adult dentate mandible; (*c*) edentulous mandible

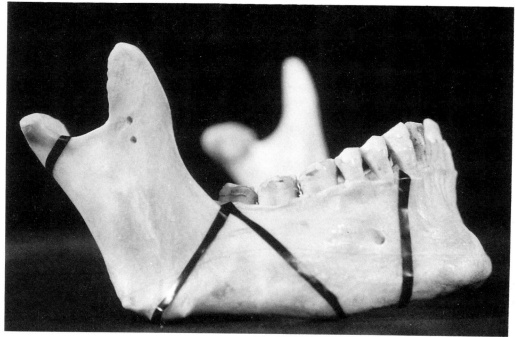

Figure 8.14 Common sites of fracture of the mandible

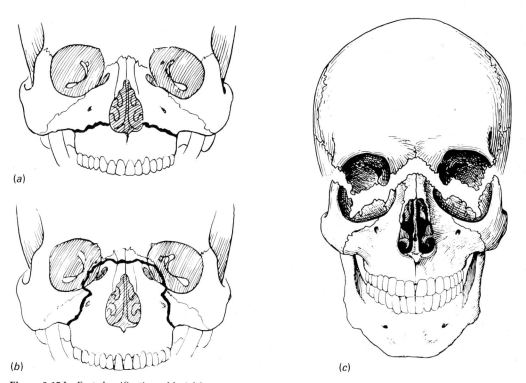

(a)

(b)

(c)

Figure 8.15 Le Fort classification of facial fractures. (a) Le Fort 1; (b) Le Fort 2; (c) Le Fort 3

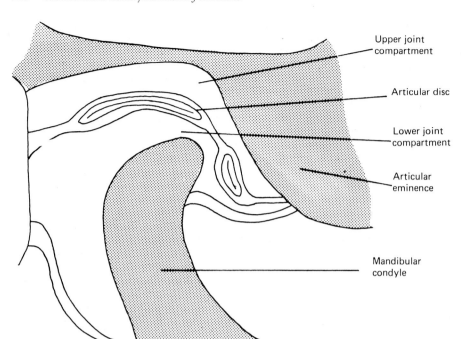

Figure 8.16 Mandibular condyle in half-open position

osteotomies, a branch of maxillofacial surgery now called *orthognathic surgery* (Killey, 1971; Archer, 1978; Laskin, 1980; Mathog, 1984).

The temporomandibular joint

The mandible can be thought of as a single long bone, articulated at both ends. However, both joints must act simultaneously with movement, which is unique in the body.

The temporomandibular joint is a synovial articulation between the head of the mandible and the glenoid fossa of the temporal bone. The joint cavity is divided into two compartments by the intervening articular disc. The movement in the lower compartment is that of a hinge joint, but in the upper compartment some anterior and posterior gliding up and down the articular eminence occurs with wider degrees of jaw opening (*Figure 8.16*).

A strong joint capsule, which is strengthened laterally and medially by sturdy collateral ligaments, is also present. The lateral ligament is called the temporomandibular ligament, which not only prevents backward displacement of the condyle but which tightens at extreme opening, thus preventing subluxation. Two accessory ligaments of the temporomandibular joint are the sphenomandibular ligament, which runs from the

spine of the sphenoid to the lingula of the mandible, and the stylomandibular ligament, which runs from the styloid process to the angle of the mandible; neither of these accessory ligaments, however, is thought to contribute significantly to the stability of the joints (*Figure 8.17*). The articular disc or meniscus is an important component of the temporomandibular joint. It consists of dense connective fibrous tissue and is moulded to the bony joint surfaces, which makes it thinner centrally than laterally, and it fills the gap produced by the disproportion between the head

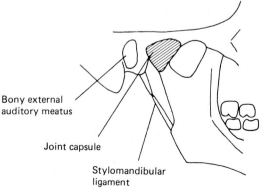

Figure 8.17 Ligaments of the temporomandibular joint

of the condyle and the glenoid fossa. Some fibres of the lateral pterygoid muscle are inserted into the anterior margin of the meniscus which is thus pulled forward with mandibular opening. Failure of coordinated movement of the articular disc may, on wide opening of the mouth, result in the head of the condyle slipping off the disc anteriorly, producing the familiar symptom of the clicking temporomandibular joint. The posterior aspect of the articular disc is rich in nerve endings concerned with proprioception in the joints (Sarnat and Laskin, 1980).

The movements of the mandible may be described as follows:

Protrusion Both mandibular condules move forward onto the articular eminences and the teeth remain in gliding contact.

Retrusion (retraction) This is the reverse process.

Opening This is partly a hinge movement and partly the result of the condyles being drawn on to the articular eminences. The mandible rotates around a horizontal axis so that, as the condyles move forward, the angles of the mandible move backwards and the chin is depressed.

Closing In this movement, the jaw may close in any number of positions. Closure in protrusion with the heads of the condyles remaining on the articular eminences, so that the lower incisors bite edge to edge with the upper incisors, is called incision. Closure with the condyles in the most backward position in the glenoid fossa, so that the teeth meet in normal occlusion, is called trituration.

Mastication requires side-to-side movements of the occlusal surfaces of the molar teeth. The condyle remains in the posterior position in the glenoid fossa on the side to which the chin is moving, and is held there by the tonic contractions of the muscle on that side; on the other side, the condyle is drawn forward and then back by the muscles of mastication on that side. The process is then repeated on the other side.

Myofacial pain dysfunction syndrome

Although the clinical symptoms associated with jaw dysfunction have long been recognized, it is only in the last 20 years that a condition previously referred to as Costen's syndrome or temporomandibular joint syndrome has been shown to be neither a primary joint disorder nor generally caused by occlusal abnormalities. Rather, it is now believed that masticatory muscle spasm is the primary factor responsible for the symptoms, for which the major causative factor is psychological stress.

The patient's symptoms are usually those of a unilateral dull ache in the ear or preauricular region that frequently radiates to the temple, to the angle of the mandible or the adjacent cervical region, or to the occiput. The pain is relatively constant but may be worse in the morning, and is exacerbated by use of the mandible.

The signs are four-fold. First, there is tenderness of the masticatory muscles to palpation; this can be elicited over the temporalis muscle but is most marked when the thumb is placed into the retromolar triangle and pressed upwards and backwards into the pterygoid muscles. Secondly, there is tenderness to firm palpation of the temporomandibular joint itself. Thirdly, there is limitation of mandibular movement and, fourthly, there is clicking of the joint. The latter two are lesser cardinal signs.

Treatments of this condition are various but most patients can be reassured that the majority of cases resolve spontaneously over a few weeks. Persistent problems require a dental opinion. Occlusal adjustments and the fitting of bite-raising appliances have been the mainstay of treatment. A very few cases may need referral to an oral surgeon for joint surgery.

The myofacial pain syndrome is commonly seen in otological practice, but the diagnosis should be entertained only after ear pathology has been eliminated following experienced examination.

Mandibular posture

At rest, there remains a gap of a few millimetres between the occlusal surfaces of the teeth, the so-called 'freeway space'. Following speech, mastication or swallowing the mandible returns to this physiological rest position. However, psychological states are known to interfere with this mechanism and the anxious individual with teeth tightly clenched is well recognized.

When establishing the occlusion of the edentulous patient for the provision of dentures, it is important to establish the physiological freeway space. An overopened occlusion on the denture produces discomfort and a 'horsey' appearance, whereas too great a freeway space produces overclosure, resulting in the sagging and falling of the soft tissues of the face, thereby mimicking or enhancing the ageing process of the face.

There has for some time been debate as to whether the temporomandibular joint is stress bearing (Hekneby, 1974). It is felt that most of the considerable stresses engendered by mastication are dispersed through the teeth and then through the well-recognized stress pathways of the facial skeleton to the skull. Some of these forces, however, must be directed through the glenoid cavity and into the temporal bone itself.

The muscles of mastication

Although other muscles also act upon the mandible, the term 'muscles of mastication' is used to describe the temporalis, the masseter and the lateral and medial pterygoid muscles. These muscles all receive their innervation from the mandibular division of the trigeminal nerve, indicating their origin from the musculature of the first branchial arch.

The *temporalis muscles* are fan-shaped muscles which take origin from the lateral aspect of the skull up to the inferior temporal line. The muscle fibres converge towards their tendinous insertions on the coronoid process of the mandible.

The *masseter muscles* may be divided into superficial and deep parts. The superficial parts arise from the lower border of the zygomatic arch and pass downwards and backwards to be inserted into the lower half of the lateral surface of the mandibular ramus. The deep parts arise from the inner surface of the lower part of the zygomatic arch and pass vertically downwards to be inserted into the mandibular ramus above the insertion of the superficial parts of the muscle.

The *lateral pterygoid muscle* has two heads, each with a separate origin: the inferior head arises from the lateral surface of the lateral pterygoid plate, and the superior head from the infratemporal surface of the greater wing of the sphenoid. The muscle fibres are inserted into the neck of the condyle and into the disc and capsule of the temporomandibular joint.

The *medial pterygoid muscle* also has two heads. The anterior head arises from the pyramidal process of the palatine bone and the posterior head from the medial surface of the lateral pterygoid plate.

Actions of the muscles of mastication

The muscles of mastication, in conjunction with other muscles, such as the mylohyoid, buccinator and digastric, initiate the movements of the mandible. The movements may be summarized as follows, with the major actions of the muscle indicated:

Elevation is produced by the masseter, medial pterygoid and anterior fibres of temporalis.
Depression is produced by the lateral pterygoids.
Protrusion is produced by the lateral and medial pterygoids.

Retraction is produced by the posterior fibres of temporalis.
Lateral excursions are produced by the medial and lateral pterygoids of both sides acting alternately (Jenkins, 1978).

Muscles of the cheeks and lips

The cheeks and lips contain some of the muscles of facial expression which are primarily muscles controlling the degree of opening and closing of the orifices of the face. The expressive functions of the facial musculature have developed secondarily.

The muscles of the face are all derived embryologically from the mesenchyme of the second branchial arch; and therefore, the motor innervation is that to the second arch, the facial nerve.

The muscle of the lip is the *orbicularis oris*, the fibres of which are divided into four parts which correspond to the four quadrants of the lips. Muscle fibres in the philtrum insert into the nasal septum. The range of movements produced by this muscle include lip closure, protrusion and pursing. The muscles which radiate from the orbicularis oris can be divided into the superficial muscles of the upper and lower lips.

Two muscles extend to the corner of the mouth, the *risorius* and the *buccinator* muscles. The risorius which lies superficial to the buccinator stretches the angle of the mouth laterally. The buccinator, which arises from the pterygomandibular raphe, inserts mostly into the mucous membrane covering the cheek, and its main function is to maintain the tension of the cheek against the teeth during mastication.

Numerous minor salivary glands line the inner surfaces of the lips and cheeks. The parotid duct pierces each buccinator muscle after passing around the anterior margin of the masseter muscle, with its orifice lying opposite the second upper molar tooth.

The soft palate

The soft palate is a fibrous aponeurosis, the shape and position of which is altered by the tensor palati muscles, the levator palati muscles, the palatoglossus and the palatopharyngeus muscles.

The tensor palati muscle arises from the scaphoid fossa of the sphenoid bone and from the lateral side of the cartilaginous part of the eustachian tube. The muscle fibres converge towards the pterygoid hamulus where they become tendinous, and bend at right angles around the hamulus to become the palatine aponeurosis. When the tensor palati muscles contract, the palatine aponeurosis becomes taut. The motor innervation is derived from the mandibular division of the trigeminal nerve.

The levator palati muscle takes origin from the petrous temporal bone and the medial side of the cartilaginous part of the eustachian tube. The muscle curves downwards, forwards and medially to form a muscular sling which, when acting against the stiffened aponeurosis, produces an upward and backward movement of the soft palate. The nerve supply to the levator palati is derived from the cranial part of the accessory nerve (*Figure 8.18*).

The paired *palatopharyngeus* muscles extend from the palate down the lateral pharyngeal walls, where they form the posterior pillars of the fauces to insert into the posterior border of the thyroid cartilage. The action of these muscles is to elevate the larynx and pharynx but they also arch the relaxed palate and depress the tensed palate. The nerve supply is from the cranial accessory nerve.

The paired *palatoglossus* muscles arise from the palatine aponeurosis and descend as the anterior pillar of the fauces to insert into the lateral margin of the tongue. Their action is to raise the tongue and narrow the oropharyngeal isthmus. They are innervated by the cranial part of the accessory nerve.

Passavant's muscle is a sphincter-like muscle which encircles the pharynx at the level of the palate. The contraction of this muscle forms a ridge against which the soft palate is elevated, and in this way the oropharynx can be shut off from the nasopharynx during swallowing and speech.

The muscles of the tongue

The muscles of the tongue are paired, and are grouped into an *intrinsic* and *extrinsic* set. The intrinsic muscle fibres of the tongue can be divided into three groups, namely the transverse, longitudinal and vertical. Their function is to alter the shape of the tongue and they are innervated by the *hypoglossal* nerve. The extrinsic muscles of the tongue are composed of four groups, namely

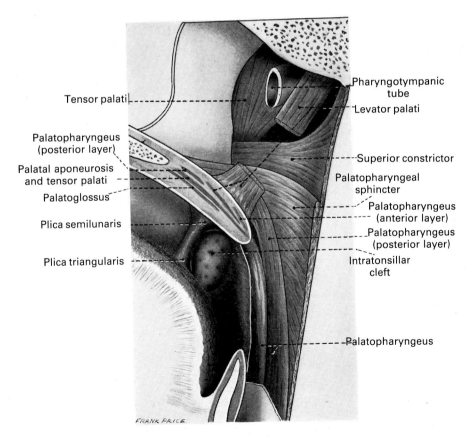

Tensor palati

Palatopharyngeus (posterior layer)

Palatal aponeurosis and tensor palati

Palatoglossus

Plica semilunaris

Plica triangularis

Pharyngotympanic tube

Levator palati

Superior constrictor

Palatopharyngeal sphincter

Palatopharyngeus (anterior layer)

Palatopharyngeus (posterior layer)

Intratonsillar cleft

Palatopharyngeus

FRANK PRICE

Figure 8.18 The muscles of the palate

the *genioglossus, hyoglossus, styloglossus* and *palato-glossus* (*Figure 8.19*).

The genioglossus is a fan-shaped muscle which arises from the upper genial tubercle and is inserted into the tongue from its tip to its root. When these muscles act together as a pair, they protrude the tongue.

The hyoglossus is a flat quadrilateral muscle arising from the greater cornu of the hyoid bone passing upwards to be inserted into the side of the tongue. When this muscle contracts, the side of the tongue is depressed.

The styloglossus arises from the styloid process and passes downwards and forwards to be inserted into the side of the tongue. The contraction of this muscle causes the tongue to be drawn upwards and backwards.

The palatoglossus arises from the aponeurosis of the soft palate and descends to the tongue as the anterior pillars of the fauces. Its action is to raise the tongue and narrow the oropharyngeal isthmus. In contrast to the other extrinsic muscles of the tongue which are innervated by the hypoglossal nerve, the palatoglossus is innervated by the cranial part of the accessory nerve.

Blood supply

The arterial supply of the head and neck is very rich and the major branches overlap and collateralize. In addition, a good cross-over exists in the midline so that the external carotid artery, which is the main supply, can be ligated without fear. The face is supplied by the facial artery which anastomoses with the vessel on the other side and also with the other vessels supplying the region – the superficial temporal artery, the infraorbital and mental branches of the maxillary artery and the nasal branch of the ophthalmic artery.

The maxilla and mandible are supplied by branches of the maxillary artery and the tongue by the lingual artery, both of which are branches of the external carotid artery.

The palate derives its blood supply from the greater and lesser palatine branches of the maxillary artery.

The veins in the head and neck have few, if any, valves. This has the advantage of allowing bidirectional flow between deep maxillary veins and intercranial venous sinuses, but has the disadvantage of also allowing bacterial emboli from superficial septic foci to enter the cranial cavity by reverse flow.

The internal jugular vein is the largest channel, beginning at the jugular foramen as a continuation of the sigmoid dural sinus. Much of the drainage from the maxilla and mandible passes backwards, by way of the pterygoid plexus of veins, into the internal jugular system.

The superficial venous system is, however, quite variable, but the facial vein draining the superficial and anterior face usually joins with the retromandibular vein to form the common facial vein. This enters the internal jugular vein and finally drains into the brachiocephalic.

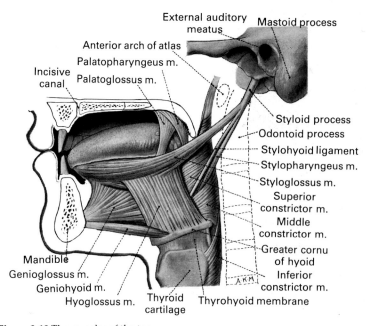

Figure 8.19 The muscles of the tongue

Lymphatic drainage

In general, the lymph from the anterior part of this region drains into the submental and submandibular nodes on the ipsilateral side and then into the deeper jugulodigastric node, whereas lymph from the posterior part drains directly into the jugulodigastric node.

The lymphatic drainage of the tongue, however, is a little more complex. Lymphatics from the anterior two-thirds of the tongue may be divided into the marginal and central vessels. The marginal vessels drain into the submandibular nodes on the same side; the central vessels at the tip of the tongue drain into the submental nodes and from further back into ipsilateral and contralateral submandibular lymph nodes. Lymphatics from the posterior third of the tongue drain directly into the jugulodigastric group of nodes (*Figure 8.20*).

The deep cervical plexus of lymphatic channels is the final common pathway for all head and neck drainage, terminating in the thoracic duct on the left and the junction of the internal jugular and subclavian veins on the right.

Nerve supply

The whole system, from the oropharynx forward, receives its sensory supply from the maxillary and mandibular division of the trigeminal nerve. The mandible, mandibular teeth, gingivae, and floor of the mouth and tongue are supplied by inferior dental, buccal, mylohyoid and lingual branches of the mandibular division.

The maxilla and maxillary teeth are served by the maxillary nerve, and by the infraorbital, pterygopalatine and anterior, middle and posterior dental nerves of the maxillary division.

The anterior hard palate is supplied by the nasopalatine nerve and the rest by the anterior and posterior palatine nerves from the maxillary division of the trigeminal nerve.

The anterior two-thirds of the tongue is supplied by the lingual nerve; the posterior one-third by the glossopharyngeal nerve (*Figure 8.21*).

The motor innervation of this region has been described previously.

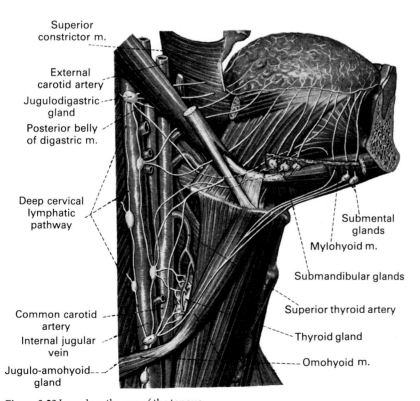

Superior constrictor m.

External carotid artery

Jugulodigastric gland

Posterior belly of digastric m.

Deep cervical lymphatic pathway

Common carotid artery

Internal jugular vein

Jugulo-amohyoid gland

Submental glands

Mylohyoid m.

Submandibular glands

Superior thyroid artery

Thyroid gland

Omohyoid m.

Figure 8.20 Lymph pathways of the tongue

222

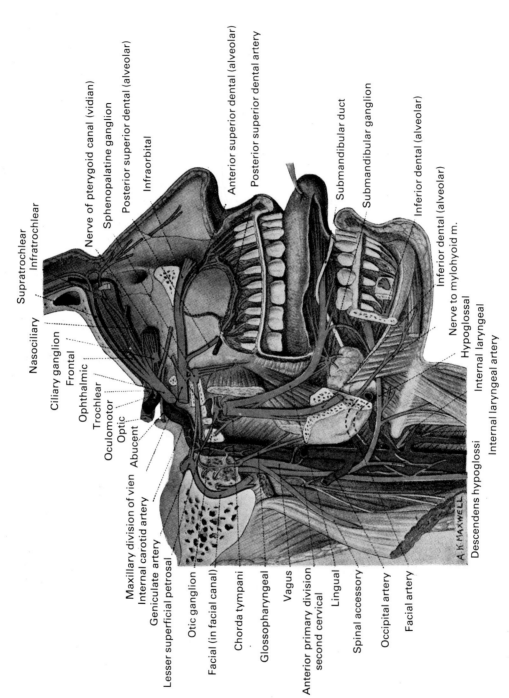

Figure 8.21 The trigeminal and the hypoglossal nerves

The fascial spaces of the head

Within the head there are anatomical spaces bounded by fascial layers, muscle, bone, skin or mucous membrane. Contained within these spaces are vessels, nerves, lymphatics and lymph nodes, and filling the unoccupied space is loose connective tissue (*Figures 8.22* and *8.23*).

These spaces or potential spaces are important because they determine the spread of infection and, to a lesser extent, of neoplasms in these areas. The most important of these spaces are:

The superficial facial compartment, which is bounded superficially by the buccinator muscle, the facial surfaces of the maxilla and mandible, and the outer surface of the masseter muscle. It is limited above by the zygomatic arch, behind by the parotid compartment, and below by the lower border of the mandible. It communicates deep to the mandibular ramus with the pterygoid space. It contains the buccal pad of fat, the duct of the parotid gland, the facial artery and vein, the buccal lymph nodes, the mental and infraorbital foramina, branches of the trigeminal and facial nerves, and the muscles of facial expression.

The sublingual compartment, which is bounded by the lingual surface of the body of the mandible, the mucous membrane of the floor of the mouth and the upper surface of the mylohyoid muscle. It contains the submandibular salivary gland, the sublingual salivary glands, and the lingual and hypoglossal nerves.

The submandibular space, which is bounded by the body of the mandible, the lower surface of the mylohyoid muscle above and the superficial layer of deep cervical fascia below. It contains the superficial part of the submandibular salivary gland, the anterior belly of the digastric muscle and the submandibular and submental lymph nodes.

The parotid compartment, which is bounded by the posterior border of the ramus of the mandible, the styloid process and its muscles, the sternomastoid and the posterior belly of the digastric muscle. It contains the parotid salivary gland and its lymph nodes.

The pterygoid space, which is bounded by the ramus of the mandible and the deep surface of the masseter on the lateral side, the skull base above and the pharynx medially. It contains the pterygoid muscles, the pterygoid venous plexus, the maxillary artery and the mandibular division of the trigeminal nerve.

The parapharyngeal space, which is bounded by the pharyngeal wall and vertebral column medially, and the deep cervical fascia and sternomastoid muscle laterally. It contains the carotid artery, the jugular vein, cranial nerves IX, X, XI, and XII, and the deep cervical lymph node chain.

The paratonsillar space, which is between the wall of the pharynx and the mucous membrane of the fauces, extends up into the soft palate.

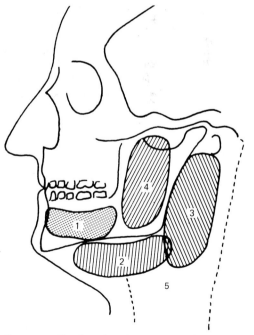

Figure 8.23 The deep fascial spaces. (1) Sublingual space; (2) submandibular space; (3) parotid space; (4) pterygoid space; (5) parapharyngeal space

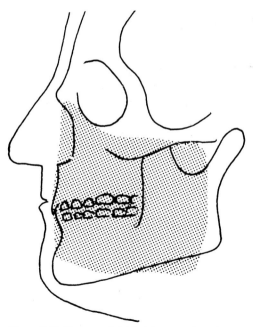

Figure 8.22 The superficial facial compartment

Taste

Taste buds, which open directly on to the lingual surface of the tongue, are present in *fungiform* papillae which cover the anterior two-thirds of the dorsum of the tongue. These papillae are circular, red, between 1 and 4 mm in diameter and number between 20 and 60. These slightly raised fungiform papillae are surrounded by the more numerous filiform papillae which do not contain taste buds. Up to eight taste buds are present within these fungiform papillae, which also contain specialized pressure, tactile and temperature receptors.

Over the posterior third of the tongue, just anterior to the V-shaped *sulcus terminalis*, lie between 8 and 20 *circumvallate* papillae which project above the surrounding lingual tissue (*Figure 8.24*). Taste buds, in numbers up to 100, are

For normal function, the taste bud receptors are exposed to the oral environment and are thought to respond to four primary stimuli: salt, sweet, sour and bitter. Differentiation of discrimination from within the various parts of the oral cavity has been observed, but the greatest number of buds respond to sweet stimuli.

Decreased taste activity is called *hypogeusia* and total loss of taste ability is known as *ageusia*. Abnormalities in the production of saliva, which is necessary for taste – such as occurs in Sjögren's syndrome, in the surgical removal of salivary glands, or after radiotherapy of the head and neck area – lead to a reduction in saliva flow and also to pathological changes in the taste buds.

Among the many pathological processes known to affect taste are vitamin deficiency, especially that of vitamins A and B$_{12}$, and zinc deficiency. Endocrine disturbances, such as hypothyroidism

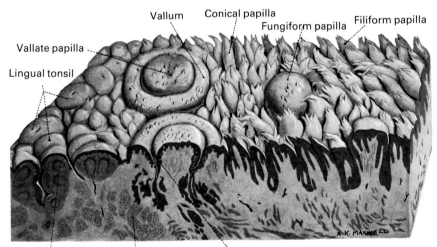

Figure 8.24 Surface view of the tongue

present in both the papillae and the crypts which surround these papillae. In the bottom of the crypts surrounding the circumvallate papillae are the Von Ebner's glands, and encircling the openings of these glands are cilia which propel the secretions into the crypts. A few taste buds may be found on the palate and lips and have even been demonstrated in the upper third of the oesophagus (Henkin, 1976).

Taste buds are made up of between 20 and 50 cells, tightly joined together by desmosomal attachments. These cells are of epithelial origin and migrate into the bud; under neural salivary influence, they differentiate into one of three cell types which undergo constant renewal. All cell types have processes which extend up into the pore region of the bud, and nerves enter and leave the taste bud through its base (*Figure 8.25*).

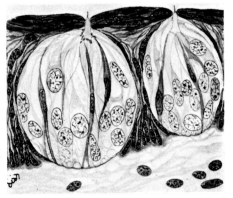

Figure 8.25 Schematic drawing of two taste buds

and Cushing's syndrome, as well as numerous drugs, such as amitriptyline and some cytotoxic agents, have been implicated.

Damage to the facial nerve in Bell's palsy, or deliberate section of the *chorda tympani* during middle ear surgery, are well known to the otolaryngologist, but one of the commonest causes of altered or lost taste sensation is postcoryzal or postinfluenzal damage, which may be accompanied by a loss of sense of smell.

Dental anatomy

Dentition

Man has two generations of teeth, namely the deciduous and the permanent.

The deciduous dentition begins to appear in the mouth at about six months of age, and the complete set of 20 teeth has erupted by about two and a half years.

The permanent dentition starts to appear in the mouth at about six years and the last of the deciduous teeth is shed at about 13 years. The permanent dentition is not complete until the third permanent molar teeth (also known as wisdom teeth) erupt at about 18–21 years. The complete permanent set of teeth numbers 32 (*Figure 8.26*).

The teeth of both dentitions are arranged in upper and lower arches, and in each arch the teeth are arranged symmetrically on either side of the median plane. The teeth are identified according to their anatomical location within each of the four quadrants. In man, the deciduous dentition has five teeth in each quadrant, comprising two incisors, one canine and two molars. The permanent dentition has eight teeth in each quadrant, comprising two incisors, one canine, two premolars and three molar teeth.

Difference between the deciduous and permanent dentitions

The deciduous teeth are smaller than their permanent successors and the crowns are more bulbous with less robust roots. The deciduous teeth are whiter than the permanent teeth, and the enamel is softer and more easily worn.

Each deciduous tooth is finally shed following the resorption of its root by the pressure of its erupting successor.

A dental shorthand is used for tooth identification. The deciduous teeth in each quadrant are labelled a to e and the permanent teeth in each quadrant numbered 1 to 8.

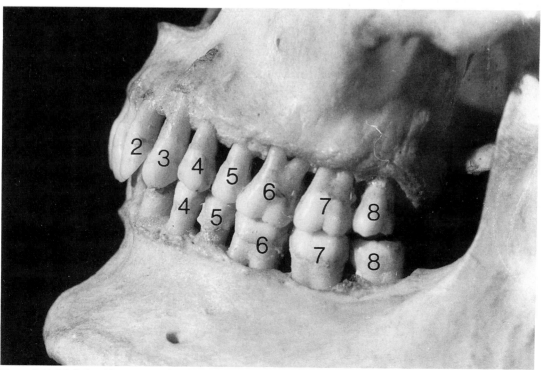

Figure 8.26 Adult dentition in normal occlusion

The symbols for the quadrants are derived from an imaginary cross imposed upon the dentition when looking at the subject.

Upper right	Upper left
Lower right	Lower left

Thus the maxillary left second molar is ⌊7 and the mandibular right deciduous first incisor is a⌉.

Definition of terms in description of tooth form

Crown   That portion of the tooth visible in the oral cavity.
Root   That portion of the tooth which lies within the alveolus.
Occlusal surface   The biting surface of a molar or premolar tooth.
Incisal margin   The cutting edge of the anterior teeth.
Cusps   The elevation in the occlusal surface of the teeth.
Fissure   Longitudinal cleft between cusps.
Buccal surface   That surface of a premolar or molar adjacent to the cheek.
Labial surface   That surface of canine or incisor which is positioned immediately adjacent to the lips.
Palatal surface   That surface of the maxillary teeth adjacent to the palate.
Lingual surface   That surface of the mandibular teeth adjacent to the tongue.
Mesial   That surface of the tooth that faces the median line.
Distal   That surface of the tooth that faces away from the median line.

Chronology of tooth eruption

Deciduous dentition

Lower incisors	b a | a b	6–9 months
Upper incisors	b a | a b	8–10 months
Upper and lower first molars	d | d / d | d	12–16 months
Deciduous canines	c | c / c | c	16–20 months
Upper and lower second molars	e | e / e | e	20–24 months

Permanent dentition

First molars	6 | 6 / 6 | 6	6–7 years
Central incisors	1 | 1 / 1 | 1	6–8 years
Lateral incisors	2 | 2 / 2 | 2	7–9 years
First premolars	4 | 4 / 4 | 4	10–12 years
Canines	3 | 3 / 3 | 3	10–12 years
Second premolars	5 | 5 / 5 | 5	10–12 years
Second molars	7 | 7 / 7 | 7	10–13 years
Third molars	8 | 8 / 8 | 8	17–21 years

Eruption times in the tables are approximate, and variations of up to six months either way are not unusual. The permanent dentition tends to be more advanced in girls than in boys.

The form of the teeth

The incisors

There are two incisors in each quadrant, upper and lower, in both deciduous and permanent dentitions. In each quadrant, the tooth nearest the midline of the dental arch is known as the central incisor and the second tooth as the lateral incisor (*Figure 8.27*). These single rooted teeth are adapted for incising and the incisal edge undergoes attrition with age. The upper incisor region is a common site for supernumerary teeth and the lower incisors are the most common teeth to exhibit crowding. A gap between the central incisors is called a *diastema*.

The canines

The name is derived from the Latin word for dog because in the dog this type of tooth is very prominent. The canines are less prominent in the human being but are still the longest rooted teeth and the crown has a sharply pointed cusp. They are the first teeth of the true maxilla, as both incisors are carried in the premaxilla.

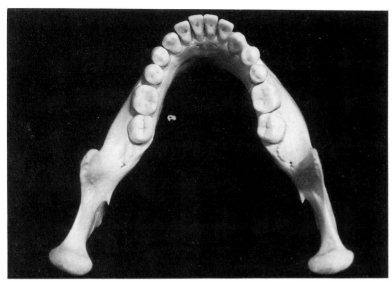

Figure 8.27 Occlusal view of an adult mandible showing the form of the teeth

The premolars

There are two premolars in each quadrant and they replace the deciduous molars.

The upper premolars have a larger buccal cusp and a smaller palatal cusp. The first premolar has two roots and the second premolar has a single root. The first premolar is the tooth most usually sacrificed to create space before orthodontic treatment. The lower premolars have a less prominent lingual cusp and are usually single rooted.

The molars

These teeth are adapted for crushing and grinding food and are multicuspid and multirooted. Upper molars have three roots and lower molars two, and they decrease in size from the largest first molar to the smallest third molar. This third molar or wisdom tooth is the most likely to be congenitally missing, and 25% of the population have one or more missing. In Caucasians, there is frequently insufficient room for the third molar to erupt so it may become impacted against the second molar in varied stages of eruption. The inability to clean the partly buried tooth, together with the sepsis that may ensue in the gingival pockets, produces discomfort in the young adult so that extraction is often necessary. The removal of these teeth, especially the mandibular impacted wisdom tooth, often requires a surgical approach because of the difficult access and the need to remove overlying bone. The apices of the roots of lower molars are usually in close relationship to

the inferior alveolar nerve which may even occasionally perforate the root.

The roots of the upper molar teeth, especially those of the first molars, are in very close proximity to the antrum. When viewed from within the antrum, these roots can be seen as elevations of the antral floor.

Periapical abscesses on these molar teeth can therefore lead to sinusitis, although this is rarely seen in present times. Certainly, as part of the treatment of maxillary sinusitis, any carious teeth or infected roots should be appropriately treated.

The bone of the floor of the antrum, which lies between the roots of the molar teeth, is thin and is therefore commonly removed still attached to the roots during dental extraction. The iatrogenic production of oroantral fistulae is certainly more common than is generally recognized. Large oroantral fistulae should be dealt with by immediate surgical closure. However, many of the unrecognized oroantral fistulae heal spontaneously, and the most important determinant is the organization of a healthy blood clot within the socket. Sepsis within the clot will cause lysis and will produce a localized osteitis in the bone. This painful condition of 'dry socket' will predispose to the formation of an oroantral fistula.

Congenital absence of all teeth is known as total anodontia and absence of some of the teeth is known as partial anodontia, although a better term is 'hypodontia'. After the wisdom teeth, the most commonly congenitally absent tooth is the upper lateral incisor. Teeth which are found in excess of the normal number are called *supernumerary* teeth (Van Beek, 1983).

Dental occlusion

Dental occlusion is the relationship of the dental arcades, set upon their bony bases, to each other. There is a recognized ideal relationship of the upper and lower dental arches which is called normal occlusion.

The guidelines for assessing the occlusion are the comparative relationships of the first permanent molars and of the upper and lower incisor teeth. To a large extent, this relationship depends on the relative sizes of the maxilla and mandible. A small set back mandible will give a distocclusion or class II relationship. A large prognathic mandible produces the opposite effect, or mesiocclusion, more commonly called a class III relationship (*Figure 8.28*).

Superimposed upon these bony bases there may also be a relative dentoalveolar disproportion, more commonly known as dental crowding. In the class I malocclusion, the bony bases are in harmony, but there is a relative crowding so that individual teeth are forced out of the dental arch.

The position that the upper incisors finally assume depends also on a balance of forces between the tongue, which tends to push them outwards, and the lower lip which counterbalances and tends to pull them back. Any 'incompetence of the lips' to become securely sealed at rest may result in the upper teeth becoming proclined outside the control of the lower lip. This produces the characteristic deformity of class II, division I. Alternatively, any over-activity of the musculature of the lower lip will tend to retrocline the upper anterior teeth, producing the deformity of class II, division II.

Treatment of these malocclusions is by means of removable or fixed appliances. These apply light but continuous forces which move the teeth through the plastic bone. This form of treatment is called orthodontics.

Severe malocclusions may have a significant adverse affect on mastication; the majority of orthodontic treatments are, however, undertaken for cosmetic reasons during the early teens.

The development of the teeth

A local proliferation of the oral epithelium in the seven-week-old embryo gives rise to the *dental lamina*. At intervals along its length, small round swellings develop which are the primitive *enamel organs* of the deciduous teeth. The primordia of the permanent dentition later develop by budding off from the deciduous enamel organs. Adjacent to the enamel organ, the mesodermal tissue proliferates to form a dense mass which becomes the *dental papillae*. The enamel organ becomes a bell-shaped structure with the dental papillae now in the hollow of the enamel organ. The inner aspect of the ectodermal enamel organ differentiates, and provokes further differentiation in the dental papilla, to form *odontoblasts*, and it begins depositing enamel upon the recently laid down dentine. The entrapped dental follicle differentiates into the dental pulp (*Figure 8.29*).

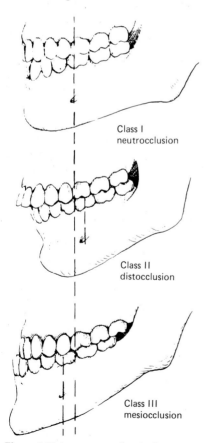

Class I
neutrocclusion

Class II
distocclusion

Class III
mesiocclusion

Figure 8.28 Assessment of occlusion

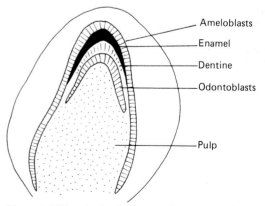

Ameloblasts

Enamel

Dentine

Odontoblasts

Pulp

Figure 8.29 Developing human tooth

When the formation of enamel is complete, the enamel epithelium extends below the cervical margin to become a two-layered structure called the *sheath of Hertwig* and this maps out the shape of the roots (Bhaskar, 1986).

When the structure of the crown is complete, the ameloblast layer will atrophy to become the reduced enamel epithelium protecting the ectodermal enamel from the mesodermal tissue in which it is buried. During eruption of the tooth, this epithelium finally unites with the epithelium of the alveolus, ensuring continuing epithelial continuity of the mucosa in spite of the eruption of the teeth (*Figure 8.30*).

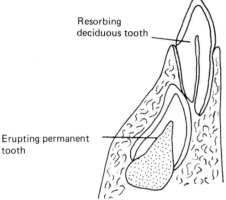

Resorbing
deciduous tooth

Erupting permanent
tooth

Figure 8.30 Resorption of deciduous incisor by erupting successor

An abnormal proliferation of odontogenic epithelium, which does not produce teeth, may occur. The proliferations may remain cellular, resulting in an *ameloblastoma*, or may lead to the production of single or multiple masses of the calcified dental tissues arranged in irregular and haphazard ways. These are known as *complex composite* and *compound composite* odontomes, respectively.

Finally, areas of epithelial dental lamina which do not differentiate into enamel organs may lie entrapped and dormant within the alveolus. These are called the *epithelial rests of Mallasez* (Ham and McCormack, 1979). Later in life, cystic conditions may occur which originate from these remnants of the dental epithelium. Among these are *cysts of eruption, dental cysts* and *dentigerous cysts*.

Structure of the teeth

In the human being, each tooth is composed of three calcified tissues, namely enamel, dentine and cementum, and contains a centrally situated soft pulp, which is the nutritive and sensory organ of the tooth.

Enamel forms the outer covering of the crown. It is grey or bluish-white in colour – its colour being modified by that of the underlying dentine – and is semitranslucent. It is the hardest substance in the body, so that it can well withstand masticatory stress, but is somewhat brittle. Enamel is highly mineralized, being 96% inorganic material, mainly in the form of hydroxyapatite crystals, 3% water and 1% organic matter. It has a crystalline prismatic structure, and each prism is the product of one ameloblast. It is ectodermal in origin, but no more enamel can be formed once the tooth has erupted.

Particular attention has recently been paid to the surface regions of enamel as it has been discovered that carious lesions within the enamel can be reversed and thereupon can reharden. Surface enamel differs both physically and chemically from subsurface enamel, in that the former is harder and less soluble. Surface enamel is rich in many trace elements, including fluorine, and it is believed that the fluoride ion incorporated in water supplies and tooth pastes has contributed to the rapid decline in the prevalence of dental caries in recent years.

Dentine, which forms the bulk of both the substances, and cementum, which covers the root, are both mesodermal in origin, that is living and capable of repair.

Dentine is composed of cells, the odontoblasts, and an intercellular substance. It is permeated by minute tubes, dentinal tubules, which contain the protoplasmic processes of the odontoblasts; the odontoblasts themselves always form a layer on the surface of the dentine. Dentine is a tissue highly sensitive to stimulation, as is commonly experienced, and although nerve fibres have been demonstrated in dentine, the odontoblasts themselves are believed to take part in the transmission of painful stimuli.

The pulp is composed of loose connective tissues richly supplied with blood vessels and nerves. The pulp is continuous with the connective tissue of the periodontal ligament and, functionally, is nutritive and sensory to the dentine. Any agent which opens up the dentinal tubules produces a reaction in the pulp. As the pulp is contained within unyielding walls of dentine, the hyperaemic and exudative changes accompanying inflammation lead to an increase in pressure inside both the pulp cavity and the vessels entering through the apical foramina, with the real risk of infarction of the pulp.

The periodontium

The periodontium is the unique attachment of the teeth to the bony bases, and includes the cementum of the tooth root, the alveolar bone and the intervening collagenous bundles of the periodontal ligament.

The most important elements of the periodontal ligament are the oblique fibres that pass from the cementum on the tooth substance to the lamina dura of the tooth socket. By the arrangement of these fibres, the tooth is suspended in its socket, and pressure upon a tooth is transformed into tension on the walls of the socket (*Figure 8.31*).

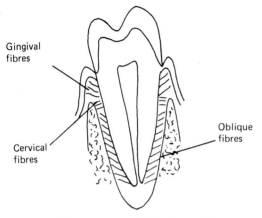

Gingival fibres

Cervical fibres

Oblique fibres

Figure 8.31 The arrangement of the fibres of the periodontal ligament

Teeth maintain their position in the arch because of a balance of the various forces acting upon each individual tooth. However, the plasticity of the alveolar bone means that teeth can move, as in eruption, or be moved by steady light pressure, and this property of the periodontium is the basis of orthodontics.

The alveolar bone, which houses the developing tooth germ and, later, the root of the tooth, is normal bone. When the teeth are lost, this bone is gradually resorbed; this process causes early problems with the fit of dentures and, with the reduction in face height, produces the ageing effect of the premature loss of the natural dentition.

The pink mucous membrane, immediately related to the teeth and firmly bound down to the alveolar bone, is called the gingiva. The gingiva follows the cervical margin of the teeth; with age, however, it physiologically moves towards the root, exposing more of the crown of the tooth, hence the expression 'getting long in the tooth'.

At the junction of the gingiva and the tooth, known as the gingival margin – representing the unique feature of a hard mineralized structure protruding through the surface integument of the body – there is a reflection of epithelium in close contact with the crown of the tooth which provides a seal at this point. Damage to this delicate seal, caused by the soft deposits of dental plaque and the calcific deposits of calculus or tartar, initiates and promotes the inflammatory process, resulting ultimately in periodontal disease, which is still the chief reason for tooth loss in adult life.

Age changes

With increasing age, the teeth undergo attrition; the enamel is worn away and the underlying dentine is exposed. The alveolar bone is progressively reduced and remodelled in those areas where the teeth have been prematurely lost. The edentulous mandible changes shape and the angle between the ramus and the body becomes more obtuse. The mental foramen comes to be closer to the upper border of the mandible where it is vulnerable to pressure.

Conclusions

As a result of changing attitudes in the UK, and of the increasing availability of innovatory methods of treatment, a greater percentage of the population are retaining their teeth for life.

Nevertheless, a substantial number of the senior adult population are edentulous and rely upon the prostheses of dentures to restore form and function.

Dental extraction is, however, still common practice and may occasionally be necessary in the course of surgical procedures undertaken by the otolaryngologist.

Surgical trainees would do well to acquaint themselves with the surgical techniques of exodontia.

References

ARCHER, W. H. (1978) *Oral and Maxillo-Facial Surgery.* Philadelphia: W. B. Saunders

BERKOVITZ, B. K. B., HOLLAND, G. R. and MOXHAM, B. J. (1977) *A Colour Atlas and Textbook of Oral Anatomy.* London: Wolfe

BHASKAR, S. N. (1986) *Orban's Oral Histology and Embryology.* St Louis: C. V. Mosby

HAM, A. W. and MCCORMACK, D. H. (1979) Histology, 8th edn. Philadelphia: J. P. Lippincott & Co

HEKNEBY, M. (1974) The load on the temporo-mandibular joint; physical calculations and analyses. *Journal of Prosthetic Dentistry,* **31**, 303–312

HENKIN, R. I. (1976) In *Taste in Scientific Foundations of Otolaryngology.* Eds R. Hinchcliffe and D. F. N. Harrison, pp. 468–483. London: Heinemann

JENKINS, G. N. (1978) *The Physiology and Biochemistry of the Mouth.* London: Blackwell

KILLEY, H. C. (1971) *Fractures of the Mandible,* 2nd edn. Bristol: Wright

KRAUS, B. S., KITAMURA, H. and LATHAM, R. A. (1966) *Atlas of Developmental Anatomy of the Face*. New York: Harper Row

LASKIN, D. M. (1980) *Oral and Maxillo-Facial Surgery*. St Louis: C. V. Mosby

LIEBGOTT, B. (1982) *The Anatomical Basis of Dentistry*. Philadelphia: W. B. Saunders

MATHOG, R. (1984) *Maxillo-Facial Trauma*. Baltimore: Williams & Wilkins

PATEN, B. M. (1953) *Human Embryology*. London: McGraw Hill

POSWILLO, D. (1975) Causal mechanisms of cranio-facial deformity. *British Medical Bulletin*, **31**, 101

SARNAT, B. G. and LASKIN, D. M. (1979) *The Temporo-Mandibular Joint*. Springfield: C. C. Thomas

SCOTT, J. H. (1967) *Dento-facial Development and Growth*. Oxford: Pergamon

SCOTT, J. H. and SYMONS, N. B. B. (1977) *Introduction to Dental Anatomy*, 8th edn. London: Churchill Livingstone

SPERBER, G. H. (1976) *Cranio-facial Embryology*, 2nd edn. Bristol: Wright

VAN BEEK, G. C. (1983) *Dental Morphology*. Bristol: Wright

9

Anatomy and physiology of the salivary glands

O. H. Shaheen

Every textbook of human physiology includes a section on the salivary glands but rarely does this provide an insight into how disturbances of function affect the individual. This is hardly surprising in view of our limited knowledge, but an awareness of the importance of the salivary glands to the health and sense of well-being of the individual is increasingly evident.

Investigations into recurrent parotitis and the sicca syndrome are but one example of how an appreciation of the mechanics of disordered function can clarify the pathological sequences, but it would not be surprising if, in the future, other subclinical entities having their basis in a physiological disturbance were to come to light.

In spite of an ever-increasing literature on the subject, much of it seemingly esoteric, our understanding of the relation of salivary physiology to disease processes remains somewhat limited. The preoccupation with tumours at the expense of non-neoplastic pathology has possibly now redounded to the detriment of the patient; attention must, therefore, be redirected towards gaining a better understanding of the salivary glands in health and in disease.

Development of the salivary glands

All the salivary glands, both major and minor, develop along the same pattern, namely as sophisticated diverticula originating from oral epithelium. The first steps in the process are a proliferation and budding of epithelium in the form of a solid cord which migrates into the subjacent mesenchyme. Subsequently, extensive branching of this diverticulum occurs and forms the template of the embryonic gland. The acquisi-

tion of a lumen proceeds through this branching system, the final arborizations representing the future acini and the principal cord linking the structure to the surface epithelium, the excretory duct. All the major glands are ectodermal in origin, but some of the minor glands, which have their origin distal to the site of the stomatodaeal plate, arise from endoderm.

The first gland to make its appearance between the fourth and sixth weeks is the parotid. As it grows back, the parotid engulfs mesenchymal structures, of which the most important will be the facial nerve, but which also include lymph follicles.

The submandibular gland arises in the sixth week and the sublingual in the eighth, the latter developing as a series of independent secretory units which ultimately fuse, while retaining their individual ducts.

Developmental anomalies relating to the salivary glands are uncommon and include congenital absences or hypoplasia, as in the Melkersson–Rosenthal syndrome, as well as ectopic collections at unusual sites.

Anomalies such as congenital cysts or fistulae, which may have an intimate relationship to structures such as the facial nerve, are of branchial origin and do not therefore represent true malformations of salivary gland development.

The parotid gland

In appearance, the lateral aspect of the parotid gland is not unlike a Welsh harp, possessing as it does a forward prolongation which overlies the masseter muscle to give off the duct, a sliver which insinuates itself into the gap between the condyle of the mandible and external meatus, and a downward extension which fills the retromandibular sulcus (*Figure 9.1*). In horizontal section, the parotid gland is broadly triangular and exhibits an external aspect, an anteromedial surface and a posteromedial surface.

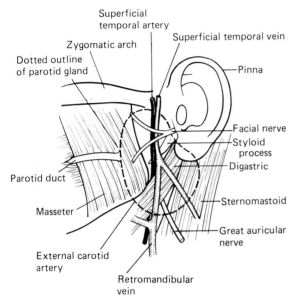

Figure 9.1 Dotted outline of parotid gland to show its relationship to adjacent structures and the associated vessels and nerves

The outer aspect of the gland is covered by an extension of the deep cervical fascia which is continuous posteriorly with the fascial envelope of the sternomastoid muscle, and anteriorly with the fascia covering the masseter muscle. This fascial covering is for the most part thick, tough and inelastic, although further forwards, where it blends with the masseteric fascia, its thickness varies and in places becomes quite thin. It sends off fibrous septa into the substance of the parotid and some of these are continuous with the fine fascial envelope surrounding the facial nerve. Superiorly, the external layer of parotid fascia is bound firmly to the zygomatic arch, while inferiorly, it blends with the deep cervical fascia anterior to the sternomastoid muscle. At the anterior and posterior borders of the gland there is a medial extension of the outer fascial covering which becomes progressively thinner the further inwards it passes, until it is no more than fine areolar tissue. The posteromedial deep extension blends with the styloid apparatus, and deep to that with the carotid sheath; however, from the

styloid process to the angle of the mandible, it condenses into a tough unyielding band called the stylomandibular ligament.

The inelastic nature of the outer layer of fascia accounts for the severe pain of which sufferers of parotitis complain, and also for the long period of time before parotid swellings become significantly obvious.

The partial absence of a definite fascial barrier on the deep aspect of the gland means that parotid suppuration may ultimately spread to the parapharyngeal space, with all the sinister connotations that such an eventuality holds for the patient. On the other hand, the presence of the tough stylomandibular ligament acts as a very definite barrier to medial extension of tumours located in the outer part of the gland, while tumours originating immediately lateral to, or in, the stylomandibular tunnel – that is between the ligament and mandible – may grow unimpeded towards the pharynx across the parapharyngeal space. If the tumours actually pass through this tunnel, they may assume a dumb-bell appearance.

A horizontal section of the gland shows that most of the gland is lodged in the retromandibular sulcus; the forward tongue of glandular tissue which overlies the masseter is but a small part of the overall volume.

The facial nerve traverses the retromandibular portion in a medial to lateral direction to subdivide the gland into a large superfacial component and a small subfacial or deep lobe, although it has been suggested that their weights are in fact roughly comparable.

The upper part of the outer aspect of the parotid gland is covered with skin and subcutaneous tissue, while the lower half of the gland is also covered with the platysma. The anteromedial surface of the gland is intimately related to the masseter, to the posterior edge of the ascending mandibular ramus, and to the back edge of the medial pterygoid muscle. Tumours arising from the deep aspect of the parotid gland and growing across the parapharyngeal space are inevitably covered on their anterior aspect with the stretched out fibres of the medial pterygoid, which are commonly mistaken for those of the superior constrictor.

The posteromedial aspect of the parotid is related to the sternomastoid, digastric, and styloid muscles, and to the bony process of the same name. At a point higher up, the relationship is with the mastoid process, cartilaginous meatus and deep meatus to which the enveloping fascia is loosely attached. There is invariably an extension of the gland back into the tympanomastoid sulcus which needs to be displaced forwards when a search is being made for the main trunk of the facial nerve.

Nerves

Nerves of sensation include the great auricular and auriculotemporal nerves.

The great auricular nerve runs upwards and slightly forwards on the deep cervical fascia covering the outer aspect of the sternomastoid to innervate the skin and fascia overlying the parotid gland. Just before it leaves the sternomastoid to enter the parotid compartment, it gives off a slender posterior branch which passes up into the postauricular region. Much is made of the need to preserve this branch during parotidectomy, as a means of trying to lessen the sensory loss, but it is by no means certain that such an objective is in fact achieved.

Loss of the great auricular nerve results in anaesthesia of the parotid area and the lower half of the pinna, which may turn into an unpleasant form of hyperaesthesia as the nerve regenerates. It is useful to preserve as much of the trunk as possible in case a graft is required, such as after parotid resection of the facial nerve.

The great auricular nerve is routinely transected during parotidectomy at the point where it leaves the sternomastoid to enter the parotid area, and it is here that an amputation neuroma may subsequently arise.

The auriculotemporal nerve which is mainly sensory to the upper pinna and side of the scalp, also carries postganglionic secretomotor fibres from the otic ganglion to the parotid. It comes into contact with the gland as it winds its way round the neck of the mandibular condyle, and then ascends anterior to the external auditory canal just behind the superficial temporal vessels. It is said to give off an anastomotic connection to the uppermost branches of the facial nerve. Its destruction does not invariably cure the syndrome of Frey, otherwise known as gustatory sweating.

This condition, which commonly occurs some months after parotidectomy, manifests itself during meals as sweating and erythema in the preauricular and subparotid areas. It is alleged to be a consequence of transected secretomotor fibres growing into the cut ends of cutaneous nerves and reinnervating sweat glands, thereby triggering off the sweating sequence when food is taken. This explanation, although currently very popular, does not accord with the fact that proximal division of the parasympathetic nerve supply fails to cure the syndrome in question.

The facial nerve exits from the stylomastoid foramen in the apex of the bony tympanomastoid sulcus some 3–4 mm deep to the rolled edge of the bony external canal. It passes forwards, downwards and outwards to bisect the sulcus, and lies in that situation immediately above the leading edge of the digastric muscle, posterolateral to the styloid process. It is enmeshed in this position by fibroareolar strands which have to be teased out at operation to reveal the trunk of the nerve. Immediately below and lateral to the facial nerve is the posterior auricular artery.

The extraparotid segment of the nerve is short, no more than 1 cm or less, but then it enters the posteromedial surface of the gland to travel in the same direction for a short distance before dividing into its two main divisions, each of which diverges sharply from the other.

The upper division proceeds upwards, forwards and very much outwards to give off temporal, upper zygomatic, lower zygomatic and buccal branches. It is stouter than the lower division and therefore better withstands handling, although the fact that its branches tend to be very sinuous in elderly or corpulent individuals means that they are more vulnerable to damage unless put on the stretch by suitable retraction.

The number of listed branches is subject to considerable variation, and no one pattern of branching prevails. However, good facial function may still be preserved even when one or two branches are eliminated because of the extensive network of fine interlacing peripheral anastomoses, although this is frequently absent between upper zygomatic and temporal fibres.

The lower zygomatic nerve has a constant relationship to the parotid duct which lies immediately below it; care must, therefore, be taken not to injure this nerve when operating to remove a calculus from the duct.

The lower division passes downwards and forwards at a deeper level to give origin to a variable number of buccal branches, a mandibular and a cervical branch. The last two emerge at the very apex of the gland, at which point the mandibular branch lies immediately anterior to the posterior facial or retromandibular vein. This constant relationship is employed when for any reason the main trunk of the facial nerve cannot be found. Once the mandibular branch is located at its point of emergence from the parotid, it can be traced cephalad to the point where it comes off into the lower division and further still to the main trunk of the nerve. In only 5% of cases does the mandibular branch have peripheral connections with the lowest buccal branch; hence damage to it is rarely compatible with spontaneous recovery of the depressor anguli oris which it supplies.

Care must always be exercised when working close to the facial nerve, but the slenderness of the lower division and its mandibular branch makes it especially vulnerable to surgical insults. It is noteworthy that the branches which are least likely to recover after injury or grafting are those to the frontalis and the depressor of the lower lip.

The sympathetic nerve supply reaches the

parotid gland from the superior cervical ganglion by way of the external carotid artery.

Blood supply

The external carotid artery enters the deep aspect of the gland just above the point where it is covered by the stylohyoid muscle. It passes vertically upwards in the deepest part of the gland, giving off the transverse facial, internal maxillary and, finally, the superficial temporal artery.

The venous drainage is mainly by means of the retromandibular or posterior facial vein which is formed by the merging of the superficial temporal and maxillary veins. This has the same direction as the artery but lies superficial to it and immediately deep to the facial nerve. It exits at the tail of the gland, at which point the mandibular branch of the facial nerve crosses immediately superficial to it before passing downwards and forwards into the submandibular triangle.

Lymphatic nodes

There are basically two groups of lymphatic tissue aggregates, namely a series of superficial nodes lying under the external parotid fascia, and about 15–20 lymph follicles embedded in the gland, superficial to the facial nerve. The deep lobe may contain one or at the very most two of these follicles.

The parotid duct

The parotid duct runs forwards from the forward prolongation of the gland along a line which is roughly equidistant from the upper and lower jaws. At the anterior border of the masseter, it curves inwards and then obliquely forwards through the buccinator to end adjacent to the second upper premolar tooth.

The submandibular gland

When viewed from the external aspect, the submandibular gland appears ovoid (*Figure 9.2*). However, its configuration in horizontal section is in fact that of an uneven U, with the limb representing the more superficial part of the gland, being considerably larger than the deep component. The gland fills the submandibular triangle and overlaps its lower boundaries, namely both bellies of the digastric muscle; but the upper edge is itself tucked away beneath the horizontal ramus of the mandible.

The superficial part of the gland is related inwardly to the mylohyoid muscle, while the junction between the deep and superficial lobes curls round the posterior free edge of that muscle. The deep part of the gland which lies sandwiched between the inner aspect of the mylohyoid and the hyoglossus muscle gives rise to the submandibular duct at its anterior extremity. The duct runs medially, forwards and upwards beneath the mucous membrane of the floor of the mouth to

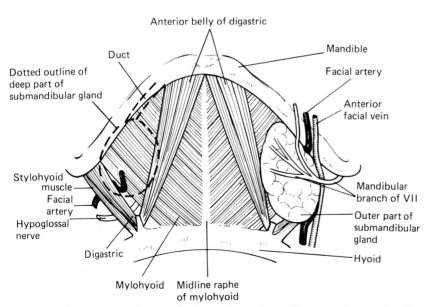

Figure 9.2 Relationships of the superficial part of the submandibular gland. Dotted outline corresponds with position of the deep part of the gland

end at the sublingual papilla close to the midline. It has on its anterolateral aspect the sublingual salivary gland, some ducts of which drain directly into it (*Figure 9.3*).

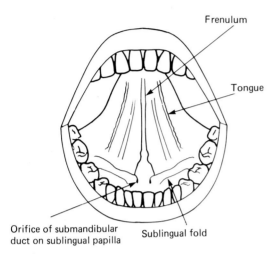

Figure 9.3 The sublingual fold corresponds with the position of the duct and the sublingual gland

The submandibular gland is covered with skin, superficial fascia, platysma, and deep cervical fascia, from which it receives a loose fine capsule. Surgical excision of the gland should always be carried out within the confines of this fine envelope in order to ensure that adjacent structures are not damaged.

Nerves

The mandibular branch of the seventh nerve, which innervates the depressor anguli oris, lies plastered to the outer aspect of the deep cervical fascia overlying the submandibular triangle; it divides into several subsidiary filaments which spread out over the whole of this compartment before heading towards the corner of the mouth. One of these filaments is often larger than the rest and would appear to provide the dominant or definitive innervation of the depressor muscle and should be safeguarded as much as possible. Incisions for the purpose of exposing and removing the submandibular gland should always, therefore, be sited over its lower border, just above the line of the hyoid bone. Elevation of the upper flap should be carried out in the plane between the gland and its surgical capsule to ensure that the mandibular branches of the facial nerve are not compromised.

The hypoglossal nerve is separated from the deep aspect of the deep lobe of the gland by a potential space and is only really vulnerable if pathological processes cause fusion of the gland and the hyoglossus on which the nerve lies.

The lingual nerve arches gently downwards just above the upper edge of the deep part of the gland to which it is attached by a ganglion. It subsequently passes forwards below the duct and curves round its outer aspect before reaching its final destination in the mucous membrane of the tongue. That part of the nerve which is closely related to the duct is very much at risk when resorting to intraoral operations for the removal of ductal calculi.

The lingual nerve carries taste and secretomotor fibres, the latter synapsing in the ganglion which lies above the deep part of the gland, and from which postganglionic fibres originate to innervate the gland. The nerve also carries tactile, thermal and pain fibres from the oral cavity, and its division therefore results in anaesthesia, agusia, paragusia and diminished salivary secretion. Sympathetic nerve fibres are carried to the submandibular gland along the facial and lingual arteries.

Blood supply

The principal arterial supply is from the facial artery which approaches the posterior edge of the gland just deep to the posterior belly of the digastric and stylohyoid muscle. This artery climbs vertically along the posterior border of the gland, or is buried within it, to reach the upper edge where it curves forwards before finally turning upwards over the lower border of the mandible.

The facial artery may be as large as the external carotid and should therefore be ligated with double ties.

Lymph nodes

A small number of nodes are present on the outer aspect of the submandibular gland, and a couple at its upper border in relation to the facial vessels. These pre- and postvascular nodes represent an important station in the lymphatic drainage of the oral cavity, and are apt to be overlooked in radical neck dissections for mouth cancer.

The sublingual gland

The sublingual gland is also ovoid in shape and roughly twice the size of an almond kernel. It lies above the mylohyoid between the inner aspect of the mandible and the genioglossus, lateral to the submandibular duct and the lingual nerve.

As many as 20 ducts may emerge from this gland, of which about half empty directly into the oral cavity and the remainder into the submandibular duct. Its nerve supply is essentially the same as for the submandibular gland, and it receives arterial blood from the sublingual branch of the facial artery.

Its lymphatics drain into the submental and submandibular lymph nodes.

The minor or accessory salivary glands

These glands, which number anything between 600 and 1000, are small, isolated and mainly numerous; each gland has its own miniscule duct. They are to be found anywhere in the mouth, but are especially concentrated in the mucous membrane of the floor of the mouth, palate and buccal areas.

Saliva

Saliva is made up of the secretion of all the aforementioned glands together with other constituents which might appropriately be regarded as contaminants. Most of the secretion comes from the parotid, submandibular and sublingual glands, but a small contribution originates in the so-called minor or accessory salivary glands.

Gingival, or as it is sometimes called crevicular fluid, forms a miniscule part of the total liquid volume of saliva, while a solid element is provided by cells of various types, notably desquamated epithelium, leucocytes, and bacteria of one kind or another.

The viscosity of saliva depends, in essence, on the interplay of the volume and rate of secretion, the relative contribution of each of the independent gland entities, and the amount of solid constituents. Recent investigations have suggested that former estimates of saliva production of 1.5 litres over 24 hours were almost certainly too high, and that a volume of between 500 and 700 ml is much more realistic. Almost half of this is produced constantly, as a so-called steady state, while the remainder appears in response to specific, although not always clearly defined, stimuli. The time of day and the nature and intensity of stimuli are important factors in determining the relative contributions of the individual glands to whole or mixed saliva.

A reasonably good assessment of the volume of resting saliva during waking hours can be arrived at by asking subjects to spit at regular intervals into a container, hence the figure of 20 ml/h. By cannulating the ducts of the major glands, the relative contribution of each can be ascertained. The submandibular gland would appear to be responsible for three-quarters of the total output, the parotid for one-fifth, and other sources for the rest.

During sleep, production of saliva by the parotid virtually ceases, whereas secretion by the submandibular gland continues as before, and the sublingual gland makes up most of the shortfall.

Under the effect of chemical stimuli, the parotid gland increases its contribution to match that of the submandibular gland, while under the influence of mechanical stimuli, the volume of parotid output may even outstrip that of the submandibular.

The contribution of the accessory glands amounts to between 6 and 7.5% of the total, depending on the absence or presence of stimulation.

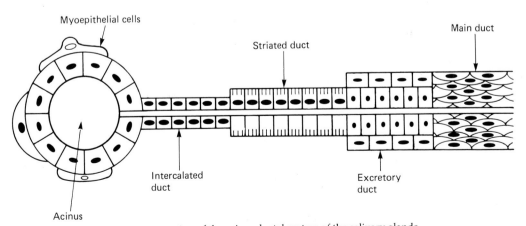

Figure 9.4 Diagrammatic representation of the acinar ductal system of the salivary glands

Microscopical anatomy of the salivary glands

A gland such as the parotid or submandibular is subdivided into lobes and lobules, comprising a multitude of basic secreting units, namely the acini and their immediate associated ducts (*Figure 9.4*).

Each acinus is composed of a circular grouping of cells surrounding a potential space which in turn leads into an intercalated duct. Beyond this is found a striated duct which joins with its counterparts from adjacent secreting units so that a succession of excretory ducts of increasing size and width are eventually formed. These ultimately merge to form the main duct of the gland.

The cells comprising the acini are backed by a basement membrane, outside of which other cells may be found; these latter cells are either secretory as in the case of the submandibular gland, or myoepithelial as those cells which surround the acini of the other major glands (*Figure 9.5*).

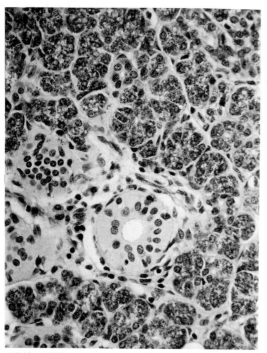

Figure 9.5 Photomicrograph of the parotid gland to show acinar secretory cells and myoepithelial cells (×400, reduced by one-quarter in reproduction)

The cells making up the acini are classified into two types depending on their staining characteristics with haematoxylin and eosin. Pink staining cells, which show a granular or vacuolated appearance, are found predominantly in the submandibular and sublingual glands, and are considered to be mucus secreting. Finely granulated cells, which stain blue, are seen mainly in the parotid but may also be seen abutting against the outer aspect of the pink-staining mucus-secreting acini of the submandibular gland.

The secretion of the parotid gland, while containing some mucoproteins and the starch-splitting enzyme amylase, is much less viscous than that produced by the other glands, hence its designation as a serous gland.

The intercalated ducts leading off the acini are short in length and lined with squat cuboidal cells with large nuclei; the striated ducts, on the other hand, are made up of taller cells exhibiting a typically striated appearance. Outside both types of duct are more of the stellate myoepithelial cells mentioned in connection with the secretory acini.

The excretory ducts are thicker than the striated ducts by virtue of an increase in the number of cell layers forming the lining epithelium, a trend culminating in the appearance of a stratified squamous epithelium in the distal part of the main duct.

Microneurohistology

Staining techniques, which permit the mapping out of nerve distributions within the salivary glands, reveal both sympathetic and parasympathetic plexus in relation to the striated and intercalated ducts, and the surface of the acini. The principal nerve trunks which activate these plexus travel along main ducts in company with blood vessels.

Electron microscopy shows both types of secretomotor fibres penetrating between individual secretory cells and also at the junction of the acini and intercalated ducts. As the fibres approach their final point of innervation, they are seen to have shed their sheaths to reveal bare axons in the immediate proximity of acinar and ductal cells.

The mechanism of secretion

Afferent stimulatory pathways

The salivary glands secrete a certain minimal volume of saliva – the so-called steady or resting state – but respond to a variety of stimuli by an outpouring of saliva. It is not clear whether or not the resting state is dependent on a background of subtle stimulation from tactile sensors within the oral cavity, but it is evident that a number of afferent pathways may be involved in the secretion of saliva.

Psychic stimuli

The thought and sight of food, or the sounds and smells associated with cooking, may be responsible for a real increase in the secretion of saliva, while, conversely, thoughts about unrelished foods may have the opposite effect. Certainly, the consequence of fear is a drying of the mouth and this cannot be exclusively a humoral effect. It is commonly believed that in some parts of the world the psychosalivatory reflex was used in courts of law to determine whether or not the accused was telling the truth.

Smell

It may be difficult to isolate purely olfactory stimuli from psychic stimuli as the one may influence the other, but experiments carried out under controlled conditions have established a relationship between olfaction and salivation. This is to be distinguished from the salivary reflex initiated by exposure of the nose to olfactory irritants.

Taste

Profuse salivation is induced by various taste stimuli, of which the most potent seems to be a mixture of acid and sugar, followed by acid, sweet and salt.

Tactile stimulation

Chewing and mastication are potent initiators of salivary production and excretion. There is some evidence to suggest that the greater the impact of touch or stretch, the greater will be the salivary response. Apart from the normal sensory endings in the oral and oropharyngeal mucosa, there are pressure sensors in the periodontal membranes of the teeth which respond to biting and chewing, and which initiate saliva production in a quantity which is related to the logarithm of the weight of the bolus. Proprioceptors in the muscles of mastication and in the temporomandibular joints also seem to activate the secretion of saliva and, together with the movements of swallowing, assist in synchronizing the ejection of saliva from the various duct orifices. By connecting a manometer to Stenson's duct, for instance, the pressure of salivary outflow is seen to rise simultaneously with swallowing, a phenomenon which is much less apparent with gustatory stimulation.

The tactile stimulating zone is very extensive for not only is the oral cavity a significant area in this respect, but the oro- and hypopharynx are both involved. Jets of saliva may be seen, for example, when the tongue is forcibly extracted or depressed, and when an oesophagoscope is passed. Equally painful conditions arising in the oral cavity, such as aphthous ulcers, toothache and quinsy, may also be responsible for salivation.

Interorgan stimuli

These stimuli are not altogether well-defined and are not thought to provide a significant stimulus to salivation. The oesophagosalivary reflex results from irritation of the distal oesophagus and has little to do with the nausea–vomiting reflex which causes much salivation. It is thought, however, that the stomach, and indeed other abdominal organs such as the liver, gallbladder and appendix, may influence salivary production using the vagus nerve as the afferent pathway.

Afferent neural pathways

The pathways thought to be at the heart of the stimulatory sequence of salivation belong in the first, fifth, seventh and ninth cranial nerves. These eventually connect through a series of synaptic links with the salivary nuclei which are responsible for the effector side of the cycle.

Central control of salivation

The cell bodies of preganglionic secretomotor neurons are the points at which incoming stimuli initiate the efferent responses to the salivary glands (*Figure 9.6*).

The parasympathetic salivary nuclei are located in the pons close to the nucleus of the facial nerve, and also in the medulla near the nucleus of the glossopharyngeal nerve. They are referred to as the superior and inferior salivary nuclei respectively, and are part of the reticular formation. The former is responsible for stimulating the submandibular and sublingual glands, and the latter for stimulating the parotid. In addition to receiving impulses from the various cranial nerves subserving the afferent side of the pathway, these nuclei are subject to influences from other parts of the brain. In this way, as mentioned before, psychic influences may either increase or decrease salivation, which will also diminish during sleep.

Certain pathological processes are known to increase salivation – for instance, rabies, encephalitis, lethargica, tabes, epilepsy, and parkinsonism – whereas rarely the reverse may occur (Rauch and McCleve, 1961).

Stimulation of the hypothalamus causes hypersialia, and may explain why excessive salivation is so often associated with nausea and vomiting.

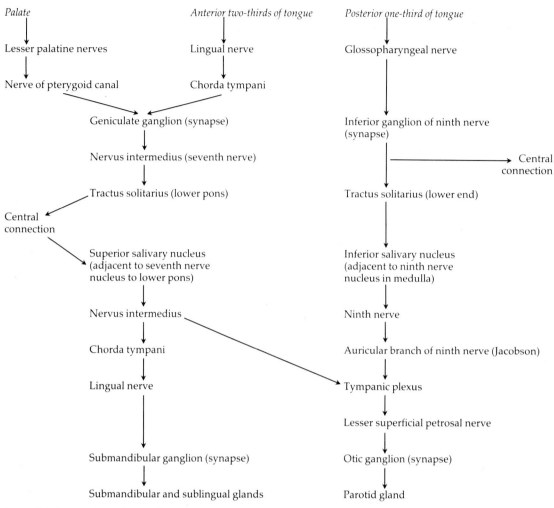

Figure 9.6 Taste and secretory pathways

The cell bodies of the sympathetic system lie in the lateral columns of the spinal cord, mainly at the level of the second thoracic nerve, and are under the control of fibres passing from the hypothalamus and medulla.

The efferent pathway

The neural control of the salivary glands is effected mainly through the parasympathetic system with preganglionic fibres being carried by the seventh and ninth cranial nerves. The facial fibres leave the seventh nerve by way of the chorda tympani and synapse in the ganglion which lies close to the submandibular and sublingual glands; their post-ganglionic fibres run a short course before reaching the salivary gland.

The glossopharyngeal fibres travel by way of the tympanic and lesser superficial petrosal nerves to synapse in the otic ganglion. The postganglionic fibres leaving the otic ganglion join the auriculotemporal nerve from which they eventually separate to innervate the parotid. The neurotransmitter released in the ganglia and at the nerve endings in the glands is acetylcholine, and it can therefore be blocked by atropine.

Sympathetic nerves also exert some control over the salivary glands. The nerve fibres in the cervical sympathetic pathway synapse in the superior cervical ganglion, whence postganglionic fibres travel in company with the nearest blood vessels to reach the salivary glands. The neurotransmitter in the superior cervical ganglion is acetylcholine, but at the glandular nerve endings it is noradrenaline.

Nerve stimulation is responsible, in general terms, for secretory activity, the rate of blood flow and the contraction of myoepithelial cells.

So far as secretion is concerned, the parasympathetic pathway would appear to play the major part although the sympathetic may also be involved. When both are employed simultaneously, the effect on secretion appears to be synergistic. It is assumed, however, that changes in the composition of saliva may be influenced by the degree of activity of each of the two neural systems at any one time.

In experimental animals, stimulation of the cervical sympathetic fibres elicits a flow of saliva from the submandibular gland exclusively, but injection of adrenaline into the ducts of all the glands produces the same effect.

The fact that large doses of atropine injected into man fail to abolish submandibular secretion supports the view that the sympathetic pathway has a secretomotor role, at least in the case of this gland.

Electron microscopical observations in man reveal the presence of parasympathetic and sympathetic fibres in proximity to the acini of both the submandibular and parotid glands, a finding which is difficult to reconcile with the view that the sympathetic has a secretory role only in the submandibular gland.

In the case of the blood supply, the parasympathetic fibres are vasodilatory whereas the sympathetic fibres have the opposite effect . Once secretion has started, bradykinin is released and causes further vasodilatation by overriding the neural mechanism.

It is not altogether clear which of the two systems is responsible for contraction of the myoepithelial cells, although there is evidence that taste stimuli may trigger off their contraction by way of the sympathetic pathway (Babkin, 1943).

Disturbances of the efferent pathways

The consequences of interrupting the parasympathetic pathways do not always accord with the predicted outcome, a situation which would seem to indicate that accepted accounts of the pathways in question may be incomplete or incorrect.

In certain instances, for example, preganglionic section of the ninth cranial nerve not only restricts parotid secretion but also causes submandibular and sublingual asialia (Dandy, 1927). One possible explanation for this invokes the existence of an anastomotic connection between Jacobson's nerve and the geniculate ganglion.

Interruption of the parasympathetic fibres at a peripheral level, such as occurs during parotidectomy, supposedly causes gustatory sweating or Frey's syndrome in consequence of the misrouting of regenerating secretomotor fibres into the cutaneous nerves which activate the sweat glands.

There are, however, reasons to doubt such a supposition. In the first place, if parasympathetic fibres transected at operation were capable of regeneration, the same would surely have to be true of the sympathetic, whose fibres are, if anything, capable of reaching the sweat glands first.

It would also appear that a condition not unlike Frey's syndrome may occur after a cervical sympathectomy and that anaesthesia or resection of the stellate ganglion will abolish it (Ashby, 1960). The fact that the division of Jacobson's nerve or of the auriculotemporal nerve fails to cure the syndrome is perhaps the strongest argument in favour of rejecting the current popular explanation for gustatory sweating.

On the other hand, it seems much more likely that the regeneration of active sympathetic fibres may be responsible for the poorly controlled or vicarious sweating which characterizes the condition.

Formation of saliva

Saliva is the end product of a process of secretion which commences in the acinus and is then modified by the activity of the intercalated and striated ducts.

The hydrostatic pressure in the capillaries surrounding the acini leads to the escape of a number of moieties from the blood stream to the adjacent interstices. These are principally water, ions, glucose, urea, amino acids and proteins of lower molecular weight.

Migration of interstitial fluid across the basement membrane of the acinar epithelium occurs by a process of diffusion resulting from the pressure gradient which exists between the capillaries and the acinar lumen. A rise in the capillary hydrostatic pressure in response to vasodilatation inevitably increases the pressure gradient and, therefore, secretion.

The acinar epithelium is freely permeable to water- and lipid-soluble substances, but less so to other products such as amino acids and glucose which can gain entry only by active diffusion.

The concentration of sodium and chloride ions within the acini is similar to that of interstitial fluid, and is important to the osmotic movement of water through these cells.

Stimulation of the secretomotor nerves causes the release of transmitter substances at the neuroepithelial termini, namely acetylcholine for the parasympathetic fibres, and noradrenaline for the sympathetic. Circulating adrenaline within local blood vessels also affects the blood supply and the functioning of the salivary glands.

The neurotransmitters act on receptors located in the surface membrane of the acini and neighbouring ductal cells, and at the same time influence the degree of contractibility of the local blood vessels. Neutralization of neurochemical mediators is brought about by specific enzymes such as acetylcholinesterase and monoamine oxidases.

The exact sequence of events which takes place within the acinus and its effluent duct in response to stimulation is the subject of controversy, but in the case of the submandibular gland it seems likely that stimulation of either the sympathetic or parasympathetic pathway increases the potential across the basal cell membrane and enhances its permeability. The immediate consequence of this is a migration of potassium ions in conjunction with interstitial fluid through the acini to their respective lumina, with a resultant increase in the level of intracellular potassium.

In the case of the parotid, however, it is possibly only the parasympathetic pathway which is capable of eliciting this sequence of events.

Salivary proteins, which are an important constituent of saliva, are synthesized by ribosomes before being assimilated into the endoplasmic reticulum from which 'granules' or 'vacuoles' are formed during the resting phase of metabolism.

A high level of intracellular calcium would appear to be necessary for the mobilization of these granules or vacuoles and their extrusion into the acinar lumen. This is brought about by a rise in the cell concentration of calcium, in response to the increased basement membrane permeability induced by acetylcholine. Calcium ions attach themselves to the secretory granules and help them to fuse with the apical or luminal membrane before their extrusion into the acinar lumen.

It is likely that the intercalated ducts modify the acinar fluid by adding further potassium ions, but major alterations occur principally in the striated ducts and result in the conversion of acinar fluid from a slightly hypertonic to a low sodium chloride hypotonic solution. Sodium ions are actively transported back from the lumen into the cells, accompanied in the process by a passive diffusion of chloride ions, while potassium ions and bicarbonate permeate in the reverse direction.

Water, on the other hand, is not reabsorbed and helps to preserve the hypotonicity of the intraluminal fluid.

Stimulation of either the sympathetic or parasympathetic pathway influences the activity of the striated ducts, in the former case by producing a small volume of saliva rich in potassium and poor in sodium.

Finally, as a result of the passage of water and potassium back into the extracellular compartment, the concentration of ions in the saliva in the excretory ducts once again begins to approach that of plasma.

Composition of saliva

Ninety-nine per cent of saliva is in the form of water, the solute being a mixture of inorganic ions and organic molecules (*Table 9.1*).

Table 9.1 Principal contents of saliva

Water

Inorganic constituents	Organic constituents
Sodium	Mucoproteins
Potassium	Serum proteins
Chloride	Enzymes
Calcium	amylase
Phosphate	lysozyme
Bicarbonate	Glycoproteins
Thiocyanate	fucose
Iodine	neuraminic acid
Bromide	mannose
Fluoride	galactose
Copper	Free sugars
Magnesium	glucose
	Blood group substances
	Lipids
	Amino acids
	Urea

Sodium appears in the acinar fluid at about the same concentration as interstitial fluid, that is to say 140–150 mm/l, but subsequently passes back through the striated ducts to leave a saliva low in sodium. However, as flow rates increase, so the concentration of sodium in saliva begins to approach that of plasma.

The concentration of extracellular potassium is low at 4–5 mm/l, whereas that in the acini and duct systems (excluding the terminal duct) is considerably higher, and varies between 20 and 80 mm/l depending on the flow rate. Stimulation brings about a sudden sharp increase in intracellular potassium with a concomitant discharge into the salivary secretion.

The reabsorption of sodium which takes place in the striated ducts is accompanied by a passive diffusion of chloride in the same direction. As the rate of secretion increases, so bicarbonate is actively expelled into the saliva, and there is a simultaneous increase in the rate of reabsorption of chloride ions to adjust the requisite ionic balance. As the flow rate increases still further, the time available for reabsorption diminishes and the concentration of chloride in saliva begins to rise again.

The pH of saliva is low when the glands are not actively secreting, but rises with faster flow rates in consequence of the outpouring of bicarbonate.

The calcium content of saliva is lowest in the parotid and highest in the accessory glands. In the resting secretion of the submandibular gland, the calcium content exceeds that of plasma; however, as the flow rate increases, it begins initially to fall, only to return gradually to a level approaching the concentration in resting saliva (3.7 mm/l). However, the amount of calcium present in mixed saliva diminishes when the flow rate increases, probably because of the dilution induced by an outpouring of low-calcium parotid secretion.

Between one-tenth and one-third of the calcium content of saliva is bound to proteins in the form of complexes, of which amylase comprises a significant proportion.

Salivary secretion involves the active transport of iodide from the plasma, so that its concentration in the glands is always higher than that of the blood stream, and the same effect is observed with the isotope technetium-99 and fluoride.

Similarly, thiocyanate is found in saliva in a higher concentration than in plasma, and this is much more apparent in smokers. The association of thiocyanate with one of the salivary proteins results in a complex which possesses some degree of bacteriostatic activity.

Salivary proteins are a mixture of glycoproteins, mucoproteins, enzymes, blood group substances and serum proteins, the sum total of which rises together with the increase in flow rates.

The gamma-globulins in saliva have received much attention in recent years because of the possibility that they may protect the host against caries and oral inflammatory disease, but this line of investigation has proved disappointing so far.

In the case of the proteins synthesized within the parotid gland, about one-third appear in the form of amylase, the enzyme by means of which starch is broken down into maltose. The proportion in submandibular or sublingual saliva is, in fact, much less and is virtually non-existent in accessory gland secretion. The concentration of amylase, particularly that of the parotid gland, increases as the flow rate goes up, but its activity in general is shortlived, and has virtually ceased by the time the food bolus has reached the stomach.

Lysozyme is an enzyme which is effective against the carbohydrate components of the cell wall of certain bacteria. It constitutes about 10% of the protein content of parotid saliva, and is found mostly in the submandibular gland.

A variety of other enzymes – including acid phosphatase, cholinesterase, ribonuclease, lipase, peroxidase and many others – is also present in saliva. Kallikrein, from which bradykinin is derived, is also an enzymatic product of the salivary glands and helps to maintain an increased blood supply following the vasodilatation induced by nerve stimulation.

Much of the protein content of saliva appears in the form of mucoproteins. For instance, 35% of parotid protein contains an appreciable quantity of associated carbohydrate, while in the case of the submandibular gland the figure is even higher. Such mucoproteins may be protective against certain viruses, but in the case of the rabies virus the role is reversed and they appear to aid its survival. They are suspected of being intimately involved in the formation of salivary calculi, by providing a matrix for the precipitation of minerals, the final product of which appears as a succession of concentric layers of salts.

Carbohydrate–protein substances corresponding to the blood group antigens are secreted by all the glands, with the exception of the parotid. Their concentration is highest in the accessory glands, followed by the sublingual and then the submandibular.

Persons harbouring blood group B seem to be the most prone to developing salivary tumours; 85% of all adenocarcinomata occur in men belonging to this blood group, and pleomorphic adenomata and papillary cystadenomata are to be found especially in people of this blood group.

A substance of protein origin, which has been given the name parotin, has been isolated from parotid saliva and is alleged to possess hormonal activity. However, its role, which appears to be directed mainly towards the maintenance of blood calcium, requires further clarification.

A number of blood-borne products – including cortisone, pilocarpine, physostigmine and even sodium and potassium chloride – may influence the function of the salivary glands.

The effect of disordered volume and composition is best illustrated by the condition of recurrent parotitis in which patients experience intermittent bouts of parotid enlargement, sometimes associated with pain.

Diminution of the secretory rate of the parotid is evident not only in the affected gland but also on the uninvolved contralateral side. In addition, the viscosity of parotid secretion will be increased, as a result of a higher concentration of proteins of all types together with the overt appearance of mucus. The net result is a significant tendency towards stasis, a state of affairs which predisposes to bacterial infection and the establishment of a progressively destructive vicious circle which can be monitored by sialography.

Hormonal influences

The reabsorption of sodium in the striated duct, in conjunction with the movement of potassium in the reverse direction, is said to be under the influence of aldosterone, whereas the reabsorption of water is affected by the antidiuretic hormone.

Salivation increases with pregnancy, testosterone and thyroxine, and decreases at the time of the menopause.

Other influences

Starvation leads to massive enlargement of the salivary glands, as seen in Greece towards the end of the Second World War. Hypoproteinaemia from other causes may also predispose to a similar hypertrophy, one example being that of the farmers in the Nile valley who are subject to chronic infestation by bilharzia or ankylostoma.

People on high protein–low carbohydrate diets are found to produce a saliva which has increased buffering power but which is deficient in amylase.

Functions of saliva

Saliva, by virtue of its glycoprotein and mucoprotein content, acts as a lubricant for ingested food. It thus serves to protect the mucous membrane from trauma caused by the food bolus while, at the same time, assisting the latter's passage into the oro- and hypopharynx.

In the absence of food in the mouth, saliva keeps the oral mucosa constantly moistened, which thereby precludes the ill-effects, namely inflammation, ulceration, hyperkeratinization, and general discomfort, resulting from dryness.

Saliva has a bacteriostatic function by virtue of the presence of lysozyme, and possibly also gamma-globulins which act against some oral bacteria. A globulin which reacts with thiocyanate is considered to be part of this protective system.

The buffering effect of saliva counters the dissolution of dental enamel by acid, and provides a source of calcium ions for recalcification.

The digestive function of saliva is limited, as amylase works best at a pH of 6.8, and after the food bolus has been swallowed, the acid environment of the stomach renders the saliva ineffective.

The role of the salivary glands in the maintenance of water balance is restricted in adults, but is possibly of greater importance in infants in whom vomiting or diarrhoea may lead to life-threatening dehydration. Antidiuretic hormone, which influences the permeability of the striated ducts to the reabsorption of water, may thus help to restrict the loss of water in saliva by producing a less hypotonic saliva.

Saliva serves as a solvent for food substances, and by virtue of its viscosity acts as an effective spreading agent, so that food is exposed to a maximum of taste buds.

Saliva also acts incidentally as an excretory organ for urea and other substances such as iodine, fluoride, thiocyanate, and bacteria. The characteristic fetor of uraemics is thus produced by the excretion of urea in saliva.

Tubercle bacilli are excreted in saliva and almost certainly account for the rare instances of cold abscess which occur in the parotid gland of both the very young and the very old.

The possible role of saliva in the aetiology of dental disease has been the subject of many investigations. However, no effect, other than that of a possible synergism with plaque formation, has yet been demonstrated.

References

ASHBY, W. B. (1960) Gustatory sweating and pilomotor changes. *British Journal of Surgery*, **47**, 406–410

BABKIN, B. P. (1943) Mechanism of secretory activity of digestive glands. *Revue Canadienne de Biologie*, **2**, 416–434

DANDY, W. E. (1927) Glossopharyngeal neuralgia (tic douloureux); its diagnosis and treatment. *Archives of Surgery*, **15**, 198–214

RAUCH, S. and McCLEVE, D. (1961) Physiopathology of neural and humoral regulation of the salivary glands. *International Dental Journal*, **11**, 376–395

10

Anatomy of the pharynx and oesophagus

P. Beasley

Embryological development

During the development of the embryo, a process of cephalocaudal and lateral folding takes place with the result that part of the endoderm-lined cavity of the secondary or definitive yolk sac is incorporated into the embryo to form the primitive gut. In the cephalic part of the embryo, the primitive gut forms a blind ending tube, the foregut, separated from the ectodermally lined stomatodaeum by the buccopharyngeal membrane (*Figure 10.1*). Towards the end of the first month (23–25 days, 10–14 somite stage), the foregut comes to lie dorsal to the developing heart tube and to the developing septum transversum (developing diaphragm). Shortly afterwards (26–27 days, 20 somite stage), the buccopharyngeal membrane ruptures and the stomatodaeum becomes continuous with the foregut. The approximate relationship between the age of the embryo and the number of somites is given in *Table 10.1*.

Table 10.1 Approximate relationship between age of embryo and number of somites

Approximate age (days)	No. of somites	Approximate age (days)	No. of somites
20	1–4	25	17–20
21	4–7	26	20–23
22	7–10	27	23–26
23	10–13	28	26–29
24	13–17	30	34–35

The endodermal lining of the foregut differentiates into a number of different structures which can be summarized as follows:

(1) part of the nasal cavities
(2) the endodermally lined part of the buccal cavity
(3) the pharynx, together with the glands and other structures derived from it, namely the anterior lobe of the pituitary gland, the thyroid, thymus and parathyroid glands, the ultimobranchial body, the pharyngotympanic (eustachian) tube, the middle ear and the tonsils

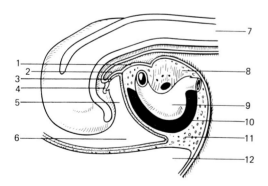

Figure 10.1 A diagram of a sagittal midline section of a 23–25 day (14 somite) embryo to show the position of the foregut and stomatodaeum, separated by the buccopharyngeal membrane

1. Tracheobronchial diverticulum
2. Foregut
3. Buccopharyngeal membrane
4. Rathke's pouch
5. Stomatodaeum
6. Amniotic cavity
7. Neural tube
8. Mesocardium
9. Heart tube
10. Pericardial cavity
11. Septum transversum
12. Yolk sac

(4) the submandibular and sublingual salivary glands
(5) the larynx, trachea, bronchi and lungs
(6) the oesophagus
(7) the stomach
(8) the duodenum as far as the liver diverticulum.

The development of the cephalic portion of the primitive gut and its derivatives will be discussed in two sections: (1) the pharyngeal gut or pharynx extending from the buccopharyngeal membrane to the tracheobronchial diverticulum; (2) the foregut, lying caudal to the tracheobronchial diverticulum from which the oesophagus develops.

Pharynx (pharyngeal gut)

The development of the branchial or pharyngeal arches in the fifth week provides one of the most characteristic external features of the head and neck region of the embryo. They consist initially of bars of mesenchymal tissue separated by deep clefts known as branchial or pharyngeal clefts. At the same time as the arches and clefts develop on the outside, a number of out-pocketings (the pharyngeal pouches) appear within the pharyngeal gut along the lateral wall. The pouches and clefts gradually penetrate the surrounding mesenchyme but, in spite of there being only a small amount of mesenchyme between the ectodermal and endodermal layers, open communication is not established. Therefore, although these developments resemble the formation of gill slits in fishes, in the human embryo real gills, or branchia, are not formed and the term 'pharyngeal arches' rather than branchial arches has been used in this description (Langman, 1981). The pharyngeal arches contribute not only to the formation of the neck and pharynx, but to the development of the head (*see* Chapters 5 and 8). By the end of the fourth week, the stomatodaeum is surrounded by the first pair of pharyngeal arches in the form of the mandibular swellings caudally, and the maxillary swellings laterally, which are the dorsal portion of the first arch. The development of the pharyngeal arches, pouches and clefts, with their derivatives, are discussed separately.

Pharyngeal arches

Each pharyngeal arch is made up of a core of mesodermal tissue covered on the outside by surface ectoderm and on the inside by epithelium derived from endoderm. The core of the arch has, in addition to local mesenchyme, substantial numbers of crest cells which migrate into the arches to contribute to the skeletal components of the face. The original mesoderm of each arch

differentiates into a cartilaginous bar and muscular component together with an arterial component. Each arch receives afferent and efferent nerves to supply the skin, musculature and endodermal lining. The muscular components of each arch have their own nerve and, wherever the muscular cells migrate, they carry their own cranial nerve component (*Figure 10.2*). In addition, each arch

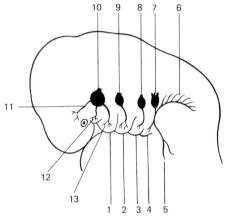

Figure 10.2 A diagram to show the cranial nerve supply to the pharyngeal arches. (Modified from Langman, J., 1981, *Medical Embryology*, 4th edn, Williams and Wilkins by courtesy of the publisher)

1. First arch (mandibular)
2. Second arch (hyoid)
3. Third arch
4. Fourth arch
5. Vagus nerve
6. Spinal root of accessory
7. Cranial root of accessory nerve
8. Glossopharyngeal nerve
9. Facial nerve
10. Trigeminal nerve and ganglion
11. Ophthalmic branch of V
12. Maxillary branch of V
13. Mandibular branch of V

receives a branch from the nerve of the succeeding arch. The arrangement of the nerve supply to each arch is a relic of the pattern found in vertebrates at a time when the nerve to the gill region was distributed cranial and caudal to the corresponding gill cleft. As a result, in man and in mammals generally, each arch receives a branch, called the post-trematic, from the nerve of its own arch; and a second branch, called the pre-trematic, from the succeeding arch. This is illustrated in *Table 10.2*.

At the end of the first month (30–32 days, 34–35 somites), the floor of the foregut shows a number of elevations produced by the mesodermal condensations and separated by depressions (*Figure 10.3*). The first arch of each side forms an elevation in the side wall of the foregut and the elevations meet in the midline. A small medial elevation, the

Table 10.2 Arch and nerve arrangement

Arch	Post-trematic nerve	Pre-trematic nerve
1st	Mandibular nerve (V)	Chorda tympani branch of VII
2nd	Facial nerve (VII)	Tympanic branch of IX (Jacobson's nerve)
3rd	Glossopharyngeal (IX)	
4th 5th 6th	Vagus (X) and accessory (XI) nerves via superior and recurrent laryngeal and pharyngeal branches	Pre-trematic nerves not well defined in man

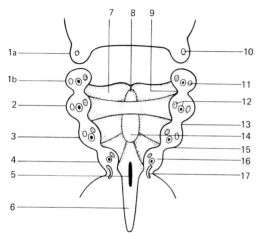

Figure 10.3 A diagram to show the arches and elevations on the floor of the foregut

1a. First arch, maxillary process
1b. First arch, mandibular process
2. Second pharyngeal arch
3. Third pharyngeal arch
4. Fourth pharyngeal arch
5. Tracheobronchial diverticulum
6. Oesophagus
7. Endodermal lining
8. Tuberculum impar
9. First pharyngeal pouch
10. Maxillary nerve
11. Mandibular nerve
12. Cartilage and artery
13. Second pharyngeal cleft
14. Hypobranchial eminence
15. Ectodermal covering
16. Mesenchyme in fourth arch
17. Superior laryngeal nerve

tuberculum impar, is seen immediately behind the middle part of the mandibular swelling. Behind the tuberculum impar is a small median depression, the foramen caecum, which marks the site of the invagination which will give rise to the median primordium of the thyroid gland. The second arch

of each side is continuous across the midline of the foregut floor. Immediately caudal to the second arch, a second and larger medial swelling develops, the hypobranchial eminence. The third and fourth arches fail to reach the midline owing to the presence of this eminence. The fifth arch makes a transitory appearance only. Caudal to the hypobranchial eminence, a tracheobronchial groove develops in the midline, the lateral boundary of which is the rudimentary sixth arch. From this groove, there develops the lining epithelia and associated glands of the larynx, trachea, bronchi and, possibly, the respiratory epithelium of the alveoli. The development of the tongue is described in Chapter 8. In the course of this development, there is a caudal migration of the hypobranchial eminence and a relative reduction in its size. At the same time, it comes to be more transversely placed behind the developing tongue, but still remains attached to the side wall of the pharynx by part of the third arch tissue, which becomes the lateral glosso-epiglottic fold of the adult. The groove between the dorsum of the tongue and the epiglottis, the glosso-epiglottic groove, is divided into the two valleculae by the appearance of a median glosso-epiglottic fold. The poorly developed swellings which lie each side of the tracheobronchial diverticulum become the arytenoid swellings.

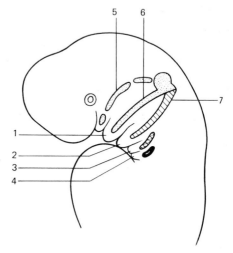

Figure 10.4 A diagram to illustrate the cartilages of the pharyngeal arches. Derivatives are indicated in *Figure 10.5*. (Modified from Langman, J., 1981, *Medical Embryology*, 4th edn, Williams and Wilkins, by courtesy of the publisher)

1. First arch
2. Second arch
3. Third arch
4. Fourth arch
5. Maxillary process
6. Meckel's cartilage
7. Reichert's cartilage

First pharyngeal arch

The cartilage of the first pharyngeal arch consists of a dorsal portion known as the maxillary process, and a ventral portion, the mandibular process or Meckel's cartilage (*Figure 10.4*). As development proceeds, both the maxillary process and Meckel's cartilage disappear except for small portions at their dorsal ends which form the incus and malleus respectively, together with the sphenomandibular ligament (*Figure 10.5*). Membranous ossification subsequently takes place in the mesenchyme of the maxillary process to give rise to the premaxilla, maxilla, zygomatic bone and part of the temporal bone. The mandible is formed in a similar way by membranous ossification in the mesenchymal tissue surrounding Meckel's cartilage.

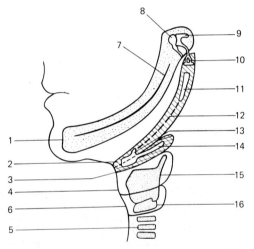

Figure 10.5 A diagram to show the derivatives of the pharyngeal arch cartilages. (Modified from Langman, J., 1981, *Medical Embryology*, 4th edn, Williams and Wilkins, by courtesy of the publisher)

1. First arch cartilage
2. Second arch cartilage
3. Third arch cartilage
4. Fourth arch cartilage
5. Tracheal rings
6. Sixth arch cartilage
7. Meckel's cartilage
8. Malleus
9. Incus
10. Stapes
11. Styloid process
12. Stylohyoid ligament
13. Lesser horn and upper body of hyoid bone
14. Greater horn and lower body of hyoid bone
15. Thyroid cartilage
16. Cricoid cartilage

The musculature of the first pharyngeal arch develops to form the muscles of mastication (temporalis, masseter, medial and lateral pterygoids), as well as the anterior belly of the digastric, the mylohyoid, the tensor tympani and tensor palati. Although the muscles are not always attached to the bony or cartilaginous components of their own arch, because of migration into surrounding regions, the arch of origin can always be traced by way of the nerve supply which comes from the original arch. In the case of the first arch, this nerve supply is provided by the mandibular branch of the trigeminal nerve (*see Figure 10.2*). The same nerve provides an afferent or sensory supply to the skin and endodermal lining of this arch.

Second pharyngeal arch

The cartilage of the second or hyoid arch (Reichert's cartilage) (*see Figure 10.4*) gives rise to the stapes, the styloid process of the temporal bone, the stylohyoid ligament and, ventrally, the lesser horn and the upper part of the body of the hyoid bone (*see Figure 10.5*). The muscles of this arch are the stapedius, the stylohyoid, the posterior belly of the digastric, the auricular muscles and the muscles of facial expression. They are supplied by the facial nerve which is the nerve of this arch.

Third pharyngeal arch

The cartilage of the third arch gives rise to the lower part of the body and the greater horn of the hyoid bone (*see Figures 10.4 and 10.5*). The caudal part of the arch cartilage disappears. The muscle of the arch is the stylopharyngeus supplied by the glossopharyngeal nerve, the nerve of the third arch.

Fourth and sixth pharyngeal arches

The remaining anterior parts of the cartilages of the fourth and sixth arches fuse to form the thyroid, cricoid, arytenoid, corniculate and cuneiform cartilages of the larynx (*see Figure 10.5*). The fifth arch only makes a transitory appearance as indicated previously. The muscles of the fourth arch are the cricothyroid, the levator palati and the constrictors of the pharynx. They are innervated by the vagus nerve, the nerve of the fourth arch, through its superior laryngeal branch and its contribution to the pharyngeal plexus. The recurrent laryngeal branch of the vagus, the nerve of the sixth arch, innervates the intrinsic muscles of the larynx.

Pharyngeal pouches

In the human embryo, there are five pairs of pharyngeal pouches, although the last one of these is often considered as part of the fourth. Each pouch has a ventral and dorsal section. The epithelial endodermal lining of the pouches gives rise to a number of derivatives that have functions very different from those of primitive gill slits.

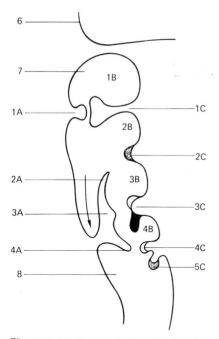
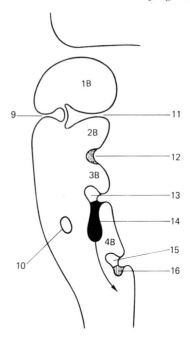

Figure 10.6 A diagram to show the development and derivatives of the pharyngeal pouches and clefts. Note the way in which the second, third and fourth clefts are buried and, if not obliterated, form the cervical sinus. (Modified from Langman, J., 1981, *Medical Embryology*, 4th edn, Williams and Wilkins, by courtesy of the publisher)

1A. First cleft	3C. Third pouch	9. External auditory meatus
1B. First arch	4A. Fourth cleft	10. Superior parathyroid gland
1C. First pouch	4B. Fourth arch	11. Pharyngotympanic tube
2A. Second cleft	4C. Fourth pouch	12. Palatine tonsil
2B. Second arch	5C. Fifth pouch	13. Inferior parathyroid gland
2C. Second pouch	6. Maxillary process	14. Thymus
3A. Third cleft	7. Mandibular process	15. Superior parathyroid gland
3B. Third arch	8. Epicardial ridge	16. Ultimobranchial body

First pharyngeal pouch

The dorsal part of the first pouch, with the adjacent pharyngeal wall and part of the dorsal portion of the second pouch, produces a diverticulum, the tubotympanic recess, which comes into contact with the ectodermal epithelial lining of the first pharyngeal cleft, the future external auditory meatus (*Figure 10.6*). The distal portion of the tubotympanic recess widens to form the primitive tympanic or middle ear cavity, whereas the proximal, stalk-like part, forms the pharyngotympanic (eustachian) tube. The ventral part of the first pouch is obliterated by the development of the tongue.

Second pharyngeal pouch

As indicated previously, only a portion of the dorsal part of the second pouch takes part in the development of the pharyngotympanic tube. The remainder of this portion is absorbed into the dorsal pharyngeal wall. The ventral portion of the second pouch is almost completely obliterated by the proliferation of its endodermal epithelial lining which forms buds that penetrate into the surrounding mesenchyme. These buds are secondarily invaded by mesodermal tissue forming the primordium of the palatine tonsil (*Figure 10.6*). Part of the pouch persists as the intratonsillar cleft or fossa. During the third to fifth months, the tonsil is gradually invaded by lymphocytes which have either arisen *in situ* or have been derived from the blood stream. A similar invasion of the endoderm of the dorsal pharyngeal wall by lymphatic tissue forms the nasopharyngeal tonsil (adenoid). The lingual tonsil is formed by aggregations of lymphatic tissue in the dorsum of the tongue (second and third arch) and the tubal tonsil by aggregations of mesenchymal cells that are later invaded by lymphocytes.

Third pharyngeal pouch

In the fifth week, the endodermal epithelium of the dorsal section of the third pouch differentiates into parathyroid tissue which will form the inferior parathyroid gland. The ventral section of the pouch gives rise to the thymus gland (*see Figure 10.6*). The primordia of both these glands lose their connection with the pharyngeal wall when the thymus migrates in a caudal and medial direction, taking the parathyroid with it (*Figure 10.7*). The main portion of the thymus gland fuses

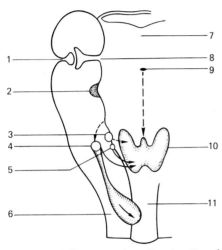

Figure 10.7 A diagram to show the migration of the thymus, parathyroid glands, and ultimobranchial body. The thyroid gland originates at the foramen caecum and descends to the level of the first tracheal ring. (Modified from Langman J., 1981, *Medical Embryology*, 4th edn, Williams and Wilkins, by courtesy of the publisher)

1. External auditory meatus	6. Thymus
2. Palatine tonsil	7. Ventral side of pharynx
3. Superior parathyroid gland from 4th pouch	8. Pharyngotympanic tube
4. Inferior parathyroid gland from 3rd pouch	9. Foramen caecum
5. Ultimobranchial body	10. Thyroid gland
	11. Foregut

with its counterpart from the opposite side when it takes up its final position in the thorax. The tail portion becomes thin and eventually disappears, although sometimes parts of it persist either within the thyroid gland or as isolated thymic cysts.

The parathyroid tissue of this pouch takes up its final position on the posterior surface of the thyroid gland as the inferior parathyroid gland.

Fourth pharyngeal pouch

The endodermal epithelium of the dorsal section of this pouch gives rise to the superior parathyroid gland. When this gland loses its contact with the

wall of the pharynx, it attaches itself, while migrating caudally, to the thyroid gland, and reaches its final position on the posterior surface of the thyroid as the superior parathyroid gland (*Figure 10.7*). The fate of the ventral section of this pouch is uncertain, although it is believed to give rise to a small amount of thymus tissue which disappears soon after its formation.

Fifth pharyngeal pouch

This is the last pharyngeal pouch to develop and is usually considered to be the ventral section of the fourth pouch. It produces the ultimobranchial body which is later incorporated into the thyroid gland (Moseley *et al.*, 1968). The cells of the ultimobranchial body give rise to the parafollicular or C cells of the thyroid gland which secrete calcitonin in the adult, a hormone involved in the regulation of the calcium level in the blood. Occasionally, the ultimobranchial body may persist and give rise to cysts.

Pharyngeal clefts

At about 5 weeks, four pharyngeal clefts can be seen on the external surface of the embryo. The dorsal section of the first cleft penetrates the underlying mesoderm and gives rise to the external auditory meatus (*see Figures 10.6 and 10.7*). The ectodermal epithelial lining of this cleft makes contact with the endodermal lining of the first pharyngeal pouch and participates in the formation of the tympanic membrane. The mesoderm of the second arch actively proliferates and moves caudally to overlap the third and fourth arches and intervening clefts before finally fusing with the epicardial ridge in the lower part of the neck (*Figure 10.8* and *see Figure 10.6*). The second, third and fourth clefts then lose contact with the outside and form a temporary cavity lined with ectodermal epithelium, the cervical sinus.

Lateral cysts and fistulae of the neck (branchial cysts and fistulae)

The cervical sinus usually disappears completely, but if it does not do so, a cervical or branchial cyst persists. If the second arch fails to fuse completely with the epicardial ridge, the cervical sinus will remain in contact with the surface and be seen as a branchial fistula. These fistulae are found on the lateral aspect of the neck anteriorly to the sternomastoid muscle. It is rare for the cervical sinus to be in communication with the pharynx internally as an internal branchial fistula. The opening of this fistula is in the tonsillar region and normally indicates that there has been a rupture of the membrane between the second pharyngeal pouch and cleft (*see Figure 10.8*).

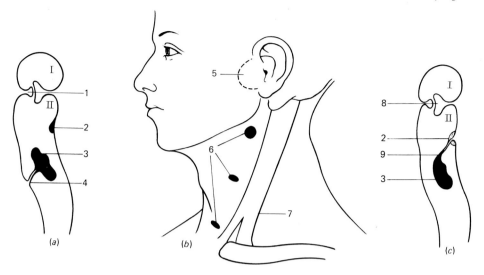

Figure 10.8 (*a*) A diagram to show a lateral cervical (branchial) cyst opening onto the surface as a fistula. (*b*) Location of cysts and fistulae anterior to the sternocleidomastoid muscle. (*c*) Internal opening of a fistula by the palatine tonsil. (Modified from Langman, J., 1981, *Medical Embryology*, 4th edn, Williams and Wilkins, by courtesy of the publisher)

1. External auditory meatus
2. Palatine tonsil
3. Lateral cervical (branchial) cyst
4. External branchial fistula
5. Region of preauricular fistulae
6. Region of lateral cervical cysts and fistulae
7. Sternocleidomastoid muscle
8. Tubotympanic recess
9. Internal branchial fistula

Foregut and oesophagus

At about 4 weeks, a small diverticulum appears on the ventral wall of the foregut at its junction with the pharyngeal gut (*see Figure 10.3*). This is the respiratory or tracheobronchial diverticulum. It is gradually separated from the dorsal part of the foregut, the developing oesophagus, by the formation of a partition known as the oesophago-tracheal septum (*Figure 10.9*). The developing oesophagus comes to lie dorsal to both the developing heart and the septum transversum (diaphragm), as a result of the folding of the anterior part of the embryo. It is embedded in visceral mesoderm without any true mesentery.

The oesophagus is at first a short tube extending from the tracheobronchial diverticulum to the fusiform dilatation of the foregut, which is to become the stomach. As the heart and lungs descend caudally, the oesophagus rapidly lengthens. The muscular coat of the oesophagus is formed from the surrounding mesenchyme and in its upper two-thirds is striated and innervated by the vagus. In the lower third, the muscle coat is smooth and innervated by the splanchnic plexus. The oesophageal endodermal lining is initially of the columnar type, but this is gradually replaced by stratified squamous epithelium.

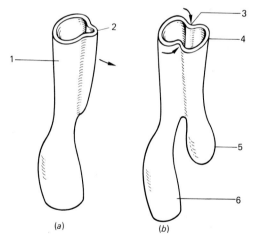

Figure 10.9 The development of the tracheobronchial (respiratory) diverticulum and oesophagus. (*a*) Laryngotracheal groove appearing in the ventral aspect of the foregut. (*b*) The lips of the groove closing in to form the oesophagotracheal septum separating the respiratory tract from the alimentary canal

1. Foregut
2. Laryngotracheal groove
3. Oesophagotracheal septum
4. Trachea
5. Lung bud
6. Stomach

Atresia of the oesophagus and oesophago-tracheal fistula are thought to occur either from a spontaneous deviation of the oesophagotracheal septum in a posterior direction, or from some other mechanical factor pushing the dorsal wall of the foregut anteriorly. The most common variety is for the proximal oesophagus to end in a blind sac and for the distal part to be connected to the trachea by a narrow canal which joins it just above the bifurcation. Occasionally, the fistulous canal is replaced by a ligamentous cord. It is very unusual for both portions of the oesophagus to open into the trachea. If the oesophageal lumen is obstructed, amniotic fluid cannot pass into the intestinal tract and thus it accumulates in the amniotic sac. This is called polyhydramnios and causes enlargement of the uterus. Once the fetus is born, atresia of the oesophagus becomes evident when drinking, resulting in overflow into the trachea and lungs.

The pharynx

General description

The pharynx forms the crossroads of the air and food passages (*Figure 10.10*). Each major road from the pharynx can be closed by a muscular sphincter. The number in *Table 10.3* corresponds to that in *Figure 10.10*.

There is a smaller turning each side from the nasal airway, above the nasopharyngeal sphincter, leading to the middle ear; it is the pharyngotympanic or eustachian tube. This tube is normally

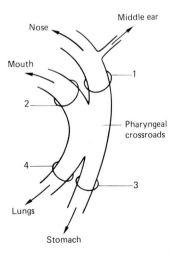

Figure 10.10 Diagram to show the pharynx as a crossroads with entrances and exits controlled by sphincters

1. Nasopharyngeal	3. Cricopharyngeal
2. Oropharyngeal	4. Laryngeal

Table 10.3 Muscles controlling the muscular sphincters in the pharynx

Sphincter	Muscles directly involved
(1) Nasopharyngeal	Levator palati Superior constrictor
(2) Oropharyngeal	Palatoglossus Horizontal intrinsic muscle of tongue
(3) Cricopharyngeal (upper oesophageal)	Cricopharyngeus (normally closed)
(4) Laryngeal	Oblique portion of interarytenoid and aryepiglottic muscles

closed, as is the cricopharyngeal or upper oesophageal sphincter.

The cavity of the pharynx is perhaps best considered as a tube flattened from front to back and with varying widths. Changes in its capacity at different levels in the resting state are best demonstrated by cross-sectional anatomy, which can now be shown by means of computerized tomographic (CT) scanning (*see* Chapter 17). The pharynx extends from the base of the skull to the level of the sixth cervical vertebra, a distance of about 12 cm, where it joins the oesophagus at the lower level of the cricoid cartilage (*Figure 10.11*). The junction is marked by the cricopharyngeus muscle which normally holds the upper oesophageal sphincter closed. The lateral and posterior walls of the pharynx are made up of muscular and fibrous tissue attached to the base of the skull superiorly. The pharynx can be in communication with the air and food passages both anteriorly and inferiorly, as indicated previously. From above downwards, these routes of communication are: the nasal cavities through the posterior nasal apertures; the middle ears through the pharyngotympanic tubes; the mouth through the oropharyngeal isthmus; the larynx through the glottis; and the oesophagus through its upper sphincter.

The interior of the pharynx and its subdivisions

The subdivisions of the pharynx described below are based on those set out in the TNM system for classification of malignant tumours published by the International Union Against Cancer (UICC) (Harmer, 1978). Where the division differs from the purely anatomical one, this has been noted.

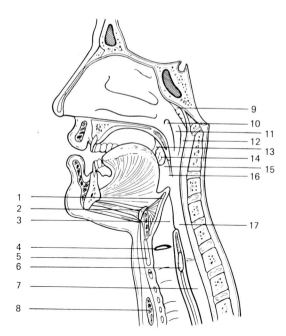

Figure 10.11 A drawing of a sagittal section through the head showing the nasal cavity, pharynx and larynx in the adult

1. Epiglottis
2. Hyoid bone
3. Aryepiglottic fold
4. Vocal cord
5. Thyroid cartilage
6. Cricoid cartilage
7. Oesophagus
8. Thyroid isthmus
9. Nasopharyngeal tonsil
10. Pharyngotympanic tube
11. Salpingopharyngeal fold
12. Nasopharynx
13. Palatoglossal fold
14. Palatine tonsil
15. Oropharynx
16. Palatopharyngeal fold
17. Hypopharynx

Nasopharynx (postnasal space)

The nasopharynx or postnasal space lies behind the nasal cavities and above the soft palate (*see Figure 10.11*). The anterior wall is formed by the openings into the nasal cavities which allow free communication between the nose and nasopharynx each side of the posterior edge of the nasal septum. Just within these openings lie the posterior ends of the inferior and middle turbinates.

The posterosuperior wall of the nasopharynx extends from the base of the skull, at the superior end of the posterior free edge of the nasal septum, down to the level of the junction of hard and soft palates. Anatomically, this lower level is often considered as being at the free edge of the soft palate. This posterosuperior wall is formed by the anteroinferior surface of the body of the sphenoid bone and basilar part of the occipital bone. These two together are termed the 'basisphenoid'. The

bony wall extends as far as the pharyngeal tubercle, but below this the wall is formed by the pharyngobasilar fascia lying in front of the anterior arch of the atlas. A collection of lymphoid tissue, the nasopharyngeal tonsil, is found in the mucous membrane overlying the basisphenoid. When the nasopharyngeal tonsil is enlarged, it is commonly referred to as 'the adenoids'. The nasopharyngeal tonsil has an oblong, rectangular shape, similar to a truncated pyramid, dependent from the roof of the nasopharynx. The anterior edge of this block of tissue is vertical and in the same plane as the posterior nasal aperture. The posterior edge gradually merges into the posterior pharyngeal wall: the lateral edges incline toward the midline.

On each lateral wall of the nasopharynx is the pharyngeal opening of the pharyngotympanic tube. It lies about 1 cm behind the posterior end of the inferior turbinate just above the level of the hard palate. The medial end of the cartilage of the tube forms an elevation shaped like a comma, with a shorter anterior limb and a longer posterior one. Behind and above the tubal cartilage lies the pharyngeal recess (fossa of Rosenmüller). This recess passes laterally above the upper edge of the superior constrictor muscle and corresponds to the position of the sinus of Morgagni. From the posterior edge of the tubal opening the salpingo-pharyngeal fold, produced by the underlying salpingopharyngeus muscle, passes downwards and fades out on the lateral pharyngeal wall. A less well-defined fold passes from the anterior edge of the tubal opening on to the upper surface of the soft palate, and is caused by the underlying levator palati muscle.

The inferior wall of the nasopharynx is formed by the superior surface of the soft palate. In the midline of this wall, there is an elevation caused by the two uvular muscles on the dorsum of the palate.

Oropharynx

The TNM system, noted previously, describes the oropharynx as extending from the junction of the hard and soft palates to the level of the floor of the valleculae. Anatomical texts describe it as extending from the lower edge of the soft palate to the tip of the epiglottis or to the laryngeal inlet. In terms of physiology, it is easier to describe the oropharynx as extending from the oropharyngeal isthmus to the level of the floor of the valleculae which is also the level of the hyoid bone. The oropharyngeal isthmus is the boundary between the buccal cavity and the oropharynx and is marked on each side by the palatoglossal fold formed by the underlying palatoglossus muscle passing from the undersurface of the palate to the

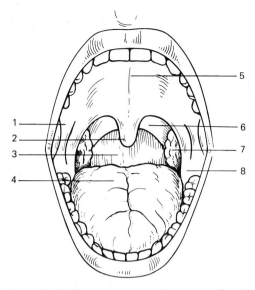

Figure 10.12 The mouth and oropharynx seen from in front

1. Pterygomandibular raphe
2. Uvula
3. Posterior pharyngeal wall
4. Tongue
5. Soft palate
6. Palatopharyngeal fold
7. Palatine tonsil
8. Palatoglossal fold

side of the tongue (*Figure 10.12*). The paired palatoglossal muscles together with the horizontal intrinsic tongue musculature form the oropharyngeal sphincter.

The anterior wall of the oropharynx is, at its upper end, in free communication with the buccal cavity. Below this, the glossoepiglottic area is formed by the posterior one-third of the tongue posterior to the vallate papillae (base of tongue). At the lower part of this anterior wall are found the paired valleculae (*Figure 10.13*). The valleculae are separated from each other in the midline by the median glossoepiglottic fold passing from the base of the tongue to the anterior or lingual surface of the epiglottis. Laterally, each is bounded by the lateral glossoepiglottic fold. The TNM system incorporates the anterior or lingual surface of the epiglottis into the oropharynx. The anterior boundary of the lateral wall of the oropharynx is drawn by the palatoglossal fold and underlying palatoglossus muscle described previously. Behind this, from the lower edge of the soft palate, the palatopharyngeal fold passes downwards and a little backwards to the side wall of the pharynx, where it fades away. Like the palatoglossal fold, this is caused by an underlying muscle, the palatopharyngeus. In the triangular space between these two folds lies the palatine or faucial tonsil. The pharyngeal surface of the tonsil is oval in shape and demonstrates a variable number of

pits or crypts. Towards the upper pole of the tonsil, but within its substance, is found the intratonsillar cleft which is much deeper than the other pits and may extend well down the deep surface of the tonsil within its capsule. A more detailed description of the structure of the tonsil and its anatomical relationships is given later.

Two folds of mucous membrane are usually described in connection with the tonsil. A thin triangular fold of mucous membrane passes backwards from the palatoglossal fold to the base of the tongue covering the lower border of the tonsil to a variable extent. A further semilunar fold of mucous membrane passes from the upper part of the palatopharyngeal fold towards the palatoglossal fold. There is wide variation in the extent to which the tonsil is set back between the palatoglossal and palatopharyngeal folds. In some cases, the tonsil seems to be very much on the surface of the lateral wall of the oropharynx giving the false impression that it is large; in other instances, it is set deeply between the folds and appears very much smaller even though its volume may be the same in both cases. Tonsils

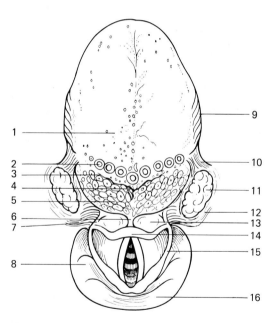

Figure 10.13 The base of tonge and valleculae from above

1. Tongue
2. Vallate papillae
3. Sulcus terminalis
4. Foramen caecum
5. Base of tongue (pharyngeal part)
6. Median glosso-epiglottic fold
7. Lateral glosso-epiglottic fold
8. Pyriform fossa
9. Folia linguae
10. Palatoglossal fold
11. Palatine tonsil
12. Palatopharyngeal fold
13. Vallecula
14. Epiglottis
15. Aryepiglottic fold
16. Posterior pharyngeal wall

that stand out into the oropharynx are better described as prominent rather than large. The palatoglossal and palatopharyngeal folds are often called the anterior and posterior faucial pillars. Between the tonsil and the base of the tongue lies the glossotonsillar sulcus.

The posterior wall of the oropharynx is formed by the constrictor muscles and overlying mucous membrane. The superior wall of the oropharynx is formed by the inferior surface of the soft palate and uvula. The soft palate is described in detail later.

Hypopharynx (laryngopharynx)

The hypopharynx is that part of the pharynx which lies behind the larynx and partly to each side, where it forms the pyriform fossae or sinuses. It is continuous above with the oropharynx and below with the oesophagus, at the lower border of the cricoid cartilage, through the cricopharyngeal sphincter.

In the anterior wall of the hypopharynx lies the larynx itself with its oblique inlet. The inlet is bounded anteriorly and superiorly by the upper part of the epiglottis, posteriorly by the elevations of the arytenoid cartilages, and laterally by the aryepiglottic folds. Below the laryngeal inlet, the anterior wall is formed by the posterior surfaces of the paired arytenoid cartilages and the posterior plate of the cricoid cartilage. To each side of the larynx lie the pyriform fossae (*Figure 10.14*). They are bounded laterally by the thyroid cartilage and medially by the surface of the aryepiglottic fold, the arytenoid and cricoid cartilages. They extend from the lateral glosso-epiglottic fold (pharyngo-epiglottic fold) to the upper end of the oesophagus. Deep to the mucous membrane of the lateral wall of the pyriform fossa lies the superior laryngeal nerve, where it is accessible for local anaesthesia.

The TNM system describes the posterior wall of this section of the pharynx as extending from the level of the floor of the valleculae to the level of the cricoarytenoid joint. This wall is formed by the constrictor muscles and overlying mucous membrane. The region below this, down to the inferior border of the cricoid cartilage, is called the pharyngo-oesophageal junction and is bounded anteriorly by the posterior plate of the cricoid cartilage and encircled by the cricopharyngeus muscle which forms the upper oesophageal sphincter.

The soft palate

The soft palate is a mobile, flexible partition between the nasopharyngeal airway and the

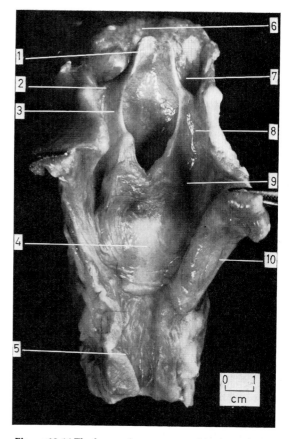

Figure 10.14 The lower pharynx, opened from behind, to show the valleculae, pyriform fossae and postcricoid regions. Note the shallow upper and deeper lower parts of the pyriform fossae

1. Epiglottis
2. Lateral glosso-
   epiglottic fold
3. Aryepiglottic fold
4. Postcricoid region
5. Cervical oesophagus

6. Base of tongue
7. Vallecula
8. Upper pyriform fossa
9. Lower pyriform fossa
10. Posterolateral
    pharyngeal wall

oropharyngeal food passage, and it can be likened to a set of points on a railway track, movement of which opens one line and closes another. It extends posteriorly from the edge of the hard palate, and laterally it blends with the lateral walls of the oropharynx. The soft palate forms the roof of the oropharynx and the floor of the nasopharynx. It lies between two sphincters: the nasopharyngeal which pulls the palate up and back to close the nasopharyngeal airway, and the oropharyngeal which pulls it down and forwards to close the oropharyngeal isthmus.

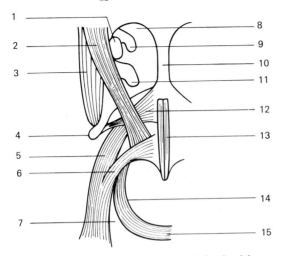

Figure 10.15 The muscles acting on the left side of the soft palate viewed from behind. (Modified from McMinn, R. M. H. and Hobdell, M. H., 1974, *Functional Anatomy of the Digestive System*, p. 25, Figure 2.16. Pitman Medical, London, by courtesy of the authors and publisher)

1. Pharyngotympanic tube
2. Levator palati
3. Tensor palati
4. Pterygoid hamulus
5. Palatopharyngeus – anterior bundle
6. Palatopharyngeus – posterior bundle
7. Tonsillar fossa
8. Posterior nasal opening
9. Middle turbinate
10. Nasal septum
11. Inferior turbinate
12. Palatine aponeurosis
13. Uvular muscle
14. Palatoglossus
15. Transverse intrinsic tongue muscle

Structure of the soft palate

The basis of the soft palate is the palatine aponeurosis formed by the expanded tendons of the tensor palati muscles which join in a median raphe (*Figure 10.15*). The aponeurosis is attached to the posterior edge of the hard palate and to its inferior surface behind the palatine crest. It is thicker in the anterior two-thirds of the palate but very thin further back. Near the midline, it splits to enclose the uvular muscle; all the other muscles of the soft palate are attached to it. The anterior part of the soft palate is less mobile and more horizontal than the posterior part and it is principally on this part that the tensor palati acts. From the posterior edge of the soft palate hangs the uvula in the midline. From the base of the uvula on each side, a fold of mucous membrane containing muscle fibres sweeps down to the lateral wall of the oropharynx (*Figure 10.16*); this is the palatopharyngeal fold, and the two folds together form the palatopharyngeal arch. More anteriorly, a smaller fold, also containing muscle

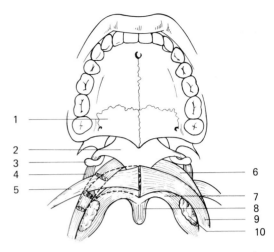

Figure 10.16 A diagram to show the five paired muscles of the soft palate from the oral (inferior) aspect. (Modified from Montgomery, W. W., 1973, *Surgery of the Upper Respiratory System*, Vol. 2, p.2, Fig.1.1 (C), Lea and Febiger, Philadelphia, by courtesy of the publisher)

1. Palatine bone
2. Palatine aponeurosis
3. Pterygoid hamulus
4. Tensor palati
5. Levator palati
6. Palatopharyngeus – anterior bundle
7. Palatopharyngeus – posterior bundle
8. Uvular muscles
9. Palatoglossus
10. Palatine tonsil

fibres, passes from the soft palate to the side of the tongue. This is the palatoglossal fold and, with its opposite number, it forms the palatoglossal arch which marks the junction of the buccal cavity and the oropharynx, the oropharyngeal isthmus. The term 'isthmus of the fauces' is sometimes used to describe both the palatal arches together.

The soft palate contains numerous mucous glands and lymphoid tissue, chiefly on the inferior aspect of the palatal aponeurosis and toward its posterior edge (*Figure 10.17*). The palate also contains the fibres of those muscles acting on it which will be described in detail later.

The mucous membrane on the superior or nasopharyngeal aspect of the palate is pseudo-stratified ciliated columnar in type, often known as 'respiratory epithelium'. On the inferior or oropharyngeal aspect, the epithelium is of the non-keratinized stratified squamous variety. The lamina propria is very vascular and contains many elastic fibres.

Muscles of the soft palate

The muscles of the soft palate are activated by swallowing, breathing and phonation (Fritzell, 1976). Deglutition is described in detail in Chapter 11.

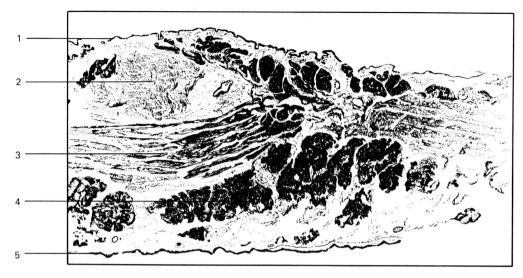

Figure 10.17 Transverse section of the soft palate showing large numbers of mucous glands, chiefly inferior to the aponeurosis and muscles

1. Pseudostratified columnar epithelium on superior (nasopharyngeal) surface
2. Transverse muscle fibres
3. Longitudinal muscle fibres
4. Mucous glands
5. Non-keratinizing stratified squamous epithelium on inferior (oral) surface

Tensor palati

The tensor palati muscle is a thin triangular muscle which arises from the scaphoid fossa of the pterygoid process of the sphenoid bone, the lateral lamina of the cartilage of the pharyngotympanic tube and the medial aspect of the spine of the sphenoid bone (*Figure 10.18*). As it descends on the lateral surface of the medial pterygoid plate, its fibres converge to form a small tendon which passes round the pterygoid hamulus of the medial plate before piercing the attachment of the buccinator to the pterygomandibular raphe and spreading out to form the palatine aponeurosis described previously (*see Figure 10.15*). There is a small bursa between the tendon and the pterygoid hamulus. The two tensor palati muscles, acting together, tighten the soft palate, primarily in its anterior part and depress it by flattening its arch. Acting alone, one tensor palati muscle will pull the soft palate to one side. This muscle is also the principal opener of the pharyngotympanic tube, assisted by the levator palati, through its attachment to the lateral lamina of the tubal cartilage.

All the muscles of the soft palate, except the tensor palati, belong to the same group as the superior constrictor and have the same nerve supply by way of the pharyngeal plexus. The tensor palati, however, is an immigrant muscle which at one time played a part in mastication. Its nerve supply comes from the mandibular division of the trigeminal nerve.

Levator palati

The levator palati is a cylindrical muscle arising by a small tendon from a rough area on the inferior surface of the petrous temporal bone immediately in front of the lower opening of the carotid canal (*see Figure 10.18*). It also arises by a few fibres from the inferior surface of the cartilaginous part of the pharyngotympanic tube. At its origin, the muscle lies inferior rather than medial to the pharyngotympanic tube and crosses to the medial side of the tube only at the level of the medial pterygoid plate. The muscle passes downwards, forwards and inwards over the upper edge of the superior constrictor muscle where it pierces the pharyngobasilar fascia, and descends in front of the salpingopharyngeus muscle to be inserted into the upper surface of the palatine aponeurosis between the two bundles of the palatopharyngeus muscle (*Figure 10.19* and *see Figure 10.15*). The muscle fibres blend with those of the levator palati from the opposite side. The action of the muscle is to raise the soft palate upwards and backwards. Its action, coupled with that of some of the upper fibres of the superior constrictor, described later, plays an important role in the closure of the nasopharyngeal isthmus during deglutition. It also assists in opening the pharyngotympanic tube by elevating the medial lamina of the tubal cartilage, but not until after the age of 7 years or so (Holborow, 1970, 1975).

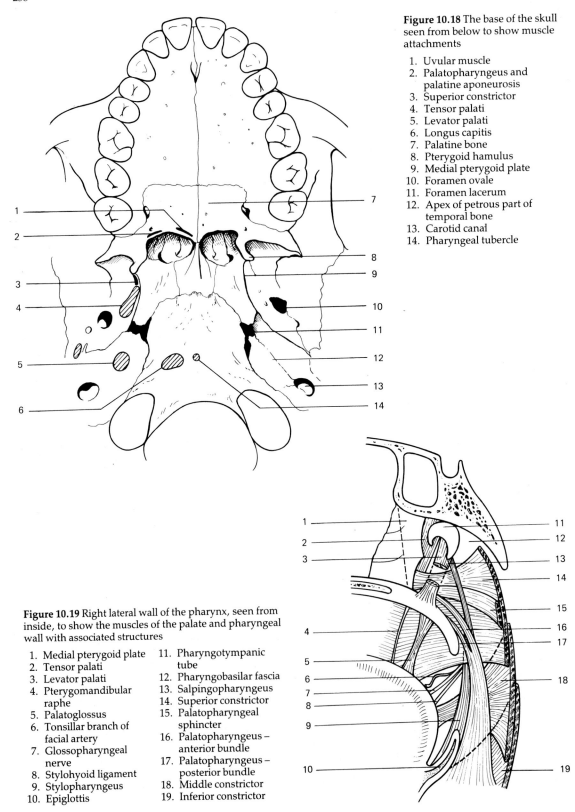

Figure 10.18 The base of the skull seen from below to show muscle attachments

1. Uvular muscle
2. Palatopharyngeus and palatine aponeurosis
3. Superior constrictor
4. Tensor palati
5. Levator palati
6. Longus capitis
7. Palatine bone
8. Pterygoid hamulus
9. Medial pterygoid plate
10. Foramen ovale
11. Foramen lacerum
12. Apex of petrous part of temporal bone
13. Carotid canal
14. Pharyngeal tubercle

Figure 10.19 Right lateral wall of the pharynx, seen from inside, to show the muscles of the palate and pharyngeal wall with associated structures

1. Medial pterygoid plate
2. Tensor palati
3. Levator palati
4. Pterygomandibular raphe
5. Palatoglossus
6. Tonsillar branch of facial artery
7. Glossopharyngeal nerve
8. Stylohyoid ligament
9. Stylopharyngeus
10. Epiglottis
11. Pharyngotympanic tube
12. Pharyngobasilar fascia
13. Salpingopharyngeus
14. Superior constrictor
15. Palatopharyngeal sphincter
16. Palatopharyngeus – anterior bundle
17. Palatopharyngeus – posterior bundle
18. Middle constrictor
19. Inferior constrictor

Palatoglossus

The palatoglossus is a small fleshy bundle of muscle fibres arising from the oral surface of the palatine aponeurosis where it is continuous with the muscle of the opposite side (*see Figure 10.16*). It passes anteroinferiorly and laterally in front of the tonsil where it forms the palatoglossal arch. It is inserted into the side of the tongue where some of its fibres spread over the dorsum of the tongue while others pass more deeply into its substance to intermingle with the transverse intrinsic muscle fibres. The action of the two muscles, together with the horizontal intrinsic fibres of the tongue, is to close the oropharyngeal isthmus by approximation of the palatoglossal arches and elevation of the tongue against the oral surface of the soft palate.

Palatopharyngeus

The palatopharyngeus arises in the palate as two bundles separated by the levator palati (*see Figure 10.15*). The anterior bundle, which is the thicker of the two, arises from the posterior border of the hard palate and from the palatine aponeurosis. It passes back between the levator and tensor palati. The posterior bundle is thinner and arises from beneath the mucous membrane of the palate and passes medial to the levator palati. The two bundles unite at the posterolateral aspect of the palate to descend in the palatopharyngeal fold before spreading out to form the inner vertical muscle layer of the pharynx and to be inserted into the posterior edge of the lamina of the thyroid cartilage (*Figure 10.20* and *see Figure 10.19*). The action of the muscle is to pull the walls of the pharynx upwards, forwards and medially, so shortening the pharynx and elevating the larynx during deglutition. Acting together, the two muscles approximate the palatopharyngeal arches to the midline and direct food and fluid down into the lower part of the oropharynx.

Uvular muscle

This is a small paired muscle arising from the palatine aponeurosis just behind the hard palate (*see Figure 10.15*). Its fibres lie adjacent to the midline between the two laminae of the aponeurosis. It passes backwards and downwards to be inserted into the mucous membrane of the uvula. Its action is to pull up and shorten the uvula and to add bulk to the dorsal surface of the soft palate which assists in closure of the nasopharyngeal opening (velopharyngeal closure) in speech and deglutition (Pigott, 1969; Azzam and Kuehn, 1977).

Nerve supply of the soft palate

All the muscles of the soft palate, except the tensor palati, are supplied by way of the pharyngeal plexus (Broomhead, 1951) with an additional supply from the facial nerve (Nishio *et al.*, 1976a,b; Ibuki *et al.*, 1978). The cell bodies of these motor nerves are found in the nucleus ambiguus and leave the brainstem in the cranial root of the accessory to join the vagus nerve and pass by its pharyngeal branch to the pharyngeal plexus. The cell bodies of the facial nerve innervation arise in the facial nucleus and pass through the geniculate ganglion, greater petrosal nerve and pterygopalatine ganglion before reaching the palatal muscles. The tensor palati is supplied by the trigeminal nerve through the nerve to the medial pterygoid, a branch of the mandibular nerve. The fibres pass through, but do not synapse, in the otic ganglion.

The sensory supply to the palate is derived from the greater and lesser palatine branches of the maxillary division of the trigeminal nerve which pass on to the surface of the palate through the greater and lesser palatine foramina. These nerves appear to be branches of the pterygopalatine ganglion but have no synaptic connection in the ganglion, the cell bodies of the sensory fibres being in the trigeminal ganglion. A sensory supply is also provided by pharyngeal branches of the glossopharyngeal nerve. The small number of taste buds on the palate are supplied by the same palatine branches, and the fibres pass up through the pterygopalatine ganglion, without synapsing, into the nerve of the pterygoid canal and the greater petrosal nerve to reach the geniculate ganglion of the facial nerve where the cell bodies are situated. The central processes enter the brainstem by way of the nervus intermedius portion of the facial nerve and end in the nucleus of the tractus solitarius. Sympathetic fibres reach the palate on the blood vessels supplying it and are derived from the superior cervical ganglion.

Blood supply of the soft palate

The blood supply of the soft palate is provided by the palatine branch of the ascending pharyngeal artery which curls over the upper edge of the superior constrictor muscle before being distributed to the palate. The ascending palatine branch of the facial artery provides an additional supply, as do the lesser palatine branches of the descending palatine branch of the maxillary artery; it runs upwards on the side wall of the pharynx and may, together with the ascending pharyngeal artery, send a branch over the upper edge of the superior constrictor muscle to the palate.

The venous drainage of the palate is to the pterygoid plexus and thence through the deep

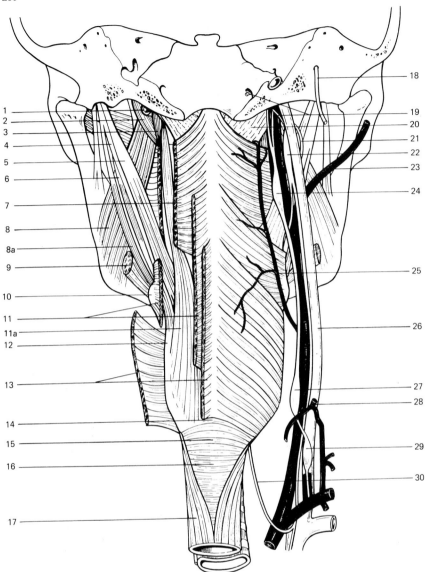

Figure 10.20 A drawing of the pharynx and associated structures as seen from the back

1. Pharyngotympanic tube
2. Tensor palati
3. Levator palati
4. Stylohyoid ligament
5. Stylopharyngeus muscle
6. Styloglossus muscle
7. Superior constrictor muscle
8. Medial pterygoid muscle
8a. Stylohyoid muscle
9. Posterior belly of the digastric
10. Greater horn of hyoid bone
11. Middle constrictor
11a. Palatopharyngeus muscle
12. Superior horn of thyroid cartilage
13. Inferior constrictor muscle – thyropharyngeus
14. Killian's dehiscence
15. Inferior constrictor muscle – cricopharyngeus
16. Circular oesophageal muscle coat
17. Longitudinal oesophageal muscle coat
18. Facial nerve
19. Hypoglossal nerve
20. Pharyngobasilar fascia
21. Accessory nerve
22. Inferior ganglion of vagus nerve
23. External carotid artery
24. Superior cervical sympathetic ganglion
25. Ascending pharyngeal artery
26. Internal jugular vein
27. Middle cervical sympathetic ganglion
28. Inferior thyroid artery
29. Inferior cervical ganglion
30. Right recurrent laryngeal nerve

facial vein to the anterior facial vein and internal jugular vein.

Lymphatic drainage of the soft palate

The lymphatic drainage of the soft palate is partly by way of the retropharyngeal nodes, but chiefly direct to the upper deep cervical group of nodes.

The pharyngeal wall

The pharyngeal wall consists of four layers which, from the inner layer outwards, are as follows:

(1) mucous membrane
(2) pharyngobasilar fascia
(3) muscle layer
(4) buccopharyngeal fascia.

Mucous membrane

The epithelial lining of the pharynx varies in accordance with differing physiological function. The nasopharynx is part of the respiratory pathway and normally only traversed by air. It is lined by a pseudostratified columnar ciliated epithelium as far as the level of the lower border of the soft palate. The oropharynx and hypopharynx are part of the alimentary tract and subject to the abrasion caused by the passage of food. These two areas have an epithelial lining of non-keratinizing stratified squamous epithelium. In the border zone between the nasopharynx and oropharynx, there may be a narrow zone of stratified columnar epithelium. Immediately beneath the epithelium, there is a connective tissue lamina propria that contains a large amount of elastic tissue and which takes the place of the muscularis mucosae found in the oesophagus.

The respiratory type of epithelium in the nasopharynx contains goblet cells. Elsewhere, the mucous membrane is pierced by ducts from glands that lie deep to it in the submucosa. These may be mucous, serous, or mixed.

The pharynx has a large amount of subepithelial or gut-associated lymphoid tissue encircling both its alimentary and respiratory openings forming Waldeyer's ring (*Figure 10.21*). There are three large aggregations of this tissue and three smaller ones. The larger are the two palatine tonsils in the oropharynx, and the nasopharyngeal tonsil on the roof of the nasopharynx. The three smaller aggregations are the tubal tonsil, above and behind the pharyngeal opening of the pharyngo-tympanic tube, the lingual tonsil, and the two lateral bands which run down posterior to the palatopharyngeal fold. The pharyngeal lymphoid tissue is described in more detail later.

Pharyngobasilar fascia

A fibrous intermediate layer lies between the mucous membrane and the muscular layers in place of the submucosa. It is thick above, where the muscle fibres are absent, and is firmly connected to the basilar region of the occipital bone and petrous part of the temporal bone medial to the carotid canal, bridging below the pharyngo-tympanic tube, and extending forwards to be attached to the posterior border of the medial pterygoid plate and the pterygomandibular raphe (*see Figure 10.19*). The pharyngobasilar fascia bridges the gap between the superior border of the superior constrictor and the base of the skull (*see Figure 10.20*). In this region it is firmly united to the buccopharyngeal fascia, forming a single layer. This fibrous layer diminishes in thickness as it descends. It is strengthened posteriorly by a strong fibrous band which is attached above to the pharyngeal tubercle on the undersurface of the basilar portion of the occipital bone, and passes

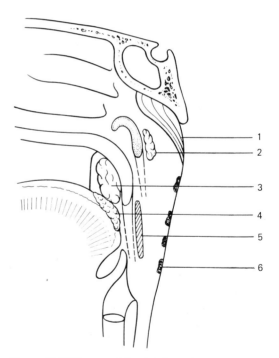

Figure 10.21 Diagram of the right lateral wall of the pharynx to show the aggregations of gut-associated lymphoid tissue that form Waldeyer's ring

1. Nasopharyngeal tonsil
2. Tubal tonsil in fossa of Rosenmüller
3. Palatine tonsil
4. Lingual tonsil on base of tongue
5. Lateral pharyngeal band of lymphoid tissue behind palatopharyngeal fold
6. Lymphoid nodules on posterior pharyngeal wall

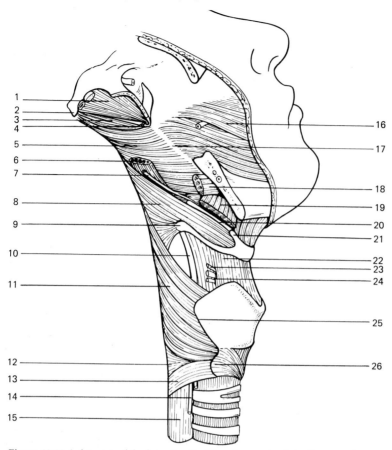

Figure 10.22 A drawing of the lateral wall of the pharynx to show the constrictor muscles and associated structures. (Modified from Williams, P. L. and Warwick, R., 1980, *Gray's Anatomy*, 36th edn, p. 1309, Figure 8.84. Churchill Livingstone, courtesy of the publishers)

1. Tensor palati
2. Spine of sphenoid bone
3. Levator palati
4. Pterygoid hamulus
5. Superior constrictor
6. Stylopharyngeus
7. Glossopharyngeal nerve
8. Middle constrictor
9. Greater horn of hyoid bone
10. Lateral thyrohyoid ligament
11. Thyropharyngeus part of inferior constrictor
12. Killian's dehiscence
13. Cricopharyngeus part of inferior constrictor
14. Right recurrent laryngeal nerve
15. Oesophagus
16. Buccinator
17. Pterygomandibular raphe
18. Styloglossus
19. Geniohyoid
20. Stylohyoid ligament
21. Lesser horn of hyoid bone
22. Thyrohyoid membrane
23. Internal laryngeal nerve
24. Superior laryngeal vessels
25. Oblique line on thyroid cartilage
26. Fascial bridge over cricothyroid muscle

downwards as a median raphe (the pharyngeal raphe), which gives attachment to the constrictors (*see Figure 10.20*). Although the pharyngeal muscles are usually described as lying external to the fibrous layer, it is formed, in reality, from the thickened, deep epimysial covering of these muscles, and the thinner external layer of the epimysium constitutes the buccopharyngeal fascia.

Muscle layer

The muscles of the pharyngeal wall are arranged into an inner longitudinal layer and an outer circular layer. The inner layer is formed by three paired muscles, namely:

(1) stylopharyngeus
(2) palatopharyngeus
(3) salpingopharyngeus.

The outer layer also has three paired muscles, namely:

(1) superior constrictor
(2) middle constrictor
(3) inferior constrictor.

Each of the constrictor muscles is a fan-shaped sheet arising on the lateral wall of the pharynx and sweeping round to be inserted into the median raphe posteriorly (*Figure 10.22* and *see Figure 10.20*). The muscles overlap each other from below upwards. Although together they form an almost complete coat for the side and posterior walls of the pharynx, their attachments anteriorly separate the edges, and it is through these intervals that structures can pass from the exterior of the pharynx towards its lumen. The interval between the upper border of the superior constrictor and the base of the skull is sometimes called the sinus of Morgagni. During deglutition, the constrictor muscles contract in a coordinated way to propel the bolus through the oropharynx into the oesophagus. The longitudinal muscles elevate the larynx and shorten the pharynx during this movement.

The superior constrictor muscle

This muscle arises from above downwards from the posterior border of the lower part of the medial pterygoid plate, the pterygoid hamulus, the pterygomandibular raphe, the posterior end of the mylohyoid line on the inner surface of the mandible, and by a few fibres from the side of the tongue (*see Figure 10.22*). The fibres pass backwards in a largely quadrilateral sheet to be inserted into the median pharyngeal raphe and, by an aponeurosis, to the pharyngeal tubercle on the basilar part of the occipital bone (*see Figure 10.18*). A band of muscle fibres arises from the anterior and lateral part of the upper surface of the palatine aponeurosis and sweeps backwards, lateral to the levator palati, to blend with the internal surface of the superior constrictor near its upper border (Whillis, 1930). This band is termed the 'palatopharyngeal sphincter' (*see Figure 10.19*). It produces a rounded ridge on the pharyngeal wall, known as Passavant's ridge, which is seen when the nasopharyngeal sphincter contracts (Calnan, 1958).

The middle constrictor muscle

This muscle arises from the posterior edge of the lower part of the stylohyoid ligament and lesser horn of the hyoid bone, as well as from the whole length of the upper border of the greater horn (*see Figure 10.22*). The fibres spread in a wide fan-shape upwards and downwards as they pass backwards to be inserted into the whole length of the median pharyngeal raphe (*see Figure 10.20*). As the upper fibres ascend, they overlap the superior constrictor; the middle fibres pass horizontally backwards, and the lower fibres descend, deep to the inferior constrictor, as far as the lower end of the pharynx.

The inferior constrictor muscle

This is the thickest of the constrictors and consists of two parts: thyropharyngeus and cricopharyngeus. The thyropharyngeus part arises from the oblique line on the lateral surface of the lamina of the thyroid cartilage, from a fine tendinous band across the cricothyroid muscle, and from a small area on the lateral surface of the cricoid cartilage at the lower edge of the above band (*see Figure 10.22*). There is also a small slip from the inferior horn of the thyroid cartilage. These fibres pass backwards to be inserted into the median pharyngeal raphe, the upper ones ascending obliquely to overlap the middle constrictor (*see Figure 10.20*). The cricopharyngeus part of the inferior constrictor arises from the side of the cricoid cartilage in the interval between the origin of the cricothyroid in front and the articular facet for the inferior horn of the thyroid cartilage behind. These fibres pass horizontally backwards and encircle the pharyngo-oesophageal junction to be inserted at the same site on the opposite side of the cricoid cartilage. They are continuous with the circular fibres of the oesophagus. Posteriorly, there is a small triangular interval between the upper edge of the cricopharyngeus and the lower fibres of the thyropharyngeus. This interval is sometimes referred to as Killian's dehiscence (*see Figure 10.20*). It is occasionally described as a point of 'weakness' in the pharyngeal wall, but this is incorrect as it is a feature of the normal anatomy of this region. However, when there is incoordination of the pharyngeal peristaltic wave, and the cricopharyngeus does not relax at the appropriate time, pressure may temporarily build up in the lower part of the pharynx, in which case the most likely place for a diverticulum to form is at Killian's dehiscence, where the additional support of the constrictor muscles is deficient.

The stylopharyngeus muscle

This muscle arises from the medial side of the base of the styloid process of the temporal bone and descends along the side of the pharynx, passing between the superior and middle constrictors, after which its fibres spread out beneath the mucous membrane, some of them merging into the constrictors and the lateral glossoepiglottic fold while others are inserted, with the palato-pharyngeus, into the posterior border of the thyroid cartilage (*see Figures 10.19* and *10.20*). The muscle is long and slender with a cylindrical shape above, flattening out below within the pharynx. It is supplied by a branch of the glossopharyngeal nerve, which winds around its posterior border before entering the pharynx alongside it to reach the tongue.

The palatopharyngeus muscle

This muscle, with its covering of mucous mem-brane, forms the palatopharyngeal fold or post-erior faucial pillar. It arises as two bundles within the soft palate. The anterior bundle, the thicker of the two, arises from the posterior border of the hard palate and from the palatine aponeurosis. It passes backwards, first anterior and then lateral to the levator palati, between the levator and the tensor palati, before descending into the pharynx. The smaller posterior and inferior bundle arises in contact with the mucous membrane covering the surface of the palate, together with the corres-ponding bundle of the opposite side in the median plane (*see Figure 10.15*). At the posterolateral border of the palate, the two bundles of muscle unite and are joined by the fibres of salpingo-pharyngeus. Passing laterally and downwards behind the tonsil, the palatopharyngeus descends posteromedial to, and in close contact with, the stylopharyngeus muscle and is inserted with it into the posterior border of the thyroid cartilage (*see Figure 10.19*). Some of its fibres end in the side wall of the pharynx attached to the fibrous coat, and others pass across the median plane to decussate with those of the opposite side.

Salpingopharyngeus

This muscle arises from the posteroinferior corner of the cartilage of the pharyngotympanic tube near its pharyngeal opening. The fibres pass down-wards and blend with the palatopharyngeus muscle (*see Figure 10.19*).

Structures entering the pharynx (*see Figure 10.22*)

Above the superior constrictor

The cartilaginous part of the pharyngotympanic tube and the tensor and levator palati muscles pass through the pharyngobasilar fascia to reach the lateral wall of the pharynx and palate respectively. The palatine branch of the ascending pharyngeal artery curls over the upper edge of the superior constrictor.

Between the middle and superior constrictor muscles

The stylopharyngeus muscle enters the pharynx at this level, as described previously, before it blends with fibres from the palatopharyngeus. It is accompanied by the glossopharyngeal nerve which supplies it before passing forward to the tongue.

Between the middle and inferior constrictor muscles

The internal laryngeal nerve and superior laryngeal vessels pierce the thyrohyoid membrane and come to lie submucosally on the lateral wall of the pyriform fossa, where the nerve is accessible for local anaesthesia.

Below the inferior constrictor

The recurrent laryngeal nerve and inferior laryngeal artery pass between the cricopharyngeal part of the inferior constrictor and the oesophagus behind the articulation of the inferior horn of the thyroid cartilage with the cricoid cartilage.

Buccopharyngeal fascia

This thin fibrous layer forms the outer coat of the pharynx and, as already indicated, probably represents the thinner external epimysial covering of the constrictor muscles. It is a coat of areolar tissue and contains the pharyngeal plexus of nerves and veins. Posteriorly, it is loosely attached to the prevertebral fascia covering the prevertebral muscles and, at the sides, is loosely connected to the styloid process and its muscles, and to the carotid sheath.

Nerve supply of the pharynx

The motor, sensory and autonomic nerve supply of the pharynx is provided through the pharyn-geal plexus, which is situated in the buccopharyn-geal fascia surrounding the pharynx. The plexus is formed by the pharyngeal branches of the glossopharyngeal and vagus nerves together with sympathetic fibres from the superior cervical ganglion. The cells of origin of the glossopharyn-geal and vagal motor branches that supply the muscles are in the rostral part of the nucleus ambiguus. The fibres leave the brainstem with the glossopharyngeal nerve and with the cranial root of the accessory nerve which joins the vagus at the level of its superior ganglion. The pharyngeal branch of the vagus carries the main motor supply to the pharyngeal plexus. All the muscles of the pharynx, with the exception of stylopharyngeus, are supplied by the pharyngeal plexus. The stylopharyngeus is supplied by a muscular branch of the glossopharyngeal nerve as it passes round the muscle to enter the pharynx with it. It is the only muscle supplied by the glossopharyngeal which is otherwise a sensory nerve. The crico-pharyngeus part of the inferior constrictor has an additional supply from the external laryngeal nerve and receives parasympathetic vagal fibres from the recurrent laryngeal nerve.

The sensory nerve supply to the pharynx is also provided by branches of the glossopharyngeal and vagus nerves, chiefly through the pharyngeal plexus. The glossopharyngeal nerve provides the supply to the upper part of the pharynx, including the surface of the tonsil, which is also supplied by the lesser palatine branch of the maxillary nerve. The posterior third of the tongue, including the vallate papillae, is supplied for both ordinary sensation and taste by the glossopharyngeal nerve. The tongue in front of the valleculae and the valleculae themselves are supplied by the internal laryngeal nerve, a branch of the superior laryngeal nerve of the vagus. A small part of the nasopharynx behind the opening of pharyngo-tympanic tube receives a sensory supply from the pharyngeal branch of the maxillary nerve. These fibres pass through the pterygopalatine ganglion without synapsing and their cell bodies are in the trigeminal ganglion.

The afferent sensory fibres of the glossopharyngeal nerve have their cell bodies in the superior and inferior ganglia of the nerve. The central processes of the unipolar nerve cells in these ganglia are received in the nucleus of the tractus solitarius for taste, and probably in the nucleus of the spinal tract of the trigeminal nerve for common sensation. In the case of the vagus nerve, the sensory fibres synapse in the inferior vagal ganglion before being received in the above brainstem nuclei.

The parasympathetic secretomotor supply to the glands of the pharyngeal mucosa, which are mainly in the nasopharynx, comes by way of the pterygopalatine ganglion. The cell bodies are in the superior salivary nucleus, and the fibres leave the brainstem in the nervus intermedius. They pass through the geniculate ganglion of the facial nerve without synapsing and leave it by the greater petrosal nerve, passing by way of the nerve of the pterygoid canal to reach the pterygo-palatine ganglion. Here they synapse with the postganglionic cell bodies whose axons reach the pharyngeal mucosa by the nasal, palatine, and pharyngeal branches from the ganglion.

Sympathetic fibres are derived from the superior cervical ganglion of the cervical sympathetic trunk. The preganglionic cell bodies are in the lateral grey column of spinal cord segments T1–T3. Their axons pass up in the sympathetic trunk to synapse in the cervical ganglia from which postganglionic fibres leave and reach the pharynx by running with its blood vessels.

The cricopharyngeal sphincter has a double autonomic innervation. Parasympathetic vagal fibres reach the muscle in the recurrent laryngeal nerve and postganglionic sympathetic fibres come from the superior cervical ganglion. Stimulation of the vagus causes relaxation and sympathetic excitation causes contraction of the sphincter.

Blood supply of the pharynx

The ascending pharyngeal artery arises from the medial side of the external carotid artery just above its origin. It passes upwards behind the carotid sheath and immediately against the pharyngeal wall. Branches are distributed to the wall of the pharynx and the tonsils. Its palatine branch passes over the upper free edge of the superior constrictor muscle to supply the inner aspect of the pharynx and the soft palate. A small branch supplies the pharyngotympanic tube. The pharynx receives a further supply of blood from the ascending palatine and tonsillar branches of the facial artery and the greater palatine and pterygoid branches of the maxillary artery. The dorsal lingual branches of the lingual artery provide an additional small contribution.

The veins of the pharynx are arranged in an internal submucous and an external pharyngeal plexus with numerous communicating branches, not only between the two plexuses but with the veins of the dorsum of the tongue, the superior laryngeal veins, and the oesophageal veins. The pharyngeal plexus drains to the internal jugular and anterior facial veins. It also communicates with the pterygoid plexus.

Lymphatic drainage of the pharynx

All the lymph vessels of the pharynx drain into the deep cervical group of lymph nodes, either directly from the tissues themselves, or indirectly after passing through one of the outlying groups of nodes. The efferents from the deep cervical group form the jugular trunk which, on the right side, may end in the junction of the internal jugular and subclavian veins or may join the right lymphatic duct. On the left side, the jugular trunk usually enters the thoracic duct although it may join either the internal jugular or the subclavian vein.

The deep cervical group of nodes lies along the carotid sheath by the internal jugular vein and is divided into superior and inferior groups. The superior group is adjacent to the upper part of the internal jugular vein, mostly deep to the sterno-cleidomastoid. Within this superior group, a smaller group consisting of one large and several small nodes is particularly to be noted. It lies in the triangular region bounded by the posterior belly of the digastric above, the facial vein, and the internal jugular vein. It is termed the 'jugulo-digastric group'.

The inferior group of deep cervical lymph nodes is also partly deep to sternocleidomastoid and extends into the subclavian triangle. It is closely related to the brachial plexus and the subclavian vessels. Within this group, one lies on, or just above, the intermediate tendon of omohyoid. It is called the jugulo-omohyoid node. The superior group of nodes drains into the inferior group. In addition to the pharynx, all of the lymph vessels of the head and neck drain into this group. The upper part of the pharynx, including the nasopharynx and the pharyngotympanic tube, drains first into the retropharyngeal lymph nodes which comprise a median and two lateral groups lying between the buccopharyngeal fascia covering the pharynx and the prevertebral fascia. These nodes are said to atrophy in childhood. Efferent vessels from them pass to the upper deep cervical nodes.

The lymphatic vessels of the oropharynx pass to the upper deep cervical group of nodes and, in particular, to the jugulodigastric group described previously. Vessels from the tonsil pierce the buccopharyngeal fascia and the superior constrictor and pass between the stylohyoid and internal jugular vein to the jugulodigastric node.

The hypopharynx drains chiefly to the inferior deep cervical group of nodes, but may also drain to paratracheal nodes which lie alongside the trachea and oesophagus beside the recurrent laryngeal nerves. Efferents from these nodes pass to the deep cervical group.

The lymphoid tissue of the pharynx

A full account of basic immunology appears in Chapter 18. This section discusses some anatomical and histological aspects of the lymphoid tissue in the pharynx.

The walls of the alimentary and respiratory tracts contain large amounts of unencapsulated lymphoid tissue, the lymphoid nodules, and these are collectively termed the 'epitheliolymphoid' or 'gut-associated lymphoid' tissue. They form part of the peripheral lymphoid organs, the other parts being the lymph nodes and similar tissues in the bone marrow and spleen. Lymphoid nodules are particularly prominent in the pharynx and include the nasopharyngeal, tubal, palatine and lingual tonsils. Further down the alimentary tract,

nodules occur in the wall of the oesophagus and large groups in the small intestine (Peyer's patches) and the vermiform appendix. There are also nodules in the trachea and bronchial tree. The prominent nodules just described, together with some less easily seen, form a ring of gut-associated lymphoid tissue around the entrance to the respiratory and alimentary tracts, known as Waldeyer's ring (*see Figure 10.21*).

In general, lymphoid nodules are situated in the lamina propria just beneath the epithelium, although when active they may extend more deeply into the submucosa and be diffused through neighbouring tissue. Although the precise form of the nodules depends on their location, there are certain features common to all sites. It is possible to distinguish within them numerous rounded follicles, similar to those seen in lymph nodes, which have germinal centres. The latter are particularly noticeable when the follicles are actively stimulated with antigens. Between the follicles lie less closely packed parafollicular lymphocytes. The follicles and intervening tissue, together with many macrophages, are supported by a fine mesh of reticulin fibres and associated fibroblasts. In some of the larger nodules, such as the palatine tonsil, there are coarser connective tissue trabeculae. In the case of the tonsil, these arise from the capsule. The surface facing the lumen is covered with epithelium pierced by glandular or other diverticula which penetrate deeply into the aggregations of lymphocytes.

The nodules have an extensive vascular network of blood vessels branching from the surrounding connective tissue to supply the follicles with a capillary plexus, which drains into postcapillary venules. This network allows free movement of lymphocytes to and from the blood stream. The lymphatic vessels associated with the lymph nodules are exclusively efferent and drain into the general network of lymphatic channels serving the area in which they are found.

Immunofluorescent studies have demonstrated that the rounded follicles contain the B lymphocytes, and the parafollicular areas contain the T lymphocytes. These cells can move either into the lymphatic system and rejoin the blood stream, or they may move out into adjacent tissues; in the case of non-stratified epithelia, they may eventually pass into the lumen of the alimentary or respiratory tracts.

The B lymphocytes are concerned with the synthesis of secretory antibodies of the IgA class, whereas T lymphocytes are concerned with cell-mediated immunity, that is they are able to kill cells infected by viruses and fungi, or neoplastic cells.

There continues to be much discussion about the exact role of the lymphoid nodules in the total lymphoid system of the body. It seems likely that these regions provide areas in which B and T lymphocytes can proliferate and act as reservoirs of defensive cells that can infiltrate the surrounding tissue to provide local defences. As already indicated, the B lymphocytes are important in the synthesis of the antibodies of the IgA class which are present in the secretions of the alimentary tract. In the lamina propria, migrating B lymphocytes are often seen to have become transformed into plasma cells, and it is these cells that secrete the antibodies in the intercellular spaces of the unicellular epithelia and into subepithelial glands. Where the epithelial lining is of the stratified squamous type, the subepithelial glands are of particular importance in enabling the antibodies to reach the lumen. In this case, certain varieties of glandular cell appear to take up the antibodies which are then modified to form the final secretory form of IgA. The role of these antibodies is of great importance in dealing with pathogenic organisms within the various tracts in which they are found.

Pathogens which have already penetrated the epithelium are dealt with by other types of antibody, IgM and IgG, secreted by plasma cells of the lamina propria. In order that this system can work efficiently, there must be a mechanism in which the lymphocytes within the lymphoid nodules can detect antigens present on the outer luminal side of the epithelium. Recently, specialized phagocytic cells have been demonstrated in the epithelium overlying lymphoid follicles, and these appear to be capable of passing particulate material to the lymphoid tissue beneath, thus providing a route for antigens to reach the immune system (Bockman and Cooper, 1973; Owen and Jones, 1974). The longitudinal clefts of the nasopharyngeal tonsil seem to be a way of presenting a bigger surface area to the incoming air in the same way as the crypts of the palatine tonsil increase the surface area presented to food and fluid passing through the pharynx. In the case of the palatine tonsil, an additional mechanism exists which may have some significance in enabling it to undertake 'sampling'. As deglutition takes place, contraction of the pharyngeal musculature, in particular that of the two palatopharyngeus muscles, draws the tonsils towards the midline and turns them forward so that the bolus travels across the surface.

The palatine tonsil

The palatine tonsil has already been briefly described, but is dealt with in more detail here because of the importance of its surgical applied anatomy.

The tonsil is an oval mass of specialized subepithelial lymphoid tissue situated in the triangular tonsillar fossa between the diverging palatopharyngeal and palatoglossal folds (*see Figure 10.12*). The medial surface of the tonsil is free and projects to a variable extent into the oropharynx, depending partly on its size but, probably more importantly, on the degree to which it is embedded into the tonsillar fossa. In late fetal life, a triangular fold of mucous membrane extends back from the lower part of the palatoglossal fold to cover the anteroinferior part of the tonsil. In childhood, however, this fold is usually invaded by lymphoid tissue and becomes incorporated into the tonsil. It is not usually possible to distinguish it clearly. A semilunar fold of mucous membranes passes from the upper part of the palatopharyngeal arch towards the upper pole of the tonsil and separates it from the base of the uvula. The extent to which this fold is visible depends upon the prominence of the tonsil.

The appearance of the tonsil, on examination of the throat, may give a misleading estimate of its size, as indicated previously. Some tonsils appear to lie very much on the surface of the throat with only a shallow tonsillar fossa; others are much more deeply buried in a deep tonsillar fossa. The upper pole of the tonsil may extend up into the soft palate and the lower pole may extend downwards beside the base of the tongue (*Figure 10.23*). At this point, the lymphoid tissue of the tonsil is continuous with the subepithelial lymphoid tissue on the base of the tongue, the lingual tonsil. A sulcus usually separates the tonsil from the base of the tongue, the tonsillolingual sulcus.

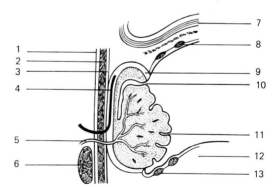

Figure 10.23 A diagram of a coronal section through the palatine tonsil to show local relationships

1. Buccopharyngeal fascia
2. Middle constrictor
3. Pharyngobasilar fascia
4. Paratonsillar vein
5. Tonsillar artery
6. Styloglossus
7. Soft palate
8. Lymphoid follicles
9. Tonsil capsule
10. Intratonsillar cleft
11. Tonsillar crypt
12. Base of tongue
13. Lingual tonsil

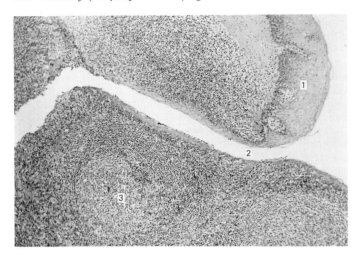

Figure 10.24 A histological section of the palatine tonsil to show mucous membrane, crypts and associated lymphoid follicles. The lymphoid tissue is slightly reactive and germinal centres can clearly be seen. Haematoxylin and eosin, × 40. (Photograph kindly provided by Dr R. H. Simpson, Senior Lecturer in Hisopathology, Exeter University)

1. Non-keratinizing squamous epithelium on the luminal surface
2. Crypt lined by similar epithelium
3. Germinal centre of lymphoid follicle

The tonsil is larger in childhood, when it is more active, and gradually becomes smaller during puberty.

Structure of the tonsil

The tonsil consists of a mass of lymphoid follicles supported in a fine connective tissue framework (*Figure 10.24*). The lymphocytes are less closely packed in the centre of each nodule, which is described as a germinal centre, because multiplication of the lymphocytes takes place in this situation. The medial surface of the tonsil, facing the lumen, is characterized by 15–20 openings, irregularly spaced over the surface, leading into deep, narrow, blind-ended recesses termed the 'tonsillar crypts'. These may penetrate nearly the whole thickness of the tonsil and distinguish it histologically from other lymphoid organs. The mucous membrane covering the luminal surface is of the non-keratinizing stratified squamous type and is continuous with that of the remainder of the oropharynx. It also dips down to line the crypts. The crypts may contain desquamated epithelial debris and cells. These plugs of debris are usually cleared from the crypts, but may occasionally remain and become hardened and yellow in appearance.

In the upper part of the tonsil, there is a deep intratonsillar cleft, much larger than the tonsillar crypts, extending laterally and inferiorly toward the lower pole of the tonsil within its capsule. This cleft lies within the substance of the tonsil. It is thought to represent a persistent part of the ventral portion of the second pharyngeal pouch. Some authorities, however, believe that the site of this part of the pouch is represented by the supratonsillar fossa, which is the area of mucous membrane above the tonsil between the palatoglossal and palatopharyngeal folds.

The deep surface of the tonsil, that is all that part not covered by mucous membrane, is covered by a fibrous capsule which is separated from the wall of the oropharynx by loose areolar tissue. This separation makes dissection of the tonsil relatively easy provided that inflammatory disease has not obliterated this space. Suppuration in this space leads to the formation of a peritonsillar abscess.

Relationships of the tonsil

The medial surface of the tonsil is free and faces towards the cavity of the oropharynx. In the act of swallowing, contraction of the musculature in this region, particularly that of the palatopharyngeus, moves the tonsil medially and turns it towards the buccal cavity.

Anteriorly and posteriorly, the tonsil is related to the palatoglossus and palatopharyngeus muscles lying within their respective folds (*Figure 10.25*). The muscles have already been described in connection with the soft palate. Some muscular fibres of the palatopharyngeus are found in the tonsil bed and are attached to the lower part of the capsule, as are fibres of the palatoglossus. Inferiorly, the capsule is firmly connected to the side of the tongue. Superiorly, the tonsil extends to a variable degree into the edge of the soft palate.

Laterally, the floor of the tonsillar fossa is formed by the pharyngobasilar fascia deep to which, in the upper part of the fossa, is the superior constrictor muscle, and below it the styloglossus muscle passing forward into the tongue (*see Figure 10.19*). Lateral to the superior constrictor is the buccopharyngeal fascia. The glossopharyngeal nerve and stylohyoid ligament pass obliquely downwards and forwards beneath the lower edge of the superior constrictor in the

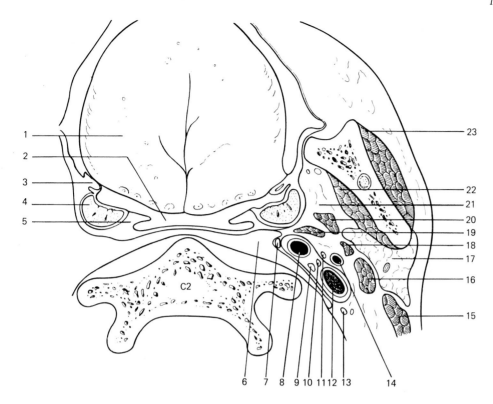

Figure 10.25 Transverse section at the level of the second cervical vertebra and tonsil to show the relations of the oropharynx including the parapharyngeal and retropharyngeal spaces

1. Tongue
2. Cavity of oropharynx
3. Palatoglossus muscle
4. Palatine tonsil
5. Palatopharyngeus muscle
6. Retropharyngeal space
7. Sympathetic ganglion
8. Internal carotid artery
9. Vagus nerve
10. Hypoglossal nerve
11. Glossopharyngeal nerve
12. Internal jugular vein
13. Accessory nerve
14. External carotid artery
15. Sternocleidomastoid muscle
16. Posterior belly of digastric
17. Parotid gland
18. Stylohyoid muscle
19. Stylopharyngeus muscle
20. Styloglossus muscle
21. Parapharyngeal space
22. Medial pterygoid muscle
23. Masseter muscle

lower part of the tonsillar fossa. A large palatine vein, the external palatine or paratonsillar vein, descends from the soft palate across the lateral aspect of the capsule of the tonsil before piercing the pharyngeal wall to join the pharyngeal plexus (*see Figure 10.23*). The tonsillar artery, a branch of the facial artery, pierces the superior constrictor and immediately enters the tonsil accompanied by two small veins. It is at this point of vascular supply that, in the course of a dissection tonsillectomy, a fibrous band will be noted between the tonsil capsule and the tonsil bed.

More distant, lateral relations of the lower part of the tonsil, outside the pharyngeal wall, are the posterior belly of the digastric muscle and the submandibular salivary gland, with the facial artery arching over them. Further laterally still are the medial pterygoid muscle and the angle of the mandible.

Nerve supply of the tonsil

The sensory nerve supply to the tonsillar region is mainly by the tonsillar branch of the glossopharyngeal nerve. The cell bodies of these fibres are in the glossopharyngeal ganglia. The upper part of the tonsil nearest to the soft palate is supplied by the lesser palatine nerves, branches of the maxillary division of the trigeminal nerve received by way of the pterygopalatine ganglia. The cell bodies of these fibres are in the trigeminal ganglion. There is no synapse in the pterygopalatine ganglion. Sympathetic fibres reach the tonsil on the arteries supplying it and are derived from the superior cervical ganglion.

Blood supply of the tonsil

The main artery of the tonsil is the tonsillar branch of the facial artery which enters the tonsil near its lower pole by piercing the superior constrictor just above the styloglossus muscle. A further arterial supply reaches the tonsil from the lingual artery, by way of the dorsal lingual branches, from the ascending palatine branch of the facial artery, and ascending pharyngeal vessels. The upper pole receives an additional supply from greater palatine vessels of the descending palatine branch of the maxillary artery.

Venous drainage of the tonsil is to the paratonsillar vein, and vessels also pass to the pharyngeal plexus or facial vein after piercing the superior constrictor. There is communication with the pterygoid plexus and drainage is eventually into the common facial and internal jugular veins.

Lymphatic drainage of the tonsil

Lymphatic vessels from the tonsil pierce the buccopharyngeal fascia and pass to the upper deep cervical group of nodes, in particular to the jugulodigastric group situated just below the posterior belly of the digastric muscle. The tonsil has no afferent lymphatic vessels.

Relationships of the pharynx

There are two important potential spaces in relation to the posterior and lateral aspects of the pharynx, and a description of these will precede an account of the other structures related to the pharynx. These spaces provide possible pathways for the spread of infection once it has entered them.

Retropharyngeal space

The potential space, known as the retropharyngeal space, lies between the prevertebral fascia posteriorly and the buccopharyngeal fascia, covering the constrictor muscles, anteriorly (*see Figure 10.25*). (The prevertebral fascia is also known as the prevertebral lamina of the cervical fascia.) The space is filled with loose areolar tissue and may contain the retropharyngeal group of lymph nodes which are present in infancy but disappear as the child grows older. The space is closed above by the base of the skull and on each side by the carotid sheath, which is a condensation of the cervical fascia in which the common and internal carotid arteries, the internal jugular vein, the vagus nerve and constitutents of the ansa cervicalis are embedded. It is thicker around the arteries than the vein. Inferiorly, it is possible to pass into the

superior mediastinum. A median partition has been described connecting the prevertebral fascia with the buccopharyngeal fascia and dividing the retropharyngeal space into two lateral spaces. However, during deglutition and movement of the head, the pharynx must be free to move and the areolar tissue that fills the space does not tether it.

Posteriorly, the prevertebral fascia covers the prevertebral muscles, longus capitis and longus cervicis, which separate it from the body and transverse processes of the cervical vertebrae. In the midline, the anterior longitudinal ligament of the vertebral column is just beneath the fascia.

Suppuration in a retropharyngeal lymph node, with the formation of pus, may push the posterior pharyngeal wall forward and present as a retropharyngeal abscess. As indicated previously, this normally occurs only in infants. It is possible, however, for such infection to spread downwards into the superior mediastinum. Infection with suppuration behind the prevertebral fascia presents laterally in the posterior triangle of the neck.

Parapharyngeal space

The potential space, filled with areolar tissue and fat, known as the parapharyngeal space and also as the lateral pharyngeal space, lies lateral to the pharynx on each side (*see Figure 10.25*). It extends from the base of the skull above, where it is widest, downwards towards the superior mediastinum. Its medial wall is formed by the buccopharyngeal fascia overlying the constrictor muscles. Its posterior wall is the prevertebral fascia. The lateral wall is formed posteriorly by the parotid gland and anteriorly by the medial pterygoid muscle overlying the angle of the mandible. The styloid process and its muscles separate, to some extent, this space from the carotid sheath, which is more posteriorly situated. In the lower part of the neck, the lateral wall is formed by the sternomastoid muscle and the infrahyoid muscles of the neck within their fascial envelope. The space contains the deep cervical group of lymph nodes. Infection may enter the space through lymphatic vessels coming to these nodes and may extend downwards toward the superior mediastinum or by way of veins to the internal jugular vein. Infection is prevented from spreading into the retropharyngeal space by the condensation of fascia around the carotid sheath.

Lateral relationships of the pharynx

The chief lateral relation running alongside the pharynx is the carotid sheath with its associated arteries, veins and nerves, together with their branches. Closely associated with the sheath are

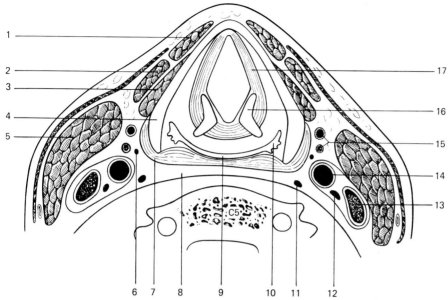

Figure 10.26 Transverse section at the level of the fifth cervical vertebra and vocal cords to show the relations of the hypopharynx and pyriform fossae

1. Sternohyoid
2. Omohyoid
3. Thyrohyoid
4. Thyroid cartilage
5. Sternocleidomastoid
6. External laryngeal nerve
7. Inferior constrictor muscle
8. Retropharyngeal space
9. Hypopharynx
10. Pyriform fossa
11. Cervical sympathetic ganglion
12. Vagus nerve
13. Internal jugular vein
14. Internal carotid artery
15. Superior thyroid artery and vein
16. Arytenoid cartilage
17. Vocal fold

the muscles and ligament arising from the styloid process. More laterally, the angles of the mandible and pterygoid muscles are related to the upper part of the pharynx anteriorly, and with the parotid gland and posterior belly of the digastric muscle more posteriorly (*see Figure 10.25*). At a lower level, the sternocleidomastoid muscle covers the carotid sheath, with the infrahyoid muscles more anteriorly and the lateral lobes of the thyroid gland interposed (*Figure 10.26*).

In particular, the superior constrictor has on its lateral surface the lingual and inferior alveolar banches of the mandibular nerve, the ascending pharyngeal artery, the ascending palatine branch of the facial artery, the stylohyoid ligament, the styloglossus and stylopharyngeus muscles and, more laterally, the medial pterygoid muscle deep to the angle of the mandible. The maxillary artery runs anteriorly to enter the pterygopalatine fossa.

The middle constrictor has on its outer surface the lingual artery, the hyoglossus muscle and the hypoglossal nerve with the tendon of the posterior belly of the digastric muscle.

The inferior constrictor has on its lateral surface the external laryngeal nerve, the thyroid gland and the sternothyroid and sternohyoid muscles together with the omohyoid.

The oesophagus

General description

The oesophagus is a muscular tube, about 25 cm in length, connecting the pharynx to the stomach. It extends from the lower border of the cricoid cartilage at the level of the sixth cervical vertebra, where it is continuous with the pharynx, to the cardiac orifice of the stomach at the side of the body of the eleventh thoracic vertebra. In passing from the pharynx to the stomach, it traverses the neck and then the superior and posterior parts of the mediastinum before piercing the diaphragm, after which it has a short abdominal course before joining the stomach.

In the new-born infant, the upper limit of the oesophagus is found at the level of the fourth or fifth cervical vertebra and it ends higher, at the level of the ninth thoracic vertebra. At birth, the length of the oesophagus varies between 8 and 10 cm, but by the end of the first year it has increased to 12 cm. Between the first and fifth years, it reaches a length of 16 cm, but growth after this is slow as it measures only 19 cm by the fifteenth year.

The diameter of the oesophagus varies according to whether or not a bolus of food or fluid is passing through it. At rest, in the adult, the diameter is about 20 mm, but this may increase to as much as 30 mm. At birth, the diameter is about 5 mm, but this dimension almost doubles in the first year, and by the age of 5 years it has attained a diameter of 15 mm. In its course from the pharynx to the stomach, the oesophagus presents an anteroposterior flexure, corresponding to the curvature of the cervical and thoracic parts of the vertebral column. It also presents two gentle curves in the coronal plane. The first begins a little below the commencement of the oesophagus and continues with a deviation to the left through the cervical and upper thoracic parts of its course, until it returns to the midline at the level of the fifth thoracic vertebra. The second coronal curve is formed as the oesophagus bends to the left to cross the descending thoracic aorta, to pierce the diaphragm and then to join the stomach.

The oesophagus is the narrowest region of the alimentary tract, except for the vermiform appendix, and it has three constrictions or indentations in its course. These are found:

(1) at 15 cm from the upper incisor teeth where the oesophagus commences at the cricopharyngeal sphincter, which is normally closed
(2) at 23 cm from the upper incisor teeth where it is crossed by the aortic arch and left main bronchus
(3) at 40 cm from the upper incisor where it pierces the diaphragm and where the lower 'physiological' oeosophageal sphincter is sited.

The oesophageal wall

The wall of the oesophagus has four layers which are, from within outwards, the mucous membrane, the submucosa, the muscle coat and an outer fibrous layer (*Figure 10.27*).

Mucous membrane of the oesophagus

The oesophagus is lined by a non-keratinizing stratified squamous epithelium which is continuous with that of the pharynx. At the junction with the stomach, however, there is an abrupt change to the columnar epithelium of that organ.

The epithelium of the oesophagus has the typical basement membrane beneath which is a loose connective tissue lamina propria containing a very fine network of elastic fibres and lymphoid nodules. At rest the mucous membrane is thrown into longitudinal folds which disappear when the organ is distended by the passage of a bolus. They can be clearly seen on a normal barium swallow (Chapter 17). Although the pharynx contains no muscularis mucosae, this layer of visceral muscle

cells makes its appearance soon after the oesophagus begins. Towards the lower end of the oesophagus, this layer becomes thicker than in any other part of the alimentary tract and, because of this thickening, it is sometimes mistakenly identified in histological preparations as part of the muscular wall.

In early embryonic life, the epithelium of the oesophagus is composed of columnar epithelium, many of the cells of which are ciliated. At the time of birth, the ciliated cells are isolated in small groups and eventually disappear. The oesophagus is now lined with stratified squamous epithelium five to six cell layers in thickness. Soon after birth, the epithelium thickens rapidly to assume its adult appearance.

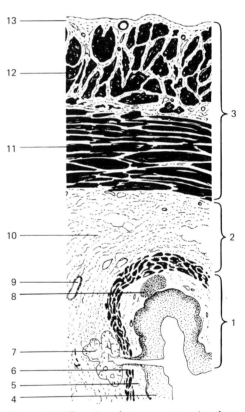

Figure 10.27 Drawing of a transverse section through the oesophageal wall. (From Hamilton, W. J., 1976, Editor, *Textbook of Human Anatomy*, 2nd edn, Figure 469, p. 359. The Macmillan Press Limited, London, by courtesy of the publishers)

1. Mucous membrane	8. Lymphoid nodule
2. Submucosa	9. Blood vessel
3. Muscle coat	10. Submucosa
4. Epithelium	11. Circular muscle
5. Lamina propria	12. Longitudinal muscle
6. Muscularis mucosae	13. Fibrous layer
7. Oesophageal gland	

The submucosa of the oesophagus

The submucosa loosely connects the mucous membrane and the muscular coat. It contains the larger blood vessels and Meissner's nerve plexus of postganglionic parasympathetic fibres, as well as the oesophageal glands which are small, compound racemose glands of the mucous type. Each gland opens into the lumen by a long duct which pierces the muscularis mucosae. These glands secrete the mucus that lubricates the passage of food through the oesophagus. The glands are distributed irregularly throughout the oesophagus. In the abdominal part of the oesophagus, near to its junction with the stomach, other glands are found which do not penetrate the muscularis mucosae and which, because structurally they resemble the cardiac glands of the stomach, are called oesophageal 'cardiac' glands. They are also found at the upper end of the oesophagus where they continue to be called 'cardiac' glands. The distal part of the duct of the oesophageal glands is lined with three or four layers of stratified squamous epithelium. Proximally, at the junction of the duct with the gland, there is a gradual transition from this stratified epithelium to a low cuboidal epithelium.

The muscular coat of the oesophagus

The muscular layer of the oesophagus is composed of an outer longitudinal and an inner circular coat. The longitudinal fibres form a complete covering for nearly the whole of the oesophagus, but at the upper end, at a point between 3 and 4 cm below the cricoid cartilage, the fibres diverge from the median plane posteriorly and form two longitudinal fasciculae which incline upwards and forwards to the front of the oesophagus where they are attached to the posterior surface of the lamina of the cricoid cartilage through a small tendon. In general, the longitudinal muscular coat of the oesophagus is thicker than the circular muscular coat.

The fibres of the circular coat are continuous superiorly with the fibres of the cricopharyngeus part of the inferior constrictor. Anteriorly, these fibres are inserted into the lateral margins of the tendon, already described, of the longitudinal fibres. Inferiorly, the circular muscle fibres are continuous with the oblique fibres of the stomach. At the lower end of the oesophagus, the circular fibres form one component of a 'physiological' sphincter which will be described later.

In the upper third of the oesophagus, the muscle fibres of both coats are striated. In the middle third, there is a gradual transition to non-striated muscle, and the lower third contains non-striated muscle only.

Fibrous layer of the oesophagus

The fibrous layer consists of an external adventitia of irregular, dense connective tissue containing many elastin fibres. The arrangement of this tissue allows expansion during swallowing and maintains the position of the oesophagus in relation to adjacent structures. In the abdominal segment of the oesophagus there is an additional covering of peritoneum. At the diaphragmatic opening, the fibrous layer attaches the oesophagus to the margins of the opening and this attachment is known as the phreno-oesophageal ligament.

The presence of this adventitial layer makes it possible for the oesophagus to be mobilized by blunt finger dissection during operations from above and below without the chest being opened. It can then be withdrawn from the thorax as, for example, in the operation of pharyngolaryngo-oesophagectomy.

Nerve supply of the oesophagus

The striated muscle in the upper third of the oesophagus is supplied by the recurrent laryngeal branches of the vagus. The cell bodies for these fibres are in the rostral part of the nucleus ambiguus. However, the chief motor supply to the non-striated muscle is parasympathetic, and the cell bodies for these fibres are in the dorsal nucleus of the vagus. They reach the oesophagus by way of the oesophageal branches of the vagus itself and through its recurrent laryngeal branches, and synapse in the oesophageal wall in the ganglia of the submucosal plexus (Meissner's) and myenteric plexus (Auerbach's), which is between the outer longitudinal and inner circular muscle layers. From these cell bodies, short postganglionic fibres emerge to innervate the muscle fibres.

The cell bodies of the preganglionic sympathetic motor fibres are found in the lateral grey column of the spinal cord in thoracic segments 2 to 6 (chiefly 5 and 6). The fibres pass out in the anterior nerve roots and reach the sympathetic trunk by way of white rami communicantes. They then run upwards to the cervical ganglia where they synapse. From these ganglia, postganglionic fibres pass down into the thorax by the superior, middle, and inferior cardiac nerves to join the cardiac plexus, which they traverse without synapsing to reach the oesophagus. Some sympathetic fibres take a more direct route to the oesophagus by way of the thoracic ganglia 2 to 6, where the synapses are situated. The cervical oesophagus receives its sympathetic supply by means of a plexus around the inferior thyroid artery. The thoracic oesophagus has branches from the sympathetic trunks which form plexuses around the blood vessels supplying this section. In the abdominal oesophagus, the plexuses form around the left gastric and inferior phrenic arteries.

Afferent fibres from the oesophagus run with the branches of the vagus and have their cell bodies in the inferior vagal ganglion from where impulses reach the dorsal vagal nucleus and nucleus of the tractus solitarius. Some of the afferent fibres that run with the sympathetic nerves convey pain sensation.

Oesophageal pain

From cervical cardiac nerves and sympathetic trunk ganglia, fibres enter the thoracic spinal nerves by way of grey rami communicantes. Although any one of the thoracic nerves may be involved, most of the pain fibres have their cell bodies in the dorsal root ganglia of thoracic spinal nerves 5 and 6. After entering the spinal cord, the fibres synapse with cell bodies in the gelatinous substance and posterior horn. The impulses are then conveyed by the lateral spinothalamic tract to the thalamus. The stimulus which seems to initiate oesophageal pain is tension in the muscular wall, resulting from either distension or muscular spasm. The mucosa is sensitive to heat and cold but not to touch. Chemical stimulation by reflux of gastric acid may, under certain conditions, cause pain.

Oesophageal pain is poorly localized and is referred to other areas. It can be severe and, if retrosternal, resembles cardiac pain. Pain produced by experimental oesophageal distension is localized anteriorly in the midline of the body in the region of the sternum. The area of reference to which the pain is projected corresponds roughly with the level of the part of the oesophagus being distended. Pain from the upper oesophagus is referred to the suprasternal region; that from the middle of the oesophagus to the retrosternal region; and that from the lower end of the oesophagus to the epigastrium.

Another variety of oesophageal pain, commonly called heartburn, is a burning, hot sensation felt under the lower part of the sternum and radiating up into the neck and jaw. The sensation may be accompanied by regurgitation of acid fluid into the throat. This pain is often ascribed to irritation of the oesophageal mucosa by acid regurgitation from the stomach. However, heartburn has been reported in patients with achlorhydria, and instillation of acid into normal oesophagus may not cause this sensation. On the other hand, a burning sensation similar to heartburn has been produced by inflation of a balloon introduced into the lower oesophagus in normal subjects. Furthermore, radiological studies have shown that during an attack of heartburn, the whole oesophagus is often in spasm. This suggests that the cause of

heartburn sensation is not primarily acid reflux, but a prolonged spastic contraction of muscle comparable to that causing the pain of intestinal colic. In some patients, where there is inflammation of the oesophageal mucosa, the pain threshold may be lowered and reflux of gastric acid may well precipitate heartburn. It is still possible, however, that the mechanism of the pain production is that the acid irritates the lower oesophageal mucosa causing muscle spasm.

Blood supply of the oesophagus

The oesophagus obtains its blood supply from adjacent vessels. In the cervical part, this is from the inferior thyroid arteries which arise from the thyrocervical trunks of the subclavian artery. In addition, a supply is obtained from the left subclavian artery. In its thoracic part, the oesophagus is supplied segmentally, either directly from the descending thoracic aorta, or by way of branches of the bronchial or upper posterior intercostal arteries. In its abdominal part, the oesophagus is supplied by the left gastric branch of the coeliac trunk and the left inferior phrenic artery direct from the abdominal aorta.

An extensive venous plexus is formed on the exterior of the oesophagus and drains in a segmental way similar to the arterial supply. In the neck, the veins drain into the inferior thyroid veins; in the thorax they drain to the azygos and hemi-azygos system; and in the abdomen into the left gastric vein. This vein is a tributary of the portal system, whereas the other veins are part of the systemic system. The lower end of the oesophagus is a site of major importance for portal–systemic anastomoses and there is free communication between the two systems. When there is portal obstruction, the multiple, small thin-walled subepithelial veins in this region become varicose and may break down and bleed heavily into the lumen.

At the upper end of the oesophagus, longitudinal submucosal oesophageal veins enter the pharyngeal/laryngeal plexus situated on the posterior and anterior walls of the pharynx at the level of the cricoid cartilage.

Lymphatic drainage of the oesophagus

Two networks of lymphatic vessels are found in the oesophagus. There is a plexus of fairly large vessels in the mucous membrane which is continuous above with those of the pharynx and below with those of the gastric mucosa. The second plexus of finer vessels is present within the muscular coat and, although this may be independent of the mucosal plexus, it drains by the same collecting vessels. The latter leave the oesophagus in two ways, either piercing the muscular coat immediately and draining into neighbouring nodes, or ascending and descending beneath the mucosa. The efferent vessels from the cervical part of the oesophagus drain into the lower group of deep cervical nodes and into the paratracheal nodes. Vessels from the thoracic part drain into the posterior mediastinal nodes and the tracheo-bronchial nodes. Vessels from the abdominal part pass to the left gastric nodes. Some vessels may pass directly to the thoracic duct.

The oesophageal sphincters

A full account of the working of the oesophageal sphincters in the course of deglutition is given in Chapter 11. This section deals with some anatomical aspects of the sphincters.

The upper oesophageal sphincter

The upper oesophageal sphincter is provided by the cricopharyngeus part of the inferior constrictor which encircles the oesophageal entrance, being attached to each side of the cricoid cartilage. This muscle has no posterior median raphe. Its fibres are continuous with the circular muscle coat of the oesophagus below. It is described in more detail above, where its nerve supply is also detailed.

This sphincter is always closed, and manometric studies demonstrate a region of raised pressure over about 3 cm in length. The pressure profile in this region shows a 1-cm zone of rising pressure proximally followed by 1 cm of peak pressure reaching about 35 mmHg. This region of peak pressure corresponds to the position of the cricopharyngeus. Beyond this is a distal 1 cm in which the pressure decreases to atmospheric pressure. These recordings demonstrate the existence of a tonic sphincter that is very competent.

The lower oesophageal sphincter

It is not possible to demonstrate a lower oesophageal sphincter histologically, on account of there being no thickening of the circular muscle coat. Manometric studies demonstrate a zone of raised pressure about 3 cm in length at the oesophagogastric junction extending above and below the diaphragm. The mean pressure here is approximately 8 mmHg higher than the intra-gastric pressure. Although this pressure is only slightly in excess of that in the stomach, regurgitation of gastric contents does not normally occur. This 'sphincter' region of the oesophagus, with an intraluminal pressure higher than the rest of the oesophagus or stomach, is regarded as one

component of a 'physiological' sphincter at the oesophagogastric zone. Radiological studies show that swallowed food is momentarily held up at the lower end of the oesophagus, before entry into the stomach. The possible components of this sphincter mechanism are as follows:

(1) An intrinsic sphincter. Present in the circular muscle fibres of the oesophagus, described previously.
(2) Pinch-cock effect of the diaphragm. The fibres of the right crus of the diaphragm split to encircle the oesophageal opening and may play an auxiliary role in achieving an effective lower oesophageal sphincter.
(3) Mucosal folds. These have been described at the lower end of the oesophagus and have been thought to exert a valvular effect (*Figure 10.28*). They may be thrown into prominence by contraction of the muscularis mucosae.
(4) Oblique muscle fibres of the stomach. The portion of the stomach adjacent to the oesophageal opening has a definite collar of muscle which is part of the innermost oblique muscle layer of the stomach. The fibres sweep up from the lesser curvature to encircle the terminal oesophagus. They may help to preserve the angle between the left edge of the oesophageal opening and the fundus of the stomach, the cardiac notch.
(5) Thoracoabdominal pressure gradient. The thoracic part of the oesophagus is subject to a negative pressure as opposed to the abdominal oesophagus which has a positive pressure applied to it. It is felt that this pressure differential may collapse the lower end of the oesophagus like a mechanical flutter valve, preventing reflux. Food and fluid passing down the oesophagus would open this valve, but it would otherwise remain closed.
(6) Oesophagogastric junction angle. It has been suggested that the sharp angle at which the left edge of the oesophagus meets the fundus of the stomach forms a fold that can act as a mechanical flap valve. A rise of intragastric pressure will compress the adjacent part of the terminal oesophagus and prevent a reflux. The higher the pressure in the stomach, the more securely will this flap valve be closed. The angle of entry of the oesophagus into the stomach is, however, very variable in humans, and patients appear to suffer reflux despite a normal oesophagogastric angle.

The way in which a competent lower oesophageal sphincter is achieved remains uncertain, but it seems that a number of mechanisms may act in concert to accomplish this (*Figure 10.29*).

276

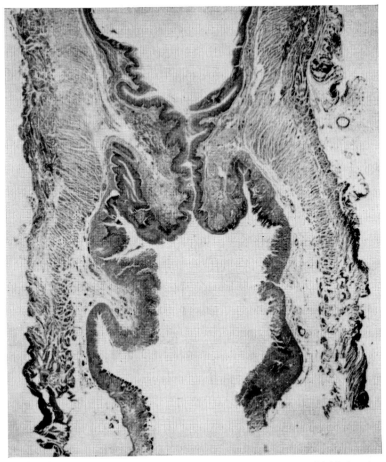

Figure 10.28 Section of oesophagogastric junction showing mucosal folds forming a valve. (From Creamer, 1955, reproduced by courtesy of the Editor of *The Lancet*)

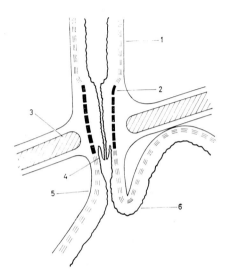

Figure 10.29 A diagram to illustrate some factors involved in the prevention of oesophagogastric reflux

1. Negative intrathoracic pressure
2. Intrinsic muscular sphincter
3. Pinch-cock effect of right crus of diaphragm
4. Mucosal folds
5. Positive intra-abdominal pressure
6. Oesophagogastric angle

Relationships of the oesophagus

The relationships of the cervical, thoracic and abdominal parts of the oesophagus will be dealt with separately. They are illustrated from anterior and lateral aspects in *Figures 10.30–10.32* and in cross-section at different levels in *Figures 10.33–10.40*.

The cervical part of the oesophagus

In the neck, the trachea lies anterior to the oesophagus attached by loose connective tissue. The recurrent laryngeal nerves ascend on each side in the groove between the trachea and oesophagus (*Figure 10.30* and *10.33*). Posteriorly, the oesophagus rests on the prevertebral fascia covering the C6–C8 vertebral bodies and the prevertebral muscles. The thoracic duct passes upwards behind the left border of the oesophagus and, at the level of C6, the duct arches laterally between the carotid and vertebral systems before opening into the junction of the left internal jugular and left subclavian veins. Laterally, on each side, lie the corresponding parts of the carotid sheath together with its contents, with the lower poles of the lateral lobes of the thyroid gland between.

Thoracic part of the oesophagus

In the superior mediastinum, the oesophagus lies between the trachea and the vertebral column, slightly to the left of the median plane. It passes behind and to the right of the aortic arch and enters the posterior mediastinum at the level of the fourth thoracic vertebra (*Figures 10.30–10.32*). It is related anteriorly to the trachea and posteriorly to the third to fourth thoracic vertebrae (*Figures 10.34–10.36*). The left recurrent laryngeal nerve is in the groove between the oesophagus and trachea on the left. The thoracic duct is behind the left oesophageal border.

Laterally, adjacent to the left border of the oesophagus, is the arch of the aorta passing from before backwards and slightly to the left, with the vagus nerve crossing the arch on its outer side and giving rise to the left recurrent laryngeal branch, which hooks beneath the ligamentum arteriosum to reach the groove between the oesophagus and the trachea. The left subclavian artery is immediately to the left of the oesophagus as the vessel arises from the aortic arch. On the right side, adjacent to the right margin of the oesophagus, is the azygos vein arching from posterior to anterior over the lung root to enter the superior vena cava. The mediastinal pleura of both sides is in contact with the oesophagus, separated on the right by the azygos vien and on the left by the aortic arch and left subclavian artery.

In the posterior mediastinum, anterior to the oesophagus, the trachea bifurcates at the level of the fifth thoracic vertebra and below this the fibrous pericardium comes into contact with the anterior surface of the oesophagus (*Figures 10.30–*

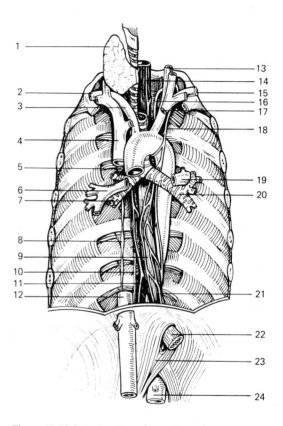

Figure 10.30 Anterior view of superior and posterior mediastinal structures to show course and relations of the oesophagus

1. Right lobe of thyroid
2. Right subclavian artery
3. Brachiocephalic artery
4. Superior vena cava
5. Azygos vein
6. Right pulmonary artery
7. Right principal bronchus
8. Sympathetic trunk
9. Right vagus nerve
10. Azygos vein
11. Thoracic duct
12. Inferior vena cava
13. Left common carotid artery
14. Left recurrent laryngeal nerve
15. Left subclavian artery
16. Thoracic duct
17. Left brachiocephalic vein
18. Left vagus nerve
19. Left pulmonary artery
20. Left principal bronchus
21. Left vagus nerve
22. Abdominal oesophagus
23. Right crus of diaphragm
24. Abdominal aorta

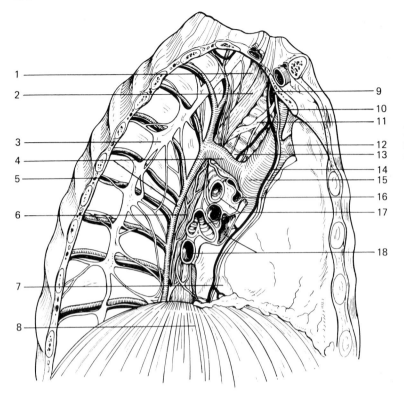

Figure 10.31 The right side of the mediastinum to show the course and relations of the oesophagus

1. Longus colli muscle
2. Oesophagus
3. Sympathetic trunk
4. Azygos vein
5. Intercostal vessels and nerve
6. Nerve plexus on oesophagus
7. Inferior vena cava
8. Dome of diaphragm
9. Brachiocephalic artery
10. Right brachiocephalic vein
11. Right vagus nerve
12. Left brachiocephalic vein
13. Trachea
14. Phrenic nerve
15. Superior vena cava
16. Right pulmonary artery
17. Right principal bronchi
18. Right pulmonary veins

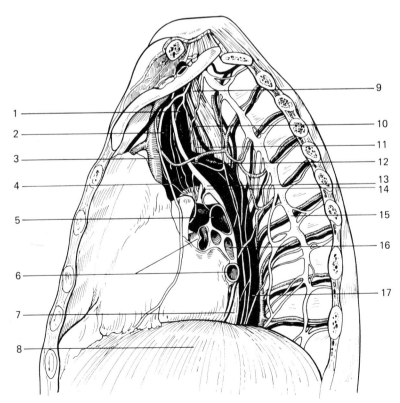

Figure 10.32 The left side of the mediastinum to show the course and relations of the oesophagus

1. Left subclavian artery
2. Left common carotid artery
3. Left brachiocephalic vein
4. Left phrenic nerve
5. Left pulmonary artery
6. Left pulmonary veins
7. Oesophagus
8. Dome of diaphragm
9. Longus colli muscle
10. Thoracic duct
11. Oesophagus
12. Aortic arch
13. Vagus nerve
14. Left recurrent laryngeal nerve
15. Sympathetic nerve trunk
16. Left principal bronchi
17. Descending thoracic aorta

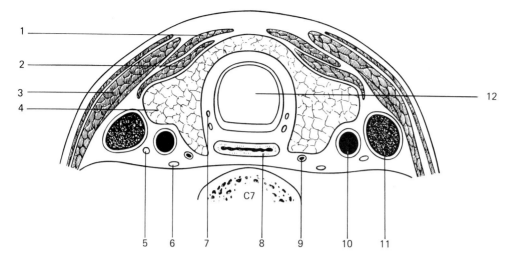

Figure 10.33 Transverse section at the level of the seventh cervical vertebra and commencement of the trachea and oesophagus to show the relations of the latter

1. Sternohyoid muscle
2. Sternothyroid muscle
3. Sternocleidomastoid muscle
4. Thyroid gland
5. Left vagus nerve
6. Cervical sympathetic ganglion
7. Left recurrent laryngeal nerve
8. Oesophagus
9. Inferior thyroid artery
10. Common carotid artery
11. Internal jugular vein
12. Trachea

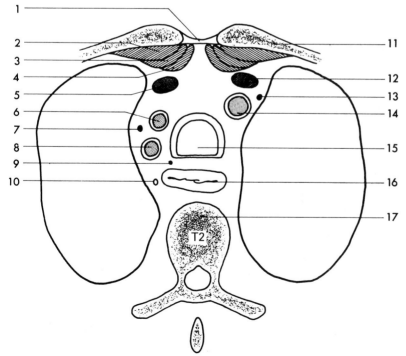

Figure 10.34 Transverse section at the level of the second thoracic vertebra and suprasternal notch to show the relationships of the lower cervical oesophagus

1. Suprasternal notch
2. Sternocleidomastoid muscle
3. Sternohyoid muscle
4. Sternothyroid muscle
5. Left brachiocephalic vein
6. Left common carotid artery
7. Left vagus nerve
8. Left subclavian artery
9. Left recurrent laryngeal nerve
10. Thoracic duct
11. Right clavicle
12. Right brachiocephalic vein
13. Right vagus nerve
14. Brachiocephalic artery
15. Trachea
16. Oesophagus
17. Second thoracic vertebra

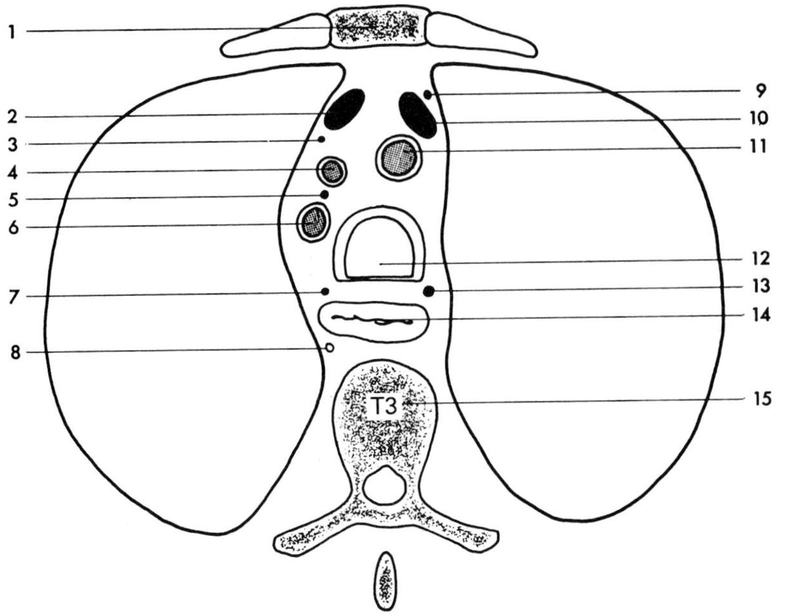

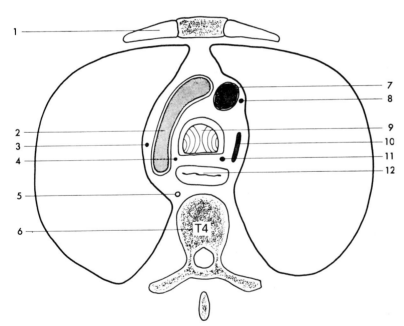

Figure 10.35 Transverse section at the level of the third thoracic vertebra just above the level of the aortic arch to show relationships of the oesophagus in the superior mediastinum

1. Manubrium sterni
2. Left brachiocephalic vein
3. Left phrenic nerve
4. Left common carotid artery
5. Left vagus nerve
6. Left subclavian artery
7. Left recurrent laryngeal nerve
8. Thoracic duct
9. Right phrenic nerve
10. Right brachiocephalic vein
11. Brachiocephalic artery
12. Trachea
13. Right vagus nerve
14. Oesophagus
15. Third thoracic vertebra

Figure 10.36 Transverse section at the level of the fourth thoracic vertebra and tracheal bifurcation to show relationships of the oesophagus at the junction of superior mediastinum with posterior mediastinum

1. Second costal cartilage
2. Aortic arch
3. Left vagus nerve
4. Left recurrent laryngeal nerve
5. Thoracic duct
6. Fourth thoracic vertebra
7. Superior vena cava
8. Right phrenic nerve
9. Tracheal bifurcation
10. Azygos vein
11. Right vagus nerve
12. Oesophagus

10.40). At the bifurcation of the trachea, the oesophagus is crossed anteriorly by the left principal bronchus passing into the left lung root beneath the aortic arch. It may indent the oesophagus anteriorly on the left. The right pulmonary artery crosses the oesophagus immediately below the tracheal bifurcation. The inferior tracheobronchial lymph nodes are inter-posed between the bifurcation of the trachea and the oesophagus. Below this, it is the left atrium of the heart that lies in front of the oesophagus, separated only by the pericardium and its oblique sinus. Lower still, the diaphragm is in front until the oesophagus enters the abdomen.

Posteriorly, in the posterior mediastinum, are the vertebral column and the long cervical

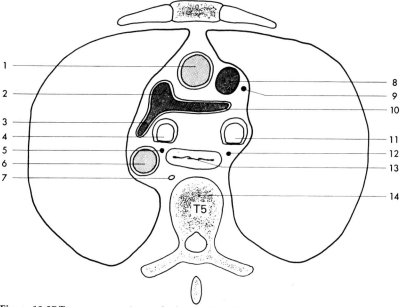

Figure 10.37 Transverse section at the level of the fifth thoracic vertebra approximately 3 cm distal to the tracheal bifurcation and just above the heart to show relationships of the oesophagus in the posterior mediastinum

1. Ascending aorta
2. Pulmonary trunk
3. Left pulmonary artery
4. Left principal bronchus
5. Left vagus nerve

6. Descending thoracic aorta
7. Thoracic duct
8. Superior vena cava
9. Right phrenic nerve
10. Right pulmonary artery

11. Right principal bronchus
12. Right vagus nerve
13. Oesophagus
14. Fifth thoracic vertebra

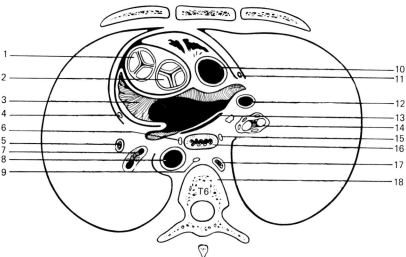

Figure 10.38 Transverse section through the mediastinum at the level of the sixth thoracic vertebra and left atrium, to show the relationships of the oesophagus in the posterior mediastinum

1. Pulmonary valve
2. Aortic valve
3. Left atrium
4. Left phrenic nerve
5. Left pulmonary artery
6. Left vagus nerve
7. Left principal bronchus

8. Descending thoracic aorta
9. Thoracic duct
10. Superior vena cava
11. Right phrenic nerve
12. Right pulmonary artery

13. Oblique sinus
14. Right principal bronchus
15. Right vagus nerve
16. Oesophagus
17. Azygos vein
18. Sixth thoracic vertebra

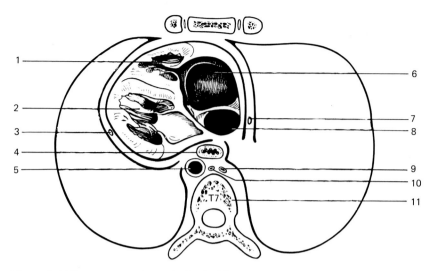

Figure 10.39 Transverse section at the level of the seventh thoracic vertebra and left ventricle to show the relationships of the oesophagus to the heart in the lower posterior mediastinum

1. Right ventricle
2. Left ventricle
3. Left phrenic nerve
4. Oesophagus with nerve plexus
5. Descending thoracic aorta
6. Right atrium
7. Right phrenic nerve
8. Inferior vena cava
9. Azygos vein
10. Thoracic duct
11. Seventh thoracic vertebra

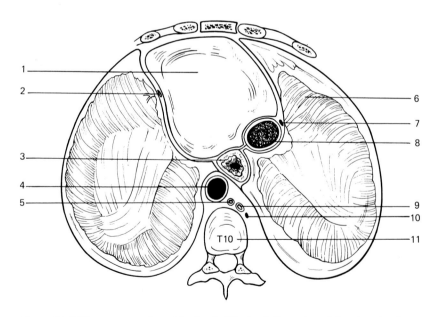

Figure 10.40 Transverse section at the level of the tenth thoracic vertebra showing the relationships of the oesophagus at the diaphragm

1. Pericardial sac
2. Left phrenic nerve
3. Oesophagus
4. Descending aorta
5. Thoracic duct
6. Dome of diaphragm
7. Right phrenic nerve
8. Inferior vena cava
9. Azygos vein
10. Splanchnic nerve
11. Tenth thoracic vertebra

muscles. The right posterior intercostal arteries arising from the descending thoracic aorta pass toward the right across the vertebral column. The thoracic duct enters the thorax through the right side of the aortic opening in the diaphragm and runs up behind the right margin of the oesophagus until, at the level of the fifth thoracic vertebra, it crosses obliquely to come to lie behind the left margin as described previously. The two hemi-azygos veins intervene between the oesophagus and the vertebral column, at the level of the seventh and eighth thoracic vertebrae, as they pass across to join the azygos vein on the right. Inferiorly, near the diaphragm, the aorta passes behind the oesophagus as the latter curves toward the left and turns forward to pass through the diaphragm to the stomach.

On the left side, in the posterior mediastinum, the oesophagus is related to the descending thoracic aorta and left mediastinal pleura (*see Figure 10.32*). On the right side, the oesophagus is related to the right pleura separated only by the azygos vein (*see Figure 10.31*). The left and right vagus nerves, having branched to form the cardiac and pulmonary plexuses, come together again as the oesophageal plexus on the oesophageal wall and then form single or multiple nerve trunks that descend with the oesophagus through the same opening in the diaphragm (*see Figure 10.30*). The left vagal fibres usually lie on the anterior surface of the oesophagus and those on the right posteriorly.

Abdominal part of the oesophagus

After the oesophagus emerges from the right crus of the diaphragm, slightly to the left of the median plane at the level of the tenth thoracic vertebra, it comes to lie in the oesophageal groove on the posterior surface of the left lobe of the liver. It curves sharply to the left to join the stomach at the cardia (*see Figure 10.30*). The right border of the oesophagus continues evenly into the lesser curvature of the stomach, while the left border is separated from the fundus of the stomach by the cardiac notch. This short abdominal section of the oesophagus is covered with the peritoneum of the greater sac anteriorly and on its left side, and with the lesser sac on the right. It is contained in the upper left portion of the lesser omentum and the peritoneum, reflected from its posterior surface to the diaphragm, is part of the gastrophrenic ligament in which the oesophageal branches of the left gastric vessels pass to the oesophagus. Behind the oesophagus at this level are the left crus of the diaphragm and the left inferior phrenic artery.

References

ANDERSON, J. E. (1983) *Grant's Atlas of Anatomy*, 8th edn. London: Williams and Wilkins

AZZAM, N. A. and KUEHN, D. P. (1977) The morphology of musculus uvulae. *Cleft Palate Journal*, **14**, 78–87

BOCKMAN, D. E. and COOPER, M. D. (1973) Pinocytosis by epithelium associated with lymphoid follicles in the bursa of Fabricus, appendix and Peyer's patches. An electron microscopic study. *American Journal of Anatomy*, **136**, 455–477

BROOMHEAD, I. W. (1951) The nerve supply of the muscles of the soft palate. *British Journal of Plastic Surgery*, **4**, 1–15

CALNAN, J. (1958) Modern views on Passavant's ridge. *British Journal of Plastic Surgery*, **10**, 89–113

CREAMER, B. (1955) Oesophageal reflux and the action of carminatives. *The Lancet*, **1**, 590–592

FRITZELL, B. (1976) Palatal function. In *Scientific Foundations of Otolaryngology*, edited by R. Hinchcliffe and D. Harrison, pp. 484–493. London: William Heinemann

HAMILTON, W. J. (ed.) (1976) *Textbook of Human Anatomy*, 2nd edn. London: Macmillan Press Limited

HARMER, M. H. (ed.) (1978) *TNM Classification of Malignant Tumours*, 3rd edn., pp. 27–32. Geneva: International Union Against Cancer

HOLBOROW, C. A. (1970) Eustachian tubal function. *Archives of Otolaryngolgy*, **92**, 624–626

HOLBOROW, C. A. (1975) Eustachian tubal function, changes throughout childhood and neuromuscular control. *Journal of Laryngology and Otology*, **89**, 47–55

IBUKI, K., MATSUYA, T., NISHIO, J., HAMAMURA, Y. and MIYAZAKI, T. (1978) The course of the facial nerve innervation for the levator palatini muscle. *Cleft Palate Journal*, **15**, 209–214

LANGMAN, J. (1981) *Medical Embryology*, 4th edn. Baltimore: Williams and Wilkins

McMINN, R. M. H. and HOBDELL, M. H. (1974) *The Functional Anatomy of the Digestive System*. London: Pitman Medical

MONTGOMERY, W. W. (1973) *Surgery of the Upper Respiratory Tract*, Vol. 2. Philadelphia: Lea and Febiger

MOSELEY, J. M., MATHEWS, E. W., BREED, R. H., GALANTE, E., TSE, A. and MacINTYRE, I. (1968) The ultimobranchial origin of calcitonin. *The Lancet*, **1**, 108–110

NISHIO, J., MATSUYA, T., MACHIDA, J. and MIYAZAKI, T. (1976a) The motor nerve supply of the velopharyngeal muscles. *Cleft Palate Journal*, **13**, 20–30

NISHIO, J., MATSUYA, T., IBUKI, K. and MIYAZAKI, T. (1976b) Roles of the facial, glossopharyngeal and vagus nerves in velopharyngeal movement. *Cleft Palate Journal*, **13**, 201–214

OWEN, R. L. and JONES, A. L. (1974) Epithelial cell specialisation within human Peyer's patches. An ultrastructural study of intestinal lymphoid follicles. *Gastroenterology*, **66**, 189–203

PIGOTT, R. W. (1969) The nasendoscopic appearance of the normal palatopharyngeal valve. *Plastic and Reconstructive Surgery*, **43**, 19–24

WHILLIS, J. (1930) A note on the muscles of the palate and the superior constrictor. *Journal of Anatomy*, **65**, 92–95

WILLIAMS, P. L. and WARWICK, R. (1980) *Gray's Anatomy*, 36th edn. London: Churchill Livingstone

11

Deglutition

W. S. Lund

Deglutition is the process whereby a bolus, liquid or solid, is transferred from the buccal cavity to the stomach. Swallowing is a complex, integrated, continuous act, involving somatic and visceral, afferent and efferent nerves together with their associated striated and smooth muscles. For simplicity of description, it is useful to divide deglutition into three phases which correspond to the three anatomical regions through which the bolus passes:

(1) oral
(2) pharyngeal
(3) oesophageal.

The initiation of the first two phases is subject to conscious control and involves striated muscles controlled by a complex of stimulatory and inhibitory signals from the brainstem. The third phase involves the smooth muscle of the oesophageal wall and depends on both central coordination and local, intramural neural arcs.

The act of swallowing has been studied from two points of view:

(1) mechanical (cineradiography and intraluminal manometry)
(2) neurophysiological, in which neural impulses are traced from afferent signals through the swallowing centre to the motor nerves in an attempt to understand the 'wiring diagram' that programmes this complex muscular response.

Oral stage

In their extensive studies of deglutition, Ardran and Kemp (1955) considered that in the first or oral stage the tongue is involved in squeezing food out of the mouth and oropharynx. When swallowing begins, the tip of the tongue is raised to the back of the incisor teeth and is then applied to the palate from before backwards, so squeezing the contents of the mouth into the pharynx. When the tail of the bolus has been expelled from the mouth, the back of the tongue arches posteriorly to meet the soft palate and pharyngeal wall. The nasopharynx is closed by the elevation of the soft palate in combination with the contraction of the superior pharyngeal constrictors.

No account of the variations in the behaviour of the tongue in swallowing can be understood without first following the movements of the hyoid bone, to which most of the extrinsic muscles of the tongue and the floor of the mouth are attached. The contraction of these muscles influences the volume and disposition of the tongue's substance relative to the mouth cavity.

Normal individuals swallow the contents of the mouth in the midline furrow in the tongue. When chewing, food may pass down the upper lateral food channels at the sides of the tongue to the valleculae, as in the rabbit.

Patients with a gap in the palate (congenital or acquired) may also divert food to the sides of the tongue and may plug the gap by raising the tongue in the midline. Patients with holes in the cheek, for example from a gunshot injury, learn to swallow on the opposite side, as do patients with unilateral weakness of the tongue. After food has been introduced into the mouth, space for it is normally made by lowering the tongue, the floor of the mouth and the hyoid bone.

During the act of swallowing, the jaws are brought together as the tongue fills the oral cavity to displace its contents and the hyoid bone is raised towards the lower border of the mandible. Maximum elevation of the hyoid bone is reached as the tail of the bolus is being expelled from the mouth, and is maintained as the tongue arches backwards to displace the bolus downwards. These movements of the hyoid bone relate to the need to adjust the volume of the tongue. As the bolus is displaced from the mouth, the tongue reoccupies its position of rest in the mouth cavity. However, as the tongue must also arch backwards to displace the bolus downwards, the volume of the tongue necessary to occlude the mouth must be further reduced by raising of the floor of the mouth. In other words, maximum elevation of the hyoid bone is indicative of maximum contraction of the mylohyoid muscle, thus reducing the mouth proper to the smallest possible size. If a large bolus is swallowed, the tongue (and hyoid bone) must be pulled well forward to provide adequate accommodation for the bolus to be taken into and through the pharynx; thus maximum displacement of the hyoid forwards relates to the degree of distension of the oropharynx.

The whole of a mouthful may not always be swallowed as a single bolus; for example, when a large mouthful is taken, the subject may elect to swallow it by means of a series of boluses. To do this, the subject releases a quantity of the content into the pharynx by parting the tongue and soft palate and then raising the tongue in the back of the mouth behind the junction of the hard and soft palates, thus cutting off the bolus in the pharynx from the rest of the contents of the mouth proper. The contents of the pharynx are then cleared by apposition of the constrictors to the back of the tongue and soft palate in the usual manner. In these circumstances, there is no oral phase of swallowing until the last mouthful is to be expelled.

Accordingly, it is possible to dissociate the forepart of the tongue from swallowing and to use it for some other purpose while swallowing is continuing. The forepart of the tongue may be lowered in the front of the mouth to create suction as occurs when drinking, or as part of the mechanism of sucking, or when the mouth is opened, as in pint-swallowing, to create a large cavity into which food can be taken or poured. With the conclusion of all these acts, it is necessary to clear the mouth either by dribbling with the head inclined forwards, or by using the whole of the tongue to swallow the contents of the mouth.

The forepart of the tongue is also used for manipulation of food in preparation for mastication and in the formation of consonants in speech; manipulation may continue during pharyngeal swallowing. The anterior third of the tongue, which corresponds with the free portion in conjunction with the lips and jaws, is mainly responsible for procedures requiring manipulation in feeding and speech. These include:

(1) taking food from a spoon or fork, for example lapping, licking etc
(2) manipulation of food in the forepart of the mouth, including cleaning the teeth and palate
(3) expressing the contents of teat or nipple, and the initial stage of swallowing
(4) forming consonants in speech, and whistling
(5) expression of emotion.

The middle third of the tongue, which corresponds to the region opposite the molar teeth, is responsible for:

(1) pressing of food on to the molars for chewing
(2) the passage of food into the upper lateral food channels at the side of the tongue
(3) the following functions when it is elevated:
   (a) cutting off the mouth cavity from the pharynx, for example, when regulating the swallowing of a large mouthful by multiple boluses
   (b) altering the shape of the oropharyngeal cavity to form vowel sounds
   (c) plugging a hole in the hard or soft palate, or cheek
   (d) compensating for a paralysed soft palate by preventing or reducing nasopharyngeal reflux in the pharyngeal phase of swallowing.

The posterior third of the tongue:

(1) acts mainly as a wedge of tissue in the pharyngeal phase of swallowing which, when opposed to the soft palate and pharyngeal constrictors, displaces the bolus downwards and helps to turn down the epiglottis
(2) in its apposition to the soft palate when the mouth is closed, normally closes off the mouth cavity at rest
(3) can be apposed to the pharyngeal wall to close off the airway to reinforce or substitute for laryngeal closure in certain circumstances; for example some normal subjects when bearing down, or in patients who can use glossopharyngeal breathing, but who cannot close the larynx.

The whole of the tongue, from before backwards, is normally involved in the coordinated peristaltic wave which squeezes food from the mouth into the lower pharynx. By a reverse response, the tongue, as it is lowered from before backwards, creates a suction mechanism, as is seen in the continuous swallowing associated with suckling or drinking.

Pharyngeal stage

When swallowing takes place in the erect position, the first half of the bolus is passed through the pharynx into the oesophagus by means of thrust from the tongue, assisted by gravity. The peristaltic wave usually commences when the tongue expressor wave reaches the soft palate. With a moderate-sized fluid bolus, the head of the bolus has often entered the oesophagus before the pharyngeal peristaltic wave has commenced.

This wave moves rapidly and smoothly downwards, clearing the pharynx of the hindpart of the bolus and pushing it through into the oesophagus. Normally, no hold-up occurs at the cricopharyngeal sphincter as the wave of relaxation, preceding the contraction of the pharynx, reduces the resting tone of the cricopharyngeal muscles. The peristaltic wave involves the sphincter as it descends, inducing tight closure of it. The sphincter subsequently relaxes and returns to its resting state after the peristaltic wave has passed.

Studies conducted by Ardran and Kemp (1961) showed that swallowing in the lower half of the pharynx occurs down the lateral lower food channels. The latter extend from the edge of the lateral pharyngoepiglottic folds downwards and backwards around the laryngeal air passage to the level of the cricopharyngeal sphincter where they fuse and become one channel continuous with the lumen of the oesophagus. These channels are functional entities and serve to transmit fluid or semifluid substances around the mouth of the larynx, thus preventing spill into the laryngeal airway. During swallowing, the bulk of a bolus is usually deflected to either side of the mouth of the larynx and comparatively little passes directly over the edge of the tongue or the epiglottis down the midline. If the bolus is large, the larynx is pulled further forward to accommodate it, and the two channels become one posteriorly.

When swallowing in the erect position, a bolus is usually directed down the midline of the tongue to the level of the median glossoepiglottic fold, whereupon it is deflected into the vallecula on either side. The epiglottis is tilted backwards towards the posterior pharyngeal wall and serves to arrest the head of the bolus as it descends on to the back of the tongue. As the bolus accumulates on the epiglottis, it spills over the lateral pharyngoepiglottic folds into the food channels on either side of the mouth of the larynx and passes forwards into the pyriform fossae; at this stage, a small quantity of fluid may spill directly over the edge of the epiglottis over the open entrance to the larynx. As the bulk of the bolus enters the upper pharynx, the larynx is raised towards the hyoid bone, the contents of the pyriform fossae are expressed upwards and backwards, and the lower part of the lateral channels is opened to allow the bolus to spill downwards and backwards towards the midline. The columns meet over the back of the cricoid cartilage at the level of the upper border of the cricopharyngeus muscles, which then open to allow the bolus to enter the oesophagus. During the descent of the two streams below the epiglottis, some fluid frequently passes behind the arytenoids joining the two columns: this part is used whenever one side is partly or completely obstructed below this level.

When the bulk of the bolus has entered the upper oropharynx, the tongue moves backwards towards the posterior pharyngeal wall and meets the contraction resulting from the pharyngeal constrictors. The tongue of the epiglottis is gradually displaced with the bolus and is bent downwards at the side so that it is arched like a monk's hood over the larynx. Each half of the epiglottis serves as a chute to deflect the bulk of the bolus to either side of the midline. A certain amount of the bolus is always displaced down the midline, but this proportion of the total bolus is small unless the amount swallowed is comparatively large, when space is made to accommodate it by taking the larynx further forwards. As the main mass of the bolus is expressed from the oropharynx, the soft palate is lowered and applied to the tongue, and the posterior pillars of the fauces are also brought forwards. The tongue of the epiglottis is pressed forward over the mouth of the larynx until its tip is over the back of the cricoid cartilage. As the tail of the bolus is expressed from the pharynx, the larynx is lowered and the lateral food channels are cleared from above downwards. Finally, the cricopharyngeus muscles contract and express the last of the bolus into the oesophagus. Only a small residue normally remains in the pharynx: this is situated over the base of the tongue on the down-turned epiglottis in what are now backward-turned valleculae. When the airway is re-established, as the larynx returns to the position of rest, the tongue of the epiglottis springs upwards; the small residue which remains on the epiglottis is either retained in the valleculae or split into the lower lateral food channels and held in the pyriform fossae.

If a person swallows with the head turned fully to one side, the bolus is deflected down the lower lateral food channel on the side opposite that to which the head is turned: the whole of an average-size bolus may be swallowed down the one lateral channel. Old people with rigidity of the spine or other lesions may not be able to turn the head enough to obstruct completely the side to which the head is turned. Many instruments, such as a test meal tube, the gastroscope and oesophagoscope, may be passed entirely down one side.

When a normal person swallows in a supine

position, the bulk of the bolus is still directed to the side of the larynx, but it takes a relatively posterolateral course; the laryngeal opening, which is situated anteriorly, is not necessarily surrounded by the bolus unless the amount swallowed is large. The course of the bolus is likewise influenced by gravity when the patient swallows lying prone, or on one side. The effect of gravity is important in consideration of the problems of management of patients with pharyngeal palsy.

The epiglottis and closure of the larynx during swallowing

Ardran and Kemp (1967) have stated that there are several components associated with the above action. In the first component, when the bolus of food begins to spill down the back of the tongue, the lumen of the laryngeal vestibule is invariably narrowed. This is in consequence of the rocking movement of the arytenoids, downwards, forwards and inwards, with resulting narrowing of the glottis, bulging inward of the vestibular folds, forward movement of the cartilages of Wrisberg and obliteration of the interarytenoid space.

The second component produces backward tilting of the leaf of the epiglottis towards the posterior pharyngeal wall. The manner in which this is brought about depends on the position of the larynx and hyoid relative to the cervical spine and lower jaw at the moment swallowing is initiated.

In normal individuals at rest in the erect position, the leaf of the epiglottis is closely approximated to the tongue. With the passage of the bolus from the mouth into the pharynx, its descent is checked by a ledge constituted by the backward-tilted epiglottis: this is the phase of vallecular arrest. At this stage, the lumen of the laryngeal vestibule is usually reduced in size, but not closed.

As the mass of the bolus accumulates on the epiglottis, the larynx and hyoid are usually elevated towards the lower jaw; the hyoid rotates so that its greater cornua become horizontal (rather than their usual oblique position), thereby producing further backward tilting of the epiglottis towards the pharyngeal wall. This may result in complete closure of any remaining gap between the epiglottis and the pharyngeal wall, thus completely checking any spill of the bolus.

With further displacement of the bolus from the mouth, the larynx and hyoid are moved forwards and further upwards. Contact between the epiglottis and the posterior wall is no longer maintained and the bolus spills over the edge of the epiglottis into the lateral food channels on either side of the laryngeal entrance. The laryngeal lumen, though narrow, is usually not completely closed and a little of the bolus may enter the vestibule at this time and pass down as far as the laryngeal ventricle. During this swallowing stage, the leaf of the epiglottis projects backwards above the entrance of the larynx into the stream of the descending bolus, and the epiglottis is raised in the middle and bent down at the side, thereby serving to deflect the bulk of the bolus to one or both sides of the larynx (*see above*).

With further descent of the bolus, the whole of the hyoid bone is approximated more closely to the thyroid cartilage. The circothyroid visor is opened which allows the arytenoid masses to be tilted bodily forward, with the various components reducing the lumen of the vestibule to about one-third of the anteroposterior diameter in quiet breathing.

At any stage during the descent of the bolus, but always when it has been expressed past the larynx, there is backward bulging of the lower part of the epiglottis into the vestibular lumen, resulting from the apposition of the thyroid cartilage to the hyoid. This, in turn, leads to further bulging of the vestibular folds and obliteration of the ventricles. The total effect of all these movements is to oppose the dorsal surface of the epiglottis to the cartilages of Wrisberg and obliterate the laryngeal lumen from the level of the vocal cord to the superior laryngeal aperture.

The final component of laryngeal closure is the sealing of the laryngeal aperture by the sudden downward turning of the leaf of the epiglottis within the column of the bolus. This action results from a number of factors, which are the sustained approximation of the thyroid to the hyoid – both structures being elevated to the lower jaw–force is transmitted to the bolus as the tongue moves backwards to the palate and posterior pharyngeal wall, the leaf of the epiglottis is pressed down by the descending peristaltic wave against the arytenoid masses and any residue of the bolus which lies beneath it is displaced from the entrance to the larynx.

In all normal individuals, the pharynx is not squeezed entirely clear of the bolus: there is always a small residue left on the dorsal surface of the down-turned leaf of the epiglottis, that is its ventral surface when erect. If the leaf of the epiglottis were not present, this residue would lie over the laryngeal entrance. When the airway is re-established, the residue is swept upwards into the valleculae as the leaf of the epiglottis rises to the erect position.

There are, of course, modifications of the foregoing sequence of events, for example when an individual swallows into a large, air-filled pharyngeal cavity, when an individual is lying supine, and so on.

Oesophageal stage

Before discussion of the final part of deglutition, some mention should be made of the cricopharyngeal sphincter which forms the junctional zone between the pharynx above and the oesophagus below. However, functionally it is probably more accurate to use the term 'oesophageal sphincter'. This sphincter is formed by the cricopharyngeus (horizontal fibres) above which are the lower oblique fibres of the inferior constrictor, and this zone is continuous below with a variable length of the circular muscle of the oesophagus.

Lund (1965) stated that the cricopharyngeal sphincter is normally closed at rest and remains so even when subjected to raised pressure from above or below. The cricopharyngeus muscles can relax, however, to allow air etc. to pass either up or down. The sphincter provides a zone of elevated pressure which is approximately 1.6 kPa (12 mmHg) above the pressure in the oesophagus.

When swallowing occurs, the sphincter initially relaxes but does not open. The bolus then passes through the relaxed sphincter by means of thrust from the tongue, assisted by gravity. The cricoid is displaced forwards by the bolus, the sphincter opening at this stage. At about the time the bolus enters the oesophagus, the peristaltic wave commences at the top of the pharynx. This moves rapidly and smoothly downwards, clearing the pharynx of the hind part of the bolus and pushing it through into the oesophagus. The peristaltic wave involves the sphincter as it descends, producing the tight closure characteristic of the second stage of the sphincter changes. After the peristaltic wave has passed, the sphincter relaxes and returns to its resting state.

However, as Goyal (1984) pointed out, part of the opening of the sphincter, with abolition of the resting pressure, is brought about by the anterior displacement of the larynx by the suprahyoid muscles. This forward and upward laryngeal movement is an early event in swallowing, with Doty, Richmond and Storey (1967) stating that mylohyoid activity is the first to appear in response to swallowing. In a sense, the suprahyoid muscle can be considered as the dilator fibres of the upper oesophageal sphincter.

Oesophagus

The oesophagus functions essentially as a conducting tube for conveying substances to, and occasionally from, the stomach. During discussion of deglutition, Slome (1971) wrote that in the intrathoracic oesophagus, the intraluminal pressure corresponds to the intrapleural pressure. However, the pressure varies considerably with inspiration and with expiration, particularly with the latter if the glottis is closed, as in coughing, straining etc. During swallowing, peristaltic waves pass down the oesophagus with waves of positive pressure reaching 6.67–13.3 kPa (50–100 mmHg). The form of the wave varies somewhat with the nature of the swallowed substance, but with liquids and semisolids there is an initial negative wave resulting from the elevation of the larynx drawing on the cervical oesophagus. This is followed by an abrupt positive wave, coinciding with the entry of the bolus into the oesophagus. Next comes a slow rise of pressure succeeded by a final, large positive pressure wave which rises and falls rapidly, this being the peristaltic stripping wave.

Secondary peristaltic waves arise locally in the oesophagus in response to distension, and they complete the transportation of bolus portions which have been left after the primary peristaltic wave. Tertiary oesophageal contractions are irregular, non-propulsive contractions involving long segments of the oesophagus, which frequently occur during emotional stress. The velocity of oesophageal transport is more rapid in the upper oesophagus than in the distal half, on account of the differences in muscle type and neural mechanism of the propagation of the peristalsis.

At the lower end of the oesophagus there is a zone of raised pressure about 3 cm in length, extending above and below the diaphragm, with a mean pressure of approximately 1 kPa higher (8 mmHg) than the intragastric pressure which can be regarded as the location of the 'physiological sphincter' of the oesophagogastric region. As with the cricopharyngeal sphincter, the oesophagogastric sphincter, which is normally in tonic contraction, undergoes relaxation before the peristalsis reaches it, with a reflex preventing the occurrence of contraction immediately the bolus has passed into the stomach.

The physical consistency of the swallowed material determines to some extent the mechanism involved in its passage through the oesophagus. When fluid is swallowed, it may be projected from the pharynx to the oesophagogastric junction in about 1 s (with the subject in a standing position), and is well ahead of the peristaltic wave. In consequence of this rapid passage, the swallowing of corrosive fluids causes burns which are often localized to the distal end of the oesophagus. When the bolus is solid or semisolid, it is passed down the oesophagus by a peristaltic contraction of the oesophageal musculature, with gravity playing little part in the process.

In the upper part of the oesophagus, peristalsis progresses rapidly; in the lower one-third, the contraction wave is more sluggish. The differences in motor activity are related to the muscular coat's being striated in the former situation and unstriated in the latter.

Oesophagogastric sphincter (the lower oesophageal sphincter)

Jewell and Selby (1982) stated that the lower oesophageal sphincter forms the major barrier to gastro-oesophageal reflux; when the muscle of the sphincter is destroyed by diseases, such as systemic sclerosis, or by cardiomyotomy for achalasia, reflux commonly occurs. The resting sphincter pressure in patients with gastro-oesophageal reflux is often subnormal but there is a wide overlap with the normal range. Many variables govern the actual pressure recorded. Radial asymmetry of pressure is present, with higher pressures being recorded towards the patient's left (Luckman and Welch, 1977). Recording technique varies and, for these and other reasons, no generally accepted normal range of lower oesophageal sphincter pressure has yet been agreed. However, it seems probable that in the protection against reflux, the capacity of the sphincter to respond to stress is more important than the resting pressure.

Circular muscle fibres from the oesophagogastric junction behave differently from those in the body of the oesophagus, in that when the former are stretched, the length–tension curve is steeper, that is they have a greater resistance to being stretched. The cause of the tone of the lower oesophageal sphincter in humans is poorly understood. It has been variously suggested either that neural influences are responsible as in the upper oesophageal sphincter, or that tone is a result of hormonal factors, or that it is an intrinsic property of the muscle fibres themselves. In the opossum, the isolated circular muscle of the sphincter retains its tone after treatment with tetrodotoxin, which blocks all nerve conduction, implying that, in this animal, tone is myogenic in origin (Goyal and Rattan, 1976). However, the tone of the lower oesophageal sphincter may certainly be influenced by neural and possibly by hormonal factors.

Neural regulation of the lower oesophageal sphincter

The vagus nerve is concerned with the regulation of lower oesophageal sphincter function. It is predominantly an afferent nerve which carries impulses from the whole alimentary tract, except for the distal large intestine, but efferent fibres influence motor and secretory activities. Vaso-vagal reflexes are poorly understood but they are known to exert both excitatory and inhibitory actions on gut motility. Section of the vagal nerve appears to have a variable effect upon the lower oesophageal sphincter in different species. In the dog, high bilateral vagotomy results in oesophageal dilatation and aperistalsis, as might be expected with denervation of striated muscle, and the lower oesophageal sphincter pressure also falls (Khan, 1981). The opossum has much more smooth muscle in the oesophagus and here a transient increase in sphincter pressure follows bilateral vagotomy, while stimulation of the peripheral end of the severed nerve causes the sphincter to relax. Stimulation of the central end causes sphincteric contraction, even when vagotomy is bilateral, which indicates that the efferent pathway for this centrally mediated mechanism lies outside the vagi (Rattan and Goyal, 1974).

In humans, gastro-oesophageal reflux is a common consequence of surgical truncal vagotomy. Resting pressure in the lower oesophageal sphincter falls to the low or low normal range. However, surgical truncal vagotomy does impair the sphincteric response to stress, and the increase in sphincter pressure normally seen after an increase in intra-abdominal pressure is thus inhibited (Angorn *et al.*, 1977). As the vagal nerve supply to the oesophagus and the lower oesophageal sphincter comes off the vagi above the level of section at truncal vagotomy, it seems probable that the operation will have severed the afferent fibres of the reflex concerned in the sphincteric response to the increased abdominal pressure. Patients with gastro-oesophageal reflux who have not undergone previous surgery, show a similar lack of sphincteric contraction in response to a rise in intra-abdominal pressure, and it appears that disruption of this reflex may well be of aetiological importance in the causation of reflux.

Much less is known about the role of the sympathetic nerve supply to the oesophagus. No gross disturbance in oesophageal function followed bilateral thoracolumbar sympathectomy when this was employed in the treatment of hypertension. This suggests that the sympathetic nerve supply to the oesophagus is not of vital importance in the regulation of motor activity.

Hormones and the lower oesophageal sphincter

Gastrin causes an increase in lower oesophageal sphincter pressure (Giles *et al.*, 1969), and this action is mediated through cholinergic mechanisms which can be blocked by atropine. There can be no doubt that this and other alimentary hormones do exert a pharmacological effect upon the sphincter. However, the evidence that these hormones are of physiological importance in the regulation of sphincter tone is much less certain. Changes in serum gastrin levels in health and disease do not correlate closely with changes in sphincteric pressure. In pernicious anaemia, the lower oesphageal sphincter pressure tends to be low, yet the serum gastrin level may be high; and in patients with the Zollinger–Ellison syndrome, the lower oesophageal sphincter pressure is certainly not increased. Although meals will influence the lower oesophageal sphincter pressure, and the rise in pressure roughly coincides with increased secretion of gastrin by the antral G cells, it seems more likely that the fluctuations in sphincteric tone are mediated by way of nervous rather than hormonal pathways.

Many other gut hormones have been shown to increase or decrease the tone of the lower oesophageal sphincter. As in the case of gastrin, it is difficult, in the present state of knowledge, to conclude that any of these play a significant part in the physiological regulation of oesophageal motility, or in the prevention of gastro-oesophageal reflux. Other agents exert a pharmacological effect on the lower oesophageal sphincter, and a number of drugs with anticholinergic actions, notably the tricyclic antidepressants, may in clinical use aggravate gastro-oesophageal reflux.

Nervous regulation of deglutition

As Mountcastle (1980) has outlined, 'the oropharyngeal phase of swallowing, completed in less than 1 second, is an intricate, stereotyped, bilaterally symmetric sequence of inhibition and excitation, involving more than 25 muscle groups and controlled by the swallowing centre of the brainstem. This complex neuroreaction pattern can be initiated by stimulation of a single efferent nerve, the superior laryngeal nerve (*Figure 11.1*). Although the initiation of swallowing is under voluntary control, in the same way as other voluntary movements, it is often effected without

conscious effort. It appears in the fetus as early as 12 weeks of gestation, long before suckling and respiratory movements occur. On average, normal adults swallow 600 times in 24 hours, with 50 swallows occurring during sleep and only 200 during eating. During the act of drinking, swallows can be repeated as frequently as 1 second but in the absence of a bolus, the frequency is greatly reduced, which is an indication that swallowing depends upon peripheral stimuli from the oropharynx as well as messages from higher centres. In fact, it would appear that swallowing can be initiated voluntarily if afferents from the pharynx are blocked by administration of a local anaesthetic. In this situation, swallowing can still be initiated by direct electrical stimulation of the superior laryngeal nerve.

In addition to the superior laryngeal nerves, other afferents which stimulate swallowing converge on the nucleus solitarius by way of the maxillary branch of the trigeminal nerve. Afferent stimuli over these same nerves also initiate other patterned responses, such as gagging, coughing and chewing. The temporal and spatial patterns of the afferent stimuli determine the patterned response that is evoked. Appropriate afferent stimuli are relayed to the swallowing centre in the reticular formation of the rostral medulla. The centre is actually two paired half centres that continue to initiate swallowing responses from the ipsilateral muscles when the connections between them are severed. Impulses from the swallowing centre then activate the appropriate motor neurons in the nucleus ambiguus and the fifth, seventh and twelfth cranial nerve nuclei. The resultant motor activity can be analysed from electromyographic tracings (*Figure 11.2*). Once the swallowing centre has been activated there is little evidence that afferent impulses play any role in modifying the oropharyngeal patterned muscular response. Activation of the swallowing centre

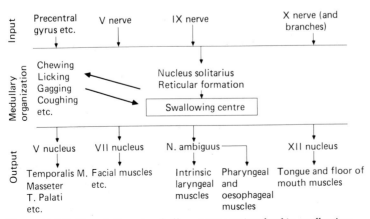

Figure 11.1 Outline of afferent and efferent systems involved in swallowing

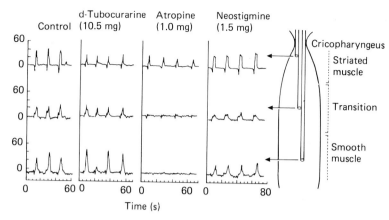

Figure 11.2 Portions of manometric recordings obtained during control period and after adminsitration of *d*-tubocurarine, atropine, and neostigmine. Amplitude of peristaltic wave is decreased in striated muscle by *d*-tubocurarine but not in smooth muscle. Atropine abolishes peristalsis in smooth muscle, but produces no further change in striated muscle. Neostigmine reverses both effects (from Kantrowitz *et al.* (1970) by permission of the publishers)

influences the activities of other centres, most notably the respiratory centre, as evidenced by an apnoeic pause of 0.5–3.5 seconds that accompanies every swallow. The continuous train of action potentials that maintains the resting tone of the upper oesophageal sphincter is interrupted, with resultant sphincter relaxation before the onset of pharyngeal peristalsis (*Figure 11.2*). Closure is effected as the neural discharge propagating the peristaltic wave passes through the sphincter and the resting tone is re-established.

It is frequently considered that the motor nerve supply to the cricopharyngeal sphincter is derived from either the recurrent laryngeal nerve or the autonomic nervous system, but there is no clinical or experimental evidence to support this view. Much more likely is that the fomer is supplied by the pharyngeal branch of the vagus.'

Lund (1965) has shown that there are experimental findings to imply that the sphincter changes are probably attributable to a reflex arc, stimulated by the peristaltic wave when it reaches the level just above the cricopharyngeal sphincter. It is likely that this 'sphincter reflex' is merely part of a series of coordinated reflexes which give rise to the peristaltic wave itself. It is suggested that the nerve supply to the cricopharyngeus muscles (a definite entity in the dog) constitutes the efferent pathway of this reflex arc. The fibres passing in these nerves are either excitatory or inhibitory, producing contraction or relaxation of the sphincter respectively. The latter change is probably a result of a reduction of the nerve impulses which normally pass continuously to the sphincter, thereby maintaining its resting tone. The arrangement of the afferent pathways is

uncertain, but it may be formed by nerve fibres in the pharyngeal wall which are derived from the pharyngeal branch of the vagus.

When a swallow is produced by stimulation of the upper pharynx, an initial wave of relaxation passes downwards. When it reaches a point just above the sphincter, the reflex arc is stimulated and the sphincter relaxes. This is followed by a contraction wave which also passes down the pharynx but, in this case, stimulates the reflex to produce contraction of the sphincter. Thus the sphincter initially relaxes and subsequently contracts, both changes being coordinated with the peristaltic wave.

When the pharynx in the dog is experimentally divided above the sphincter, the peristaltic wave is unable to pass downwards in the normal way. As a result, the afferent pathway is not stimulated and the normal sphincter changes do not occur, even though the nerve supply to the cricopharyngeus muscles is intact. Similarly, the sphincter again fails to function normally if the nerve supply to the cricopharyngeus muscles is divided, but the pharynx is continuous with the sphincter. In this case, it is the efferent pathway which has been destroyed.

Sphincter actions, therefore, depend upon the integrity of the nerve supply to the cricopharyngeus muscles and also on continuity being maintained between the pharynx above and the sphincter below.

A distinction has been made between primary and secondary peristalsis. Mountcastle (1980) pointed out that 'it was originally believed that primary peristalsis, which is initiated by swallowing, was mediated by impulses originating from the swallowing centre, whereas secondary peristalsis, which is initiated by a bolus in the oesophagus, was mediated by local intramural neural pathways. Secondary peristalsis serves to return material, following its reflux into the oesophagus, to the stomach, or to carry material to the stomach that has been left behind by an ineffectual peristaltic wave. Secondary peristalsis can be produced experimentally by inflation and deflation of a balloon in the oesophagus. It now appears that the designations 'primary' and 'secondary' peristalsis should be used only to indicate how peristalsis is initiated as both central and local neural pathways appear to be involved, regardless of the means of initiation. The initial event in oesophageal peristalsis is stimulation of the longitudinal muscle of the oesophagus followed by segmental activation of circular muscle and inhibition of the distal oesophagus.

The stimulation of the longitudinal muscle is cholinergic (atropine sensitive). The circular muscle displays a different response in that it does not contract until after the end of the electrical stimulus (off-response) and is not inhibited by antagonists to any of the known autonomic neurotransmitters. It has been suggested that vagal non-cholinergic non-adrenergic inhibitory nerves hyperpolarize the circular muscle by an as yet unidentified neurotransmitter. When the source of stimulation is turned off, rebound depolarization leads to contraction. Oesophageal peristalsis will not be understood until the relation between the longitudinal and circular muscle activity is clarified and the nature of the mediator of the vagal inhibitory nerve is identified. The ability of anticholinergic drugs to block peristalsis in the oesophagus (*Figure 11.2*) may be through their action on the cholinergically innervated longitudinal muscle.

With increasing age, the frequency of 'misfires' and abnormal segmental, non-progressive contractions in the smooth muscle segment increases (tertiary contractions). If, instead of a single swallow, the subject takes a series of swallows – as in drinking a glass of water – each swallow initiates the complete oropharyngeal sequence, but peristalsis in the oesophagus is inhibited until the last swallow of the series. The cricopharyngeal sphincter relaxes and closes with each swallow, whereas the cardiac sphincter opens with the first swallow and closes only when the peristaltic wave enters the sphincter. Secondary peristalsis, initiated by balloon distension of the body of the oesophagus, can be inhibited by a swallow. These observations are best interpreted as an indication of the inhibition of distal neuromuscular activity during that of the proximal segments, presumably mediated through the swallowing centre. In addition, local afferent impulses from the oesophagus alter oesophageal peristalsis, for example the course of the peristaltic contraction is proportional to the size of the bolus. On the other hand, swallows of hot liquid increase the speed and amplitude of oesophageal peristalsis, whereas cold swallows decrease speed and amplitude and finally abolish peristalsis altogether. Acid swallows cause disorder and delay of oesophageal peristalsis. Recent studies suggest that afferent impulses of local origin may not only modify the pattern of oesophageal peristalsis, but may indeed be essential for its normal propagation. In conscious dogs, with a cervical oesophageal cannula in place, it was found that with the cannula closed oesophageal peristalsis occurred after 90% of water swallows, while with the cannula open and the water swallows diverted to the outside, no peristalsis was recorded in the lower oesophagus. These findings may be relevant to oesophageal function in humans for transection of the smooth muscle portion of the oesophagus in the monkey interferes with primary peristalsis. It appears that primary and secondary peristalsis both depend on descending neural activity originating in the swallowing centre, as well as on sequential afferent input from the oesophagus.

Innervation of the oesophagus

Although knowledge of the afferent innervation of the oesophagus is of great importance to an understanding of its motor function, very little is known at present. Neither the location and characteristics of the sensory receptors nor the functional significance of the afferent impulses that are found in the vagus and sympathetic nerves have been defined. Electrical records from the nodose ganglion in the cat show two kinds of afferent signals arising from the oesophagus in response to balloon distension. One is a continuous discharge for the duration of the distension, and the other is an 'on–off' signal firing one burst after inflation and another after deflation of the balloon.

Although the striated portion of the oesophagus appears to have the same innervation as that of other striated muscles, it contracts slowly, remains contracted for 1–2 seconds, and then relaxes slowly.

The motor innervation of the smooth muscle portion of the oesophagus is believed to be from the vagal oesophageal plexus. The preganglionic parasympathetic fibres synapse in the myenteric plexuses with postganglionic neurons that innervate the oesophageal smooth muscle. Exactly how the peristaltic wave is propagated is not understood, but it is unlikely that it is mediated by serial excitation of cells in the motor nuclei of the vagus. Distension of isolated segments of the opossum oesophagus – which, like the human oesophagus, has smooth muscle in its distal half – produces peristalsis. This peristalsis is neural rather than myogenic in origin because it is blocked by tetrodotoxin, a pharmacological agent that selectively depresses transmission along nerve fibres. Studies of this preparation suggest that there are motor nerves in the oesophagus that are neither cholinergic nor adrenergic, the so-called non-adrenergic inhibitory nerves.

The contribution of the adrenergic nerves to oesophageal motor function is still undefined. It seems clear, however, that the classic view that cholinergic impulses are excitatory and adrenergic impulses are inhibitory is an over-simplification.

In summary, deglutition, or swallowing, is a complex neuromuscular operation initiated consciously but carried to completion by an integration of afferent impulses and central nervous system efferent impulses, organized both in the swallowing centre and in local intramural arcs, the latter act on a muscular tube made up of both striated and smooth muscle. The oesophagus is separated from the pharynx above and the stomach below by a pair of sphincters, the upper and lower oesophageal sphincters, which maintain a resting intraluminal pressure greater than the adjacent segments. Swallowing may be viewed as a relaxation of the swallowing tube to receive the swallowed bolus, followed by caudally progressing muscular contracture, the peristaltic wave, sweeping the bolus before it. Relaxation is most obvious in those segments with a high resting tone, namely the sphincters, whereas the progressive nature of the peristaltic wave is most obvious in the remaining segments that exhibit a low resting tone. It is possible that the sphincters are differentiated from adjacent segments, not so much by special neural arrangements, but rather by an increased sensitivity of the neuromuscular elements of the sphincters to the neurohumoral determinants of motor function.'

Applied physiology of deglutition

Pharyngeal paralysis

The cranial nuclei, containing the cell bodies of the neurons which supply the muscles in swallowing, lie close together in the medulla. Lesions in this region, such as those of bulbar poliomyelitis, motor neuron disease, or thrombosis of the posterior inferior cerebellar artery, may cause dysphagia. The palatal and pharyngeal muscles may be paralysed, but, interestingly, the cricopharyngeal sphincter is usually unaffected and will relax normally. A complete hold-up of the bolus at the level of the sphincter may occur very rarely in a total pharyngeal palsy, but after an

interval of time, the bolus normally passes through successfully by virtue of thrust by the tongue and gravity in the erect position. Nasal regurgitation and laryngeal spill with coughing can occur on attempted swallowing. In these cases, a cricopharyngeal myotomy may be indicated in progressive neurosurgical disorders; however, it should be remembered that there is a risk of a reflux of the oesophageal contents upwards through the divided sphincter, particularly if the oesophagus is also paralysed.

As already mentioned, the opening of the oesophageal sphincter results from two separate mechanisms, that is the central inhibition of the ongoing activity in the cricopharyngeal constrictors, together with active contraction of the suprahyoid muscles. Abnormalities in the opening of the upper sphincter may be due, therefore, to involvement of either the cricopharyngeus or the suprahyoid muscles, or both, as suggested by Goyal and Cobb (1981).

A lump in the throat

If local and distant (gastro-oesophageal junction) causes have been excluded, the lump in the throat symptom will usually be a consequence of spasm or failure of the cricopharyngeal sphincter to relax.

Although cineradiography is of enormous help in assessing these patients, in a review of 100 consecutive cine films, Lund (1965) found no radiological abnormality in 85 patients. In the remaining 15 patients, the commonest irregularity was gastro-oesophageal reflux.

Watson and Sullivan (1974) would seem to confirm this aetiology as they found high resting upper oesophageal sphincter pressures in patients with 'globus sensation' to the order of 140–220 mmHg, as compared with pressures of 70–140 mmHg in their control subjects.

Lane (1980) also believed that incompetence of the lower oesophageal sphincter is relevant in that it reduces the pH in the oesophagus; this, in turn, initiates incoordinated peristaltic movements, with reflex production of alkaline saliva which the patient continually swallows. It is the latter which exacerbates the feeling of a lump in the throat.

The posterior pharyngeal or Zenker's diverticulum

This condition occurs posteriorly between the upper and lower halves of the inferior constrictor muscles, that is the thyro- and cricopharyngeal muscles respectively. The pouch arises as a result of a combination of early closure of the cricopharyngeal sphincter and weakness or incoordination of the pharyngeal peristaltic wave.

If the peristaltic wave in a normal swallow is likened to the smooth, progressive squeezing of a toothpaste tube (held upside down) from the bottom to the top, then a similar analogy can be drawn to describe the formation of these early pouches. If the toothpaste is first squeezed down from the bottom of the tube (the peristaltic wave sweeping down the pharynx) and then suddenly, with the other hand, pressure is applied in front (the cricopharyngeal muscles contracting), a bulge will appear in the tube between the two flattened portions (this is the equivalent of the pouch). Thus the pouch is formed when the sphincter is closing and not when it is relaxing, with relaxation generally being adequate. This explanation is supported by the manometric findings of Ellis *et al.* (1969) in which all patients showed an abnormal temporal relationship between pharyngeal contraction and termination of sphincter relaxation, as the sphincter contraction occurred before completion of contraction in the pharynx.

Oesophageal motility

Bouchier *et al.* (1984) maintained that the three indices of normal oesophageal motility (peristalsis, sphincter tone and sphincter relaxation) may be disturbed in several ways in oesophageal motility disorders. The peristaltic nature of the contraction wave may become lost. This often results in pressure waves, which develop simultaneously or in a non-sequential way at different levels of the oesophagus and, as such, are deprived of much of their propulsive force. The contraction may also be too strong and last too long, resulting in painful spasm or dysphagia. Contractions that are too weak will have little or no propulsive force. Other manifestations of disordered motility are 'spontaneous' motor activity (not elicited by swallowing) and repetitive contractions in response to a single swallow. Sphincters may be hypotensive and relax inappropriately, thus allowing reflux. They may be hypertensive and produce pain, or they may fail to relax sufficiently so that dysphagia ensues and stasis develops proximally. In most cases of disordered motility, several of these abnormalities are combined. However, the combination is not always sufficiently typical and specific to be pathognomonic.

Oesophageal motility disorders have been classified as primary and secondary. In primary motor disorders, the oesophagus is the site of major involvement; this group includes achalasia, diffuse oesophageal spasm and related motor disorders, as well as the conditions termed 'presbyoesophagus' and 'symptomatic (or hypertensive) peristalsis' (nutcracker oesophagus). In secondary motor disorders, oesophageal abnormalities are caused by more generalized nervous, muscular, or systemic diseases, metabolic disturbances, or to inflammatory or new growth lesions of the oesophageal wall. Examples in this secondary group are systemic sclerosis, various muscle diseases such as myotonia dystrophica, and lesions of the central nervous system involving the brainstem.

References

ANGORN, E. B., DIMOPOULOS, G., HEGARTY, M. M. and MOSHAL, M. G. (1977) The effect of vagotomy on the lower oesophageal sphincter: a manometric study. *British Journal of Surgery*, **64**, 466–469

ARDRAN, G. M. and KEMP, F. H. (1955) A radiographic study of movements of the tongue in swallowing. *The Dental Practitioner*, **5**, 252–261

ARDRAN, G. M. and KEMP, F. H. (1961) The radiology of the lower lateral food channels. *Journal of Laryngology and Otology*, **75**, 358–370

ARDRAN, G. M. and KEMP, F. H. (1967) The mechanism of the larynx. Part II. The epiglottis and the closure of the larynx. *British Journal of Radiology*, **40**, 372–389

BOUCHIER, I. A. D., ALLAN, R. N., HODGSON, H. I. F. and KEIGHTLEY, M. R. B. (1984) The oesophagus; motor disorders. In *Textobook of Gastroenterology*, edited by R. N. Allen, H. I. F. Hodgson and M. R. B. Keighley, pp. 26–38. London: Balillière Tindall

DOTY, R. W., RICHMOND, W. H. and STOREY, A. T. (1967) Effect of medullary lesions on coordination of deglutition. *Experimental Neurology*, **17**, 91–106

ELLIS, F. H., SCHLEGEL, J. F., LYNCH, V. P. and SPENCER PAINE, M. D. (1969) Crico-pharyngeal myotomy for pharyngeo-esophageal diverticulum. *Annals of Surgery*, **170**, 340–349

GILES, G. R., MASON, M. C., HUMPHRIES, C. and CLARK, C. G. (1969) Action of gastrin on the lower oesophageal sphincter in man. *Gut*, **10**, 730–734

GOYAL, R. K. (1984) Disorders of the cricopharyngeus muscle. *Otolaryngologic Clinics of North America*, **17**, 115–130

GOYAL, R. K. and COBB, B. W. (1981) Motility of the pharynx, esophagus and esophageal sphincters. In *Physiology of the Gastro-intestinal Tract*, edited by L. Johnson *et al.*, pp. 359–391. New York: Raven Press

GOYAL, R. K. and RATTAN, S. (1976) Genesis of basal sphincter pressure: effect of tetrodoxin on lower oesophageal sphincter pressure in opossum *in vivo*. *Gastroenterology*, **71**, 62–67

JEWELL, D. P. and SELBY, W. S. (eds) (1982) Physiology of the oesophagus. In *Topics in Gastroenterology*, pp. 42–45. Oxford: Blackwell Scientific Publications

KANTROWITZ, P. A. *et al.* (1970) Response of the human esophagus to *d*-tubocurarine and atropine. *Gut*, **11**, 47

KHAN, T. A. (1981) Effect of proximal selective vagotomy on the canine lower esophageal sphincter. *American Journal of Surgery*, **141**, 219–221

LANE, J. L. (1980) Lump in the throat. *South African Medical Journal*, **58**, 243–245

LUCKMAN, K. and WELCH, R. W. (1977) The significance of lower oesophageal sphincter pressure asymmetry in man and its correlation with a new measure of closure strength. *Gastroenterology*, **72**, 1091 (abstract)

LUND, W. S. (1965) A study of the cricopharyngeal sphincter in man and in the dog. Arris and Gale lecture. *Annals of the Royal College of Surgeons,* **37,** 225–246

MOUNTCASTLE, V. B. (ed.) (1980) The motility of the alimentary canal. In *Medical Physiology,* pp. 1322–1332. St Louis: C. V. Mosby Co.

RATTAN, S. and GOYAL, R. K. (1974) Neural control of the lower esophageal sphincter: influence of the vagus nerve. *Journal of Clinical Investigation,* **54,** 899–906

SLOME, D. (1971) Physiology of the mouth, pharynx and oesophagus. In *Scott-Brown's Diseases of the Ear, Nose and Throat,* 3rd edn. edited by J. Ballantyne and J. Groves, pp. 235–302. London: Butterworths

WATSON, W. C. and SULLIVAN, S.N. (1974) Hypertonicity of the cricopharyngeal sphincter: a cause of globus sensation. *The Lancet,* **2,** 1417–1419

12

Anatomy of the larynx and tracheobronchial tree

Neil Weir

Development of larynx, trachea, bronchi and lungs

During the fourth week of embryonic development, the rudiment of the respiratory tree appears as a median laryngotracheal groove in the ventral wall of the pharynx (*Figure 12.1*). The groove subsequently deepens and its edges fuse to form a septum, thus converting the groove into a splanchnopleuric laryngotracheal tube. This process of fusion commences caudally and extends cranially but does not involve the cranial end where the edges remain separate, bounding a slit-like aperture through which the tube opens into the pharynx.

The tube is lined with endoderm from which the epithelial lining of the respiratory tract is developed. The cranial end of the tube forms the larynx and the trachea, and the caudal end produces two lateral outgrowths from which the bronchi and right and left lung buds develop. These grow into the pleural coelomata and are thus covered with splanchnic mesenchyme from which the connective tissue, cartilage, nonstriated muscle and the vasculature of the bronchi and lungs are developed.

Larynx and trachea

The primitive larynx is the cranial end of the laryngotracheal groove, bounded vertically by the caudal part of the hypobranchial eminence and laterally by the ventral folds of the sixth arches. The arytenoid swellings appear on both sides of the groove and as they enlarge they become approximated to each other and to the caudal part of the hypobranchial eminence from which the

epiglottis develops. The opening into the laryngeal cavity is at first a vertical slit or cleft, which becomes T-shaped with the appearance of the arytenoids. However, the epithelial walls of the cleft soon adhere to each other and the aperture of the larynx is thus occluded until the third month when its lumen is restored. The arytenoid swellings grow upwards and deepen to produce the primitive aryepiglottic folds. This, in turn, produces a further aperture above the level of the primitive aperture which itself becomes the glottis. During the second month of fetal life, the arytenoid swellings differentiate into the arytenoid and corniculate cartilages (derivatives of the sixth arch), and the folds joining them to the epiglottis become the aryepiglottic folds in which the cuneiform cartilages are developed as derivatives of the epiglottis. The thyroid cartilage develops from the ventral ends of the cartilages of the fourth branchial arch, appearing as two lateral plates, each with two chondrification centres. The cricoid cartilage and cartilages of the trachea develop from the sixth branchial arch during the sixth week. The trachea increases rapidly in length from the fifth week onwards.

The branchial nerves of the fourth and sixth arches, namely the superior laryngeal and recurrent laryngeal nerves, supply the larynx (*Figure 12.2*).

Each visceral arch is traversed by an artery (aortic arch). Each aortic arch connects the ventral and dorsal aortae of its own visceral arch. The primitive recurrent laryngeal nerve enters the sixth visceral arch, on each side, caudal to the sixth aortic arch. On the left side, the arch retains its position as the ductus arteriosus and the nerve is found caudal to the ligamentum arteriosum in the adult. On the right side, the dorsal part of the sixth

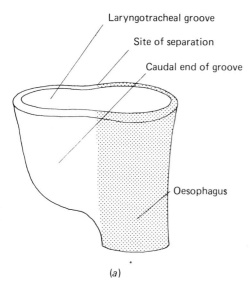

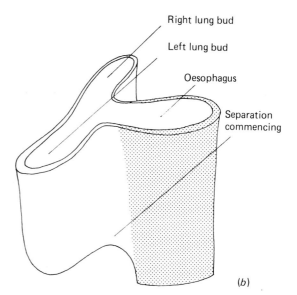

Figure 12.1 Diagrams to show the closure of the laryngotracheal groove and its separation from the oesophagus in the latter part of the fourth week

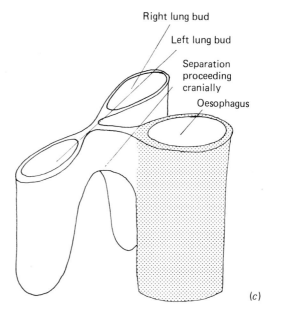

aortic arch and the whole of the fifth arch disappear. The nerve is, therefore, found on the caudal aspect of the fourth aortic arch, which becomes the subclavian artery.

Bronchi and lungs

The right and left lung buds appear before the laryngotracheal groove is converted into a tube. They grow out into the pleural passages caudal to the common cardinal veins and divide into lobules, three appearing on the right and two on the left. It is uncertain whether lung budding determines the septal pattern or whether the development of the connective tissue septa controls the final form of the lung (Emery, 1969). Each primary bronchus continues to divide dichotomously until by birth some 18–23 generations of divisions have appeared which are not necessarily equal in the individual lobes.

Three periods of development of the lung are described: a 'glandular' period, when the primitive bronchi ramify through the mesenchyme (up to 4 months); a 'canicular' period when the primitive respiratory bronchioles are generated from the terminal bronchi (4–6 months); and an 'alveolar' period from 6 months onwards when further respiratory bronchioles and the terminal alveoli, which will be the functional airspaces with their blood–air barriers, are formed.

There has been considerable discussion as to how much of the subsequent development of the bronchi and alveoli occurs after birth. The current views are summarized by Reid (1967) in her three 'laws' of lung development:

(1) the bronchial tree is fully developed by the sixteenth week of intrauterine life
(2) alveoli, as commonly understood, develop after birth, increasing in number until the age of 8 years, and in size until growth of the chest wall is complete
(3) blood vessels are remodelled and increase in number, certainly while new alveoli are forming.

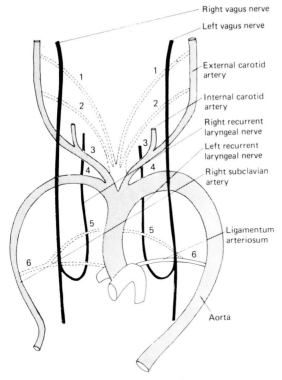

Right vagus nerve

Left vagus nerve

External carotid artery

Internal carotid artery

Right recurrent laryngeal nerve

Left recurrent laryngeal nerve

Right subclavian artery

Ligamentum arteriosum

Aorta

Figure 12.2 The branchial arteries and recurrent laryngeal nerves

During the course of their development, the lungs migrate in a caudal direction, so that by birth the bifurcation of the trachea is opposite the fourth thoracic vertebra. As the lungs grow, they become enveloped in pleura derived from the splanchnic mesenchyme.

For further reading on development of the trachea and lungs, consult Boyden (1972), O'Rahilly and Boyden (1973) and Reid (1976).

The larynx

Comparative anatomy and modification for olfaction and deglutition

The prime reason for the existence of the larynx is not to make phonation possible, but to provide a protective sphincter at the inlet of the air passages. This can be seen in a lung fish, where the larynx takes the form of a simple muscular sphincter surrounding the opening of the air passage in the floor of the pharynx. In birds, the rima glottidis in the floor of the mouth shuts to close the air inlet but it makes no sound; phonation occurs from a dilatation, the syrinx, at the lower end of the trachea just above its bifurcation.

The first breathers of air, the amphibia, do however phonate. They achieve this by 'swallowing' air which, as there is no separate nasal cavity, is drawn in through valvular 'nostrils' opening anteriorly into the roof of the mouth. In mammals, a nasal cavity develops with the appearance of a palate. The separation of a respiratory and olfactory chamber from the mouth has considerable advantages: predatory mammals can still breathe while the mouth is obstructed by prey, and herbivorous prey can still sense warning odours while feeding. In aquatic vertebrates, such as crocodiles, dolphins and whales, an intranarial larynx has been developed where the inlet of the larynx is suspended within the nasopharynx and clasped by the sphincter of the nasopharyngeal inlet (the palatopharyngeus). Thus respiration and olfaction can continue at the water surface even with the mouth submerged, open and ready for prey.

The larynx of man is still an essential sphincter, preventing the entry of swallowed food and other foreign bodies, and providing a blockade to build up pressure for coughing or for aiding extreme muscular efforts. However, man differs from other mammals in the ability to produce speech by the highest integrations of the nervous and locomotive systems.

Descriptive anatomy

The larynx is situated at the upper end of the trachea; it lies opposite the third to sixth cervical vertebrae in men, while being somewhat higher in women and children. The average length, transverse diameter and anteroposterior diameter are, in the male, 44 mm, 43 mm and 36 mm, and, in the female, 36 mm, 41 mm and 26 mm, respectively.

There is little difference in the size of the larynx in boys and girls until after puberty when the anteroposterior diameter in the male almost doubles.

The skeletal framework of the larynx (*Figures 12.3 and 12.4*) is formed of cartilages, which are connected by ligaments and membranes and are moved in relation to one another by both intrinsic and extrinsic muscles. It is lined with mucous membrane which is continuous above and behind with that of the pharynx and below with that of the trachea.

The infantile larynx is both absolutely and relatively smaller than the larynx of the adult. The lumen is therefore disproportionately narrower. It is more funnel-shaped and its narrowest part is at the junction of the subglottic larynx with the trachea. A very slight swelling of the lax mucosa in this area may thus produce a very serious obstruction to breathing. The laryngeal cartilages

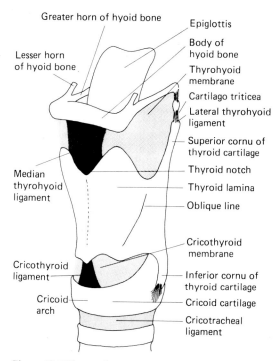

Greater horn of hyoid bone
Epiglottis
Body of hyoid bone
Lesser horn of hyoid bone
Thyrohyoid membrane
Cartilago triticea
Lateral thyrohyoid ligament
Superior cornu of thyroid cartilage
Median thyrohyoid ligament
Thyroid notch
Thyroid lamina
Oblique line
Cricothyroid membrane
Cricothyroid ligament
Inferior cornu of thyroid cartilage
Cricoid arch
Cricoid cartilage
Cricotracheal ligament

Figure 12.3 The cartilages and ligaments of the larynx

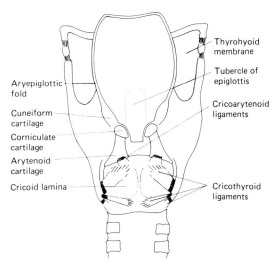

Aryepiglottic fold
Cuneiform cartilage
Corniculate cartilage
Arytenoid cartilage
Cricoid lamina
Thyrohyoid membrane
Tubercle of epiglottis
Cricoarytenoid ligaments
Cricothyroid ligaments

Figure 12.4 Ligaments, membranes and cartilages of the larynx seen from behind

are much softer in the infant and therefore collapse more easily in forced inspiratory efforts. The infantile larynx starts high up under the tongue and with development assumes an increasingly lower position.

Laryngeal cartilages

The thyroid cartilage

This shield-like cartilage (*see Figures 12.3 and 12.4*) is the longest of the laryngeal cartilages and consists of two laminae which meet in the midline inferiorly, leaving the easily palpable thyroid notch between them above. The angle of fusion of the laminae is about 90° in men and 120° in women. In the male, the fused anterior borders form a projection, again easily palpable, which is the laryngeal prominence or 'Adam's apple'. A small narrow strip of cartilage, the intrathyroid cartilage, separates the two laminae anteriorly in childhood. Posteriorly, the laminae diverge and the posterior border of each is prolonged as two slender processes, the superior and inferior cornua. The superior cornu is long and narrow and curves upwards, backwards and medially, ending in a conical extremity to which is attached the lateral thyroid ligament. The inferior cornu is shorter and thicker and curves downwards and medially. On the medial surface of its lower end

there is a small oval facet for articulation with the cricoid cartilage.

On the external surface of each lamina, an oblique line curves downwards and forwards from the superior thyroid tubercle, situated just in front of the root of the superior horn, to the inferior thyroid tubercle on the lower border of the lamina. This line marks the attachments of the thyrohyoid, sternothyroid and inferior constrictor muscles. The inner aspects of the laminae are smooth and are mainly covered by loosely attached mucous membrane. The thyroepiglottic ligament is attached to the inner aspect of the thyroid notch, and below this, and on each side of the midline, the vestibular and vocal ligaments, and the thyroarytenoid, thyroepiglottic and vocalis muscles are attached. The fusion of the anterior ends of the two vocal ligaments produces the anterior commissure tendon which is of importance in the spread of carcinoma.

The superior border of each lamina gives attachment to the corresponding half of the thyrohyoid ligament. The inferior border of each half is divided into two by the inferior tubercle. The cricothyroid membrane is attached to the inner aspect of the medial portion of the inferior border of the thyroid cartilage.

The cricoid cartilage

The cricoid cartilage (*see Figures 12.3 and 12.4*) is the only complete cartilaginous ring present in the air passages. It forms the inferior part of the anterior and lateral walls and most of the posterior wall of the larynx. Likened to a signet ring, it comprises a deep broad quadrilateral lamina posteriorly and a narrow arch anteriorly. Near the junction of arch and lamina, an articular facet exists for the inferior cornu of the thyroid cartilage. The lamina has sloping shoulders, which carry articular facets for the arytenoids. These joints are synovial with capsular ligaments. Rotation of the cricoid cartilage on the thyroid cartilage can occur about an axis passing traversely through the joints. A vertical ridge in the midline of the lamina gives attachment to the longitudinal muscle of the oesophagus and produces a shallow concavity on each side for the origin of the posterior cricoarytenoid muscle. The entire surface of the cricoid cartilage is lined with mucous membrane.

The arytenoids and small cartilages

The two arytenoid cartilages (*see Figure 12.4*) are placed close together on the upper and lateral borders of the cricoid lamina. Each is an irregular three-sided pyramid with a forward projection, the vocal process, attached to the vocal folds, and also a lateral projection, the muscular process to which are attached the posterior cricoarytenoid and lateral cricoarytenoid muscles. Between these two processes is the anterolateral surface which is irregular and divided into two fossae by a crest running from the apex. The upper triangular fossa gives attachment to the vestibular ligament and the lower to the vocalis and lateral cricoarytenoid muscles. The apex is curved backwards and medially and is flattened for articulation with the corniculate cartilage to which is attached the aryepiglottic folds. The medial surfaces are covered with mucous membrane and form the lateral boundary of the intercartilaginous part of the rima glottidis. The posterior surface is covered entirely by the transverse arytenoid muscle.

The base is concave and presents a smooth surface for articulation, with the sloping shoulder on the upper border of the cricoid lamina. The capsular ligament of this synovial joint is lax, allowing both rotary and medial and lateral gliding movements. In man the cylindrical articulating surfaces permit a greater range of gliding than of rotary movement, and the shape of the open human glottis resembles a V. A firm posterior cricoarytenoid ligament prevents forward movement of the arytenoid cartilage.

The corniculate and cuneiform cartilages

The corniculate cartilages (*see Figure 12.4*) are two small conical nodules of elastic fibrocartilage which articulate as a synovial joint, or which are sometimes fused, with the apices of the arytenoid cartilages. They are situated in the posterior parts of the aryepiglottic folds of mucous membrane.

The cuneiform cartilages are two small elongated flakes of elastic fibrocartilage placed one in each margin of the aryepiglottic fold.

The cartilage of the epiglottis

The epiglottis is a thin, leaf-like sheet of elastic fibrocartilage which projects upwards behind the tongue and the body of the hyoid bone (*see Figure 12.4*). The narrow stalk is attached by the thyroepiglottic ligament to the angle between the thyroid laminae, below the thyroid notch. The upper broad part is directed upwards and backwards; its superior margin is free. The sides of the epiglottis are attached to the arytenoid cartilages by the aryepiglottic folds of mucous membrane which, together with the free edge of the epiglottis, form the anterior boundary to the inlet of the larynx. The posterior surface of the epiglottis is concave and smooth but a small central projection, the tubercle, is present in the lower part. The bare cartilage is indented by numbers of small pits into which mucous glands project. The anterior surface of the epiglottis is free and is covered with mucous membrane which is reflected on to the pharyngeal part of the tongue and on to the lateral wall of the pharynx, forming a median glossoepiglottic fold and two lateral glossoepiglottic folds. The depression formed on each side of the median glossoepiglottic fold is the vallecula. An elastic ligament, the hyoepiglottic ligament, connects the lower part of the epiglottis to the hyoid bone in front. The space between the epiglottis and the thyrohyoid membrane is filled with fatty tissue. The epiglottis is not functionally developed in man in that respiration, deglutition and phonation can take place almost normally even if it has been destroyed. In neonates and infants, however, the epiglottis is omega-shaped. This long, deeply grooved, 'floppy' epiglottis more closely resembles that of aquatic mammals and is more suited to its function of protecting the nasotracheal air passage during suckling.

Calcification of the laryngeal cartilages

The corniculate and cuneiform cartilages, the epiglottis, and the apices of the arytenoids consist of elastic fibrocartilage, which shows little tendency to calcify. The thyroid, cricoid and greater part of the arytenoids consist of hyaline cartilage which begins to calcify in the person's late teens or early twenties. Calcification of the thyroid cartilage starts in the region of the inferior cornu and proceeds anteriorly and superiorly until the entire rim is involved. A central translucent window persists into old age. Calcification of the posterior part of the lamina of the cricoid and of the posterior part of arytenoid may be confused at radiology with a foreign body (*see also under* Applied anatomy of larynx). Calcification of the body and muscular process of the arytenoid begins later but the vocal process tends not to ossify.

The ligaments

Extrinsic ligaments

The extrinsic ligaments (*see Figures 12.3, 12.4 and 12.5*) connect the cartilages to the hyoid and trachea.

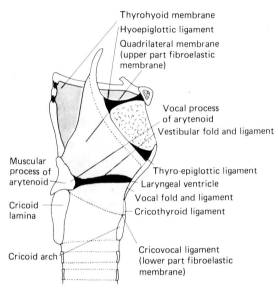

Thyrohyoid membrane
Hyoepiglottic ligament
Quadrilateral membrane (upper part fibroelastic membrane)
Vocal process of arytenoid
Vestibular fold and ligament
Muscular process of arytenoid
Thyro-epiglottic ligament
Laryngeal ventricle
Vocal fold and ligament
Cricoid lamina
Cricothyroid ligament
Cricoid arch
Cricovocal ligament (lower part fibroelastic membrane)

Figure 12.5 Ligaments and membranes of the larynx seen laterally

The thyrohyoid membrane stretches between the upper border of the thyroid and the upper border of the posterior surfaces of the body and greater cornua of the hyoid bone. The membrane is composed of fibroelastic tissue and is strengthened anteriorly by condensed fibrous tissue called the median thyrohyoid ligament. The posterior margin is also stretched to form the lateral thyrohyoid ligament which connects the tips of the superior cornua of the thyroid cartilage to the posterior ends of the greater cornua of the hyoid. The ligaments often contain a small nodule, the cartilago triticea. The membrane is pierced by the internal branch of the superior laryngeal nerve and by the superior laryngeal vessels.

The cricotracheal ligament unites the lower border of the cricoid cartilage with the first tracheal ring.

The hyoepiglottic ligament connects the epiglottis to the back of the body of the hyoid.

Intrinsic ligaments

The intrinsic ligaments (*Figure 12.5*) connect the cartilages themselves, and together they strengthen the capsules of the intercartilaginous joints and form the broad sheet of fibroelastic tissue, the fibroelastic membrane, which lies beneath the mucous membrane of the larynx and creates an internal framework.

The fibroelastic membrane is divided into an upper and lower part by the laryngeal ventricle. The upper quadrilateral membrane extends between the border of the epiglottis and the arytenoid cartilage. The upper margin forms the frame of the aryepiglottic fold which is the fibrous skeleton of the laryngeal inlet; the lower margin is thickened to form the vestibular ligament which underlies the vestibular fold or false cord. The lower part is altogether a thicker membrane, containing many elastic fibres. It is commonly called the cricovocal ligament, cricothyroid ligament or, by a more loose term, the conus elasticus. It is attached below to the upper border of the cricoid cartilage and above is stretched between the midpoint of the laryngeal prominence of the thyroid cartilage anteriorly and the vocal process of the arytenoid behind. The free upper border of this membrane constitutes the vocal ligament, the framework of the vocal fold or true cord. Anteriorly, there is a thickening of the membrane, the cricothyroid ligament, which links the cricoid and the thyroid cartilages in the midline. (For laryngotomy, *see under* Applied anatomy of the larynx.)

The interior of the larynx

The cavity of the larynx extends from the pharynx at the laryngeal inlet to the beginning of the lumen of the trachea at the lower border of the cricoid cartilage and is divided by the vestibular and vocal folds into three compartments. The superior vestibule is above the vestibular folds, the ventricle or sinus of the larynx lies between the vestibular and vocal folds, and the subglottic space extends from the vocal folds to the lower border of the cricoid cartilage (*see Figure 12.5*). The fissure between the vestibular folds is called the rima vestibuli and that between the vocal folds is the rima glottidis or glottis. The paraglottic and pre-epiglottic spaces, which are of importance in the spread of tumours, lie within the larynx.

The laryngeal inlet is bounded superiorly by the free edge of the epiglottis and on each side by the aryepiglottic folds. Posteriorly, the inlet is completed by the mucous membrane between the two arytenoid cartilages. There is a plentiful supply of mucous glands in the margins of the aryepiglottic folds.

The superor vestibule lies between the inlet of the larynx and the level of the vestibular folds. It narrows as it extends downwards and the anterior wall, which is the posterior surface of the epiglottis, is much deeper than the posterior wall which is formed by mucous membrane covering the anterior surface of the arytenoid cartilages. The lateral walls are formed by the inner aspect of the aryepiglottic folds.

The pre-epiglottic space is a wedge-shaped space lying in front of the epiglottis and is bounded anteriorly by the thyrohyoid ligament and the hyoid bone. Above a deep layer of fascia, the hyoepiglottic ligament connects the epiglottis to the hyoid bone. It is continuous laterally with the paraglottic space which is bounded by the thyroid cartilage laterally, the conus elasticus and quandrangular membrane medially and the anterior reflection of the pyriform fossa mucosa posteriorly. It embraces the ventricles and saccules.

The middle part of the cavity (and ventricle) lies between the vestibular and vocal folds which cover the ligaments of the same name. On each side, it opens, through a narrow horizontal slit, into an elongated recess, the laryngeal ventricle or sinus. From the anterior part of the ventricle, a pouch, the saccule of the larynx, ascends between the vestibular folds and the inner surface of the thyroid cartilage. It may extend as far as the upper border of the cartilage; indeed, in some monkeys and apes, it extends even further into the neck, as far as the axilla. In man, the saccule occasionally protrudes through the thyrohyoid membrane. The mucous membrane lining the saccule contains numerous mucous glands, lodged in submucous aveolar tissue. Fibrous tissue surrounds the saccule and a limited number of muscle fibres pass from the apex of the arytenoid cartilage across the medial aspect of the saccule to the aryepiglottic fold. The muscle is presumed to compress the saccule and to express the secretion of its mucous glands over the surface of the vocal folds.

The vestibular folds are two thick, pink folds of mucous membrane, each enclosing a narrow band of fibrous tissue, the vestibular ligament, which is fixed in front to the angle of the thyroid cartilage, just below the attachment of the epiglottic cartilage, and behind to the anterolateral surface of the arytenoid cartilage, just above the vocal process.

The vocal folds are two sharp, white folds of mucous membrane closely attached to the vocal ligaments which extend from the middle of the angle of the thyroid cartilage to the vocal processes of the arytenoid cartilages. The vocal ligaments are the free upper margins of the cricovocal membrane and consist of a band of yellow elastic tissue, related on the lateral side to the vocalis muscle; the

ligaments are, therefore, capable of stretching and their alteration in shape is fundamental to the production of voice. The vocal folds are covered with stratified squamous epithelium. As a result of the absence of a submucous layer and blood vessels, the vocal fold is a pearly white colour in the living subject.

The rima glottidis or glottis is an elongated fissure between the vocal folds anteriorly, and the vocal processes and bases of the arytenoid cartilages posteriorly. It is limited behind by the mucous membrane between the arytenoid cartilages, at the level of the vocal folds. The region between the vocal folds accounts for three-fifths of the length of the aperture and is termed the 'intermembranous part'. The remainder lies between the vocal processes and is called the intercartilaginous part. The average length of the glottis varies between 23 mm in the male and 16–17 mm in the female. In the resting state, the vocal processes are usually 8 mm apart. The glottis alters shape with phonation and respiration.

The lower part of the laryngeal cavity or subglottic space extends from the level of the vocal folds to the lower border of the cricoid cartilage. Its upper part is elliptical in form, but its lower part widens and becomes circular in shape and continuous with the cavity of the trachea. It is lined with mucous membrane, and its walls consist of the cricothyroid ligament above and the inner surface of the cricoid cartilage below.

The muscles

The muscles of the larynx may be divided into extrinsic, which attach the larynx to neighbouring structures and intrinsic, which move the various cartilages of the larynx.

Extrinsic muscles

The extrinsic muscles are the sternothyroid, thyrohyoid and inferior constrictor of the pharynx. In addition, a few fibres of the stylopharyngeus and palatopharyngeus reach forward to the posterior border of the thyroid cartilage.

The sternothyroid muscle arises from the posterior surface of the manubrium sterni and from the edge of the first, and occasionally the second, costal cartilage, and is inserted into the oblique line on the anterolateral surface of the thyroid lamina. It is supplied by the ansa cervicalis (C2,3), and depresses the larynx.

The thyrohyoid muscle arises from the oblique line of the thyroid lamina and is inserted into the inferior border of the greater cornu of the hyoid bone. It is supplied by C1 fibres by way of the hypoglossal nerve. This muscle either elevates the larynx if the hyoid is fixed, or depresses the hyoid if the larynx is fixed.

The inferior constrictor muscle is divided into two parts, namely cricopharyngeus and thyropharyngeus, and is described fully in Chapter 10. Although it is attached to the laryngeal cartilages, this muscle has no direct action on laryngeal movement.

The stylopharyngeus muscle arises from the inner surface of the base of the styloid process, passes between the superior and middle constrictors and spreads out beneath the mucous membrane to blend with the inferior constrictors and palatopharyngeus. Some fibres are inserted into the posterior border of the thyroid cartilage. This muscle is supplied by the glossopharyngeal nerve and helps to elevate the larynx.

The palatopharyngeus muscle is described in Chapter 10. It is inserted into the posterior border of the thyroid cartilage and is supplied by the accessory nerve through the pharyngeal plexus. Although its main action is to raise and shorten the wall of the pharynx, this muscle probably helps in the forward tilting of the larynx, thus enabling food to pass straight into the oesophagus during the act of swallowing.

Because the larynx is attached to the hyoid bone by the thyrohyoid membrane, any muscle which elevates the hyoid, such as the mylohyoid, geniohyoid and stylohyoid, will also elevate the larynx, while the sternohyoid and omohyoid will depress it.

The actions of the extrinsic laryngeal muscles can, therefore, be summarized into two categories: elevators of the larynx which include the thyrohyoid (if hyoid is fixed), stylopharyngeus, palatopharyngeus, mylohyoid, geniohyoid and stylohyoid muscles; and depressors of the larynx which include the sternothyroid, sternohyoid and omohyoid muscles.

Intrinsic muscles

The intrinsic muscles of the larynx (*Figures 12.6 and 12.7*) may be divided into: first, those that open and close the glottis, namely the lateral and posterior cricoarytenoids and the transverse and oblique arytenoids; second, those that control the tension of the vocal ligaments, namely the thyroarytenoids, the vocalis and the cricothyroids; and third, those that alter the shape of the inlet of the larynx, namely the aryepiglotticus and the thyroepiglotticus. With the exception of the transverse arytenoid, all these muscles are paired.

The lateral cricoarytenoid arises from the superior border of the lateral part of the arch of the cricoid cartilage and is inserted into the front of the muscular process of the arytenoid. It adducts the

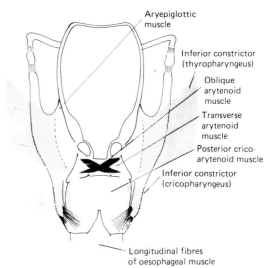

Figure 12.6 Intrinsic muscles of the larynx seen from behind

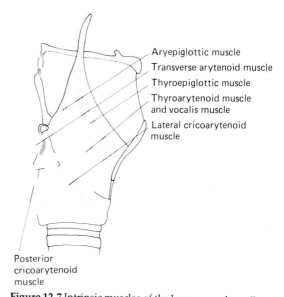

Figure 12.7 Intrinsic muscles of the larynx seen laterally

vocal ligaments by rotating the arytenoid cartilages medially.

The posterior cricoarytenoid muscle, which is the only muscle to open the glottis, arises from the lower and medial surface of the back of the cricoid lamina and fans out to be inserted into the back of the muscular process of the arytenoid cartilage. Its upper fibres are almost horizontal, while its lateral fibres are almost vertical. The horizontal action rotates the arytenoids and moves the muscular processes towards each other, thus separating the vocal processes and abducting the vocal ligaments. The vertical action (lateral fibres) draws the arytenoids down the sloping shoulders of the cricoid cartilage, thus separating the arytenoids from each other. These actions occur simultaneously, although in man there is a greater proportion of vertical movement, thus opening the glottis in a V shape. An additional action of the posterior cricoarytenoid muscle is to brace back the arytenoids during phonation, thus preventing the vocal processes from tilting forwards. The weight of the abductor muscles of the larynx is not more than 25% of that of the adductors (Bowden and Sheuer, 1960), which may explain the greater vulnerability of the abductors in the event of partial injury to the recurrent laryngeal nerve. In a study of the intrinsic muscles of 54 normal postmortem larynges, it was observed that while no significant alterations had occurred in the cricothyroid, interarytenoid, lateral cricoarytenoid or thyroarytenoid muscles, all the larynges from patients 13 years old or over revealed microscopical changes in the posterior cricoarytenoid muscle, and in many of those from patients over 46 years old there had also been some necrosis and associated reactive changes to this (Guindi *et al.*, 1981). Because the posterior cricoarytenoid muscle is the sole abductor of the vocal folds, the changes may be a manifestation of the continuous activity of this muscle. The changes start with the deposition of coarse lipofuscin granules near the sarcolemma. Similar granules are found in tongue muscle and in myocardial fibres from an early age. Only in the posterior cricoarytenoid muscle, however, does concomitant muscle and other sarcoplastic change take place.

The interarytenoid muscles comprise the paired oblique arytenoid muscles and the unpaired transverse arytenoid muscle. Each acts as adductor of the vocal folds by approximating the arytenoid cartilages. The transverse arytenoid muscle arises from the posterior surface of the muscular process and the outer edge of one arytenoid and passes to similar attachments on the other cartilage. The oblique arytenoid muscles lie superficial to the transverse arytenoid muscle and pass from the posterior aspect of the muscular process of one arytenoid cartilage to the apex of the other; they, therefore, cross each other. Some of the fibres pass round the apex of the arytenoid cartilage and are prolonged into the aryepiglottic fold as the aryepiglottic muscle which acts as a rather weak sphincter of the laryngeal inlet.

The thyroarytenoid muscles arise from the lower posterior aspect of the junction of the thyroid laminae and from the cricothyroid ligament below. They are inserted into the anterolateral surface of each arytenoid cartilage. Each muscle is in the form of a broad sheet which passes lateral to the vocal ligaments and the cricovocal membrane. The lower part of the muscle is thicker and forms a distinct bundle called the vocalis muscle which is attached posteriorly to the vocal process of the arytenoid and to the lateral surface of the body of the cartilage. It is generally thought that many of the fibres arise from the vocal ligament and do not extend as far forwards as the thyroid cartilage, but this is disputed by some who believe that all its fibres extend from the thyroid cartilage to the arytenoid (Tautz and Rohen, 1967). The muscle is thus more pronounced posteriorly. Contraction of the vocalis pulls up portions of the cricovocal membrane, thereby increasing the vertical depth of the opposing surfaces of the vocal folds. The action of the thyroarytenoid muscles is to draw the arytenoid cartilages towards the thyroid cartilage and thus to shorten the vocal ligaments. At the same time, they rotate the arytenoid cartilages medially and approximate the vocal folds. A considerable number of fibres of the thyroarytenoid are prolonged into the aryepiglottic fold, some continuing to the margin of the epiglottis as the thyroepiglottic muscle which tends to widen the inlet of the larynx by pulling the aryepiglottic folds slightly apart. Occasionally, there is present a very fine muscle, the superior thyroarytenoid, which lies on the lateral surface of the main mass of the thyroarytenoid and extends obliquely from the angle of the thyroid cartilage to the muscular process of the arytenoid cartilage.

The cricothyroid muscle (*Figure 12.8*) is the only intrinsic laryngeal muscle which lies outside the cartilaginous framework. It is fan-shaped and

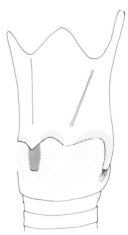

Figure 12.8 The cricothyroid muscle

arises from the lateral surface of the anterior arch of the cricoid cartilage. Its fibres then diverge and pass backwards in two groups. The lower, oblique fibres pass backwards and laterally to the anterior border of the inferior cornu of the thyroid cartilage, and the upper, straight fibres ascend to the posterior part of the lower border of the thyroid lamina. The cricothyroid muscle rotates the cricoid cartilage about the horizontal axis passing through the cricothyroid joint (*Figure 12.9*). The question of whether the thyroid

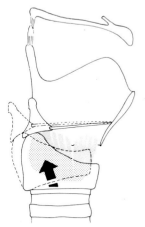

Figure 12.9 Movements of the cricothyroid muscle

cartilage moves on a fixed cricoid cartilage, as in phonation when the cricoid cartilage is held immovably against the vertebral column by the action of cricopharyngeus, or whether the cricoid cartilage moves on the thyroid cartilage, as in swallowing, is immaterial because the action of the cricothyroid in each case is to lengthen the vocal ligaments by increasing the distance between the angle of the thyroid cartilage and arytenoids.

Movements of the vocal folds and the anatomy of speech

The understanding of the movements of the vocal folds during phonation was enhanced by the high-speed film made by the Bell Telephone Laboratories in 1940. This classic film, shot at 4000 frames per second, has been analysed by many observers (Farnsworth, 1940; Pressman, 1942). Other methods of observing vocal fold movements during phonation include frontal tomography (Fink and Kirschner, 1958; Hollien and Curtis, 1960) and stroboscopy (Smith, 1954).

In quiet respiration, the intermembranous part of the glottis is triangular, and the intercartilaginous part is rectangular as the medial surfaces of the arytenoids are parallel (*Figure 12.10a*).

In forced respiration (*Figure 12.10b*), the vocal folds undergo extreme abduction; the arytenoid cartilages are rotated laterally and their vocal processes move widely apart. The glottis is thus rhomboid in shape.

Abduction of the vocal folds (*Figure 12.10c*) is effected by the pull of the posterior cricoarytenoid muscles. The arytenoids are laterally rotated and thus the glottis becomes triangular.

Preparatory to phonation, the intermembranous and intercartilaginous parts of the glottis are reduced to a linear chink by the adduction of the vocal folds and adduction and medial rotation of the arytenoid cartilages. The crude adduction is effected by the cricothyroid and lateral cricoarytenoid muscles (*Figure 12.10d*), and the fine tension of the vocal fold is produced by the tonic contraction of the thyroarytenoid muscle. The interarytenoid muscles, by pulling the arytenoid cartilages together, complete adduction by closing the posterior glottic chink (*Figure 12.10e*).

The vocal folds are lengthened by the cricothyroid muscles. Because of the nature of the felted membrane of fibroelastic tissue within the vocal folds, squares of this network are converted into diamonds by increasing the length of the vocal folds without a corresponding increase in tension. The tension of the vocal fold is a function of the tonic contraction of the thyroarytenoid muscle

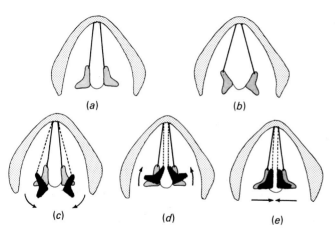

Figure 12.10 Diagrams to show the different positions of the vocal folds and arytenoid cartilages. (*a*) Position at rest in quiet respiration. (*b*) Forced inspiration. (*c*) Abduction of the vocal folds. (*d*) Adduction of the vocal folds. (*e*) Closure of the posterior glottic chink

which is well designed to produce a wide range of tension in many small steps (Zenker, 1964).

Changes in length and tension control the pitch of the voice and occur normally only when the vocal folds are in contact for phonation.

Three forces act to bring the vocal folds in contact with each other. They are: first, the tension in the fold; second, the decrease in subglottic air pressure which occurs with each vibratory opening of the glottis; and third, the sucking-in effect of escaping air (the Bernoulli effect). The result of this rapidly repeating cycle of opening and closing at the glottis is the release of small puffs from the subglottic air column which form sound waves.

Frontal tomography shows that the area of vocal fold surface in contact with its partners varies according to pitch; at low pitches, the cross-sectional area of the vocal folds is large, but as the pitch rises, the folds become thinner (Hollien and Curtis, 1960).

Stroboscopy demonstrates the presence of both transverse and longitudinal waves in the vocal folds and also the points of contact of the vocal folds.

The function of the vocal folds is to produce sound varying only in intensity and pitch. This is then modified by various resonating chambers above and below the larynx and is ultimately converted into phonemes by the articulating action of the pharynx, tongue, palate, teeth and lips.

Techniques of spectral analysis of the voice show that the vocal tract (larynx, pharynx, mouth and nasal cavities) acts as an intricately selective filter and resonator which propagates a remarkably similar pattern irrespective of the fundamental frequency. This is essential to speech as it ensures that, in spite of a continuously varying tone of voice, a constant quality or timbre is maintained.

Consonants of speech are associated with particular anatomical sites, from which they usually take their designations in the terminology of phonetics; for example, 'p' and 'b' are labials, 't' and 'd' are dentals, and 'm' and 'n' are nasals. These sites have two factors in common. They cause a partial obstruction or constriction at some level in the vocal tract, and they produce an aperiodic vibration or noise which is superimposed on or interrupts the flow of laryngeal tones. For example, dental consonants result from apposition of the top of the tongue to the back of the teeth. This momentarily constricts the passage of escaping air, modifies the resonant parameters of the 'vocal tract' and also generates local noise.

The extreme complexity of speech is reflected in the multiplicity of laryngeal, pharyngeal, hyoid, palatal, lingual and circumoral muscular movements which are combined in rapidly changing combinations to produce phonation and articulation.

Mucous membranes of the larynx

The mucous membrane lining the larynx is continuous above with that of the pharynx and below with that of the trachea. It is closely attached over the posterior surface of the epiglottis, over the corniculate and cuneiform cartilages, and over the vocal ligaments. Elsewhere, it is loosely attached and therefore liable to become swollen.

The epithelium of the larynx is either squamous, ciliated columnar or transitional. The upper half of the posterior surface of the epiglottis, the upper part of the aryepiglottic folds and the posterior commissure are covered with squamous epithelium. The vocal folds, which have a fusiform outline, are also covered with squamous epithelium. The height of the vocal fold diminishes towards the anterior commissure mainly because the inferior edge of the vocal fold slopes upwards. The lower edges of the anterior end of the folds form the apex of the triangular fixed part of the subglottis. Thus a tumour reaching or spreading across the anterior commissure might involve the subglottic space (Stell, Gregory and Watt, 1978).

The remainder of the epithelium of the laryngeal mucous membrane is ciliated columnar, except that islands of squamous metaplasia have been found in the subglottic space in 50% of post-mortem larynges taken from non-smokers (Stell, Gregory and Watt, 1980).

Mucous glands are freely distributed throughout the mucous membrane and are particularly numerous on the posterior surface of the epiglottis, where they form indentations into the cartilage, and in the margins of the lower part of the aryepiglottic folds, and in the saccules. The vocal folds do not possess any glands, and the mucous membrane is lubricated by the glands within the saccules. The squamous epithelium covering the vocal folds is therefore vulnerable to desiccation. Scanning electron microscopy has demonstrated the existence not only of microvilli, but also of microridges (microplicae) on the surface cells of the epithelium of the folds and elsewhere in the larynx (Andrews, 1975; Tillmann, Peitsch-Rohrscheider and Hoenges, 1977). Such features have been observed in other epithelia subjected to drying out (for example, the corneal epithelium), and microplicae are regarded as being conducive to the retention of surface secretions.

Some taste buds, similar to those in the tongue, are scattered over the posterior surface of the epiglottis, and in the aryepiglottic folds.

Blood supply

The blood supply is derived from the laryngeal branches of the superior and inferior thyroid arteries and the cricothyroid branch of the superior thyroid artery. The superior thyroid artery arises from the external carotid artery, and the inferior thyroid artery arises from the thyrocervical trunk of the first part of the subclavian artery. On the left side, the thoracic duct is an important relation to the commencement of the inferior thyroid artery. It lies in front of either the artery or the thyrocervical trunk, crossing them from medial to lateral side.

The superior laryngeal artery arises from the superior thyroid artery. It passes deep to the thyrohyoid muscle and, together with the internal branch of the superior laryngeal nerve, pierces the thyrohyoid membrane to supply the muscles and mucous membrane of the larynx and to anastomose with branches of its opposite side and with those of the inferior laryngeal artery. The latter arises from the inferior thyroid artery at the level of the lower border of the thyroid gland and ascends on the trachea, together with the recurrent laryngeal nerve. It enters the larynx beneath the lower border of the inferior constrictor muscle and supplies the muscles and mucous membrane. The cricothyroid artery passes from the superior thyroid artery, across the upper part of the cricothyroid ligament and anastomoses with the branch of the opposite side.

The veins leaving the larynx accompany the arteries; the superior vessels enter the internal jugular vein by way of the superior thyroid or facial vein; the inferior vessels drain by way of the inferior thyroid vein into the brachiocephalic veins. Some venous drainage from the larynx is by way of the middle thyroid vein into the internal jugular vein.

Lymphatic drainage

The lymphatics of the larynx are separated by the vocal folds into an upper and lower group. The part of the larynx above the vocal folds is drained by vessels which accompany the superior laryngeal vein, pierce the thyrohyoid membrane and empty into the upper deep cervical lymph nodes; whereas the zone below the vocal folds drains, together with the inferior vein, into the lower part of the deep cervical chain often through the prelaryngeal and pretracheal nodes.

The vocal folds are firmly bound down to the underlying vocal ligaments and this results in an absence of lymph vessels, a fact which accounts for the clearly defined watershed between the upper and lower zones.

Nerve supply

The nerve supply of the larynx is from the vagus by way of its superior and recurrent laryngeal branches.

The superior laryngeal nerve arises from the inferior ganglion of the vagus and receives a branch from the superior cervical sympathetic ganglion. It descends lateral to the pharynx, behind the internal carotid and, at the level of the greater horn of the hyoid, divides into a small external branch and a larger internal branch. The external branch provides motor supply to the cricothyroid muscle while the internal branch pierces the thyrohyoid membrane above the entrance of the superior laryngeal artery and divides into two main sensory and secretomotor branches. The upper branch supplies the mucous membrane of the lower part of the pharynx, epiglottis, vallecula and vestibule of the larynx. The lower branch descends in the medial wall of the pyriform fossa beneath the mucous membrane and supplies the aryepiglottic fold and the mucous membrane down to the level of the vocal folds.

The internal laryngeal nerve also carries fibres from neuromuscular spindles and other stretch receptors in the larynx. The nerve ends by piercing the inferior constrictor muscle of the pharynx, and unites with an ascending branch of the recurrent laryngeal nerve. This branch is called Galen's anastomosis or loop and is purely sensory.

The recurrent (inferior) laryngeal nerve on the right side leaves the vagus as the latter crosses the right subclavian artery and then loops under the artery and ascends to the larynx in the groove between the oesophagus and trachea. On the left side, the nerve originates from the vagus as it crosses the aortic arch. It then passes under the arch and the ligamentum arteriosum to reach the groove between the oesophagus and trachea. In the neck, both nerves follow the same course and pass upwards accompanied by the laryngeal branch of the inferior thyroid artery, deep to the lower border of the inferior constrictor, and enter the larynx behind the cricothyroid joint. The nerve then divides into motor and sensory branches.

The motor branch has fibres derived from the cranial root of the accessory nerve with cell bodies lying in the nucleus ambiguus; these supply all the intrinsic muscles of the larynx with the exception of the cricothyroid. The sensory branch supplies the laryngeal mucous membrane below the level of the vocal folds and also carries afferent fibres from stretch receptors in the larynx.

As the recurrent laryngeal nerve curves round the subclavian artery or the arch of the aorta, it gives off several cardiac filaments to the deep part of the cardiac plexus. As it ascends in the neck, it gives branches – which are more numerous on the right than the left – to the mucous membrane and the muscular coat of the oesophagus and trachea, and some filaments to the inferior constrictor.

Applied anatomy of the larynx

Surface anatomy and laryngotomy

In the midline from above downwards, it is possible to palpate the hyoid bone, the thyroid cartilage with the laryngeal prominence (Adam's apple), the cricoid cartilage and the trachea. The level of the vocal folds is approximately at the midpoint of the anterior of the thyroid cartilage. By rolling the finger upwards over the cricoid cartilage, it is possible to feel a soft depression between the cricoid and thyroid cartilages. This is the cricothyroid ligament (*Figure 12.11*) and is the site at which to perform a cricothyrotomy or laryngotomy to relieve upper airway obstruction.

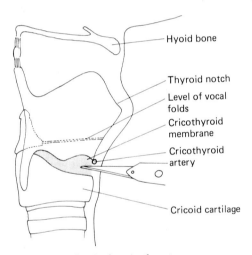

Figure 12.11 The site for cricothyrotomy

This is preferable, as an emergency procedure, to a tracheostomy because of the increased depth of soft tissue associated with an approach to the trachea and the greater likelihood of bleeding from the thyroid isthmus.

Laryngoscopic examination

The larynx and surrounding structures can be examined by either indirect or direct laryngoscopy. With a cooperative patient, indirect laryngoscopy (*Figure 12.12*), using the laryngeal mirror, will give a good view of the back of the tongue, the valleculae, the epiglottis (which is seen foreshortened), the pyriform fossae and the structures of the larynx. If the patient will not tolerate the laryngeal mirror, there are two options open to the

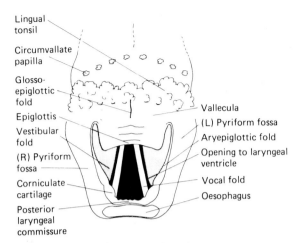

Figure 12.12 Larynx seen on indirect laryngoscopy

examiner. First, the flexible fibreoptic nasolaryngoscope can be passed along the floor of a previously locally anaesthetized nasal cavity and then suspended above the larynx to give a direct view. This technique affords an excellent view of the nose and nasopharynx as well as of the larynx and adjacent structures. The laryngeal position is natural in that the patient's tongue is not being pulled out, and the examination is well tolerated by the patient. Second, if a pathological lesion is seen or suspected and a biopsy or removal of tissue is required, then direct laryngoscopy with or without microscopy under general anaesthesia is recommended. This technique will afford a better view of the laryngeal ventricles and of the subglottis.

Radiology

A good lateral cervical radiograph (*Figure 12.13*) will give a wealth of information about the state of the upper airway, signs of obstruction or the presence of foreign bodies. Oedema of the epiglottis or supraglottic structures will be visible, as will stenosis of the subglottis or upper trachea. The normal ventricle is seen as a clear horizontal area. Care must be taken not to confuse fine lines of calcification in the arytenoid cartilages or the posterior aspect of the thyroid cartilage with foreign bodies (*Figure 12.14*). Tomography, computerized tomography (CT) scanning, and contrast laryngography can all aid the diagnosis of laryngeal lesions.

Injuries to the laryngeal nerves

There is an intimate and important relationship between the nerves which supply the larynx and the vessels which supply the thyroid gland. In a

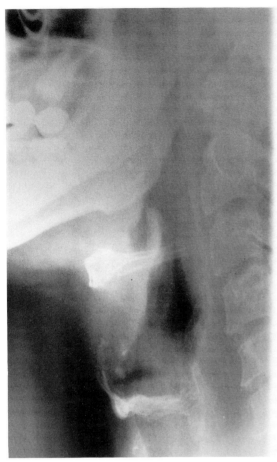

Figure 12.13 Lateral cervical radiograph

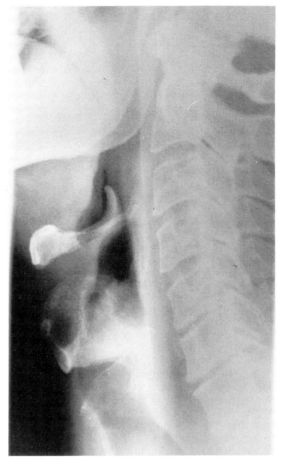

Figure 12.14 Lateral cervical radiograph showing calcification in cartilages not to be confused with foreign bodies

postoperative study of voice function in 325 patients who had undergone thyroidectomy, Kark *et al.* (1984) found that permanent changes occurred in 35 (25%) after a subtotal thyroidectomy, and in 19 (11%) after lobectomy. The commonest cause of voice change appeared to be injury to the external laryngeal nerves on one or both sides. Damage to the recurrent laryngeal nerve, which was routinely identified and protected, was rarely a cause. They found that when the external laryngeal nerve – which descends over the inferior constrictor muscle immediately deep to the superior thryoid artery and vein as these pass to the superior pole of the gland – was identified and preserved, permanent voice changes occurred in only 5% of cases (*Figure 12.15*). This was similar to an incidence of 3% in control patients after endotracheal intubation alone. The functional effect of damage to the external laryngeal nerve is a lower pitched, husky voice that is easily fatigued and has a reduced range. The laryngoscopic changes are much less obvious than those which occur after palsy of the recurrent laryngeal nerve, and their identification may be helped by the use of a stroboscopic light. The edge of the affected vocal fold may be irregular or wavy and usually lies at a lower level, producing an oblique glottic aperture. Recovery after palsy of the external nerve is poor and prognosis is not good (Arnold, 1962).

The recurrent laryngeal nerve comes into close relationship with the inferior thyroid artery as the latter passes medially, behind the common carotid artery, to the gland. The artery may cross posteriorly or anteriorly to the nerve, or the nerve may pass between the terminal branches of the artery (*Figure 12.16*). On the right side, there is an equal chance of locating the nerve in each of these three situations; on the left, the nerve is more likely to lie posterior to the artery (Bowden, 1955).

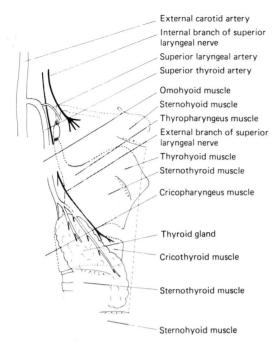

Figure 12.15 label list:
External carotid artery
Internal branch of superior laryngeal nerve
Superior laryngeal artery
Superior thyroid artery
Omohyoid muscle
Sternohyoid muscle
Thyropharyngeus muscle
External branch of superior laryngeal nerve
Thyrohyoid muscle
Sternothyroid muscle
Cricopharyngeus muscle
Thyroid gland
Cricothyroid muscle
Sternothyroid muscle
Sternohyoid muscle

Figure 12.15 Anatomy of the external branch of the superior laryngeal nerve

Injury to the recurrent nerve is enhanced by its displacement from the normal anatomical location by the diseased thyroid gland.

Apart from injury occurring at thyroidectomy, the nerve can also be affected by benign or malignant enlargement of the thyroid gland, by enlarged lymph nodes or by cervical trauma. Paralysis of the left nerve, by virtue of its intrathoracic course, is twice as likely to occur as that of the right. It may be involved by malignant tumours of the lung or oesophagus, by malignant

or inflamed nodes, by an aneurysm of the aortic arch, or by left atrial hypertrophy associated with mitral stenosis.

The functional effect of damage to one recurrent laryngeal nerve is hoarseness, which later resolves itself almost completely in 50% of patients (Watt-Boolsen *et al.*, 1977), either by a return of function on the affected side or by compensatory over-adduction of the opposite normal vocal fold. Bilateral paralysis, however, results in complete loss of vocal power and a marked inspiratory stridor, usually necessitating tracheostomy. Respiratory obstruction following a thyroidectomy can also result from the collapse of the tracheal cartilages (tracheomalacia) associated with a large goitre or with carcinoma of the thyroid.

External pressure on the trachea from postoperative haemorrhage can also lead to respiratory obstruction.

It is generally accepted that the concept embodied in Semon's law, namely that the abductor nerve or muscle fibres are generally more susceptible to injury, is no longer valid. The 'law', after several amendments, stated: 'In the course of a gradually advancing organic lesion of a recurrent nerve or its fibres in the peripheral trunk of the recurrent nerve, three stages can be observed. In the first stage, only abductor fibres are damaged and the vocal folds approximate in the midline and adduction is still possible. In the second stage, additional contracture of the adductors occurs so that the vocal folds are immobilized in the median position. In the third stage, the adductor becomes paralysed and the vocal fold assumes the cadaveric position'.

Descriptions of multiple positions assumed by paralysed vocal cords still cause confusion.

The hypothesis, attributed to Wagner (1890) and Grossman (1897) – which states, first, that total paralysis of the recurrent nerve immobilizes the vocal fold in the paramedian position because of the adductive action of the intact cricothyroid

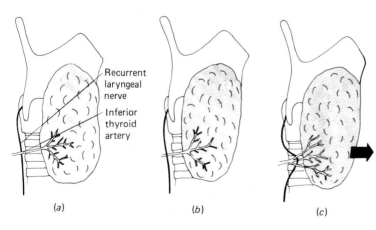

(a)   (b)   (c)

Recurrent laryngeal nerve
Inferior thyroid artery

Figure 12.16 Variations in the relationship of the recurrent laryngeal nerve and the inferior thyroid artery (after Bowden, 1955). (*a*) The nerve may cross posteriorly to the artery, (*b*) anterior to the artery, or (*c*) through the branches of the artery. The lateral lobe of the thyroid has been pulled forward as it would be during thyroidectomy

muscles, and, second, that a 'combined' recurrent laryngeal nerve and superior laryngeal nerve paralysis causes the cord to be immobilized in the intermediate (open or cadaveric) position – is the one preferred by present day laryngologists (Dedo and Dedo, 1980).

This hypothesis is supported by electromyographic and photographic studies of both the human and canine larynx. It is confirmed that the adduction and lengthening effect of an intact cricothyroid muscle is the primary force that holds a paralysed vocal fold in the paramedian position. A vocal fold in the paramedian position is, therefore, paralysed only by a defective recurrent laryngeal nerve, while a vocal fold immobilized in the intermediate position is usually paralysed by a lesion affecting both recurrent and superior laryngeal nerves (*Figure 12.17*). The apparent small variations of positions can be attributed to compensation provided by the normal vocal fold crossing the midline, or to atrophy and scarring of the paralysed vocal fold.

Kirchner (1982) stated that if the ipsilateral vagus nerve, as well as the recurrent laryngeal nerve, were injured, the vocal fold might assume the intermediate position because of the loss of the adductor function of the cricothyroid muscle brought about by the interruption of vagal afferent fibres originating in pulmonary stretch receptors. These receptors exert a monitoring effect on the respiratory centre which, in turn, allows reflex adjustments of laryngeal resistance in breathing.

Trachea and bronchi

The trachea

The trachea is a cartilaginous and membranous tube, about 10–11 cm in length, which extends from its attachment to the lower end of the cricoid cartilage, at the level of the sixth cervical vertebra, to its termination at the bifurcation at the level of the upper border of the fifth thoracic vertebra, or more easily the second costal cartilage or the manubriosternal angle. The bifurcation moves upwards during the act of swallowing, and downwards and forwards during inspiration, often to the level of the sixth thoracic vertebra. The trachea lies mainly in the median plane, although the bifurcation is usually a little to the right of the midline. The diameter of the air passages increases appreciably during inspiration, and decreases during expiration.

In the child, the trachea is smaller, more deeply placed and more movable than in the adult, and the bifurcation is at a higher level until the age of 10–12 years.

The trachea is D-shaped in cross-section, with incomplete cartilaginous rings anteriorly and laterally, and a straight membranous wall posteriorly. The rings of the trachea can easily be seen endoscopically in outline beneath the mucosa, as they cause a slight elevation and pallor of the mucosa. The transverse diameter is greater than the anteroposterior (about 20 mm compared with 15 mm in the adult male).

Measurements of the internal diameter of the trachea vary from study to study but those given in *Table 12.1* (after Engel, 1962) are representative.

The main bronchi and branches

In the adult, the trachea bifurcates into the right and left main bronchi at the level of the second costal cartilage. The main bronchi are separated at their origin by a narrow ridge which, in view of its resemblance to the keel of an upturned boat, is called the carina. The carina always contains cartilage, although the actual dividing ridge is frequently membranous.

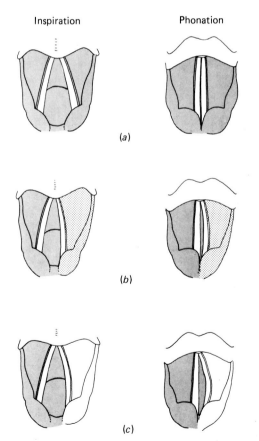

Inspiration   Phonation

(a)

(b)

(c)

Figure 12.17 Vocal fold positions in inspiration and phonation. (*a*) Normal, (*b*) paramedian and (*c*) intermediate

Table 12.1 The internal dimensions of the trachea (after Engel, 1962)

Age	Average length (cm)	Average diameter (mm)	
		Sagittal	Coronal
0–1 months	3.8	5.7	6.0
1–3 months	4.0	6.5	6.8
3–6 months	4.2	7.6	7.2
6–12 months	4.3	7.0	7.8
1–2 years	4.5	9.4	8.8
2–3 years	5.0	10.8	9.4
3–4 years	5.3	9.1	11.2
6–8 years	5.7	10.4	11.0
10–12 years	6.3	9.3	12.4
14–16 years	7.2	13.7	13.5
Adults	9.15	16.5	14.4

The right main bronchus

The definition (to be used in this chapter) of the extent of the right main bronchus is that portion from the tracheal bifurcation to the orifices of the right middle lobe bronchus and the apical segment of the right lower lobe. The right main bronchus (*Figure 12.18*) is about 5 cm in length. It is wider, shorter and more vertical than the left main bronchus. It has a posterior membranous wall and a series of cartilage rings which, although smaller in size, are very similar in structure to those of the trachea. The average angle made by the right main bronchus with the trachea is 25–30°. The coronal diameter of the right main bronchus is about 17 ± 4 mm in the male and about 15 ± 4 mm in the female; the corresponding diameter on the left side is 2–3 mm less. The right pulmonary artery is at first below and in front of the right main bronchus and the azygos vein arches over it. The right upper lobe bronchus is given off 2.5 cm along the course of the main bronchus which, on entering the hilum of the lung, divides into a middle and lower lobe bronchus.

The right upper lobe bronchus (1, 2 and 3)

The right upper lobe bronchus arises from the right lateral aspect of the parent bronchus about 12–20 mm from the carina. It runs superolaterally to enter the hilum of the lung. It is about 1 cm in length and divides into three segmental bronchi which supply the apical, posterior and anterior segments of the upper lobe (*see Figures 12.18 and*

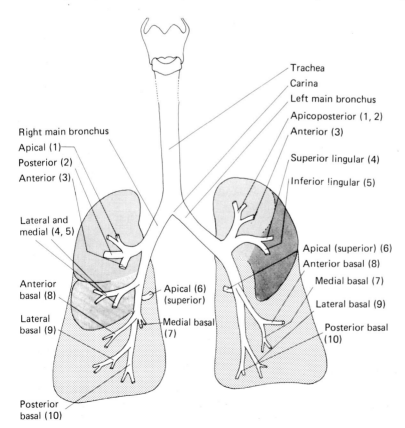

Right main bronchus
Apical (1)
Posterior (2)
Anterior (3)

Lateral and medial (4, 5)

Anterior basal (8)

Lateral basal (9)

Apical (6) (superior)

Medial basal (7)

Posterior basal (10)

Trachea
Carina
Left main bronchus
Apicoposterior (1, 2)
Anterior (3)
Superior lingular (4)
Inferior lingular (5)

Apical (superior) (6)
Anterior basal (8)
Medial basal (7)
Lateral basal (9)
Posterior basal (10)

Figure 12.18 Anterior view of trachea, bronchi and bronchopulmonary segments

12.19). All these can be seen bronchoscopically with a right-angled telescope or with a fibreoptic bronchoscope. This subdivision is a remarkably constant pattern. The most notable of the few variations that do occur is that of an apical segment supplied by a 'tracheal' bronchus which arises from the right lateral aspect of the trachea just above the carina. Its chief clinical importance is that of the confusion it may cause during the resection of a lung, in the case, for example, of carcinoma.

The apical segmental bronchus (1) passes upwards. After about 1 cm, it divides into apical and anterior subsegmental branches.

The posterior segmental bronchus (2) serves the posterior–inferior part of the superior lobe of the lung and runs backwards and somewhat upwards. It divides into lateral (or axillary) and anterior subsegmental bronchi.

Left lung		Right lung	
1.	Apical	1.	Apical
2.	Posterior	2.	Posterior
3.	Anterior	3.	Anterior
4.	Superior lingular	4.	Lateral (of middle lobe)
5.	Inferior lingular	5.	Medial (of middle lobe)
6.	Apical (superior)	6.	Apical (superior)
7.	Medial basal	7.	Medial basal
8.	Anterior basal	8.	Anterior basal
9.	Lateral basal	9.	Lateral basal
10.	Posterior basal	10.	Posterior basal

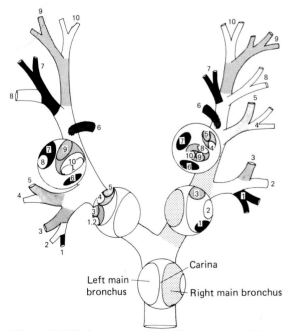

Figure 12.19 Endoscopic anatomy of tracheobronchial tree

The anterior segmental bronchus (3) runs anteroinferiorly to supply the rest of the superior lobe. After a short distance, it divides into lateral (or axillary) and anterior subsegmental branches.

The right middle lobe bronchus (4 and 5)

The right middle lobe bronchus arises about 2.5 cm beyond the origin of the right upper lobe bronchus from the anterior aspect of the bronchus. It is directed forwards, downwards and laterally, and after a short distance divides into lateral (4) and medial (5) subsegments.

The right lower lobe bronchus (6, 7, 8, 9 and 10)

The right lower lobe bronchus is the continuation of the principal stem beyond the origin of the middle lobe bronchus. It supplies five segments of the lung.

The apical (superior) segmental bronchus (6) arises from the posterior aspect of the termination of the right main bronchus. Its orifice is opposite to and only a short distance lower than that of the right middle lobe. It subsequently divides into medial, superior and lateral branches, the former two usually arising from a common stem.

In over 50% of right lungs, a subapical (subsuperior) segmental bronchus arises from the posterior surface of the right lower lobe bronchus between 1 and 3 cm below the apical (superior) segmental bronchus. This is distributed to the region of lung between the apical (superior) and posterior basal segments.

The medial basal (cardiac) segmental bronchus (7) has a higher point of origin than the other basal bronchi. It runs inferomedially parallel to the right border of the heart. The lower lobe bronchus then divides into an anterior basal segmental bronchus (8) which descends anteriorly, and a trunk which divides into lateral (9) and posterior (10) basal segments.

The left main bronchus

The left main bronchus is 5.5 cm long and, because it supplies the smaller lung, is narrower than the right main bronchus. In order to reach the hilum of the lung, the main bronchus has to extend laterally beneath the aortic arch. Its angle to the trachea averages 45°. The bronchus crosses anterior to the oesophagus, thoracic duct and descending aorta; the left pulmonary artery lies at first anterior and then superior to it. At the level of the sixth thoracic vertebra, it enters the hilum of the lung and divides into the upper and lower lobe bronchus.

The left upper lobe bronchus (1, 2, 3, 4 and 5)

The left upper lobe bronchus arises from the anterolateral aspect of the parent bronchus about 5.5 cm from the carina. It curves laterally for a short distance and then divides into two bronchi, which correspond to the branches of the right main bronchus to both apical (superior) and middle lobes of the right lung. They are both distributed to the apical (superior) lobe of the left lung, which does not possess a separate middle lobe. The cranial division acsends for about 10 mm before giving off an anterior segmental bronchus (3). It then continues upwards for a further 1 cm as the apicoposterior segmental bronchus (1 and 2), which subsequently subdivides into apical and posterior branches.

The caudal division descends anterolaterally to be distributed to the anteroinferior part of the superior lobe of the left lung. This part of the lung is called the lingular area. The lingular bronchus divides into superior lingular (4) and inferior lingular (5) segmental bronchi.

The left lower lobe bronchus (6, 7, 8, 9 and 10)

The left lower lobe is smaller than the right. The apical (superior) segmental bronchus (6) takes its origin posteriorly from the left lower lobe bronchus about 1 cm below the upper lobe orifice. The inferior lobe bronchus continues for a further 1–2 cm before dividing into two stems, an anteromedial and a posterolateral stem. The medial basal segmental bronchus (7) arises in common with the anterior basal segmental bronchus (8) from the former; the lateral basal segmental bronchus (9) arises in common with the posterior basal segmental bronchus (10) from the latter.

There has not always been recognition of the medial basal segmental bronchus on the left side because of its common origin with the anterior basal segment. However, in 10% of lungs it arises independently from the lower lobe bronchus, and in all cases it supplies a territory similar to its opposite number on the right side.

A subapical (subsuperior) segmental bronchus arises from the posterior surface of the left lower lobe bronchus in as many as 30% of lungs.

Bronchopulmonary segments

The lung is divided functionally into a series of bronchopulmonary segments, each with its own bronchus and its own blood supply from the pulmonary artery. Each segment is surrounded by connective tissue, continuous with that of the visceral pleura, and forms a separate respiratory unit of the lung. Modern lung resection surgery,

Table 12.2 The bronchopulmonary segments

Right lung		Left lung	
Right upper lobe		Left upper lobe	
apical segment	(1)	apicoposterior	
posterior segment	(2)	segment	(1 + 2)
anterior segment	(3)	anterior segment	(3)
Right middle lobe		Lingula	
lateral segment	(4)	superior segment	(4)
medial segment	(5)	inferior segment	(5)
Right lower lobe		Left lower lobe	
apical segment	(6)	apical segment	(6)
medial basal segment	(7)	medial basal segment	(7)
anterior basal		anterior basal	
segment	(8)	segment	(8)
lateral basal		lateral basal	
segment	(9)	segment	(9)
posterior basal		posterior basal	
segment	(10)	segment	(10)

postural drainage and chest radiology are based on the detailed anatomy of these segments (*see* Applied anatomy of trachea and bronchi).

The segments which have been described in detail previously are summarized in *Table 12.2*, and also in *Figure 12.19*. For further details of bronchopulmonary segmentation, consult Brock (1943, 1954), and Boyden (1955).

Structure of trachea and major bronchi

The trachea and extrapulmonary bronchi consist of a framework of incomplete rings of hyaline cartilage, united by fibrous tissue and non-striated muscle. They are lined by mucous membrane (*Figure 12.20*).

The cartilages

The number of cartilages in the trachea varies from 16 to 20. The cartilages are incomplete rings which stiffen the wall of the trachea both anteriorly and laterally. Behind, where the 'rings' are deficient, the tube is flat and is completed by fibrous and elastic tissue and non-striated muscle fibres. The cartilages measure about 4 mm vertically and 1 mm in thickness. They are placed horizontally one above the other, and are separated by narrow intervals; two or more of the cartilages often unite, partially or completely, and are sometimes bifurcated at their extremities. They are highly elastic, but may become calcified in advanced life. In the extrapulmonary bronchi, the cartilages are shorter, narrower, and rather less regular than those of the trachea, but otherwise they have a similar arrangement.

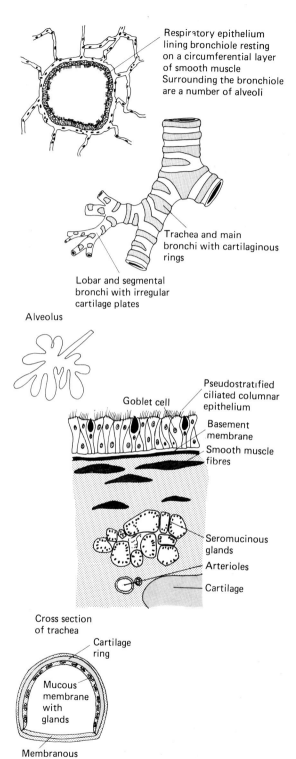

Respiratory epithelium lining bronchiole resting on a circumferential layer of smooth muscle Surrounding the bronchiole are a number of alveoli

Trachea and main bronchi with cartilaginous rings

Lobar and segmental bronchi with irregular cartilage plates

Alveolus

Goblet cell

Pseudostratified ciliated columnar epithelium

Basement membrane

Smooth muscle fibres

Seromucinous glands

Arterioles

Cartilage

Cross section of trachea

Cartilage ring

Mucous membrane with glands

Membranous wall with trachealis muscle

Figure 12.20 Diagrams to illustrate the histological structure of the trachea, bronchus and bronchiole

The first tracheal cartilage is broader than the rest and is sometimes blended with the cricoid cartilages to which it is connected by the crico-tracheal ligament. The last tracheal cartilage is thick and broad in the middle where its lower border is prolonged into a triangular process which curves downwards and backwards between the two bronchi forming a bridge called the carina. The C-ring structure persists in the extrapulmonary portion of the bronchial tree where the walls need to be relatively rigid. In the extrapulmonary bronchi, the walls are supported by numerous cartilaginous plates of very varied shape and size. Here the walls need to be relatively mobile and have less tendency to collapse (Vampeperstraete, 1973).

The fibrous membrane

Each of the cartilages is enclosed in a perichondrium, which is continuous with a sheet of dense irregular connective tissue forming a fibrous membrane between adjacent 'rings' of cartilage and at the posterior aspect of the trachea and extrapulmonary bronchi where the cartilage is incomplete. The fibrous layer of the perichondrium and the fibrous membrane are composed mainly of collagen intermingled with some elastic fibres. The fibres cross each other diagonally, allowing changes in diameter of the enclosed airway, and the elastic component provides the property of elastic recoil when the membrane is stretched.

Non-striated muscle fibres occur within the fibrous membrane at the back of the tube. Most of these fibres are transverse and are inserted into the perichondrium of the posterior extremities of the cartilages (in the trachea, they are known as the trachealis muscle). Contraction of these fibres, therefore, alters the cross-sectional area of the trachea and bronchi. A few longitudinal muscle fibres lie external to the transverse fibres. The relative thickness of the muscle increases as the branching bronchi become narrower.

The mucous membrane

The mucous membrane is continuous with, and similar to, that of the larynx above and the intrapulmonary bronchi below. It consists of a layer of pseudostratified ciliated columnar epithelium with numerous goblet cells resting on a broad basement membrane. The cilia beat the overlying layer of mucus upwards to the larynx and pharynx. Deep to the epithelium and its basement membrane are: first, a lamina propria, rich in longitudinal elastic fibres; second, a submucosa of loose irregular connective tissue in which are situated larger blood vessels, nerve trunks and most of the tubular glands and patches of lymphoid tissue; and third, the perichondrium and fibrous membrane, lying deep to the submucosa.

The outer fibrous and muscular layer of the trachea and bronchi is continuous with the fascial planes of surrounding muscles and the oesophagus, and also with the loose areolar tissue of the mediastinum.

The structure of the smaller bronchi

With increased branching of the segmental bronchi, the epithelial lining becomes thinner and, ultimately, single-layered. There are fewer goblet cells, on a narrower basement membrane, in the smaller air passages. The cartilage plates also gradually become smaller and fewer in number, and are not found in the cartilages of smaller bronchi. Circular muscle fibres almost completely surround the tube inside the cartilages, replacing the fibroelastic layer found in the trachea. The muscle fibres contain numerous elastic fibres and are arranged in an interlacing network, partly circular and partly diagonal, so that their contraction constricts and shortens the tube.

The branched tubuloracemose glands are less numerous in the smaller bronchi and are not present in the bronchioles. Lymphoid tissue is found diffused throughout the mucosa of the bronchi, often in solitary nodules and particularly at points of bifurcation.

Blood supply

The blood supply of the trachea is derived mainly from branches of the inferior thyroid arteries. However, the thoracic end is supplied by bronchial arteries which anastomose with the inferior thyroid arteries and also supply the oesophagus in this region. The tracheal veins drain into the thyroid venous plexus.

The bronchi, from the carina to the respiratory bronchioles, lung tissue, visceral pleura and pulmonary nodes are all supplied by the bronchial arteries, which are usually three in number, one for the right lung and two for the left. The left bronchial arteries usually arise from the anterior aspect of the descending thoracic aorta. The right is more variable; it may arise from the aorta, the first intercostal artery, the third intercostal artery (which is the first intercostal branch of the aorta), the internal mammary artery, or the right subclavian artery. The arteries lie against the posterior walls of their respective bronchi.

The bronchial veins form two distinct systems (Marchand, Gilroy and Wilson, 1950). The deep bronchial veins commence as a network in the intrapulmonary bronchioles and communicate freely with the pulmonary veins; they eventually join to form a single trunk which terminates in a main pulmonary vein or in the left atrium. The superficial bronchial veins drain the extrapulmonary bronchi, the visceral pleura and the hilar lymph nodes. They terminate in the azygos vein on the right side, and in the left superior intercostal vein or the accessory (superior) hemiazygos vein on the left side. The bronchial veins do not receive all the blood conveyed to the lungs by the bronchial arteries for the reason that some enters the pulmonary veins.

Lymphatic drainage

The tracheal lymphatics drain to the pretracheal and paratracheal groups of nodes.

The lung has an abundant lymphatic supply which exists as two systems.

The superficial or pleural system forms a plexus of lymphatics beneath the pleura and is provided with numerous valves. These lymphatics unite and drain into the hilar lymph nodes. The deep or alveolar system accompanies the pulmonary and bronchial arteries and conveys lymph from the interior of the lung to the hilar nodes. There are few valves, except at points of anastomoses with pleural lymphatics, and at the hilum. The bronchial lymph vessels originate in plexuses beneath the mucous membrane. They then penetrate the muscle coat and form a second plexus in the outer fibrous coat, often incorporating nodules of lymphoid tissue.

The distribution of tracheal and bronchial lymph nodes is shown in *Figure 12.21*. These are pulmonary groups of nodes around the smaller bronchi, with bronchopulmonary nodes being mainly beneath the points of division of the intrapulmonary air passages, inferior tracheobronchial nodes being beneath the divisions of the larger bronchi, and a subcoronal group of nodes being beneath the bifurcation of the trachea.

All these nodes subsequently drain to either the right or the left paratracheal nodes by way of the right and left superior tracheobronchial nodes. The right superior tracheobronchial nodes drain the whole of the right lung and also have communications with the left upper lobe. The left superior tracheobronchial nodes drain the greater part of the left lung. The inferior tracheobronchial (subcarinal) group of nodes is important in that these nodes drain lymph from both lungs and, in turn, drain to both right and left paratracheal nodes. Clinically, if these nodes become enlarged, they will cause widening of the carina which will be visible on bronchoscopy. If the nodes are involved in metastatic spread then curative surgery is not feasible.

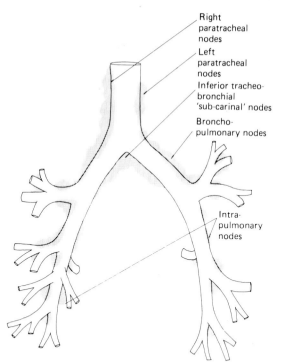

Right
paratracheal
nodes

Left
paratracheal
nodes

Inferior tracheo-
bronchial
'sub-carinal' nodes

Broncho-
pulmonary nodes

Intra-
pulmonary
nodes

Figure 12.21 The distribution of pulmonary and tracheobronchial lymph nodes

Lymphatics from the right and left paratracheal nodes unite with vessels from the internal thoracic and brachiocephalic lymph nodes to form the right and left bronchomediastinal trunks which drain either into the right lymphatic duct and left thoracic duct respectively, or independently into the junction of the internal jugular and subclavian veins of their own side.

Nerve supply

The muscle fibres of the trachea, including the trachealis muscle, are innervated by the recurrent laryngeal nerves which also carry sensory fibres from the mucous membrane. Sympathetic nerve fibres are derived mainly from the middle cervical ganglion and have connections with the recurrent laryngeal nerves.

The lungs are supplied from the anterior and posterior pulmonary plexuses situated at the hilum of each lung. The parasympathetic fibres, carried in the vagus nerve, are afferent (cell bodies in the inferior ganglion) and efferent (cell bodies in the dorsal nucleus with relay in the bronchial mucosa). The vagal efferents are bronchoconstrictor to the bronchial muscles, and secretomotor and vasodilator to the bronchial mucous glands. Afferent fibres are involved in the cough reflex. The efferent sympathetic fibres are postganglionic branches of the second to fifth thoracic ganglion, with an occasional contribution from the first (stellate) ganglion. They are dilator (inhibitory) to the bronchi and pulmonary arterioles. The afferent sympathetic fibres have their cells of origin in the ganglion on the posterior roots of the second to fifth thoracic spinal nerves.

Relations of cervical trachea (*Figure 12.22*)

Anterior

The central part of the trachea is covered anteriorly by skin, superficial and deep fascia and by the sternohyoid and sternothyroid muscles. The isthmus of the thyroid gland covers a variable number of uppermost rings, usually the second to the fourth. There are thus a large number of layers between skin and trachea that have to be divided, in a tracheostomy operation, in spite of the fact that in a thin subject the trachea is easily palpated in the neck. The trachea in the lower part of the neck is crossed by a communicating band between the anterior jugular veins, as well as by the inferior thyroid veins and, when present, by the thyroidea ima artery which ascends from the arch of the aorta or from the brachiocephalic artery.

Lateral

The right and left lobes of the thyroid gland, which descends to the level of the fifth and sixth tracheal cartilages, lie on either side of the trachea, as does the carotid sheath enclosing the common carotid artery, the internal jugular vein and the vagus nerve. The inferior thyroid artery lies anterolaterally.

Posterior

The oesophagus lies behind the trachea, and in the groove between them is the recurrent laryngeal nerve. Behind the oesophagus are the prevertebral fascia and the vertebral column.

Relations of the thoracic trachea (*Figure 12.23*)

Anterior

As the trachea descends through the superior mediastinum, it is related anteriorly to the manubrium sterni, the origins of the sternohyoids and sternothyroids and the thymus gland – the latter of which is usually small and insignificant in the adult, but quite large and fleshy in the infant – the inferior thyroid veins, the left brachiocephalic vein, the arch of the aorta, the brachiocephalic and left common carotid arteries, the deep part of the

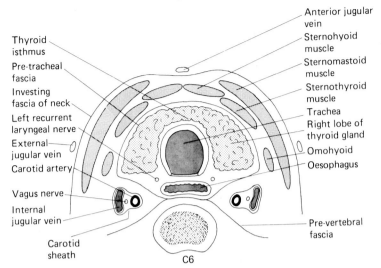

Figure 12.22 Relations of the cervical trachea as shown by transverse section of the neck at the level of the sixth cervical vertebra

cardiac plexus and a variable number of pre-tracheal and paratracheal lymph nodes.

It should be noted that in infants the brachiocephalic artery is higher and crosses the trachea just as it descends behind the suprasternal notch. The left brachiocephalic vein may project upwards into the neck to form an anterior relation of the cervical trachea and a potential hazard during tracheostomy.

Lateral

On the left side are the left common carotid and left subclavian arteries, the left vagus nerve and the descending part of the arch of the aorta. The left recurrent laryngeal nerve passes upwards deep to the arch of the aorta and then into the groove between the trachea and oesophagus.

On the right side, the trachea is related to the pleura and upper lobe of the right lung, the right brachiocephalic vein, the superior vena cava, the right vagus nerve and the azygos vein.

Posterior

The trachea is related to the oesophagus and, behind it, to the vertebral column. To the left and posterior to the oesophagus lies the thoracic duct.

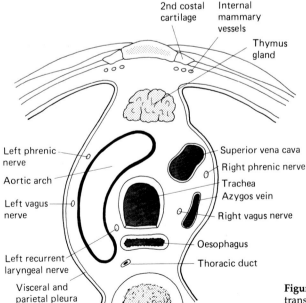

Figure 12.23 Relations of the thoracic trachea as shown in transverse section at the level of the fourth thoracic vertebra

Relations of lung root (*Figure 12.24a, b*)

The root or hilum of the lung transmits the following structures within a sheath of pleura: the pulmonary artery, the two pulmonary veins, the bronchus, the bronchial vessels, the lymphatics, the lymph nodes and the nerves. The bronchi are situated posterior to the pulmonary vessels. The pulmonary arteries lie above the veins. The bronchial vessels hug the posterior surface of the bronchus. All these structures lie between anterior and posterior pulmonary plexuses. The right side differs from the left in one respect, namely that there is an additional upper lobe bronchus which lies above ('eparterial'), but still posterior to, the pulmonary vessels.

The following are the relationships of the lung roots themselves.

Anterior

On the left is the phrenic nerve, and on the right are the superior vena cava and the phrenic nerve.

Posterior

On the left are the descending aorta and vagus nerve, and on the right is the vagus nerve.

Superior

On the left is the aortic arch, and on the right the azygos vein.

Inferior

The pulmonary ligaments are merely a sleeve of slack pleura allowing the necessary freedom of 'dead space' for the structures of the lung root.

Applied anatomy of the trachea and bronchi

Surface anatomy of trachea and main bronchi and relationship to tracheostomy

The trachea, which lies about 2 cm under the skin, extends from the cricoid cartilage almost vertically downwards in the median plane as far as the sternal angle, after which it inclines very slightly to the right. The right main bronchus runs from the lower end of the trachea downwards and to the right for 2.5 cm, to reach the hilum of the lung opposite the sternal end of the right third costal cartilage. The left main bronchus runs at a smaller angle from the lower end of the trachea for 5 cm to the left and downwards to reach the hilum of the lung behind the left third costal cartilage, 3.5 cm from the median plane.

In order to increase the proportion of cervical trachea before a tracheostomy, the head is extended maximally by placing a sandbag between the shoulders. The cricoid cartilage is palpated and the skin incision in the adult is placed approximately 2.5 cm below this level. From the cosmetic point of view, a short collar skin incision is

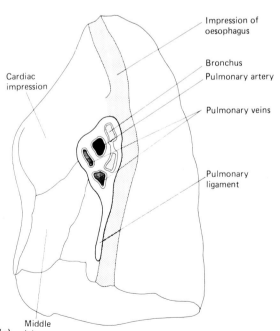

Cardiac impression

Impression of oesophagus

Bronchus
Pulmonary artery

Pulmonary veins

Pulmonary ligament

Middle lobe

(*a*)

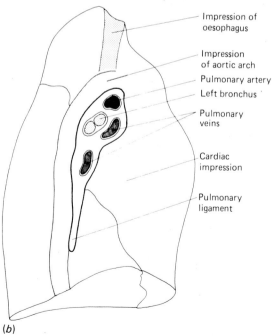

Impression of oesophagus

Impression of aortic arch

Pulmonary artery

Left bronchus

Pulmonary veins

Cardiac impression

Pulmonary ligament

(*b*)

Figure 12.24 (*a*) Root of right lung. (*b*) Root of left lung

preferable to a vertical one. By staying exactly in the midline, danger to the major vessels in the neck is avoided. The pretracheal muscles are separated and the thyroid isthmus is either displaced upwards or downwards or divided. The trachea is opened between the second and third rings. In the adult, a window is cut out of the front of the trachea by removing a part of the second and third, or the third and fourth rings. In the child, the cartilages are very soft and a vertical incision is sufficient to introduce a tube. Care must always be taken not to damage the first tracheal ring. As mentioned previously, the left brachiocephalic vein may project up into the neck in children, and the close relationship of the brachiocephalic artery to the trachea has led to a sudden profuse haemorrhage in consequence of the tracheal wall's being eroded by a tracheostomy tube.

Examination of trachea and bronchi by tracheoscopy and bronchoscopy, and clinical significance of bronchopulmonary segments

Tracheoscopy and bronchoscopy (*see Figure 12.19*)

Tracheoscopy and bronchoscopy can be performed under local or general anaesthesia using either rigid or fibreoptic instruments. At the present time, the most common method is probably that of fibrescopic instrumentation under local anaesthesia combined with controlled sedation. Examination of the trachea and bronchi enables pathological states to be studied and biopsies for histology to be taken, foreign bodies to be removed, or accumulation of fluid to be removed by suction.

Bronchoscopy is an exercise in the practical knowledge of the bronchopulmonary segments.

The trachea is a glistening tube which has a white appearance where there are rings of cartilage and a reddish appearance in the areas between them. The tube appears slightly flattened where it is crossed by the aortic arch, and pulsations are visible. The tracheal bifurcation or carina lies slightly to the left of the midtracheal line because of the more vertically placed right main bronchus. It is consequently easier to advance initially down this bronchus. With the aid of the retrograde telescope or, alternatively, by bending the tip of the fibrescope, the orifices of the anterior, posterior and apical branches of the right upper lobe can be seen. Further advance will reveal a horizontal ridge marking the anteriorly placed orifice of the middle lobe bronchus, below which the lower lobe bronchus lies. Posteriorly, the latter's apical branch orifice can be seen; then the medial (cardiac) orifice appears and, finally, placed close together, from above downwards,

appear the anterior, lateral and posterior basal orifices. If the instrument is now withdrawn into the trachea and advanced along the left main bronchus, the first impression is that of the greater length of the bronchus before the appearance of the left upper lobe in the lateral wall. The mouth of the lingula bronchus can best be seen through a retrograde telescope or by bending the tip of the fibrescope. The advance along the lower lobe bronchus brings the apical and medial basal branches into view posteriorly and then, beyond this, the cluster of orifices of the anterior, lateral and posterior basal bronchi.

Clinical significance of bronchopulmonary segments

The right main bronchus is more nearly in line with the trachea than is the left. It is easier, therefore, for inhaled foreign bodies or fluids, such as gastric contents, to enter the right rather than the left bronchial tree. If the patient is lying on his side, such material enters the lateral (or 'axillary') subsegments of the anterior and posterior segments of the lobe (*Figure 12.25a*). They are thus a frequent site for the development of inhalational pneumonitis, segmental collapse or of a lung abscess.

If the patient is supine then the apical (superior) segmental bronchus, which arises from the posterior aspect of the right or left lower lobe bronchi, is the most likely part of the lung for aspirated

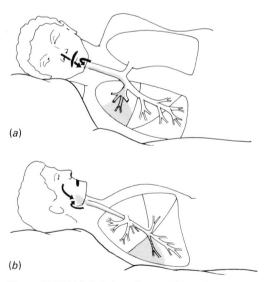

(a)

(b)

Figure 12.25 (*a*) Inhalation of material into the anterior and posterior segmental bronchi of the right upper lobe by an unconscious patient lying on the right side. (*b*) Inhalation of material into the apical bronchus of the right lower lobe by an unconscious patient lying in the supine position

material to collect (*Figure 12.25b*). It was formerly, also, a not uncommon site for a tubercular cavity.

When inhaled, foreign bodies may, according to their size, obstruct either a main, lobe, segmental or smaller bronchus.

While pathological conditions, such as bronchiectasis, and certain infective processes may be restricted to one or more bronchopulmonary segments, malignant neoplasms and tuberculosis break through from one segment to adjacent ones.

If appropriate, surgical resection of a single bronchopulmonary segment can be undertaken. More radical procedures include the removal of a number of segments, of a whole pulmonary lobe (lobectomy), or of a complete lung (pneumonectomy).

Acknowledgement

The illustrations for this chapter were drawn by Mr Stephen Metcalfe, FRCS.

References

ANDREWS, P. M. (1975) Microplicae. *Journal of Cell Biology*, **67**, 11a

ARNOLD, J. E. (1962) Vocal rehabilitation of paralytic dysphonia. *Archives of Otolaryngology*, **75**, 549–570

BOWDEN, R. E. M. (1955) The surgical anatomy of the recurrent laryngeal nerve. *British Journal of Surgery*, **43**, 153–157

BOWDEN, R. E. M. and SHEUER, J. L. (1960) Weight of abductor and adductor muscles of the human larynx. *Journal of Laryngology and Otology*, **74**, 971–980

BOYDEN, E. A. (1955) *Segmental Anatomy of the Lungs*. New York: McGraw-Hill

BOYDEN, E. A. (1972) Development of the human lung. In *Brennemann's Practice of Paediatrics*, Volume 4. Chapter 64. New York: Harper and Row

BROCK, R. C. (1943) Observations on the anatomy of the bronchial tree, with special reference to the surgery of lung abscess. *Guy's Hospital Reports*, **92**, 35–37

BROCK, R. C. (1954) *The Anatomy of the Bronchial Tree*. London: Oxford University Press

DEDO, D. D. and DEDO, H. H. (1980) Vocal cord paralysis. In *Otolaryngology Volume III*, edited by M. M. Paparella and D. A. Shumrick, pp. 2489–2503. Philadelphia: W. B. Saunders

EMERY, J. (1969) (Editor) *The Anatomy of the Developing Lung*. London: Heinemann

ENGEL, S. (1962) *Lung Structure*. Springfield, Ill: Thomas

FARNSWORTH, D. W. (1940) High speed motion pictures of human vocal cords. *Bell Laboratories Records*, **18**, 203–213

FINK, B. R. and KIRSCHNER, F. (1958) Observations on the acoustical and mechanical properties of the vocal folds. *Folia Phoniatrica (Basel)*, **11**, 167–175

GROSSMAN, M. (1897) Experimentelle Beitrage zur Lehre von der 'Posticuslähmung'. *Archiv für Laryngologie und Rhinologie*, **6**, 282–360

GUINDI, G. M., MICHAELS, L., BANNISTER, R. and GIBSON, W. (1981) Pathology of the intrinsic muscles of the larynx. *Clinical Otolaryngology*, **6**, 101–109

HOLLIEN, H. and CURTIS, J. (1960) A laminographic study of vocal pitch. *Journal of Speech and Hearing Research*, **3**, 157–165

KARK, A. E., KISSIN, M. W., AUERBACH, R. and MEIKLE, M. (1984) Voice changes after thyroidectomy: role of the external laryngeal nerve. *British Medical Journal*, **289**, 1412–1415

KIRCHNER, J. A. (1982) Semon's law a century later. *Journal of Laryngology and Otology*, **96**, 645–657

MARCHAND, P., GILROY, J. C. and WILSON, V. H. (1950) Anatomical study of bronchial vascular system and its variations in disease. *Thorax*, **5**, 207–221

O'RAHILLY, R. and BOYDEN, E. A. (1973) The timing and sequence of events in the development of the human respiratory system during the embryonic period proper. *Zeitschrift für Anatomie und Entwicklungsgeschichte*, **141**, 237–250

PRESSMAN, J. J. (1942) Physiology of vocal cords in phonation and respiration. *Archives of Otolaryngology*, **35**, 355–398

REID L. (1967) In *Development of the Lung*. (Ciba Foundation Symposium), p. 109. London: Churchill

REID, L. (1976) Visceral cartilage. *Journal of Anatomy*, **122**, 349–355

SMITH, S. (1954) Remarks on the physiology of the vibrations of the vocal cords. *Folia Phoniatrica (Basel)*, **6**, 166–171

STELL, P. M., GREGORY, I. and WATT, J. (1978) Morphology of the epithelial lining of the human larynx. I. The glottis. *Clinical Otolaryngology*, **3**, 13–20

STELL, P. M., GREGORY, I. and WATT, J. (1980) Morphology of the human larynx. II. The subglottis. *Clinical Otolaryngology*, **5**, 389–395

TAUTZ, C. and ROHEN, H. W. (1967) Über den Konstruktiven Bau des M. vocalis beim Menschen. *Anatomischer Anzeiger (Jena)*, **120**, 409–429

TILLMAN, B., PEITZCH-ROHRSCHEIDER, I. and HOENGES, H. L. (1977) The human vocal cords surface. *Cell Tissue Research (Berlin)*, **185**, 279–283

VAMPEPERSTRAETE, F. (1973) The cartilaginous skeleton of the bronchial tree. *Advances in Anatomy, Embryology and Cell Biology*, **48**, 3–10

WAGNER, R. (1890) Die medianstellung der stimmbander bei der Rekurrenslähmung. *Archiv für Pathologische Anatomie und Physiologie*, **120**, 437–459

WATT-BOOLSEN, S., BLICHERT-TOFT, M., HENSE, J. B., JORGENSEN, S. J. and BOBERG, A. (1977) Late voice function after injury to the recurrent nerve. *Clinical Otolaryngology*, **2**, 191–197

ZENKER, W. (1964) Vocal muscle fibres and their motor endplates. In *Research Potentials in Voice Physiology*, edited by D. W. Brewer, pp. 256–271. New York: New York State University Press

13

Physiology of respiration

Michael Apps and Guy Kenyon

The rhythmic act of quiet breathing entails an active inspiratory movement in which the diaphragm and the chest wall is pulled outwards by active contraction of the external intercostal muscles. In this way, the volume of the thoracic cage is increased and air is drawn into the airway. The primary function of the lung is to provide a site for gaseous exchange so that oxygen can enter the circulation and carbon dioxide can be eliminated. This gaseous exchange occurs in the terminal branches of the bronchial tree in both the respiratory bronchioles and alveoli, while the remainder of the tracheobronchial tree acts simply as a conduit for air passing to and from these exchange sites (*Figure 13.1*).

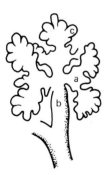

Figure 13.1 Diagram of termination of respiratory bronchiole. a = atrium; b = respiratory bronchiole; c = alveolus

The system has necessarily evolved sophisticated mechanisms to ensure that air inspired through the nose, mouth and pharynx is adequately filtered, and the added protection of the pharyngeal reflexes and the sphincter action of the larynx ensure that food and other large particles do not enter the airway. In addition, the bronchial tree is continually cleansed by ciliated epithelium with an overlying mucous layer which traps fine particulate matter and clears the airway. Adequate respiratory function also demands complex control mechanisms to ensure that oxygenation of the blood is achieved in a variety of different circumstances while allowing for minor irregularities of flow caused by speed and swallowing.

It is the purpose of this chapter to expand and discuss some of the outlines given of the physiology of respiration together with those respiratory function tests in common clinical usage, and to describe the common abnormalities of respiration seen in upper airway disease and in disorders of the tracheobronchial tree.

Pathophysiology of respiration

Mechanics of ventilation and blood flow

Chest wall and respiratory muscles

Quiet breathing entails an active inspiratory movement in which the diaphragm descends and the chest wall is expanded by active contraction of the external intercostal muscles. This results in the generation of a profound negative intrapleural pressure and causes a rapid expansion of lung volume which draws air into the lungs. In contrast, expiration is largely a passive movement which relies on the elastic recoil of lung substance and chest wall.

Downward displacement of the diaphragm results from contraction of the diaphragmatic crura, and this is supplemented by flattening of the hemidiaphragms caused by the contraction of muscle fibres running from the costal margin to the central fibrous tendon. During quiet breathing there is little movement of the chest wall or activity in the intercostal muscles, and most muscle activity emanates from the diaphragm alone; in these circumstances, any intercostal muscle activity serves to prevent inward collapse of the chest wall during diaphragmatic descent. However, where there is an increased workload and more active respiration is required, the external intercostal muscles are recruited. These muscles pass downwards and medially from one rib to another causing, by their actions, upward and outward movement of the ribs which, at the same time, become more horizontal. Where there is a requirement for maximum ventilation (such as occurs during extreme exercise), the accessory muscles of respiration are also utilized. These muscles – including the sternomastoid, the trapezius and the scalene group – help to expand the upper ribs and thereby increase further the intrathoracic volume.

In the presence of diseases of the lung parenchyma, the work of breathing is increased by the concomitant loss of lung elasticity and, in some states such as chronic obstructive airway disease, the problem is compounded by air trapping with flattening of the diaphragms. As a result there is loss of diaphragmatic muscle efficiency. Narrowing of the airway increases the airway resistance and this also increases the work of breathing. Where increased work is required, the metabolic load placed on the respiratory muscles is enhanced; in the presence of coexistent hypoxia, hypokalaemia, hypocalcaemia or hypomagnesaemia, muscle fatigue is accelerated and the likelihood of respiratory failure therefore increased.

In disease states with an increased airway resistance, expiratory movements may also become dependent on active muscle contraction. In such circumstances, the internal intercostal and abdominal wall muscles may be required to expel air from the bronchial tree. In other patients, such as those with kyphoscoliosis and ankylosing spondylitis, respiratory embarrassment results from loss of chest wall mobility and expansion of the lungs becomes more dependent on diaphragmatic movement. In contrast, patients with neurological diseases or muscle dystrophies (such as occur in poliomyelitis or the myasthenia of the Guillain–Barré syndrome) have marked diaphragmatic weakness, and in these circumstances those actions of the accessory and intercostal muscles that are preserved assume a great importance.

Lung volume and dead space

The major subdivisions of lung volume are shown in *Figure 13.2*. The tidal volume is the volume of air breathed in or out during quiet respiration, and is approximately 500 ml, with a resting respiratory rate of 15–20 breaths per minute. The inspiratory reserve volume represents the maximum volume of air which can be inspired after completing a normal tidal respiration, that is inspired from the end-inspiratory position (2000–3000 ml), and the expiratory reserve volume represents the maximum volume capable of being expired after a normal tidal expiration, that is expired from the end-expiratory position (750–1000 ml). As the lung volume decreases on expiration, there is a progressive narrowing of the small airways; these eventually close, trapping air in the distal airway. Even on forced expiration some air remains, and this is termed the 'residual volume' (1200 ml).

One of the most frequently measured parameters in clinical work is the vital capacity. This is the maximal volume of air which can be expelled from the lungs by a forceful effort following maximal inspiration. The vital capacity averages 4.8 litres in the male and 3.2 litres in the female, but is related to the size and age of the subject. It is reduced in older people and also in diseases of the respiratory tract such as respiratory obstruction, pleural effusion, pneumothorax, pulmonary fibro-

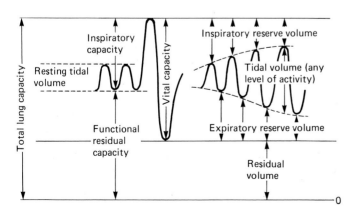

Figure 13.2 Diagram of principal lung volumes and capacities. (Redrawn from Pappenheimer, J. R. *et al.* (1980) *Federation Proceedings*, Vol. 9, p. 602)

sis, emphysema and pulmonary oedema. If the vital capacity is measured by means of a spirometer, the volume of air expelled can be timed. Normally, 75% of the vital capacity should be expired in the first second, which is termed the 'forced expiratory volume' (FEV_1). Such a measurement provides a much more sensitive index of obstruction in the airway than does measurement of the vital capacity alone. Studies of vital capacity and its subdivisions are used to assess pulmonary function and are particularly useful prior to surgery in assessing the risks of general anaesthesia.

Also shown in *Figure 13.2* are: the total lung capacity (TLC); the inspiratory capacity, which is the maximal volume of gas which can be inspired from the resting expiratory level; and the functional respiratory capacity (FRC), which is the volume of gas remaining in the lungs at the resting expiratory level. Most of these lung volumes and capacities can be measured by using a simple spirometer, but residual volume, and hence the functional residual capacity and total lung volume, can be assessed only by measurements of nitrogen washout (in a patient breathing pure oxygen), by whole body plethysmography or, most commonly, by helium dilution. Alternatively, radiological techniques may be applied.

As has already been observed, the respiratory tract is divided into conducting passages and gas exchange surfaces. The latter, formed by the respiratory bronchioles and alveoli, comprise a surface area of some 70–80 m^2 in the adult. Therefore, although much of the surface area of the respiratory system is used for gas exchange, some of the inspired air (about 150 ml) merely fills the conducting air passages between the mouth and nose and respiratory bronchioles; this is called the anatomical dead space. The physiological dead space comprises this volume and also the volume of inspired gas which ventilates alveoli in excess of that which is required to oxygenate blood in the adjacent pulmonary capillaries. In a healthy state, this additional volume is negligible, but in disease states (where there are unequal ventilation/perfusion ratios in parts of the lung) the physiological dead space may greatly exceed that of the anatomical dead space and only a very small volume of the inspired air is then available for gas transfer.

Air flow

In the respiratory tract, air flows through a rapidly branching system which progressively narrows. The resistance to air flow in such a tubular system is inversely proportional to the fourth power of the radius. Therefore, in the normal upper airway and larynx, resistance is low and the flow of air is fast; but if there is narrowing at these sites, turbulence together with a considerable rise in airway resistance will result. As the airway divides, the diameter becomes progressively smaller and hence the resistance to air flow tends to increase. However, this effect is mitigated because the number of airways also rapidly increases and the overall resultant rise in airway resistance is not large. In fact, only 20% of air flow resistance is situated in the small airways and 60% of the overall resistance is found in the medium-sized airways between 2 and 6 mm in diameter.

In the normal subject, minor changes in airway resistance result during different phases of the respiratory cycle. In extrathoracic sites, inspiration tends to collapse the airway, although normal muscle tone and the structure of the airway oppose such forces in order to keep the airway patent. During expiration, the same part of the airway tends to expand as expired air flows from the lungs. In contrast, the major intrathoracic airways expand as the volume of the chest increases during inspiration, and are then compressed by the diminution of lung volume during the expiratory phase. Thus any defect in the extrathoracic airway leads to an increase in the inspiratory resistance, whereas problems in the intrathoracic airways tend to be more acute in expiration. Air passing down the larger airways is therefore subject to some fluctuation in resistance, but as airway radius decreases, the resistance becomes less phase variable and more dependent on airway diameter alone. Eventually, at about the eleventh generation of bronchi (each generation implying an airway division), bulk flow of air ceases and oxygen and carbon dioxide diffuse to the remainder of the lower part of the pulmonary tree.

Gas exchange

Once the inspired air reaches the respiratory bronchioles and alveoli, gas exchange by diffusion across the alveolar membranes and into the pulmonary capillaries occurs. It follows that for this exchange to take place, the blood in the capillaries must be in close proximity to ventilated alveoli, and the transport of oxygen and carbon dioxide will be impaired if there is any mismatch between ventilation and perfusion. In a normal person, both the major air flow and perfusion are to the lower lobes since expansion is maximal in the lower part of the chest and pulmonary arteriolar pressure is low at the bases. Many disease processes produce a mismatch: lobar pneumonia (where there is consolidated lung which has a good blood supply but minimal ventilation) and pulmonary embolus (where there is adequate ventilation but poor perfusion) are extreme examples of conditions which produce imbalance, but many lesser degrees of the same phenomenon may occur.

The transport of oxygen across the basement membrane is limited by the poor solubility of this gas, and as its solubility is considerably less than that of carbon dioxide, a ventilation perfusion imbalance tends to lead to hypoxia, without resulting in decreased carbon dioxide transfer and hypercapnia.

Pulmonary circulation and oxygen transport

Blood returning from the periphery drains to the vena cavae and hence into the right side of the heart. This is a low pressure circulation with a mean arterial pressure of only 25 mmHg, and a maximum pressure of less than 50 mmHg. This low pulmonary vascular pressure means that when the subject is erect most of the blood flow is diverted to the lower lobes of the lungs and very little reaches the apices where the arterial pressure may be as low as 5–10 mmHg.

The pulmonary circulation may be deranged in a variety of ways. One of the most common is a pulmonary embolus which occurs when detached thrombus passes from a large peripheral vein and traverses the right side of the heart to become lodged in part of the pulmonary arterial tree. This event produces a decrease in local lung perfusion in the presence of normal ventilation, with an increase in pulmonary vascular resistance and increased right ventricular work and strain. The rise in pulmonary artery pressure which accompanies a pulmonary embolus may lead to the opening up of arteriovenous anastomoses, and hence to the shunting of blood to the left atrium, with concomitant bypassing of the lungs; this may produce additional hypoxia.

Occasionally, pulmonary artery pressure rises as the result of a shunt of blood from the left to the right side of the heart: such an event occurs in the presence of an atrial or ventricular septal defect. Such a shunt initially produces dilatation of the pulmonary arteries, but this is followed by pulmonary artery vasoconstriction and a subsequent fixed narrowing of the pulmonary arterioles with thickening of the vessel walls. As a consequence, there is a diminution of pulmonary perfusion. Conversely, when there is increased back pressure from the heart, as occurs in left ventricular failure, mitral regurgitation or mitral stenosis, the pulmonary veins become overfilled with blood. Initially, there is no accompanying rise in pulmonary venous pressure, but as the system is further filled the pressure rises and, as a result, the postcapillary pressure is elevated. As in the systemic circulation, fluid balance in the pulmon-

ary capillaries obeys Starling's law; thus fluid normally leaves the capillary circulation at the high pressure arterial end and is reabsorbed at the distal end where the luminal pressure is lower and the oncotic pressure of the blood is sufficient to encourage fluid to return. However, if the pulmonary pressure is raised there is a net movement of fluid into the parenchyma of the lung and pulmonary oedema with decreased lung compliance and hypoxia will result.

Changes in haemoglobin concentration also affect oxygen transport. A reduced concentration of haemoglobin clearly allows less oxygen to be carried in the blood; conversely, an increase in the concentration causes increased blood viscosity with a rise in pulmonary vascular resistance, a reduction in pulmonary capillary perfusion and a diminution in the efficiency of gas transport in the lung. This is particularly likely to occur if the packed cell volume of the peripheral blood exceeds 55% of the total blood volume as this causes a marked rise in viscosity; however, if the packed cell volume remains below 50%, the viscosity of the blood is seldom a limiting factor in gas transport.

The binding of oxygen to, and the dissociation of oxygen from, haemoglobin can be plotted on a dissociation curve (*Figure 13.3*). As the partial pressure of oxygen in the tissues falls, oxygen is released from haemoglobin which, as it passes through the alveolar capillaries, is reoxygenated to form oxyhaemoglobin. The oxygen dissociation curve is altered by changes in the acidity of the environment, with a decrease in pH leading to a decreased affinity of haemoglobin for oxygen. The

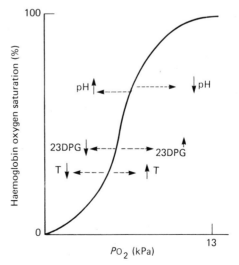

Figure 13.3 Haemoglobin oxygen dissociation curve. T = temperature; pH = acidity/alkalinity; 23DPG = 2,3-diphosphoglycerate

position of the curve is also affected by the concentration of 2,3-diphosphoglycerate in the red cells. This metabolite is produced from cells engaged in active metabolism and is reduced in old cells and particularly in those which have been stored; as a result, transfused blood has a low concentration of diphosphoglycerate which causes a shift in the dissociation curve to the left. A large transfusion, therefore, limits the amount of oxygen which can be delivered to the tissues.

Carbon monoxide also binds to haemoglobin to form carboxyhaemoglobin. This reaction proceeds with an avidity which is more than 250 times the affinity for oxygen. As a result, the binding of this gas is irreversible in practical terms, and any haemoglobin which is linked to carbon monoxide is unavailable for oxygen transport. This becomes clinically relevant in patients who are hypoxic with lung disease and who continue to smoke. Such subjects already have difficulty with ventilation as a consequence of damaged lung tissue, and clearly there will be an added difficulty in providing adequate tissue oxygenation if between 5 and 10% of their circulating haemoglobin is unavailable for oxygen transport on account of its conversion to carboxyhaemoglobin.

Ventilatory regulation

Breathing patterns are under both voluntary and automatic control (*Figure 13.4*). Automatic control is localized in the 'respiratory centre' which comprises a pool of neurons in the grey matter of the pons and upper medulla. Evidence from stimulation testing in experimental preparations has made it possible to delineate separate areas within this group which are responsible for inspiration and expiration, but there is close interaction so that inspiration is associated with inhibition of expiratory neurons in the medulla and expiration with reciprocal inhibition of spinal cord neurons. It is also known that feedback from muscle spindles in the intercostal and abdominal muscles, as well as from the accessory muscles of respiration, acts with the input from pulmonary stretch receptors, 'J' receptors (junctional receptors in bronchial walls) and irritant receptors by way of the vagus nerves to moderate this activity. Although these centres will develop rhythmic discharge when isolated from the upper brainstem and from afferent input, their activity is usually moderated by both the higher brainstem and by phasic impulse traffic in the vagal nerves.

Experimental evidence has also suggested that activity in these centres is moderated by other parts of the pontine reticular formation. Stimulation of the lateral part of the middle and lower pons induces a sustained inspiratory effort, and this 'apneustic centre' is thought to exert a tonic discharge upon the medullary inspiratory centre to promote a more sustained respiratory effort. In turn, this tonic activity is controlled and lessened by vagal afferents, and by an upper pontine centre called the pneumotaxic centre. Even after vagal transection, this latter centre will hold the apneustic centre in check.

It is thought that this somewhat complicated system acts in the following way. The inspiratory centre, under the influence of the stimulus provided by the arterial P_{CO_2} and the tonic activity of the apneustic centre, discharges through the spinal cord to the anterior horn cells in the cervical and thoracic regions that are responsible for promoting diaphragmatic and chest wall movements; inspiration then occurs. At the same time, the inspiratory centre provokes the pneumotaxic centre and this discharges inhibitory impulses to the apneustic centre. This latter centre is therefore exposed simultaneously to these inhibitory impulses and to inhibition relayed by way of the vagus nerve from the pulmonary stretch receptors. In turn, this inhibition reduces activity in the medullary inspiratory centre. This centre then stops discharging and expiration follows passively. It is assumed that the pneumotaxic centre relays excitatory impulses from higher centres to the expiratory centre when active expiration is required.

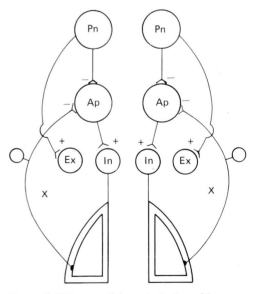

Figure 13.4 Diagram of the organization of the respiratory centres. Pn = pneumotaxic centre; Ap = apneuristic centre; In = inspiratory centre; Ex = expiratory centre; X = vagus afferent from the lung parenchyma

Response to changes in oxygen and carbon dioxide tension

A lack of oxygen or an excess of carbon dioxide in the arterial blood affects respiration, with both hypoxia and hypercapnia causing a rise in the respiratory rate. Chemosensitive areas for this reaction are located in the brainstem and in the carotid and aortic bodies. Thus a decrease in the arterial partial pressure of oxygen causes increased discharge in fibres of the glossopharyngeal and vagus nerves serving the peripheral chemoreceptors, while an increase in oxygen tension (above 27 kPa or 200 mmHg) leads to an abolition of activity in the cells in these organs that are sensitive to hypoxia. Similarly, a rising arterial carbon dioxide tension leads to a parallel rise in hydrogen ion concentration in the peripheral chemoreceptors and this, in turn, results in increased activity in this system. Although the response to hypoxia and hyperoxia is mediated solely through peripheral receptors, the greatest response to a rising carbon dioxide level comes from central chemoreceptors located in the base of the fourth ventricle. These cells are responsive to changes in the hydrogen ion concentration in the surrounding cerebrospinal fluid. They contain a high concentration of the enzyme carbonic anhydrase which catalyses the reaction binding the carbon dioxide and this directly influences the local hydrogen ion concentration by way of the formation of carbonic acid.

Effects of the reticular activating system

The reaction of the respiratory neurons is related to the rest of the brainstem so that a depression of brainstem activity, as is seen in sleep or during anaesthesia, results in a reduction in responsiveness to hypoxia and hypercarbic drives. During sleep, the decrease in these drives is most marked in rapid eye movement (REM) sleep; in this phase, the arterial carbon dioxide in the normal subject may rise by 1 kPa (5–8 mmHg) and the arterial oxygen may fall by 4%. It follows that any patient with a severe respiratory disability, who is only just able to clear carbon dioxide and provide adequate oxygenation when awake, may suffer severe hypoxia and hypercapnia when asleep or anaesthetized.

Higher control of breathing

The respiratory neurons in the brainstem, together with the peripheral receptors and receptors in the fourth ventricle, act in concert to provide a constant arterial oxygen Po_2 and Pco_2 by adjustment of the respiratory rate, respiratory volume and length of the different phases of respiration. If brainstem function is normal, respiration is regular and quiet with a constant pattern of inspiration and expiration. If there is damage to the relevant parts of the brain then this pattern becomes deranged, and either the periodic waxing and waning of Cheyne–Stokes respiration or an irregular gasping pattern of respiration becomes apparent. Superimposed upon the normal patterns of respiration are voluntary and semi-automatic control systems. Therefore, the act of speaking, which requires the coordination of the larynx, pharynx and mouth, and delivery of the correct volume of air to the glottis at an adequate pressure, is not totally involuntary, but necessitates superimposed semi-automatic control which results from coordination learned in childhood. Central organization of this control requires the basal ganglia, cerebellum and cerebrum to act by imposing the desired respiratory pattern upon automatic control while maintaining Po_2 and Pco_2 levels within normal limits. When this system breaks down, words are produced, but there are difficulties in controlling the volume or tone of the speech; such abnormalities are commonly seen after cerebrovascular accidents. In addition, a few patients have been reported with complete cerebromedullary disconnection. Such subjects also experience an inability to superimpose upon automatic respiration the irregularities of respiration associated with voluntary control. Thus in the normal patient, voluntary, semi-automatic and automatic respiration are superimposed during waking hours, but during sleep semi-automatic and voluntary control is lost and respiration becomes totally automatic. As a result, some patients with deranged brainstem control, but normal semi-automatic and voluntary mechanisms, have normal respiration when awake but show severe respiratory dysrhythmias during sleep. For example, in the Shy–Drager syndrome, abnormalities of central autonomic function cause fluctuations in cardiovascular and respiratory control and irregular and disorganized respiration during sleep, with frequent apnoeic episodes. In some subjects, brainstem control is so severely disrupted that sleep results in total cessation of normal breathing (Ondine's curse).

Respiratory failure

Respiratory failure, with its attendant lowering of the arterial Po_2 to less than 8 kPa, may occur with damage to the respiratory system at any level. In most cases, there is inadequate gas exchange as a result of lung damage due to either chronic obstructive airway disease or to pulmonary fibrosis. Initially, the resultant high carbon dioxide levels cause an increased respiratory drive, but responsiveness gradually diminishes and tolerance develops. Carbon dioxide drive is usually the major determinant of ventilatory volume and when this fails the P_{O_2} rises. When levels exceed 10 kPa, carbon dioxide acts as a narcotic and the resultant drowsiness and fluctuating consciousness further depress the respiratory drive. A major problem resulting from this decrease in carbon dioxide responsivenes is the increased reliance on hypoxic drives. Such patients are therefore at risk when given high concentrations of inspired oxygen, for a further reduction in ventilatory drive may result in an additional rise in carbon dioxide tension and consequent unconsciousness. It is for this reason that controlled oxygen therapy is used in patients with chronic obstructive airway disease, and blood gases must be checked regularly to ensure that such therapy does not result in carbon dioxide retention. The respiratory depression caused by sedative drugs, narcotics, strong analgesics or anaesthetic agents can exacerbate this situation and lead to high P_{CO_2} levels and severe hypoxia.

Respiratory control of the upper airway

Coordination of muscle activity in the oral cavity, pharynx and larynx depends upon normal central control in the brainstem and intact pharyngeal wall receptors with normal innervation (provided by the glossopharyngeal and vagus nerves). Defects in this system lead to a loss in patency of the upper airway which may be exacerbated by drug ingestion. This problem will be considered in subsequent sections of this chapter where upper airway disease is discussed.

Breathlessness

Breathlessness is a subjective sensation which does not always correspond with objective evidence of a compromised respiratory system. To some subjects, breathlessness implies tachypnoea whereas to others it implies the physical difficulty of getting air into or out of the chest, with or without an attendant feeling of distress. These differing views result from the various pathologies which give rise to a perception of breathlessness.

If a subject is asked to hold his breath for as long as possible after maximum inspiration, the resulting sensation of distress will rapidly become severe, which will force the person to exhale and resume a normal breathing pattern; this is called the break point. Such holding of breath after the inspiration of a mixture with a low P_{O_2} or a high P_{CO_2} leads to a shortened breath holding time and an earlier break point. Thus hypoxia and hypercapnia clearly influence breathlessness. However, the duration also depends on lung volume, since the duration of breath hold from total lung capacity is much longer than from functional residual capacity or residual volume. It is known that chest wall muscle receptors (which provide information to the central nervous system about the work of breathing and the volume of the chest) also contribute directly to the sensation of breathlessness, as chest wall paralysis causes breath holding to lose its element of respiratory distress. All of these factors interact and are in turn overlayed by psychological elements.

Exercise limitation is often the first sign of respiratory insufficiency. The degree of limitation depends on the respiratory reserve, and a subject with only mild pulmonary disease may not notice any abnormality unless he is forced to exert himself maximally; accordingly, there is no complaint of breathlessness. However, when the respiratory reserve has been lost, even mild exertion will cause dyspnoea, and it is usually at this point that there is an objective realization of breathlessness by the patient. Even so, in some cases the patient's awareness of a respiratory problem may be limited in the face of objective evidence of quite severe disease.

Respiratory toilet and defences

The nose

Air passes through the passages of the nose during quiet respiration and is warmed and humidified. Any large particles are trapped on the nasal mucosa and are expelled either by the nasal cilia or by sneezing. Inhaled gases, such as chlorine, cause irritation in the nose, and this produces reflex rhinorrhoea and sneezing before affecting the rest of the airway to produce coughing. The cilia of the nose and the mechanisms of their action in the nose and tracheobronchial tree are identical and will be considered later.

The pharynx

There are a large number of irritant receptors in the pharyngeal wall and these can be blocked by topical anaesthesia. These receptors act to protect the airway from noxious fumes or foreign bodies by initiating an expulsive cough when stimulated. Patients with brainstem disease or decreased levels of consciousness may suffer suppression of their pharyngeal cough reflex and this leads to the easier passage of foreign material into the tracheobronchial tree. Functionally, the pharynx, larynx and oesophagus are closely coordinated so that breathing and swallowing can occur without allowing excess aerophagia or aspiration of gastric or oesophageal contents into the bronchial tree. Acid reflux or incoordination in the oesophagus (especially at the level of the cricopharyngeus) is liable to cause aspiration, and this is a particular feature of pseudobulbar and bulbar palsy, and may also be a feature of cerebellar disease. Coordination is also often poor at the extremes of life, and young children and the elderly are therefore prone to choke on food or quietly to aspirate gastric contents while asleep.

The larynx

The laryngeal inlet acts as a sphincter to protect the airway. In addition, the closure of the laryngeal sphincter during expiration allows increased intrathoracic pressure to develop, and this manoeuvre aids the development of a large explosive force of expired air which acts to clear the tracheobronchial tree during coughing. Glottic closure also fixes the chest and diaphragm and allows increased abdominal pressure to be produced when the abdominal muscles contract; this aids defaecation, micturition and parturition.

During swallowing, an elevation of the larynx towards the base of the tongue is effected by contraction of the inferior constrictor and palato-pharyngeus and stylopharyngeus muscles; this also brings the pharyngo-oesophageal opening towards the bolus of food. At the same time there is a cessation of air flow as a result of reflex central inhibition, and laryngeal closure occurs at both the glottic and supraglottic levels to prevent food passing into the trachea. As the bolus passes, the epiglottis passively tilts and the shape of its upper surface assists in guiding the swallowed material towards the oesophagus.

The laryngeal sphincters are arranged in three tiers. The first layer is formed by the aryepiglottic folds and epiglottis, the second by the false cords and the third by the true vocal cords. The aryepiglottic sphincter lies almost vertically and consists of a thick band formed by the thyro-arytenoid and interarytenoid muscles. This sphincter closes the pharynx above from the laryngeal vestibule, and sphincteric closure is completed anteriorly by the tubercle of the epiglottis and posteriorly by the bodies of the arytenoid cartilages.

The false cords lie above the true cords from which they are separated by the laryngeal ventricle. Each fold has a free medial border, and the folds extend from the thyroid cartilage anteriorly to the anterolateral surface of the arytenoid cartilages posteriorly. The main substance of the folds consists of a mixture of fibrous and elastic tissue which is covered with pseudostratified columnar epithelium containing mucous glands. At rest, these folds do not project as far medially as the true cords, but when the muscle fibres external to these ventricular bands contract, the bodies of the arytenoid cartilages are approximated.

The true cords extend from the angle between the laminae of the thyroid cartilages to the vocal processes of the arytenoid cartilages. The fibrous element is condensed at the medial border of these folds with the elastic tissue of the upper border of the conus elasticus; the muscle element is provided by fibres of the thyroarytenoid muscle. The upper surface of this cord is flat but the lower surface shows a downward concavity. This shape provides a more efficient valve than a simple sphincter for preventing air entry during inspiration, and the dome-shaped undersurface of the cord concentrates the infraglottic air pressure onto the sloping free margins of the folds, which has the effect of abducting the cords during expiration.

During closure of the laryngeal sphincters, the true vocal cords are the first to approximate and these establish contact progressively from the front backwards. This is followed by a similar adduction and closure of the false cords, with short segments at the posterior commissure being the first to close as the arytenoid cartilages adduct and rotate medially under the influence of the interarytenoid, thyroarytenoid and lateral crico-thyroid muscles. The remaining parts of the false cords then close from the front backwards, and closure is finally completed by the forward tilt of the arytenoids.

The trachea and bronchial tree

The trachea and bronchial tree are lined with a ciliated epithelium which contains mucous cells. Between 100 and 200 ml of mucus are produced each day and this contains small quantities of sialic acid, neutral polysaccharides, albumin, secretory immunoglobulin (IgA) and lysozyme, together with water which forms 95% of the total volume. Air which has passed through the nose is humidified and is 90–95% saturated with water vapour, but the presence of mucus in the bronchial tree serves to diminish any water loss in the lower airways as well as providing a surface protection against inhaled chemicals, organisms and other irritants. In chronic bronchitis there is an increase in the number of mucus-producing cells with a resultant increase in bronchial secretions; this mucus may be difficult to cough up as there may also be a simultaneous reduction in cilial beating.

Normally, the cilia which are present in the trachea, the larynx and the nose move mucus in streams away from the lower airways towards the pharynx where it can be swallowed. Cilial structure is shown in *Figure 13.5*. Each cilium consists of two central fibres enclosed in a sheath and these are connected to nine pairs of peripheral

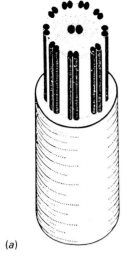

(a)

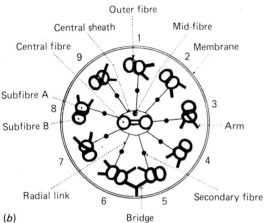

(b)

Figure 13.5 (a) Simplified diagrammatic representation of structure of cilium; (b) diagrammatic representation of transverse section of cilium showing detail of internal fibre organization

fibres which are interlinked with dynein arms. Radial secondary fibres connect the central and peripheral fibres and the whole is enclosed in an outer membrane. The cilia move with a beating motion and this provides the mucous escalator which traps particular matter. Inflammation, cigarette smoke and other irritants all reduce cilial activity, but in a small number of patients the cilia are immobile as a result of structural abnormalities. Whatever the cause, reduced clearance of mucus leads to pooling with secondary infection and bronchial damage which predisposes to bronchiectasis. In the case of the nose, the consequence is chronic inflammatory changes with sinusitis. The clinical picture is seen in patients with Kartagener's syndrome, where immobile cilia are responsible for a clinical picture which includes sinusitis and bronchiectasis, as well as infertility attributable to immobility of the spermatozoa.

Although small particles are cleared by the cilial escalator, larger debris is cleared by coughing. Stimulation of irritant receptors in the bronchial tree passes by way of the vagus to the brainstem and an inspiratory effort then results, which is followed by forced expiration initiated with the glottis closed to raise the intrathoracic pressure. With relaxation of the laryngeal sphincters, a rapid flow of air up the trachea results and the irritant is expelled. In the presence of bronchial hyper-reactivity there is a decreased threshold for activation of irritant receptors, and spasmodic coughing may therefore occur spontaneously or after minimal simulation, (for example by cold air).

Measurement of respiratory function
Measurement of lung volume

The early measurements of lung volume were carried out by means of a wet spirometer. The subject was asked to inspire maximally and then to exhale through a tube into a bell that contained air floating in a bath of water; air entry caused the bell to rise and thus allowed measurement of the vital capacity to be made. Today, dry spirometers are employed with a bellows which are expanded by the gas blown into it, and of these the most commonly used in the UK is the Vitalograph (*see Figure 13.6*). The subject breathes in to total lung capacity and then exhales to his residual volume. Most spirometers plot the volume of expired gas against time and this allows the forced expiratory volume in one second (FEV_1) to be taken from the trace. In turn, this can be used as a measure of air flow limitation. A severe diminution in vital capacity which is below that predicted for the individual on the basis of his sex, height and age is an indication that blood gases should be checked. As a guideline for surgery, a vital capacity of less than 1200 ml is often associated with an increase in anaesthetic and postoperative complications.

Lung volumes may also be measured by using the dilution of gas mixtures to assess the residual volume. In the single breath transfer test, one measured inhalation of a helium and air mixture is taken, held for 10 seconds, and then exhaled. The helium and air mixture is diluted with air already present in the alveolae, and only a proportion of the helium which is breathed in will be blown out, the remainder being left behind in the residual volume. The difference in concentration between the inspired and expired helium allows calculation of the residual volume of the lung and, as the vital capacity was the volume of the gas inspired, the total lung volume may then be calculated.

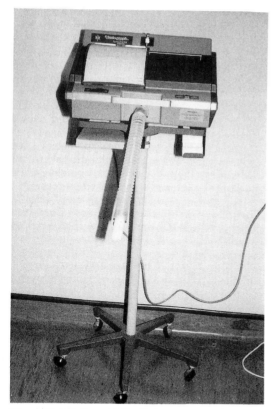

Figure 13.6 Vitalograph Dry Spirometer used for measuring vital capacity and FEV

This single breath method of measuring lung volume is limited as the subject may not take a breath equal to vital capacity, and there may be unequal mixing of gases in the lung. For this reason, rebreathing of a fixed volume of helium and air mixture with compensation for oxygen consumption and absorption of CO_2 is a more accurate method of assessment, and this test should be available in most respiratory function laboratories. Once adequate mixing has had time to occur and the helium concentration in the system has become constant, this method enables a calculation of helium dilution to be performed. At this point, the subject exhales and this allows the measurement of both the vital capacity and the inspiratory and expiratory reserve volumes. Calculation then allows an assessment of the functional residual capacity and residual volume so that the total lung volume may be computed. Full lung volume measurement with body box plethysmography is also possible, but is available in only a limited number of centres and is rarely required clinically. Vital capacity measured with a Vitalograph is usually all that is needed for routine clinical work and more comprehensive measure-

ments are used only for monitoring the progression of disease or for monitoring the effects of treatment.

Air flow

Peak flow

Peak flow measurement is the most commonly performed respiratory function test, and cheap reliable peak flowmeters are readily available on most hospital wards. The peak expiratory flow rate measured by these machines is the maximum air flow which is maintained for a period of at least 10 ms. In this test, the subject is requested to breathe in to total lung capacity and then to breathe out as fast as he/she can, but unless there is good effort, and unless the expiration starts at maximum lung volume, the peak flow measured will be reduced and inaccurate. A common error with this method, especially with the mini-Wright peak flowmeter, occurs if the subject places his fingers over the slide indicating the peak flow and prevents or reduces its movement; in spite of these limitations, the peak expiratory flow is readily performed in most subjects and is easily repeatable. Measurements of peak flow allow obstructive airway disease from any case to be easily assessed; for example, peak flow is reduced in asthma but rises after treatment with a bronchodilator. In patients with upper airway narrowing, measurement of peak flow allows the conditions of variable intrathoracic obstruction and fixed upper airway obstruction to be assessed with ease. However, if there is variable extrathoracic airway obstruction, the expiratory flows will be normal, and reliance must then be placed on maximum inspiratory flows to detect the abnormality. These conditions and the change in peak flow associated with them will be considered in the section on abnormalities of upper airway function.

Forced expiratory volume

When a spirometer is used to measure vital capacity, the expiratory spirogram is usually plotted as volume against time. This allows the volume of air exhaled in the first second of forced expiration (FEV_1) to be measured. FEV_1 provides information on air flow in large and medium-sized airways and is reduced in asthma and upper airway disease. With disease of the trachea or larynx, the FEV_1 is reduced less than the peak flow, and this forms the basis of the Empey Index which is the FEV_1 (in ml) divided by the peak flow (in l/min). In the normal subject, this ratio is less than 10. In the presence of upper airway disease, the peak flow is reduced more than the FEV_1, and the Empey Index will rise; if the Empey Index exceeds 10, this would suggest that there is fixed airway or variable intrathoracic airway narrowing. Variable extrathoracic airway narrowing only reduces inspiratory flows and does not affect the Empey Index (*see* later).

Flow–volume loops

Measurements of the peak flow are limited as they provide recordings of flow obtained at only one lung volume. The flow–volume loop provides information on the maximum flows obtained at all lung volumes, both in inspiration and expiration. In this test, flow is measured with a pneumotachograph or is obtained by differentiation of the volume signal from a dry spirometer. Flow is plotted on the y axis and lung volume on the x axis of a graph, with total lung capacity at the origin and residual volume on the right. By convention, expiratory flows are plotted as positive and inspiratory flows as negative values (*Figure 13.7*).

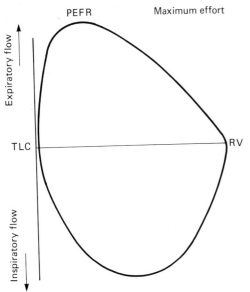

Figure 13.7 Normal flow–volume loop. PEFR = peak expiratory flow rate; TLC = total lung capacity; RV = residual volume

This investigation allows a large amount of physiological information to be obtained and is particularly useful in the management and investigation of patients with upper airway or tracheal disease. As in any lung function test, the cooperation of the subject and the production of a maximum effort are necessary for a meaningful result. If there has been a breath of subvital capacity volume or of inadequate effort, this can often be identified from the trace so that unwarranted diagnosis and conclusions are not made.

Flow–volume loop measurement is available in most district general hospitals, and the details of the different loops obtained in different airway pathologies are discussed in the final section of this chapter.

Other tests

Body plethysmographic methods are available for the measurement of airway resistance and conductance. Forced oscillation methods allow measurement of the resistance to air flow of both the lungs and chest wall, and measurement of transpleural pressures allows the compliance of the lung to be assessed. A detailed examination of the flow–volume loop obtained with a pneumotachograph can be made by using a computer analysis. All of these methods of assessment are available in only a limited number of centres and are of little value in clinical management. Measurements of peak flow and FEV_1, in combination with recordings of the flow–volume loop, allow sufficient physiological information to be assembled in most instances.

Gas transfer

The simplest method of measuring gas transfer in the lungs is to measure the concentrations of oxygen and carbon dioxide carried in the arterial blood. Hypoxia in a patient breathing room air implies that the transfer of oxygen across the lungs is reduced. If the patient is already breathing oxygen-enriched air, subtraction of the arterial P_{O_2} from the inspired P_{O_2} (obtained by calculation) allows the alveolar/arterial gradient to be estimated and this reflects the efficiency of the lungs. Similarly, comparison of the arterial P_{CO_2} with that in the environment allows the efficiency of clearance of CO_2 to be assessed and an estimate of the efficiency of respiratory drives and control to be made.

The most commonly used method for assessing the transfer of gas across the lung is the single breath carbon monoxide transfer test. A mixture of air, helium and carbon monoxide is inhaled and held in the lungs for 10 seconds before being expired. Helium is not absorbed across the lung basement membrane, but some helium mixes with the residual volume and thus the concentration expired is lower than that which is inspired. Knowledge of the concentration of gas inspired and its volume allows the residual volume of the lung to be calculated and hence the total lung volume (vital capacity plus residual volume) to be derived. The gas mixture contains a small quantity of carbon monoxide and this crosses the basement membrane of the lung and is bound strongly to haemoglobin. If the concentration of carbon monoxide, which is inspired and expired, is measured, the quantity of carbon monoxide absorbed (as ml/min per mmHg) can be calculated; this is the transfer factor and depends on the size of the lung as well as on its efficiency in gas transfer. Correction for the alveolar volume allows the transfer coeffficient (K_{CO}) to be assessed.

The transfer coefficient is reduced if there is pulmonary oedema, pulmonary fibrosis or ventilation perfusion mismatch, but it can also be increased if there is intrapulmonary haemorrhage as carbon monoxide will be bound to intrapulmonary haemoglobin and will appear to have transferred into the circulation. As only a single breath is used for this test there are many sources of potential error; certainly, if the breath is not held adequately or if inspiration is not to vital capacity the efficiency of the test will be impaired.

Exercise testing

Many patients with altered lung function are limited in their capacity to exercise. However, most lung function tests measure respiration at rest, and these tests correlate only moderately well with exercise tolerance. A major disadvantage of any test of lung function is that it cannot allow for limitations of exercise capacity caused by other factors such as cardiac failure or angina, previous cerebrovascular disease or musculoskeletal disorders. All of these may increase the work for a given amount of exercise.

Exercise testing can vary from the very simple to the extremely complex. This section describes currently available methods of testing in order of increasing complexity.

Clinical assessment

The patient may be able to quantify, in terms of yards or of number of stops for a measured distance, how far he/she can walk before stopping. Alternatively, the number of steps or flights of stairs that the patient can climb before he/she needs to stop can be recorded. However, as most subjects have difficulty in quantifying distance, this limits the usefulness of these questions. In towns, the distance between lamp posts is usually 25 metres and this represents a measured distance which may be of use in the assessment of exercise tolerance. The ability to climb the stairs to an out-patient clinic was for many years used by cardiothoracic surgeons as a measure of respiratory function; if a patient could easily ascend two flights of stairs then he would be able to withstand cardiothoracic surgery.

Walking

McGavin and his colleagues in Edinburgh introduced a timed walk as a measure of exercise tolerance. They asked patients to walk as fast as they could for 6 min (resting when necessary) and then measured the distance covered during the time. They found that this test correlated well with lung function and with the patients' symptoms, and that it gave a repeatable measure of exercise limitations. Several forms of these tests have now been tried, using a 12-min walk, a 2-min walk or the time to walk 100 metres.

Treadmill exercise testing

The testing of a patient on a treadmill, while walking either at a constant speed or with increasing speed, allows exercise ability to be quantified. If blood gases can be measured before and after the exercise, the degree of hypoxia caused by exercising can be assessed, which will provide an indication of the efficiency of the lungs for a given exercise load.

In the case of patients who have cardiac dysrhythmias or angina, exercise testing by means of the treadmill allows the exercise to be carried out with constant monitoring of the patient. This type of test has the obvious advantage that patients may be observed more closely than when they are undertaking an unsupervised walk up and down a hospital corridor.

Physiological measurement

The most complicated of all exercise tests comprises a full physiological assessment of respiration on exercise. In these tests, such factors as ventilation, oxygen consumption, oxygen saturation and carbon dioxide production can be measured to assess the physiological response to exercise. These tests are usually carried out by using an exercise cycle, and they provide a considerable amount of information concerning the exercise capacities of the subject. However, because such tests require a large amount of equipment and are expensive to perform, they are available in only a few centres. Such complex measurements of respiratory function are rarely indicated in the routine assessment of patients, and are much more part of research into respiratory disease and its effects than of an overall assessment which would be of use to the clinician.

The most useful assessment of exercise is that of the history combined with either the 6-min or the 2-min walk. This combination usually gives a good assessment of the patient's functional abilities.

Abnormalities of upper airway function

Introduction

Phase variation in airway resistance has been described in a previous section. During inspiration, the intrathoracic airway is held patent as the chest and lungs expand, but during expiration the lungs are in a state of collapse, resulting in external compression of the trachea. Therefore, in disorders of the trachea or bronchi, obstruction tends to be most marked during expiration, and this produces expiratory wheezing. In contrast, inspiration induces a negative pressure in the pharynx, larynx and extrathoracic trachea which leads to collapse of the airway in the absence of mechanisms to ensure patency. Patency during inspiration is ensured as follows: the pharynx is kept open by protrusion of the tongue resulting from the action of the genioglossus, the pharyngeal circumferential muscle contracts similarly to prevent inward flopping of the pharyngeal wall and the vocal cords are abducted. In addition, the tracheal rings keep the trachea patent and prevent collapse. On the other hand, expiration leads to an increase in upper airway air pressure which tends to keep the extrathoracic airway patent.

Snoring and obstructive apnoea

During sleep there is a decrease in the tone of the genioglossus and the circumferential pharyngeal muscles which maintain upper airway patency. This allows the tongue to fall back and the pharynx to collapse inwards during inspiration, with partial air flow obstruction and inspiratory snoring. Such partial pharyngeal obstruction occurs most commonly when the person is supine as gravity itself causes the tongue to fall back. Snoring is therefore most common in the supine position, and can often be prevented by turning the person on their side; waking the person also increases respiratory drives and muscle tone, and hence helps to remove obstruction. Snoring may be aggravated by the use of sedatives and muscle relaxants and, of these agents, alcohol is the most common offender as it leads to sedation, reduction in respiratory drive, and acts as a muscle relaxant. Any lesion causing a partial blockage of the extrathoracic airway will tend to predispose to upper airway collapse and may thus lead to snoring.

A more complete obstruction to air flow occurs in obstructive sleep apnoea, where there are episodes of complete cessation of air flow resulting from collapse of the pharynx during inspiration. Once obstruction to air flow occurs in the awake person there is respiratory distress, and increased muscle tone ensures pharyngeal patency. In light sleep, the respiratory drives are partially reduced and airway obstruction tends to lead to arousal and waking; however, in rapid eye movement sleep, the respiratory drives are all reduced to a considerable extent and there is an additional reduction in muscle tone.

During rapid eye movement sleep, obstruction to the upper airway does not necessarily produce instant arousal and wakening. However, as the duration of air flow obstruction continues, hypoxia and hypercapnia will result, leading to an increase in pulmonary artery pressure and a parallel increase in systemic blood pressure. Inspiration against a closed or obstructed upper airway (the Müller manoeuvre), as occurs in obstructive sleep apnoea, leads to an increase in vagal activity which produces bradycardia. Vagal overactivity in the presence of hypoxia also may be associated with the development of cardiac dysrhythmias, and these may be both atrial and ventricular in origin and lead potentially to asystole and sudden death.

In spite of these effects, obstructive apnoea rarely leads to death. More commonly, after a period of upper airway collapse and apnoea with hypoxia, there is arousal with increased respiratory drives and the relief of obstruction. A patient with obstructive sleep apnoea will thus suffer the problems of both hypoxia and vagal overactivity combined with frequent wakening. Rapid eye movement sleep and even light sleep can become so fragmented that the patient will sleep extremely poorly (possibly less than 60 min per night) and will experience sleep deprivation, which in itself can lead to a reduction in respiratory drives and cause the episodes of obstruction to occur even more frequently. The patient will also suffer from daytime hypersomnolence. In turn, recurrent hypoxia leads to an increase in pulmonary artery pressure and pulmonary vascular resistance, which culminates in fixed pulmonary hypertension with cor pulmonale. If hypoxia is prolonged there will be an increase in erythropoietin production with a concomitant increase in red cell production and thus an increased red cell mass and polycythaemia. This picture of cor pulmonale, polycythaemia and severe hypoxia with cardiac dysrhythmia is seen only in patients with frequent and prolonged obstructive sleep apnoea.

The severity of the sleep apnoea syndrome depends both on the number of apnoeic attacks and on their duration. Obstructive sleep apnoea syndrome is said to be present only if there are more than 30 episodes of obstruction each of which lasts more than 10 seconds during 6 hours of sleep. Even this number of apnoeic attacks is unlikely to produce more than frequent wakening with tiredness and possibly daytime sleepiness. Many patients who demonstrate the more severe sequelae of obstructive apnoea show, by contrast, several hundred apnoeic attacks per night (severe hypoxia with haemoglobin oxygen saturations of less than 50% with each apnoeic attack longer than a minute in duration and terminated by wakening and hyperkinetic activity).

Causes of upper airway obstruction
(*Figure 13.8*)

Nose

In obligate nose breathers, such as a feeding baby, nasal obstruction may lead to severe respiratory embarrassment. In most people, nasal obstruction produces only partial upper airway problems as breathing through the mouth alone provides adequate compensation. However, a partial obstruction may lead to snoring and occasionally to sleep apnoea; thus snoring is common with upper respiratory tract infection and rhinitis, and obstructive sleep apnoea has been reported in patients with deviation of the nasal septum or polyps and can be produced with nasal packing.

Mouth and pharynx

Partial occlusion of the oropharynx during sleep has already been discussed. The enlarged tongue seen in acromegaly, Down's syndrome, and occasionally in hypothyroidism, may also cause sleep apnoea as may shortening of the anteroposterior diameter of the oropharynx (which occurs with the bird-like face of the Pierre–Robin, Treacher Collins, Prader–Willi and Kearns–Sayre syndromes, and, occasionally, in patients with temperomandibular joint subluxation). This also predisposes to obstructive sleep apnoea. In these cases, lengthening of the lower jaw with bilateral osteotomy reduces or removes the obstruction and prevents obstructive apnoea.

Inflammation of the tonsils, adenoids and epiglottis may also lead to airway narrowing and obstruction, as can simple tonsillar and adenoidal hypertrophy. Patients with myxoedema, acromegaly and the mucopolysaccharidoses deposit myxoid material around the pharynx, and this circumferential narrowing of the airway also causes partial airway obstruction. Similarly, extremely obese patients deposit fat around the pharynx, and the consequent narrowing of the airway can be seen on computerized tomographic (CT) scanning of the neck. Retropharyngeal

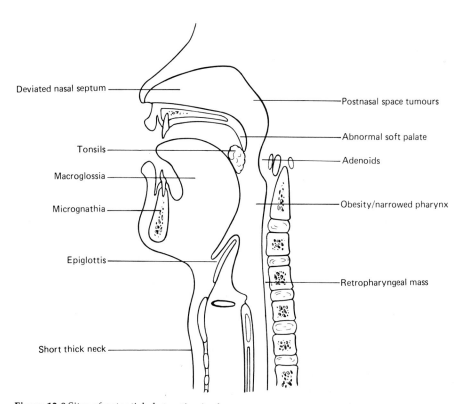

Figure 13.8 Sites of potential obstruction in sleep apnoea

masses caused by tumour, enlarged lymph nodes or abscesses also reduce the pharyngeal size and may produce airway obstruction. Some patients have a very large uvula and soft palate with large mucosal folds which may close off the entrance to the pharynx and lead to air flow obstruction, snoring and obstructive apnoea. In these cases, removal of the uvula and trimming of the redundant soft palate (uvulopalatopharyngoplasty), will reduce obstruction and may cure sleep apnoea in 60–70% of the patients. The short fat neck may also be associated with upper airway obstruction as there is a reduction in the length of the pharynx from nasopharynx to larynx, and the lateral and posterior walls of the pharynx tend to bulge into the lumen. If obesity also develops and fat is deposited around the pharynx, these subjects are especially at risk of developing severe snoring and obstructive apnoea.

The larynx

The larynx is the narrowest point in the upper airway and fixed narrowing of the larynx leads to upper airway obstruction and stridor. Recurrent laryngeal nerve palsy also compromises the larynx, causing loss of laryngeal dilatation in inspiration, and predisposing to stridor and obstructive apnoea. Polychondritis (where the cartilage becomes infiltrated with inflammatory cells and destroyed by anticartilage antibody) destroys cartilage in both the larynx and trachea, and the resulting laryngeal stenosis may produce a floppy trachea which collapses during maximum inspiration.

Trachea

As noted in the introduction to this section, extrathoracic airway obstruction becomes worse in inspiration and characteristically causes stridor. In contrast, the intrathoracic airway is smallest during expiration, and narrowing typically produces wheezing. The trachea, passing as it does from the extrathoracic larynx down into the thoracic cavity, may show either or both of these abnormalities. Fixed tracheal stenosis, as occurs with an enlarged thyroid or mediastinal mass pressing upon the trachea, leads to a reduction in both inspiratory and expiratory flow. Variable tracheal narrowing, which occurs with a floppy trachea following polychondritis or with a pedunculated tumour, will produce differing symptoms, depending on its size. There may be stridor from extrathoracic collapse during inspiration, or wheezing from intrathoracic obstruction; this may be confused with the wheezing of obstructive airway disease. Although post-tracheostomy scarring produces some fixed obstruction, the cartilage destruction associated with such a stoma allows variable tracheal collapse during inspiration and therefore produces signs compatible with both fixed and variable airway narrowing.

The investigation of upper airway disease

Plain X-rays of the neck, thorax and thoracic inlet allow the upper airway to be measured and should show the site of fixed airway narrowing. Tomography and CT scanning of the neck allow greater accuracy in identification of mass lesions and will also identify peripharyngeal deposits of fat. None of these techniques will necessarily allow a laryngeal site of obstruction to be identified. Examination of the upper airway by direct vision, by indirect or direct laryngoscopy and by bronchoscopy enable fixed areas of narrowing to be seen and a biopsy to be made, but a floppy trachea or a pharynx which collapses will not necessarily be identified.

Respiratory function tests allow both identification of the physiological nature of an upper airway obstruction and characterization according to whether the latter is fixed or variable, intrathoracic or extrathoracic. However, more precise identification is not possible. Occasionally, muscle weakness or chest wall stiffness may produce a similar flow–volume loop appearance to upper airway obstruction.

Although when taken individually, neither direct vision, radiology nor respiratory function tests will provide all the answers in the examination of a patient with upper airway disease, when taken together, the site, nature and severity of the lesion may usually be reasonably ascertained.

Spirometry and the Empey Index

Air flow is fast in the upper airway, and obstruction therefore limits the maximum possible flow. The peak expiratory flow rate (PEFR) may thus be reduced to a greater extent than the forced expiratory volume in one second (FEV_1). A fixed airway narrowing reduces expiratory flows in both the extrathoracic and intrathoracic large airways, whereas a variable airway narrowing reduces expiratory flow only in the intrathoracic airway. Therefore, measurements of peak expiratory flow rate and the FEV_1 are useful in the assessment of intrathoracic variable airway obstruction, and in both intrathoracic and extrathoracic fixed obstruction. The greater reduction in peak expiratory flow rate when compared to the forced expiratory volume in one second is made use of in the Empey Index (FEV$_1$ in ml; PEFR in l/min). If there is a significant fixed upper airway narrowing or intrathoracic variable airway narrowing there will be a FEV$_1$/PEFR ratio of greater than 10. However, the test will be useless in identifying extrathoracic variable airway disease, for which examination of the inspiratory flow pattern is necessary. In spite of its limitations, the Empey Index is easy to measure and can be of considerable use in following the progress of a patient with upper airway disease.

Flow–volume loop

It is possible to display flow and volume recorded by a pneumotachograph or obtained by differentiation of the volume recording from a spirometer, in order to produce synchronous flow and volume measurements which can be used to examine the air flow through the upper airway. Flow–volume loops which display only the expiratory portion of a maximum effort are of limited use as they do not provide information on airway collapse during inspiration. Both the shape of the trace and any irregularity of flow are useful. If there is a variable airway narrowing, as occurs with a collapsible pharynx, the oscillation of both inspiratory and expiratory flows gives a sawtooth appearance on the trace. Such a sawtooth pattern

is seen in *Figure 13.9* and is from a patient with obstructive sleep apnoea. In this latter condition, the variable collapse of the upper airway results in such a sawtooth pattern in 60% of subjects, and this is superimposed on the flow–volume loop appearance of variable extrathoracic obstruction. The flow–volume loop appearance in fixed intrathoracic and extrathoracic obstruction, and in variable intrathoracic and extrathoracic obstruction, is shown in *Figure 13.10*.

Fixed extrathoracic obstruction

Fixed extrathoracic obstruction is found in laryngeal stenosis or pharyngeal stenosis caused by a mass lesion. There is a fixed obstruction of air flow which occurs in both inspiration and expiration, and curves for maximum inspiration and expiration are therefore reduced. As a result, the flow–volume loop has a flattened appearance (*Figure 13.10a*) and the Empey Index is raised. This appearance is partially duplicated if there is severe muscle weakness, such as occurs in muscular dystrophy, myasthenia and polyneuritis, although

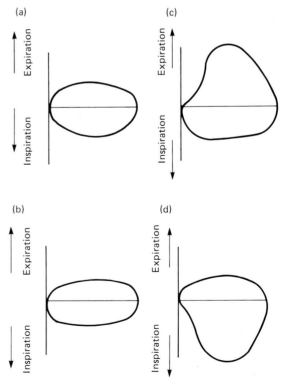

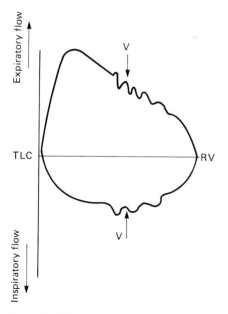

Figure 13.9 Flow–volume loop in obstructive apnoea; variation in expiration and inspiration. TLC = total lung capacity; RV = residual volume; V = variation in flow

Figure 13.10 Flow–volume loop appearances in upper airway obstruction. (*a*) Fixed extrathoracic obstruction; (*b*) fixed intrathoracic obstruction; (*c*) variable extrathoracic obstruction; (*d*) variable intrathoracic obstruction

in these instances inspiratory flows usually exceed those achieved in expiration and the resultant curves are therefore asymmetrical.

Fixed intrathoracic obstruction

Fixed intrathoracic obstruction may be caused by tracheal stenosis but is more commonly a result of extrinsic compression of the trachea from an intrathoracic mass. In such circumstances, the flow–volume loop shows a pattern which is similar to that which is found in fixed extrathoracic obstruction (*Figure 13.10b*) and the Empey Index is again raised. However, if only one main bronchus is affected the pattern is normal. It therefore follows that, if there is a flattening of the flow–volume loop, the obstruction must be in the upper airway above the carina.

Variable extrathoracic obstruction

The most common cause of variable extrathoracic obstruction is pharyngeal collapse. Variable obstruction also occurs if the trachea collapses as the result of tracheomalacia; this may follow a tracheostomy where the tracheal wall has been permanently scarred, or in polychondritis where the tracheal cartilages are absent or floppy. Occasionally, tracheal or laryngeal obstruction may be the result of a pedunculated tumour, and flow will be reduced over only part of the respiratory cycle. In this group of patients, the Empey Index is normal but the flow–volume loop shows a cut-off of the inspiratory limb with reduced maximum inspiratory flow as the trachea collapses (*Figure 13.10c*).

This pattern may also be seen in inspiratory muscle weakness and bilateral diaphragmatic paralysis. It is also reproduced in those subjects who have a fixed chest wall with limited inspiratory excursion, but who are able to retain expiratory flows by diaphragmatic movement. Such fixation of the chest wall should be obvious

and not difficult to differentiate from extrathoracic variable airway obstruction. However, muscle weakness may be much less apparent unless maximum inspiratory and expiratory pressures are measured.

Intrathoracic variable obstruction

Intrathoracic variable obstruction tends to obstruct air flow during expiration, but inspiration is unaffected since the intrathoracic contents, including the major airways, are expanded as the thorax enlarges. A reduction of expiratory flow results with a normal inspiratory pattern. The flow–volume loop is again characteristic (*Figure 13.10d*) and this, in conjunction with the Empey Index (*see above*), should allow definition of the site of obstruction and its degree of variability.

Further reading

COMROE, J. H. J. (1962) *The Lung*. Chicago: Year Book Publishers

COTES, J. E. (1979) *Lung Function*. Oxford: Blackwell

EMPEY, D. W. (1972) Assessment of upper airway obstruction. *British Medical Journal*, **3**, 503–505

GREEN, N. and MOXHAM, J. (1983) Respiratory muscles. In *Recent Advances in Respiratory Medicine 3*, edited by D. C. Flenley and T. L. Petty. Edinburgh: Churchill Livingstone

HORNBEIN, T. F. (Ed.) (1981) *Lung Biology in Health and Disease*. Vol. 17, *Regulation of Breathing*. New York: Marcel Dekker

SAUNDERS, N. A. and SULLIVAN, C. E. (Eds) (1984) *Lung Biology in Health and Disease*. Vol. 23, *Sleep and Breathing*. New York: Marcel Dekker

SHIM, C., CORRO, P., PARK, S. S. and WILLIAMS, M. H. (1972) Pulmonary function studies in patients with upper airway obstruction. *American Review of Respiratory Disease*, **106**, 233–238

WEST, J. B. (1979) *Respiratory Physiology – The Essentials*. Oxford: Blackwell

WEST, J. B. (1979) *Pulmonary Pathophysiology – The Essentials*. Oxford: Blackwell

14

The generation and reception of speech

Adrian Fourcin and Michael Gleeson

This chapter gives a brief overview of the aspects of the generation and reception of speech that are capable of being given the quantitative treatment associated with modern phonetic studies. The daily clinical availability of microprocessor computing facilities now makes it possible for results which were previously restricted for the use of specialist workers commanding the resources of well-equipped laboratories, to be made available for the practical management of the communication-impaired patient. After a brief review of the phonetic bases of speech sound description, examples are given of the application of these techniques both to the production of speech with particular reference to voice, and to the perception of speech with particular reference to the use of speech synthesis techniques in the interactive evaluation of speech processing ability. The emphasis is on the quantitative use of presently available methods and the relation of these results to our greater understanding of the processes of normal and abnormal speech development in the child, voice and speech pathology in the adult, and the use and design of prostheses.

Linguistic systems

All methods of communication depend on the use of readily communicable differences – contrasts between transmitted signals. For example, in morse code, where a single dimension is used, the presence or absence of a tonality provides the basis of communication. Speech, however, has a large number of dimensions involving the definition of its essential contrasts. All natural languages have the common property that their systems use contrasts which are hierarchically structured, that

is to say that the systems include small units which are combined together to form units of the next higher level, and so on. The sound sequences of speech can be regarded as being made up of elements which are combined in a hierarchically structured, patterned form, and speech is only acceptable and intelligible when it is produced and perceived according to its patterned structured rules.

We perceive and produce speech sound sequences rather than separate sounds, but it is very convenient and relevant to describe the basic components of speech in terms of separate elements. The 'phone' level is concerned with the nature of the sounds, and the 'phoneme' level is concerned with the use of sounds to convey meaning. It is important to distinguish between the physical nature of the sounds, sound sequences of speech and their more abstract linguistic representation. Physically and phonetically we are concerned with the nature of the utterance. Linguistically the concern is with the use of the utterance for the purposes of communication. For example, a child and a man may both produce totally acceptable and linguistically identical sound sequences, although quite obviously their detailed physical analysis and their phonetic representations may be very different one from the other.

Table 14.1 gives an overview of the main contrastive sound classes used for communication in English. Using the International Phonetic Alphabet (IPA) symbols, for example, from the first column on the left, the word 'bat' produced by an individual speaker would be represented as [bæt]. In this particular example, three phones are used to represent the individual nature of this particular utterance. The 'b' phone here is in a

Table 14.1 A listing of the sounds of English represented in three different ways

Keyword IPA*		Keyed as	ASCII
Vowels			
1 *bead*	iː	iː	105, 58
2 *bid*	ɪ	I	73
3 *bed*	e	e	101
4 *bad*	æ	&	38
5 *card*	ɑː	A:	65, 58
6 *cod*	ɒ	Q	81
7 *cord*	ɔː	O:	79, 58
8 *good*	u	U	85
9 *food*	uː	u:	117, 58
10 *bud*	ʌ	V	86
11 *bird*	ɜ	3:	51, 58
12 *allow*	ə	@	64
13 *day*	eɪ	eI	101, 73
14 *know*	əʊ	@U	64, 85
15 *eye*	aɪ	aI	97, 73
16 *cow*	au	aU	97, 85
17 *boy*	ɔɪ	OI	79, 73
18 *beer*	ɪə	I@	73, 64
19 *bare*	eə	e@	101, 64
20 *tour*	uə	U@	85, 64
Consonants			
sing	ŋ	N	78
thin	θ	T	84
then	ð	D	68
shed	ʃ	S	83
beige	ʒ	Z	90
etch	tʃ	tS	116, 83
edge	dʒ	dZ	100, 90
yet	j	j	106

p t k b d g m n f v s z r l w h
– keyed as normal ASCII

*IPA refers to the symbolism of the International Phonetic Alphabet. The keyed input relates simply to the representation which is equivalent to IPA, but when only a standard typewriter is available. Finally, the new standard computer in the change format for these standard alphabetic IPA equivalents is shown.

particular context at the beginning of a word and immediately preceding the vowel 'æ'. All phones in this context can be grouped together to form an allophone and all the possible allophonic variations associated with a particular sound of speech are grouped together to produce a phoneme class. When the phoneme level of representation is involved, the sound sequence is enclosed between slanting brackets. The phoneme version of the previous particular utterance is /bat/. Phonetic symbols are not generally available on typewriters or in computer output terminals and, in order to overcome this difficulty, this sequence can be represented here, for example, as /b&t/ using the

symbols of the centre column which are dependent on a machine representation of numbers of the form shown in the third column (Wells, 1986).

It is possible to draw up a complete inventory of the phonemic classes in a language by systematically going through the possible substitutions in phoneme sequences. For instance, in addition to the sequence /bæt/, the sequences /bæd/, /bæg/, and so on, also occur in which a substitution has been made in the third position in the sequence. Further possibilities are found by making a change in the first place, as in /pæt/, /sæt/, and so on, or in the second place, as in /bɪt/, /bet/. The vocal tract settings, or articulations, for these basic sounds of English are outlined in *Table 14.2*. They form the heart of the system of classification used in phonetics but, as will be discussed, there are other important levels of representation.

Sequences of phonemes make up the morphemes, which are the next order of units and which have a grammatical function. It is important to realize that each type of linguistic unit is distinguished by its function rather than its form. The word 'bat' was used as an example in the phoneme system. This is one of the words which consists of only one morpheme; in fact there are two English morphemes /bæt/, one which functions as a noun and one which functions as a verb. The latter may have another morpheme added to it, for example the morpheme /ɪn/, in the sentence 'He's been batting for an hour'; or the morpheme /ɪd/, in the sentence 'He batted for an hour'. In this way morphemes are put together to make words, which are the next order of units, but there are a great many cases in which one morpheme also forms a word in English and, in addition, there will be a small number of morphemes which do not constitute words. The total number of English words in use at any one period is very large; Daniel Jones' *English Pronouncing Dictionary*, for example, lists about 55 000 words.

It is one of the features of the economy of natural languages that a small basic repertory of phonemic units is used to give a very large store of words. This is an important fact in the learning of a language. By the time he is 5 or 7 years old, a child has learned the whole of the phonemic system, and for the rest of his life has no need to add to his inventory of phonemes (as far as his native language is concerned), yet he will continually add to his stock of words, and has yet to complete his knowledge of the detailed forms of contrastive sounds. The stringing together of words to make sentences only needs the comment at this stage that, in the spoken language, any complete remark constitutes a sentence, on the basis of a complete programming of its constituent elements at the levels of both sound and intonation. It is very common even for a single word to

Table 14.2 Classification of English vowels and consonants

	Front	*Central*	*Back*
Vowels			
Close	i:		u:
Half-close	i		u
Half-open	e	ɜ , ə, ʌ	ɔ:
Open	æ		ɑ:

Consonants

Manner of articulation	*Place of articulation*						
	Bilabial	*Labiodental*	*Dental*	*Alveolar*	*Palatal*	*Velar*	*Glottal*
Plosive	p b			t d		k g	
Affricate				tʃ dʒ			
				tr dr			
Fricative		f v	θ ð	s z			h
				ʃ ʒ			
Nasal	m			n		ŋ	
Lateral				l			
Semi-vowel				r	j	w	

function as a sentence, on a basis of the knowledge of the contrastive constraints involved.

Knowledge of a language, then, means first of all a knowledge of the units that are available at the various levels; but it also means a knowledge of the rules governing the combination of units on one level into units on the next level. At the phonemic level, the language-user knows the complete inventory of phonemes and knows the sequences of phonemes that are likely to occur in the composition of morphemes and words; the English speaker knows, for example, that a word may well begin with the sequence /pr/ but that it will certainly not begin with the sequence /pf/. He also knows which morphemes may or may not follow each other in his own language. The village child who was heard to say: 'Er bain't a-calling we, us don't belong to she', was applying rules of morpheme combination just as surely as another child brought up in a different language environment who might say, 'She's not calling us, we don't belong to her'. That is to say, the word 'rules' in this connection is related not to any notion of 'correctness', but only to usage.

In a similar way, most of the information concerning the sentence-level is stored in the form of rules for combining words into sequences that are possible in the language.

On the morpheme and word levels, the language-user will have a fairly large vocabulary of units which he can recognize (his passive vocabulary) and a much more restricted list of units which he himself will utter (his active vocabulary).

No communication by speech is possible without recourse to the kind of information that has just been briefly sketched. The first operation on the part of the speaker is to formulate what he has to say in language form. He chooses certain key words (content words) which embody the substance of what he wants to say, and intersperses them with words that settle the grammatical form of the sentence (form words). The choice of words in itself implies the choice of the proper morphemes, and this in its turn dictates the string of phonemes to be selected. Phoneme selection is a vital part of the process of speech-generation, because on it depend the operating instructions fed forward to the muscles used in speech.

Basic to these instructions are the operations of vocal tract control which subserve the acoustic aims of the speaker. These involve two essential aspects of speech: excitation and response. Excitation is dependent on the control and use of air flow and includes phonation or voice. Response is dependent on vocal tract adjustment and includes what is commonly referred to as articulation.

Voice input

Phonation is the activity which produces voice, and voice is the input to the vocal tract – normally coming from the vibration of the vocal folds within the larynx – which gives speech its characteristic pitch and enables the contrasts of intonation to be produced. In all languages of the world, the voiced sounds are the most important in regard to the functional contrastive load that they carry. Developmentally, voice productive skills are the first acquired and, physically, the voice input to the vocal tract is the most efficient basis for the definition of the contrastive resonances which carry linguistically important information. In speech, voice itself is contrasted with silence, and with whisper and frication. While voice is essentially dependent on a regular periodic acoustic input to the vocal tract, whisper and frication come from the random noise-like turbulent motion of the air stream. Although the dynamics of laryngeal activity differ in respect of the overall characteristics of control between speakers, so that the characteristic pitch or register, the range or extent of frequency variation of laryngeal vibra-

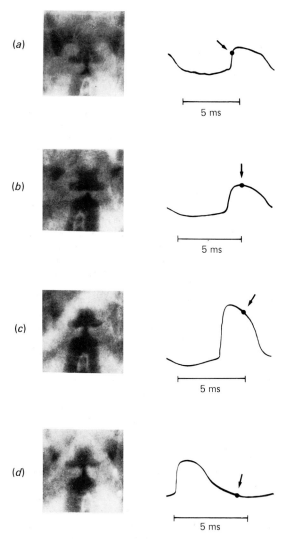

(a)

5 ms

(b)

5 ms

(c)

5 ms

(d)

5 ms

Figure 14.1 Flash X-ray radiographs. Four separately recorded instants in the cycle of vibratory activity for a single adult male speaker are shown, together with the triggering instants on the associated laryngograph waveform, *Lx*

tion, and the quality of voice, which will be discussed later on, all vary appreciably from listener to listener and in important respect from language to language, the essential characteristics of vocal fold activity for normal voice are identical.

Many different studies have sought to correlate phonatory activity with different aspects of the mechanisms of vocal fold vibration. Direct laryngoscopic views of the vibrating vocal folds have been obtained using stroboscopic techniques, (for example Lecluse, 1977) or by the measurement or inference of air flow between the vibrating vocal folds using inverse filtering techniques, (for example Fourcin, 1974; Childers and Kirshnamurthy, 1985), or by using strobolaminographic techniques (Hollien, Curtis and Coleman, 1968).

Figure 14.1 gives a brief indication of another way of observing these phenomena which has the advantage of providing a frontal view of the vibrating vocal folds at particular unique instants during normal voice production. A simple electrolaryngograph waveform, *Lx*, has been obtained by the use of electrodes lightly placed superficially in contact with the speaker's neck at the level of the alae of the thyroid cartilage (Fourcin, 1971). An *x*-flash source operating at approximately 300 kV with a flash duration time of 1.5×10^{-9} seconds has been synchronized with this laryngograph waveform so that any predetermined instant in the *Lx* waveform can be used to trigger a frontal irradiation of the speaker's vocal folds. In speech terms, the duration of this burst of radiation is essentially instantaneous. In this way, in *Figure 14.1a*, the vocal folds have been arrested in their phonatory movement towards closure immediately before the peak of the *Lx* waveform. The ventricular folds can be seen very clearly and the superior edges of the vocal folds themselves can just be perceived. It should be remembered here that the image results from the total contribution of all the soft tissue involved. The somewhat laminographic effect associated with the radiograph is due to the relatively greater penetrating power of these high voltage X-rays. The associated shorter wavelength reduces the relative opacity of cartilaginous and bony tissues and the soft water-containing tissues have a greater stopping power, and show up in a more enhanced fashion (the total dosage for one flash is less than 100 nGy) (Noscoe *et al.*, 1983).

In *Figure 14.1b*, the closure cycle has been completed and the vocal folds are shown at their maximum contact. The speaker for all of the four images shown in this figure has been phonating normally to produce the vowel [*a*] in the centre of his larynx frequency range. The fairly slight maximal contact which is shown is typical for ordinary phonation. The massive contact which is ordinarily shown diagrammatically is not obtained in practice, although obviously, as with a laryngoscopic view, one can see that the covers of the two vocal folds do interact quite extensively during the peak of closure. In *Figure 14.1c* the vocal folds are beginning to separate, and the different shape of the separating vocal folds from that which is obtained at *Figure 14.1a* is typical of ordinary phonatory activity. In *Figure 14.1d* the vocal folds are essentially maximally separated. The glottal area is at its greatest and the output from the laryngograph electrodes is near to its minimum since the electrical impedance presented by the vibrating vocal folds is at its greatest as opposed to the minimal impedance condition associated with *Figure 14.1b*.

While these X-rays are typical of what is found with a variety of speakers producing normal voice, the individual flashes were not triggered in very rapid succession, but with a break between utterances, while the high voltage source was allowed to recharge. The very low radiation doses associated with the examinations and the possibility of having a relatively clear picture of the internal surfaces of the normally, or abnormally, vibrating vocal folds, make this approach of potential clinical value, although, as yet, it is not applied. In the present discussion, a particular utility of this presentation is in regard not only to its illumination of the stages of vocal fold vibratory activity in a normal cycle of closures, but also in respect of its establishment of the intrinsic usefulness of the *Lx* waveform itself. These radiographs in effect provide a calibration of the output of the electrolaryngograph which, together with previous calibrations obtained by strobolaryngoscopic and inverse filtering techniques makes it possible to use the *Lx* waveform for the study of both normal and abnormal phonatory activity.

The vibration of the normal vocal folds, illustrated in *Figure 14.1*, is maintained by the energy associated with the egressive pulmonic air flow which is ordinarily associated with voice production. In normal phonation, vocal fold closure occurs very much more rapidly than vocal fold separation. This is illustrated both in the *Lx* waveforms of *Figure 14.1* and also in the *Lx* waveform of *Figure 14.2b*, which is associated with the production of a different vowel from that in *Figure 14.1*, but by the same speaker. This rapid closure of the vocal folds is an essential characteristic of normal voice production and is of major consequence to our use of speech as a primary means of communication.

The total energy in the air particles flowing through the glottis depends on two factors – velocity and pressure. Once adduction of the vocal folds is initiated, the associated reduction in glottal area necessarily causes an increase in particle velocity. This increase in velocity is, by definition, the source of an increase in the energy associated with particle movement and, in consequence, since total energy is constant, there must be a complementary reduction in the air pressure associated with the particles. In this way, the reduction in energy associated with pressure complements the increase in energy associated with velocity. External atmospheric pressure is constant, so the reduction of glottal air pressure will be associated with a positive feedback process in which further glottal area reduction gives rise to a concomitant increase in air particle velocity. This, in turn, is necessarily associated with a further decrease in glottal pressure, and a further inward movement of the adapting vocal folds as the result of the external air pressure and the intrinsic tension of the vocalis muscles.

The process is highly complex, but progress is being made towards the detailed modelling of vocal fold vibration, to an extent which makes it feasible for the shape of the laryngograph waveform and of the associated glottal air volume velocity to be predicted, so that the model gives results closely approximating those which are shown in the particular example of *Figure 14.2b* and *c* (Titze and Talkin, 1979). The part of the vocal fold closure cycle which is effective in producing the pressure change responsible for the main acoustic excitation of the resonances of the vocal tract takes place in only a few tenths of a millisecond, and the complete closure of the vocal tract which is associated with the maximum degree of possible contact between the opposing vocal folds is accomplished in only a slightly longer time interval.

The mucosal cover of the vocal folds is normally bathed in low viscosity fluid and it is this which is responsible for the rapidity with which the air flow is arrested in the final stages of vocal fold closure. A typical, often transient, interference with normal vocal fold vibration arises when longer molecular chain antibodies are incorporated in this fluid, since the consequent increase in viscosity interferes with the normal process of vocal fold closure and separation. The fluid is the third component which must always be considered in conjunction with the body and cover descriptors used by Hirano (1981). In physical terms, the vocal folds can be regarded as a non-sinusoidal relaxation oscillator and, in the final stage of closure, the source of sustaining energy associated with the actual flow of air particles in the glottis is removed, and the temporary relaxation of the closing forces enables the vocal folds to separate and their whole cycle of movement to begin again.

The rapid adduction of the vocal folds which terminates each vocal fold cycle is a positive feedback process which gives a shock excitation

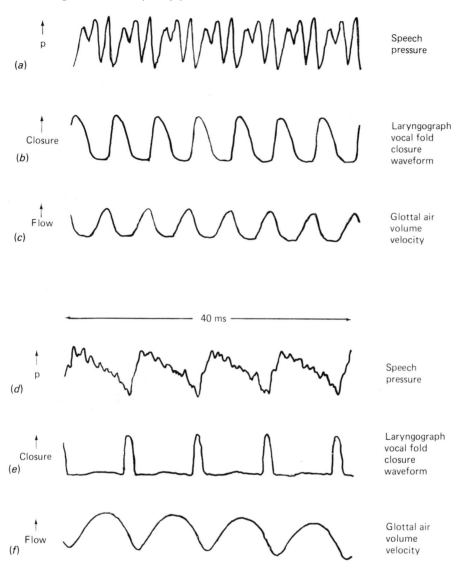

Figure 14.2 Sustained [ɜ:] vowel in the normal adult. (a)–(c) Normal voice quality; (d)–(f) breathy voice quality

acoustically to the vocal tract. Immediately follow-ing this shock excitation there is a period during which the vocal folds remain closed together thus effectively separating the supraglottal resonators from the subglottal cavities. The resulting acoustic response of the vocal tract for a typical vowel sound (the neutral vowel [ɜ:]) is illustrated in *Figure 14.2a*. Each rapid vocal fold closure elicits a corresponding rapid response with a positive pressure peak in the acoustic output from the vocal tract, delayed by the separation acoustically between the larynx and the lips of the speakers. The oscillatory response of the vocal tract resona-tors clearly follows the sharply defined closure of the vocal folds and this response continues during the vocal fold closure phase. During the open phase, however, the coupling of the subglottal cavities to the vocal tract changes the resonances and reduces their acoustic response. While the conditions for normal vocal fold vibration are shown in *Figures 14.2a, b* and *c,* the conditions relating to breathy voice are shown in *Figure 14.2d, e* and *f.* Here, the increased length of the open phase introduces a marked increase in vocal tract damping due to the enhanced coupling between the subglottal and supraglottal cavities, and the resonances of the vocal tract are in consequence far less well defined. Breathy voice is associated not only with an increased open phase, but with a reduced rapidity of vocal fold closure, so that the higher resonances are auditorily absent or less well defined, both as the result of the slowness of closure and of the increased subglottal damping. These effects, of course, also influence the definition of the lower resonances.

Good voice production depends on three factors which are clearly shown in *Figure 14.2.* First, there must be a sharply defined closure of the vocal folds in order adequately spectrally to illuminate the resonances of the vocal tract. Second, closure must be maintained for an appreciable proportion of the vibratory cycle so that the coupling of the subglottal cavities to the supraglottal cavities does not interfere unduly with the damping of the supraglottal resonators. Third, the closure of the vocal folds must occur regularly so that the pitch of the voice is clearly defined. These features are crucial to the understanding of the production of both good and abnormal pathological voice conditions.

These main features of good normal voice production are summarized in *Figure 14.3a.* Following the rapid contact of the vocal folds, there is what may be described as a 'hold' phase; this

corresponds to the interval of time during which the vocal folds are essentially in contact and thus isolating the supraglottal from the subglottal cavities. During this period, the pressure waveform is very much less damped than during the rest of the laryngeal cycle. As described above, the hold phase corresponds to the positive peak of the *Lx* waveform. The trough of the *Lx* waveform is produced by the separation of the vocal folds. The two sketches of the ventricular and vocal fold outlines in *Figure 14.3a* have been derived from *Figures 14.1a–d,* and *Figure 14.3b* indicates the position relative to the 'open' phase, during which there is substantial coupling between the supraglottal and subglottal cavities of the vocal tract. Sustained departure from these basic voice characteristics in continuous speech will inevitably entail a corresponding departure from normal voice quality.

In *Figure 14.4b,* a voice condition, which is a typical aspect of normal speech production, but only of transient occurrence, is illustrated. Creaky voice is associated with the flaccid adjustment of the vocal folds and their irregular vibration. It occurs typically, for example, at the end of a fall in the pitch of the voice. *Figure 14.4b* shows the laryngograph waveform corresponding to a brief sample of creaky voice excitation produced by the same speaker with the same vowel quality as in *Figures 14.1, 14.2* and *14.3.* Typically, in British

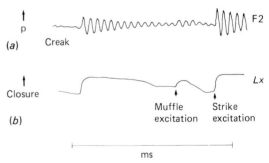

Figure 14.4 Characteristic features of a creaky voice. (*a*) speech pressure waveform for the isolated second formant; (*b*) *Lx* waveform

English, creaky voice is associated with doublets of vocal fold closure, with the first closure being fairly well defined and with a long hold period, while the second closure is less well defined, more variable in its moment of occurrence, and with a shorter hold phase. The flaccid adjustment of the vocal folds necessarily introduces an overall irregularity in the temporal organization of the closure sequences. In order to illustrate the important acoustic effects of different aspects of vocal fold vibration, the single resonance associated with the second formant is shown (analysed

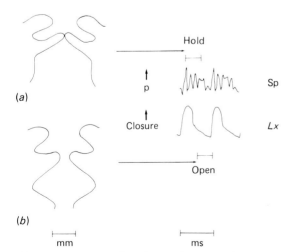

Figure 14.3 Features of good normal voice production. (*a*) Closed phase; (*b*) open phase

out – by signal 'dissection') in *Figure 14.4a*. The relationship between laryngeal input and acoustic output is clarified in this way, since the individual closures, hold and open phases in *Figure 14.4b*, have their correlates clearly indicated in *Figure 14.4a*. The first closure in *Figure 14.4b* produces an obvious damped response in respect of the isolated *F2* resonance. This is followed by a second response corresponding to the minor closure. Finally, in this figure, the last closure in *Figure 14.4b* has the biggest response in *Figure 14.4a*, and it is noteworthy that this last closure occurs more rapidly than all the others. This is called here a 'strike' excitation, in contrast to the other inputs to the vocal tract from this sequence and this strike excitation tends to be characteristic of the major closures in creak. The immediately preceding 'muffle' excitation corresponds to a less rapid closure of the vocal folds.

These effects, which are found occasionally in normal speech, are of crucial consequence in interpreting the departures from normality which are characteristic of pathological conditions. A brief hold phase introduces extra damping and this can be seen to a degree in the sequence following the muffle excitation peak. The muffle

excitation peak itself, because it is not well defined in terms of rapidity and amplitude of closure, produces a small acoustic output. Irregularity in the closure sequence produces a corresponding irregularity in the final auditory percept of the pitch of the speaking voice. Within this single sequence there are three sorts of excitation each giving their own colouration to the final output of the speaker's vocal tract, and it is worth noting even at this point that the auditory analytical capabilities of the ear appear to be well able to cope with the timbre changes which are potentially available as the result of these excitation differences from moment to moment. Further aspects of the effects of differing laryngeal input are shown in *Figure 14.11* and discussed below.

Regular vocal fold closure not only gives a coherent excitation to the resonances of the vocal tract, but also defines the speaking and singing voice. *Figure 14.5* illustrates the way in which the controlled adjustment of the laryngeal musculature by a normal adult male speaker can result in changes in vocal fold frequency which are significant in speech. On the left, a citation question form is shown corresponding to a rising voice pitch while, on the right, a falling statement form is shown. These apparently smooth curves are obtained by the direct, unsmoothed measurement of successive vocal fold periods derived by measurement from the closures detected in the speaker's laryngograph waveforms. The creaky voice example of the previous figure would produce a much more irregular curve with marked step-like changes from period to period being shown.

This technique of measurement provides a very accurate basis for the measurement of the frequency, *Fx*, with which the vibrating vocal folds excite the resonances of the vocal tract, and the combination of precision and simplicity makes the laryngograph a useful tool for both clinical work

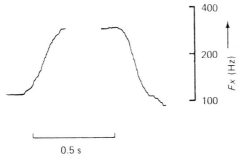

0.5 s

Figure 14.5 Adult male rise–fall intonation contrast measured directly from *Lx* waveforms

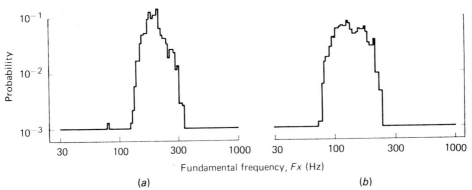

(*a*)   (*b*)

Figure 14.6 Normal voice frequency distributions obtained from long recordings of *Lx* waveforms. (*a*) Adult female (50 s voice time); (*b*) adult male (25 s voice time)

and research. The apparatus is routinely employed for therapy and examples of its application and the results obtained are discussed later in this chapter. It is also possible to provide a basis for the quantitative assessment of treatment by the use of the laryngograph technique. Speech and Lx recordings are made on standard audio two-channel (stereo) recorders and the Lx information analysed to provide a quantitative basis for the assessment of the patient's voice condition which may be included in the case notes. (The advent of microcomputers has made it possible for these quantitative measures to be made available simply and economically in the clinic and put into the case notes.)

A particularly simple and useful representation of this type is shown in *Figure 14.6*. *Figure 14.6a* shows the distribution of larynx frequencies in the speech of a normal woman, while *Figure 14.6b* displays the results of a similar analysis for a normal adult male speaker. These distributions are typical of normal phonation; the range of Fx is compact and, within each speaker's register, there are well defined modes. This type of analysis can be obtained while the speaker is talking normally without constraint and, since it depends on the laryngograph waveform, is unaffected by ambient noise. The measurements are simply determined from the observation of successive larynx closures as defined by the Lx waveform, the positive edge of which sharply defines the beginning of each period as has been seen in the previous figures. The probability ordinates in these figures simply relate to the probability of occurrence of laryngeal periods corresponding to the fundamental frequency abscissa. This method of representation gives rather more importance to the higher frequency components in the voice than would be obtained, for example, if the probability simply related to the speaking time at any given fundamental frequency. This larynx period representation is a basic form from which others can be derived.

In *Figure 14.7a*, a first example of a derivation from the basic distribution of *Figure 14.6* is given. On the left, the basic larynx frequency distribution, Fx, of the previous figure is shown for a normal woman speaker. This speaker is using a very expressive voice and has, in consequence, greater range. She is also within her phonation making much greater use of creaky voice contrasts than was the case for the speaker in *Figure 14.6a*, and this is shown by the small irregular double-peaked low frequency tail to the main distribution. On the right-hand side of *Figure 14.7a*, a third order, Fx, larynx frequency distribution is shown. This has been derived by counting only those larynx periods in speech which are associated with the immediately succeeding occurrence of two

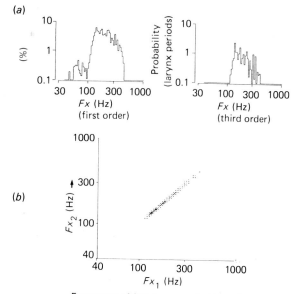

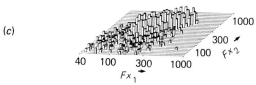

Figure 14.7 Long-term laryngograph based analyses from a normal woman speaking with an expressive intonation. (*a*) First and third order larynx period distributions. (*b*) Diagram larynx period scatter plot – intensity proportional to log probability. (*c*) Diagram plot as in (*b*) with height proportional to log probability

effectively identical laryngeal periods in the analysis. The frequency range between 10 and 1000 Hz has been divided into 100 logarithmically equal intervals and, if a larynx period falls within one of these intervals, it contributes to the count in that interval. Here, then, the restriction has been that three successive intervals must fall within a 'bin' in order to be represented. This third order analysis provides a coarse indication of the degree of regularity in the speaking voice, enhances modes which are dominant, and discards information relating to irregular laryngeal activity. In consequence, the double-peaked low frequency tail of the main first order distribution is missing in the third order representation of the data.

In *Figure 14.7b*, a further development of this method of assessing laryngeal regularity and irregularity is shown. Along the horizontal ordinate the frequency of the first larynx period in any pair is represented, and vertically the frequency of the second member of any pair is shown. On the figure itself the bins which result from this division of the whole frequency range are shown in terms of black dots, the density of which corresponds to the number of occurrences at that pair of larynx frequencies. In this way, for an ideally regular voice there will only be a narrow diagonal line shown across, since if the voice has the characteristics of *Figure 14.5*, there will be a very close relationship between the frequencies of successive vocal fold vibrations. Where there is irregularity as in, for example, *Figure 14.4* or in the low frequency range as shown in *Figure 14.7a* on the left, in the creaky voice component, then there will be significant departures from the diagonal line. Here, creaky voice is exemplified by the parallel lines which are on either side of the main diagonal and by the very low frequency components in the bottom left hand part of the figure. The main concentrations of dark filled bins in *Figure 14.7b* correspond to the modes which can be seen in the peaks of the distributions in *Figure 14.7a*.

Another way of illustrating the relationship between successive vocal fold closures using exactly the same data is shown in *Figure 14.7c*. Here the number of occurrences within any particular bin on the 'scatter' plot is shown by the vertical extent of the trace. Now, the height of the vertical line corresponds to the logarithm of the probability of the occurrence. These representations are increasingly used in the evaluation of pathological conditions, and make it possible for the disability and progress of a patient, in regard to phonatory ability, to be seen easily and to be followed over a period of time by the inclusion of plots, readily available at present using simple microcomputer techniques, which can be incorporated into the case notes.

It is not infrequent in clinical practice that a patient can report voice production difficulty and yet on examination appear to have no pathology. In *Figure 14.8*, the analyses relate to the speech output of a young woman of the same age as the one in *Figure 14.7*. The patient was a television producer who was beginning to suffer from voice abuse and was obliged to restrict her range of laryngeal activity in order to control its regularity. In *Figure 14.8a*, the vocal fold closure irregularity which is associated with an attempt to produce a large pitch excursion is shown. The *Lx* waveform obviously has gross irregularities. This is only a very small sample taken from a much larger whole where, by and large, the vocal fold vibration is regular, but here the alternate peaks of large closure are quite abnormal and indicative of the closure and period irregularities which are characteristic of differing sorts of pathology. The two distributions in *Figure 14.8b* correspond to the first and third order analyses of vocal fold vibration

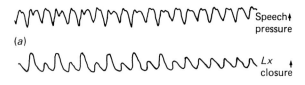

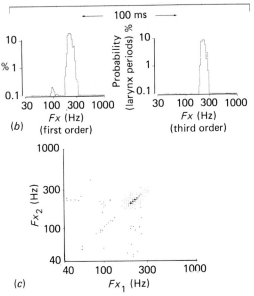

Figure 14.8 Vocal fold abuse in an adult female. (*a*) Vocal fold vibratory irregularity occurs primarily in rapidly changing sequences; (*b*) narrow range and high correlation between first and third order distributions; (*c*) relatively large scatter for a small range in the diagram distribution

and here the third order distribution is almost of the same height as the first, as the result of the patient's using a very narrow range in an attempt to produce regular voice. *Figure 14.8c* shows the diagram distribution and here the very small diagonal length, compared for example with that in *Figure 14.7*, corresponds to this restricted range and the relatively greater scatter around this small diagonal corresponds to the irregularities associated with voice abuse. Therapy properly directed can, in these cases, lead to the re-establishment of a greater range and smaller closure irregularity and avoid the need for possible surgical intervention later.

In *Figure 14.9*, a 50-year-old male speaker with oedematous vocal folds illustrates the extent to which there may be an extremely low correlation between laryngeal vibrational activity and corresponding speech pressure response in the vocal tract. Direct observation of vocal fold vibration can

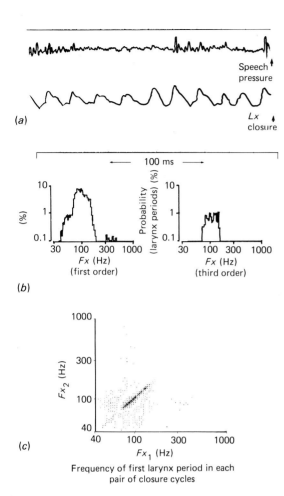

(a)

(b)

(c)

Frequency of first larynx period in each
pair of closure cycles

Figure 14.9 Reinke's oedema in an adult male.
(*a*) Irregular vocal fold closures with a low correlation
between speech pressure and vocal fold vibration;
(*b*) frequency irregularity shown by the width of the first
order distribution and small height of the third order;
(*c*) large dispersion in diagram distribution

pitch of this voice is one of extreme irregularity. In *Figure 14.9b*, the intrinsic aperiodicity of vibrational movement is responsible for the fairly low probability of the peaks in the third order triplet distribution, compared with the modal values in the first order distribution. The large excursion of the low frequency skirt of the first order distribution in *Figure 14.9b* is associated with extreme irregularity. This irregularity is also responsible for the difference in the width between the first and third order distributions and for the large difference in their heights.

The scatter distribution in *Figure 14.9c* clearly indicates the degree to which there is, on occasion, a very low correspondence between successive vocal fold periods. Treatment of the oedema can substantially reduce this scatter and reduces very markedly the low frequency components of the first order distribution shown in *Figure 14.9b*, and gives an increase in the heights of the modal values in the third order distribution. These factors are readily available as indicators of success of treatment.

This discussion has concentrated on the temporal analysis of closure features of vocal fold vibration since these are of immediate clinical value, bearing as they do as directly on the perceived pitch of the voice and on the intrinsic condition of the vibrating vocal folds themselves. The approach, however, has much greater longer-term interest. This is because the direct availability of closure information in synchrony with the acoustic signal makes it possible to provide far more complete analyses of both normal and pathological conditions than is ever likely to be feasible by more indirect single acoustic waveform techniques – especially when using, for example, simple spectral or linear predictive coefficient analyses of the sort which are currently employed in more industrially orientated speech analysis work.

Figure 14.10 shows the sequence of *Fx* histograms recorded from an 11-year-old girl before, and at intervals after, endotracheal intubation with a cuffed Portex tube. The preoperative histogram has a small low frequency irregular tail due to the creaky voice components which are sometimes found in adult speech. In this case and many other normal children's speech, however, this is more the product of a diplophonic (octave jumps accompanied by temporal irregularity) rather than a creaky voice. The diplophonic speech is a feature of the immature larynx. After intubation, the range of the girl's voice became restricted with many more pitch breaks. These features are shown in the histogram obtained on the first postoperative day by a bimodal peaking with narrowing of the main lobe of the distribution. Resolution of this functional abnormality to

yield information which it is difficult to obtain using other means. Auditorily the voice is irregular, breathy and of poor timbre so far as the speech quality is concerned. The physical nature of the origin of these effects, however, cannot be easily determined auditorily, although a visual inspection obviously defines the main source of difficulty. When vocal fold closure is not sufficiently well defined in regard to its rapidity and duration, then, although there may be very large movements of the vocal folds, there will not necessarily be a concomitant large acoustic output. The swollen oedematous masses of the vocal folds in the case of this speaker produced closures of the glottis which, since they very often occur slowly, do not always produce large corresponding acoustic outputs. The perceptual quality of the

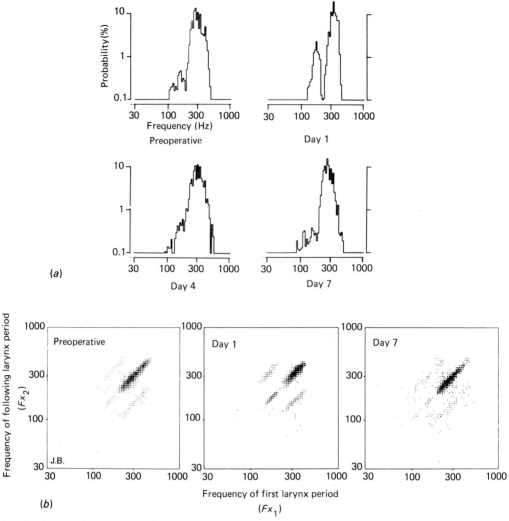

Figure 14.10 Laryngeal trauma secondary to intubation. (*a*) Sequential *Fx* histograms showing low frequency irregularity in preoperative recording, bimodal tracing produced by octave pitch breaks immediately after intubation, and slow recovery over 1 week. (*b*) Scatter plot analysis showing restriction of range and increased irregularity on day 1 and increased range together with loss of irregularity on day 7

the initial condition took one week. The main modal frequency value of the subsidiary peak in the first day is half that of the peak of the main body of the histogram. The *Fx* contours associated with this postoperative condition, instead of being smooth, are interrupted by prolonged octave pitch break jumps. Scatter plots of this sequence of events also show the restricted range, increased vibratory irregularity, and the presence of largely octave jumps. Similarly, the scatter plots also indicate the essential resolution of the condition by the end of the first week. Similar, but less pronounced, changes have been documented following intubation with non-cuffed tubes (Gleeson and Fourcin, 1983).

Acoustic output and auditory input

The vocal tract extends from the larynx to the lips and nostrils. It can be regarded as a set of tubes of irregular shape, varying intrinsically both as a function of the anatomy of the speaker and the setting of the articulators. Although in English the lips, tongue and soft palate are the primary articulators – the means of control of the shape of the vocal tract used by the speaker – in other language environments additional articulators are employed, for example the epiglottis and the body of the larynx itself. In all languages, however, the whole ensemble of the vocal tract can be conveniently regarded as an acoustic filter which operates

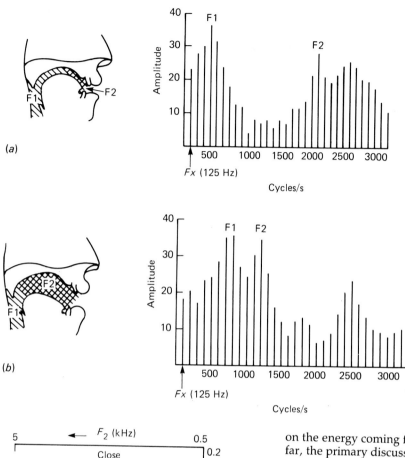

(a)

(b)

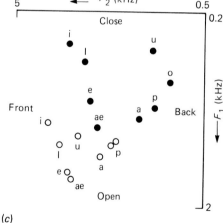

(c)

Figure 14.11 (*a*) Shape of the vocal tract and sound sm17pectrum of the vowel /i/; (*b*) shape of the vocal tract and sound spectrum of the vowel /a:/. (*c*) British English vowel formants approximately related to articulation. The average formant frequencies of adult men (●) are compared with the average formant frequencies for 4-year-old children (○). Although this is only a simple presentation of the data, the partial emergence of the same formant patterning in the children as is present for the men may be seen

on the energy coming from an excitation input. So far, the primary discussion in respect of the means of excitation of the vocal tract has centred on the acoustic energy coming from the larynx as the result of the regular and irregular vibrations of the vocal folds in a normally egressive air stream, but, as will be discussed, other sources of excitation are also possible. Voiced excitation is, however, the primary source of contrastive linguistic information in all speech systems.

Figure 14.11 illustrates two contrastive settings of a hypothetical vocal tract. In *Figure 14.11a*, this vocal tract is adjusted for the production of the close front vowel [i]. Here, the volume of the oropharyngeal cavity is fairly big and the volume immediately between the lips and the point of maximum constriction is relatively small compared with other vowel settings. In general, it is not appropriate to refer to separate parts of the vocal tract as being totally responsible for particular resonances in its response. However, when there is a very close constriction, then, to a first approximation, this representation of different parts of the vocal tract as being associated with different resonances is acceptable, and it is certainly convenient as a very approximate description of the contribution of the vocal tract to the shaping of the overall spectrum of its output. In the case of [i], the large back cavity produces a low first formant, and the small front cavity produces a high second formant. This vowel in consequence tends to be characterized by a wide separation between the first and second formants, or resonances of the vocal tract. These resonances serve as frequency regions which are associated with the best transmission of energy from the laryngeal source. Intervening frequencies are not so well transmitted simply because the impedance acoustically presented by the vocal tract is greater to the laryngeal source at points on the overall frequency response distant from the resonances. Changing the shape of the vocal tract by the adjustment of the articulators changes the resonances, and the response curve, correspondingly. The relationship is highly complex in physical terms, but one which is learned by the child in the first months and years of life. For the vowel [a:] the oral cavity is very much larger than for the close front vowel [i], and the back cavity is smaller. This adjustment, to a gross first approximation, makes the second formant lower in frequency and the first formant higher in frequency, and this is illustrated in *Figure 14.11b*.

Both *Figures 14.11a* and *14.11b* are best interpreted in terms of the frequency response of a vocal tract which is characterized by its resonant frequencies, and with an input coming from a regularly vibrating vocal fold source which imparts to the response of the vocal tract a final output composed only of harmonics of a fundamental frequency determined by the rate of vibration of the vocal folds. In these two examples the vocal folds vibrate at 125 Hz and, in consequence, the resonances of the two vocal tracts are in effect illuminated by harmonics which are whole number multiples of this fundamental frequency of 125 Hz. The potential range of larynx frequencies is dependent upon the construction of the individual speaker's vocal tract and larynx. In going from one speaker type to another, both larynx frequency modes and formant frequency values for particular vowels will differ very markedly.

In *Figure 14.11c*, the relationships between the first two resonant frequencies, F1 and F2, for an adult male capable of producing the particular vowel tokens of *Figures 14.6a* and *14.6b* are illustrated for the range of southern British vowels discussed phonetically at the beginning of this chapter. Immediately under the full circles defining the formant frequencies for the typical adult male, there are open circles which have been obtained from measurements made on the speech of 4-year-old children. Two important aspects of these different distributions of formant frequencies should be noted. First, for the children the

formant values are uniformly higher, corresponding to their smaller vocal tracts. Second, the relative disposition of the formant frequencies for the children is largely similar to that for the adults. Two factors are at issue here. First, the children necessarily are employing a contrastive system which corresponds to that employed by the adults. Second, the children are still at the stage of learning how best to produce these contrasts and, in consequence, they are not as completely organized as they will be at a later stage of development. Auditorily, the normal listener is capable of making adjustments for both of these factors. First, it is possible to interpret the widely different formant frequencies as being associated with the same phonetically definable vowel qualities by a process of inference which is called 'normalization'. Second, allowance is made for an inadequate system of contrasts produced by the immature speaker.

In *Figure 14.12*, the representations are different in two main respects. First, they relate to another way of displaying the acoustic information relating to a speech utterance. In this figure time is shown along the horizontal axis and frequency along the vertical axis. At any point in this frequency–time plane, the darkness of the trace indicates the energy acoustically associated with the utterance. In *Figure 14.12* these 'spectrograms' have the additional property that they represent utterances which intrinsically change with time. They would be produced by the articulations of *Figure 14.11* being set so that they alter from one position to another while the larynx excitation illuminates the changing resonances produced by the alteration. If, for example, the lips of the speaker were closed at the beginning of the utterance and then rapidly separated, the spectrograms at the top of *Figure 14.12* for [b] and [p] would be obtained, dependent upon whether for [b] the larynx excitation occurred immediately following the opening of the speaker's lips or, as in [p], if there were a slight delay. For this figure there is one additional variation, the steady state portion of the utterance, which follows the initial release of the closure produced at the top of the figure by the speaker's lips, is associated with the vowel [ɜ:], a central vowel both in regard to articulatory setting and in respect of the formant frequencies which would be plotted in the type of representation shown in *Figure 14.11c*. Changing the steady setting of the speaker's vocal tract changes the formants and, in consequence, the steady vowel quality, but generally in speech these constant settings are never found.

Speech is essentially a dynamic process, the characteristics of its contrasts being determined by the nature of their temporal change. The nature of the temporal change for progressively different

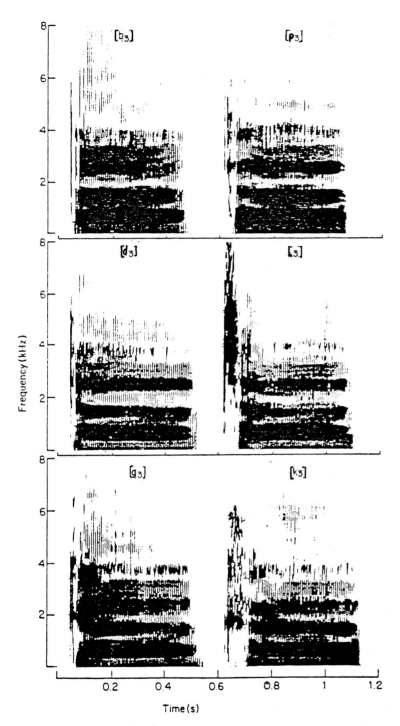

Figure 14.12 Spectrographic (frequency–intensity–time) characteristics associated with minimal plosive consonant contrasts in English

initial closure settings is illustrated in *Figure 14.12*. Working from top to bottom, the closure is first at the level of the lips, second at the level of the alveolar ridge with the tongue closing off the vocal tract immediately behind the teeth, and finally in the lowest pair of spectrograms with the tongue closing off the vocal tract immediately before the soft palate. In each of these cases, following initial closure a rapid release with, on the left-hand side, larynx excitation immediately following the release and, on the right-hand side, larynx excitation following the release with some delay in voice production, characterizes the dynamic sequence associated with the sound in two main ways. First, for the left column, working from top to bottom, voicing occurring early is an important characteristic, compared with the right-hand column where voicing occurs later than the release. This first main difference is characterized by the essential absence of low frequency energy in all of the spectrograms in the right-hand column, and by the presence of random fricative energy acoustically produced by the turbulent random air flow in the constriction associated with the closure point immediately following its release. The second main dynamic feature associated with these spectrograms relates to the character of the change in time associated with the resonances of the vocal tract. As the speaker's tongue moves from the closure setting to the steady setting for the vowel, the vocal tract's resonances change in a systematic fashion which signals to the listener the essential phonetic nature of the contrast produced.

In the initial introduction the main phonetic characteristics defining class divisions in the sounds of English were referred to primarily in terms of the vocal tract settings with which they were associated. Here, the spectrograms simply show the acoustic pattern differences associated with these phonetically contrastive classes. In the case of the normal speaker, there is a relatively close correspondence between articulatory setting and acoustic pattern form. In pathology, however, this is not necessarily so; for example a patient who has had a glossectomy may well seek to achieve comparable acoustic outputs by the use of articulatory settings and movements which differ from those which would be produced by the normal speaker. If, however, the patient is capable of imitating normal acoustic pattern forms sufficiently well with a different articulation, he will, nevertheless, be able to communicate satisfactorily. Patterns of the type shown in *Figure 14.12* provide a key to the understanding of how effective communication can be re-established, both by a speaker who has a vocal tract pathology to combat, and by a listener who has a hearing disability to circumvent. In both cases, either the production or the inference of acoustic pattern

forms, with reference to phonetic contrasts, provides the key to adequate communication. Acoustically, the pattern features which the listener normally seeks in respect of the phonetic contrast in *Figure 14.12* relate to three factors: the nature of the acoustic burst; the characteristics of the following aspiration (the term applied to the turbulent energy which immediately precedes voicing); and the nature of the transitions (the formant frequency changes which occur in time, leading into or from the steady vowel setting). If these burst and transition characteristics are capable of being simulated adequately, even in part, then the listener has the basis for the inference of a sufficient definition of the phonetic components necessary for communication.

Dynamic effects

In *Figure 14.13*, the complete progression is made from the steady forms of *Figure 14.11* and the citation forms of *Figure 14.12* to a complete dynamic sequence with, as before, frequency of the acoustic components shown vertically and time displayed horizontally. The waveform displayed in *Figure 14.13a* relates to the pressure changes produced as the output of the speaker's vocal tract and which are basic to the analysis shown immediately below. Running through the spectrogram, vertical lines can easily be seen for all of the voiced parts of the utterance. Each vertical line corresponds, as seen previously, to an individual closure of the speaker's vocal folds, and the resonances which follow the leading edge of the vertical line occur primarily during the closure phase of the vocal fold vibratory cycle. Spacing of adjacent vertical lines corresponds to the laryngeal period, at the end of the utterance for the word 'book' for example, the spacing is very much greater than it is during the higher pitched vowel [æ] in 'began'.

These intonational changes are used by the speaker to signal to the listener how the sentence itself is structured and are employed essentially as a means of giving an indication of the overall grammatical form and semantic consequence of the utterance. At the very beginning of the sentence, however, there are no organized vertical lines, striations, associated with laryngeal vibration. For the consonant at the beginning of 'she', the excitation in the vocal tract is produced by the turbulent energy acoustically associated with the passage of air through the tongue–palato-alveolar constriction. This voiceless fricative has one characteristic of vowel sounds in that it is capable of being sustained, and is different in this respect from the voiceless sounds which have just been discussed with reference to *Figure 14.12*, associ-

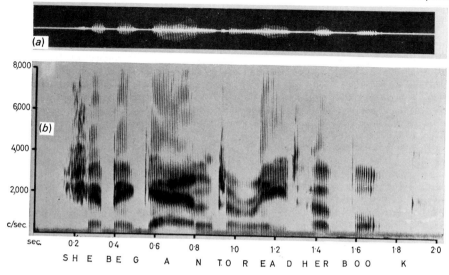

Figure 14.13 (*a*) Oscillogram of the sentence: 'She began to read her book'; (*b*) spectrogram of the sentence: 'She began to read her book' (filter bandwidth 300 Hz)

ated with [p], [t] and [k]. The [t] burst of energy associated with 'to' in this sentence is quite apparent, and is obviously of longer duration than the burst of energy associated with the release for the [g] in 'began' and the [b] in 'book'. With reference to the earlier discussion on laryngeal excitation, it is worth noting the irregularity in laryngeal vibration immediately prior to the [k] in 'book', a characteristic 'signing off' at the end of a voiced utterance. The changes in amplitude signalled by the darkness of the traces in the vowel [æ] in 'began', are the result of variations in larynx excitation and the 'cutback' in $F2$ and $F3$ compared with $F1$ in [n], immediately prior to the 'to'.

In going from the gross overall pattern of the difference between voiceless and voiced energy, the gross shaping of the spectra in terms of the formant resonances and their transitions, to these final subtle points, one travels through a series of successive approximations which make the difference between speech which is barely intelligible and speech which is totally natural. These steps can be followed in the process of the artificial synthesis of speech sequences by both machine and man. In the case of pathology, whether productive or receptive, the gross features adequately processed can be used as the basis, in the presence of contextual clues, to provide a satisfactory means of communication. Systematic attention to the reduction of the salient differences between the expectations of the ordinary listener and the productions of the speaker can make for substantial improvements in communicative competence. These factors are capable of being explored by the use of speech analysis and

synthesis techniques, and exploration can be applied both to the sequences of normal speech acquisition and to the assessment of acquisition in deviant situations – for the handicapped child and adult.

Clues to speech contrasts

When changes in the vocal tract occur, there are necessarily both alterations in formant patterns and in the patterns of excitation – whether voiceless or with a combination of voiced and voiceless excitation present simultaneously. The acoustic features of normal speech have been presented in a sequence going from the level of larynx input where the basis of intonation – fundamental frequency structuring – is established, to the level at which the main resonances of the vocal tract are defined with respect to the steady state vowel-like contrasts and continuing to the discussion of the all-important transitions. The underlying concept is one of changing structures of acoustic/auditory patterns resulting from formant frequency variations corresponding to vocal tract articulatory alterations.

This sequence of levels of description is associated not only with basic productive simplicity and salience but also with acoustic prominence. The component of larynx excitation which is responsible for the voiced components of speech must exist in order for the most important contrasts of all language speech systems to be viable. This laryngeal component is also associated with the most dominant auditory characteristic of speech, that which determines pitch of the speaking voice.

A developing child not only must learn how to control vocal fold vibration in order to produce an effective cry, but must also learn how to perceive changes in intonation. At the very beginning of the apprenticeship in speech, the development of cry and intonation control are the first speech skills that are acquired. These are linked to the ability to control vowel contrasts and intrinsically are associated with the abilities to produce labial voiced consonants, alveolar consonants, and velar consonants approximately in this order of acquisition. Very largely, in the early speech–phonological development associated with the normal child's acquisition of language skills, articulatory complexity and the intricacies of acoustic pattern contrasts are in a high degree of correspondence. Where there are differences, however, they appear to depend on a dominance of acoustic pattern or auditory pattern complexity rather than articulatory control. There is, for example, an early ability to produce labial voiceless contrasts which are acoustically auditorily salient, although the cooperative activity of both larynx and vocal tract presents considerable productive difficulty.

This early ordering of speech development gives an insight into the way in which the receptive ability of both adults and children can be analytically investigated. For example, in *Figure 14.14*, the simple contrast of rising and falling intonation contours, which was first shown from a natural utterance in *Figure 14.5*, has been arranged so that it can provide the basis for the assessment using synthetic speech techniques of perceptual contrastive receptive ability. In the contour (1) in *Figure 14.14a* the set of intonation contrasts is a maximum rise and in the contour (9) in *Figure 14.14a*, in the same sequence, is a maximum fall. These two contrasts provide redundant information in regard to the opposition between the question and statement forms that can often be encountered in normal citation form English. In the rise, the contour shape gives an indication that it is a question and similarly the falling countour indicates a statement. However, there is, in addition, a shift in fundamental frequency between these two contours which also signals whether the speaker is operating at the upper or lower ends of his/her fundamental frequency range. Although these contours, (1) and (9), have been modelled on natural utterances, as in *Figure 14.5*, the intermediate contours in *Figure 14.14* have been artificially determined by equal logarithmic interpolation. By presenting these contours superimposed on the diphthong [əu], it is possible to determine the listeners' receptive ability in respect of both the contrastive power of the individual contours and of the individual listeners' discriminative capacity.

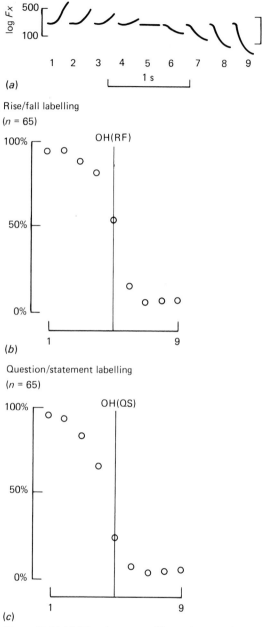

(a)

Rise/fall labelling (n = 65)

(b)

Question/statement labelling (n = 65)

(c)

Figure 14.14 (a) Stimulus range, (b) psychoacoustic, (c) linguistically based labelling for voice pitch changes

The lower part of *Figure 14.14* shows two results of the application of this type of synthetic speech receptive assessment technique to a group of 65 listeners. On the left, the listeners have responded to the stimuli labelling them as though they were either rising or falling. This is a purely psychoacoustic assessment. On the right, the listeners have responded, appraising the stimuli as though they were either questions or statements. It will be noted that there is, in each case, a characteristic sigmoid labelling response function associated with the average of the listeners' responses. There is a significant difference between the two labelling tasks. Where rise–fall is the criterion the sigmoid response is symmetrical over the stimulus range. Where question–statement is the labelling response used by the listeners, the response curve is significantly biased so that it is necessary for the listeners to be presented with a markedly rising contour in order for it to be classified as being associated with a question. Running through speech there is this essential difference between the modes of

psychoacoustic response and the modes of phonological interpretation which the listener may place on the complex stimuli presented to him. In work for the hearing-impaired these two factors provide a key to the understanding of how speech patterns can be used for assessment and in connection with the design of new prostheses – but they are also of importance in the management of productive pathologies.

The two modes of response are illustrated in quite different contexts in *Figure 14.15*. Here, the stimuli have been presented to a profoundly deaf child at a comfortable listening level in an assessment of the child's ability to profit from the

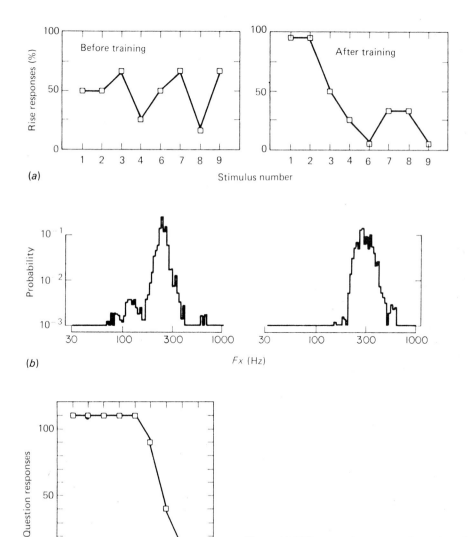

Figure 14.15 Perceptual response of a profoundly deaf child to random presentations of stimuli 1–4 and 6–9 of *Figure 14.14a*. (*a*) Before and after training; (*b*) the change in voice characteristics; (*c*) *Fx* labelling by a totally, postlingually, deaf patient for the full range of *Figure 14.14* with electrical presentation of the stimuli

receptive and productive training, associated with a Voiscope® display (Fourcin, 1979). Before training, the child's ability to discriminate between rise and fall responses is essentially random but after 6 weeks' work, involving approximately 10 minutes a day, receptive ability is very significantly improved and the child can now confidently make rise–fall judgements on the basis of simple contrastive intonation contours.

The display work involved the simultaneous auditory and visual presentation of the speech fundamental frequency contours and the child's responses were associated both with production as well as reception. As a result of the productive training, the larynx frequency distribution of the type discussed earlier in this chapter, which is shown before training on the left, has very markedly improved in the analysis shown on the right.

In *Figure 14.15c*, a quite different stimulus response situation is involved. A postlingually deaf adult woman has been given electrocochlear stimuli associated with the use of constant current round window stimulation, having fundamental frequency contours corresponding precisely to those of *Figure 14.14*. No training was involved of any sort in respect of the actual presentations associated with these stimuli. In the same way as for the deaf child, only general work with the Voiscope® had been undertaken with the patient. The extremely well-defined grouping of the stimuli into question and statement response categories gives a striking example of the way in which an artificially presented speech pattern element is capable of being recognized linguistically. It also indicates the striking fashion in which

the transmission of temporal information is capable of providing a useful basis for single channel electrocochlear stimulation. It is likely that the child already discussed is also operating as a result of learning how to process purely temporal information. With an average pure-tone loss of 90 dB between 125 and 500 Hz, he is likely to have extremely wide auditory filtering and be essentially unable to respond to changes in the frequency spacing of harmonic components.

A similar stimulus presentation to that employed for the labelling results of *Figure 14.15* is shown in *Figure 14.3* of Volume 2. It is particularly important to note, however, that in *Figure 14.3*, Volume 2, the synthetic rise–fall stimuli have the same mean frequency throughout the range and so it is quite impossible to interpret the labelling responses which have been obtained both by normal listeners and by those receiving electrocochlear stimulation (who are otherwise totally deaf) in terms of a discrimination simply of mean frequency as opposed to changing direction of intonation contour. While this result is of importance in its own right in respect of the use of temporal processing ability by the electrocochlear patients for the labelling of speech-like stimuli, it is also of more general consequence in indicating the way in which speech synthetic techniques can be utilized so as to investigate a single aspect of receptive processing ability by normal individuals as well as the hearing impaired.

In *Figure 14.16*, the sequence previously used in *Figure 14.15* has been employed for the study of the perceptual processing development of a profoundly deaf boy during a period in which he was given daily speech therapy using the interac-

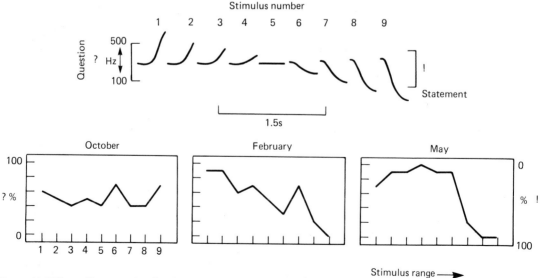

Figure 14.16 Prosodic contrastive development in a 14-year-old deaf child

tive visual 'intonation contour' laryngograph display, the Voiscope®, coupled with the use of an auditory presentation of the associated speech (work by Yvonne Paris at Mary Hare School for the Deaf). Three main stages in perceptual development over the period of months can be discerned: first, the random level of response which was previously displayed for the younger child in *Figure 14.15a*; second, a period of progressive labelling in which essentially only the extremes are confidently responded to; and in the third and final stage, the beginnings of true categorical labelling are evident. Together with this acquisition of better labelling ability, the same improvement in productive ability as was previously obtained for the younger child was also found. In general, in the limited experience that the authors have with this work, the same basic situation is obtained for all profoundly hearing-impaired children who have usable residual hearing. Training improves perception and production, and the two go hand in hand. If, however, there is no effective residual hearing capable of providing the basis for categorization, then the random labelling characteristic is maintained, although some improvement in productive ability with visual training can be expected. While the older child may take a year or more to achieve satisfactory performance, the younger child below the age of 10 years may well be expected to achieve comparable results both productively and receptively in a matter of only 2 months, with considerable variation from child to child depending upon circumstances and intrinsic capacity.

In the normal child it is possible to hypothesize three levels of development which are basic to the establishment of the capacity to make phonological distinctions. First, at the level of the peripheral hearing mechanism, the anatomical structures and physiological mechanisms which subserve acoustic signal processing must exist. Second, the signal processing capacity, provided by the interaction between the mechanical response of the peripheral hearing mechanism and the neural innervation, must be developed so that primary speech pattern features can be resolved. Third, the cognitive development which makes it feasible for the complexes of patterns to be given adequate phonetic/phonological interpretation must be achieved. Of course, these are broad aspects of a highly complex situation and little experimental evidence is currently available either to justify these assertions or to throw light upon their detailed form. However, with regard to the second level source, some studies on animals are beginning which indicate the important interactions which definitely appear to exist in respect of the efferent system's ability to influence peripheral auditory development (Dodson *et al.*, 1986).

Contrastive phonetic ability must develop early in order for the normal child to begin to interact adequately with its speaking environment. Phonologically, the earliest speech pattern component is associated with intonational contrasts and these are already being employed within the first year of life of the normal child. Controlled testing is difficult at this age, thus it is not readily possible to arrive at the analytical investigation of intonation contrastive development in the normal child in the way that one can with the hearing-impaired child who may well be going through a process of speech development at the age of 6 or 7 years or even much later, that the normal child has totally mastered by the age of 18 months. Other aspects of speech pattern contrastive ability are developed, however, much later in the normal child and in *Figure 14.17* the receptive development

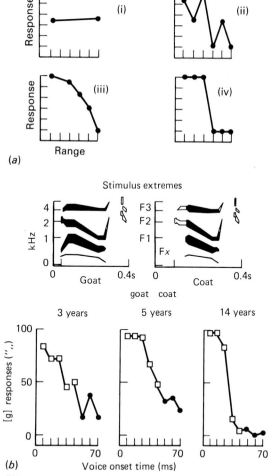

Figure 14.17 Normal developmental sequences: (*a*) progression (i–iv) in the normal child with idealized representations; (*b*) stimuli used in an experimental progression as in *Figure 14.14a*

sequence for the velar voiced–voiceless consonantal development of [g]–[k] in normal English children is delineated. The speech patterns involved are shown at the top of the figure, two main acoustic pattern features serve the phonetic contrast in this situation. On the left, the black filled in formants indicate the presence of voice excitation, while on the right, the initial open formant patterning for F2 and F3 indicates the presence of voiceless, turbulent energy, excitation. Physically the main difference between the initial [g] and (ɦ) is associated with the contrasts between periodic or aperiodic vocal tract excitation (*see Figure 14.12*).

There is, however, another important pattern difference. Auditorily, the first formant in the voiceless 'coat' exemplar is not excited at the beginning of the transition. This makes it possible to interleave two types of speech pattern form into the stimuli which are used for the labelling experiments run with these children. Using synthetic speech techniques it is possible to produce sounds which cannot be obtained from the normal human vocal tract and the 'goat' stimuli have also been synthesized with a flat F1 onset. In this situation, voicing starts early but with an unnatural formant patterning, in fact the younger children are not significantly able to respond to the difference between these two stimuli, while for the older children and normal adults the flat F1 onset receives a much worse response than that associated with the normal

transition, although the voicing onset is itself perfectly normal. This indicates once more the importance of cognitive interpretation in respect of basic speech pattern forms. The first work on these experiments is discussed elsewhere (Simon and Fourcin, 1976), but the main importance of this particular presentation lies in the way in which it shows how the development sequence obtained for deaf children, discussed briefly in *Figures 14.15* and *14.16*, can be seen to have close correspondences with an aspect of normal development in respect of ordinary phonological acquisition with children having good hearing.

In *Figure 14.17*, the receptive developmental sequence going from random to progressive to established categorical labelling is of the same overall patterning as that which was discussed previously for hearing–impaired children. The development of profoundly hearing–impaired children has been followed over a period of years using the same type of stimuli. *Figure 14.18* shows the corresponding type of phonological development to that exemplified in *Figure 14.17* for normal individuals. The very profoundly hearing–impaired child is capable of following a path of development which, although very much delayed, is not necessarily deviant. Some aspects of the acoustic patterning of the complex contrasts in speech will not be available for the profoundly hearing–impaired ear to transmit for subsequent cognitive appraisal. Those features which are saliently available, however, are evidently proces-

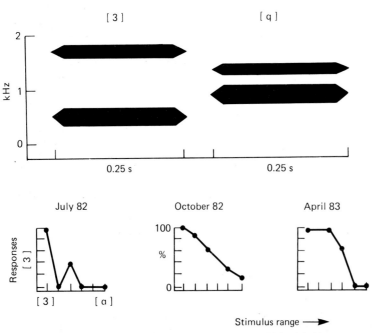

Figure 14.18 Vowel contrastive development in a 7-year-old deaf child

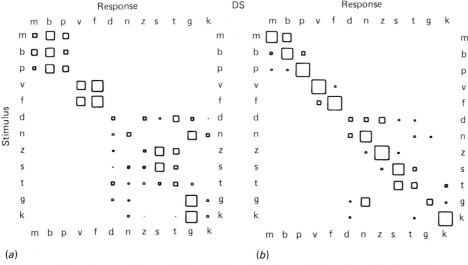

Figure 14.19 Speech pattern interpretation. (*a*) Lipreading alone; (*b*) lipreading with electrical stimulation

sed and can lead to effective labelling ability in these experiments and, from parallel work in studying the speech productive ability of these children, to effective use in speech communication (Abberton, Fourcin and Hazan, 1986; Hazan, 1986).

Saunders (Volume 2, Chapter 14) comments on the use of speech pattern assessment techniques coupled with voice therapy in work with patients receiving cochlear stimulation. It is important to note that tests based on the use of synthetic speech in ordinary clinical practice should precede therapy sessions. The improvements in receptive and in productive development that have been reported have always been based on measurements made prior to speech therapy sessions so that the patient is making use of previously acquired skills not those which have recently been refreshed.

Figure 14.19 shows an aspect of speech pattern interpretation which is based upon the joint use of features which come from the visual observation of the speaking face. Lipreading skills, when they are the only basis of speech information, can provide important place disambiguating information, but are not capable of providing accurate voice contrastive ability. In *Figure 14.19* confusion matrices are shown which are based on the use of random vowel–consonant–vowel presentations in which the vowel is fixed but the consonant is varied. The stimulus in a lipreading situation can in consequence evoke responses which will depend on the interpretation of the lipread information on the face of the speaker by the viewer and when acoustic information is provided, on the combination of the auditory with the

visual patterns. In the absence of acoustic/auditory information, while place information can be fairly readily assessed, voice and manner information, as previously discussed at the beginning of the chapter, are inadequately transmitted. In consequence, confusion can result with the necessary grouping together of responses in terms of their place, so that for example /b/, /p/ and /m/ form a grouping quite distinct from /d/, /t/ and /s/ and /n/. The provision of voice only (*Fx*) pattern information can begin to resolve these ambiguities and reduce the scatter associated with the lipreading alone situation. *Figure 14.19* shows the result for a cochlear stimulation patient receiving only this combination of *Fx* and visual information (Fourcin *et al.*, 1984; Abberton *et al.*, 1985; Rosen *et al.*, 1985).

Tests employing the presentation of vowel–consonant–vowel combinations of this sort are necessarily a little removed from the ordinary communication circumstances that the patient experiences, and while they can provide valuable information in respect of the analytical ability conferred by different aids, their remoteness from ordinary conversational situations is a disadvantage. In *Figure 14.20*, another method of assessment which is complementary to that used in *Figure 14.19* is applied in the assessment of an associated acoustic hearing aid. Sito, the sine voice aid, is essentially an acoustic laryngograph (Rosen and Fourcin, 1983; Walliker, Rosen and Fourcin, 1986). In the assessment of lipreading when continuous speech is used, for 'discourse tracking', as described by Saunders (Volume 2, Chapter 14), a more representative test of a real-life situation is obtained. In this present

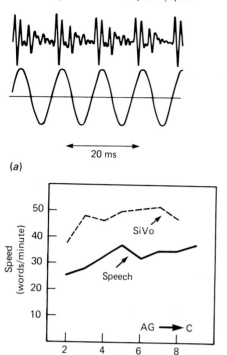

20 ms

(*a*)

(*b*)

Figure 14.20 (*a*) Speech sound pressure waveform (top) and acoustic output (bottom) from 'SiVo' for the token 'ah'. (*b*) Three-point smoothed results from connected discourse tracking, comparing the degree to which the lipreading is helped, either by an ordinary hearing aid, or the 'SiVo' device in the 'Mapitch' (−50 Hz) mode

aid is excellent, for a large number of profoundly hearing-impaired adults and children a different approach may eventually be of greater practical value. At present the possibility of analysing out a restricted set of speech pattern features so that their presentation can be associated with greater perceptual clarity and greater relevance, in the case of the child, to speech developmental needs is not yet practicable. In the next decade, however, it will be. The speech pattern receptive tests which have been described here, the speech pattern training display which complements these tests and the development of the equipment itself are beginning to be quite well established. They are likely soon to find regular clinical use with adults.

In work with children, however, although this new generation of techniques for assessment, therapy and hearing aid design will make for radical improvements in respect of the profoundly hearing-impaired child's chances of being integrated into normal society. However they can only be achieved with thoroughly informed management. This is primarily because the use of 'aids for stages' of development depends on the close association of otological/audiological assessment with educational/developmental need.

example, the rate at which lipreading can be achieved in a discourse tracking test is shown when the patient is dependent upon lipreading alone compared to the situation in which the patient is making use both of the visual input and of a single auditory pattern derived only from the intonational component of the acoustic output of the speaker. A pure sinewave is used, matched so that it is at a comfortable listening level, whatever larynx frequency is analysed. It provides disambiguating information in respect of voiced–voiceless contrasts and, more importantly for continuous speech, the overall intonation pattern structure of the speech sequences.

The advent of new microprocessor devices which are capable of low power consumption and more comprehensive signal analysis makes it possible to contemplate the situation in the future in which patients will fairly readily be able to make use of a prosthesis giving simplified pattern presentations which will enhance their ability to make phonetically important discriminations in normal conversation. While for those who have a moderate degree of loss, the conventional hearing

References

ABBERTON, E., FOURCIN, A. J. and HAZAN, V. (1986) Phonological competence with profound hearing loss. In *Speech, Hearing and Language, Work in Progress*, Vol. 2, edited by A. J. Fourcin and D. Howard, pp. 1–14. London: University College

ABBERTON, E., FOURCIN, A. J., ROSEN, S., WALLIKER, J. R., HOWARD, D. M., MOORE, B. C. J. *et al.* (1985) Speech perceptual and productive rehabilitation in electro-cochlear stimulation. In *Cochlear Implants*, edited by R. A. Schindler and M. M. Merzenich, pp. 527–537. New York: Raven Press

CHILDERS, D. and KRISHNAMURTHY, A. K. (1985) A critical review of electroglottography. *CRC Critical Reviews in Biomedical Engineering*, **12**, 131–161

DELATTRE, P. C. (1966) *Studies in French and Comparative Phonetics*. The Hague: Mouton

DELATTRE, P. C., LIBERMAN, A. M. and COOPER, F. S. (1955) Acoustic loci and transitional cues for consonants. *Journal of the Acoustical Society of America*, **27**, 769

DENES, P. B. and PINSON, E. N. (1963) *The Speech Chain*. New Jersey: Bell Telephone Laboratories

DODSON, H. C., WALLIKER, J. R., FRAMPTON, S., DOUEK, E. E., FOURCIN, A. J. and BANNISTER, L. H. (1986) Structural alterations of the hair cells in the contralateral ear resulting from extracochlear electrical stimulation. *Nature*, **30**, 65–67

FANT, G. (1960) *Acoustic Theory of Speech Production*. The Hague: Mouton

FLETCHER, H. (1953) *Speech and Hearing in Communication*. New York: van Nostrand

FOURCIN, A. J. (1971) First applications of a new laryngography. *Medical and Biological Illustration*, **21**, 172–182

FOURCIN, A. J. (1974) Laryngographic examination of vocal fold vibration. In *Ventilatory and Phonatory Control Systems*, edited by B. Wyke, pp. 315–333. London: Oxford University Press

FOURCIN, A. J. (1976) Speech pattern test for deaf children. In *Disorders of Auditory Function*, edited by S. D. G. Stephens, pp. 197–208. London: Academic Press

FOURCIN, A. J. (1979) Auditory patterning and vocal fold vibration. In *Frontiers of Speech Communication Research*, edited by B. Lindblom and S. Ohman, pp. 167–176. London: Academic Press

FOURCIN, A. J. (1980) Speech pattern audiometry. In *Auditory Investigation: the Scientific and Technical Basis*, edited by H. A. Beagley, pp. 170–208. Oxford: Academic Press

FOURCIN, A. J. and ABBERTON, E. (1976) The laryngograph and voiscope in speech therapy. *Proceedings of XVIth International Congress Logopedics and Phoniatrics*, edited by E. Loebell, pp. 116–132. Basel: Karger

FOURCIN, A. J., DOUEK, E., MOORE, B., ABBERTON, E., ROSEN, S. and WALLIKER, J. (1984) Speech pattern element stimulation in electrical hearing. *Archives of Otolaryngology*, **110**, 145–153

FRY, D. B. (1963) Coding and decoding in speech. In *Signs, Signals and Symbols*, edited by S. E. Mason. London: Methuen

FRY, D. B. (1964) The correction of errors in the reception of speech. *Phonetica*, **11**, 164

FRY, D. B. (1966a) The development of the phonological system in the normal and the deaf child. In *The Genesis of Language*, edited by Frank Smith and George A. Miller, Cambridge, Mass.: M.I.T. Press, *Society of America*, **29**, 117

FRY, D. B. (1966b) The control of speech and voice. In *Regulation and Control in Living Systems*, edited by H. Kalmus. London: John Wiley

FRY, D. B. (1968) Prosodic phenomena. In *Manual of Phonetics*, edited by Malmberg. Amsterdam: North Holland

GLEESON, M. and FOURCIN, A. J. (1983) Clinical analysis of laryngeal trauma secondary to intubation. *Journal of the Royal Society of Medicine*, **76**, 928–932

GOLDMAN-EISLER, F. (1958) The predictability of words in context and the length of pauses in speech. *Language and Speech*, **1**, 226

GOLDMAN-EISLER, F. (1961) Continuity of speech utterance its determinants and its significance. *Language and Speech*, **4**, 220

GOLDMAN-EISLER, F. (1968a) Hesitation and information in speech. In *Information Theory*, edited by C. Cherry. London: Butterworths

GOLDMAN-EISLER, F. (1968b) *Psycholinguistics: Experiments in Spontaneous Speech*. London: Academic Press

GRAY, G. W. and WISE, C. M. (1959) *The Bases of Speech*. New York: Harper

HAZAN, V. (1986) Speech pattern audiometric assessment of hearing-impaired children. *Unpublished PhD Thesis*, University of London

HAZAN, V., FOURCIN, A. J. and ABBERTON, E. (1985) Speech pattern audiometry for hearing-impaired children. *Proceedings of the International Congress on Education of the Deaf*, Manchester

HIRANO, M. (1981) *Clinical Examination of Voice*. Vienna: Springer-Verlag

HOLLIEN, H., CURTIS, J. F. and COLEMAN, R. F. (1968) Stroboscopic laminography of the larynx during phonation. *Acta Oto-Laryngologica*, **65**, 209–215

LECLUSE, F. (1977) Elektroglottografie. *MD Thesis*, Erasmus University, Rotterdam. Utrecht: Drukkerijein Kwijk BV

LEE, B. S. (1950) Effects of delayed speech feedback. *Journal of the Acoustical Society of America*, **22**, 824

LIBERMAN, A. M. (1957) Some results of research on speech perception. *Journal of the Acoustical Society of America*, **29**, 117

NOSCOE, N. J., FOURCIN, A. J., BROWN, N. J. and BERRY, R. J. (1983) Examination of vocal fold movement by ultra-short pulse X radio *British Journal of Radiology*, **56**, 641–645

POTTER, R. K., KOPP, G. A. and GREEN, H. C. (1947) *Visible Speech*. New York: van Nostrand

ROSEN, S. M. (1979) Range and frequency effects in consonant categorisation. *Journal of Phonetics*, **7**, 393–402

ROSEN, S. and FOURCIN, A. J. (1983) When less is more: further work. *Speech, Hearing and Language: Work in Progress*, 1, pp. 207–212. London: University College London

ROSEN, S. and FOURCIN, A. (1986) Frequency selectivity and the perception of speech. *Frequency Selectivity in Hearing*, edited by B. C. J. Moore, pp. 373–487. London: Academic Press

ROSEN, S. M., FOURCIN, A. J., ABBERTON, E., WALLIKER, J. R., HOWARD, D. M., MOORE, B. C. J. et al. (1985) Assessing assessment. In *Cochlear Implants*, edited by R. A. Schindler and M. M. Merzenich, pp. 479–498. New York: Raven Press

SIMON, C. and FOURCIN, A. J. (1976) Differences between individual listeners in their comprehension of speech and perception of sound patterns. In *Speech and Hearing*, pp. 94–125, May. London: University College

STEVENS, K. N. and HOUSE, A. S. (1955) Development of a quantitative description of vowel articulation. *Journal of the Acoustical Society of America*, **27**, 484

TITZE, I. R. and TALKIN, D. T. (1979) A theoretical study of various laryngeal configurations on the acoustics of phonation. *Journal of the Acoustical Society of America*, **66**, 60–74

WALLIKER, J., ROSEN, S. and FOURCIN, A. J. (1986) Speech pattern prostheses for the profoundly and totally deaf. *International Conference on Speech Input/Output Techniques and Applications*, IEE Conference Publication no.258, pp. 194–199

WECHSLER, E., NEIL, W. F. and FOURCIN, A. J. (1976) Laryngographic analysis of pathological vocal fold vibration. *Proceedings of the Institute of Acoustics*, Edinburgh, 2-16-1/2-16-4

WELLS, J. C. (1962) A study of formants of the pure vowels of British English. *MA Thesis*, University of London

WELLS, J. C. (1986) A standardised machine-readable phonetic notation. *International Conference on Speech Input/Output Techniques and Applications*, IEE Conference Publication No.258, pp. 134–137

WHETNALL, E. and FRY, D. B. (1964) *The Deaf Child*. London: Heinemann

WHETNALL, E. and FRY, D. B. (1970) *Learning to Hear*, edited by R. B. Niven. London: Heinemann

15

Surgical anatomy of the skull base

C. M. Bailey

This chapter presents the surgical anatomy of the undersurface of the skull as it relates to the practice of otolaryngology; the intracranial aspect of the skull base is not discussed.

The description falls into two sections: first, a systematic topographical description of the anatomy of the skull base and structures beneath it; and second, an account of the anatomical basis of the lateral surgical approach to the skull base.

Overall topography of the skull base

The inferior aspect of the skull base is bounded in front by the upper incisor teeth, behind by the superior nuchal line of the occipital bone, and laterally by the remaining upper teeth, the zygomatic arch and its posterior root, and the mastoid process.

The region may be divided into posterior, central and anterior parts. The posterior part is separated from the central part by an arbitrary line drawn transversely through the anterior margin of the foramen magnum. The boundary between the central and anterior parts is the posterior border of the hard palate.

The *posterior skull base* comprises the occipital (muscular) area.

The *central skull base* can be subdivided into different bone areas that correspond to compartments underneath (van Huijzen, 1984) (*Figure 15.1*). It contains the pharyngeal, tubal, neurovascular, auditory and articular areas, and the infratemporal fossa.

The *anterior skull base*, on a lower level than the part behind, is formed by the hard palate and alveolar arches. It is part of the faciomaxillary structure, and will not be described further here (*see* Chapters 5 and 8).

Osteology of the skull base

Behind the faciomaxillary bones, the cranial base is made up of the occipital bone, temporal bones and part of the sphenoid bones.

Occipital bone

The occipital bone is convex posteriorly and encloses the foramen magnum, through which the cranial cavity communicates with the vertebral canal. The broad, curved plate behind and above the foramen magnum is termed the squamous part; the occipital condyle on each side of the foramen arises from the lateral part; and the thick, square piece in front of the foramen is the basi-occiput.

The *foramen magnum* is oval in shape, with its long diameter lying anteroposteriorly. The fibrous dura mater is attached to the margins of the foramen; below, it is projected down the spinal canal as the spinal dura mater (theca); above, it sweeps up into the posterior cranial fossa. Within the dural sheath in the subarachnoid space, passing through the foramen, lie the lower medulla with the cervical roots of the spinal accessory nerves, the spinal arteries and veins, and the vertebral arteries.

The anterior margin of the foramen magnum gives attachment to a number of ligaments ascending from the axis: the membrana tectoria, vertical limb of the cruciform ligament, and the apical and pair of alar ligaments of the odontoid peg. The anterior atlanto-occipital membrane is attached to a ridge that joins the anterior poles of the occipital condyles; the posterior atlanto-occipital membrane is attached to the posterior edge of the foramen magnum.

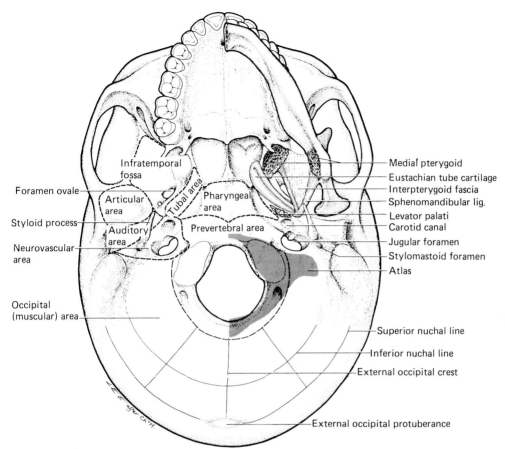

Figure 15.1 The skull base viewed from below. On the right half of the skull are indicated the regions of the central base; in the left half the mandible has been added in occlusion, with the interpterygoid fascia and eustachian tube in position. (From van Huijzen, 1984, with permission of the publishers, S. Karger)

The *squamous part* of the occipital bone gives attachment to the muscles of the back of the neck, and is described further in the section on the occipital (muscular) area of the skull base.

The *lateral part* gives rise to the occipital condyle on each side. Each condyle has a convex surface covered in hyaline cartilage which articulates with the concave surface of the atlas; these atlanto-occipital joints permit nodding only, rotation being the function of the atlantoaxial joints. Behind the condyle is a shallow fossa often perforated by the tiny posterior condylar canal, carrying a vein from the sigmoid sinus to the suboccipital venous plexus. In front of the condyle, just medial to the jugular foramen, lies the anterior condylar canal through which passes the twelfth nerve.

The *basiocciput* is an oblong block of bone which extends forward from the foramen magnum and fuses with the basisphenoid just behind the nose. The pharyngeal tubercle is a small protuberance in the midline, one-third of the way from the anterior margin of the foramen magnum to the posterior edge of the nasal septum. In front of the tubercle, the bone forms the roof of the nasopharynx and lies in the 'pharyngeal area' described in a following section. Behind it are attached the uppermost prevertebral muscles, with the longus capitis lying in front of the rectus capitis anterior. Separating the nasopharynx from the prevertebral region is the pharyngobasilar fascia with the prevertebral fascia just behind it.

Temporal bone

The temporal bone is made up of four parts which ossify separately and later fuse. The squamous part contributes the 'articular area' to the skull base, but most of it is in the temporal fossa on the side of the skull. The petromastoid part forms an important and complicated portion of the skull base lateral to the occipital bone. The tympanic plate, rolled like a tube open at the top, lies below the petrous and squamous parts, and just behind it the styloid process projects from the petrous bone.

The *squamous temporal bone* contains the hollow of the glenoid fossa, with, in front, the convex eminentia articularis joined laterally to the zygomatic process. This area lies almost wholly within the temporomandibular joint, with only a small triangular part anterior to the joint forming part of the infratemporal surface of the skull.

The *petromastoid bone* projects forwards and medially at 45°, wedged between the basiocciput and the greater wing of the sphenoid; at the apex of the wedge the three bones do not quite meet, leaving a gap termed the 'foramen lacerum' which is closed by dense fibrocartilage and transmits nothing other than a few minute vessels.

More laterally, along the junction between the petrous bone and the greater wing of the sphenoid, lies the cartilaginous portion of the eustachian tube, running posterolaterally into the bony part of the tube where it is overhung by the spine of the sphenoid. Just posterior to this is the carotid foramen, separated by a ridge of bone from the jugular foramen behind.

Lateral to the carotid and jugular foramina lies the *tympanic bone*. Laterally, it forms the bony part of the external auditory canal, articulating with the squamous bone of the glenoid fossa in front (squamotympanic fissure) and the mastoid bone behind (tympanomastoid fissure). Medially, it forms the floor of the hypotympanum. The medial part of the squamotympanic fissure becomes divided by a thin flange of petrous bone (the projecting margin of the tegmen tympani), so creating a petrosquamous fissure in front and a petrotympanic fissure behind.

Lateral to the jugular foramen, and tucked in close behind the tympanic bone, projects the *styloid process*, which is of very variable length. Behind its base lies the stylomastoid foramen, and further posteriorly the mastoid bone is indented by the digastric notch, medial to which there is a groove for the occipital artery.

Sphenoid bone

The greater wing of the sphenoid, with the medial and lateral pterygoid plates, contributes to the base of the skull.

The *greater wing* articulates with the squamous temporal bone to form the roof of the infratemporal fossa. Anteriorly, this infratemporal surface ends in the inferior orbital fissure behind the maxilla. Medially, the greater wing is edge-to-edge with the petrous bone, perforated by the foramen ovale anteriorly and the foramen spinosum posteriorly; in front, it ends in the pterygoid plates, and behind, in the spine of the sphenoid which is an important surgical landmark. Occasionally two smaller foramina exist as well: the foramen of Vesalius (medial to the foramen ovale) and the innominate foramen (posterior to the foramen ovale).

The *medial pterygoid plate* projects back from the lateral margin of the choanal opening, where it articulates with the vertical plate of the palatine bone. Inferiorly, it ends in the pterygoid hamulus, superiorly in the pterygoid tubercle which projects back into the foramen lacerum. Halfway up the posterior edge is a spur, from which a ridge runs upwards and laterally towards the opening of the bony eustachian tube, enclosing the concave scaphoid fossa lateral to the pterygoid tubercle.

The *lateral pterygoid plate* extends back and laterally into the infratemporal fossa. Its only purpose is to give attachment to the pterygoid muscles.

Occipital (muscular) area

The superior nuchal line is a rather faint ridge that runs from the mastoid process to the external occipital protuberance, in a curve concentric with the foramen magnum (*see Figure 15.1*). Halfway between the superior nuchal line and the foramen magnum, and concentric with them, is another ill-defined ridge, the inferior nuchal line. The external occipital crest separates the two sides of the occipital area, running from the foramen magnum to the external occipital protuberance. Each half is then bisected by a very vague line radiating outwards from the foramen magnum to the superior nuchal line.

Thus each half of the occipital region is subdivided into four areas. The two alongside the foramen magnum receive the recti. The medial area receives the rectus capitis posterior minor, which arises from the posterior arch of the atlas, is supplied by the posterior primary ramus of C1, and acts to extend the head. The lateral area receives the rectus capitis posterior major, which arises from the spinous process of the axis, is also supplied by C1, and acts to extend and rotate the head.

Between the superior and inferior nuchal lines, the medial area receives the semispinalis capitis, which arises from the transverse vertebral processes of C4–C7 and T1–T6, is supplied segmentally by posterior primary rami of the spinal nerves, and is the chief extensor of the head. The lateral area receives the superior oblique muscle, which arises from the lateral mass of the atlas, is supplied by C1, and acts primarily as a lateral flexor of the head; this muscle is covered laterally by the posterior parts of the insertions of splenius and sternomastoid into the superior nuchal line.

Pharyngeal area

Situated centrally in the skull base, this area forms the roof of the nasopharynx, and its boundaries are formed by the line of attachment of the pharyngeal wall. The pharyngeal constrictor muscles do not extend right up to the base of the skull but are attached to it by a rigid membrane, the pharyngobasilar fascia, and it is this which makes up the wall of the nasopharynx.

The *pharyngobasilar fascia* is attached to the skull base and medial pterygoid plates (that is to the back of the nose), and is thickened posteriorly into a pharyngeal ligament that continues inferiorly as the pharyngeal raphe. It is separated from the prevertebral muscles posteriorly by the prevertebral fascia. The origin of the pharyngobasilar fascia can be traced laterally from the pharyngeal tubercle across the basiocciput, to the petrous temporal bone just in front of the carotid foramen (*see Figure 15.1*). It then swings anteromedially, its attachment running along the cartilaginous eustachian tube to reach the sharp posterior edge of the medial pterygoid plate, to which it is attached all the way down to the hamulus. The lower edge of the pharyngobasilar fascia lies at the level of the hamuli and hard plate, within the superior constrictor muscle.

It will be seen that the apex of the petrous bone (and the foramen lacerum) lies within a lateral recess of the nasopharynx, the fossa of Rosenmüller. The levator palati muscle arises here and is, therefore, intrapharyngeal, covered medially by mucous membrane. A postnasal carcinoma involving the fossa of Rosenmüller may invade upwards through the foramen lacerum, sometimes producing a lateral rectus palsy by compressing the sixth nerve where it crosses the apex of the petrous bone and enters the cavernous sinus.

Tubal area

The tubal area lies just lateral to the pharyngeal area, and simply comprises the region occupied by the eustachian tube (*see Figure 15.1*). Anteriorly, it includes the scaphoid fossa at the base of the medial pterygoid plate, from where it runs posterolaterally along the slit that lies between the petrous bone and the greater wing of the sphenoid until the bony eustachian tube is reached just in front of the carotid canal.

The bony part of the *eustachian tube* is about 1 cm long, and tapers down from the anterior wall of the middle ear to its junction with the cartilaginous part of the tube. This junction, the isthmus, is the narrowest part of the tube and lies just medial to the spine of the sphenoid. The cartilaginous part of the eustachian tube (2 cm long), runs forwards and medially at 45° and downwards at 30°, to open into the nasopharynx by way of a trumpet-shaped orifice attached to the back of the medial pterygoid plate just above the pharyngobasilar fascia. The eustachian tube cartilage is an important landmark in base of the skull anatomy. Along its lateral aspect, a straight line passes from the lateral pterygoid plate along the medial lip of the foramen ovale to the foramen spinosum and into the petrotympanic fissure (Bosley and Martinez, 1986).

The *salpingopharyngeus* muscle arises from the posterior margin of the tubal orifice and runs vertically down inside the pharynx to be inserted into the posterior border of the thyroid cartilage and the adjacent pharyngeal wall. It is supplied by way of the pharyngeal plexus by the pharyngeal branch of the vagus, and its contraction assists in opening the tube.

The pharyngobasilar fascia is attached to the undersurface of the tube, and the two 'paratubal' muscles arise one on each side of it. The levator palati arises medially (within the pharynx) and the tensor palati arises laterally (outside the pharynx). Both muscles are partly attached to the tube, and so open it during the act of swallowing. The paratubal muscles are fully described in the section on the parapharyngeal space.

Neurovascular area

Posterior to the tubal area lies the neurovascular area, containing the structures of the carotid sheath and styloid apparatus, as well as the facial nerve (*see Figure 15.1*).

Carotid sheath

The carotid sheath itself is not a membranous fascia, but a dense feltwork of areolar tissue that surrounds the internal carotid artery and vagus nerve; it is virtually absent over the internal jugular vein, however, which is thus able to expand greatly during periods of increased blood flow. The carotid sheath is attached to the skull base around the carotid foramen, and continues downwards as far as the aortic arch.

In the neck, the carotid sheath, together with

the pretracheal fascia, is firmly attached anteriorly to the deep surface of sternomastoid. Posteriorly, it is not attached to the prevertebral fascia, but is free to slide over it. This means that pus tracking laterally from a parapharyngeal abscess passes behind the sheath and behind the sternomastoid, to point in the posterior triangle.

The *internal carotid artery* passes vertically upwards from the carotid bifurcation in the neck to enter the carotid foramen (*Plate 2*). It has no branches, but carries with it the carotid plexus of sympathetic nerves from the superior cervical ganglion.

The jugular foramen is divided by two transverse septa of fibrous dura (which may ossify) into three compartments. The anterior compartment is occupied by the ninth cranial nerve and the inferior petrosal sinus; the middle compartment is shared by the tenth and eleventh nerves; and the posterior compartment is filled by the emerging internal jugular vein. The ninth and eleventh nerves lie more laterally than the tenth in the foramen.

The *internal jugular vein* descends from the jugular bulb to lie behind the internal carotid artery on the lateral mass of the atlas (*Plate 3*); just below the base of the skull, it receives the inferior petrosal sinus. As it descends, it passes across on to the lateral side of the internal carotid artery, receiving tributaries from the pharyngeal plexus of veins, and crossed on its lateral side by the accessory nerve. Also on the lateral side of the vein lie the deep cervical lymph nodes.

The *glossopharyngeal nerve* (IX) lies lateral to the inferior petrosal sinus as it emerges from the anterior part of the jugular foramen (*Plates 4 and 5*). The nerve passes down on the lateral surface of the internal carotid artery and then gently curves forward around the lateral side of stylopharyngeus, medial to the external carotid artery towards the tongue.

The *vagus nerve* (X) emerges from its superior ganglion in the middle compartment of the jugular foramen and runs straight down in the back of the carotid sheath between the carotid artery and jugular vein (*Plates 4 and 5*). Just below the skull base, it is dilated into its inferior ganglion, where it receives a connection from the accessory nerve carrying fibres from the nucleus ambiguus.

The *accessory nerve* (XI) is just lateral to the vagus in the middle compartment of the jugular foramen (*Plates 4 and 5*). It immediately begins to curve away posteriorly across the lateral surface of the internal jugular vein, medial to the styloid process and posterior belly of the digastric, giving a branch to the sternomastoid before piercing the muscle to gain the posterior triangle.

The *hypoglossal nerve* (XII) emerges from the anterior condylar foramen, medial to the carotid sheath, and spirals in a lateral direction behind the vagus between the internal jugular vein and internal carotid artery (that is through the carotid sheath) (*Plates 4 and 5*). It then swings forward lateral to the carotid arteries, deep to the styloid muscles and digastric, on its way to the tongue.

The *cervical sympathetic trunk* lies behind the carotid sheath in front of the prevertebral fascia, just medial to the vagus nerve. It ends superiorly at the superior cervical ganglion.

Styloid apparatus

From the tip of the styloid process, the stylohyoid ligament passes downwards and forwards to the lesser cornu of the hyoid bone. All these structures are derived from the second branchial arch cartilage. The stylomandibular ligament is not a distinct structure, but merely a condensation of the deep layer of the parotid fascia between the base of the styloid process and the angle of the mandible almost directly below it.

Three muscles diverge from the styloid process: the stylopharyngeus, the stylohyoid and the styloglossus (*Plate 6*). All three have a different nerve supply, but all three participate in the mechanism of swallowing.

The *stylopharyngeus* arises from the deep aspect of the base of the styloid process, slopes down across the lateral aspect of the internal carotid artery, and is inserted into the thyroid cartilage and side wall of the pharynx. It is supplied by the ninth nerve, and elevates the larynx and the pharynx.

The *stylohyoid* arises from the back of the base of the styloid process, and slopes downwards and forwards to be inserted by two slips (which pass on either side of the intermediate tendon of the digastric) into the base of the greater cornu of the hyoid. It passes lateral to the external carotid artery. It is supplied by the seventh nerve, and elevates and retracts the hyoid.

The *styloglossus* arises from the front of the styloid process and upper part of the stylohyoid ligament. It crosses lateral to the internal carotid artery and then swings forward medial to the lingual nerve to reach its insertion into the side of the tongue. It is supplied by the twelfth nerve, and retracts the tongue.

The external carotid artery is closely adjacent to the muscles of the styloid apparatus. It runs up deep to the stylohyoid (and the digastric), but lies superficial to stylopharyngeus and styloglossus, on its way to enter the parotid gland. The retromandibular vein, on the other hand, runs down superficially to all elements of the styloid apparatus.

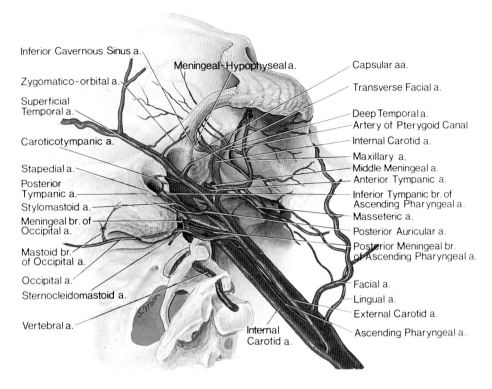

Plate 2 The arteries of the central skull base.
(From Goldenberg, 1984, with permission of the author and publishers, *The Laryngoscope*)

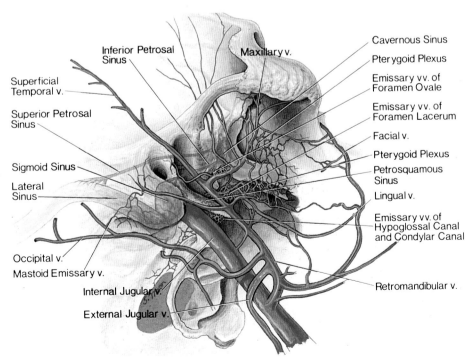

Plate 3 The veins of the central skull base.
(From Goldenberg, 1984, with permission of the author and publishers, *The Laryngoscope*)

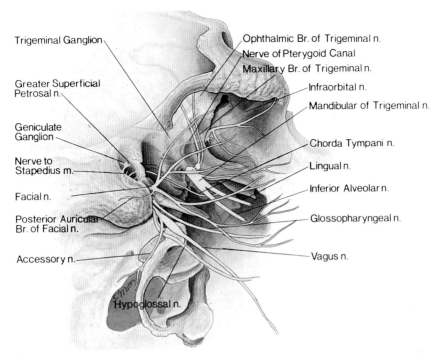

Plate 4 The nerves of the central skull base.
(From Goldenberg, 1984, with permission of the author and publishers, *The Laryngoscope*)

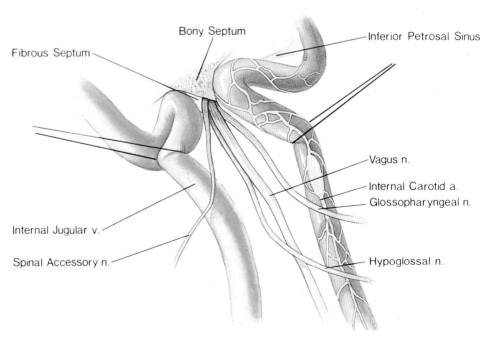

Plate 5 The structures in the jugular foramen.
(From Goldenberg, 1984, with permission of the author and publishers, *The Laryngoscope*)

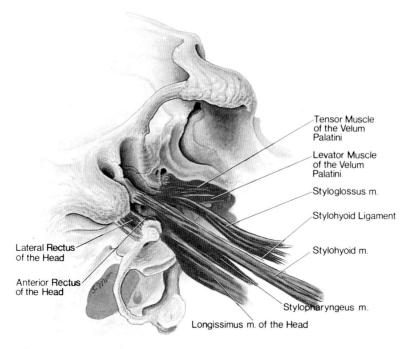

Tensor Muscle
of the Velum
Palatini

Levator Muscle
of the Velum
Palatini

Styloglossus m.

Stylohyoid Ligament

Stylohyoid m.

Lateral Rectus
of the Head

Anterior Rectus
of the Head

Stylopharyngeus m.

Longissimus m. of the Head

Plate 6 The deep muscles of the central skull base.
(From Goldenberg, 1984, with permission of the author and publishers, *The Laryngoscope*)

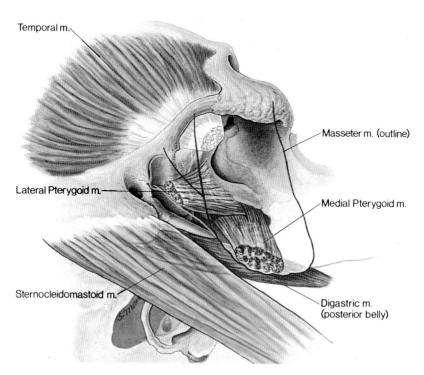

Temporal m.

Masseter m. (outline)

Lateral Pterygoid m.

Medial Pterygoid m.

Sternocleidomastoid m.

Digastric m.
(posterior belly)

Plate 7 The superficial muscles of the central skull base.
(From Goldenberg, 1984, with permission of the author and publishers, *The Laryngoscope*)

Facial nerve (VII)

The stylomastoid foramen transmits the facial nerve and the stylomastoid artery. As soon as it emerges from the foramen, the facial nerve gives off the posterior auricular nerve (supplying the occipital belly of occipitofrontalis) and a muscular branch (supplying posterior belly of digastric and stylohyoid). It then swings forward into the parotid gland, dividing as it does so into upper and lower divisions which then redivide to form the plexus of the pes anserinus within the substance of the gland.

Auditory area

This small area anterolateral to the neurovascular area comprises the steeply sloping face of the tympanic bone, forming as it does the floor and anterior wall of the external auditory canal and middle ear.

At the anteromedial edge of the area lies the petrotympanic fissure of Glaser (already described in the section on the osteology of the temporal bone). This transmits the chorda tympani and anterior tympanic branch of the maxillary artery, and the corresponding veins which drain into the pterygoid plexus.

The *chorda tympani* emerges from the petrotympanic fissure and indents the spine of the sphenoid before joining the lingual nerve 2 cm below the skull base.

Articular area

This area, immediately in front of the auditory area, is the surface on which the head of the mandible articulates (by way of an intervening fibrocartilaginous disc). It is bordered by the attachment of the joint capsule, anteriorly just in front of the eminentia articularis, posteriorly to the squamotympanic fissure, and medially and laterally to the margins of the mandibular fossa.

Infratemporal fossa

The infratemporal fossa lies below the middle cranial fossa, between the ramus of the mandible and the lateral wall of the pharynx (*Figures 15.2, 15.3 and 15.4*).

Its roof is the infratemporal area of the skull base, which is made up by the greater wing of the sphenoid with a small triangular contribution posteriorly from the squamous temporal bone. It has no anatomical floor and continues down into the neck. Anteriorly lies the posterior wall of the maxilla with the pterygomaxillary and inferior orbital fissures; posteriorly, it is bounded by the carotid sheath and styloid apparatus. The fossa is limited medially by the medial pterygoid muscle and interpterygoid fascia, and laterally by the mandible.

The contents of the fossa are the lateral and medial pterygoid muscles, the maxillary artery and its branches, the pterygoid venous plexus and maxillary veins, and the branches of the mandibular nerve.

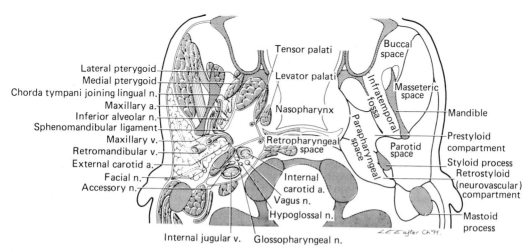

Figure 15.2 Central part of a horizontal section of the head passing through the foramen magnum, between the eustachian tube and the palate. In the left half all relevant structures have been drawn; on the right the different compartments are indicated as they appear at this level. (From van Huijzen, 1984, with permission of the publishers, S. Karger)

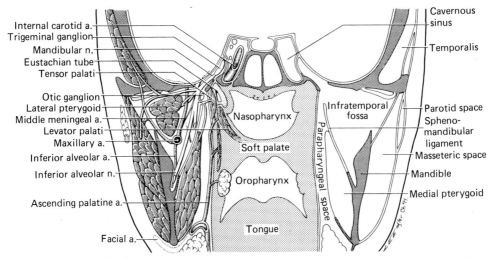

Figure 15.3 Coronal section of the head passing through the foramen ovale. On the left all relevant structures are illustrated; on the right the main compartments are shown. (From van Huijzen, 1984, with permission of the publishers, S. Karger)

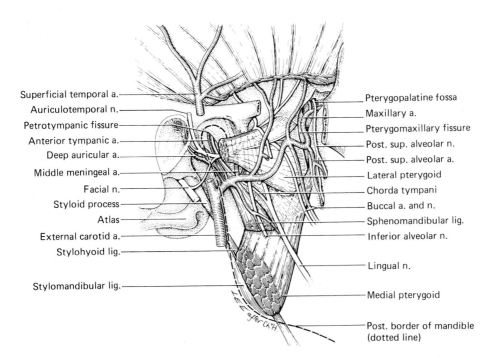

Figure 15.4 The structures of the infratemporal fossa, viewed from laterally. The veins have been omitted in order to permit a better view of the other structures. Part of the zygomatic arch has been removed. The posterior border of the mandible is indicated and the plane of attachment of both pterygoid muscles to the mandible can be seen. (From van Huijzen, 1984, with permission of the publishers, S. Karger)

Lateral pterygoid muscle

This muscle arises from two heads: the upper head from the whole infratemporal surface of the skull, and the lower head from the outer surface of the lateral pterygoid plate. The heads converge posteriorly into a tendon which is inserted into the pterygoid pit at the medial end of the mandibular condyle (*Plate 7*). It is supplied by the fifth nerve (mandibular division), and acts in opening the mouth by pulling the condyle forwards onto the eminentia articularis.

Medial pterygoid muscle

The medial pterygoid arises from the medial surface of the lateral pterygoid plate and the fossa between the two plates; a small slip joins from the tuberosity of the maxilla and tubercle of the palatine bone. It passes outwards, down and back at 45° to its insertion into the angle of the mandible (*Plate 7*). It is supplied by the fifth nerve (mandibular division), and acts to close the mouth and move the mandible towards the opposite side in chewing.

Maxillary artery

The external carotid artery has two terminal branches, the superficial temporal and the maxillary (*see Plate 2*). The maxillary artery enters the infratemporal fossa between the sphenomandibular ligament and the neck of the mandible, and passes forward either lateral or medial to the lateral pterygoid muscle. If it takes the medial course, the artery then turns laterally again to emerge between the two heads of the muscle. It leaves the infratemporal fossa through the pterygomaxillary fissure to enter the pterygopalatine fossa.

The artery is traditionally described in three parts: before, on and beyond the lateral pterygoid muscle, with five branches coming from each part. From the first and third parts, the five branches all enter foramina in bones; from the second part, none of the branches go through bony foramina (Last, 1973).

The *first part* gives off the inferior alveolar, middle meningeal, accessory meningeal, deep auricular and anterior tympanic arteries. The inferior alveolar artery passes down to join the inferior alveolar nerve and enter the mandibular foramen. The middle meningeal artery passes straight up through the foramen spinosum, while the accessory meningeal artery goes through the foramen ovale. The deep auricular artery passes up to supply the external auditory canal, and the anterior tympanic artery enters the petrotympanic fissure on its way to the middle ear (Davies, 1967).

The *second part* of the maxillary artery gives off five branches to the soft tissues: the lateral and medial pterygoid muscles, the temporalis muscle, the lingual and long buccal nerves.

The *third part* of the artery divides into the pterygopalatine fossa and will not be described further here.

The pterygoid plexus and maxillary veins

The pterygoid plexus of veins lies within and on the lateral surface of the lateral pterygoid muscle, and receives tributaries corresponding to the branches of the maxillary artery. The plexus drains into two short, large maxillary veins which pass horizontally backwards deep to the neck of the mandible to join the superficial temporal vein and form the retromandibular vein (*see Plate 3*).

The pterygoid plexus has three important communicating veins. The inferior ophthalmic veins pass to it through the inferior orbital fissure; a connecting vein passes vertically down from the cavernous sinus by way of the foramen ovale or, when present, the foramen of Vesalius; and the deep facial vein runs forward beneath the zygoma to join the anterior facial vein. These connections can allow infection from the face to spread by way of the pterygoid plexus to produce a cavernous sinus thrombosis.

The mandibular nerve

The mandibular nerve drops down through the foramen ovale and, after a short course just deep to the upper head of the lateral pterygoid muscle, the main trunk divides into anterior and posterior divisions (*see Plate 4*). Before it does so, the *main trunk* gives off the sensory nervus spinosus (which re-enters the middle fossa through the foramen spinosum), and the motor nerve to the medial pterygoid, which also supplies the tensor palati and tensor tympani.

The *anterior division* is motor except for the long buccal nerve. The latter passes between the heads of the lateral pterygoid to swing forwards and downwards on the deep surface of the temporalis muscle, and then pierces the buccinator to supply the mucous membrane of the cheek. The motor branches supply the temporalis, masseter (by a branch which emerges through the mandibular notch) and the lateral pterygoid.

The *posterior division* is sensory except for the mylohyoid nerve. The auriculotemporal nerve springs from two roots which pass either side of the middle meningeal artery, and passes backwards between the sphenomandibular ligament and neck of the mandible. The inferior alveolar nerve swings downwards on the surface of the medial pterygoid muscle, passes between the sphenomandibular ligament and neck of the mandible, and gives off the mylohoid nerve before entering the mandibular foramen. The lingual nerve is joined by the chorda tympani 2 cm below the base of the skull and passes downwards and forwards on the medial pterygoid, grooving the mandible before entering the mouth.

The *otic ganglion* lies close to the mandibular nerve just below the foramen ovale, between the nerve and the tensor palati muscle. It relays secretomotor fibres for the parotid gland, which it receives by way of the lesser superficial petrosal nerve and transmits to the auriculotemporal nerve. The lesser superficial petrosal nerve leaves the middle fossa through the foramen ovale, or sometimes through its own foramen, the foramen innominatum.

The sphenomandibular ligament

The sphenomandibular ligament is a fibrous band joining the spine of the sphenoid to the lingula of the mandibular foramen. It is derived from the first branchial arch (Meckel's) cartilage. Anterior-ly, it blends into the interpterygoid fascia, which separates the lateral and medial pterygoid muscles, stretching forward as a sheet to be attached to the posterior edge of the lateral pterygoid plate.

Parotid space

The space enclosed within the capsule of the parotid gland lies partly superficial to the mandible, and extends through the retromandibular space behind the infratemporal fossa to abut against the parapharyngeal space (*Figure 15.5* and *see Figure 15.2*). The parotid space is described in Chapter 9.

Parapharyngeal space
Prestyloid compartment

This compartment contains the two palati muscles, and two arteries, the ascending palatine and ascending pharyngeal (*Figure 15.6* and *see Figures 15.2* and *15.3*).

The *tensor palati muscle* arises from the skull base in a line from the scaphoid fossa along the edge of the greater wing to the spine of the sphenoid, and is also attached to the lateral side of the eustachian tube. It tapers down to a tendon which takes a

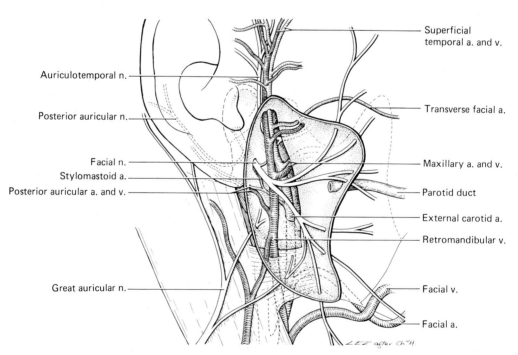

Figure 15.5 The structures of the parotid space viewed from the lateral side. The parotid gland has been removed from its capsule, leaving the vessels and nerves intact. (From van Huijzen, 1984, with permission of the publishers, S. Karger)

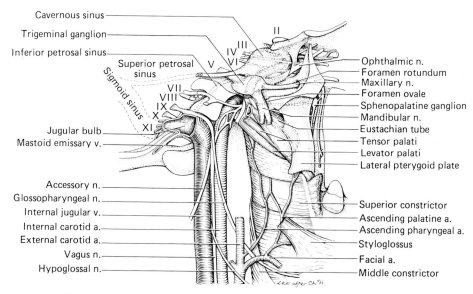

Cavernous sinus
Trigeminal ganglion
Inferior petrosal sinus
Superior petrosal sinus
Sigmoid sinus
Jugular bulb
Mastoid emissary v.
Accessory n.
Glossopharyngeal n.
Internal jugular v.
Internal carotid a.
External carotid a.
Vagus n.
Hypoglossal n.

II
III
IV
VI
V
VII
VIII
IX
X
XI

Ophthalmic n.
Foramen rotundum
Maxillary n.
Foramen ovale
Sphenopalatine ganglion
Mandibular n.
Eustachian tube
Tensor palati
Levator palati
Lateral pterygoid plate
Superior constrictor
Ascending palatine a.
Ascending pharyngeal a.
Styloglossus
Facial a.
Middle constrictor

Figure 15.6 The structures of the pharyngeal space and of the skull base above it, seen from laterally in a sagittal section passing through the foramen ovale. (From van Huijzen, 1984, with permission of the publishers, S. Karger)

right-angled turn around the hamulus to enter the pharynx, where it broadens into a flat aponeurosis; this triangular sheet blends with its counterpart on the opposite side and is attached to the posterior edge of the hard palate (the crest of the palatine bone). It is supplied by the fifth nerve by way of the nerve to the medial pterygoid. The action of this muscle is to tense the palate so that other muscles can raise and lower it.

The *levator palati muscle* arises from the petrous apex anterolateral to the carotid foramen and from the medial end of the tubal cartilage, and is inserted into the upper surface of the palatal aponeurosis. Supplied by the tenth nerve by way of the pharyngeal plexus, it acts to raise the soft palate and close off the nasopharynx.

The *ascending palatine artery*, a branch of the facial artery, ascends close to the pharyngeal wall to supply the soft palate and tonsil.

The *ascending pharyngeal artery*, a branch of the external carotid artery, ascends a little more posteriorly along the superior constrictor to supply the pharynx, the middle ear and the meninges. Often it is a major feeding vessel to a glomus tumour.

Retrostyloid compartment

This corresponds to the neurovascular space, and contains the carotid sheath (*see* previous section).

Structures within the skull base

The *internal carotid artery* curves forwards in the petrous bone from the carotid foramen, and then curves upwards into the upper part of the foramen lacerum in the middle fossa, emerging at the apex of the petrous bone and immediately entering the cavernous sinus. It lies in front of the cochlea and middle ear cavity, separated from the middle ear and eustachian tube by a thin plate of bone which may be dehiscent. It gives off some small intrapetrous branches, including the caroticotympanic artery, which may enlarge as feeding vessels for a glomus tumour.

The *jugular bulb* is the point at which the sigmoid sinus feeds into the upper end of the internal jugular vein. It usually lies below the posterior part of the floor of the middle ear, although its bony covering may be dehiscent, with only mucosa separating it from the middle ear cavity. However, its position is extremely variable and it may intrude right up into the middle ear ('high jugular bulb') (Graham, 1977). The inferior petrosal sinus joints the jugular bulb at the skull base; it emerges from the skull in the anterior part of the jugular foramen and crosses either lateral or medial to the ninth, tenth and eleventh nerves to enter the bulb. It is variable and may consist of three or more channels (Goldenberg, 1984).

The internal carotid artery diverges from the jugular bulb beneath the middle ear, leaving a wedge of bone between the two vessels (*see Plate 5*) which is clearly shown on lateral hypocycloidal polytomography. Erosion of this 'keel' of bone is an early finding in patients with a glomus jugulare tumour.

The paths of the ninth, tenth and eleventh *cranial nerves* in the jugular foramen, and of the twelfth nerve at this level, have already been described (*see* subsection on the carotid sheath).

The greater superficial petrosal nerve enters the foramen lacerum from the middle fossa and is joined there by the deep petrosal nerve, which is a branch of the sympathetic carotid plexus. The two nerves unite to form the nerve of the pterygoid canal (vidian nerve) which leaves the foramen lacerum in the pterygoid canal and runs forward to the pterygopalatine ganglion.

The tympanic branch of the ninth nerve (Jacobson's nerve) leaves the glossopharyngeal nerve at the petrous ganglion and passes through a canaliculus in the keel of petrous bone between the jugular and carotid foramina to supply the middle ear (tympanic plexus).

The auricular branch of the tenth nerve (Arnold's nerve) passes behind the internal jugular vein and enters the mastoid canaliculus on the lateral wall of the jugular foramen, from which it emerges by way of the tympanomastoid fissure to supply the skin of part of the external auditory meatus.

The anatomy of the ear within the petrous temporal bone is described in Chapter 1.

Muscles superficial to the lateral skull base

Four muscles lying laterally, superficial to the base of the skull, are important in achieving surgical exposure of the area, and are, therefore, briefly described in the following (*see Plate 7*).

The *masseter muscle* arises from the zygomatic arch and is inserted into a wide area on the lateral aspect of the mandible from the angle forwards along the lower border, and upwards over the lower part of the ascending ramus. It is supplied by the fifth nerve by way of the masseteric branch from the anterior division of the mandibular nerve, and its action is to close the jaws.

The *temporalis muscle* arises from the temporal fossa on the side of the skull, and from this large origin it converges in the shape of a fan to be inserted into the coronoid process of the mandible, mainly on its inner surface. It is supplied by the fifth nerve by way of the deep temporal branches of the anterior division of the mandibular nerve. It acts to close the jaws, and its posterior fibres also retract the mandible.

The *sternomastoid muscle* arises from two heads: from the manubrium and clavicle. It is inserted into a curved line extending from the tip of the mastoid process to the superior nuchal line of the occiput. It is supplied by the eleventh nerve and its main action is to protract the head (moving it forwards while keeping it vertical with a horizontal gaze).

The *digastric muscle* arises from the digastric notch on the medial surface of the mastoid process. This posterior belly narrows into an intermediate tendon which passes through a fibrous sling on the hyoid near the lesser cornu, and then expands into the anterior belly which runs beneath the mylohyoid to its insertion into the digastric fossa on the lower edge of the mandible. The posterior belly is supplied by the seventh nerve (nerve to digastric) and the anterior belly by the fifth nerve (mylohoid nerve). Its action is to depress and retract the chin.

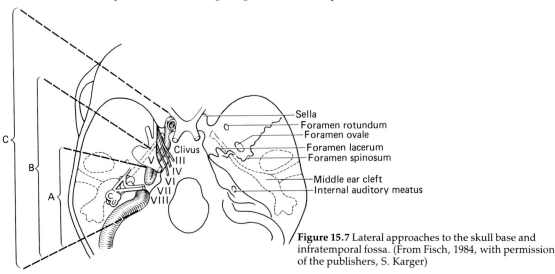

Figure 15.7 Lateral approaches to the skull base and infratemporal fossa. (From Fisch, 1984, with permission of the publishers, S. Karger)

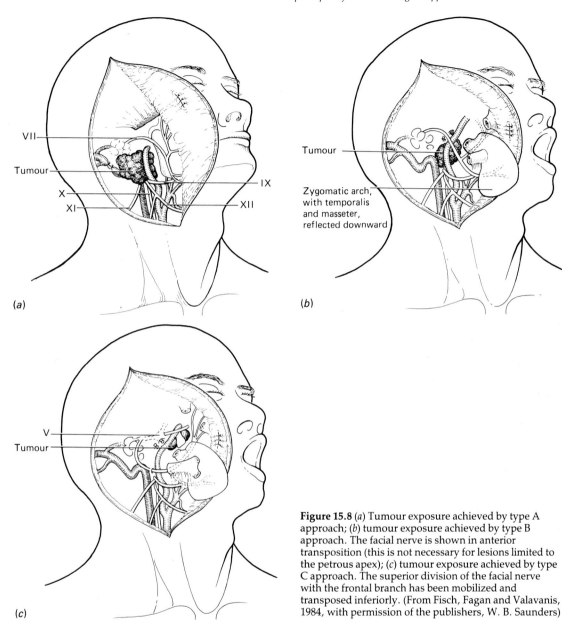

Figure 15.8 (*a*) Tumour exposure achieved by type A approach; (*b*) tumour exposure achieved by type B approach. The facial nerve is shown in anterior transposition (this is not necessary for lesions limited to the petrous apex); (*c*) tumour exposure achieved by type C approach. The superior division of the facial nerve with the frontal branch has been mobilized and transposed inferiorly. (From Fisch, Fagan and Valavanis, 1984, with permission of the publishers, W. B. Saunders)

Anatomical principles of the lateral surgical approach to the skull base

Several different surgical approaches have been employed in order to reach lesions in the rather inaccessible region of the skull base (Sasaki, McCabe and Kirchner, 1984). However, it is the lateral approach that has recently become established as the approach of choice for most surgeons who work in this area (Goldenberg, 1984).

The main difficulty in creating adequate expo-sure has been the long, tortuous course of the facial nerve, which prevents direct access. Howev-er, the technique of anterior transposition of the nerve demonstrated by Fisch (1977) has provided the access necessary for control of the internal carotid artery and internal jugular vein, and so has permitted satisfactory exploration of the skull base from the lateral approach. Fisch has developed three variants of this lateral approach, which he loosely terms the 'infratemporal fossa approach' (Fisch, 1984) (*Figures 15.7* and *15.8*).

The type A approach provides access to the temporal bone right up to the petrous apex. The type B involves a more anterior approach which allows dissection to proceed across the petrous apex to the basiocciput and clivus. The type C approach takes the exposure even further forward, allowing the surgeon to remove lesions in the nasopharynx and parasellar region.

Type A approach

This technique is employed primarily for the removal of glomus jugulare tumours, and involves the now classic manoeuvre of anterior facial nerve transposition.

A long postaural incision is extended down into the neck, and if necessary up into the temporal region (*Figure 15.9*). The dissection begins in the

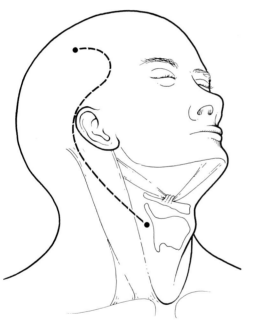

Figure 15.9 Skin incision for type A approach. (From Fisch, 1984, with permission of the publishers, S. Karger)

neck with identification of the great auricular nerve where it lies on the surface of the sternomastoid; it is preserved for later use as a facial nerve graft, if needed. The accessory nerve is identified where it emerges from the posterior border of the sternomastoid, and the carotid sheath is then exposed. Control tapes are passed round the external and internal carotid arteries, and the ascending pharyngeal and occipital arteries are identified; the latter are usually major

feeding vessels for the tumour and may, therefore, need ligation.

The internal jugular vein is ligated and divided at the level of the carotid bifurcation, elevated and dissected up towards the jugular foramen.

The hypoglossal nerve is identified as it crosses lateral to the external carotid artery. The sternomastoid is divided at its insertion into the mastoid tip, preserving and tracing out the accessory nerve as the muscle is turned down. The internal jugular vein can then be dissected right up to the skull base, where cranial nerves IX, X, XI and XII are identified at the jugular foramen, and the internal carotid artery is exposed as it enters the carotid canal.

The intratemporal part of the operation can now commence, as a widely bevelled cortical mastoidectomy with transection of the cartilaginous external auditory canal, which is closed by suture as a blind-ending sac. The vertical portion of the facial nerve is identified, and the posterior bony canal wall is taken down with removal of the mastoid tip. The tympanic membrane, malleus and incus are removed, and the tympanic bone in the anterior hypotympanum is drilled away to expose the lateral aspect of the jugular bulb. The facial nerve is mobilized from the geniculate ganglion to its division in the parotid, and is then transposed anteriorly into a new fallopian canal created in the anterior attic (*Figure 15.10*). The sigmoid sinus can then be exposed with the drill from the sinodural angle downwards and anteriorly to the jugular bulb; the sinus is then either packed or ligated superiorly.

The next step is obliteration of the eustachian tube at the isthmus. In the case of a large tumour extending forwards into the carotid canal, the internal carotid artery must next be identified at the medial wall of the protympanum, and its intratemporal portion exposed by further removal of tympanic bone. Fisch then breaks off the styloid process and introduces a special infratemporal fossa retractor to displace the ascending ramus of the mandible forward, and permit separation of the anterior pole of the tumour from the internal carotid artery. The caroticotympanic artery usually feeds the tumour and requires coagulation.

The superior and posterior tumour poles are then separated from the otic capsule and posterior fossa dura. Separation from posterior fossa dura is achieved by opening the ligated sigmoid sinus and following its lumen down to the tumour.

Finally, the inferior pole of the tumour is approached at the jugular foramen and separated from cranial nerves IX, X, XI and XII. The whole jugular bulb can then be removed together with the tumour. There is brisk haemorrhage from the inferior petrosal sinus, which is packed and obliterated.

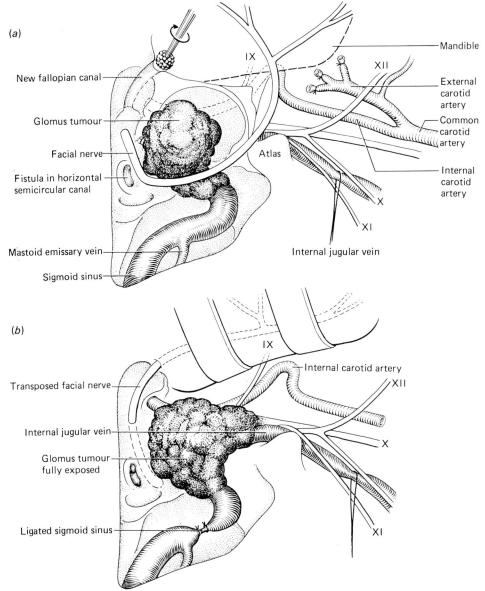

(a)

New fallopian canal

Glomus tumour

Facial nerve

Fistula in horizontal
semicircular canal

Mastoid emissary vein

Sigmoid sinus

IX

XII

Atlas

Mandible

External
carotid
artery

Common
carotid
artery

Internal
carotid
artery

X

XI

Internal jugular vein

(b)

Transposed facial nerve

Internal jugular vein

Glomus tumour
fully exposed

Ligated sigmoid sinus

IX

Internal carotid artery

XII

X

XI

Figure 15.10 (*a*) Exposure of glomus jugulare tumour by type A approach; (*b*) exposure of glomus jugulare tumour by type A approach, after transposition of the facial nerve and ligation of the sigmoid sinus. (From Fisch, 1984, with permission of the publishers, S. Karger)

Large glomus jugulare tumours with intradural extension demand a neurosurgical approach to remove the intradural portion of the lesion once the extradural part has been excised.

Type B approach

For exposure of the clivus to remove a chordoma or petrous apex cholesteatoma, the type A approach is extended forward into the infratemporal fossa. Anterior facial nerve transposition may not be necessary, but its frontal branch must be dissected free from the parotid as far forward as the lateral rim of the orbit, permitting it to be displaced inferiorly.

The zygomatic arch is divided at each end. The temporalis muscle is then raised off the squamous temporal bone and reflected downwards together with the zygomatic arch and attached masseter.

The bone of the glenoid fossa is drilled away to expose the temporomandibular joint, and this allows the mandibular condyle to be displaced inferiorly using the Fisch infratemporal fossa retractor. Some surgeons prefer to divide the ascending ramus of the mandible in order further to improve access.

The horizontal segment of the intratemporal portion of the internal carotid artery is exposed by drilling away the tympanic bone lateral and anterior to it. The cartilaginous eustachian tube is detached, and drilling may then proceed through the petrous apex to the foramen lacerum.

The middle meningeal artery is identified, coagulated and divided where it enters the foramen spinosum just anteromedial to the spine of the sphenoid. The mandibular nerve is identified next as it exits through the foramen ovale; this is readily done by following the posterior edge of the lateral pterygoid plate up to the skull base, where it leads directly to the foramen.

For extensive lesions of the basiocciput, it may be necessary to section the mandibular nerve and drill away the pterygoid tubercle. The tensor palati and cartilaginous eustachian tube are displaced inferiorly to complete the exposure.

Type C approach

This approach can be employed for very anteriorly placed lesions in the nasopharyngeal, parasellar, retromaxillary and paratubal regions. A subtotal petrosectomy is carried out as for the type A and type B approaches, but anterior transposition of the facial nerve is not required.

The surgery is completed as for a type B approach, and then continues with detachment of the upper head of the lateral pterygoid to expose the lateral pterygoid plate. Both pterygoid plates are removed and the maxillary nerve is sectioned at the foramen rotundum. The internal carotid artery can then be followed upwards as far as the cavernous sinus. Next, the pterygopalatine fossa is entered and, after division of the vidian nerve, the maxillary sinus, nasopharynx and sphenoid sinus may be exposed.

References

BOSLEY, J. H. and MARTINEZ, D. McN. (1986) Practical surgical anatomy of the skull base. *Ear, Nose and Throat Journal*, **65**, 52–56

DAVIES, D. V. (ed.) (1967) *Gray's Anatomy*, 34th edn. London: Longmans

FISCH, U. (1977) Infratemporal fossa approach for extensive tumors of the temporal bone and base of the skull. In *Neurological Surgery of the Ear*, edited by H. Silverstein and N. Norrell, pp. 34–53. Birmingham: Aesculapius

FISCH, U. (1984) Infratemporal fossa approach for lesions in the temporal bone and base of the skull. *Advances in Oto-Rhino-Laryngology*, **34**, 254–266

FISCH, U., FAGAN, P. and VALAVANIS, A. (1984) The infratemporal fossa approach for the lateral skull base. *Otolaryngologic Clinics of North America*, **17**, 513–552

GOLDENBERG, R. A. (1984) Surgeon's view of the skull base from the lateral approach. *The Laryngoscope*, **94** (Suppl. 36), 1–21

GRAHAM, M. D. (1977) The jugular bulb: its anatomic and clinical considerations in contemporary otology. *The Laryngoscope*, **87**, 105–125

LAST, R. J. (1973) *Anatomy, Regional and Applied*, 5th edn. London: Churchill Livingstone

SASAKI, C. T., McCABE, B. F. and KIRCHNER, J. A. (1984) (eds) *Surgery of the Skull Base*. Philadelphia: Lippincott

VAN HUIJZEN, C. (1984) Anatomy of the skull base and the infratemporal fossa. *Advances in Oto-Rhino-Laryngology*, **34**, 242–253

16

Neuroanatomy and applied neurophysiology for the otolaryngologist

John Philip Patten

Although this chapter is included in the basic sciences volume, the applied aspect is of such importance in differential diagnosis of diseases affecting neuro-otolaryngological function that some licence has been taken to indicate, whenever possible, the signficance of both anatomy and physiology in disease states and differential diagnosis.

In some instances, gross anatomy is of great importance and in others, complex central connections require detailed elaboration to illustrate and explain clinical disorders. The following account is always biased in the direction of practical applications, and information of limited or dubious clinical importance has been excluded.

The cranial nerves fall into three major groups on the basis of both functional and gross anatomical similarities, and they share common anatomical relationships and pathology. Differing patterns of involvement within these groups allow very accurate differential diagnoses to be advanced, based on both the sequencing and ultimate extent of damage in these groups. The advent of computer-assisted tomography, which until recently was available only in slice format, has added a remarkable dimension to our ability to confirm or refute a clinically based diagnosis in this hitherto investigational no man's land. The recent ability to reconstruct slice scans in both sagittal and coronal planes has further transformed diagnostic accuracy. Interpretation still requires a very good grasp of gross anatomical relationships of the intracranial and extracranial courses of the cranial nerves, and these features will form the bulk of this chapter. The groupings are:

(1) cranial nerves I, II, III, IV and VI and the final distribution of the cervical sympathetic nerve

(2) cranial nerves V, VII and VIII
(3) cranial nerves IX, X, XI and XII and the cervical components of the sympathetic chain.

The influences of cerebellar, pyramidal, extrapyramidal and corticobulbar dysfunction on these nerves, and peripheral evidences of disordered brainstem function, will be detailed at the end of the chapter, or where appropriate.

Group one

In the first group, the close relationship between the olfactory and optic nerves and the varying relationships between the three nerves supplying the extraocular muscles are considered. The relationships of the first division of the fifth nerve, which traverses the orbit, to these structures, must also be noted, although the detailed anatomy of this nerve is dealt with in group two.

The olfactory nerve (I)

Anatomy (*Figure 16.1*)

The olfactory epithelium lies in the olfactory cleft which occupies the upper 10 mm of the nasal septum, the roof of the nasal cavity and down the lateral wall towards the origin of the superior concha. In man its total surface area is some 5 cm^2 and it is a yellowish colour. In other species, increasing pigmentation is associated with increased sensitivity to odours. The mucosa is bathed in a lipid-rich secretion from the epithelial Bowman's glands, indicating that lipid solubility may be a critical factor in odour detection. The olfactory receptor cells lie on the basal epithelium and extend vertically to the surface, from which

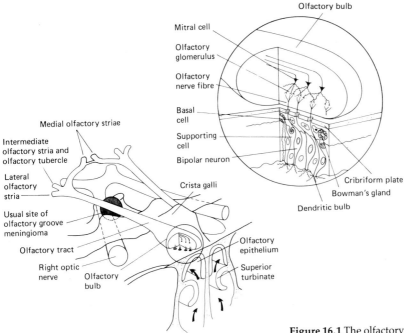

Figure 16.1 The olfactory pathways

the terminal enlargement protrudes and gives rise to 8–20 olfactory cilia. Although these have the 9+2 fibril arrangement of mobile cilia in other areas, they are thought to be non-motile and form a dense mat of fibrils lying on the surface of the epithelium. Pinocytic vacuoles have been demonstrated in the terminal enlargement of the receptor cells, but their functional significance is uncertain (Fitzgerald, 1985).

The receptor cells are derived from ectoderm and are unique in being replaced from stem cells every 30 days. They also enter the central nervous system (CNS) as non-myelinated axons without synapsing. These axons become grouped and ensheathed by Schwann cells forming some 20 fasciculi which, invested by pia and arachnoid mater, pass through the orifices of the cribriform plate to enter the olfactory bulbs, lying each side of the crista galli in the floor of the anterior cranial fossa. These axons synapse with dendrites of the large mitral cells in the olfactory glomeruli and each glomerulus receives axons from a wide area of the epithelium – there appears to be no functional grouping of axons. This allows a relatively small number of receptor cells to distinguish a large number of different odours. The axons of the mitral cells form the bulk of the olfactory tract, but centrifugal axons of uncertain origin pass to the olfactory bulb and undoubtedly modify activity in the olfactory glomeruli, perhaps by both inhibitory and facilitatory action.

The olfactory tracts pass posteriorly and slightly

laterally crossing the floor of the anterior cranial fossa and the optic nerves; and immediately above the optic chiasm, just in front of the anterior perforated substance, each divides into medial, intermediate and lateral olfactory striae.

The termination of the medial striae is uncertain. Many fibres decussate to the opposite medial striae and these may become the centrifugal fibres of the opposite olfactory tract, having both facilitatory and inhibitory effects on the opposite olfactory bulb. The intermediate striae terminate in the olfactory tubercle, but the latter's further functional anatomy is unknown. The lateral olfactory striae synapse with neurons in the lateral anterior perforated substance, the lateral olfactory gyrus, the prepyriform cortex and the medial group of amygdaloid nuclei – a group of tissues which, in man, represents the primary olfactory cortex. These are the *only* sensory pathways in man that do not relay in the thalamus. The distribution in the limbic system then contributes to both the pleasurable and unpleasant consequences of odour detection at a conscious level, and the appropriate autonomic responses by way of the hypothalamus. This is related to activity in a secondary olfactory cortex in the entorhinal complex including the uncus and a tertiary olfactory cortex in the posterior orbitofrontal cortex. Descending pathways from these areas enter the pontine reticular formation in the brainstem, and mediate reflex activity such as salivation (Tanabe, Iino and Takagi, 1975).

Physiology

The receptor proteins lie in the olfactory cilia, and it is likely that many different types of protein are involved. A smell must be volatile to enter the cavity, actively sucked into the area of the olfactory epithelium by sniffing, to create turbulent flow in the nasal passages, and also lipid soluble to facilitate access to the fluid-bathed cilia.

Once stimulated, the activity in the neuron is difficult to study. Attempts at single fibre analysis are technically almost impossible and such studies as are available demonstrate no similarities in evoked potentials between similar groups of substances or stimuli. There is considerable evidence that some odours inhibit as well as excite, in addition to which an anatomical arrangement allows not only local inhibition and excitation but crossed and possibly centrally mediated control by both lateral and negative feedback mechanisms. This enables the human being to identify some 3000 different odours. The central pathways clearly allow for further discrimination and perhaps clarification of odour recognition. A contrast can be found in the remarkable process of adaptation, by means of which continuous exposure to an unpleasant smell diminishes perception to such a degree that the smell no longer registers.

Several theories exist which seek to explain odour appreciation. One theory is based on receptor site configuration but it seems unlikely that sufficient variation in shape exists to explain the full range of odours. Furthermore, the lack of structural similarity between chemicals that smell the same makes this explanation improbable as a sole mechanism (Amoore, 1963). A second theory has been proposed which is based partly on structural chemical considerations combined with molecular vibration, and some support for this can be found in the fact that there is a similarity of smell between chemicals with a similar frequency of vibration but a different chemical structure (Wright, 1964). The most acceptable theory, however, suggests that a dissolved molecule of specific size and shape is adsorbed on to and penetrates the receptor membrane, leaving a temporary hole, which allows local depolarization of a size, rate and duration proportional to the molecule characteristics. Even this cannot explain all the features of olfaction and it is probable that a combination of all three possibilities is involved (Davies and Taylor, 1959).

Applied anatomy and physiology

Of immediate otolaryngological concern are simple mechanical factors interfering with access of the odour to the receptors, with simple airway obstruction, complicated by oedema or drying up of the mucosa as the most common causes of trouble. Mechanical destruction or blockage of the nasal passages by pathology ranging from allergic rhinitis to complex vascular diseases such as Wegener's granulomatosis can occur. Simple polyps, deviated nasal septum and foreign bodies all have similar effects.

Many drugs and generalized medical conditions that can damage or interfere with a highly metabolically active tissue, with a 30-day turnover rate, can also affect smell. These include generalized metabolic disorders such as renal failure, hepatic failure, endocrine disorders, including diabetes, and influenza. Drugs affecting membrane moistness (antihistamines), cell turnover (antibiotics, antimetabolites) and cell function (anti-inflammatory agents, antithyroid drugs) may all affect both smell and taste (Schiffman, 1983).

Traumatic lesions of the olfactory fasciculi are caused by the shearing effect of brain movement when the head decelerates during a head injury. This complicates some 30% of serious head injuries, particularly where immediate anteroposterior forces are applied to the head, so that a fall squarely on to the occiput is especially likely to result in this complication. In such cases, little or no recovery can be anticipated. Severe injury of this type may also tear the arachnoid cuffs and lead to cerebrospinal fluid rhinorrhoea with a significant risk of subsequent meningitis.

Experimental evidence is available that viral infections may gain access to the meninges by means of the same route, even in the absence of prior injury, with herpes simplex encephalitis being a notable example. In the latter condition, the initial localization of the infection to the anterior temporal lobes gives support to this theory of aetiology, the virus presumably gaining access along the olfactory tract, although there is no definite evidence that this is the case (Johnson and Mims, 1978).

Inside the skull, tumours of the olfactory groove, notably meningiomata, will produce unilateral anosmia, usually unrecognized by the patient. On account of the local anatomy, progressive visual loss in the same eye will follow – also often unrecognized by the patient. It is very important to test the sense of smell in any patient with suddenly discovered loss of vision in one eye.

At central level, disorders of smell appreciation are not recognized. Most patients who complain of a constant awful smell sensation or altered smell appreciation are suffering from a depressive or psychotic illness. The most identifiable centrally based disorder is uncinate epilepsy in which an epileptic event originating in the temporal lobe is preceded by the production of hallucinatory phenomena embracing sensation of unpleasant smell and, occasionally, unpleasant taste. These olfactory hallucinations are characterized by being both unpleasant and of extremely short duration, usually only a matter of seconds, often insufficient to enable the patient to identify the odour as other than unpleasant – burning rubber or rotting rubbish being the commonest descriptions volunteered.

Considerable degeneration of the olfactory glomeruli occurs with age. Olfaction is the first sensory modality to be impaired with age and is possibly responsible for decreasing appetite and interest in food in the elderly (Schiffman, 1979).

The optic nerve (II)

The orbit is entirely surrounded by structures of otolaryngological significance, and only the lateral border is relatively safe from possible infection or invasive pathology. The frontal ethmoid, maxillary sinuses and the lateral wall of the nose bound the orbit superiorly, inferiorly and medially and are all prone to infection or malignant pathology.

The optic nerve enters the orbit through a tight canal – the optic foramen. The nerve is a direct extension of the brain and is invested with glial derived tissue to the back of the globe, consisting of three membranes. The inner pial sheath invests the nerve and sends septae into the nerve itself, dividing the nerve into a bundle of fasciculi. The intermediate arachnoid sheath is very delicate, with a potential subarachnoid space inside it and a subdural space outside. These are covered by a thick extension of the dura which merges with the sclera at the back of the globe. These membranes form a direct means of communication with the intracranial space and are responsible for the transmission of raised intracranial pressure to the optic disc causing papilloedema, although the exact mechanism of the disc swelling remains uncertain.

The myelinated fibres of the optic nerve are derived from the rods and cones of the retina. As these cell processes form the most superficial layer of the retina, they are normally non-myelinated until they enter the disc. Occasional patches of myelination of these fibres as they cross the retina produce a characteristic fundal appearance and a field defect which is unnoticed by the patient, in the same way as there is unawareness of the normal blind spot. The important papillomacular fibres conveying macular vision lie in the medial part of the nerve, assuming their central position in the nerve only at the optic foramen. In spite of this anatomy, extrinsic compression of the nerve in the orbit and the canal specifically affects these fibres, producing a central scotoma rather than a defect spreading in from the periphery, as might be expected purely on anatomical grounds (*Figure 16.2*).

There are 1.2 million fibres in each optic nerve, just over half of which decussate in the optic chiasm. The fibres which cross are the fibres from the nasal retina, covering the temporal half field, and enter the contralateral optic tract. The temporal half fibres (the nasal field) pass into the ipsilateral optic tract.

Lesions in the orbit tend to produce mechanical displacement of the globe with proptosis and diplopia. The optic nerve itself is remarkably resistant to damage by pressure and displacement in the orbit, although an infective process may be more damaging by vascular mechanisms (Forrest, 1949; Font and Perry, 1976).

Lesions in the optic canal, however, readily cause visual disturbance and a central scotoma is often the first evidence of a lesion, followed by extraocular nerve palsies and, very much later, proptosis. Meningiomata or neurofibromata of the optic nerve sheath are perhaps the most common tumours in the posterior orbit, but neoplastic infiltration from the paranasal sinuses and

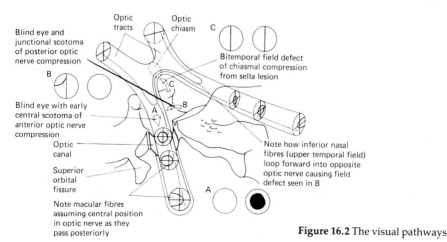

Blind eye and junctional scotoma of posterior optic nerve compression

Optic tracts

Optic chiasm

C

Bitemporal field defect of chiasmal compression from sella lesion

B

Blind eye with early central scotoma of anterior optic nerve compression

Optic canal

Superior orbital fissure

Note macular fibres assuming central position in optic nerve as they pass posteriorly

Note how inferior nasal fibres (upper temporal field) loop forward into opposite optic nerve causing field defect seen in B

Figure 16.2 The visual pathways

nasopharynx can occur and metastatic spread from remote sites such as the prostate or suprarenal is well recognized. In general, the rate of development of the signs and the presence or absence of pain will indicate the likely diagnosis (Takashi, 1956).

Involvement of the optic nerve at the intracranial part of the optic foramen may produce bilateral visual problems. The inferior nasal fibres of the opposite optic nerve not only cross in the chiasm but sweep forwards into the optic nerve before turning sharply and heading posteriorly. They can be damaged by a lesion just anterior to the chiasm. A meningioma of the tuberculum sellae is the lesion most likely to be responsible. This can produce a blind eye, an upper temporal field defect in the other eye (called a junctional scotoma) and, if large, can cause loss of smell on the side of the blind eye and papilloedema in the opposite eye; disc swelling in the blind eye is prevented by the compressing lesion. This condition is the famous, but extremely rare, Foster–Kennedy syndrome.

The optic chiasm itself lies more posteriorly than is generally appreciated – it lies above and behind the pituitary gland, not on the groove in front of the pituitary fossa seen on the skull. Pathology in the pituitary region includes not only pituitary tumours but neoplasia arising in the ethmoid and sphenoid sinus, mucocoele of the sphenoid sinus and a variety of aneurysms around the circle of Willis or arising from the great vessels themselves. The importance of excluding vascular anomalies or aneurysms *before* a transnasal approach to the pituitary fossa is perhaps even more important than in the days of the frontal approach when unrecognized aneurysms were encountered with occasional fatal results. Lesions extending up from the pituitary region damage the underside of the chiasm anteriorly. This produces a bitemporal hemianopia which comes down from the upper temporal field (the lower fibres derived from lower retinal cells, therefore upper field), although the field defect is rarely appreciated by the patient at this stage or, indeed, occasionally even when complete. When testing the temporal fields, particular attention should be paid to the upper temporal field to avoid missing a junctional scotoma (*see* previous section) or a developing bitemporal hemianopia. In contrast, lesions damaging the chiasm from above and behind tend to affect the lower fields first; these include craniopharyngiomata, hypothalamic tumours and a dilated third ventricle.

Because there are many situations in which the visual fields are of help in otolaryngological diagnosis, it is worth describing simple field examination at the bedside. Carefully examined fields, using a red and white hatpin, should be as accurate as screen testing and should take only a few minutes. The examiner should sit in front of the patient (in the traditional otolaryngological position) about 1 m (3 ft) from the patient. The patient should cover one eye. A white 5 mm hatpin, preferably mounted on the handle of a tendon hammer, should be brought into the patient's field of vision on four arcs, upper and lower temporal and upper and lower nasal, respectively. If all are seen at the periphery, no field cut is likely. The pin should then be brought across from the temporal field on a horizontal meridian, with the patient keeping the examiner's pupil in view. The blindspot should be detected without difficulty and can be compared with that of the examiner, with both parties losing the object in the same area. Following across into the nasal field, any small scotoma will be indicated by the pin disappearing again. The size and shape of the scotoma can then be readily explored and even a small scotoma can be easily confirmed by this technique. At a more sophisticated level, the very earliest evidence of a field defect can be found with the red pin. Care must be taken not to mistake the normal loss of brightness of a red object in the temporal half field for an indication of an early field defect.

Differential diagnosis of the painful red eye
(Sergott, 1983)

Otolaryngologists are often involved in cases where blurred vision and diplopia occur in the setting of an inflamed, proptosed eye, and they may well be the first doctors to see the patient. Diagnosis falls into four main groups of disorders – inflammatory, vascular, infective and neoplastic.

Inflammatory causes

Acute thyroid exophthalmos

The eye is often injected with chemosis. Lid lag is especially noticeable on downward gaze. There may be diplopia caused by globe displacement, although paralysis of the superior and lateral rectus muscles is not uncommon. The condition is usually unilateral. Vision may be threatened and high dose steroids may be of value in treatment. A computerized tomographic (CT) scan will show swelling of the extraocular muscles.

Pseudotumour of the orbit

This is an immunologically based inflammatory disorder affecting all tissues in the orbit. It can complicate sarcoid, systemic lupus erythematosus (SLE), tuberculosis, Wegener's granulomatosis, polyarteritis nodosa or the Tolosa–Hunt syndrome. Proptosis, pain and diplopia, associated with a very high sedimentation rate, might all seem to indicate infection. As steroids will be indicated, urgent exclusion of infective disease in the paranasal sinuses is vital. CT scans show normal extraocular muscles in the midst of oedematous orbital contents. The condition occurs in two main age groups: between 10 and 30 years and in the over 60s.

Vascular causes

Acute caroticocavernous fistula

This condition usually follows known trauma but occasionally an aneurysmal dilatation of the carotid may rupture into the cavernous sinus, producing acute pulsating exophthalmos with marked arterial pulsation in the fundal veins. Carotid ligation or embolization is the procedure of choice.

Cavernous haemangioma

This produces a gradual exophthalmos with proptosis aggravated by bending or straining. There is usually no diplopia or field defect and little pain.

Infective causes

Local infections can readily spread into the orbit. Small boils on the nose, eyelids or face had lethal potential in the preantibiotic era. Paranasal sinus infection, especially of the ethmoids, can easily extend directly into the orbit and frontal sinusitis, usually causing oedema of the eyelid and ptosis. In the diabetic patient, all these infections carry even greater risk and additional specific problems such as mucormycosis and other rare fungal infections. The first vesicles of herpes zoster ophthalmicus usually erupt in the eyebrow after several days of severe pain and the acute red eye and oedematous lids may be mistaken for bacterial infection until the vesicles appear.

Neoplastic causes

Any primary or secondary neoplasm may involve the orbit, the latter by direct extension or from remote sites. Usually, chemosis and injection are not marked. In the elderly, pseudotumour of the orbit can be a presenting symptom of lymphoma and, as always, the importance of a general physical examination must be emphasized.

The benign primary orbital tumours which are most often seen are lipomata, angiomata and haemangiomata. Less frequently, fibromata, myxomata and leiomyomata may be encountered.

Malignant primary orbital tumours are usually rhabdomyosarcomata which are locally invasive and normally occur in childhood. It is rare for fibrosarcoma, myxosarcoma, liposarcoma, chondrosarcoma, osteogenic sarcoma and haemangioendothelioma to occur. Lacrimal gland tumours of variable malignancy do occur and they tend to be locally invasive through the roof of the orbit into the intracranial cavity.

Metastatic tumours in the orbit are, in 50% of cases, caused by carcinoma of the breast. Tumours originating in the lung and kidney account for the rest. Malignant melanoma has been reported but is hard to distinguish from a primary melanoma of the ciliary body, or retina. In children with neuroblastoma, orbital metastases occur in 20–50% of cases (Farnarier, Saracco and Blane, 1972).

Pupillary abnormalities

As the main determinant of pupil size is the incident light, it is appropriate, at this stage, to discuss the major pupillary abnormalities.

In a blind eye, assuming that the cause of blindness has not simultaneously damaged the iris mechanism, the pupil will dilate or constrict in proportion to the light falling on the unaffected eye. The direct light reaction will be absent but the consensual light reflex from the opposite eye will be intact. No consensual reflex in the normal eye will be seen when the affected eye is stimulated. This is quite a useful check for non-organic claimed loss of vision in one eye.

In acute retrobulbar neuritis, the pupil reaction may be incomplete and the pupil may dilate in spite of a constant light source (pupillary escape phenomenon). In a patient with eye pain, aggravated by movement with blurred vision, this Marcus–Gunn pupil reaction is strongly indicative of demyelinating disease. The postulated mechanism is a decrease in fibres conveying light sensation.

In third nerve lesions, damage to the efferent pupilloconstrictor fibres will produce a fixed dilated pupil even though the patient perceives light normally. Incomplete lesions may merely cause a slightly dilated pupil with a sluggish reaction – an important stage in the evolution of a third nerve palsy in a patient who is deteriorating following a head injury. A useful clue in a conscious patient with a third nerve lesion is the almost constant accompanying ptosis of varying degree, followed by diplopia caused by paralysis of the superior rectus muscle (*see* next main section). Argyll Robertson pupils resulting from meningovascular syphilis have become a great rarity. This is a small pupil, usually irregular, that does not react to light but does react to accommodation (Loewenfeld, 1969).

A sympathetic nerve lesion (Horner's syndrome) will be detected by only the most alert clinician. On account of the loss of the less important pupillodilator fibres, a slightly smaller pupil is found showing a normal light reaction; this is because the light reflex pathway mechanisms are unaffected. A modest and variable degree of ptosis will occur which rarely goes lower than the edge of the pupil. As the cervical sympathetic pathway courses in and out of otolaryngological territory, a full understanding of the syndrome is essential to the otolaryngologist (*see also* section on cranial nerves IX, X, XI and XII) (Jaffe, 1950).

A Holmes–Adie (myotonic) pupil may present as severe eye pain because the pupil fails to constrict in bright light. The affected pupil may be larger or smaller than the other, depending on whether the incident light produces a slower constriction or a slower dilatation of the affected pupil. If the light reaction is very slow, definite constriction followed by slow dilatation may best be demonstrated by maintained forced convergence for about one minute. If the patient sits in a dark room before entering the clinic, the pupil will stay very large, but if the patient enters from a bright sunlit room, the affected pupil may at first be *smaller* than the normal pupil (Loewenfeld and Thompson, 1967).

The nerve supply to the extraocular muscles

The three nerves supplying the extraocular muscles and controlling eye movements have complex central control mechanisms and run peripheral courses that render them vulnerable, both individually and as a group, to a wide range of surgical and medical disorders. They are of special interest to otolaryngologists because of their involvement in local neoplastic disease and in infective processes originating in paranasal sinuses, nose and nasopharynx.

The oculomotor nerve (III) (*Figures 16.3, 16.4* and *16.5a*)

The third nerve exits from the brainstem in the interpeduncular fossa and runs forwards and slightly downwards in the subarachnoid space diverging towards the roof of the cavernous sinus. In its distal subarachnoid course, it runs parallel to the posterior communicating artery, hence its unique susceptibility to damage by aneurysms which commonly arise at either end of this vessel. It enters the roof and then the lateral wall of the cavernous sinus in between the two layers of dura, dividing into two branches before entering the superior orbital fissure. In the wall of the sinus, it picks up sympathetic fibres from the plexus on the carotid artery, and additional parasympathetic fibres from the ophthalmic division of the fifth nerve.

The superior ramus supplies the levator palpebrae superioris and the superior rectus muscle. The inferior ramus supplies the medial and inferior recti and the inferior oblique, and it carries the sympathetic and parasympathetic elements to the ciliary ganglion by way of the branch to the inferior oblique.

The anatomy of the pupillary fibres in the nerve itself is of great significance. The fibres appear to lie dorsolaterally in the periphery of the nerve. They are thought to have a blood supply derived from the pial plexus on the surface of the nerve,

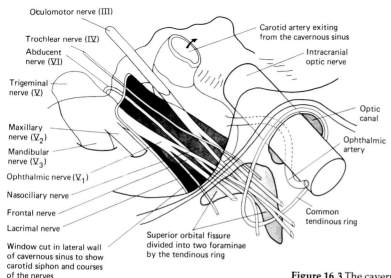

Oculomotor nerve (III)
Trochlear nerve (IV)
Abducent nerve (VI)
Trigeminal nerve (V)
Maxillary nerve (V₂)
Mandibular nerve (V₃)
Ophthalmic nerve (V₁)
Nasociliary nerve
Frontal nerve
Lacrimal nerve
Window cut in lateral wall of cavernous sinus to show carotid siphon and courses of the nerves
Superior orbital fissure divided into two foraminae by the tendinous ring
Carotid artery exiting from the cavernous sinus
Intracranial optic nerve
Optic canal
Ophthalmic artery
Common tendinous ring

Figure 16.3 The cavernous sinus and orbital foramina

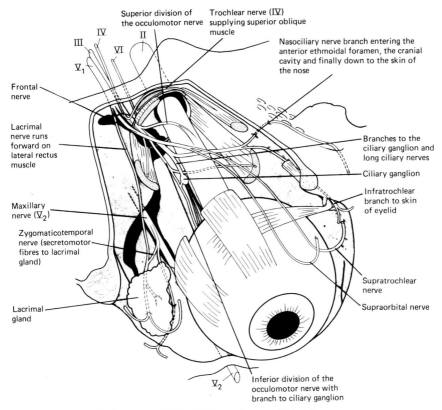

Figure 16.4 The orbital contents (right orbit from above and lateral)

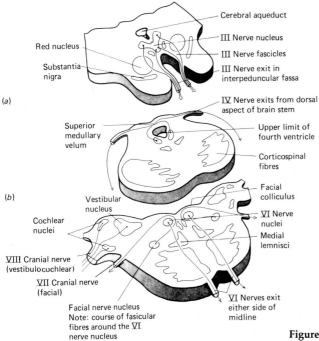

Figure 16.5 Brainstem connections of the extraocular nerves

the core being supplied by a vasa nervorum. If this latter vessel is occluded by vascular disease (diabetes, arteriosclerosis, arteritis), the peripheral pupillary fibres are spared. Conversely, if the nerve is damaged from without by a surgical lesion (aneurysm, tumour, abscess), the pupillary fibres are readily involved. In third nerve lesions, the involvement or otherwise of the pupil is a major diagnostic pointer. Pain tends to be a feature of surgical lesions; therefore, a painful onset of a third nerve lesion with pupil involvement is almost certain to indicate a compressive lesion. No pain and a spared pupil is almost certain to indicate a medical cause (Wray, 1983).

Central anatomy (*Figure 16.5a*)

The controversial anatomical features of the oculomotor nucleus are beyond the scope of the present text. The nucleus is shaped like an inverted V, straddling the midline. The lateral nuclear columns supply the eyelid and the four extraocular muscles, the superior, medial and inferior rectus and the inferior oblique. The midline nuclei have mainly parasympathetic function, especially the upper midline Edinger–Westphal nucleus which is the main central control mechanism for pupil size. The fasciculi of the third nerve fan out and traverse the red nucleus and substantia nigra and then converge to form the main nerve trunk as it emerges just lateral to the midline in the interpeduncular fossa.

The trochlear nerve (IV) (*see Figures 16.3, 16,4 and 16.5b*)

The fourth nerve is unique in two ways. It arises from the dorsal aspect of the brainstem at the level of the inferior colliculus and decussates in the superior medullary velum, so that the right nucleus supplies the left superior oblique muscle and vice versa. It also has the longest intracranial course of any cranial nerve and is very slender, both of which are properties that possibly protect it from damage by external pressure around the brainstem and in the subarachnoid space. It enters the wall of the cavernous sinus beneath the third nerve, but crosses it to reach a higher position as it enters the superior orbital fissure to supply the superior oblique muscle. The nerve is almost never damaged in isolation in cavernous sinus lesions, the third and sixth nerves being much more vulnerable. Vascular lesions of the nerve caused by diabetes are probably the commonest cause of pure fourth nerve lesions. Of particular importance to the otolaryngologist is the small fibrocartilaginous loop attached to the trochlear fossa in the upper medial orbit, through which the

muscle tendon passes. Accidental or surgical trauma easily damages the tendon in this region and produces an apparent fourth nerve palsy (Burger, Kalvin and Smith, 1970).

The abducent nerve (VI) (*see Figures 16.3, 16.4 and 16.5c*)

The sixth nerve arises from the pontomedullary junction, the most medial of the three nerves arising from this groove, and ascends on the front of the pons, angles forwards across the top of the petrous bone to enter the cavernous sinus in which it lies free in close relationship to the intracavernous portion of the carotid artery. The long subarachnoid and meningeal course of the nerve renders it particularly susceptible to damage in acute and chronic meningitis and any meningeal process, including remote or direct spread of malignancy. Its angulated entry into the cavernous sinus renders it vulnerable to stretch when the brainstem is pushed downwards by raised supratentorial pressure causing false localizing sixth nerve palsies, which nearly always become bilateral. The nerve may be involved in inflammation of the petrous bone secondary to otitis media. This is often combined with severe pain in the fifth nerve territory and loss of hearing, a condition referred to as Gradenigo's syndrome. Inflammatory disease of the cavernous sinus and aneurysmal dilatation of the carotid siphon are particularly likely to involve the sixth nerve early on. The third and fourth nerves are almost always involved at a later stage by way of the same process. Nerve trunk infarction caused by diabetes, arteritis and arteriosclerosis also occurs exactly as for the third and fourth nerves, as discussed previously. Intracranially, both cholesteatomata and acoustic neuromata may involve the nerve, but this is a relatively rare occurrence. As it enters the orbit, the nerve occupies a lateral position in order to reach its single muscle, the lateral rectus (*see Figure 16.3*). At this point, it is particularly susceptible to damage by carcinoma infiltrating the orbit through the inferior orbital fissure from the nasopharynx (Rucker, 1966).

Central anatomy (*see Figure 16.5c*)

The nucleus of the sixth nerve lies in the floor of the fourth ventricle just lateral to the midline. The fibres of the facial nerve sweep round it. Although derived from the same nuclear column as the third and fourth nerve nuclei, it has migrated during the massive enlargement of the pons, but remains intimately linked by the medial longitudinal bundle discussed in the following. The fasciculi of the nerve have to traverse the whole depth of the

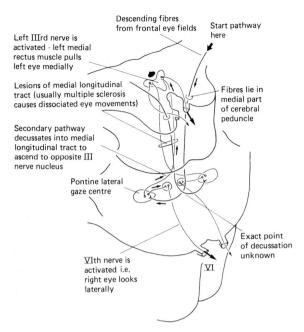

Left IIIrd nerve is activated - left medial rectus muscle pulls left eye medially

Descending fibres from frontal eye fields

Start pathway here

Fibres lie in medial part of cerebral peduncle

Lesions of medial longitudinal tract (usually multiple sclerosis causes dissociated eye movements)

Secondary pathway decussates into medial longitudinal tract to ascend to opposite III nerve nucleus

Pontine lateral gaze centre

Exact point of decussation unknown

VIth nerve is activated i.e. right eye looks laterally

VI

Figure 16.6 The internuclear pathways. (Pathway shown moves both eyes to the right side)

pons to reach the point of emergence on the pontomedullary junction. It lies in close relationship to the medial lemniscus and corticospinal pathways.

Central mechanisms of nerves III, IV and VI
(Figure 16.6)

The central control mechanisms for eye movement comprise a complex group of pathways which adjust eye position to movement and posture, mainly by vestibular and extrapyramidal pathways.

There are two forms of voluntarily controlled eye movements:

(1) visual pursuit where a specific target is fixed and followed, using parietal gaze centres closely integrated with the adjacent visual cortex

(2) the ability to select a new target and relocate vision to suit by way of frontal gaze centres more allied to direct pyramidal motor pathway mechanisms.

Damage in either of these areas causes conjugate gaze palsies.

At brainstem level, the need to integrate eye movements mediated by three different cranial nerves, widely spaced in the brainstem, requires complex and extremely rapidly conducting internuclear pathways. The most critical of these is the

medial longitudinal fasciculus. Damage in this pathway causes internuclear ophthalmoplegias, with disconjugate gaze palsies. The cortical influences have final relays bilaterally in the brainstem in the pons – the lateral gaze centres. There are also four gaze centres in the midbrain, two on each side; that is one to look up and one to look down. Eye movements occur in saccades, a series of little jerk movements without overshoot or undershoot, until the new position is reached. This is achieved by rapid bursts at 1000 cycles/s by cells in the gaze centres. These bursts are initiated by voluntary information from the frontal eye fields by way of the anterior limb of the internal capsule. Automatic movements, such as occur in reading, are closely allied to visual information relayed by way of the optic tract without projection to the visual cortex. Feedback from stretch receptors in the ocular muscles is also of great importance in this type of movement. Tracking movements are controlled mainly by the superior colliculi, once the object to be followed has been located, using stereo-optic control. Vergence mechanisms require the voluntary frontal eye fields to work in conjunction with the parietal cortex with simultaneous inhibition of those brainstem mechanisms which normally prevent convergence and divergence. Only those animals with binocular stereoscopic vision have the need to converge to focus close objects.

Parietal lobe lesions

Poor object following or pursuit gaze problems are often difficult to demonstrate clinically as lesions in these areas also tend to cause a hemianopic field defect, so that the following movement is lost as the object moves into the blind half field. If, however, the object is kept in sight, a full range of pursuit movement is usually achieved. A tendency to ignore objects on one side (an attention defect) may be related to the inability of the eye to scan peripherally as a result of lack of sensory input.

Frontal lobe lesions

An irritative lesion such as a tumour or abscess in the frontal pole will drive the eyes away from the lesion. A right frontal tumour, therefore, will often cause a fit with movement of the head and eyes to the left-hand side before the patient loses consciousness. A destructive lesion, such as surgical extirpation or a cerebrovascular accident, will allow the eyes to gaze preferentially towards the side of the lesion because of the unopposed push from the intact side.

Midbrain lesions

Midbrain visual mechanisms are concerned mainly with upward and downward gaze. The classical
lesion causing Parinaud's syndrome is a pineal
tumour damaging the superior colliculus and the
region of the posterior commissure. This also
blocks the light reflex relays producing fixed
dilated pupils, impared upward gaze and loss of
convergence. Lesions of the inferior colliculus
impair downward gaze. In some instances, the
ineffectual movements of the extraocular muscles
in an attempt to achieve upward and downward
gaze may pull the eyeball in and out of the socket,
producing retractory nystagmus.

Lesions affecting the thalamic nuclei, both
structural and pharmacological, may cause fixed
deviations of upward or downward gaze (an
oculogyric crisis). Sometimes divergence with one
eye up and one eye down (skew deviation), with
see-saw nystagmus on attempted lateral eye
movement, may occur with lesions in this area. A
haemorrhage between the third nerve nuclei
produces a divergent squint, with both eyes at the
extremes of lateral gaze with intact upward and
downward gaze limited only by mechanical factors
at this extreme position.

Disorders affecting the midbrain

Anteriorly, aneurysms of the upper basilar artery
or a tortuous basilar artery (basilar ectasia) may
damage and distort the emergent third nerves.
Posteriorly, pineal tumours, distortion and dilatation of the posterior end of the third ventricle,
resulting from aqueduct stenosis, cause Parinaud's syndrome. Infiltration of the superior
medullary velum by direct spread of a medulloblastoma may cause bilateral fourth nerve lesions
and impaired downward gaze. Intrinsic lesions,
resulting from vascular occlusion, haemorrhage,
demyelinating disease and tumour, cause anterior
internuclear ophthalmoplegia, that is a divergent
squint with loss of convergence.

There are three named vascular syndromes of
the midbrain which are caused by combinations of
third nerve lesions and local pathway damage.

Nothnagel's syndrome: a third nerve lesion with
ipsilateral ataxia resulting from infarction of the
superior cerebellar peduncle.

Benedikt's syndrome: a third nerve lesion with
contralateral cerebellar movement disorder resulting from a lesion of the red nucleus.

Weber's syndrome: a third nerve lesion with
contralateral hemiparesis resulting from a lesion of
the basis pedunculi.

Pontine lesions

The pontine lateral gaze centres are often damaged by vascular lesions and demyelinating

disease. This results in loss of gaze to the same
side as the lesion, as their descending pathways
have already decussated. In a drowsy or unconscious patient, this will result in the eyes deviating
towards the good side.

Disorders affecting the pons

Anteriorly, because of their long meningeal
course, the sixth nerves are often involved in
bacterial, fungal or malignant meningitis. Pontine
tumours may involve the nerve nuclei or fascicular
fibres and the posterior internuclear pathways.
These tumours usually occur in children or adults
with neurofibromatosis. Tumours blocking or
infiltrating the fourth ventricle cause headache
and vomiting as a consequence of cerebrospinal
fluid pathway block, and sixth nerve palsies in
consequence of stretching by raised intracranial
pressure. If the sixth nerve palsy is caused by
direct tumour infiltration, the seventh nerve
should also be involved. These tumours include
ependymoma, medulloblastoma, cerebellar
astrocytoma or haemangioblastoma. Conditions
such as multiple sclerosis, haemorrhage and
infarction, metabolic disorders (vitamin B deficiency), drug intoxication and fluid balance disturbance may all cause either a conjugate gaze palsy if
damaging the lateral pons, or an internuclear
ophthalmoplegia with nystagmus if the lesion is in
the central pons. Vascular occlusive lesions tend to
cause unilateral internuclear ophthalmoplegia, as
the lesion extends only to the midline. There are
numerous named vascular syndromes of the pons
which are a consequence of a variety of combinations of damage to the sixth and seventh nuclei
and their fasciculi, and to the sensory, motor and
cerebellar pathways. There is no special advantage
in learning these by heart, but the named
syndromes include those of Millard Gubler,
Foville, Grenet, Raymond-Cestan, Marie-Foix and
Gasperini (Loeb, 1962). As a cautionary note, any
hint of variability in diplopia should always raise
the possibility of myasthenia gravis. If combined
with variable dysarthria or swallowing difficulty, a
brainstem lesion may be incorrectly suspected.
This is a very difficult diagnostic trap into which
even experienced neurologists may fall.

Internuclear lesions (*see Figure 16.6*)

Internuclear lesions are caused by multiple sclerosis (bilateral) or vascular disease (strictly unilateral unless haemorrhagic). In these instances, the
lateral gaze centre is intact and abducts the
ipsilateral eye normally – the relay to the opposite
third nerve nucleus is blocked and the inward
looking eye cannot adduct to match it. With a
bilateral lesion, neither eye adducts while the

abducting eye moves normally, and shows marked nystagmus. This picture is almost diagnostic of multiple sclerosis. The integrity of the upper brainstem can be demonstrated by intact vertical gaze and convergence, unless the lesion affecting these pathways actually lies between the third nerve nuclei.

Nystagmus

A detailed account of nystagmus is given in Chapter 4. From a simplistic neurological point of view, it is a less valuable physical sign than is often believed. The differentiation into the various types – jerk, pendular, rotatory etc. – is often less easy to make than is suggested in most descriptions. Ultimately, a breakdown in the vestibular mechanisms as they affect the smoothness and stability of eye movements, is being witnessed. Weak support from vestibular mechanisms will lead to poor maintenance of gaze (slow phase) and a quick restorative movement (the jerk phase) which is the feature used to define the direction of nystagmus. This is maximal when looking away from the side of vestibular lesion, be it in the end organ, the eighth nerve or in the vestibular nuclear connections. A controlling influence over vertical eye movements is also apparent in the phenomenon of vertical nystagmus which occurs with a structural or metabolic lesion of the brainstem. It is important to note that vertical nystagmus means vertical displacement of the eyes and *not* side-to-side nystagmus which is also seen when attempting upward and downward gaze. As defined, vertical nystagmus always indicates brainstem damage. Another feature of brainstem disease is jelly nystagmus, which is probably a consequence of the failure of inhibitory 'pause' neurons which normally stop the 'burst' neurons from producing visible little saccades.

Cerebellar lesions, especially those affecting the flocculonodular lobes, cause nystagmus as a result of the loss of the stabilizing effect of input from head posture receptors. In general, the fast phase of cerebellar nystagmus is towards the side of a cerebellar lesion.

Group two

The second major grouping of cranial nerves includes those lying in the cerebellopontine angle. The medial extent of the angle is defined by the sixth nerve, the upper extent by the fifth nerve and the lower extent by the ninth nerve. The seventh and eighth nerves pass in close proximity across the subarachnoid space to enter the internal auditory canal at the start of their long intraosseous courses.

The trigeminal nerve (V)

The trigeminal nerve is the largest cranial nerve. It arises from the middle of the pons and passes forwards and laterally across the subarachnoid space. Its large ganglion lies over the tip of the petrous bone where the nerve divides into its three divisions.

The ophthalmic nerve (V₁) (*see Figures 16.3 and 16.4*)

The first division of the fifth nerve lies below the sixth nerve in the lateral wall of the cavernous sinus and is liable to damage by the same pathologies. Because of its extensive sensory distribution, severe pain in the forehead, nose and scalp, back as far as the vertex may result from such damage.

The nerve divides into three branches as it enters the superior orbital fissure.

(1) The lacrimal nerve runs along the lateral rectus muscle to the lacrimal gland. It supplies the skin over the lateral eyelid and brow. It picks up secretomotor fibres from the zygomaticotemporal nerve which it conveys to the lacrimal gland. In the skin it receives proprioceptive filaments from the facial nerve.
(2) The frontal nerve divides into two nerves, the supratrochlear and supraorbital nerves, which supply the skin of the forehead and scalp to the vertex. They are liable to damage by minor injuries over the brow, and a causalgic syndrome may follow local trauma.
(3) The nasociliary nerve has the important autonomic and cutaneous functions:
 (a) The main trunk traverses the orbit and enters the anterior ethmoidal foramen into the intracranial cavity, runs across the cribriform plate and exits from the skull through a slit in the crista galli to enter the nose. It supplies the mucosa of the nasal cavity and emerges at the lower end of the nasal bone to supply the skin over the tip of the nose, ala and vestibule.
 (b) In the orbit, the nasociliary nerve gives off branches to the ciliary ganglion and two or three long ciliary nerves which carry the pupillodilator sympathetic fibres, and convey sensation from the cornea. This is of cardinal importance to the protection of the very delicate cornea.
 (c) The infratrochlear branch is given off just behind the anterior ethmoidal foramen and lies on the medial wall of the orbit. It supplies the skin of the upper medial eyelid and upper side of the nose.

The corneal reflex

It is essential that otolaryngologists know how to elicit this reflex correctly. The afferent limb of the reflex is by way of the nasociliary nerve as previously described, and the efferent limb is via the facial nerve. A pointed wisp of cotton wool should be used. The patient should be asked to look upwards, whereupon, while resting the hand on the patient's cheek, the wisp should be applied to the lower cornea; care must be taken not to bring it into vision or a blink reflex will result. The patient will flinch, the eyeball will roll up and the eye will attempt to close. Even if the seventh nerve is paralysed, the eyeball will roll up and the discomfort will be felt. The opposite eyelid will also close as this is a consensual reflex. Absence of the corneal reflex is often the first clinical evidence of fifth nerve damage.

The maxillary nerve (V₂) (*Figure 16.7*)

The middle branch of the fifth nerve ganglion lies in the extreme lower lateral wall of the cavernous sinus and exits by way of the foramen rotundum. It passes through the pterygopalatine fossa and enters the floor of the orbit by way of the inferior orbital fissure. At first, it lies in a groove in the orbital floor and then enters the short canal and exits on to the face by way of the infraorbital foramen. It then supplies the skin of the cheek, midlateral nose and lateral part of the alar, lower eyelid and the mucous membranes of the cheek and upper lip. In its course, it gives off the following branches:

(1) meningeal branches to the floor of the meningeal fossa
(2) two branches to the sphenopalatine ganglion conveying the secretomotor fibres destined for the lacrimal gland
(3) the zygomatic nerve which lies in the floor of the orbit and divides into the zygomatico-temporal nerve (secretomotor to the lacrimal gland and cutaneous sensation to the temporal area) and the zygomaticofacial nerve which, after penetrating the zygomatic bone, supplies cutaneous sensation to the prominence of the cheek
(4) the three alveolar nerves which supply the teeth, gums and adjacent palate by way of the superior dental plexus; the anterior superior branch is the largest and supplies not only the incisor and canine teeth, but also the lateral nasal wall, nasal septum, the lower eyelid and the skin of the upper lip.

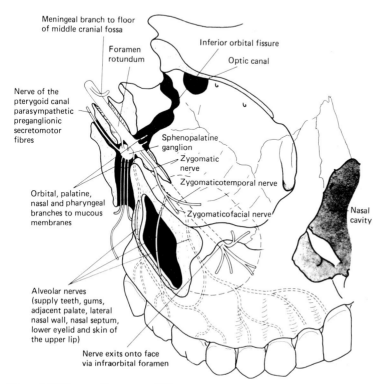

Figure 16.7 The maxillary nerve (V₂)

The pterygopalatine (sphenopalatine) ganglion

This very large ganglion is suspended from the maxillary division, deep in the pterygopalatine fossa. It receives its main connection from the nerve of the pterygoid canal. This carries pre-ganglionic parasympathetic fibres from the nervus intermedius (seventh nerve) and sympathetic elements from the middle meningeal artery. Both groups of fibres are then relayed by way of their complex course to the lacrimal gland. The main outflow, however, is by way of the orbital, palatine, nasal and pharyngeal nerves to the mucous membranes of the orbit, nasal passages, pharynx, palate and upper gums.

The mandibular nerve (V₃) (*Figure 16.8*)

This is the largest branch of the fifth nerve and includes the main motor component of the nerve. It exits from the skull by way of the foramen ovale; the main sensory trunk is joined by the much smaller motor root, in Meckel's cave, just outside the skull. A meningeal branch re-enters the skull with the middle meningeal artery through the foramen spinosum and supplies the lateral, middle and anterior cranial fossae. A small branch, the nerve to the medial pterygoid, supplies the medial pterygoid, tensor tympani and tensor veli palatini.

The main nerve then divides into anterior and posterior trunks. The anterior trunk conveys the bulk of the motor root to supply the masseter, temporalis and the lateral pterygoid. The main branch of the anterior trunk is the buccal nerve which merges with the buccal branches of the facial nerve to supply the skin over the buccinator, the mucous membranes of the cheek and the posterior part of the buccal surface of the gum.

The posterior trunk is mainly sensory and divides into three main nerves.

(1) The auriculotemporal nerve passes behind the temporomandibular joint to join the facial nerve with which it is distributed to the skin over the tragus, helix, auditory meatus and tympanic membrane, and, by way of superficial temporal branches, to the skin over temporalis. It also conveys secretomotor fibres to the parotid gland and fibres derived from the tympanic branch of the glossopharyngeal nerve by way of the otic ganglion (*see* the following).

(2) The lingual nerve supplies sensation to the presulcal tongue, the floor of the mouth and lower gums. It carries the taste fibres of the chorda tympani to the mucous membranes of the tongue. It also conveys secretomotor fibres from the submandibular ganglion to the sublingual and anterior lingual glands. It communicates with the hypoglossal nerve.

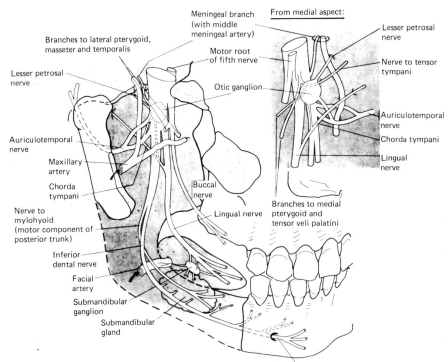

Figure 16.8 The mandibular nerve (V₃)

(3) The inferior alveolar (dental) nerve enters the mandibular canal running forwards in the mandible to re-emerge on the chin at the mental foramen dividing into the incisive and mental branches, supplying the skin and mucous membrane of the lower lip, jaw, incisor and canine teeth. The motor component of the posterior trunk leaves the inferior alveolar nerve, just before it enters the mandibular canal, as the mylohyoid nerve supplying mylohyoid and the anterior belly of digastric.

Central mechanisms of the fifth nerve (*Figure 16.9*)

The central anatomy of the fifth nerve is very complicated. The small motor nucleus lies in a mid-position in the upper lateral pons opposite the nerve root. It receives bilateral supranuclear innervation by way of corticobulbar fibres leaving the main pyramidal pathways at the same level. Direct connections from proprioceptive fibres in the main sensory nucleus allow a simple stretch reflex for mastication to operate. The jaw jerk tests the integrity of this pathway and, if greatly enhanced, indicates a bilateral upper motor neuron lesion above midpontine level, the highest stretch reflex that can be elicited (McIntyre and Robertson, 1959).

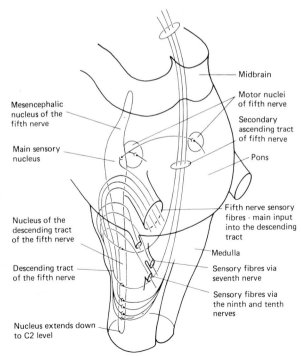

Figure 16.9 Central sensory pathways

Labels on figure:
- Midbrain
- Motor nuclei of fifth nerve
- Secondary ascending tract of fifth nerve
- Pons
- Fifth nerve sensory fibres - main input into the descending tract
- Medulla
- Sensory fibres via seventh nerve
- Sensory fibres via the ninth and tenth nerves
- Mesencephalic nucleus of the fifth nerve
- Main sensory nucleus
- Nucleus of the descending tract of the fifth nerve
- Descending tract of the fifth nerve
- Nucleus extends down to C2 level

The sensory nucleus is very extensive. The cell bodies of the sensory fibres lie in the gasserian ganglion at the petrous apex. At least 50% of the fibres do not enter the main sensory nucleus but are concerned with reflex activity. The other fibres form ascending and descending branches. The ascending fibres enter the mesencephalic nucleus of the fifth nerve. Their subsequent course and function is not understood. The descending fibres convey pain and temperature sensation and form a synapse in the nucleus of the descending tract of the fifth nerve which lies parallel to the descending tract and extends as low as C2 cord level. The sensory fibres derived from the facial, glossopharyngeal and vagus nerves all end in the same tract and are relayed in the nucleus. The secondary ascending pathway swings across the brainstem, ventral to the central canal to form the secondary ascending tract of the fifth nerve which is closely associated with the medial lemniscus, adding sensation derived from the face to that of the arm and leg. In the decussation, these fibres are very vulnerable to damage by midline lesions, such as syringomyelia and syringobulbia, producing a sensory deficit extending forwards from the back of the head.

Clinical aspects of the fifth cranial nerve

Damage to the fifth cranial nerve is very important to the otolaryngologist. Branches of the nerve and its associated ganglia lie in areas often involved by otolaryngological disease, especially oropharyngeal and nasopharyngeal neoplasms.

Involvement of the motor root of the fifth nerve is quite rare as it seems to be resistant to pressure or distortion. If damaged, the wasting of the masseter is usually easy to see and palpate on teeth clenching. The pterygoids are tested by attempted jaw opening against resistance, the jaw deviating towards the paralysed side.

Painless or painful loss of sensation over any part of the face, but particularly V_2, is a very ominous finding and malignant disease in the antrum or nasopharynx is the most likely pathology. Repeated examination and biopsy of the nasopharynx is vital in such cases to establish the cause. Involvement of V_1 is usually painful and nearly always accompanied by extraocular nerve palsies. It is most commonly caused by lesions in and around the cavernous sinus, but may also be involved by malignant disease entering the orbit by way of the inferior orbital fissure.

Nasopharyngeal tumours most commonly arise in the fossa of Rosenmüller or near to the eustachian tube and are commonly anaplastic squamous cell carcinomata. Tumours originating in the maxillary antrum or ethmoids are usually squamous cell or adenocarcinomata. Forty per cent of such tumours present as neurological problems. In 70% of cases the fifth nerve is involved; in 50% of cases nerves III, IV and VI are involved. Visual pathways are affected in 8.5% of cases, and the lower cranial nerves in 10%. The favourite routes of entry into the skull are through the inferior orbital fissure or by way of the foramen lacerum with the carotid artery (Godt-fredsen, 1944).

The V_2 division runs across the mouth of the eustachian tube and the fossa of Rosenmüller, through the orbital floor just above the antrum and on to the face. Nasopharyngeal and antral carcinomata are particularly likely to damage this division and seem to cause loss of sensation more frequently than pain. The surface branches of both V_1 and V_2 are easily damaged by blunt trauma around the orbit and cheek, or divided by lacerations. V_3 is involved in oropharyngeal, tonsillar and mandibular tumours; and, as noted previously, painless numbness over the chin may be the presenting symptom, rather than pain.

Trigeminal sensory neuropathy is a very rare condition in which painless numbness over the fifth nerve territory progressively develops, usually starting in the second division and becoming bilateral. Only the passage of time and failure to demonstrate a responsible lesion allow this diagnosis to be entertained (Spillane and Wells, 1959).

The sensory root of the fifth nerve is very sensitive to distortion and pressure, and loss of the corneal reflex is an important early sign of a lesion in the cerebellopontine angle. It is rare for extensive loss of sensation over the face to be the presenting symptom of an acoustic neuroma.

Trigeminal neuralgia

Trigeminal neuralgia is probably the most painful condition known, in contrast to the cause, which would appear to be minor ageing changes in the nerve or minor irritation by adjacent arteries. From a practical anatomical point of view, the very strict localization of the pain into fifth nerve territory is vital. There is no such entity as atypical trigeminal neuralgia and it is not acceptable to allow the pain to radiate behind the ear, on to the neck, or across the midline, and the exact distribution is the linch-pin of diagnosis. The pain usually occurs in two characteristic distributions. The first runs from the lower canine tooth along the lower jaw to just in front of the ear and sometimes round into the upper jaw, that is it involves both V_3 and V_2. The second less frequent type runs from the upper incisor or canine, up the side or inside the nose and encircles the eye, involving both V_2 and V_1. It is probably this spread over two divisions that makes simple peripheral branch section unsuccessful in managing the condition, although

triggering can occasionally be reduced. Although it is claimed that transient sensory deficit may follow a spasm of pain, any evidence of sensory loss, impaired corneal reflex or fifth nerve motor weakness, should invalidate the diagnosis. Although trigeminal neuralgia may complicate multiple sclerosis, it is very rare as a presenting symptom of the latter disease. The condition is dealt with in greater detail in Volume 4.

Herpes zoster ophthalmicus

Most patients with this condition develop severe pain in the distribution of V_1. The pain lasts 4–5 days. During this time, the diagnosis of ruptured aneurysm, cranial arteritis or acute frontal sinusitis may all have to be seriously considered. The vesicles usually appear in the medial part of the eyebrow. They then involve the entire distribution of the nerve branch. Severe chemosis of the eye and extraocular nerve palsies may further complicate the picture.

Aneurysmal dilatation of the carotid artery

This is the other major condition in the elderly that can cause very severe pain in a V_1 distribution, with chemosis, extraocular nerve palsies and even blindness. The onset is usually very sudden, and the condition typically occurs in elderly females with long-standing hypertension.

The facial nerve (VII) *(Figure 16.10)*

The seventh nerve is primarily motor to the muscles of facial expression. It also conveys the important taste fibres from the tongue by way of the chorda tympani and taste from the palate by way of the nerve of the pterygoid canal. A small but clinically important cutaneous supply to the skin of the external ear is mediated in fibres carried by way of the vagus. These sensory fibres are contained in a separate trunk, the nervus intermedius, which runs with the eighth nerve rather than the seventh nerve in the subarachnoid space. The cell bodies of the sensory root lie in the geniculate ganglion. The nervus intermedius also carries preganglionic parasympathetic secretomotor fibres to the submandibular and sublingual salivary glands. These fibres originate in the superior salivatory nucleus. Several important branches arise from the intrapetrous part of the nerve.

(1) The greater petrosal nerve arises from the geniculate ganglion. It carries taste fibres from the palate, and it conveys preganglionic parasympathetic fibres to the pterygopalatine

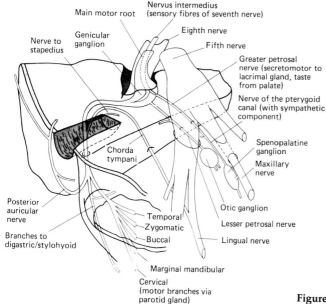

Figure 16.10 The facial nerve

ganglion, and, by way of the zygomatico-temporal and lacrimal nerves, to the lacrimal gland. It is joined by the deep petrosal nerve (derived from the sympathetic plexus on the carotid artery) to form the nerve of the pterygoid canal.

(2) A branch from the ganglion joins the lesser petrosal nerve and thence the otic ganglion. This conveys secretomotor fibres to the parotid gland which reach it by way of the auriculo-temporal nerve. It also carries sympathetic fibres derived from the carotid artery to the blood vessels of the gland.

(3) A small twig, the nerve to stapedius, arises 6 mm above the stylomastoid foramen.

(4) The chorda tympani arises at the same level and runs forward across the middle ear and enters a canal in the petrotympanic fissure, grooves the spine of the sphenoid and joins the lingual branch of the fifth nerve with which it is distributed to the presulcal part of the tongue.

(5) At the stylomastoid foramen, twigs join both the vagus and glossopharyngeal nerve.

(6) The posterior auricular nerve supplies the muscles of the ear and occipital belly of occipitofrontalis.

(7) The branches to the muscles of facial expression are from above downwards – namely the temporal, zygomatic, buccal, mandibular and cervical – passing through the parotid gland.

(8) Cutaneous fibres are distributed with the auricular branch of the vagus supplying the skin on both sides of the auricle and part of the external auditory canal and tympanic membrane.

The submandibular ganglion

The submandibular ganglion lies on the lingual nerve. Its preganglionic fibres are derived from the superior salivatory nucleus, and reach it by way of the facial nerve, chorda tympani and lingual nerve. These fibres are secretomotor to the submandibular and sublingual glands. The sympathetic components are derived from the plexus on the facial artery and pass uninterrupted through the ganglion to the blood vessels of the same glands.

The central connections of the facial nerve (*see* *Figure 16.5*)

The nucleus lies in a deep position in the central pons. The dorsal part of the nucleus receives bilateral supranuclear innervation, whereas the lower part of the nucleus receives mainly contra-lateral supranuclear innervation. This has important consequences for the clinical varieties of seventh nerve lesions. The nucleus is closely related to the fifth nerve and this provides a suitable arrangement for the important corneal reflex and its own reflex activity by way of the nucleus of the tractus solitarius. The fascicular course of the nerve is unusual in that the fibres course towards the floor of the fourth ventricle, wrap around the nucleus of the sixth nerve, producing a visible enlargement on the floor of the ventricle (the facial colliculus), and then retrace their course across the entire depth of the pons to exit at the pontomedullary junction. This complex arrangement is thought to result from the migration of the nucleus from an original position in the floor of the fourth ventricle to achieve its close relationship to the nucleus of the fifth nerve and the nucleus of the tractus solitarius.

Taste mechanisms (*Figure 16.11*)

Taste is mediated by means of taste buds–some 50 cells arranged in a pear-like cluster. These are

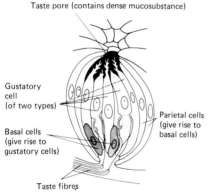

Taste pore (contains dense mucosubstance)

Gustatory cell (of two types)

Parietal cells (give rise to basal cells)

Basal cells (give rise to gustatory cells)

Taste fibres

Figure 16.11 The taste bud

found on the tongue, undersurface of the palate, palatoglossal folds, posterior wall of the pharynx, posterior surface of the epiglottis and the upper third of the oesophagus. They are most numerous on the lateral tongue and decrease in number with age by about 1% per annum. Each taste bud opens on the surface of the mucous membrane as a pore. The buds are found in the vallate, fungiform and foliate papillae. The lifespan of these cells, which are renewed from epithelial cells surrounding the bud, is about 10 days. They are, therefore, very vulnerable to factors inhibiting rapid cell turnover.

Two main receptor cells have been identified, although they are possibly different types of the same cell. Some receptor cells have receptor sites for afferent neurons and small presynaptic vesicles; others contain larger vesicles and have more definite ciliary processes at their tip, just inside the pore. There is evidence of considerable cross-innervation of taste buds which may indicate inhibitory and facilitatory control similar to that seen in the smell receptors. It is thought that patterns of taste over a wide area of receptors are critical in perceiving different tastes, rather than

specific receptors being responsible for specific tastes.

The neural connections of the taste receptor cells are the unipolar processes of cells in the geniculate ganglion of the seventh nerve, the inferior ganglion of the ninth nerve and the inferior ganglion of the tenth nerve. The central processes of these cells form the tractus solitarius and they synapse in the adjacent nucleus of the tract. These fibres then ascend in the medial lemniscus to the opposite nucleus ventralis posterior medialis of the thalamus. The final pathway is by way of the internal capsule to the sensory cortex and insula. Some information from the pons relays to the hypothalamus for autonomic reflex purposes. The anatomy of the peripheral taste pathways is complex and, for practical purposes, the supply of the anterior two-thirds of the tongue is mediated by means of the chorda tympani but distributed in the lingual branch of the mandibular division of the fifth nerve. The facial nerve, by way of the greater petrosal nerve and the nerve of the pterygoid canal, also conveys sensation from the taste buds on the palate, through the middle and posterior palatine nerves. Taste sensation from the vallate papillae, pharyngeal tongue and palato-glossal folds is conveyed by fibres carried in the ninth nerve. Taste sensation from the lowest part of the tongue, epiglottis and hypopharynx is carried by the vagus by way of its superior laryngeal branch.

Free nerve endings of the fifth nerve are also widespread, conveying somatic sensation from these areas. Furthermore, they undoubtedly contribute to the perception of extremely strong stimuli, such as curry powder, carbonated drinks and acid substances; modifications of this pattern of gustatory and simple physical stimuli can alter taste sensation, heightening the unpleasant features of such highly flavoured compounds. It is clear that taste mechanisms are rather more complex than the generally accepted permutations of sweet, bitter, salt and sour. Parallel smell appreciation adds savour to taste. Patients with loss of smell describe all food as tasting like cardboard and only highly spiced or flavoured foods make any impact, often not a pleasant one. Once again, adaptation plays a role. The modification of fruit juice flavours by the previous use of mint toothpaste is a universally appreciated phenomenon. Because of the vital role of smell in taste appreciation, and the frequent simultaneous impairment of smell, it is difficult to isolate specific taste disorders. For example, in Bell's palsy, patients identify tastes as having a metallic flavour in spite of the lesion being strictly unilateral and with no impairment of smell. Chemicals and systemic diseases that modify taste and smell are listed in the previous section on smell.

Clinical disorders of the seventh nerve

The seventh nerve is frequently damaged by diseases of otolaryngological origin inside the skull, in the petrous bone and in the parotid gland (Tschiassny, 1953).

For reasons noted previously, a cortical lesion affecting the seventh nerve function, such as a vascular lesion or tumour in the motor strip, will cause weakness maximal in the lower face which is mainly contralaterally innervated. The upper face, in particular forehead movement and eye closure, will be relatively unaffected, on account of bilateral supranuclear innervation. This is an upper motor neuron facial weakness, and in many instances is more apparent during spontaneous smiling and speaking than during deliberate attempts to move the face to command.

Lesions affecting the whole facial nucleus or peripheral part of the nerve should cause total weakness. In some instances, if weakness is more marked in the lower face – which may occur in the early or recovery phase of a simple Bell's palsy – an upper motor neuron lesion may be incorrectly identified. Much less commonly, a very dense upper motor neuron lesion may occur and mimic a lower motor neuron lesion. These difficulties are being stressed because the distinction is of immense diagnostic importance and mistakes are easily made.

Lesions in the brainstem usually also involve the sixth nerve on account of the intimate anatomical relationship, and long tract signs may also be detected on careful examination.

Where the nerve crosses the subarachnoid space and enters the auditory foramen, it lies in very close relationship with the eighth nerve; this is the cerebellopontine angle. An acoustic neuroma is the most frequent lesion found in this area. Acoustic neuromata, although grossly distorting the seventh nerve, very rarely present as a seventh nerve palsy. If there is clinical evidence of a cerebellopontine angle lesion, and if the seventh nerve *is* involved, alternative pathology is likely (Thomsen, 1976). Permanent damage following surgical removal of an acoustic neuroma is very common.

In the facial canal, the nerve is liable to ischaemic damage and this is the probable mechanism of Bell's palsy in which the nerve is thought to be damaged by the inflammatory response to an antecedent viral infection. In nearly all cases, very severe pain in the ear occurs in the 24 hours before the onset of the Bell's palsy. It is particularly severe and persistent if herpes zoster is responsible (Ramsay Hunt syndrome). The pain and local swelling may suggest bacterial infection until the vesicles appear 3–4 days later. The facial paralysis is usually complete on the second day and includes occipitofrontalis and platysma. Hear-ing distortion caused by paralysis of the stapedius, and impaired taste resulting from involvement of chorda tympani, do not always occur, and in mild cases the lower half of the face may be more severely affected than the upper half, as discussed previously (Taverner, 1955).

Seventy-five per cent of patients make a good recovery over 3–6 weeks, with or without treatment. Twenty per cent make an acceptable but slow recovery, complicated by the development of facial synkinesis. This is a consequence of nerve sprouting with subsequent loss of fine control which can turn a smile into a snarl and eye closure into a distorted grimace. Five per cent of cases make little or no recovery and may ultimately require plastic surgical repair. In some cases, aberrant regeneration may lead to lacrimation instead of salivation on eating, so-called crocodile tears (Chorobski, 1951). It is most important that patients with Bell's palsy are not told that they have had a small stroke. Exclusion of underlying hypertension, diabetes, sarcoidosis and inflammatory arterial disease is important.

Middle ear infection especially if associated with cholesteatoma carries a considerable risk of damaging the nerve by similar mechanisms. There is a 1% risk of damage to the facial nerve during mastoid surgery. Fractures through the petrous bones are often complicated by facial nerve palsy. Those of immediate onset are usually caused by nerve laceration. Those of delayed onset, usually 2–3 days after trauma, are caused by oedema and carry an excellent prognosis. Trauma to the nerve as it emerges from the stylomastoid foramen is a well recognized complication of forceps delivery.

Benign hemifacial spasm can occur in either sex and at any age, but seems to be more common in elderly hypertensive females. Since the advent of scanning, a surprising number of underlying lesions have been found in this condition, such as cholesteatoma, acoustic neuromata, meningiomata, or aneurysms of the basilar artery. Many regard CT scanning as a necessary investigation. The symptoms consist of a constant flickering and twitching of the facial muscles. This usually starts around the eye producing involuntary winking and later extends to involve the mouth. It is usually worse in company but continues 24 hours a day. The condition may respond to carbamazepine (Tegretol) but, if the patient's age and condition allow, posterior fossa exploration to identify vascular irritation by a small vessel and exclude other lesions is indicated (Ehni and Woltman, 1945).

Clinical testing of the seventh nerve

A standard sequence of movements should be tested. Wrinkling the forehead, followed by forced eye closure will usually reveal weakness in the upper half of the face. The ability to flare the nostrils and wrinkle the nose should be tested, followed by a forcible showing of the teeth and an attempt to blow out the cheeks. Eversion of the lower lip is difficult to achieve but it is a means of testing the perioral muscles and does produce striking contraction in platysma. It should take only about 30 seconds to perform these tests. Hearing loss is not usually detected by simple clinical testing, although the patient may report distorted hearing. In the same way, formal testing of taste with standard test flavours may be carried out but often the patient's own perception of altered taste will be adequate for diagnostic purposes.

Whenever the seventh nerve is damaged, it is important to exclude coexistent fifth nerve damage, in particular the presence of the corneal reflex. Not only will this exclude a simple Bell's palsy, but the considerable danger to an unprotected and anaesthetic cornea will be identified. Eye movements should be carefully tested to exclude a sixth nerve lesion, which would indicate brainstem damage. Simple clinical tests of hearing should also be performed, particularly if the corneal reflex is depressed, as simultaneous involvement of these three nerves would indicate a lesion in the cerebellopontine angle. It should be remembered that herpes zoster may affect several cranial nerves simultaneously and can cause severe pain which, when accompanied by multiple cranial nerve palsies, can present a very difficult diagnostic situation until the vesicles appear.

The vestibulocochlear nerve (VIII)

The anatomy and physiology of the specialized end organs of the eighth nerve are discussed in the first four chapters of this volume. Therefore, discussion here is confined to the role of hearing impairment and balance disorders in the diagnosis of neurological disease.

Because of the anatomical proximity of the seventh and eighth nerves, simultaneous involvement under all circumstances would seem likely. In reality, such damage is quite unusual, with the exception of acute traumatic lesions of the petrous bone in which both nerves are lacerated simultaneously. These peculiarities are of considerable clinical importance.

The cerebellopontine angle syndrome (*Figure 16.12*)

The most frequent tumour found in the angle is an acoustic neuroma. Although arising on the vestibular division of the nerve, growth is usually so

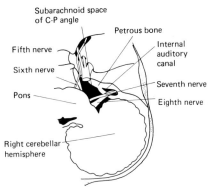

The angle is bounded by the petrous bone anteriorly, the pons medially, and the cerebellum posteriorly

Figure 16.12 The cerebellopontine angle

insidious that a purely vestibular presentation is extremely unusual. Gradual and often unrecognized impairment of hearing is the rule. Similarly, the seventh nerve may become grossly distorted but facial hemispasm or weakness as a presenting symptom is also unusual. In contrast, minimal pressure on the fifth nerve root as the tumour extends upwards, or perhaps stretching of the fifth nerve root as the pons is displaced, regularly produces impairment of the corneal reflex. In spite of this, frank pain or numbness in the face is also very unusual. An acoustic nerve tumour may obviously present as facial hemispasm, facial weakness, facial numbness or a trigeminal neuralgia-like syndrome. In all such instances, however, a cholesteatoma or meningioma in the cerebellopontine angle is a more likely diagnosis. If the clinical picture has evolved extremely rapidly, either metastatic carcinoma or lymphoma could be responsible. Less frequently, and usually in a younger age group, pontine glioma or cerebellar medulloblastoma can extend into the cerebellopontine angle to produce the typical combination of nerve lesions. The age of the patient, usually between 5 and 15 years, should provide a strong clue to these diagnostic possibilities.

Balance disorders and vertigo

Unsteadiness is a common symptom for referral to otolaryngological or neurological clinics. The most important consideration is that of establishing what the patient means by the complaints of being 'off balance', 'giddy', or 'dizzy'. Often, close questioning will reveal that the patient means 'light headed', 'floaty' or 'woozy', all non-specific symptoms usually resulting from anxiety. The patient will not have the illusion of his own movement or that of his surroundings, which is an indication of true vertigo and, therefore, a justification for extensive otoneurological investigation to define the cause.

Disorders of balance, such as Menière's disease, vestibular neuronitis and benign positional vertigo, will be discussed in detail elsewhere. The frequency with which vertigo occurs as a symptom in migraine attacks also deserves a mention. A feature of all these situations is that the attacks are episodic or provoked by change of position.

Disorders of balance caused by structural organic disease in the central nervous system tend to produce both continuing difficulty with balance and non-stop vertigo. The most frequent causes are multiple sclerosis and cerebral vascular accidents, affecting vestibular and cerebellar connections in the brainstem. Pure cerebellar lesions are less likely to produce vertigo unless they distort the brainstem. They usually produce impaired coordination or a tendency to veer to one side while walking, rather than the drunken reeling with vertigo which is seen in patients with brainstem lesions.

For further discussion, readers are referred to the first four chapters of this volume and later volumes in the series.

Group three

The final group of cranial nerves are not only anatomically bunched at their major exit, the jugular foramen, but share common nuclear origins. They also have peripheral cross-connections for final distribution that make for poor physiological distinction of function as well as complex anatomy. Only the hypoglossal nerve, with its discrete nuclear origin and separate hypoglossal canal, can be discussed in isolation. Even then, its peripheral course brings it into close anatomical relationship with the other three nerves.

The glossopharyngeal nerve (IX) (*Figures 16.13. 16.14* and *16.15*)

The glossopharyngeal nerve has sensory, motor and autonomic components. The sensory ganglion cells lie in the superior and inferior ganglia of the nerve, and the central processes pass to the nucleus of the tractus solitarius, conveying taste sensation, and to the nucleus of the spinal tract of the fifth nerve conveying somatic sensation. The motor nucleus is the upper part of the nucleus ambiguus which receives bilateral supranuclear innervation from corticobulbar fibres. This nucleus supplies the stylopharyngeus. The autonomic parasympathetic fibres arise in the inferior salivatory nucleus. These fibres reach the lesser petrosal nerve by way of the tympanic branch and relay in the otic ganglion. The postganglionic fibres are distributed to the parotid gland by way of the auriculotemporal nerve.

The glossopharyngeal nerve emerges from the brainstem in line with the vagus and accessory nerves and exits from the skull by way of the jugular foramen. It descends between the jugular vein and carotid artery picking up sympathetic fibres from the carotid plexus as it loops forwards and medially to reach the soft tissues of the oropharynx, posterior tongue and palate. In its course, it gives off the tympanic (Jacobson's) nerve, conveying the secretomotor fibres for the parotid gland to the otic ganglion by way of the tympanic plexus and lesser petrosal nerve. An

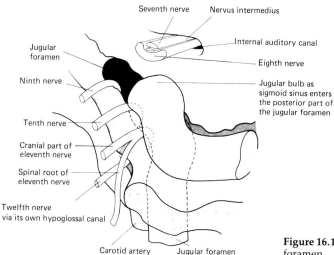

Seventh nerve
Nervus intermedius
Jugular foramen
Internal auditory canal
Ninth nerve
Eighth nerve
Jugular bulb as sigmoid sinus enters the posterior part of the jugular foramen
Tenth nerve
Cranial part of eleventh nerve
Spinal root of eleventh nerve
Twelfth nerve via its own hypoglossal canal
Carotid artery   Jugular foramen

Figure 16.13 Schematic diagram of internal jugular foramen

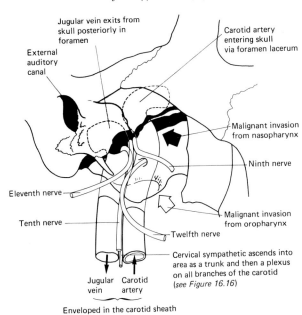

Figure 16.14 Schematic diagram of external jugular foramen

important nerve, the carotid branch, innervates the carotid body and carotid sinus conveying, respectively, chemoceptor and stretch reflex information centrally for respiratory and circulatory reflex function. The final branches are the pharyngeal tonsillar and lingual branches, conveying

general sensation and taste from the appropriate areas.

The otic ganglion

The otic ganglion lies just below the foramen ovale, attached to the mandibular nerve but functionally conveying information from the glossopharyngeal nerve. The parasympathetic fibres relay in it and supply the parotid gland by way of the auriculotemporal nerves. Sympathetic fibres from the middle meningeal artery pass through the ganglion and are distributed to the blood vessels of the parotid gland in the same nerve.

Glossopharyngeal neuralgia

This is a rare condition occurring at about one-tenth the frequency of trigeminal neuralgia. It consists of excruciatingly severe pain in the palate, throat and external auditory canal, locations demonstrating the somatic sensory distribution of the nerve. The pain has the typical burning, electric shock quality of neuralgia and is mainly triggered by swallowing. The incidence of underlying lesions inside the skull is thought to be very much higher than in trigeminal neuralgia. Both phenytoin and carbamazepine may control the pain. CT scanning would seem a wise precaution in all instances, but small lesions may be missed and intracranial root exploration is necessary if medical treatment fails. Peripheral glossopharyngeal section has little to commend it, and can

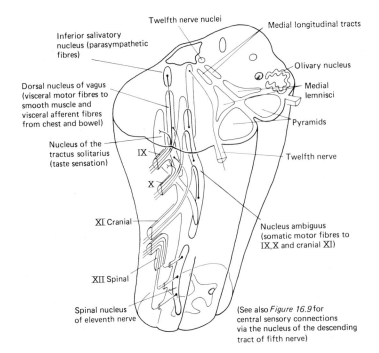

Figure 16.15 Central connections of nerves IX, X, XI and XII (viewed anterolaterally from the right side)

seriously interfere with normal swallowing mechanisms (Ekbom and Westerberg, 1966).

The vagus nerve (X) (see Figures 16.13, 16.14 and 16.15)

The vagus nerve (the wanderer) is the most widely distributed cranial nerve, hence only those aspects essential to otolaryngologists will be detailed.

The central connections are similar to the ninth nerve.

(1) The dorsal nucleus of the vagus contains motor and sensory components. The motor fibres are general visceral efferent to the smooth muscle of the bronchi, heart, oesophagus, stomach and intestine. The sensory fibres are general visceral afferent originating in the oesophagus and upper bowel with cell bodies in the superior and inferior vagal ganglia.
(2) The nucleus ambiguus gives origin to fibres controlling the striated muscle of the pharynx and intrinsic muscles of the larynx. It has a bilateral supranuclear innervation.
(3) The nucleus of the tractus solitarius is shared with the glossopharyngeal nerve and receives fibres from the taste buds of the epiglottis and vallecula.
(4) The spinal nucleus of the fifth nerve receives general somatic afferent fibres from the pharynx and larynx.

Because of these extensive nuclear connections, multiple rootlets emerge from the brainstem and form a flat cord which enters the jugular foramen. The superior and inferior ganglia lie both in the foramen and just below it, identical to the glossopharyngeal nerve. Both ganglia make connections with the accessory and hypoglossal nerves and the sympathetic plexus on the carotid artery. Below the inferior ganglion, the cranial root of the accessory nerve merges into the vagus nerve which distributes its fibres to the pharynx and larynx.

The vagal branches of practical importance are as follows.

(1) A meningeal branch supplying the dura of the posterior fossa is given off in the jugular foramen.
(2) The auricular branch arises from the superior ganglion. It is joined by a branch from the glossopharyngeal and is distributed to the skin of the external ear with the branch of the facial nerve. These fibres all enter the nucleus of the descending tract of the fifth nerve.
(3) The pharyngeal branch arises just above the inferior ganglion and distributes the accessory components to the pharyngeal plexus, supplying the pharynx and palate.
(4) The superior laryngeal nerve comes off the inferior ganglion and divides into two branches. The internal laryngeal nerve which supplies sensation to the mucous membrane of the larynx and proprioceptive information from the neuromuscular spindles and stretch receptors of the larynx; and the external laryngeal nerve which supplies the cricothyroid and contributes to the pharyngeal plexus, and which is of considerable importance in speech mechanisms.
(5) The recurrent laryngeal nerve has differing courses on each side. On the right it loops under the subclavian artery and on the left under the aortic arch. On both sides it then ascends on the side of the trachea. It supplies all the muscles of the larynx, except the cricothyroid, and carries sensory fibres from the mucous membranes and stretch receptors of the larynx.

The spinal accessory nerve (XI) (see Figures 16.13, 16.14 and 16.15)

The cranial part of this nerve is a detached portion of the vagus and the spinal part is motor to the sternocleidomastoid and trapezius.

The cranial portion arises from the lower part of the nucleus ambiguus and a small component from the dorsal efferent nucleus of the vagus. The nerve rootlets emerge in line with the vagus, are joined by the ascending spinal component and then run laterally to enter the jugular foramen. The cranial portion merges with the vagus at the level of the inferior vagal ganglion and is then distributed in the pharyngeal and recurrent laryngeal branches of the vagus. These fibres probably supply the muscles of the soft palate.

The spinal root arises from the ventral horn cells from C1 to C5. The fibres emerge from the cord laterally between the anterior and posterior spinal nerve roots to form a separate nerve trunk ascending into the skull through the foramen magnum. It then exits from the skull by way of the jugular foramen in the same dural sheath as the vagus. It runs posteriorly as soon as it emerges to supply the sternocleidomastoid and the upper part of trapezius, and it receives a major contribution from branches of the anterior roots of C3 and C4 to form a plexus which supplies the cervical musculature. Surgical evidence suggests that these root components make important contributions, as upper cervical root section is required to denervate completely the sternocleidomastoid and trapezius. The peripheral portion of the nerve is easily damaged in lymph node biopsy and other operations in the posterior triangle of the neck (Eisen and Bertrand, 1972).

The accessory nerve is unusual in that clinical evidence indicates that its supranuclear innervation is ipsilateral. In hemiparetic vascular lesions, the weakness in sternocleidomastoid is on the *same* side as the lesion. In epileptic fits originating in the frontal pole, the head turns away from the side of the lesion, that is the *ipsilateral* sternocleidomastoid is contracting. If there is a failure to recognize this distribution, the symptoms may seem to indicate that a patient with a left hemiparesis has a right accessory nerve lesion, and hence a lower brainstem lesion, rather than a simple capsular cerebrovascular accident. This is an easy mistake to make.

The hypoglossal nerve (XII) (Figures 16.13, 16.14 and 16.15)

The hypoglossal nerve arises from a nuclear column in the floor of the fourth ventricle derived from the same cell groups as the nuclei of nerves III, IV and VI. In the same way as nerves III and VI, the fascicular fibres have to traverse the full sagittal diameter of the medulla to exit from the ventral surface of the medulla between the pyramid and olive. The numerous rootlets combine and become two main fasciculi with their own dural sleeves, and exit by way of the hypoglossal canal just below the jugular foramen. The nerve, therefore, emerges deep to the other structures and has to course downwards and anteriorly to emerge between the jugular vein and carotid artery, cross the inferior vagal ganglion and then course upwards and anteriorly on the hyoglossus, distributing branches to all the muscles of the tongue. It receives sympathetic fibres from the superior cervical ganglion, some fibres from the vagus and the motor roots of C1 and C2 by way of the ansa cervicalis. Numerous filaments connect to and are distributed with the lingual nerve.

Fibres derived from the hypoglossal nucleus supply the styloglossus, hyoglossus, geniohyoid and genioglossus. The fibres derived from the C1 components are distributed to the sternohyoid, sternothyroid, omohyoid, thyrohyoid and geniohyoid. Although a twelfth nerve lesion paralyses one side of the tongue as its most obvious feature, the larynx is also pulled across to the opposite side on swallowing, in consequence of the failure of hyoid elevation on the paralysed side.

The supranuclear innervation of the hypoglossal nucleus is usually bilateral but can be mainly contralateral. The nerve is particularly vulnerable to surgical trauma in operations on the neck for malignant disease and during carotid endarterectomy (Dehn and Taylor, 1983). Paralysis following central venous catheterization has also been reported (Whittet and Boscoe, 1984).

The cervical sympathetic nerve (Figure 16.16)

Horner's syndrome is caused by damage to the cervical sympathetic nerve and is one of the most frequently missed physical signs in medicine. In the present context, its detection is of vital importance.

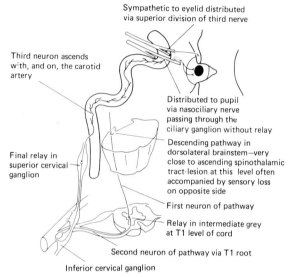

Figure 16.16 Schematic course of the cervical sympathetic

The cervical sympathetic nerve originates in the ipsilateral hypothalamus, runs through the entire dorsolateral brainstem to the cervical spinal cord at T1 level. The fibres leave the cord, by way of the ventral root, join the sympathetic chain and ascend through the various ganglia to end as a plexus on the carotid artery, on which they re-enter the intracranial cavity. It supplies sympathetic fibres to all the cranial nerves innervating the pupil, glands and blood vessels of the head and neck.

There are said to be several external evidences of Horner's syndrome which are as follows:

(1) enophthalmos is rarely visible and of dubious authenticity
(2) loss of sweating over the face and forehead is rarely noted unless specifically tested by warming the patient
(3) ptosis of the eyelid may be very subtle and somewhat variable, as the nerve endings become sensitized to circulating adrenaline caused by denervation hypersensitivity; the lid rarely drops lower than the edge of the pupil
(4) pupilloconstriction, or more accurately a failure of pupillodilatation, leads to an entirely

normally reactive pupil to light and accommodation, but through a smaller range

(5) congenital Horner's syndrome can occur and is associated with failure of pigmentation of the affected iris which remains blue.

Causes of Horner's syndrome

The causes of Horner's syndrome are as follows:

(1) lesions in the dorsolateral brainstem, especially vascular lesions in the medulla, multiple sclerosis at any level, or pontine glioma

(2) lesions in the central cervical cord, syringomyelia, ependymoma, glioma or traumatic damage

(3) lesions of T1 roots, apical carcinoma of the lung, cervical rib, aortic aneurysm or avulsion of the lower brachial plexus

(4) lesions of the sympathetic chain in the neck, thyroid carcinoma, thyroid surgery, neoplastic lesions, local trauma, accidental surgical damage or surgical extirpation for various vascular syndromes of the arm

(5) lesions of the carotid plexus, carotid artery surgery, carotid artery thrombosis, migrainous spasm, local neoplastic destruction in the skull base or involvement by aneurysm or malignancy in the region of the carotid siphon.

Clinical evaluation of the last four cranial nerves

Multiple involvement of the last four cranial nerves is extremely common, so that the symptoms and signs of individual nerve lesions can be difficult to isolate, both from looking at the history and on examination. Disorders of swallowing, speaking, coughing and pain syndromes are the usual presenting symptoms.

A glossopharyngeal nerve lesion will cause impaired taste sensation over the posterior third of the tongue, but this is usually asymptomatic, and impossible to test. The loss of somatic sensation over the palate and oropharynx will cause impaired swallowing reflexes as the initial stimulus to deglutition is the arrival of the bolus against the palate. This will lead to occasional choking on food and fluids. Pain in the throat and ear may occur with sensory fibre irritation and true glossopharyngeal neuralgia may result. This characteristically will be triggered by swallowing.

Sensation over the palate should be tested by touching the palate with an orange stick and if sensation appears blunted, this can be confirmed using a long hatpin. A further check can be made by touching the posterior pharyngeal wall while the patient says, 'Ah', to elevate the palate.

A vagal nerve lesion at brainstem or jugular foramen level will affect the palate and vocal cords. Unilateral weakness of the palate causes nasal speech and a tendency for food to come back up the nose. Vocal cord paralysis will cause a hoarse soft voice and prevent explosive coughing. The failure adequately to protect the airway, as swallowing is initiated, leads to spluttering of food and fluids, with secondary regurgitation through the nasal passages. Pain in the ear may result from irritation of the sensory fibres in the nerve. In a peripheral recurrent laryngeal nerve lesion, the palate will not be affected, but the voice symptoms will be similar and a tendency to choke on fluids will still be seen. It has recently been recognized that the external laryngeal nerve and its supplied muscle, the cricothyroid, has a greater effect on speech than previously realized. Damage causes more severe and lasting speech problems than results from a recurrent laryngeal nerve lesion (Kark *et al.*, 1984).

The integrity of the vagus can be assessed by the patient's voice, ability to cough, direct inspection of the palate and indirect or fibreoptic laryngoscopy.

An accessory nerve lesion is really a spinal root lesion as the cranial part of the nerve is distributed with the vagus. Weakness and wasting of the sternocleidomastoid and the upper part of trapezius is readily demonstrable, provided that it is carefully sought. In the same way as with Horner's syndrome, this is a physical finding that is easily missed.

A hypoglossal nerve lesion produces paralysis of the intrinsic musculature of the tongue on the same side. This causes surprisingly little disability and is often discovered accidentally by the patient or his dentist. Once recognized, some slight difficulty with chewing may become apparent.

On examination at rest, the affected side of the tongue will be shrivelled and fasciculating. On attempted tongue protrusion, the tongue will deviate towards the affected side.

Clinical involvement of nerves IX, X, XI, XII and cervical sympathetic nerve (*see Figures 16.14* and *16.16*)

As the last four cranial nerves lie in close proximity to one another inside the skull and even closer to one another outside the skull, multiple involvements are the rule and a variety of named syndromes have been reported. Of immediate practical importance are four major anatomical features.

(1) The proximity in the brainstem of the nucleus of IX, X and XI to the spinothalamic tract and descending cervical sympathetic produces multiple nerve involvement, sparing XII and affecting spinothalamic sensation on the oppo-

site side of the body and associated with an ipsilateral Horner's syndrome.

(2) The twelfth nerve lies in a different brainstem vascular territory and the nerve emerges lateral to the pyramid. A vascular lesion of this area will produce a twelfth nerve lesion with contralateral hemiplegia and contralateral impairment of posture sense and touch. As the nerve exits through a separate foramen, it is often spared by a lesion involving the jugular foramen structures from above.

(3) Outside the skull, all four nerves lie so close together that the twelfth nerve is less likely to be spared and is often the first structure affected by lesions infiltrating the area from the oropharynx. Any mass in this region is often palpable.

(4) As the cervical sympathetic has ascended into the region, its involvement (provided that there is no evidence of a brainstem lesion) is certain evidence of an external jugular foramen lesion.

The named syndromes

Eponymous syndromes have been applied to almost every conceivable permutation of nerve and tract involvement affecting the last four cranial nerves. Those terms in regular use are as follows:

Vernet's syndrome (of the internal jugular foramen) is characterized by the involvement of nerves IX, X and XI only (an identical syndrome has been attributed to Schmidt).

Avellis' syndrome (of the brainstem) involves nerve X and the contralateral spinothalamic tract (loss of pain and temperature only).

Tapia's syndrome involves nerves X and XII. It is difficult to see how this syndrome occurs at either brainstem or peripheral level in view of the anatomical reasons above. Presumably this would be a chance association.

Jackson's syndrome is characterized by the involvement of nerves X, XI and XII. Again, it is difficult to see how this combination could occur on any logical basis; presumably, as a consequence of a chance peripheral combination of lesions.

Collet–Sicard syndrome (of the posterior lacerocondylar space). This is basically an external jugular foramen syndrome involving nerves IX, X, XI and XII but sparing the cervical sympathetic nerve.

Villaret's syndrome (of the posterior retropharyngeal space). This is involvement of nerves IX, X, XI and XII *and* the cervical sympathetic nerve and is diagnostic of an external jugular foramen syndrome.

Wallenberg's syndrome (infarction of the dorsolateral medulla). This consists of lesions of nerves IX and X, the cervical sympathetic nerve, contralateral spinothalamic loss in the limbs, ipsilateral spinothalamic loss over the face and severe vertigo, vomiting and hiccoughs.

Causes (excluding cerebrovascular accidents affecting brainstem)

Intracranial lesions

Neuromata of nerve XII, less frequently of nerves IX, X and XI, and rarely an acoustic neuroma may extend down into the internal jugular foramen.

Meningioma of the lateral recess.

Cholesteatoma (particularly likely to affect VII and IX).

Meningitis (especially malignant or chronic).

Fracture of the skull base.

Extracranial lesions

Thrombosis of the jugular bulb.

Metastatic tumour in the carotid sheath lymph nodes.

Retropharyngeal abscess or neoplasm.

Glomus jugulare tumour. This may start externally and erode through the petrous bone, or start within the vein in the petrous bone and erode through the skull base.

The presenting symptoms in these cases may be the following:

(1) persistent occipital headache, often resembling a migraine
(2) persistent otalgia, which may be aggravated by swallowing
(3) hoarse voice, pain in the throat or persistent sore throat
(4) difficulty in swallowing, choking or nasal regurgitation.

Computerized tomographic scanning has revolutionized the investigation of these syndromes. Previously, plain skull films, tomography, and carotid angiography were used and often failed to establish a diagnosis. CT scanning will reveal very early evidence of skull base erosion or infiltration by tumour.

Bulbar palsy

The differential diagnosis of lower cranial nerve lesions includes those conditions destroying motor nuclei in the brainstem. Poliomyelitis has, fortunately, become a condition of the past, and the commonest cause now is motor neuron disease. The presenting symptoms consist of a tendency to cough and splutter, initially on fluids but then extending to include all consistencies.

Nasal regurgitation and aspiration are common. Speech becomes progressively unintelligible and the patient typically arrives in the clinic clutching a handkerchief to his mouth, with a written list of complaints. In the early stages, poor palatal movements, poor tongue movements and weakness of jaw closure and opening may be found, but the symmetry of involvement may make it difficult to identify mild disability. Fasciculation may be seen in the tongue and facial muscles, or palpated in the masseter. Long tract signs are important and a brisk jaw jerk, increased reflexes and extensor plantars would provide strong supporting evidence for the diagnosis. Myasthenia gravis of the bulbar type is the most important differential diagnosis. Although variability ought to be the hallmark of this disorder, continuing disability occasionally produces a confusing picture. This is further compounded by the occurrence of myasthenia gravis in this particular form in elderly males – the same group who tend to develop motor neuron disease.

Pseudobulbar palsy

It has been noted in earlier discussion that certain motor cranial nerve nuclei have equal bilateral upper motor neuron innervation; only the part of the facial nerve nucleus controlling the lower face shows a major variation, as it has mainly contralateral supranuclear innervation. Both the palate and tongue are sometimes visibly affected by upper motor neuron lesions, suggesting a variable pattern of supranuclear innervation. The accessory nerve is unique in having mainly ipsilateral supranuclear innervation. The significance of these variations is in the occurrence of pseudobulbar palsy. This is usually consequent on vascular disease but occasionally occurs in motor neuron disease and in the Steele–Richardson syndrome. These latter conditions produce symmetrical bilateral supranuclear degeneration. In vascular disease, a unilateral lesion will usually cause little or no dysfunction of the lower cranial nerves (Willoughby and Anderson, 1984). An upper motor neuron facial weakness and ipsilateral weakness of sternocleidomastoid and upper trapezius may be detected. A transient weakness of the palate and tongue may be detected on careful examination in the early hours following the incident. Some time later, a stroke on the opposite side will deprive the lower cranial nerves of the residual 50% of their supranuclear innervation. This will result in acute inability to speak and swallow, and is often accompanied by severe emotional lability. In stroke-related disease, these problems will always be of acute onset. In degenerative disease, such as the Steele-Richardson syndrome or motor neuron disease of the upper motor neuron type, the onset is insidious.

Extrapyramidal disease

Fine control of articulation, swallowing and the facial movements associated with speech are all achieved by extrapyramidal mechanisms.

Parkinson's disease

The loss of spontaneous facial expression and infrequent blinking constitute two of the cardinal features of this disease. In the later stages, hypophonic, tachyphemic speech is characteristic, with the short, sharp whispered phrases being virtually unintelligible. The act of chewing food is extremely laboured and the patient may seem to lack the will to initiate swallowing. If to this is added the slowness of cutting up and transporting food to the mouth, then the occasional cathectic state of terminal parkinsonian patients is easy to understand. The apparent sialorrhoea of Parkinson's disease actually represents a decreased swallowing rate with a normal production of saliva; it is not a consequence of excessive secretion.

Choreiform syndromes

Choreiform movements of the tongue, palate and mouth conspire to produce spluttering, slurred, explosive speech. This may be seen in Sydenham's chorea as a transient phenomenon, but it constitutes a severe and progressively disabling problem in Huntington's chorea.

Dyskinetic syndromes

The so-called buccal–lingual–masticatory syndrome is usually seen as a complication of prolonged neuroleptic therapy but can occur in mental subnormality and dementia. In these conditions, the movements do not seem to interfere with speech or swallowing as the movements subside while speaking and eating. They are mainly a feature when the patient is at rest.

The oromandibular syndrome (Meige's syndrome) with slow dystonic opening of the jaw and mouth in association with tongue protrusion and blepharospasm, usually occurs without neuroleptic provocation. In this condition, attempts to talk and eat, if anything, aggravate the movements.

Another possibly related dystonic syndrome is spasmodic dysphonia, a disorder characterized by choking of the voice while speaking, normally as a result of a laryngeal spasm, especially on initial vowel sounds. The patient can usually whisper, hum and sing normally. During the choking phase, spasms in the face and neck muscles, and blepharospasm may be observed (Bicknell, Greenhouse and Pesch, 1968).

Cerebellar disorders

Dysarthria is a feature of generalized cerebellar disease. It typically consists of a slurred spluttering type of dysarthria as breathing mechanisms are desynchronized with speech. There is also incoordination of tongue, palatal and facial movements. Inherited cerebellar degeneration and multiple sclerosis are the commonest causes, although in the latter condition the disability is compounded by coexistent spastic dysarthria, producing the typical scanning dysarthria of the disease. Cerebellar neoplasms rarely seem to produce definite speech disturbances.

Conclusion

Although much clinical material has been included in this chapter to emphasize the salient features of the anatomy and physiology of the cranial nerves in the clinical situation, the coverage is by no means comprehensive. It is hoped that the clinical physiology of cranial nerve function included here will enable the reader to perform a competent clinical examination of the cranial nerves in those otolaryngological conditions in which there is a high probability of anatomical damage occurring to these structures.

References

AMOORE, J. E. (1963) Stereochemical theory of olfaction. *Nature*, **198**, 271–272

BICKNELL, J. M., GREENHOUSE, A. H. and PESCH, R. N. (1968) Spastic dysphonia. *Journal of Neurology, Neurosurgery and Psychiatry*, **31**, 158–161

BURGER, L. J., KALVIN, N. H. and SMITH, J. L. (1970) Acquired lesions of the fourth cranial nerve. *Brain*, **93**, 567–574

CHOROBSKI, J. (1951) The syndrome of crocodile tears. *Archives of Neurology and Psychiatry*, **65**, 299–318

DAVIES, J. T. and TAYLOR, F. H. (1959) The role of adsorption and molecular morphology on olfaction. *Biology Bulletin of Maine Biology Laboratory, Woods Hole*, **117**, 222–238

DEHN, T. C. B. and TAYLOR, G. W. (1983) Cranial and cervical nerve damage associated with carotid endarterectomy. *British Journal of Surgery*, **70**, 365–368

EHNI, G. and WOLTMAN, H. W. (1945) Hemifacial spasm – a review of 106 cases. *Archives of Neurology and Psychiatry*, **53**, 205–213

EISEN, A. and BERTRAND, G. (1972) Isolated accessory nerve palsy of spontaneous origin – a clinical and electromyographic study. *Archives of Neurology*, **27**, 496–502

EKBOM, K. A. and WESTERBERG, C. E. (1966) Carbamazepine in glossopharyngeal neuralgia. *Archives of Neurology*, **14**, 595–596

FARNARIER, G., SARACCO, J. B. and BLANC, P. (1972) L'action du traitement medical sur les carcinomes secondaires oculo-orbitaires. *Archives d'Ophthalmologie*, **32**, 29–40

FITZGERALD, M. J. T. (ed.) (1985) Smell and taste. In *Neuroanatomy basic and applied*. Ch. 27 pp. 190–193. London: Baillière-Tindall

FONT, R. L. and PERRY, A. P. (1976) Carcinoma metastatic to the eye and orbit. III: A clinical pathologic study of 28 cases metastatic to the orbit. *Cancer*, **38**, 1326–1335

FORREST, A. W. (1949) Intraorbital tumours. *Archives of Ophthalmology*, **41**, 198–232

GODTFREDSEN, E. (1944) Ophthalmologic and neurologic symptoms of malignant naso-pharyngeal tumours: a clinical study comprising 454 cases with special reference to histopathology and the possibility of early recognition. *Acta Psychiatrica et Neurologica*, Suppl. 34, 1–323

JAFFE, N. S. (1950) Localisation of lesions causing Horner's syndrome. *Archives of Ophthalmology*, **44**, 710–780

JOHNSON, R. T. and MIMS, C. A. (1978) Pathogenesis of virus infections of the nervous system. *New England Journal of Medicine*, **278**, 23–30

KARK, A. E., KISSIN, M. W., AUERBACH, R. and MEIKLE, M. (1984) Voice changes after thyroidectomy: role of the external laryngeal nerve. *British Medical Journal*, **289**, 1412–1415

LOEB, C. (1962) *Strokes due to Vertebrobasilar Disease*. Springfield, Ill: Charles C. Thomas

LOEWENFELD, I. E. (1969) The Argyll Robertson pupil: a re-evaluation. *Survey of Ophthalmology*, **14**, 199–299

LOEWENFELD, I. E. and THOMPSON, H. S. (1967) The tonic pupil: a re-evaluation. *American Journal of Ophthalmology*, **63**, 46–89

McINTYRE, A. K. and ROBINSON, R. F. (1959) Pathway for the jaw jerk in man. *Brain*, **82**, 468–471

RUCKER, C. W. (1966) The causes of paralysis of the third, fourth and sixth cranial nerves. *American Journal of Ophthalmology*, **62**, 1293–1298

SCHIFFMAN, S. S. (1979) Changes in taste and smell with age. In *Sensory Systems and Communication in the Elderly*, edited by J. M. Ordy and K. R. Brizzee, pp. 227–246. New York: Raven Press

SCHIFFMAN, S. S. (1983) Taste and smell in disease. *New England Journal of Medicine*, **308**, 1275–1279, 1337–1343

SERGOTT, R. C. (1983) Neuro-ophthalmic evaluation of the red orbit syndrome. *Neurology Clinics*, **1**, 897–908

SPILLANE, J. D. and WELLS, C. E. C. (1959) Isolated trigeminal neuropathy. A report of 16 cases. *Brain*, **82**, 391–393

TAKASHI, M. (1956) Carcinoma of the paranasal sinuses: its histogenesis and classification. *American Journal of Pathology*, **32**, 501–520

TANABE, T., IINO, M. and TAKAGI, S. F. (1975) Discrimination of odours in olfactory bulb, pyriform amygdaloid areas and orbito-frontal cortex of monkey. *Journal of Neurophysiology*, **38**, 1284–1296

TAVERNER, D. (1955) Bell's palsy – a clinical and electromyographic study. *Brain*, **72**, 209–215

THOMSEN, J. (1976) Cerebellopontine angle tumours other than acoustic neuromas. Report of 34 cases. *Acta Oto-Laryngologica*, **82**, 106–111

TSCHIASSNY, U. (1953) Eight syndromes of facial paralysis and their significance in localising the lesion. *Annals of Otology and Laryngology*, **62**, 677–685

WHITTET, H. B. and BOSCOE, M. J. (1984) Isolated palsy of the hypoglossal nerve after central venous catheterisation. *British Medical Journal*, **288**, 1042–1043

WILLOUGHBY, E. W. and ANDERSON, N. E. (1984) Lower cranial nerve motor function in unilateral vascular lesions of the cerebral hemisphere. *British Medical Journal*, **289**, 791–794

WRAY, S. H. (1983) Neuro-ophthmalmologic diseases. *The Clinical Neurosciences*, edited by R. N. Rosenberg, vol. 2, Chap. 20, pp. 797–840. New York: Churchill Livingstone

WRIGHT, R. H. (1964) *The Science of Smell*. London: Allen and Unwin

17

Radiography and imaging in otolaryngology

P. D. Phelps

Ever since their discovery around the turn of the century, X-rays have been used with variable success for the investigation of diseases of the ear, nose and throat. In the first half of the century, such imaging was limited to plain radiographic demonstration of bony structures of the petromastoid, sinuses and skull base, and to the assessment of normally air-filled structures in the upper aero-digestive tract. This was assisted by the administration of positive contrast agents, especially those containing barium, to show the pharynx and oesophagus. Air encephalography was the only means of demonstrating intracranial structures and lesions, but as vascular and intrathecal contrast agents became less toxic, angiography began to play a greater part.

Tomography, or sectional imaging, was a useful addition to these techniques, demonstrating specific anatomy and lesions without overlap of other bony structures. The highest refinement of this process is complex motion tomography using a spiral or hypocycloidal movement of the X-ray tube; and for small bony structures and canals of the ear, this method remains unsurpassed. In spite of many claims to the contrary, polytomography still gives a lower radiation dose to the eyes than any other craniofacial radiological technique. Unfortunately, polytomography requires expert interpretation, and the low photographic contrast of the pictures is hard to reproduce in the form of illustrations. Hence, for the figures in this account, computerized tomography sections have been used predominantly.

It is computerized tomography (CT) which has, in the last few years, made the most important contribution to radiology in otolaryngology. Initially, CT represented a great advance in soft tissue imaging because of its greatly improved density resolution. Recently, improved spatial resolution for structures of high inherent contrast, such as bone, has meant that high resolution CT pictures have given good demonstration of fine bone detail equivalent to polytomography. The ability of CT to show soft tissue abnormalities with clear air-soft tissue interface and excellent surrounding bone detail makes this the optimum means of investigating soft tissue masses in the middle ear cavity, the sinuses and the postnasal space, while making contrast nasopharyngography and laryngography redundant.

More important than showing the outline of the nasopharynx is the new found ability to demonstrate tissue planes on either side in the infratemporal fossa and the parapharyngeal region. Air meatography – an examination whereby a few millilitres of air are introduced by lumbar puncture and CT is used to show the contents of the cerebellopontine angle and internal auditory meatus – is the definitive investigation for demonstrating or excluding small acoustic neuromata. In the future, magnetic resonance, which has already been shown to be superior to CT for demonstrating the posterior cranial fossa, may well replace it for the demonstration of all acoustic neuromata, whether large or small.

Reconstruction of an image from a set of measurements, rather than a direct recording of the image on film, is now a feature of many imaging techniques, especially that of CT. Proton magnetic resonance (MR) is used to produce sectional images not unlike those of CT, and the reconstruction methods are virtually identical. However, MR differs from CT in not using an external source of ionizing radiation. MR images are derived from radio signals emitted by substances in the body in response to an alternating applied magnetic field. This technique will almost certainly have a much wider application in the future.

Barium studies with fluoroscopic screening have for a long time been a standard means of investigation of the upper digestive tract and are particularly good at demonstrating lesions below the cricopharyngeus. It is believed by some that any complaint of a 'lump in the throat', as well as of true dysphagia, warrants a barium swallow (*Figure 17.1*), but it should never be forgotten that lesions of the oesophagus, hiatus hernia and even gastric neoplasms may present with unexpected symptoms. Lesions below the cricopharyngeus are

whereas in the case of other tumours, it is probably only of value for those which show contrast enhancement with CT. The use of two relatively new angiographic techniques is increasing. These are as follows:

(1) digital subtraction angiography, also called digital vascular imaging, provides a less detailed, but more convenient demonstration of vascular anatomy, often as an outpatient procedure
(2) embolization techniques carried out preoperatively to reduce the blood supply to vascular tumours such as glomus jugulare and juvenile nasopharyngeal angiofibroma.

Imaging equipment and techniques

Plain radiography

It is possible to obtain good plain film views of the head and neck by using almost any basic radiographic unit; however, for maximum detail and contrast, a specialized skull unit, which keeps the film and incident X-ray beam central, is a distinct advantage. High energy X-ray tubes, with a fine focus and with small cones to limit the field size, also improve resolution. There are now advanced skull units available (*Figure 17.2*) which allow the X-ray tube to be adjusted to any point on the surface of a sphere. The X-ray film is located

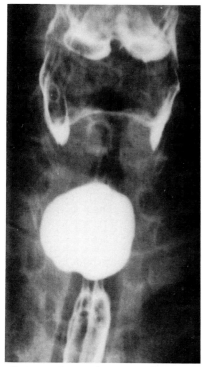

Figure 17.1 Routine barium swallow on a patient with vague dyspeptic symptoms. This anteroposterior projection shows a large unsuspected pharyngeal pouch. Above this, barium can be seen in the piriform fossae and the valleculae

more clearly demonstrated. Dynamic studies of swallowing using cine radiography have added a new dimension to the investigation of dysphagia and are further discussed in Volume 5, Chapter 2, but a barium swallow is of rather dubious value in the identification of ingested foreign bodies.

Angiography has a limited subsidiary role in radiology in otolaryngology, especially now that CT gives a more satisfactory demonstration of the location and extent of tumours. Only for glomus jugulare tumours is angiography mandatory,

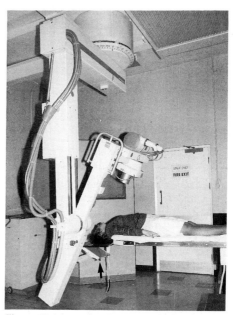

Figure 17.2 A modern isocentric skull unit. The patient is in position for a submentovertical view; this is the only projection for which the head needs to be moved from the fixed supine position. The arrow indicates the tray for the cassette

opposite and perpendicular to the central beam, and the part of the skull to be investigated is positioned in the centre of the sphere. With the skull immobilized in the supine position, accurate angulation in three reference planes is easily reproduced and there is constant magnification with no distortion of the radiographs. For a base view, however, the head has to be extended from the fixed supine position, and the advantages of the fixed reference planes are forfeited if a special table is not used or if the examination is not done with the head supine. Mathematically, accurate positioning can be achieved using the reference planes, and a full description of the technique has been given by the Swedish authors, Radberg and Thibaut (1971).

Lines and planes used in basic skull radiography (*Figure 17.3*) are as follows.

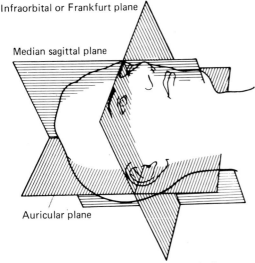

Figure 17.3 Lines and planes used in basic skull radiography. The orbitomeatal baseline (not shown) is close to the Frankfurt plane

Radiographic baseline – orbitomeatal baseline

This is a line drawn from the outer canthus of the eye to the centre of the external auditory meatus. In the neutral position it is regarded as being always perpendicular to the film. It is raised by extending the head and lowered by flexing it. The base line is always kept at 90° to the film unless stated otherwise.

Infraorbital plane (also known as the Frankfurt plane)

This passes through the lower orbital margins and the roofs of the external auditory canals. An angle of 10° exists between the orbitomeatal baseline and the Frankfurt plane.

Auricular plane

This is at right angles to the infraorbital plane, and passes through the external auditory canals.

Median sagittal plane

A vertical plane running anteroposteriorly which bisects the skull into two equal halves. It must be aligned at right angles to the film for antero-posterior projections, and parallel to it for lateral projections. Rotation of the head around the vertical axis is referred to as rotation of the sagittal plane – the face being turned to whichever side is indicated.

Coronal plane

This is a vertical plane at right angles to the median sagittal plane, parallel to the film in anteroposterior projections. The meatal or auricular plane is a coronal plane passing through the external auditory meatuses.

Tube angulation

This refers to the direction followed by the central ray emerging from the tube, which can be either 'cephalically', towards the head, or 'caudally', towards the feet. If fluid levels are being sought, a horizontal beam should be used, regardless of whether the patient is in a sitting or recumbent position.

Radiographic positions

These are named according to the direction of the central ray, with the part in contact with the film being positioned last; for example, 20° occipito-frontal means the central ray is angled 20° caudally, and directed through the occiput to emerge through the frontal bone positioned against the film.

Immobilization

The head must always be carefully immobilized, with either head bands or special clamps, and respiration must be arrested during exposure to reduce lack of sharpness caused by movement.

Film quality

Film definition (a combination of detail and contrast) is improved if:
(1) a Potter–Bucky diaphragm or grid is used, to reduce the amount of scattered radiation reaching the film
(2) the beam is collimated to include only the structures under examination

(3) the patient's head is immobilized to prevent movement during exposure

(4) the smallest focal spot is used compatible with acceptable exposure times, optimum exposure factors, and tube focus loading

(5) suitable intensifying screens are used for optimum resolution consistent with the tube or generator output available. Rare earth screens may improve the diagnostic result if exposure factors are limited.

Conventional tomography

The basic radiograph is an image of the entire part being X-rayed with the result that structures of varying density through that body area are superimposed on each other. The tomograph consists of a radiograph visualizing just a horizontal slice of the area in question with the overlying and underlying structures blurred out by motion. This generally means that the tube and the film are the moving components while the patient remains still.

The simplest type of movement, which also has the shortest exposure time, is the linear. The linear is, therefore, most suitable for the larynx, which together with the tracheobronchial tree are the only areas examined by the present author using the linear mode.

Complex motion of the X-ray tube, either hypocycloidal or spiral, gives the most uniform blurring of structures outside the plane of the section, as well as producing thinner sections of 1–2 mm thickness.

The Polytome continues to be used for routine demonstration of the petrous temporal bone (*Figure 17.4*), as this specialist unit gives the best

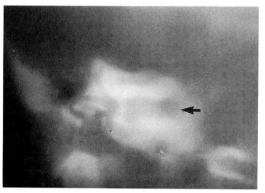

Figure 17.5 Hypocycloidal coronal section tomogram of the temporal bone at the level of the vestibule and internal auditory meatus (arrow). The oval window is particularly well shown

and most convenient demonstration of bone detail, especially of the internal auditory meatus, more cheaply and with less radiation to the patient's eyes than either plain films or computerized tomography (*Figure 17.5*). However, good radiographic technique and positioning are required, as well as the use of the optimum film/screen combination which, if a 0.3 mm focal spot tube is used, would appear to be the limiting factor to spatial resolution with the inherent low contrast of the picture. Various new general purpose X-ray machines have a built-in facility for spiral tomography and, if access to CT is limited, they may be used for sectional demonstration of fine bone detail in the head.

Computerized tomography

Computerized tomography is the reconstruction by computer of a tomographic plane of an object (section or slice). It is developed from multiple absorption or attenuation measurements made around the periphery of the object (a scan). CT scanners use a highly collimated X-ray beam, but the radiographic film of conventional imaging has been replaced by a battery of ionization detectors which enable the required information to be obtained with maximum dose efficiency. The small volumes (voxels) of tissue, for which an attenuation value is derived, have a cross-sectional area normally less than 1 mm^2 and a depth equal to the thickness of the slice, which may be from 0.5 to 13 mm depending on the machine and the type of examination. The picture elements (pixels) are a two-dimensional reconstruction in the scan plane, displayed as a grey-scale picture on a television monitor. Computerized mathematical techniques are required to give accurate determination of the

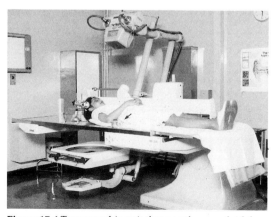

Figure 17.4 Tomographic unit that uses hypocycloidal movement of the X-ray tube. Note the enlargement tray for the cassette, which can be tilted to give angled views and the lead eye shields (arrow) which are used to reduce the radiation dose to the orbits

attenuation values at all points of the matrix within the section. These, as well as further considerations of how scanners function, are beyond the scope of this account. However, a brief consideration of image quality and limitation, as they affect radiology in otolaryngology, would seem to be pertinent.

The success of CT has been on account of the great sensitivity of the method for very small changes in X-ray attenuation. This is known as contrast resolution. The quality of the CT image, however, depends on a complex relationship between radiation dose, spatial resolution, contrast resolution and noise. Noise is the mottling or granularity which affects the image when there is insufficient information from the detectors available for asssessment. To some extent, therefore, there is a trade-off between optimum contrast resolution and optimum spatial resolution (raising the radiation dose to unacceptable levels still only partially overcomes this problem). In practice, most scanners have two options for image production, namely standard resolution for optimum density discrimination, as when demonstrating brain tumours, and high resolution for fine detail discrimination, especially that of small bony structures in sinus and temporal bone. With the new rotate-only scanners, it is possible to obtain images in both soft tissue and bone resolution, using the same raw data, but, inevitably, the reprocessing increases the length of the examination.

Twenty years ago, the demonstration of fine detail in the ear was considered the ultimate achievement of polytomography. In some respects the same is now true of high resolution CT, and a brief consideration of some of the limiting factors of this technique for the examination of regions such as the middle ear seems desirable.

(1) Partial volume averaging is a phenomenon that occurs with CT when the dimensions of the object being imaged are smaller than the slice thickness and the individual voxel. Non-representative attenuation values may be generated when all the densities within an individual voxel are averaged to produce a single attenuation coefficient. Bone or air in a voxel depicting soft tissue will significantly raise or lower the averaged attenuation reading of that voxel.

(2) Soft tissue silhouetting is the silhouetting of small dense structures which may occur when soft tissue densities such as normal adjacent brain, haemorrhage, tumour or fluid envelope are contiguous with a structure usually bordered by air. The difference in density between the structures and the background density may be insufficient for their visualiza-

tion. This phenomenon is an even greater problem with the low contrast images of polytomography and is important in the evaluation of ossicular abnormalities in conjunction with soft tissue masses or small erosions. Some practical aspects of these two phenomena are demonstrated in *Figure 17.6*.

High resolution CT: partial volume averaging

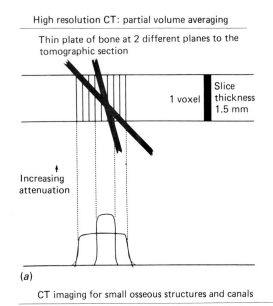

(a)

CT imaging for small osseous structures and canals

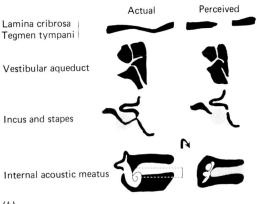

(b)

Figure 17.6 (*a*) The difficulties of imaging a thin plate of bone. At certain angles to the X-ray beam the plate will appear thicker than it should and averaging of attenuation values may mimic soft tissue. (*b*) Some practical aspects of problems with CT imaging in otolaryngology. Thin bony plates may not be demonstrated and may be thought to be eroded or dehiscent. Small canals may not be shown, and may be considered to be obliterated. A soft tissue mass surrounding thin bony structures may obscure the bone detail, as in a cholesteatoma around the incudostapedial joint, and partial volume averaging may suggest a soft tissue mass within the internal auditory meatus at air meatography

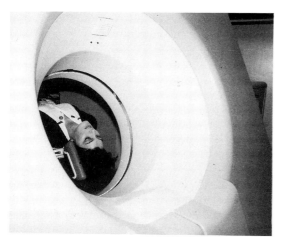

(a)

Figure 17.7 (a) Coronal CT on a modern scanner, with the patient in the 'head hanging' position and the scanner gantry tilted 20°. (b) Coronal CT scan at the level of the cochlea (arrow) in a case of right-sided hemifacial microsomia; this section on a high resolution setting and a window width of 4000 Hounsfield units also shows the deformed ossicles in the air-containing right middle ear, but does not adequately demonstrate the soft tissues below the temporal bones. (c) A similar coronal CT section in another case of right hemifacial microsomia, showing the hypoplastic muscles; picture on a narrow window setting has many artefacts because the high resolution mode for bone detail was used

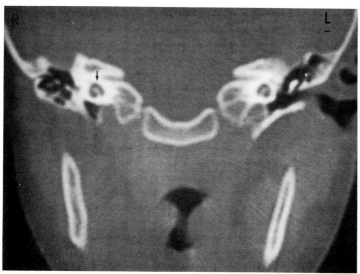

(b)

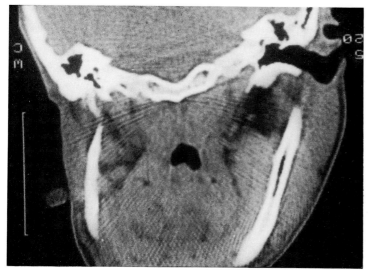

(c)

The standard axial or horizontal sections are used for almost all CT imaging in the ear, nose and throat, but further coronal views are often desirable, particularly for the sinuses and temporal bones. These may be obtained directly by elevating the patient's chin or by putting the head back (*Figure 17.7*). Direct CT imaging is not often used in other planes, but several projections for the temporal bones have been described in the literature (Zonnefeld *et al.*, 1984). The alternative to direct imaging is reconstructed imaging from the raw data obtained from multiple axial sections. This can be done in any desired plane (*Figure 17.8*), but multiple axial images and, therefore, considerable extra irradiation are required. For the temporal bone, intervals of 1 mm are recommended. Even then, however, the quality of the 'reformatted' pictures will be inferior to direct imaging because of the interpolation process between adjacent slices and the problems of patient movement.

Administration of iodine-containing contrast agents, as used for many routine radiological investigations, such as excretion urography, was found in the earliest days to improve the demonstration of many intracranial pathological processes, especially that of tumours. 'Contrast enhancement', as it will henceforth be called, is still necessary for the demonstration of masses in the posterior cranial fossa. No brain scan investigation for suspected acoustic neuromata is complete without contrast enhancement. This enhancement is mainly a result of two factors:

(1) increased opacification of vessels
(2) extravasation into the extracellular spaces.

Outside the cranial cavity, the second phenomenon, in particular, is less apparent. Recently, the timing and degree of enhancement have been used in an attempt to differentiate tumours with little stroma, such as glomus tumours – which show instant enhancement in the vascular phase followed by rapid washout – from other vascular tumours, such as meningioma, where there is no such rapid enhancement, but a more pronounced and persistent opacification beyond the initial vascular phase (Mafee *et al.*, 1983). Such rapid scans of the same slice, followed by a plot of time versus attenuation, are known as 'dynamic CT' (*Figure 17.9*). Because CT imaging involves computer assessment of X-ray attenuation, it is relatively easy to obtain attenuation values for any particular structure or discrete lesion, provided that partial volume averaging is avoided. It was hoped that this would be useful for differential diagnosis, but the results with or without contrast enhancement have been most disappointing.

Radiotherapy planning

Computerized tomography images provide accurate information on the extent and location of tumours, which would be difficult or impossible to detect with conventional X-ray apparatus. Until recently, the information obtained had to be entered manually into the planning system with the inevitable losses in time and accuracy. Various planning systems, which enable the CT slice data to be entered directly, have been developed. A sophisticated dose calculation model provides accurate calculation and optimization of the three-dimensional dose distribution. This appears to be particularly useful in the area of the paranasal sinuses and nasopharynx where, in one series, 86% of patients had the planned field enlarged on the basis of the CT planning scan (Adam *et al.*, 1984). However, unless therapy scans can be taken in the treatment plane, they

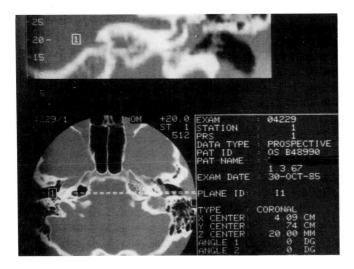

Figure 17.8 The left-sided glomus jugulare tumour has eroded the jugular fossa and extended into the middle ear cavity. A coronal reconstruction was done in the plane shown by the dotted line, and the resultant 'reformatted' coronal image shows the soft tissue mass in the lower part of the middle ear cavity below the lateral semicircular canal as well as air in the external auditory and in the attic

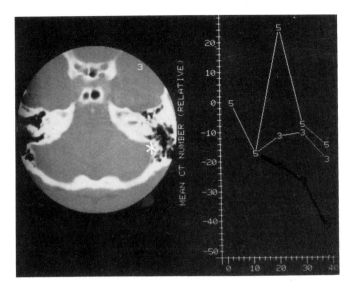

Figure 17.9 The same case of glomus jugulare as in *Figure 17.8*. A graph of attenuation versus time was made through the middle ear mass and shows the rapid enhancement that occurred after the injection of contrast. Control measurements through part of the brain show no such peak. The asterisk shows the enhancement in the sigmoid sinus

have little advantage over diagnostic CT scans which can be used to reconstruct the tumour limits on a simulator film. If the CT scans are to be used within a radiotherapy planning computer, it is important that the diagnostic images are taken with the same section orientation as will be used on the therapy equipment.

Magnetic resonance

Just as CT proved initially to be a valuable technique for imaging the brain, so proton magnetic resonance (MR) imaging has shown its main worth in the demonstration of neurological disease (*Figure 17.10*). A high level of contrast and

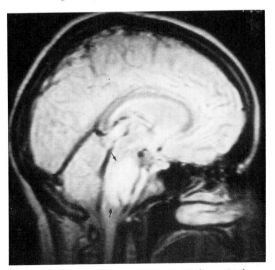

Figure 17.10 Magnetic resonance scan in the sagittal plane showing a brainstem glioma (arrows)

an absence of artefacts characterize, in particular, the posterior cranial fossa, where MR is now proving superior to CT, especially as it makes possible direct coronal and sagittal imaging. Spatial resolution is improving rapidly, although it continues to be inferior to CT in most instances, and a particular disadvantage is that bone is not well demonstrated. Thus, CT is superior in the imaging of the temporal bone and sinuses because of its special ability to demonstrate soft tissue abnormalities together with fine bone detail. Magnetic resonance appears more useful for the infratemporal fossa and the parapharyngeal regions, where tumours are well demonstrated (Lloyd and Phelps, 1986). The relationship of masses to the various major blood vessels is better shown by MR than by contrast-enhanced CT (*Figure 17.11*). MR imaging relates almost exclusively to the behaviour of hydrogen protons. When the radiofrequency field which has disturbed a sample of protons is terminated, the protons return to their state of equilibrium and, in so doing, give a measurable MR signal. The magnitude of the signal is an indication of the number of protons affected and is referred to as the proton density. Only those hydrogen protons which are part of highly mobile molecules are affected; hence, at present, the technique is effectively limited to the display of water and mobile lipids. In most body tissues, it is the hydrogen of water which provides the biggest component of the MR signal. The other properties are the T_1 or longitudinal relaxation time, and T_2 or transverse relaxation time of these same protons.

Perhaps a more effective 'tissue characterization', so unsatisfactory with CT, may be possible with magnetic resonance using T_1 and T_2 relaxation times, together with proton density and other

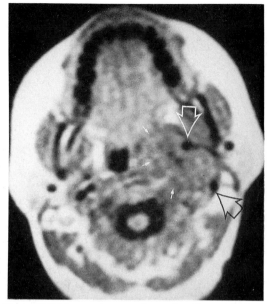

Figure 17.11 A parapharyngeal mass (small arrows) displaces the carotid artery forwards (open white arrow) and the internal jugular vein laterally (open black arrow)

MR observable properties. As with CT, partial volume averaging is an additional problem affecting characterization of normal and abnormal tissues, and it does not seem that there will be much practical application of tissue characterization techniques in the near future. Meanwhile, magnetic resonance, in common with other sectional imaging, requires a profound knowledge of anatomy for an effective interpretation of the image.

Angiography

Apart from the recently developed digital vascular imaging, almost all angiography of the head and neck is now done by catheterization of the femoral artery, followed by manipulation of the tip of the catheter into the appropriate vessel under fluoroscopic control. High resolution image intensification together with rapid automatic film changing and advances in catheter technology have led to selective and super-selective examination of the area of interest (*Figure 17.12*). The success of computerized tomography has superseded the diagnostic role of angiography in some conditions and modified it in others. Angiography is now used principally in cases of cerebral ischaemia and of intracranial haemorrhage, and in the diagnosis of aneurysm and angiomatous malformation. It still has an important role for vascular tumours, particularly glomus jugulare; and there has recently been an increased therapeutic application, particularly in the treatment of glomus tumours. The types of investigation may be listed as follows:

(1) Arch aortography. This is used – although rarely now – for a demonstration of the major vessels of the neck.
(2) Common carotid injection.
(3) Internal carotid injection. This is used mainly for intracranial lesions.
(4) External carotid injection. This is used principally for lesions of the face, and for demonstrating the blood supply of meningiomata (*Figure 17.13*). Super-selective demonstration of branches of the external carotid, particularly the ascending pharyngeal and the maxillary artery, is important for embolization techniques. Anastomoses with the internal carotid supply can also be demonstrated.

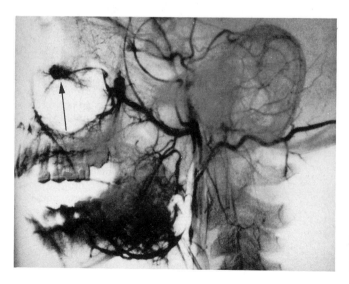

Figure 17.12 External carotid angiogram with subtraction demonstrates Little's area (arrow)

(5) Vertebral angiography. This was formerly used for diagnosing lesions in the posterior cranial fossa. Although it is no longer used in the diagnosis of acoustic neuromata, this type of investigation is considered advisable by many surgeons for showing the vascular architecture preoperatively.

(6) Retrograde jugulography. This is occasionally used to confirm the diagnosis of a glomus jugulare tumour and to show its lower limits. The sigmoid sinus and the jugular bulb can often be shown in the venous phase of a carotid angiogram.

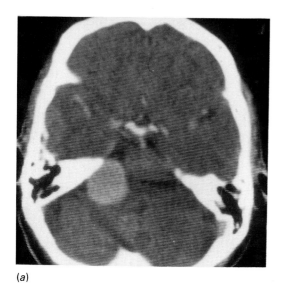

(a)

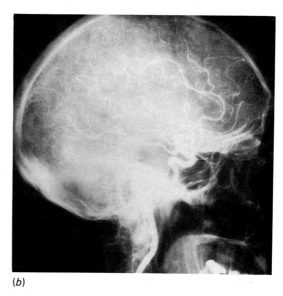

(b)

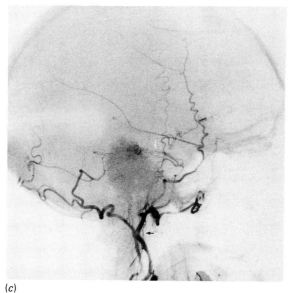

(c)

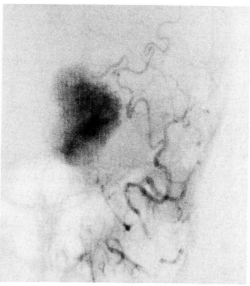

(d)

Figure 17.13 (a) Posterior fossa CT scan with contrast shows a dense homgeneously enhancing round mass in the posterior cranial fossa with the typical appearances of a meningioma. (b) The internal carotid angiogram shows no abnormality. (c) The external carotid angiogram with subtraction shows the pathological vessels of the tumour and its supply from the ascending pharyngeal artery (black arrow), and from the middle meningeal artery (white arrow). (d) Another view of the tumour showing blood supply from branches of the external carotid artery. (Courtesy of Dr Anthony D. Lloyd)

Digital angiography

Digital subtraction angiography is a modified form of the subtraction technique used in vascular imaging. The essential difference between digital subtraction angiography and photographic subtraction lies in the digitization of the video signals from an image intensifier/television system. This is followed by subtraction contrast enhancement and reconversion to analogue signals, which are subjected to further enhancement by windowing and grey-scale manipulation methods similar to those used for viewing CT images. In some systems, image enhancement is performed digitally and the resultant data are subsequently converted into analogue form for the television display.

It was hoped initially that intravenous digital subtraction would completely replace intra-arterial procedures, but such techniques necessitate large doses of contrast agent, and movement by the patient is a problem. Movement downgrades the quality of the images recorded, but the problem can be partially overcome by what is called 're-registration' of the patient, whereby further views for the subtraction process are made during the examination.

The main applications of intravenous digital subtraction angiography are in the study of the extracranial cerebral arteries, of certain intracranial lesions, such as large aneurysms, and of arteriovenous malformations, and in the diagnosis of cerebral venous sinus disease.

Intra-arterial digital subtraction angiography allows a low concentration of contrast medium and finer catheters to be used, reducing the risk of arterial damage. The rapid subtraction with real time display and the ability to study selected frames make this an ideal preliminary to interventional studies, although the inferior resolution for small vessels can be a problem. The efficacy of embolization and any alterations of flow which might take place can be immediately assessed. Undoubtedly, the use of digital imaging for angiography will increase rapidly, although, at present the intra-arterial techniques (*Figure 17.14*) appear more satisfactory than the intravenous ones, and are especially useful for children, where strict limitation of contrast dose is necessary.

Embolization techniques

Embolization is a technique of intravascular occlusion in which catheters are selectively manipulated into a pathological vascular territory for the purpose of injecting occlusive or embolic agents. Detachable balloons have been used to obliterate large vascular fistulae, and a great variety of embolic agents – such as Gelfoam,

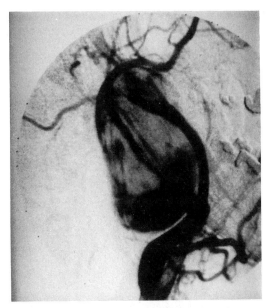

Figure 17.14 Arterial digital vascular imaging showing an aneurysm arising from the carotid system

silicone spheres, tantalum powder and various chemical agents – have been used to obliterate feeding vessels of tumours, usually as a prelude to surgery. Super-selective catheterization is an essential preliminary. Occlusion of the nidus of the lesion, and not merely of the feeding pedicle, should be performed, and the distal migration of the emboli to the venous circulation, and beyond it, must be prevented. Such procedures should be carried out only in a few specialist neuroradiological centres.

Subsidiary imaging techniques

Radiological and other imaging investigations, which are sometimes used in otolaryngology but whose main application is in related specialties, will be briefly described.

Xeroradiography

A conventional source of X-rays is used for this technique; however, instead of recording on film, use is made of specially charged selenium plates to produce an image. Tomography can be used in the same way as with radiographic methods. Low contrast detail within the soft tissues is improved by the phenomenon of edge enhancement, providing a good demonstration of the air/soft tissue interface in the pharynx and larynx (*Figure 17.15*).

The wide exposure latitude provides, in the same image, good detail of both soft tissue and bone, and xerotomography of the larynx has been advocated for radiotherapy planning of the treatment volume of laryngeal and related neck carcinomata (Julian, Noscoe and Berry, 1981). The disadvantages of xeroradiography are those of the increased radiation dose, which must be considered when examining children, the increased cost,

and some loss of bone detail. Practical experience has shown that the improvement in soft tissue detail is useful in examining the pharynx and larynx, but there is little call for the technique in other areas, such as the sinuses, and therapy planning is now probably better done with CT.

Panoramic radiography (orthopantomography)

Synchronous and reciprocal movement of the X-ray tube and film cassette around the lower part of the head of the patient constitutes the basic design of the panoramic X-ray machine. The curved focal plane is engineered to correspond to the size and shape of the average dental arch. It is possible to achieve, on one film, a complete demonstration of all bony structures in upper and lower jaws, as well as of all teeth, both erupted and unerupted. These machines are now widely available, especially in dental clinics where their main use is for dental surveys; they are particularly useful to the orthodontist in the case of children with developmental abnormalities, as a comparison between the two sides can easily be made. The patient is examined standing or sitting when using the commonest type of orthopantomograph. A bite block or jaw support automatically positions the jaws within the focal plane, but some repositioning may be necessary to obtain views of the antra and the temporomandibular joints. Spring loaded or movable head-clamps are normally used because of the long X-ray exposure times (between 15 and 22 s).

A quick and simple demonstration of the temporomandibular joints and parotid regions can be achieved (*Figure 17.16*), although the slightly

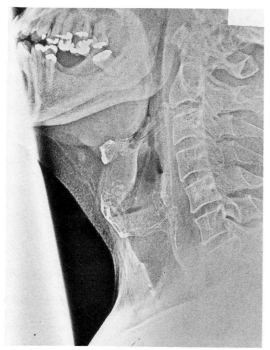

Figure 17.15 Lateral xerogram of the soft tissues of the neck showing the outlines of pharynx and larynx as well as the hyoid bone and laryngeal cartilages

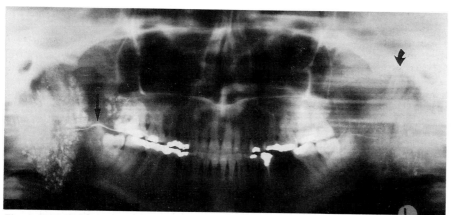

Figure 17.16 Orthopantomograph of a bilateral parotid sialogram. The main duct (straight arrow) and gland on the right are well demonstrated, but on the left the gland architecture has largely emptied of contrast. There is a punctate sialectasis. The curved arrow points to the temporomandibular joint on the left side

oblique view of the temporomandibular joint demonstrates the neck and condyle of the mandible better than the articular fossa and eminence. A 'reversed orthopantomograph', an option available only on certain types of orthopantomograph, gives a rather better demonstration of the joint (*Figure 17.17*). However, the best demonstration of

standard anode film distance of 152 cm (60 inches); the patient's head should be stabilized to produce a true lateral projection and the soft tissue profile of the face must be seen in addition to the skeletal structures. Such cephalometric methods have been used to estimate the size of the adenoid pad (Maw, Jeans and Fernando, 1981).

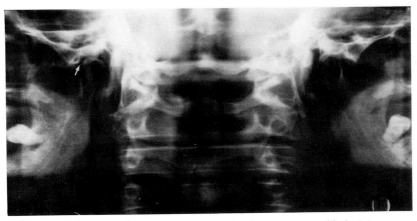

Figure 17.17 Reversed orthopantomograph to show the temporomandibular joints

bone detail in the temporomandibular joint is by lateral complex motion tomography, but CT, MR or arthrography are necessary to show the state of the intra-articular disc.

The patient is examined in the supine position on a sophisticated and versatile, but more expensive, development of the basic panoramic X-ray machine. The panoramic image comes from a combination of linear and circular movements of the X-ray tube around the patient's head. The exposure is made throughout or during only certain segments of the tube movement and planned programmes for the middle third of face anatomy; temporomandibular joints (lateral view), cervical vertebrae, optic foramina and dentition are available. There is no need to turn or move the supine patient during the examination, and a good demonstration of facial anatomy makes this an excellent apparatus for assessing a badly injured patient. However, for dental surveys and demonstrations of the temporo-mandibular joints, this technique has no advantage over simpler panoramic X-ray machines. Other options available – such as views of the temporal bones – are, in the opinion of the author, of little value.

Attachments for cephalometric skull radiography are sometimes added to panoramic machines for use in dental clinics. Cephalometric radiographs are used primarily by orthodontists and oral and maxillofacial surgeons in the evaluation of facial growth and development. The lateral and posteroanterior radiographs are made at a

Ultrasonography

Although ultrasound has been used for the investigation of sinus disease, its practical value in otolaryngology is very limited and depends on its ability to identify fluid-filled cavities. Ultrasound may help, therefore, to confirm the cystic nature of masses in the neck – particularly in or around the thyroid gland – in the salivary glands and branchial cysts. A typical cystic lesion which proved to be vascular is shown in *Figure 17.18*.

Isotope scanning

The introduction of radioactive tracer materials, especially the technetium phosphate analogues, together with improved camera techniques and better diagnostic image resolution, have today resulted in the ready adaptation of bone scanning to the diagnosis of a variety of clinical problems. The major role of bone scanning in medicine generally remains that of the search for occult bony metastases in patients harbouring cancers known to have a predilection for the bony skeleton (that is breast, lung and prostate). The bone scan demonstrates areas of increased osteoblastic activity; however, this is a non-specific finding which may indicate a variety of disease processes including fracture, osteomyelitis, arthropathy, bone dysplasia, or primary or secondary tumour in bone. Carcinoma of the oral cavity, and

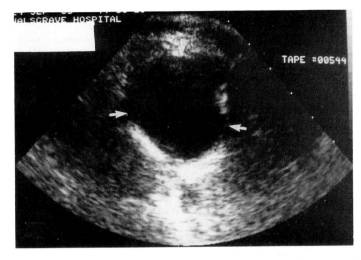

Figure 17.18 An ultrasound scan of a cystic mass in the neck, which proved to be an aneurysm. In the neck, ultrasound is only of value in confirming the fluid-filled nature of the mass

particularly of the floor of the mouth, frequently invades the mandible subclinically before there is any evidence of bone destruction on plain films or orthopantomography. The extent of surgical resection depends greatly on whether or not there is bone involvement by the tumour; osteoblastic reaction on delayed bone scanning is often the earliest indication (*Figure 17.19*).

Formerly, radionuclide studies had an important role in neuroradiology, where they were able to demonstrate approximately 80% of brain tumours. However, these investigations have now been almost completely superseded by computerized tomography and magnetic resonance. Dynamic and functional studies of the cerebro-spinal fluid pathways, using labelled proteins or labelled inorganic chelating agents, still have a place; but CT, combined with cerebrospinal fluid water-soluble contrast agents, has the advantage of morphological display. Similarly, radionuclide cisternography has been used with variable success in the evolution of cerebrospinal fluid leaks – particularly rhinorrhoea. This technique is even less satisfactory for demonstrating fistulae through the ear, and it is not required if a congenital deformity of the labyrinth is demonstrated by tomography or CT and the discharge of cerebrospinal fluid is confirmed by analysis of the fluid or the use of fluorescein or other tracers (*see* Volume 6, Chapter 2).

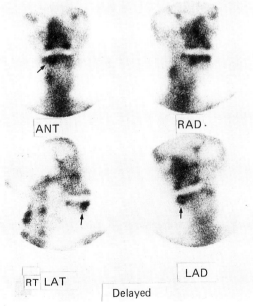

(*a*)

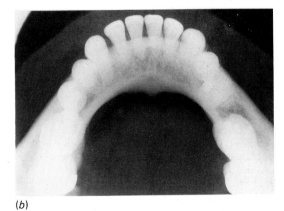

(*b*)

Figure 17.19 (*a*) A technetium-based isotope scan of the jaws showing an area of increased uptake in the anterior part of the mandible (arrow). The patient had a carcinoma of the floor of the mouth and the bone scan confirms that the mandible was involved. This was proved at surgery. (*b*) An intraoral view of the anterior part of the mandible shows no evidence of any involvement by this tumour. (Courtesy of Dr Arnold M. Noyek, Toronto)

Temporomandibular joint disorders can be usefully assessed by bone scanning. Most discomfort and/or pain in or about the temporomandibular joint relates to altered muscle tension about the joint by the powerful muscles of mastication, probably on account of dental malocclusion which causes a change in bite dynamics. Isotope studies have also been used for the assessment of facial fractures and osteomyelitis or to predict the likely growth rate of osteomata. The salivary glands normally concentrate technetium-99m sodium pertechnetate. Originally, this was considered to be a nuisance on brain scans, but it is now used for the functional assessment of the gland parenchyma. Hyperfunction is seen in acute sialadenitis, granulomatous diseases, lymphoma and the sialoses; decreased activity with Sjögren's syndrome and most primary and metastatic tumours. Exceptions are Warthin's tumours and oncocytomata which intensely accumulate the radionuclide. The larynx is another organ which has been investigated with radioactive isotopes. Anterior extension of laryngeal cancer into the pre-epiglottic space is an important finding which may affect management of the disease. Extensive pre-epiglottic space involvement, sufficient to reach the hyoid bone, will incite a delayed osteoblastic response on the bone scan. For an account of this and other aspects of radionuclide scanning in otolaryngology, the reader is referred to the work of Noyek (1979).

Dacrocystography

Ultrafluid Lipiodol injected into the inferior canaliculus through a very fine catheter is used to demonstrate the patency of the canaliculi, lacrimal sac and the nasolacrimal duct. When disease is present, the site and degree of obstruction and the presence of fistulae, diverticula and concretions are shown. The exposure of the films is made during the actual injection of the contrast medium, and in normal patients will produce an image which is continuous throughout the duct system (*Figure 17.20*). Subtraction studies are particularly useful for demonstrating the common canaliculus. Common canaliculus blocks are characterized by the regurgitation of contrast medium through the upper punctum, and the outlining of both the upper and lower canaliculi on the radiographs, without filling of the lacrimal sac if the obstruction is complete. Complete or partial obstruction distally in the sac or nasolacrimal duct usually shows as dilation or 'mucocoele' of the lacrimal sac; it may be caused by congenital stenosis, inflammatory processes, trauma or neoplasms.

Sialography

Injection of radiopaque contrast medium into Stenson's or Wharton's duct to demonstrate the glandular ductal system is still the principal means of investigation into diseases of the parotid and submandibular salivary glands.

Before the contrast medium is introduced, plain films are obtained to demonstrate any radiopaque calculi or calcification within the gland. For the parotid gland, lateral and oblique views should be obtained in the open mouth position. The lateral view for the submandibular gland should be taken with the floor of the mouth depressed by the patient's finger or a wooden spatula pressing the tongue downwards. An intraoral occlusal film is necessary to exclude a stone in Wharton's duct.

For the injection, either a water soluble or an oily contrast medium may be used. The present

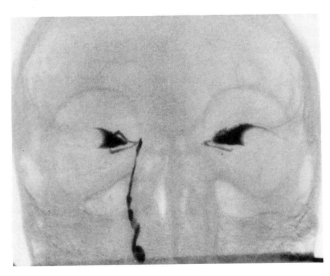

Figure 17.20 Bilateral dacrocystogram shows normal appearances on the right and a blockage of the common canaliculus on the left

author uses ultrafluid Lipiodol, which allows good filling of the smallest calibre salivary ducts, and, being more viscid than the water-soluble agents, is easier to keep in the ductal system. This is a desirable feature if, after the conventional sialogram, a CT sialogram is to be performed. A detailed description of the technique is given by Som and Saunders (1984) and only a brief account is given here.

The opening of Stenson's duct of the parotid gland is opposite the second molar tooth. The orifice of Wharton's duct of the submandibular

gland lies under the tip of the tongue on the sublingual papilla, and is smaller than that of Stenson's duct. In either case, the opening needs to be gently dilated with suitable dilators of the lacrimal type. Cannulation is by catheters or sialographic cannula, and a hand injection technique is used. A sialogram can be considered in three phases – ductal filling, acinar filling, and evacuation. Acinar filling can be accomplished in most patients. The patient should be warned that discomfort will be felt in the region of the injected gland (*Figure 17.21*), and should be told to signal when this occurs.

Conventional sialography is still the best examination for the duct architecture and for diseases of the duct system, such as sialectasis. It is less satisfactory for the demonstration of mass lesions, which appear as filling defects in the normal sialogram. Tumours within the parotid gland are better demonstrated and outlined by CT. The parotid glands usually show lower attenuation than the adjacent muscles, and this feature also occurs with intraparotid tumours. Parotid sialography may give a better demonstration of the situation and extent of such a mass; however, with the improved resolution of the latest scanners, it is now less necessary than it previously was.

Arthrography of the temporomandibular joint

The best demonstration of the bony components of the temporomandibular joint, that is condyle of mandible and articular fossa and eminence, is obtained with lateral complex motion tomography. Plain film views and panoramic tomography are less satisfactory, especially for showing the articular fossa. However, none of these conventional techniques will show the thin fibro-cartilaginous disc that divides this synovial joint into an upper and lower compartment. Recently, CT has been used to delineate the soft tissues of the temporomandibular joint, but positioning is difficult for direct sagittal sections and the definition of reformatted images is not really adequate. Magnetic resonance has also been used to show the disc.

In the meantime, arthrography, although not widely used, can be performed to provide evidence of disc displacement, disc perforation or both. The examination is most helpful diagnostically in those cases which have little or no bony abnormality shown on the tomograms, but in which the clinical features nevertheless suggest disc derangement. Either or both joint spaces may be injected, but usually just the lower compartment is opacified (*Figure 17.22*), although disc

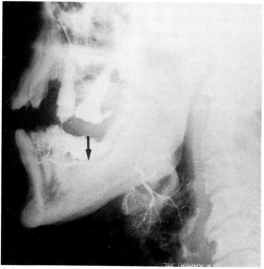

(a)

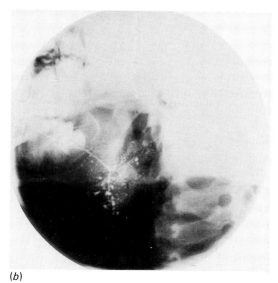

(b)

Figure 17.21 (a) Submandibular sialogram. The arrow points to the main duct. (b) Parotid sialogram with some degree of punctate sialectasis

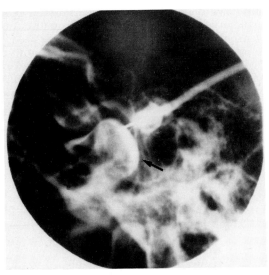

Figure 17.22 Temporomandibular joint arthrography. Contrast is in the inferior compartment (arrow). (Courtesy of Dr Ferraro)

perforation will allow the upper compartment to fill as well. Further elaboration of the technique can be achieved by use of tomography, double contrast (using air as well as water-soluble contrast agents), fluoroscopy and cineradiography.

Conclusions

The foregoing is an account of the imaging techniques which are, or can be, used in the practice of otolaryngology for the demonstration of normal and abnormal anatomy; for showing the situation and extent of disease processes; and, in some instances, for indicating the nature of the lesion. Few, if any, should be considered routine examinations, and they should be requested only after an adequate clinical examination has been made. Most hospitals in the UK have open access to radiographic facilities for general practitioners, but whether such otolaryngological radiographic investigations should be ordered by general practitioners is debatable. A barium swallow is perhaps the only satisfactory investigation that may be undertaken without a prior otolaryngological opinion. The most frequent examination requested is that of plain film views of the sinuses in cases referred from general practitioners, otolaryngologists and other specialities, for a variety of symptoms, some of which are quite non-specific. Clear sinus X-rays not uncommonly exist in the presence of a nasopharyngeal carcinoma; which can result in a false sense of security unless this is appreciated. The author believes that a radiological examination of the petrous bone

should be requested only by a specialist in this field. Radiographs of the cervical spine in the case of dizziness in an elderly patient serve no purpose.

The greatest change in the last 5 years has been the development of computerized tomography, particularly in the high resolution mode. Radiologists can now demonstrate not only the bony changes that are produced by abnormalities of the head and neck, but also the soft tissue changes. The deep extent of a lesion can be shown by CT and not just the encroachment on the adjacent lumen. CT is now the optimum imaging mode for most aspects of otolaryngolgy, although its widespread application is still limited by cost and availability of equipment. CT is the optimum means of showing the soft tissue and bone abnormalities in sinus disease and in the middle ear; however, the author continues to use polytomography on account of its unsurpassed demonstration of bone detail in the inner ear. Demonstration of enlargement of the internal auditory meatus is still the best screening investigation for small acoustic neuromata (schwannomata). High resolution CT is now becoming available at district general hospital level, and the greatly improved demonstration of bone and soft tissue structures in the head and neck gives an added impetus for radiologists and otolaryngologists to become familiar with the sectional anatomy displayed.

The subsidiary techniques listed previously have only occasional application in otolaryngology and, depending on availability, need to be used after discussion with a radiologist in the attempt to solve a specific problem. The latest computer-assisted methods can readily be used to measure certain properties of the normal and abnormal tissues being imaged, particularly X-ray attenuation by CT, and proton density and relaxation times by magnetic resonance. However, the attempts to chart a limited range of such values without overlap and to provide a means of 'tissue characterization' have so far proved largely unsuccessful.

What of the future of imaging in otolaryngology? The rapid advance of new technology during the last 5 years is indicative of certain trends. The limitations of plain radiographs, the cost of silver and the problems of storage of X-ray film probably mean that the traditional imaging methods will be used less. Tomographic methods will have increasing application. The demand for increasing the spatial resolution in CT means increasing the number of detectors and, simultaneously, the concomitant radiation exposure of the patient. A possible solution to this problem is provided by partial scanning. The mathematical reconstruction is made over a limited target volume or all detectors are directed towards a limited region of interest within the body, and only this region is scanned. The procedure reduces X-ray exposure, and all the detectors can be used to provide a high-resolution image of the scanned region. However, slice reconstruction does pose some problems. Another solution is to use imaging with non-ionizing radiation. The ionizing effect of X-rays restricts their usefulness in diagnostic imaging, in view of the need to limit the radiation exposure received by the patient. Hence all kinds of imaging with non-ionizing radiation are attractive alternatives, provided that acceptable image quality can be achieved. In this context, image quality mainly means spatial resolution, a process which for magnetic resonance is being rapidly improved, although, generally speaking, the latter remains inferior to CT.

Digital radiography, the manipulation of digital data storage and the retrieval of pictorial information, will be increasingly used as a consequence of the availability of powerful small computers, very fast dedicated image processors and large storage capacity. The latest digital storage media could be the nucleus of an overall information system within a hospital. This could incorporate one year's image storage. The picture source can be any kind of imaging system, such as CT or ultrasound, and even conventional X-ray film can be converted into digital data, making basements full of 'old films' a thing of the past.

References

ADAM, E. J., BERRY, R. J., CLITHEROW, S. and BEDFORD, A. (1984) Evaluation of the role of computed tomography in radiotherapy treatment planning. *Clinical Radiology*, **35**, 147

JULIAN, W. L., NOSCOE, N. J. and BERRY, R. J. (1981) Xeroradiographic tomography of the larynx. *Clinical Radiology*, **32**, 577

LLOYD, G. A. S. and PHELPS, P. D. (1986) The demonstration of tumours of the parapharyngeal space by magnetic resonance imaging. *British Journal of Radiology*, **59**, 675–683

MAFEE, M. F., VALVASSORI, G. E., SHUGAR, M. A., YANNIAS, D. A. and DOBBEN, G. D. (1983) High resolution and dynamic sequential computed tomography. *Archives of Otolaryngology*, **109**, 691

MAW, A. R., JEANS, W. D. and FERNANDO, D. C. J. (1981) Inter-observer variability in the clinical and radiological assessment of adenoid size, and the correlation with adenoid volume. *Clinical Otolaryngology*, **6**, 317

NOYEK, A. M. (1979) Bone scanning in otolaryngology. *The Laryngoscope*, **89** (Suppl. 18)

RADBERG, C. and THIBAUT, A. in collaboration with DELVAUX G. (1971) *Supine Skull Radiography with Orbix*. Sölna, Sweden: Elema Schonander AB

SOM, P. M. and SAUNDERS, D. E. (1984) The salivary glands. In *Head and Neck Imaging*, edited by R. T. Bergeron, A. G. Osborne, and P. M. Som, p. 186. St Louis: C. V. Mosby Co.

ZONNEVELD, F. W., VAN WAES, P. F. G. M., DAMSMA, H., RABISCHONG, P. and VIGNAUD, J. (1984) Direct multiplanar CT of the petrous bone. *Head and Neck Imaging*, **16**, 754–778

18

Basic immunology

Lee S. Rayfield and Stephen J. Challacombe

Immunology is the study of the immune system and has its historical foundations in the way the body combats infectious disease. Long before the principles of microbiology and immunology were understood, it had been recognized that not all individuals became ill during an epidemic, and that those who recovered were resistant to future outbreaks. This state was termed 'immunity', meaning exemption.

In order effectively to resist an invading organism, whether virus, bacterium, fungus, protozoan or worm, the immune system has to be able to distinguish between the body's own constituents ('self') and those of the invader ('non-self'). Normally an individual fails to respond to (is tolerant of) self, but in autoimmune disease this tolerance breaks down. In immunodeficiency there is a partial or complete failure of some part of the immune system, which results in recurrent, and sometimes life-threatening, infections. In transplantation reactions, the graft, which is desirable to the body, is nevertheless rejected because it is foreign.

Damage to the surrounding tissues during the course of an immune response may sometimes exceed the potential benefits. Such exaggerated responses are termed 'hypersensitivity reactions'.

As immunological processes are involved in the majority of human diseases, including those of the ear, nose and throat, an understanding of the cellular and molecular basis of the immune system is essential. This chapter summarizes fundamental immunological mechanisms and their role in defence and disease states.

Immunity to infection

The means by which the body protects itself from invasion and infection can be broadly classified into two types. Those where prior exposure to the particular organism enhances a second immune response, namely specific, acquired or adaptive immunity, and those which are only minimally affected, namely non-specific, innate or natural immunity. Innate immunity is the more primitive type and will be considered first.

Innate immunity

A variety of factors contribute to innate immunity. The most obvious obstacle to a potential invader is perhaps the physical barrier provided by the skin and mucous membranes. Although these surfaces are by no means impervious, the severe infections found in patients suffering from burns show just how important this primary mechanical barrier is. Secretions which bathe mucosal surfaces, cleanse and hamper colonization by microorganisms. The cilia of the lungs and the motility of the gastrointestinal tract contribute to expulsion. A number of inhibitory or microbicidal substances are present on the skin and in seromucous secretions, including lactic acid, saturated and unsaturated fatty acids and basic polypeptides.

In saliva and milk, lactoferrin inhibits bacterial growth by chelating the available iron. Lactoperoxidase, in the presence of hydrogen peroxide and thiocyanate ions, kills bacteria. Lysozyme is an enzyme which splits the mucopeptides of the bacterial cell wall by cleaving N-acetylmuramic acid from N-acetylglucosamine. It is found in tears, nasal secretions, saliva, blood and on the skin. Lysozyme is particularly toxic to Gram-positive bacteria, and it can also kill Gram-negative organisms if the cell wall is damaged to allow the enzyme access.

Non-pathogenic, commensal or symbiotic organisms constitute the normal mucosal flora. In addition to providing essential nutrients (for example vitamin K), they prevent colonization by virulent organisms through competition or by the production of microbicidal agents.

If a potentially pathogenic organism breaches the external barriers and enters the blood, two vital second lines of non-specific defence are provided by phagocytic cells and the complement system.

Phagocytic cells

Phagocytosis (literally 'cell-eating') involves the recognition, engulfment, killing and digestion of particulate matter. The latter may be whole cells or debris, and of foreign or host origin; phagocytes are thus not only defenders but also scavengers. The task is principally undertaken by two, morphologically distinct populations of bone-marrow derived leucocytes. Neutrophils are part of the granulocyte lineage and comprise between 45 and 70% of the adult leucocyte population. They are short-lived, lasting about 2 days, and have a high turnover rate in the bone marrow. They have a diameter of 12–14 µm and a characteristic multilobed nucleus. Within the cytoplasm there are many azurophilic granules (lysosomes), which hold a battery of proteolytic and hydrolytic enzymes (*Figure 18.1a*).

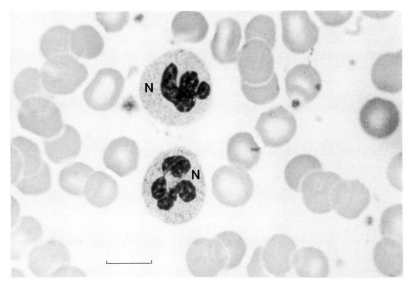

(a)

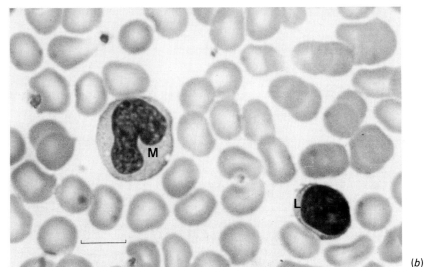

(b)

Figure 18.1 Blood films stained by May–Grunwald/Giemsa method. (*a*) Neutrophils (N); (*b*) monocyte (M) and a lymphocyte (L). Scale measures 10 µm. (Courtesy of Dr V. Sljivic)

In contrast to neutrophils, which are relatively uniform in appearance, the second group of phagocytes, monocytes and macrophages, form a heterogeneous collection of cell types. Both monocytes and macrophages derive from a common precursor, the promonocyte, but the macrophage is generally regarded as a terminally differentiated cell.

Fixed tissue macrophages comprise the mononuclear phagocyte system or reticuloendothelial system and function as an extremely effective filter. The Kupffer cells of the liver, alveolar and peritoneal macrophages, histiocytes of the skin, sinusoidal lining cells of the spleen, bone osteoclasts and, possibly, the microglia of the brain all belong to the mononuclear phagocyte system. Monocytes and macrophages are long-lived, having a lifespan of many weeks. They range in size from 15 to 40 μm and possess potent cytocidal and digestive substances within the small membranous lysosomes of the cytoplasm. Monocytes make up between 2 and 8% of normal peripheral blood leucocytes and are distinguished by their indented, horseshoe-shaped nucleus (*Figure 18.1b*).

Stages in phagocytosis

Phagocytosis can be divided into several distinct phases (*Figure 18.2*).

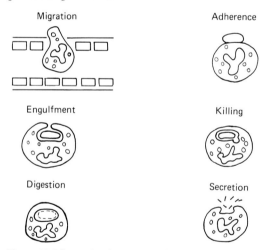

Figure 18.2 Stages in phagocytosis by neutrophils, monocytes and macrophages

Migration

Blood-borne neutrophils and monocytes are attracted to sites of inflammation where the integrity of the tissues has been disturbed and a variety of pharmacological mediators have been activated, including chemotactic factors (*see below*). Vasoactive substances, such as histamine and serotonin (5-hydroxytryptamine), cause the blood vessels to become leaky and facilitate the adherence of phagocytes to the endothelium. The phagocytes form pseudopodia, which push between the endothelial cells and allow the cell to squeeze through the vessel wall.

Adherence

Contact between the particle to be engulfed and the phagocyte results in adherence to the cell membrane. This adherence may be greatly enhanced by the presence of opsonins, which coat the particle and bind to specific receptors on the phagocyte surface (*see below*). In the absence of opsonins, adherence most probably results from electrostatic interactions between particle and membrane. Whatever the nature of the binding, adherence triggers a metabolic or respiratory burst and the formation of a plethora of oxygen-dependent and highly microbicidal agents within the lysosomes.

Engulfment

Spreading of the initial site of attachment to the cell continues until the particle is completely surrounded by membrane. This is then pinched off to form an intracellular vacuole known as a phagosome.

Killing

The lysosomes fuse with the phagosome to form a phagolysosome, releasing toxic and digestive substances into the vacuole. Of the oxygen-dependent mechanisms activated during the respiratory burst, the generation of hydrogen peroxide (H_2O_2) and the formation of free oxygen radicals, such as superoxide anions (O_2^-), singlet oxygen ($^1O_2$) and hydroxyl groups (OH), are perhaps the most significant.

Digestion

Breakdown of phagocytosed particles may be brought about by the action of hydrogen peroxide and myeloperoxidase, and by proteolytic and hydrolytic enzymes.

Secretion

Following killing and digestion, the contents of the phagolysosome are expelled from the cell after fusion with the cell membrane. Macrophages, but not neutrophils, may retain some of the breakdown products on the cell membrane and present them to lymphocytes (this interaction will be dealt with more fully later). The secretion of active enzymes or radicals may cause damage to other microorganisms that have not been phagocytosed. However, local tissue damage may also result.

The complement system

The complement system consists of a series of glycoproteins (*Table 18.1*) that circulate in the extracellular fluid compartment. They participate in a triggered enzyme cascade which comprises an initiation phase, amplification and the assembly of a membrane attack sequence. It involves a precise, sequential activation of inactive components, called proenzymes. These, in turn, act enzymatically on components further along the pathway and cause the release of biologically active portions of the components (cleavage fragments). The process is one of amplification because an initial stimulus can cause the activation of millions of later components.

There are two major pathways of complement activation: the classical pathway, which was discovered first, and the alternative pathway, which is probably the more primitive phylogenetically. Both pathways lead to the formation of an enzyme (convertase) which splits the third complement component C3, the lynch-pin of the complement system. Both pathways also share a terminal sequence (or attack sequence) involving the components designated C5, C6, C7, C8 and C9. Biologically, the triggering of the complement cascade by either pathway leads to the activation of cells, opsonization and the lysis of complement coated cells. A simplified representation of the cascade is shown in *Figure 18.3*.

Complement activation by the classical pathway

The components of complement that take part in the classical pathway are C1, C4, C2 and C3 (*Figure 18.3a*) – because the numbers were assigned to the components as they were discovered, the activation sequence does not follow the numerical order. Furthermore, C1 consists of three subunits: C1q, C1r and C1s. The major initiating stimulus for the classical pathway is the binding of C1q to an antigen–antibody complex. However, in the absence of antibody the pathway can be activated by lipid A – a constituent of the cell wall of certain bacteria – and by the envelope of oncornaviruses.

Table 18.1 Components of the complement system

Pathway	Component	Fragments	Molecular weight (kilodaltons)	Activity
Classical	C1q		410	Binds to C1r and C1q receptors on T and B cells
	C1r		170	Activates C1s
	C1s		85	With C1q and r cleaves C4 and C2
	C4		210	
		C4a	10	Anaphylatoxin
		C4b	200	Complexed with C2b splits C3, weak immune adherence via CR1
	C2		115	
		C2a	35	None
		C2b	80	Complexed with C4b splits C3
Alternative	Factor B		93	Binds to C3b
		Ba	30	? None
		Bb	63	Complexes with C3b to form convertase
	Factor D		25	Cleaves factor B
	Properdin		184	Stabilizes C3bBb complex
Terminal common pathway	C3		195	
		C3a	9	Anaphylatoxin
		C3b	186	Immune adherence via CR1 on phagocytes
	C5		205	
		C5a	11	Anaphylatoxin, chemotaxin
		C5b	195	
	C6		128	Binds to C5b
	C7		121	Binds to C5bC6, complex attaches to lipid membranes
	C8		155	Polymerizes C9
	C9		75	Forms channel in membrane
Regulation	C1 INH		100	Inhibits C1r and C1s
	Factor H		150	Competes with factor B
	Factor I (C3 INA)		100	Converts C3b to inactive C3bi

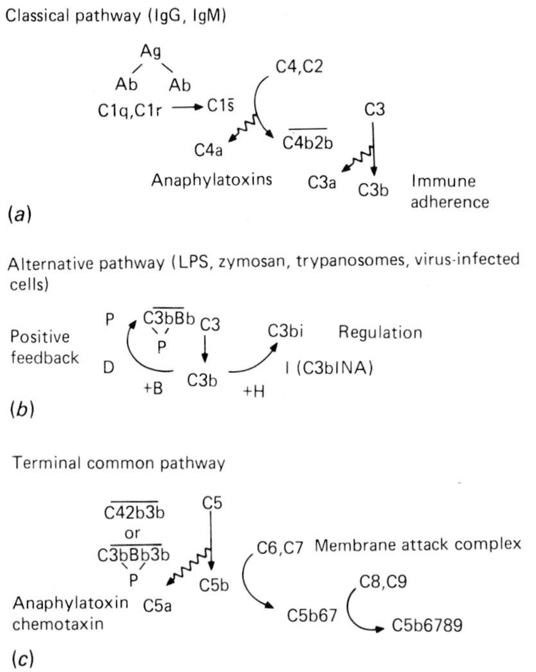

Classical pathway (IgG, IgM)

(a)

Alternative pathway (LPS, zymosan, trypanosomes, virus-infected cells)

(b)

Terminal common pathway

(c)

Figure 18.3 The activation of complement. A bar over a component, by convention, indicates an active enzyme. (Adapted from K. A. Joiner, E. J. Brown and M. Frank (1984) *Annual Review of Immunology*, Vol. 2, pp. 461–491)

Once activated, C1q converts C1r to an enzymatically active molecule capable of activating C1s. The $\overline{C1q,r,s}$ complex (also known as C1 esterase, $\overline{C1s}$) binds and cleaves C4 into two: a large fragment C4b, which can covalently couple with the surface of a particle, and a smaller fragment C4a. C4b will bind C2 which is then cleaved by C1 esterase to produce a complex of C4b2b. It is this complex which acts as the C3 convertase.

C3, the most abundant of the complement components, is split into two fragments, C3a and C3b (*see Table 18.1* and *Figure 18.3a*). The smaller fragment, C3a, is a peptide which causes the degranulation of mast cells and the consequent release of a variety of pharmacologically active substances. These include histamine, serotonin, a slow-reacting substance of anaphylaxis (SRS-A now renamed leukotriene C) and eosinophil chemotactic factor. C3a is termed an anaphylatoxin because of its effect on mast cells (*see* section on hypersensitivity). C3a causes smooth muscle contraction, both directly and through the substances released by mast cells, and the release of hydrolytic enzymes from neutrophils. It has recently been found that C4a also has anaphylatoxic properties.

Immune adherence

C3b, the larger cleavage fragment of C3, can covalently couple with cell surfaces around the site of complement activation. Such an interaction can lead to the cleavage of more C3 by the alternative pathway (*see below*). Bound C3b is the ligand for a receptor found on the surface of phagocytic cells – the C3b receptor (also known as CR1). Particles coated with C3b are therefore readily phagocytosed by neutrophils and macrophages and are said to be opsonized (made ready for eating). Binding of C3b opsonized particles to the C3b receptor is called immune adherence.

The C4b2b complex is not very efficient in activating C3 but many hundreds of molecules are split by a single complex because of the abundance of C3 in plasma. However, only one C3b molecule combines directly with C4b2b to activate C5 and initiate the terminal sequence.

Complement activation by the alternative pathway

C3 spontaneously degrades to C3b in the plasma at a low level. In the presence of an initiator of the alternative pathway, the following events take place (*see Figure 18.3b*). C3b binds to factor B to produce a C3bB complex. This is susceptible to the action of another enzyme called factor D. Cleavage of factor B leaves a potent C3 convertase, C3bBb, capable of fixing additional C3b to the activating surface which leads subsequently to the formation of more C3bBb. As the formation of C3b by the alternative pathway produces more C3b, there is said to be positive feedback. The C3bBb complex is stabilized by another cofactor, properdin, which increases the half-life of the molecule from about 5 to 30 minutes.

Positive feedback by C3b to create more C3b would clearly exhaust C3, and later components of the pathway, if left unchecked. To prevent this happening there are a number of regulatory proteins (*see Table 18.1*). Factor H binds to C3b and inhibits its interaction with factor B; factor I (or C3b-INA) then rapidly cleaves the C3b to produce an inactive C3bi fragment. Although incapable of activating further C3, the C3bi is still bound to the activating surface and can interact with C3bi receptors (termed CR3), on the surface of the phagocytes. Further slow, proteolytic digestion eventually leads to a C3d fragment remaining on the surface.

The alternative pathway is initiated by cell wall polysaccharides of yeast (zymosan) and Gram-negative bacteria (lipopolysaccharide or endotoxin), bacterial dextrans and levans, parasites such as trypanosomes and schistosomes, and some virally transformed cells.

The terminal sequence of complement activation

Activation of the terminal complement components C5–C9 (*see Figure 18.3c* and *Table 18.1*) results in the formation of a membrane attack complex. This causes cell lysis when inserted in the lipid bilayer of cell membranes. The first step in this common pathway is the cleavage of C5 by the C4b2b3b convertase, classical, or the C3bBb properdin convertase, alternative, to generate C5b and C5a fragments (*see Figure 18.3c*). The smaller fragment, C5a, is a potent anaphylatoxin and has similar effects to C3a. In addition, C5a is itself chemotactic and attracts granulocytes and monocytes. The large fragment, C5b, associates with C6 to form a C5b6 complex which can non-covalently interact with biological membranes. C7 is then added to the complex.

It is possible for the C5b67 complex to become attached to membranes distinct from the activator surface where the complement system has been triggered. This can lead to the fixation of a membrane attack complex on bystander cells (reactive lysis). Membrane bound C5b67 binds one molecule of C8 and six of C9; although fixation of C8 can bring about some lysis, the addition of C9 vastly increases its efficiency. The final components (C8 and C9) result in the formation of a channel through the lipid bilayer and perturbation of osmotic stability.

The role of complement and phagocytic cells

Although phagocytes are perhaps the humblest of the cells involved in immunity, they have a central role in virtually all types of immune response, as will become clear in later sections. Deficiencies in one or both classes of phagocytic cells lead to recurrent and life-threatening infections (*see* section on immunodeficiency). Nevertheless, in isolation, neutrophils and monocytes remove blood-borne parasites only poorly and certain microorganisms have developed antiphagocytic properties.

Many bacteria possess hydrophobic capsules which fail to adhere to the phagocyte cell membrane; often only the encapsulated variants of a bacterial species are virulent. These capsules may be polysaccharide in nature (for example pneumococci) or composed of polypeptides (for example *Bacillus anthracis*). The M-protein found on the surface of β-haemolytic streptococci (*Streptococcus pyogenes*) is antiphagocytic, and the production of coagulase by *Staphylococcus aureus* (*Staph. pyogenes*) promotes the deposition of fibrin around the bacterium. Lipoprotein antigens of the plague bacillus *Yersinia pestis* and lipopolysaccharides in the cell wall of *Salmonella typhi* also inhibit adherence to the phagocyte membrane.

Activation of the alternative pathway of complement by cell wall constituents greatly enhances phagocytosis. The specific interactions between complement receptors, notably CR1, and opsonized particles are far more effective than electrostatic interactions. Furthermore, the release of inflammatory and chemotactic factors facilitate migration and intra- and extracellular killing.

Although phagocytic cells in combination with complement form a formidable barrier to invading organisms, they cannot deal with parasites which fail to activate complement or adhere to the phagocyte membrane; nor can they deal adequately with organisms which produce toxins or are resistant to the killing mechanisms of the phagocytes and take up residence with the cell, such as mycobacteria.

It is the adaptive or acquired immune system which meets this threat and provides a means by which any potential invader can be recognized and eliminated.

Acquired immunity

Acquired immune responses have the following characteristics:

(1) they show memory – initial exposure to an infectious organism leads to a primary response; encountering the organism again produces an accelerated secondary response which persists (*Figure 18.4*)
(2) they show specificity – the development of resistance following exposure to one organism does not confer resistance to unrelated organisms
(3) they can be divided into responses which are mediated by humoral factors (antibodies) and those mediated by specifically sensitized cells.

In practice, development of resistance generally involves both types of response, although the relative importance of antibody or cell-mediated immunity varies for individual organisms.

Antibody-mediated immunity

The structure of antibodies

Antibodies are proteins (immunoglobulins) found predominantly in the γ-globulin fraction of serum. There are five major classes of immunoglobulin (Ig): G, A, M, D and E. Although there are differences in molecular size, serum concentration, valency and function, the basic structure of these classes is similar, consisting of four chains: two identical heavy chains and two identical light chains (*Figure 18.5*). The heavy chain distinguishes the particular Ig classes and is denoted by a Greek

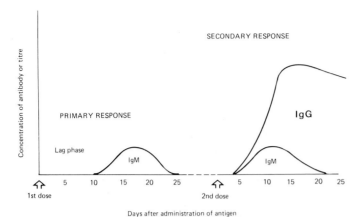

Figure 18.4 Production of immunoglobulins during primary and secondary immune responses

letter (*Table 18.2*). The heavy (H) chains are composed of three (IgG, IgA, IgD) or four (IgM, IgE) constant domains (C_H) and a single variable domain (V_H). These domains each comprise a loop of about 110 amino acid residues with an intrachain disulphide bond. As the name implies, constant domains are identical from one Ig molecule to another, provided that the molecules are of the same type.

Interchain disulphide bonds link heavy chains with one another and with light (L) chains; the precise number varies with different Ig classes. Light chains possess only two domains, one constant (C_L) and one variable (V_L); two kinds of L chain class exist, kappa (κ) and lambda (λ), and either one may associate with an H chain to form a functional Ig molecule.

Some Ig classes have subclasses (*see Table 18.2*) that contain slightly different amino acid sequences within their C regions. Four subclasses of human IgG, two of IgA and two of IgM have been recognized. Another name given to Ig classes and subclasses is isotype.

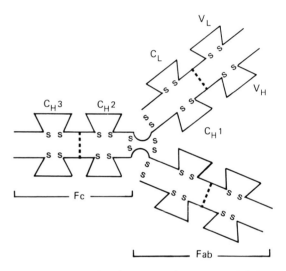

Figure 18.5 Generalized structure of an immunoglobulin molecule, based on human IgG1. The portion where the disulphide bonds hold the H chains together is the hinge region. The dotted lines mark the extent of the domains

Table 18.2 Immunoglobulin isotypes

Class	Heavy chain	Light chain	Molecular structure	Subclasses	Average molecular weight (daltons)	Concentration in serum (mg/ml)	Serum Ig (%)	Average half-life (days)
IgG	γ	κ or λ	H_2L_2	4	150 000	8–16	70–75	20–21 (7 for IgG3)
IgA	α	κ or λ	H_2L_2 $(H_2L_2)_2$ $(H_2L_2)_3$	2	160 000	1.5–4	15–20	6
IgM	μ	κ or λ	$(H_2L_2)_5$	2	900 000	0.5–2	10	10
IgD	δ	κ or λ	H_2L_2	1	160 000	0–0.4	1	3
IgE	ε	κ or λ	H_2L_2	1	170 000	<0.0005	trace	2

Variable regions

Although antibodies of a single isotype are virtually identical in terms of protein structure, they are capable of binding to a wide range of different antigens – an antigen being defined here as any substance to which an antibody can bind. This discrimination is a function of the V regions, and variation between molecules of the same subclass is known as idiotypic variation.

It is the idiotype which determines the specificity for antigen. A comparison of the amino acid sequences of several different V regions highlights defined areas, called complementarity determining regions or hypervariable regions. These areas show the greatest variation and provide the molecular basis for interaction with antigen.

Fc and Fab fragments

IgG molecules can be cleaved into fragments by certain enzymes. Papain splits the molecules into three: two antigen-binding fragments (Fab) which retain the capacity to recognize antigen, and a third crystallizable 'tail' fragment (Fc; *see Figure 18.5*). The Fab fragments are dimers of H and L chain constant and variable regions; Fc fragments are dimers of the second and third constant regions Cγ2 and Cγ3. Pepsin cleaves IgG to leave a F(ab')$_2$ fragment, two Fab fragments linked by the disulphide bridges at the hinge region; the rest of the molecule is degraded into small peptides.

Functions of immunoglobulins

These can be divided into Fab dependent and Fc dependent (or adjunctive) properties.

Binding of Fab portions of an Ig molecule to antigenic determinants (epitopes) on distinct particles leads to the formation of aggregates. If the epitopes are present on whole cells, this leads to agglutination; if the epitopes are on soluble elements, formation of large complexes leads to precipitation. Some bacteria, including the causative agents of diphtheria (*Corynebacterium diphtheriae*), tetanus (*Clostridium tetani*), cholera (*Vibrio cholerae*) and scarlet fever (*Strep. pyogenes*) produce toxins which cause local or systemic pathological changes. Immunoglobulins neutralize toxins by blocking the active site, either directly or by inducing a conformational change in the toxin molecule. Neutralization is also important in preventing infection, in this case the site of action is the receptor of the virus or bacterium for cell surface structures (for example influenza virus haemagglutinin). The adjunctive properties of Ig molecules depend upon an intact Fc region and vary with isotype (*see below*).

Complement fixation by way of the classical pathway is initiated, following antigen-binding, when two or more Fc regions are in close proximity. Receptors for the Fc portions facilitate phagocytosis (opsonize), allow cells to bind to antigen and release cytotoxic or inflammatory agents, and permit the passive transfer of antibody (IgG) from mother to fetus.

Role of different immunoglobulin isotypes

IgG is the principal Ig species found in blood and the extracellular spaces. Of the four human IgG subclasses, it is IgG1, IgG3 and, to a lesser extent, IgG2 which activate complement through the classical pathway and bind to the Fcγ receptor on phagocytic cells; IgG can thus opsonize directly or through the generation of C3b. A population of leucocytes, defined functionally as K cells (for killer), can attach by way of Fcγ receptors to IgG-coated cells and, through the release of cytotoxins, bring about cell lysis. The phenomenon has been termed antibody-dependent cellular cytotoxicity, or ADCC for short. In addition to K cells, neutrophils and monocytes, eosinophils and platelets bear receptors for antigen-bound IgG and can cause damage to opsonized microorganisms by the release of cytotoxic agents, enzymes or mediators of inflammation. IgG is the only Ig class to be transferred across the placenta (*see* section on passive immunization) and is generally the major immunoglobulin synthesized during a secondary immune response (*see Figure 18.4*).

IgA is the second most abundant Ig in blood where it is found mainly as a monomer, although about 15% is present as dimers and trimers: two or three IgA molecules of identical antigen specificity are joined together at the Fc region by J chain, a 15 kilodalton (kD) polypeptide. There are two subclasses of IgA. In blood, IgA1 represents about 80% of the total IgA, but in secretions, IgA2 is predominant (about 60%). The functions of serum IgA are unclear, but may be immunoregulatory as many IgG functions can be modulated by serum IgA.

IgA in secretions differs from serum IgA and is called secretory IgA (SIgA). The IgA molecules in secretions are almost entirely dimeric and are independent of serum IgA. Sometimes referred to as mucosal paint, SIgA antibodies are found in the secretions covering mucosal surfaces, including gastric, bronchial and nasal secretions, colostrum, milk, tears and saliva. In viral infections of the middle ear, the concentration of specific IgA is two to six times higher than that of the IgG.

In addition to J chain, dimers of secretory IgA (*Figure 18.6*) are complexed with another protein, namely the 70 kD secretory component (SC or secretory piece), which is synthesized by epithelial cells and acts as a vehicle for the transport of IgA

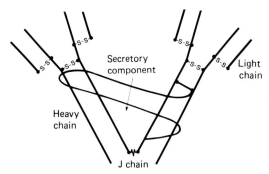

Figure 18.6 Schematic structure of a secretory IgA molecule showing the J chain and secretory component

from serum to mucosa (*see* section on the secretory immune system).

SIgA does not rely on opsonization or complement fixation for its biological activity; its main actions are neutralization of viruses, inhibition of adherence and growth of microorganisms on epithelial and other surfaces, neutralization of toxins, and antigen exclusion by preventing the access of antigen to the systemic immune system.

IgM exists in the blood as a pentamer and is the largest Ig species, sometimes known as macroglobulin, and diffuses only poorly into extravascular spaces. Its high valency for antigen and the proximity of five Fc portions make IgM antibodies very efficient agglutinins and activators of the classical complement pathway. During a primary response, IgM is the major class of Ig synthesized (*see Figure 18.4*). The five monomers in IgM are joined by a single J chain. IgM can be complexed with secretory component and act as a secretory antibody.

IgD is a monomeric Ig found at a low concentration in the blood. Its principal role appears to be as a cell surface receptor on the antibody forming cell (*see below*).

IgE is normally found in only trace amounts (*see Table 18.2*), but in certain conditions, such as atopic allergy or during the course of infection with a parasitic worm, the level may be raised. Mast cells and basophils possess Fcε receptors which bind monomeric IgE molecules. This stabilization of the IgE increases its half-life from 2.5 days to around 12 weeks. Cross-linking, brought about by the simultaneous binding of antigen to adjacent IgE molecules, causes the rapid release of the contents of cytoplasmic granules into the surrounding medium. This is termed 'degranulation'. The vasoactive and inflammatory constituents include histamine, serotonin, eosinophil chemotactic factor, platelet aggregating factor and slow reacting substance of anaphylaxis (SRS-A) (*see also* section on hypersensitivity). Eosinophils also possess Fcε receptors

and can bind to IgE-coated worms in the gut and contribute to parasite expulsion. IgE, like IgA, seems to play a major role in protecting external surfaces.

Some tests for antigen and antibody reactions

Precipitation of immune complexes forms the basis of some immunological tests for antibody or antigen, as outlined in *Figure 18.7*. If an antigen has two or more epitopes, antibody can cross-link antigen molecules. In gross antigen excess, each Fab binds to a separate antigen and causes formation of small complexes. As the concentration of antibody is increased, bigger, insoluble complexes form. At equivalence, all the antigen and antibody are complexed in a lattice structure. At antibody excess, the complexes tend to become smaller and more soluble because antibody fails to cross-link epitopes on different antigen molecules.

A rather different type of test for detecting antibody is the complement fixation test which is performed in two stages. In the first stage, the test serum is serially diluted and a constant amount of antigen is added, together with a source of complement. In the second stage, following incubation, antibody-coated red blood cells are added to indicate whether complement has been consumed in the first stage. If there is sufficient complement, these indicator cells will be lysed. If they are not, complement components must have been exhausted in the first stage by the formation of immune complexes. Hence antibody must have

Double diffusion (Ouchterlony method)

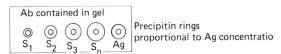

Single radial diffusion (Mancini method)

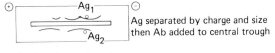

Immunoelectrophoresis

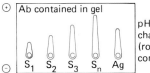

Rocket electrophoresis

Figure 18.7 Some tests for antigen and antibody reactions

been present in the test serum. Radioimmunoassay and enzyme-linked immunosorbent assay (ELISA) techniques, which are extremely useful, are described in the section on diagnosis of autoimmune disease.

B lymphocytes and the synthesis of immunoglobulins

Antibodies are produced by lymphocytes; that is by B lymphocytes, which differentiate, at least in mammals, in the bone marrow. The earliest B lymphocytes, pre-B cells, possess IgM molecules within the cytoplasm. Immature or primary B cells have both cytoplasmic and surface membrane-bound (monomeric rather than pentameric) IgM. The latter functions as a receptor for antigen because the antigen-binding Fab regions are exposed to the external environment. The genes on only one of the two parental chromosomes are transcribed (allelic exclusion) and each B lymphocyte is committed to synthesizing immunoglobulin molecules with a single specificity. Mature B lymphocytes express IgM and IgD and possibly one other from IgG, IgA or IgE. All of the isotypes expressed as receptors have the same specificity for antigen.

During primary stimulation with antigen, mature B lymphocytes expand clonally to produce more cells capable of producing antibody. Some of the cells transform into plasma cells which are end cells and which secrete large quantities of immunoglobulin. There may be a switch in the class of Ig produced before the plasma cell is formed so that an isotype other than IgM is synthesized. A proportion of the B lymphocytes develop into memory cells which, on re-exposure to antigen, permit a more rapid response than unprimed cells (*see Figure 18.4*).

Monoclonal antibodies

The fusion of a B lymphocyte with a tumour derived from a plasma cell (plasmacytoma) has made it possible to create antibody secreting cells (hybridoma) which will divide indefinitely in culture and produce vast amounts of completely pure, monospecific antibody. These monoclonal antibodies have revolutionized diagnostic and research procedures because of their specificity, lack of batch-to-batch variation and ease of production.

The secretory or mucosal immune system

Many of the mucous membranes of the body are constantly exposed to microorganisms, and the secretions which bathe epithelial surfaces play a major role in the local defence against such microorganisms (*see* previous section). The secretory immune system is a system of local immunity which protects mucosal surfaces and which can be stimulated independently of systemic immunity.

The system comprises the secretions which bathe the mucous membranes of the body and their associated glands. The organs involved include the eyes, middle ear, salivary glands, lungs, gastrointestinal tracts, genitourinary tract and the mammary glands. Specialized lymphoid tissue is associated with the secretory system in the gut (gut-associated lymphoid tissue or GALT) and in the lungs (bronchial-associated lymphoid tissue or BALT; *see* section on lymphoid tissues).

Stimulation of the secretory immune system

Antibodies can be induced in secretions by local immunization or, alternatively, by stimulation of gut-associated lymphoid tissue either by ingestion of antigen, or by deposition in the small bowel. Antigen in the gut leads to the release of IgA precursor cells from Peyer's patches, which selectively migrate to (or are selectively retained in) mucosal tissues. These IgA plasma cell precursors are released into the local lymphatics where they migrate sequentially to the mesenteric lymph nodes, to the thoracic duct and into the blood stream, before migrating to the lamina propria of the gut and other secretory tissues, including the mammary glands. Local immunization leads to a proliferation of these cells, recruitment of others and an enhanced local SIgA response.

Synthesis and transport of SIgA

Plasma cells in the lamina propria (the connective tissue adjacent to the epithelium) secrete dimeric IgA, including one unit of J chain. This molecule has an affinity for secretory component which is produced by, and found on, the cell membrane of the epithelial cells. The secretory component acts as a receptor for dimeric but not monomeric IgA. The whole complex is taken up into the cells and secreted into the lumen of the gland as SIgA (*see* section on secretory IgA). The secretory component confers a resistance to proteolysis on the IgA, which probably allows it to function in a hostile environment for longer periods.

Cell-mediated immunity

Although antibody provides an effective adaptive defence mechanism in the blood, in extracellular fluid and at the external surfaces, it is virtually ineffective once a microorganism has established intracellular residence. In the case of budding viruses, antibody may control the level of viraemia but it cannot eradicate the source. Macrophages and monocytes may provide a habitat for bacterial or protozoal parasites that are not killed during phagocytosis. The cell-mediated arm of the acquired immune system is suited to deal with intracellular parasites.

T lymphocytes and antigen recognition

The term 'cell-mediated' has been applied to immunity which is transferable with living cells, but not with serum from sensitized animals, and is mediated by lymphocytes that have differentiated under the influence of the thymus. These T lymphocytes, like B lymphocytes, are specific for a single antigen. Stimulation of T cells transforms them into activated T lymphocytes or lymphoblasts which have a much higher cytoplasm:nucleus ratio, a lower density and a greater diameter. Memory T cells are also generated during the course of clonal expansion.

In contrast to B lymphocytes, T lymphocytes neither recognize nor bind to antigen directly. They require the antigen to be presented on another cell in association with products of the major histocompatibility complex (MHC) which function as markers of self-identity. This major histocompatibility complex restriction enables sensitized T lymphocytes to distinguish cells which bear foreign antigens from those which are free from infection. (A special case where T cells do not require the presence of self-histocompatibility markers is the recognition of tissue transplants, and this will be discussed later.)

The receptor for antigen is not Ig but a structurally related polypeptide dimer formed between non-identical α and β chains, each of 40–50 kD in size. Both chains comprise a constant region, shared between T cells of different specificities, and a variable region which determines antigen/major histocompatibility complex specificity. A third glycoprotein complex, T3, is required for insertion of the αβ heterodimer into the cell membrane.

T lymphocytes confer immunity through the production of lymphokines and the generation of cytotoxic cells.

Lymphokines is the generic term given to a variety of T-lymphocyte products (factors), which recruit other cell types, modulate their action or lead to cell lysis (*Table 18.3*). Chemotactic factors attract monocytes and macrophages, and migration inhibition factors ensure that the recruited cells stay in the locality. Gamma interferon and macrophage-activating factor greatly enhance the capacity of macrophages to engulf and kill microorganisms; these lymphokine-activated cells are called angry macrophages. Transmission of virus particles between cells is blocked by the action of interferon and the cytotoxic potential of natural killer cells (*see below*) is increased. T cells themselves release lymphotoxins which kill some kinds of tumour cells.

T lymphocytes provide the main resistance to infections with obligate or facultative intracellular bacteria and protozoans, and to fungi. Organisms such as the tubercle and leprosy bacilli, *Brucella*, *Legionella* and *Toxoplasma* spp. are all susceptible to destruction by lymphokine-activated macrophages. In chronic infections, aggregates of macrophages form foci called granuloma.

Cytotoxic T lymphocytes are generated in response to viral infection or following the transplantation of histoincompatible tissue grafts. Cytotoxic T lymphocytes bind specifically to the infected or foreign cells and cause lysis.

The distinction between the two arms of the acquired immune response is useful in defining which protective mechanisms are most relevant in the case of particular infections. However, in the majority of infections, humoral and cell-mediated immunity both play a role in eliminating the organism (*Figure 18.8*), and this is most apparent when the regulatory interactions between T and B lymphocytes are examined. For this it is necessary to understand, in more detail, the role of the major histocompatibility complex.

Table 18.3 A few lymphokines and their functions

Lymphokine	Function
Migration inhibition factor (MIF)	Localizes monocytes/macrophages at the antigenic site
Macrophage-activating factor (MAF)	Enhances phagocytic properties (probably identical to γ-interferon)
Chemotactic factor for macrophages (CFM)	Recruits monocytes/macrophages to antigenic site
Leucocyte inhibition factor (LIF)	Localizes neutrophils and other granulocytes
Interleukin 2 (IL-2)	Regulates T-lymphocyte, and possibly B-lymphocyte, responses
B-cell growth factors	Regulate B-lymphocyte differentiation and antibody production
Lymphotoxin	Kills some types of tumour cell
γ-Interferon	Activates macrophages, regulates T- and B-lymphocyte responses

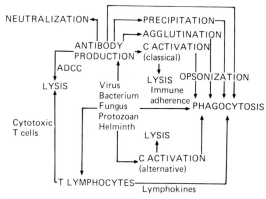

Figure 18.8 The interrelationship between various immune mechanisms

Cellular interactions between lymphocytes

The major histocompatibility complex

If skin grafts are transplanted between non-identical members of a species (allografts) or between members of different species (xeno-grafts), there is an immunological reaction which results in destruction of the graft. Those antigens eliciting the strongest reactions are encoded by the major histocompatibility complex of a species, which in man is designated HLA, for human leucocyte antigen, and is located on the short arm of chromosome 6. The HLA is a complex because several genes or loci are clustered together over a relatively short distance (*Figure 18.9*). The complex can be divided into regions and subregions which encode functionally or biochemically distinguishable molecules.

Class I and class II histocompatibility molecules

The HLA-A, -B, and -C loci all code for class I histocompatibility molecules (*see Figure 18.9*). Structurally, they are composed of a 44-kD heavy α chain which associates with a light chain, β_2 microglobulin, encoded by a gene on chromosome 15. Class I α chains possess three, Ig-like domains (*see Figure 18.9*) and are found on almost all nucleated cells, but they are absent from human erythrocytes.

The HLA-D region, containing DP, DQ and DR subregions, codes for class II histocompatibility molecules. These are integral, membrane-bound dimers formed between a 34-kD α chain and a 29-kD β chain; each chain has two domains (*see Figure 18.9*). DP,DQ and DR subregions contain genes for both α and β chains but the products only associate with complementary chains from the same subregion – for example DPα forms dimers with DPβ but not with DQβ or DRβ. Products of the subregions are codominantly expressed on selective cell types which are, in general, cells of the immune system – principally B lymphocytes, macrophages and other antigen presenting cells (*see below*) – and activated T cells. Gamma interferon induces class II expression on some cell types, such as thyrocytes. The class II histocompatibility molecules are sometimes referred to as I-region associated, Ia, antigens by analogy with the equivalent molecules in the mouse. The genes for classical and alternative complement components C2, C4 and factor B (Bf) are also found within the HLA complex and have been termed 'class III histocompatibility molecules'. They have no clear role in cellular recognition by T lymphocytes and are unrelated to the class I and class II molecules.

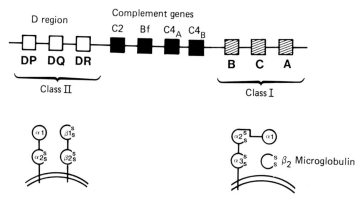

Figure 18.9 The HLA complex on chromosome 6 and the molecular structure of class I and class II histocompatibility antigens

Detection of major histocompatibility antigens

Individuals who have received deliberate or therapeutic blood transfusions develop antibodies to the histocompatibility antigens on leucocytes. Repeated pregnancies by the same father immunize mothers to paternal antigens carried by the fetus. By using such antisera, polymorphic forms of class I or II molecules can be serologically defined.

Class II antigens can also be detected by culturing lymphocytes from one individual with those of another, to form a mixed lymphocyte culture (MLC). If the cells express different class II antigens, the result will be a mixed lymphocyte reaction (MLR) and a clonal expansion of the reactive T cells. The reaction can be made one-way if the lymphocytes from one donor are pre-treated so that they cannot proliferate. The magnitude of proliferation can be quantified by the addition of tritiated thymidine, which is taken up in dividing but not in static cells. Polymorphisms in class II antigens detected in this way are lymphocyte defined. The use of antibodies or lymphocytes to detect histocompatibility antigens forms the basis of tissue typing (*see* section on transplantation).

Polymorphism

When there is more than one allele for a gene, the gene is said to be polymorphic. A minimum of 20 HLA-A, 42 HLA-B and 8 HLA-C specificities have so far been defined serologically, indicating the remarkable degree of polymorphism within the HLA complex. Each allele is designated by a letter and a number – for example A1 and B7 – and the combination of alleles expressed by an individual is known as a haplotype. Because HLA genes are inherited from both parents, a haplotype consists of up to six different class I alleles plus two D region specificities. There is a low frequency of recombination within HLA on account of the close genetic distance of the loci; thus haplotypes tend to be inherited *en bloc*.

Immune responses and their regulation

T-cell dependency of antibody responses

Although B lymphocytes are the only cells capable of synthesizing Ig, the antibody response to most antigens involves T lymphocytes. Congenital absence of the thymus impairs antibody production, particularly secondary responses, to many different types of antigen, and these have been termed 'thymus-dependent' (TD) antigens. A minority of antigens trigger B cells in the absence of T cells, and these are the so-called thymus-independent (TI) antigens. Two types of thymus-independent antigen have been described, which nevertheless share a common feature in their both being large, polymeric molecules with a recurring structure. Often thymus-independent antigens stimulate polyclonal production of Ig, so that B lymphocytes other than those specific for the antigen are activated.

The cells which assist B lymphocytes to secrete Ig are helper or inducer T lymphocytes (T_H); they are specific for the same antigen as the B cell they help. The determinants to which T_H cells respond are termed 'carrier epitopes'. Cross-linking of Ig molecules on the surface of the B cell in the case of thymus-dependent antigens is a necessary but insufficient signal for antibody production. T_H cells provide a second activation signal, probably by way of direct cell-to-cell contact and the release of growth and differentiation promoting lymphokines (*see Table 18.3*). Antigen-specific and non-specific factors may be secreted. For optimal T–B-cell cooperation, the T_H and B lymphocytes must share HLA-D region polymorphism, so there is a major histocompatibility complex restriction through class II histocompatibility molecules.

Subsets of T lymphocyte

T lymphocytes are functionally heterogeneous, and several distinct T-cell subsets have been defined, including T_H (*Table 18.4*). Cytotoxic T lymphocytes (T_C), which kill virally infected cells, recognize viral antigens in the context of class I molecules. As for B lymphocytes, the precursors of T_C require specific T_H cells which recognize other viral determinants in association with class II molecules. Interleukin 2, a lymphokine, is very important in the expansion of antigen-reactive T cells. The T lymphocytes responsible for delayed-type hypersensitivity (*see below*) represent another effector subset. In addition to subsets which enhance T- or B-cell responses, there are cells

Table 18.4 Functions of T-lymphocyte subsets

Subset	Function
T_H helper (inducer)	Enhance antibody production and cell-mediated immunity
T_C cytotoxic	Kill foreign or virally infected cells
T_S suppressor	Suppress antibody production and cell-mediated immunity
T_D delayed-type hypersensitivity	Elicit delayed-type hypersensitivity reactions

which suppress them, namely suppressor T lymphocytes (T_S). Suppression may be non-specific, that is affecting many different clones, or specific, thereby inhibiting only those that respond to the same antigen as T_S. The T_S lymphocytes can act both by soluble factors and cell-to-cell contact. Various types of T_S lymphocyte have been described which either induce suppression, effect suppression or inhibit suppression.

Antigen presentation

Because T lymphocytes do not recognize antigen without compatible major histocompatibility complex molecules, there is a requirement for a cell to present antigen to the T cell. A number of cell types can perform this function, notably macrophages, dendritic cells and Langerhans cells. Antigens are endocytosed non-specifically and degraded (processed) into smaller fragments before expression on the cell surface. B lymphocytes can present antigen to T cells also, and in this case the uptake of antigen is specific as it occurs through the antigen-binding surface Ig.

Organization of lymphoid tissues

Lymphocytes in common with other blood cells are derived from the self-renewing pluripotent haemopoietic stem cells found in the fetal yolk sac and liver, and in the adult bone marrow. Lymphopoiesis, the generation of lymphocytes, takes place in the primary lymphoid organs: immature precursors multiply and produce more mature cells for release into the peripheral circulation and subsequent residence within secondary lymphoid organs.

Whether a precursor develops along the T- or B-lymphocyte lineage depends on the primary lymphoid organ to which it migrates, and this appears to be pre-programmed ('determined').

Primary lymphoid organs

Thymus

At about the sixth week of gestation, the thymus develops from the third and fourth pharyngeal pouches; it is seeded by lymphoid precursors, and lymphopoiesis begins around the eighth week. T lymphocytes are exported from the thymus from 12 weeks, but they are not yet fully functional. Within the thymus, T cells begin to express a variety of surface markers, some of which are unique to T cells, and characterize distinct subsets (*Table 18.5*). Anatomically, the thymus comprises two lobes which are subdivided into lobules; each

Table 18.5 Some surface markers of human peripheral blood T lymphocytes

Marker	Expression on peripheral blood T lymphocytes
T1 (CD5)	~100%; also on some B lymphocytes
T3 (CD3)	~100%; non-covalently linked to T-cell antigen receptor
T4 (CD4)	~65%; predominantly on T helper/inducer cells
T8 (CD8)	~35%; predominantly on T suppressor/cytotoxic cells
T11 (CD2)	~100%; binds sheep erythrocytes and phytohaemagglutinin

has an outer cortex and an inner medulla. The more mature thymocytes probably migrate from the medulla.

Bone marrow

The fetal liver together with the bone marrow of both fetus and adult provide a lymphopoiesis-inducing microenvironment for B lymphocytes. Because birds have a specialized organ in which B cells differentiate, namely the bursa of Fabricius, the bone marrow and fetal liver of mammals are described as bursal equivalent tissues. Immature B lymphocytes, bearing surface IgM, can be found in the liver after 9 weeks of gestation. IgG and IgA are not normally produced until after birth. IgM synthesis begins shortly before birth to reach 10% of the adult value at birth, but it is dramatically increased if the fetus is congenitally infected (for example with Toxoplasma or rubella).

Secondary lymphoid organs

T and B lymphocytes are not fully mature when they leave the primary lymphoid organs and migrate to the secondary lymphoid organs, that is the lymph nodes, spleen and mucosal-associated lymphoid tissues (MALT). They home to particular areas of the organs and establish T-dependent and B-dependent regions.

Lymph nodes

The T-dependent paracortical zone lies within the B-dependent outer cortex (*Figure 18.10*). Lymphoid follicles contain B lymphocytes: primary follicles are unstimulated, while secondary follicles are larger with germinal centres and have been activated by antigen. The medullary region contains a mixture of T and B lymphocytes, and plasma cells which secrete antibody lie along the chords. The lymph nodes draining the external ear are the superficial parotid nodes (tragus and anterior area), retroauricular nodes (posterior and cranial aspects) and superficial cervical nodes (lobule). The lymphatic vessels of tympanum and mastoid antrum drain into the parotid and upper deep cervical lymph nodes.

Spleen

The leucocyte-rich white pulp is situated within an erythrocyte-rich red pulp. The T-dependent periarteriolar sheath surrounds the splenic arterioles, and outside this is a B-dependent marginal zone containing follicles and plasma cells.

Mucosal-associated lymphoid tissue

Mucosal-associated lymphoid tissue may be of the organized or diffuse type. Examples of mucosal-associated lymphoid tissue include the tonsils (*see Figure 18.10*), appendix, the Peyer's patches which lie along the gut, and the bronchial-associated lymphoid tissue. Unlike other secondary lymphoid organs, mucosal-associated lymphoid tissue is not encapsulated and has no afferent lymphatic vessels.

The primary and secondary lymphoid organs, with their connecting blood and lymphatic vessels, collectively make up the lymphon. A proportion of lymphocytes, after maturation in lymph node, spleen or mucosal-associated lymphoid tissue, recirculate through these organs. B-and T-lymphocyte responses take place within the secondary lymphoid organs; antigens may be carried on antigen presenting cells from local sites to the draining lymphoid tissue.

Immunization

The induction of immunity to particular infectious agents is known as immunization. This can be accomplished by the transfer of antibodies from one individual to another, called passive immunization, or by the administration of vaccines containing avirulent antigenic material to provoke an immune response, called active immunization.

Passive immunization

The transfer of immunoglobulins to fetus and neonate represents a natural form of passive immunization. In the former, antibodies of the IgG isotype are transported across the placenta by way of Fcγ receptors during the second and third trimesters. The process is selective; other Ig isotypes or proteins of similar molecular size to IgG do not cross the placenta. Up to about 6 months after birth, therefore, the fetus receives protection against a variety of potential pathogens that the mother has encountered. The protective effect is lost as a result of gradual catabolism. In some cases, transplacental passage of IgG can be harmful and cause autoimmune disease and rhesus haemolytic disease (*see below*).

The newborn infant receives additional protective antibodies from the mother in the colostrum and milk. In the first few days after birth this is very rich in SIgA, which coats the gut mucosa. Failure to provide secretory antibodies has been implicated in the development of food allergy.

Pooled γ-globulin fractions of normal human serum can be used to give temporary protection when needed – for example, to protect premature infants who have failed to receive their full measure of maternal IgG or patients who are immunosuppressed for therapeutic reasons (such as transplant recipients), or individuals with immunodeficiency syndromes (*see below*). Preparations of γ-globulins are administered intramuscularly to avoid anaphylactic shock, as aggregated Ig could activate the complement cascade by way of the classical pathway.

Pooled γ-globulin fractions from other species (heterologous or xenogeneic γ-globulins) are used infrequently nowadays because of adverse reactions such as serum sickness (*see below*). Specific antibodies can be raised in animals (for example in horse) and given to non-immune individuals who

LYMPH NODE

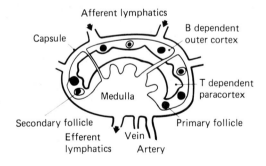

TONSIL

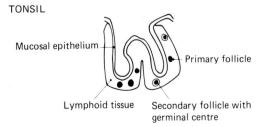

Figure 18.10 Schematic representation of lymph node and tonsil

have come into contact with the infective organism. If passive immunization with heterologous antibodies is necessary (for example, as an antitoxin), it should always be accompanied by a schedule of active immunization. Protection afforded by passive immunization is rapid but transient because of normal catabolism of the Ig molecules.

Active immunization

Active immunization or vaccination involves the production of protective antibodies before natural infection and the provision of memory populations of T and B lymphocytes which will respond with second set kinetics when the appropriate organism is encountered. There are several different kinds of vaccine; generally the best are those which most closely mimic the natural infection.

Non-replicating vaccines

Killed organisms

For these vaccines to be successful, the treatment employed to kill the microorganism – usually by means of heating and fixation with formalin or phenol – must preserve the antigenic structures necessary to establish immunity. Examples include the bacterial vaccines for whooping cough (*Bordetella pertussis*) and typhoid fever (*Salmonella typhi, Salmonella paratyphi*), the rickettsial vaccine for typhus fever and the killed polio virus vaccine (Salk type).

Protective antigens derived from whole organisms

Toxoids are toxins that have been denatured and inactivated by treatment with formaldehyde. Some of the most successful vaccines, notably diphtheria and tetanus toxoids, have been produced by this means. These are particularly useful when the disease is caused by a toxin rather than by invasion of the organism.

Non-infectious subunits or components of the microorganism may be suitable vaccines; examples include the hepatitis B virus surface antigen and the pneumococcal polysaccharide vaccines. Although relative safe and stable, the major disadvantage of non-replicative vaccines is that they have to be given in large doses by way of an unnatural (parenteral) route. They may be only weakly immunogenic and, as such, may require an adjuvant, a substance which boosts the immune response without necessarily inducing an antibody response to itself.

Live vaccines

Cross-protective organisms

A variant of the cowpox virus, vaccinia virus, is antigenically related to smallpox virus (variola) but, in the main, causes a mild local skin eruption in humans. Inoculation with vaccinia raises antibodies which cross-react with variola and confer immunity. The vaccine has been so effective that the smallpox virus, whose only reservoir is man, has been eradicated. Because vaccinia can occasionally produce complications, such as generalized vaccinia infection or encephalomyelitis, it is no longer ethical to vaccinate unless there is a clear risk of smallpox infection. Cross-protective vaccines are used for some animal diseases, for example human measles virus for canine distemper.

Attenuated organisms

Culture or treatment of infectious organisms, to render them avirulent yet able to induce protective immunity, is known as attenuation. There are numerous examples including the viral vaccines for German measles (rubella) and polio (Sabin type), and the bacillus of Calmette–Guérin (BCG), an attenuated strain of *Mycobacterium tuberculosis*. A novel approach to vaccine design – which is as yet at the research stage – is to construct attenuated viral vectors (such as vaccinia) which have been genetically engineered to contain important antigens of other viruses (for example hepatitis B, Epstein–Barr virus).

The great advantage of live vaccines is that they can be administered in small doses and can mimic natural infections to provide both local and systemic immunity. Indeed, cytotoxic T lymphocytes, which are crucial to the elimination of many viruses, are induced only by live viruses. Set against the advantages are the potential risks that organisms might re-acquire virulence, or that other viruses, possibly oncogenic, might contaminate the preparation. Even with attenuated organisms there may be a risk of disease if the inoculated individual is immunologically compromised.

Hypersensitivity reactions

An exaggerated or inappropriate immune response which damages host tissues is termed a 'hypersensitivity reaction'. Four main types of hypersensitivity, I–IV, have been classified by Coombs and Gell (1975): the first three cover hypersensitivity associated with antibodies, the fourth is mediated by T lymphocytes.

It is important to bear in mind that the mechanisms responsible for hypersensitivity are the same as those used in defence, the difference being that damage to the host outweighs the benefits.

Type I: immediate or reaginic hypersensitivity

The term 'immediate hypersensitivity' was originally applied because reactions occurred within minutes after exposure to a particular antigen. The principal mediators of immediate hypersensitivity or anaphylaxis are antibodies of the IgE isotype (so-called reaginic antibodies), and mast cells.

Local anaphylaxis

Atopic allergy, encompassing hay fever and some kinds of asthma and eczema, affects about 10% of the British population. By means of mechanisms that are poorly understood, repeated exposure of these individuals to an antigen (allergen) leads to the production of specific antibodies of IgE isotype. Common allergens include pollens and proteins of the housedust mite. By way of receptors for Fcε, the antibodies bind to the surface of mast cells or basophils within the skin, and to mucosal membranes. Contact with the allergen leads to cross-linking of IgE molecules and explosive degranulation of the cell, with the release of the inflammatory mediators already alluded to in the section on the role of antibody. Vasodilatation, platelet aggregation, increased capillary permeability and the leakage of blood fluids (extravasation) produce an oedematous red wheal and flare reaction. Inflammation of the ducts draining the tears causes the eyes to run. In the lungs, slow-reacting substance of anaphylaxis brings about a gradual but long-lasting bronchoconstriction.

Systemic anaphylaxis

When an allergen is introduced directly into the bloodstream, degranulation can take place in any organ or tissue where there are sensitized mast cells. In man, the shock organs, which are most prone to anaphylactic responses, are the respiratory and circulatory systems. Anaphylactic shock is rare but very dangerous if not treated by injection of adrenaline; in extreme cases, an individual begins wheezing, and can collapse and die in a matter of minutes. Sensitivity to antibiotics or other drugs could lead to local or systemic anaphylaxis.

Type II: antibody dependent, cytotoxic hypersensitivity

The specific binding of antibody to the surface of a cell can lead to destruction by one of a number of different pathways: activation of complement, phagocytosis and targetting of cytotoxic macrophages, neutrophils, eosinophils or K cells.

Blood transfusion reactions

Human erythrocytes carry carbohydrate molecules which constitute the ABO blood group antigens. The alleles for these molecules are codominantly expressed, and phenotypically the red cells may be A, B, AB, or O. Group A individuals have in their serum antibodies to group B and vice versa. These natural antibodies are found in the absence of previous transfusion; they are of the IgM class and are called isohaemagglutinins. (Similar antigens to the ABO substances have been found on bacteria and it is thought that sensitization by way of the gut induces antibodies which cross-react with human erythrocytes.)

Group O individuals possess only a backbone sugar molecule, substance H, and do not express A or B group antigens. For this reason, O blood is a universal donor because it can be given to any recipient. Conversely, AB individuals behave as universal recipients as they have antibodies to neither A nor B in their serum. If a blood transfusion is accidentally given to an incompatible recipient, an immediate and severe reaction ensues. The isohaemagglutinins agglutinate erythrocytes and fix complement. Symptoms include acute tubular necrosis of the kidneys, resulting from the sudden haemolysis, fever, hypotension, nausea and vomiting. Antigens other than those of the ABO system can elicit transfusion reactions, including those on leucocytes.

Rhesus haemolytic disease of the newborn

Erythrocytes also carry molecules encoded by the rhesus (Rh) system, of which the RhD antigen is the strongest and the only one of clinical significance. There are two alleles at the RhD locus, D and d; expression of D is dominant and about 85% of the British population are RhD$^+$. If a RhD$^-$ woman becomes pregnant by a RhD$^+$ father, the fetus may be RhD$^+$. At parturition, a significant leakage of fetal cells into the maternal circulation occurs, which immunizes the mother to RhD. In the course of a second pregnancy with a RhD$^+$ fetus, a small number of fetal erythrocytes leak across the placenta and induce a secondary response in the mother. IgG antibodies to RhD cross the placenta, giving rise to haemolysis and jaundice. In severe cases, exchange blood transfusion with RhD$^+$ blood is necessary *in utero* or following premature delivery.

To prevent sensitization of the mother, *postpartum* anti-RhD antibodies are given prophylactically. This has dramatically reduced the incidence of rhesus haemolytic disease in the newborn, presumably because the anti-RhD antibodies remove fetal cells before they sensitize the mother. The decreased chance of rhesus haemolytic disease when the mother and fetus are ABO incompatible can probably be explained in a similar fashion. The mechanisms involved in type II hypersensitivity reactions may contribute to autoimmune diseases in which organ-specific autoantibodies are generated.

Type III: immune complex-mediated hypersensitivity

Immune complexes formed between antigen and antibody activate the complement cascade; type III hypersensitivity responses have immuno-pathological consequences.

Local, Arthus-type reactions

In 1903, Arthus and Breton found that the intradermal injection of horse serum into hyper-immunized rabbits induced a red oedematous lesion after about 6–8 hours. This Arthus reaction is brought about by the deposition of immune complexes in and around the local venules. Activation of complement produces chemotactic and anaphylatoxic factors. Neutrophils infiltrate the site and, unable to phagocytose trapped immune complexes, release their lysosomal enzymes, thereby causing damage and necrosis. Farmer's lung and pigeon fancier's disease are the result of type III hypersensitivity responses to inhaled antigen, with actinomycetes of mouldy hay being responsible for the former and serum proteins in the droppings of birds for the latter.

Systemic reactions

Following parenteral administration of a large dose of antigen to immune recipients, immune complexes may be deposited at many sites, notably the kidneys, heart, joints and skin. When passive immunization with horse γ-globulins was used in the treatment of diphtheria, formation of antibodies to the circulating heterologous proteins precipitated serum sickness. Small complexes, formed in conditions of antigen excess, are cleared only slowly by the mononuclear phagocyte system. Type III hypersensitivity reactions are mainly responsible for the pathology seen in non-organ-specific autoimmune disease (*see below*).

Type IV: delayed-type hypersensitivity

In 1890, Koch described a local erythematous indurated lesion in the skin of tuberculosis (TB) patients after the injection of tuberculin, an extract of *M. tuberculosis*. Because the reaction took between 24 and 72 hours to develop, he called it delayed. Delayed-type hypersensitivity reactions are mediated exclusively by T lymphocytes and are characterized by a mononuclear cell infiltration of lymphocytes (10–20%) and monocytes (80–90%); it is this dense cellular infiltration that gives the lesion a solid feel (induration). The release of lymphokines, and the recruitment and activation of monocytes, cause local tissue damage and vasodilatation.

The term 'delayed-type hypersensitivity reaction' is often used incorrectly to describe a protective immune response. Although the mechanisms involved in delayed hypersensitivity are part of the normal cell-mediated repertoire, a delayed-type hypersensitivity reaction does not necessarily indicate protective immunity. In some experimental models, immunity can be transferred with T lymphocytes independently of delayed-type hypersensitivity reactivity. Moreover, the immunopathology of diseases such as tuberculosis, and some kinds of leprosy, results from ineffective T-cell responses. In tuberculosis, the formation of granuloma in the lungs and other organs produces cavitation. In leprosy, the importance of T-lymphocyte responses in immunity to *M.leprae* is evident; weak T-cell reactivity is associated with many organisms (lepromatous type) and strong reactivity with a few (tuberculoid type). Borderline leprosy in the middle of the scale is associated with moderate T-cell reactivity, moderate *M.leprae* infection, but with severe granulomatous lesions.

A particular form of delayed-type hypersensitivity reaction, which has no apparent relevance to protective immunity, is that of contact sensitivity. Simple chemicals (haptens) that in isolation are non-immunogenic, can be absorbed through the skin to form immunogenic complexes with free or cell bound proteins. When the chemical is reapplied, a delayed-type hypersensitivity-like lesion develops. Nickel, constituents of rubber, clothing dyes and materials, and plant oils (for example, poison ivy in the USA) can all elicit contact sensitivity.

Autoimmune disease

The immune system does not normally respond to the body's own antigens because there is normally an immunological tolerance to self-antigens. If this tolerance is broken, autoimmune responses against self-antigens can produce disease. Most autoimmune diseases are associated with the production of antibodies (autoantibodies), but autoreactive T lymphocytes may also be involved. A spectrum of autoimmune disease has been described, with organ-specific and non-organ-specific disorders at either ends of the spectrum.

In an archetypal organ-specific disease, auto-antibodies are formed to antigens found in a single organ. Autoimmune diseases of the thyroid gland – such as Hashimoto's thyroiditis and thyrotoxicosis (Grave's disease) – would be cardinal examples (*Table 18.6*). Goodpasture's syndrome, in which autoantibodies react to a common antigen on glomerular and alveolar basement membranes, and myasthenia gravis (autoantibodies to the acetylcholine receptor at the neuromuscular junction of voluntary muscles), represent less absolute organ-specific diseases.

At the opposite end of the spectrum is systemic lupus erythematosus. The disease gets its name from the wolf (lupus)-like appearance of the facial rash. Systemic lupus erythematosus is associated with a plethora of autoantibodies (those to double-stranded DNA being of particular diagnostic value) and lesions in a variety of systems. Skin and joints are most commonly affected, but there may also be pulmonary, renal, cardiac, neurological and haematological involvement. Many of the non-organ-specific diseases are rheumatological, affecting joints and muscles.

Towards the middle of the spectrum are diseases where autoantibodies to an antigen present in many tissues, nevertheless damage a rather specific target – for example primary biliary cirrhosis – or where relatively specific autoantibodies cause systemic effects, for example autoimmune haemolytic anaemias.

Autoantigens and mechanisms of self-tolerance

Theoretically, any antigen can behave as an autoantigen, for example plasma proteins, cell-membrane components and receptors, extracellular antigens and intracellular constituents (*see Table 18.6*). In general, autoantibodies to antigens found at high concentrations throughout the body lead to non-organ-specific disease, while localized antigens are associated with organ-specific disorders. Autoantibodies are not confined to a single isotype. For example, in rheumatoid arthritis, IgG, IgA and IgM autoantibodies to IgG (rheumatoid factors) have all been described, although IgM is most common. The aetiology of the majority of autoimmune diseases remains unknown. In the normal state, self-tolerance is maintained by several mechanisms.

Lack of autoreactive cells

During lymphocyte development there is selection against cells which respond to self-antigens. Thus, potentially autoreactive T and B lymphocytes are functionally deleted from the immune system. It has been shown experimentally that the introduction of foreign antigens early in ontogeny induces long-lasting specific unresponsiveness to those antigens.

Table 18.6 Some autoimmune diseases

Condition	Autoantibodies to	Target organ(s)	Effects
Hashimoto's thyroiditis	Thyroglobulin, thyroid microsomes	Thyroid	Hypothyroid (myxoedema)
Grave's disease	TSH receptor	Thyroid	Thyrotoxicosis
Pernicious anaemia	Intrinsic factor	Gut	Malabsorption of vitamin B_{12}
Goodpasture's disease	Glomerular and alveolar basement membrane	Kidneys, lungs	Nephritis, alveolitis
Myasthenia gravis	Acetylcholine receptor	Voluntary muscles	Muscular weakness
Pemphigus vulgaris	Intercellular substance	Skin	Bullous formation
Sympathetic ophthalmitis	Ocular proteins	Eye	Destruction of healthy eye
Primary biliary cirrhosis	Mitochondria	Small bile duct	Liver damage
Sjögren's disease	Salivary duct	Mouth, eyes, joints	Sicca complex, arthritis
Rheumatoid arthritis	IgG	Joints, skin, blood vessels, kidneys, heart	Arthritis, skin lesions, vasculitis, nephritis, etc.
Systemic lupus erythematosus	Double-stranded DNA, nuclear proteins, mitochondria, leucocytes	Skin, blood vessels, joints, kidneys, heart	Skin lesions, vasculitis, arthritis, nephritis, thrombocytopenia, etc.

Lack of antigen presentation

Although self-reactive T and B lymphocytes may be present, they fail to respond because the antigen is sequestered and does not come into contact with lymphoid cells. This mode of tolerance operates for ocular proteins. Damage to one eye and the release of proteins into the circulation induce clones of self-reactive T and B lymphocytes which attack the other healthy eye and cause sympathetic ophthalmitis. The expression of class II histocompatibility molecules can allow cells to present self-antigens directly to self-reactive T lymphocytes. Such inappropriate class II expression has been implicated in autoimmune diseases of the thyroid.

Lack of T-lymphocyte help

In the case of T-dependent autoantigens, autoantibodies will not be produced if autoreactive T_H cells are absent. However, this requirement can be bypassed if the autoantigen is presented on an immunogenic carrier (the carrier determinants are those recognized by T cells). Drugs which chemically modify red cell or platelet antigens provide helper determinants in drug-induced autoimmune haemolytic anaemia and thrombocytopenia respectively. Agents which activate B cells polyclonally, such as the Epstein–Barr virus, could elicit autoantibody formation without T-cell cooperation.

Lack of suppression

A key question is whether autoreactive T and B lymphocytes are always present but not triggered, or whether new autoreactive clones are generated. It would seem that, for many self-antigens, autoreactive lymphocytes are present but are not activated on account of the control by T-suppressor cells. One of the reasons for the increased prevalence of autoimmune diseases with age may be a decreased efficiency of T suppression. Gross defects in T_S function have been implicated in the aetiology of systemic lupus erythematosus and may play a role in other autoimmune diseases.

Pathogenesis

Autoantibodies can damage cells by various hypersensitivity reactions; in autoimmune disease, the immune response is inappropriate because the antigens are self components. Organ-specific lesions involve antibody-dependent, cytotoxic mechanisms (type II hypersensitivity) while non-organ-specific lesions are mediated by immune complexes (type III hypersensitivity). The injection of many types of autoantibodies can be shown by experiment to induce organ-specific pathology. Although most of the damage in autoimmune diseases is mediated by antibody, it is likely that T-cell-mediated damage is also present in many organ-specific diseases, as autoreactive T lymphocytes have been able to transfer the disease in experimental models. Further, lymphocyte transformation *in vitro* to autoantigens in sympathetic ophthalmitis and pernicious anaemia, and the demonstration of autoreactive T lymphocytes in Grave's disease, would suggest a role for type IV hypersensitivity in these diseases *in vivo*.

Stimulatory hypersensitivity

In autoimmune disease, a special form of antibody-mediated hypersensitivity, sometimes called type V or stimulatory hypersensitivity, has been described. Many patients with Grave's disease have in their serum an antibody which mimics the action of the thyroid stimulating hormone (TSH) by binding to the TSH receptor on thyrocytes. Unlike TSH, the autoantibody, the long-acting thyroid stimulator, is not subject to negative feedback by way of the hypothalamus and thus causes excess production of thyroxine (thyrotoxicosis). In myasthenia gravis and a rare form of insulin-resistant diabetes (associated with acanthosis nigricans), antireceptor antibodies stimulate receptor turnover, leading to long-term depletion of the receptor.

Autoimmune diseases with head and neck manifestations

Sjögren's disease

Patients with Sjögren's disease usually present with sicca complex, a combination of dry mouth (xerostomia) and dry eyes (keratoconjunctivitis sicca). Autoantibodies to salivary duct antigens are present. An association between any non-organ-specific autoimmune disease, in particular rheumatoid arthritis, and sicca complex, is diagnostic of Sjögren's syndrome.

Behçet's syndrome

This syndrome is a chronic, multisystem disease which involves the mouth, genital organs, skin, blood vessels, nerves, gut and joints. Oral ulceration is the most common presenting feature, and autoantibodies which bind to extracts of oral mucosa and other tissues are found in 70–80% of patients. Immune complexes are found in the serum of about 60%.

Pemphigus vulgaris

Pemphigus vulgaris is a serious blistering condition which had a mortality rate of about 50% before the advent of steroid therapy. Flaccid blisters, bullae, develop within the epidermis of mouth and scalp, rapidly disseminating over the body. Autoantibodies to the intercellular cement of the skin epithelium are present in serum.

Diagnosis of autoimmune disease

Autoantibodies present in serum may be detected by immunofluorescence, agglutination, radioimmunoassays, enzyme-linked immunosorbent assays (ELISA) and complement fixation tests.

Immunofluorescence

After incubation with normal tissue specimens, autoantibodies in serum are demonstrated by means of fluorochrome-conjugated antibody to human Ig. Autoantibodies already fixed to the tissue can be detected in biopsy sections.

Agglutination

Autoantibodies to red blood cell antigens (for example rhesus D) which bind to but do not directly agglutinate the cells, can be shown by adding an anti-human Ig to the patient's red cells which then agglutinate (Coombs' test). Agglutination by antibodies of erythrocytes coated with antigen is known as passive haemagglutination. It forms the basis of the Rose–Waaler test for rheumatoid factor, although Latex beads coated with IgG may be used in place of red blood cells.

Radioimmunoassay

A radioactively labelled antigen or secondary antibody (anti-human Ig) is used to detect autoantibodies to intrinsic factor, acetylcholine receptors, double-stranded DNA and glomerular basement membrane.

Enzyme-linked immunosorbent assay

In ELISA, serum from a patient is incubated with the relevant antigen, and any autoantibodies present are detected by means of an anti-human Ig conjugated to an enzyme. Addition of the appropriate enzyme substrate causes a colour change which is quantified by spectrophotometry and is proportional to the amount of autoantibody present.

Complement fixation

Complement fixation tests detect complement consumption by antigen–autoantibody complexes (*see* section on tests for antigen and antibody reactions).

Management of autoimmune disease

Treatment of autoimmune disease depends upon its clinical severity. Many organ-specific disorders can be treated by metabolic control – for example, patients with Hashimoto's disease are given thyroxine, those with myasthenia receive anticholinesterase drugs, and patients with pernicious anaemia are supplemented with vitamin B_{12}. Immunosuppressive therapy is necessary in severe myasthenia gravis, pemphigus vulgaris, systemic lupus erythematosus and immune complex-mediated nephritis. Inflammation can be reduced in rheumatoid arthritis and related diseases by anti-inflammatory agents including indomethacin and salicylates. Plasma exchange (plasmapheresis) is helpful in life-threatening immune complex-mediated arteritis. Antimitotic agents, such as methotrexate, cyclophosphamide and azathioprine, have been used in the treatment of chronic active hepatitis, autoimmune haemolytic anaemia and systemic lupus erythematosus.

Immunodeficiency

Failure of one or more elements of the immune system causes immunodeficiency. Innate or acquired immune responses may be compromised and this may be either genetically determined, a primary immunodeficiency, or be secondary to another disease process. Recurrent infections with common pathogens or with opportunistic organisms which take advantage of the lowered defences typify immunity deficiency and characterize the particular defect (*Table 18.7*).

Primary deficiencies of innate immunity

Phagocytic cells may show a reduced capacity to kill, for example chronic granulomatous disease, or may fail to migrate to chemotactic stimuli, for example lazy leucocyte syndrome. Natural killer (NK) cells are mononuclear, lymphocyte-like cells which are not readily characterized as either B or T lymphocytes and have been termed 'null cells'. They are cytotoxic for a variety of tumour cell lines *in vitro* but display no clear specificity or memory pattern and are, therefore, considered to be an innate immune mechanism. In patients with Chediak–Higashi disease, neutrophils, monocytes

Table 18.7 Infections associated with deficiencies in innate or acquired immunity

	Innate immunity		Acquired immunity	
	Complement defects	*Phagocyte defects*	*T-lymphocyte defects*	*B-lymphocyte defects*
Viruses			Polioviruses Echoviruses Vaccinia Mumps Epstein–Barr virus Cytomegalovirus	
Bacteria	Staphylococci Streptococci H. influenzae Neisseria	*Serratia* *Klebsiella* *Salmonella*	*Mycobacteria* *Legionella* *Listeria* *Nocardia asteroides*	Staphylococci Streptococci (pneumococci meningococci)
Protozoa			*Pneumocystis carinii* *Toxoplasma gondii* *Giardia lamblia*	
Fungi		*Candida*	*Candida*	

and natural killer cells possess abnormal giant lysosomes which inhibit locomotion and cytotoxic potential. These patients are particularly susceptible to bacterial infections and have a tendency to develop lymphomata. The latter observation supports the concept that natural killer cells play a role in surveillance against tumours.

Deficiencies in complement components can be broadly divided into those affecting the classical pathway, C3, or the terminal lytic sequence.

(1) Deficiencies of C1, C2 or C4 are associated with increased risk of bacterial infection. More significantly, there is an increase in immune-complex-mediated hypersensitivity lesions, presumably as a result of decreased clearance of antigen–antibody complexes. A deficiency of C1 inactivator causes hereditary angio-oedema in which sudden oedema occurs in the deep dermis, subcutaneous or mucous membranes of skin, intestine or larynx.

(2) C3 may be reduced directly or by defects in the C3 inactivator, with both cases being characterized by acute life-threatening infections.

(3) Absence of a component of the terminal lytic sequence predisposes to infection with *Neisseria* species, *N.meningitides* or *N.gonorrhoeae*. Lysis of *Neisseria* seems to be necessary for effective clearance of the organism.

Table 18.8 Severe combined immunodeficiency (SCID) syndromes

Condition	Defect	Inheritance
SCID with leucopenia (reticular dysgenesis)	Absence of all leucocytes, erythrocytes and platelets present	Autosomal recessive
SCID ('Swiss type' agammaglobulinaemia)	Absence of T and B lymphocytes	Autosomal recessive or X-linked
SCID with adenosine deaminase deficiency	Enzyme lacking or inactive	Autosomal recessive (chromosome 20)
Cellular immunodeficiency with immunoglobulins (Nezelof's syndrome)	Normal B-lymphocyte numbers but low Ig levels	Autosomal recessive or X-linked
Bare lymphocyte syndrome	No HLA class I molecules on lymphocytes	Familial

Primary deficiencies of acquired immunity

Severe combined immunodeficiency

Failure of both antibody production and cell-mediated immunity results in severe combined immunodeficiency. Several subtypes have been classified (*Table 18.8*), most of which present with diarrhoea and failure to thrive in early infancy.

Deficiencies of T lymphocytes

Aberrant differentiation of the thymus results in the Di George syndrome. In the complete syndrome there is aplasia and involvement of heart and parathyroid glands. Partial Di George syndrome patients possess a hypoplastic thymus.

A defect in purine nucleoside phosphorylase, an enzyme of the purine salvage pathway, reduces cell-mediated immunity; some T-cell subpopulations may be more susceptible to this deficiency than others, for example cytotoxic T cells. Other disorders which have a predominant effect on T lymphocytes are shown in *Table 18.9*. The distinction between deficiencies of cell-mediated immunity and antibody are somewhat blurred by the T-cell dependency of many antibody responses. For example, in late onset or common variable hypogammaglobulinaemia there is a profound decrease in Ig levels, and plasma cells are absent. Although the syndrome is heterogeneous, it is likely that the hypogammaglobulinaemia is a consequence of aberrant T-cell function, either increased suppressor or decreased helper activity.

Deficiencies of B lymphocytes

The first immunodeficiency syndrome was described by Bruton in 1952. In congenital or Bruton's aggammaglobulinaemia, the concentration of all Ig isotypes is diminished, although it is most marked for IgM and IgA. Repeated infections with pyogenic bacteria and an opportunistic protozoan, *Pneumocystis carinii*, are observed from about 6 months *postpartum* when the protective effect of maternal IgG has waned. The lymphoid tissue is hypoplastic with no plasma cells and germinal centres, but T-cell reactivity is normal. Bruton's disease is X-linked and is treated by administration of whole plasma or γ-globulins.

There are a number of disorders with selective deficiencies in one or more Ig isotypes. The most common is selective IgA deficiency, with an incidence of about one in 800. It is associated with recurrent infections of the respiratory tract and paranasal sinuses. Allergic, type I hypersensitivity reactions may cause gastrointestinal damage if food antigens, normally neutralized by SIgA, trigger mast cell degranulation. The irritant effects of antigen in the lungs or gut may promote tumour growth or autoimmune disease. Autoantibodies to IgA are frequently present in selective IgA deficiency, but it is not clear whether they cause the disorder or whether they arise because tolerance, in the absence of IgA, is lost. The clinically observed effects of IgA deficiency might be expected from its role as a defender of mucosal surfaces. Nevertheless, a significant proportion of individuals are healthy and in many of these an increase in secretory IgM compensates for the loss of SIgA.

Secondary immunodeficiency

Most immunodeficiencies are secondary and result from immunosuppression, or increased loss or catabolism of Ig. There are a variety of causes,

Table 18.9 Primary immunodeficiencies predominantly affecting T lymphocytes

Condition	Defect	Inheritance

Di George syndrome
  complete
  partial
	Thymic aplasia
	Thymic hypoplasia
	Cardiovascular abnormalities
		Non-familial

Purine nucleoside phosphorylase deficiency	Enzyme lacking or inactive	Autosomal recessive (chromosome 14)
Wiskott–Aldrich syndrome	Slightly reduced T-cell numbers, T cells functionally abnormal, platelets and neutrophils decreased, elevated eosinophil levels	X-linked
Ataxia telangiectasia	Embryonic thymus, T-cell number reduced, loss of coordination, dilatation of capillaries in skin and eye, defective DNA repair	Autosomal recessive

including protein or calorie malnutrition, lympho-proliferative diseases, radiotherapy or chemotherapy, and the use of immunosuppressive drugs.

Some organisms depress, rather than stimulate, the immune response. Perhaps the most extreme example is the virus responsible for the acquired immunodeficiency syndrome (AIDS). This virus, designated human immunodeficiency virus (HIV), is cytopathic for T lymphocytes bearing the T4 surface marker, the majority of which are involved in inducing antibody or effector T-lymphocyte responses (*see Table 18.5*). In full-blown AIDS, the immunodeficiency mimics that of clinical immunosuppression and is so profound that rare opportunistic organisms, including *Pneumocystis carinii* and *Mycobacterium avium intracellulare*, can establish intractable infections. Infection with other viruses, including cytomegalovirus, rubella, Epstein–Barr virus and hepatitis B virus, can lead to immunosuppression.

Some tests for immunity and immunity deficiency

Grossly abnormal numbers of neutrophils, monocytes or lymphocytes can be detected by using routine haematological methods. Abnormalities in lymphocyte numbers can be investigated further by employing phenotypic markers of B and T cells (*Table 18.10*). All B lymphocytes express surface Ig (IgM for the majority of primary, blood-borne cells). Immunofluorescence with fluorochrome-conjugated anti-human Ig antibodies can be used to quantify the proportion.

T lymphocytes bear a variety of markers which can be detected with immunofluorescence, and these define functionally distinguishable T-cell populations (*see Tables 18.5 and 18.10*). In addition, human T lymphocytes spontaneously form rosettes with sheep erythrocytes by way of the T11 surface glycoprotein, and this can be used to enumerate T-cell numbers microscopically.

Mitogens are substances which induce polyclonal expansion of lymphocytes, and they can be used to test the ability of lymphocytes to proliferate normally. Pokeweed mitogen (PWM) is mitogenic for T and B lymphocytes, and it elicits Ig secretion. Phytohaemagglutinin (PHA) and concanavalin A are T-lymphocyte mitogens.

In vitro lymphocyte transformation to mitogens, allogeneic cells (MLR), or specific recall antigens to which the patient has previously been exposed, is evaluated by the incorporation of tritiated thymidine. Immunity to recall antigens can be assessed *in vivo* by the response to intradermal injection of antigen. A panel of common antigens is employed, including PPD (a purified protein derivative of *M.tuberculosis*), streptokinase-streptodornase, *Candida albicans*, mumps virus and trichophyton. In children and infants, active induction of contact sensitivity by the application of dinitrochlorobenzene can be used to test for primary T-cell deficiency.

Clinical aspects of human leucocyte antigen (HLA)

Disease associations

A wide variety of diseases show an association with particular HLA specificities or haplotypes. The most striking is that of ankylosing spondylitis with the HLA-B27 specificity. Approximately 90% of patients with the disease are positive for B27. This association does not mean that all B27 individuals will develop the disease, but that there is an increased risk of their doing so. An association between a disease and an allele may be very significant statistically yet carry little relative risk. Associations between HLA antigens and diseases related to infection (for example arthritis following *Salmonella* infection), autoimmune disease and even psychoses such as manic depression have been reported. A few of the disease associations are shown in *Table 18.11*.

It is not clear why there is such an association. One possibility is that the HLA product behaves as an immune response gene. According to this explanation, certain HLA specificities regulate whether there is a heightened or reduced response to a particular antigen. Therefore, an exaggerated response to an antigen might provoke an autoimmune disease or hypersensitivity state, whereas a weak response to a pathogen will permit infection. It is also possible that the histocompatibility

Table 18.10 Some tests for immunity

Total leucocyte numbers
    proportion of surface Ig bearing cells
    proportion of T-lymphocyte subpopulations,
        for example T4:T8
Serum immunoglobulin levels
    different subclasses
    specific antibodies, for example isohaemagglutinins,
        anti-*Escherichia coli*
Lymphocyte transformation
    to mitogens, for example Con A, PHA
    to specific antigens, for example allogeneic cells
        (MLR, PPD)
In vivo tests
    to recall antigens, for example *Candida*, PPD (Mantoux,
        Heaf tests)
    to contact sensitizing agents
    of toxin neutralization, for example Schick test, Dick
        test

Table 18.11 Associations between HLA and certain diseases

Condition	HLA	Frequency (%)		Relative risk
		Patients	Control	
Hodgkin's disease	A1	40	32.0	1.4
Behçet's disease	B5	41	10.1	6.3
Ankylosing spondylitis	B27	90	9.4	87.4
Reiter's disease	B27	79	9.4	37.0
Psoriasis vulgaris	Cw6	87	33.1	13.3
Multiple sclerosis	D/DR2	59	25.8	4.1
Goodpasture's syndrome	D/DR2	88	32.0	15.9
Dermatitis herpetiformis	D/DR3	85	26.3	15.4
Sicca syndrome	D/DR3	78	26.3	9.7
Grave's disease	D/DR3	56	26.3	3.7
Myasthenia gravis	D/DR3	50	28.2	2.5
Systemic lupus erythematosus	D/DR3	70	28.2	5.8
Rheumatoid arthritis	D/DR4	50	19.4	4.2
Pemphigus (Jews)	D/DR4	87	32.1	14.4
Hashimoto's thyroiditis	D/DR5	19	6.9	3.2
Pernicious anaemia	D/DR5	25	5.8	5.4

Data adapted from Svejgaard, A., Platx, P. and Ryder, L. P. (1983). *Immunological Reviews*, **70**, 193–218.

antigen acts as a receptor for an infective agent so that the disease is limited to certain specificities.

An alternative possibility is that the gene responsible for the disease is not HLA itself, but a gene in linkage disequilibrium with it. An allele is said to be in linkage disequilibrium with another if, at genetic equilibrium, the two alleles occur less or more frequently than would be expected from the frequencies of the individual alleles in the population. Linkage disequilibrium implies either a positive or negative selection for a combination of alleles, depending on whether there is a higher or lower frequency, respectively, than is to be expected. Where different HLA specificities are associated with the same disease in different populations, linkage disequilibrium is suspected as the cause of the association, for example Grave's disease is associated with B8 in Caucasians but with Bw35 in Japanese.

Transplantation

Transplantation of tissue grafts between unrelated individuals results in rejection of the graft. In the special case of bone marrow transplantation, the graft itself contains immunologically reactive cells which may respond to the recipient's antigens and elicit a graft versus host disease. Although antigens coded for by the HLA on their own elicit strong transplantation reactions, a number of loci outside the HLA complex code for minor histocompatibility antigens which, in combination, induce rejection comparable to HLA disparity.

Transplantation reactions are mediated by T lymphocytes, and T-deficient individuals or animals show impaired rejection responses. Indeed, athymic nude mice, the murine equivalent of Di George patients, accept skin xenografts. In the same way as for conventional antigens, re-exposure to histocompatibility antigens provokes accelerated or second-set rejection.

Antibody can play a role in hyperacute rejection, for instance of kidney allografts; high titres of antibody induced by multiple transplantation cause a type II hypersensitivity reaction and rapid necrosis of the transplant. Chronic rejection may also be brought about by antibodies.

The importance of the various HLA region products on the outcome of cadaver kidney transplants has been evaluated. At the HLA-A and -B loci, the recipient and graft may differ (mismatch) by up to four specificities; the greater the number of mismatches, the greater the incidence of rejection. More striking differences are seen with mismatches at the HLA-D locus, indicating a greater need for compatibility at this locus during transplantation.

Blood transfusion

Paradoxically, it has been found that the administration of a blood transfusion prior to kidney graft transplantation increases the chance of allograft acceptance and suppresses the reactivity of the recipient. In fact, the transfusion effect is so marked that it obviates the need for matching HLA-A and -B loci, although HLA-D matching is still beneficial.

Typing for HLA-D

Two methods are used to type cells for HLA-D antigens, and both make use of one-way mixed lymphocyte reaction (*see* section on the HLA complex). The first involves the use of homozygous typing cells as the stimulator cell. A panel of cells homozygous for HLA-D specificities are cultured with the lymphocytes that are to be typed. If there is a positive reaction, the responder cells are not tolerant of the HLA-D antigens expressed by the homozygous stimulator cell and do not, therefore, possess that particular HLA-D polymorphism. If they fail to respond, it implies that they carry that HLA-D specificity.

The second test, primed lymphocyte typing, is more reliable because the presence of an HLA-D allele is demonstrated by a positive reaction. In primed lymphocyte typing, lymphocytes that have been primed to a particular HLA-D product are the responders, and the cells to be typed are the stimulators. If the stimulator cells bear the HLA-D antigen to which the responders are primed, the latter respond rapidly and strongly. The two typing techniques complement one another. HLA-D typing requires from 2 to 6 days to obtain a result and it is therefore not always practical to use it – for instance, in the case of cadaver organs. Typing for HLA-DR serological specificities is performed using antibody. It correlates well with HLA-D typing (*see Figure 18.8*) and can be used in isolation, where necessary. HLA-D, as well as some serologically defined HLA antigens, sometimes include the w designation, for example HLA-Dw6. This indicates that the final specificity is yet to be internationally agreed.

Immunology in otolaryngology

The contribution of the immune response to diseases of the ear, nose and throat has, in the case of some disorders such as diphtheria and allergic rhinitis, been recognized for many years. More recently, however, immunological mechanisms have been suspected in a number of other conditions. These include type I and type IV hypersensitivity reactions in otitis media, with effusion and immune-complex deposition in hearing loss associated with Wegener's granulomatosis. Sensorineural hearing loss has been obtained in experimental animals following the induction of autoimmunity. Also immunomanipulation, by the administration of lymphokines, has been used in the treatment of juvenile laryngeal papillomatosis. It seems likely that the interface between the disciplines of immunology and otolaryngology will lead to advances in our understanding of the aetiology of diseases of the ear, nose and throat, and will also facilitate the development of new therapies.

Further reading

CHAPEL, H. and HAENEY, M. (1984) *Essentials of Clinical Immunology*. Oxford: Blackwell Scientific Publications

COOMBS, R. R. A. and GELL, P. G. H. (1975) Classification of allergic reactions responsible for clinical hypersensitivity and disease. In *Clinical Aspects of Immunology*, 3rd edn, edited by P. G. Gell, R. R. A. Coombs and P. J. Lachmann, pp. 761–781. Oxford: Blackwell Scientific Publications

KLEIN, J. (1982) *Immunology: The Science of Self–Nonself Discrimination*. New York: John Wiley and Sons

LACHMANN, P. J. and PETERS, D. K. (1982) (Editors) *Clinical Aspects of Immunology*, 4th edn. Oxford: Blackwell Scientific Publications

LEE, K. J. (1985) (Editor) Immunology and Allergy. *Otolaryngologic Clinics of North America*, **18**, 627–832

McCONNELL, I., MUNRO, A. and WALDMANN, H. (1981) *The Immune System: A Course on the Molecular and Cellular Basis of Immunity*, 2nd edn. Oxford: Blackwell Scientific Publications

ROITT, I. M., BROSTOFF, J. and MALE, D. K. (1985) *Immunology*. London: Churchill Livingstone

19

Microbiology of the ear, nose and throat

R. Y. Cartwright

The battle against microorganisms, in their role as a primary cause of disease as well as of a cause of the infective complications of medical and surgical techniques, has not lessened in spite of modern antimicrobial therapy. The interaction between one biological system, the host, and another, the parasite, is both complex and infinitely variable. Nevertheless, infection and infectious disease can be kept under control if both the basic principles underlying the host–parasite relationship and the basic properties of the pathogenic microorganisms are understood. Infection must not, however, be considered solely in terms of an individual host, as the successful parasite will travel from host to host. The communicable property of microbial disease is important in the ward or hospital and in the outside community.

Infections of the ear, nose and throat are still a major cause of morbidity. Major killing diseases, such as diphtheria, have been controlled by immunization; however, although the incidence of streptococcal sore throats remain common, although the incidence of rheumatic fever and acute glomerulonephritis has been greatly reduced; middle ear infections associated with a range of bacteria and viruses are still an important childhood affliction, while the major respiratory virus infections, such as influenza and the common cold, remain unconquered.

The widespread use of antimicrobial agents has been associated with the emergence of multiple resistant strains of bacteria which can cause both primary and postoperative infections. The use of corticosteroids and immunosuppressive agents has been associated with the emergence of opportunistic infections by organisms not previously regarded as pathogenic to man.

The emergence of a new virus, the human immunodeficiency virus (HIV), formerly known as the human T-cell lymphotropic III virus (HTLV III)

which causes the acquired immune deficiency syndrome (AIDS), has implications for all branches of clinical medicine.

Although an increasing range of pathogens has been recognized, there has been a simultaneous growth in the understanding of the importance of the normal flora and its role in preventing infection.

This chapter will consider the normal flora, the main pathogens both past and present, the principles of antimicrobial therapy and, finally, the use of the clinical microbiology laboratory.

Normal flora

Only a few genera and species of microorganism are pathogenic for man. This is equally true for microorganisms in the ear, nose and throat. In common with other external surfaces, the skin and mucous membrane coverings have a prolific normal flora. The constituent microorganisms of this normal flora are either ignored or their importance in ensuring and maintaining 'normality' is not understood. The normal must be known and understood before the abnormal can be fully recognized and assessed.

The living nature of both the host site and its flora ensures that any studies thereof are invariably snapshots of the situation at a given moment in time. The snapshots put together reveal a kaleidoscope of variations and fluctuations among a population that is constantly changing while tending to modulate about a mean. The population relates not only to the host but also to its own constituent members which compete for favoured sites with varying degrees of success. The microorganisms of the normal flora are generally non-pathogenic to man, although some may be opportunistic pathogens giving rise to disease when host defence mechanisms are diminished. While some recognized pathogens may reside in the ear, nose or throat without causing an infection, their spread to other body sites or to other hosts may result in the development of an infection. Some bacteria, such as *Neisseria meningitidis*, may form part of the normal flora in only a small percentage of persons who have had previous contact with meningococcal disease, yet in outbreak situations the incidence of carriage without disease may rise to as high as 88%. Following an infection, *Corynebacterium diphtheriae* may persist in the throat for considerable periods of time, with no clinical signs. In this carrier state, the bacterium acts as part of the normal flora.

The normal flora in any site is affected by a variety of natural factors, such as temperature, humidity and pH. Disease processes may result in local microenvironmental changes which lead, in turn, to an altered local flora. Major changes in the normal flora can frequently be observed following medical treatment either with drugs or by surgical techniques.

Acquisition of normal flora

The fetus *in utero* does not have a normal flora but colonization occurs rapidly within the first few days of life. Babies delivered by the vaginal route may acquire skin organisms during delivery. Sarkany and Gaylarde (1968), by means of contact plates, sampled skin immediately after birth; the sample skin sites were on the head, the scapular region, axilla, periumbilical region and the groin. Staphylococci were present in all the babies and diphtheroids were isolated in 60% of them. Coliform organisms and streptococci were isolated from some babies. A study by Evans, Akpata and Baki (1970) examined babies within 2.5 hours of delivery. In only half the infants were they able to demonstrate the existence of bacteria on the skin and in the nose. The carriage of organisms in the nose increased in the first three days of life. *Staphylococcus epidermidis* was the most common organism, with non-haemolytic streptococci the second most common. Full-term babies were colonized more rapidly than preterm ones. *Pseudomonas aeruginosa* was isolated more frequently from the nose of preterm babies.

The microorganisms which affect the baby are acquired from the mother, attendants and the environment. Studies on the acquisition of *Staph. aureus* have shown the significance of other infants in a nursery (Parker and Kennedy, 1949; Rountree and Barbour, 1950). Members of staff may act both as a source (Baldwin *et al.*, 1957) and as carriers of staphylococci from other babies (Love *et al.*, 1963).

Studies of the upper respiratory tract of infants indicate that *Streptococcus pneumoniae* and *Haemophilus influenzae* establish themselves more frequently than streptococci of the viridans and non-haemolytic type (Laurell, Tunevall and Wallmark, 1958; Box, Cleveland and Willard, 1961.)

Temporary colonization in conjunction with other organisms may occur. If the mother develops an infection of the liquor, the infecting organisms will be present at birth on the baby's skin. Although the organisms will generally die rapidly and be replaced by normal flora, some may persist in the external auditory meatus. The external auditory meatus of sick neonates should always be examined microbiologically, with special reference to *Listeria monocytogenes* and Group B streptococci.

Children have a varied bacterial flora over the skin, in the nose and in the throat. Nasal carriage of *Staph. aureus*, *Strep. pneumoniae* and Gram-negative bacteria is commoner in children than in adults.

Adenoviruses have been isolated from the tonsils and adenoids of children even in the absence of any clinical infection, but whether the virus was being carried following an infection or whether it can exist as part of the normal flora is unclear. Equally, the Epstein–Barr virus and the herpes simplex virus may be present in the throat and nasopharynx of persons without clinical infection.

With the onset of puberty, changes of both a physiological and anatomical nature occur. In the skin, sebum and cerumen producing glands become more active, thereby increasing the local concentrations of fatty acids. Fatty acids constitute more than 40% of the total lipid present in cerumen. They do not, however, appear to inhibit organisms to any great extent (Perry and Nichols, 1956).

Various investigators agree that the commonest bacteria in the healthy ear are micrococci and diphtheroids. *Staph. aureus* and streptococci are not uncommon. Although Enterobacteriaciae, such as *Escherichia coli* and *Proteus* spp., were found in a small proportion of ears, the percentage is increased in diseased ears. Respiratory tract *Neisseria* have also been isolated from the ears.

Yeasts and *Ps. aeruginosa* are very rare inhabitants of the healthy ear and, if present, are in very small numbers.

The flora of the nasal passages has been intensively studied. In a quantitative study (Herzo *et al.*, 1981) of carriers and non-carriers of *Staph. aureus*, *Staph. xylosus*, *Staph. hominis* and anaerobic *Propionibacterium* spp., especially *P. acnes*, were usually present in most subjects. Yeasts were often present in significant numbers. Streptococci and Gram-negative rods were not common.

Incidence studies indicate that between 35 and 50% of normal adults carry a strain of *Staph. aureus* in the anterior nares. Repeated swabbing of the same population shows that 20–35% of persons are persistent carriers, 30–70% intermittent carriers and 10–40% are never carriers (Williams, 1963). Persistent carriers usually have the same strain for long periods. The presence of large numbers of one strain prevents the implantation of other strains. This bacterial interference is the rationale of instilling a 'safe' strain into the nose when attempting to control outbreaks of staphylococcal infection. The nasal carriage of group A streptococci occurs in 1–4% of children.

In the nasopharynx and down into the throat, the normal flora changes with an increasing presence of streptococci and *Neisseria* sp. The streptococci are primarily α-haemolytic or non-haemolytic. Group A haemolytic streptococci can be isolated from the throat of normal persons not in contact with epidemic streptococcal infection. The frequency in children varies between 10 and 25% (Quinn, Denny and Riley, 1957) and in adults between 2 and 8%, with the determinants being age, season and geographical location. A study of 2400 London children by Holmes and Williams (1954) showed a total incidence of 21%, although within individual school or nursery units, rates varying between 0 and 79% were observed. The highest carriage rate was in the 3–4 year age group. The rate in children with tonsils was 28% whereas it was only 8% in those without tonsils. Seasonal variation was observed by Ross (1971) with the highest incidence in the winter months.

The number of children carrying group A streptococci in both their nose and throat lies at 1–4%. The nasal carrier rate often exceeds that of the throat in tropical areas where tonsillitis is uncommon but impetigo is prevalent.

Neisseria meningitidis can be isolated from 2–4% of normal persons. During an investigation by the author of 42 young people, of whom two had developed group B type 15 meningococcal meningitis, eight carriers were identified. In three of these, the isolate was indistinguishable from the meningitis strains; in four, it could not be grouped; and in one, it belonged to group B but could not be ascribed to type. All the carriers were free of symptoms.

Haemophilus influenzae is carried in the nasopharynx by up to 80% of normal people. However, only 2–4% carry capsulated type B and 1–2% other capsulated strains.

Functions of the normal flora

The importance of maintaining the normal flora has been recognized not so much from understanding its function as from observing the consequences of upsetting the normal balance. Gram-negative bacilli, especially *Ps. aeruginosa* and yeasts such as *Candida albicans*, may be present in low numbers; if the balance is upset, it is these organisms, in particular, which proliferate and may be the cause of symptoms in the patient. The interactions between microorganisms of the same and different species, both qualitative and quantitative, are complex and, as such, not well understood.

The potential capacity of one bacterial strain to interfere with another has been recognized, and it was the ability of one strain of *Staph. aureus* to prevent colonization with another strain which was used by Shinefield *et al.* (1963) to control outbreaks of staphylococcal sepsis in nurseries. Outbreaks of skin and systemic infections, caused by staphylococci of the group I (52, 52A, 80, 81) bacteriophage complex, were difficult to control. *Staph. aureus* 502A belonging to the group III bacteriophage complex, and regarded as 'avirulent', was instilled into the nares of neonates. Colonization with this strain prevented subsequent colonization with the outbreak strain, which was effective in reducing the frequency of sepsis in a number of nurseries suffering from outbreaks of staphylococcal infection. The mode of action of this bacterial interference is not known, although the production of bacteriocins has been postulated. However, the growth inhibition of staphylococcal strains by 502A cannot be demonstrated *in vitro*; particularly as 502A colonization made no impact on an outbreak of impetigo caused by type 55/71 staphylococci belonging to bacteriophage group II. Staphylococcal interference is most effective between strains of the same groups. Group II strains have less affinity to strains of group I or III, than strains of group I and III have with one another.

Wickman (1970), by using guinea-pig models, has demonstrated the inhibitory effect of *Staph. epidermidis* on the subsequent colonization of *Staph. aureus*.

Martin and White (1968) showed that nasal carriers of coagulase-negative cocci and diphtheroids resisted recolonization by *Staph. aureus*. If, however, the nasal flora had been reduced with antimicrobical chemotherapy, recolonization occurred readily.

Observations on skin flora have shown that the suppression of normal diphtheroids and skin staphylococci is followed by replacement with Gram-negative flora.

Studies *in vitro* of interactions between organisms found in the normal ear, nose and throat include the classic requirement of *H. influenzae* for haematin and coenzyme A. On a blood agar plate, coenzyme A can be supplied by a colony of *Staph. aureus*. Surrounding colonies of *H. influenzae* are larger than those elsewhere on the plate. This phenomenon of satellitism has been known since 1898.

The production of antistaphylococcal substances by viridans streptococci was described by Myers (1959) and Noble and Somerville (1974). Sprunt and Redman (1968) found that α-haemolytic streptococci produce a factor which has an inhibitory effect on other organisms in the throat. Inhibition is often related to specific strains. *Staph. aureus* strains of group II produce antibacterial substances active against *Corynebacterium* and *Streptococcus* species. Type 71, in particular, produces a protein or polypeptide which acts against streptococci of Lancefield groups A, C, and D, pneumococci and *Co. diphtheriae*.

Antigenic similarities between the normal flora and the pathogenic organisms may provide a further protective mechanism. Local antibody produced against antigenic determinants in the normal flora may also act against various pathogens. It has been postulated that the ability of pneumococci, meningococci and *H. influenzae* to produce IgA1 proteases may facilitate mucosal colonization (Turk, 1984; Falcone and Campa, 1981).

Transient flora with pathogenic organisms which briefly colonize but do not cause a clinical infection may, nevertheless, stimulate local immunity. This would explain why during respiratory virus outbreaks not all those exposed develop clinical illness yet they have protection against future attacks with the production of specific antibodies.

Factors influencing the normal flora

Changes in normal flora throughout life are observed in the different age groups – the neonate to the child, then through puberty to adult life and finally the elderly. Changes in the microbial flora reflect the alteration in the microenvironments which are crudely measured in terms of pH, moisture and chemical substances, such as fatty acids. Anatomical development also affects the microenvironment. Age-related environmental and social factors will affect exposure to microorganisms which may colonize the ear, nose and throat. In clinical practice, the major changes are observed in relation to disease and the treatment of disease. The use of antimicrobial agents affects not only the pathogens against which they are directed but also the normal flora. The majority of bacteria constituting the normal flora of the ear, nose and throat are susceptible to the main groups of antibacterial drugs. The use of the latter to treat an infection anywhere in the body causes a varying suppression of part or all of the normal flora. This in turn allows resistant bacteria to

multiply during therapy and affects the recolonization pattern after the therapy has ceased. Gram-negative bacilli and in particular strains of the *Proteus* and *Klebsiella* species and *Ps. aeruginosa* and the yeast *C. albicans* flourish in these circumstances.

The changed flora is usually dependent on a continued antibacterial pressure, and when that pressure is discontinued the normal pattern will eventually be re-established. However, the Gram-negative bacilli and yeasts may become so dominant that, if there is an underlying abnormality or disease of the ear, nose or throat, they may themselves be the cause of symptoms or they may occasionally persist. The treatment of chronic otitis externa with various locally applied antibacterial compounds will frequently result in *Ps. aeruginosa*, *Proteus* spp. or *C. albicans* becoming firmly established in the patient's auditory canal, with the altered microenvironment brought about by the repeated application of ear drops aiding, in particular, the more resistant Gram-negative bacteria. Careful local cleansing and drying is often all that is required to re-establish a healthy ear with a normal flora.

Similarly, patients with chronic sinus problems, who have received multiple courses of antibacterials, have an altered flora in the nose and nasopharynx with a preponderance of Gram-negative bacilli.

Microorganisms associated with infections in the ear, nose and throat

This section could include almost all known bacteria, viruses and fungi, as the ability to keep immunosuppressed patients alive for longer periods has led to a concomitant increase in the incidence and range of organisms causing 'opportunistic' infections. Therefore, those organisms which are described here are the recognized major pathogens, past and present, and those whose study elucidates important principles in the understanding of the host–parasite relationship. It is not possible, however, to discuss in detail every aspect of each organism, and this information can be obtained from textbooks on microbiology.

Bacteria

Bacterial species and genera are defined and described within an overall bacterial classification, and each is represented by a type culture maintained by one or more of the major type collections. There is an internationally agreed nomenclature which should always be followed to avoid confusion. Some organisms, the names of which vary according to country, now have an accepted official name. For example, *Clostridium perfringens*, an organism causing gas gangrene, was for many years referred to as *Clostridium welchii* in the UK.

The full identification of a bacterium depends initially on defining a range of characteristics including morphology, cultural appearances, growth requirements, biochemical reactions, resistance to physical and chemical conditions, antigenic structure, chemical analysis and composition and homology of the deoxyribonucleic acid (DNA). Numerical coding and weighting of individual characteristics has, with the use of computers, enabled organisms to be grouped and sorted – a classification termed 'numerical taxonomy'.

In routine clinical practice, it is generally sufficient to undertake only a few discriminating tests in order to place a pathogenic bacterium in one of the main groups of medically important organisms. Further detailed tests in hospital laboratories are usually undertaken for epidemiological rather than taxonomic purposes.

It is essential to identify the microorganisms which are causing the infection if the particular infection process and the spread of the infection, both within and between hosts, is to be understood.

Corynebacterium and other coryneform organisms

The diphtheria bacillus was first observed by Klebs in 1883, in a diphtheritic false membrane. In 1884, Loeffler cultivated the organism and described its characteristics. Over the years, several other organisms have been included in the genus *Corynebacterium* and they are often described as diphtheroids. The application of numerical taxonomy and DNA studies have now enabled differences to be recognized. The group of coryneform or Gram-positive, non-mycelial, non-sporing bacteria that exhibit a pleomorphic morphology includes the genera *Corynebacterium*, *Arthrobacter*, *Brevibacterium*, *Microbacterium*, *Cellulomonas*, *Listeria*, *Erysipelothrix*, *Mycobacterium* and some species of *Nocardia*. The term 'diphtheroid' is descriptive and refers both to organisms in the genus *Corynebacterium* and to some organisms which are erstwhile members of the genus but are now excluded. The latter organisms include '*Corynebacterium*' *pyogenes* and '*Co.*' *haemolyticum*.

Corynebacterium

Type species: Corynebacterium diphtheriae

The main pathogen to man is *Co. diphtheriae*. *Co. ulcerans* can cause tonsillitis. '*Co*'. *haemolyticum* and '*Co*'. *pyogenes* can be isolated from the throats of human patients with a disease associated with a scarlatiniform rash (Ryan, 1972).

Morphology

This organism is characteristically pleomorphic in spite of the name being derived from the description 'coryneform' or club-shaped cells. It is generally a slender bacillus with rounded or swollen ends, although shorter stubby forms may occur. The morphology will vary with the culture media and the age of the culture. The uptake of aniline dyes and methylene blue is erratic and frequently it is described as Gram-variable, although it is Gram-positive. A characterizing feature is the presence of metachromatic granules. These granules are coloured reddish purple when a film preparation is stained with methylene blue. They are routinely demonstrated by means of a differential stain described by Neisser, or Albert. Granule production is enhanced by culturing on a medium which is deficient in iron.

The arrangement of the bacilli in a film preparation is also very characteristic. Cells tend to lie at an angle to each other, forming an L or V; groups of such pairs acquire the appearance of Chinese letters, or of cuneiform writing. True branching is also observed with *Co. diphtheriae*.

Other species within the genus have a similar appearance, although their ability to retain dyes is more effective.

Cultural characteristics

Members of the genus grow well on ordinary nutrient agar. Growth is improved by the addition of animal protein, and Loeffler's serum is a popular medium for growing *Co. diphtheriae*. When grown on tellurite blood agar, three types of *Co. diphtheriae* – gravis, intermedius and mitis – can be recognized from the colonial appearance. Other diphtheroid bacilli grown on tellurite blood agar form colonies which are distinctly different from those of *Co. diphtheriae*. The morphology and colonial appearances are well described in standard textbooks but depend to a large extent on the actual medium used. A tellurite medium using a brain heart base with 10% blood and 0.03% potassium tellurite readily grows *Co. diphtheriae* from clinical specimens within a 24-hour period. The potassium tellurite is inhibitory to streptococci, staphylococci and micrococci.

Biochemical reactions

In clinical laboratories, members of the genera and other diphtheroids are differentiated mainly by their ability to ferment glucose, maltose, sucrose and starch, and to effect the hydrolysis of urea and the reduction of nitrate to nitrite.

Toxin production

Co. diphtheriae is capable of producing a powerful exotoxin which is the main cause of the symptoms in patients suffering from diphtheria. It is produced by young, rapidly growing cells and liberated from the bacterial cells.

Not all strains of *Co. diphtheriae* are toxin producers and the ability to produce the toxin is associated with the presence of a bacteriophage in the bacterial cell. A close parallel has been demonstrated between toxin production and the synthesis of new phage particles.

The production of toxin by an isolate of the diphtheria bacillus can be demonstrated by guinea-pig inoculation and by a gel diffusion technique. If a guinea-pig is inoculated subcutaneously with a virulent culture or a toxic filtrate, an area of soft oedema appears at the injection site within 12–18 hours, and gradually spreads. The ill animal becomes progressively worse, dying after 18–36 hours according to the dose of culture or filtrate administered. A post-mortem examination will reveal a characteristic extensive area of gelatinous haemorrhagic oedema at the site of inoculation, regional lymph nodes are swollen, the adrenal glands are swollen and congested, and body cavities contain exudates which may be blood-stained.

The production of toxin *in vitro* from colonies adjacent to antitoxin containing strips embedded in the agar, can be demonstrated by the development of precipitation lines in the agar. Unknown strains are tested adjacent to known strong and weak toxin-producing strains. The fusion of diffusion lines from known and unknown strains confirms toxin production. The composition of the test medium is important if diffusion lines are to develop within 24–36 hours, although usually 48 hours are required.

Strains of 'Co'. *ulcerans* also produce a toxin indistinguishable from that of *Co. diphtheriae*.

Suitable treatment with formalin converts the toxin into a toxoid which is no longer toxic and can be used to stimulate antitoxin production in animals. In the immunization of infants against diphtheria, the toxoid usually adsorbed onto aluminium phosphate is used.

Resistance

Co. diphtheriae is readily killed by heat and by the usual disinfectants. Although some studies suggest that it is relatively resistant to drying, survival in the environment is not an important link in the chain of infection. Most strains are highly sensitive to erythromycin and penicillin.

Clinical microbiology

If a clinical diagnosis of diphtheria is suspected, the microbiology laboratory must be informed immediately, and throat and nose swabs should be taken. The swabs will be inoculated onto tellurite blood agar, a Loeffler's serum agar slope and ordinary blood agar. A presumptive bacteriological confirmation of the diagnosis can usually be given in 18–24 hours, but demonstration of toxin production may take a further 24–48 hours. It is important, therefore, that initial treatment should be carried out on the basis of a clinical diagnosis.

Streptococcus

Streptococci are Gram-positive cocci that divide in one plane to form chains or pairs. They cause a variety of diseases in both humans and animals.

Although many different species of streptococci form part of the normal flora of the upper respiratory tract, relatively few of them are pathogenic to man. *Streptococcus pyogenes* Lancefield group A is the major cause of acute sore throats and tonsillitis. Local infection may also be followed by late sequelae rheumatic fever and acute glomerulonephritis. *Streptococcus pneumoniae* may cause sinusitis. The other streptococci which can be isolated from the throat are not usually associated with local infection, although they may be carried to a damaged heart valve and cause bacterial endocarditis.

Streptococcus pyogenes

Streptococcus pyogenes was described by Rosenbach in 1884 to define an organism which had been isolated from suppurative lesions in man and which grew in chains. This organism was the cause of classic puerperal fever; it can cause severe suppurative wound infections; it is the cause of impetigo, scarlet fever and erysipelas; it remains a common cause of tonsillitis and pharyngitis; and infection resulting from it may be followed by rheumatic fever or acute glomerulonephritis.

Morphology

The usual morphology is that of Gram-positive cocci arranged in chains. Capsulated strains have been described but are uncommon.

Cultural characteristics

The organism does not grow well on basic culture medium unless the culture medium is enriched with blood, serum or glucose. Colonies on blood agar are usually 0.8–1 mm in diameter following incubation at 37 °C for 18–24 hours. If horse blood is used in the medium, the colonies are sur-rounded by a clear zone of haemolysis (β-haemolysis). The area of haemolysis is improved by anaerobic incubation.

Biochemical reactions

In clinical laboratories, the identification of *Strep. pyogenes* does not rely on biochemical reactions. In situations where it is necessary to differentiate *Strep. faecalis*, use is made of the ability of the latter species to hydrolyse aesculin in the presence of bile salts.

Toxin production

Strep. pyogenes is a potent producer of extracellular toxins: streptolysin O and streptolysin S are both haemolysins. 'O' is oxygen labile and 'S' serum soluble. The presence of antistreptolysin O anti-bodies in serum is commonly used to detect recent streptococcal infection. Streptolysin S does not stimulate antibody production. The production of an erythrogenic toxin was originally thought to cause the erythematous lesions of scarlet fever, although there is now considerable evidence that the rash is the consequence of a hypersensitivity reaction. Deoxyribonuclease and ribonuclease are formed by all strains of *Strep. pyogenes*. Other extracellar toxins and enzymes include strepto-kinase, proteinase, hyaluronidase, nicotinamide adenine dinucleotidase and neuraminidase.

Antigenic structure

Most of the pyogenic streptococci can be divided into groups according to specific polysaccharide or teichoic acid antigens. Streptococci in groups A, B, C, E, F and G have a polysaccharide antigen, whereas groups D and N have a teichoic acid antigen. The group antigens do not stimulate protective immunity. Group A streptococci can be divided according to the presence or absence of M, T and R antigens. The M antigen is closely linked to an associated protein, and anti-M associated protein antibodies are usually higher in rheumatic fever than in either nephritis or uncomplicated streptococcal respiratory infection. The M protein is an essential pathogenicity factor, as in its absence streptococci do not survive in normal human blood. The M antibody is type protective. T and R antigens, although useful for typing strains for epidemiological studies, have no other known function.

Resistance

The group A streptococcus is remarkable in its persistent sensitivity to penicillin, whereas resis-tance to erythromycin, tetracycline and analogues,

and chloramphenicol is not infrequent. For clinical purposes, the streptococci are resistant to amino-glycosides. A useful laboratory test is the sensitiv-ity of group A streptococci to bacitracin. The organism is capable of surviving in dust for many weeks, especially if protected by dried secretions. Cross-infection of wounds can occur by way of this route, although drying reduces the ability of the organism to cause respiratory tract infection.

Clinical microbiology

Swabs from infected wounds or throats should be sent to the laboratory in a transport medium. A blood agar plate is inoculated and incubated at 37 °C preferably in an atmosphere of 7–10% carbon dioxide. Typical colonies are visible within 18 hours; and if a bacitracin identity disc has been placed on the culture plate, a presumptive group A identification can be made. Confirmation of the group is normally undertaken by slide agglutina-tion using specific monoclonal antibodies.

Streptococcus pneumoniae

This streptococcus, which is often referred to as pneumococcus, is easily distinguishable from other members of the genus. This organism has a characteristic morphology, it is soluble in bile and is sensitive to Optochin.

Morphology

The organisms are normally arranged in pairs or in very short chains. Many strains develop capsules which, in stained film preparations, show as clear haloes around the bacteria.

Cultural characteristics

The organisms will grow on basic culture media. Growth is stimulated by blood and glucose. Some strains from clinical material require the presence of 5–15% carbon dioxide for initial isolation. On blood agar, the colonies are surrounded by an area of α-haemolysis when grown aerobically. The solubility of pneumococci in a solution of bile can be demonstrated on the culture plate or in a suspension of the organism.

Antigenic structure

The capsular polysaccharides are antigenic and thus enable pneumococci to be typed. More than 80 types are recognized. In Europe, 14 types are associated with the most serious pneumococcal infections. The antibodies produced are protec-tive, and this factor forms the basis of a pneumococcal vaccine.

Resistance

Pneumococci, in the same way as the group A streptococci, are sensitive to penicillin, although a degree of resistance in some strains has been reported. Resistance to tetracycline and erythromycin is related to their use in the community.

Pathogenicity

The pneumococcus causes lobar pneumonia, sinusitis, otitis media, meningitis, pyogenic arthritis and peritonitis. Virulence is associated with the polysaccharide capsule.

Clinical microbiology

As with group A streptococci, the pneumococcus is readily grown from clinical specimens. Identification is by means of assessing its sensitivity to Optochin or by its bile solubility.

Other streptococci

Group B streptococci are associated with neonatal sepsis and vaginal infection. Groups C and G may be isolated from the throat and have been associated with tonsillitis. A range of streptococci, known colloquially as α-haemolytic streptococci on account of the nature of their appearance on blood agar plates, can be isolated from the oropharynx. They do not cause local infections but are causes of bacterial endocarditis. They can be divided biochemically and include *Strep. mitor*, *Strep. sanguis*, *Strep. milleri*, *Strep. mutans* and *Strep. salivarius*. *Strep. faecalis* belongs to group D; it is found mainly in the large bowel and referred to as the faecal streptococcus.

Staphylococcus

Staphylococci are Gram-positive cocci which, when divided, form clusters. They were recognized in pus by Koch in 1878 and were cultured by Pasteur in 1880. *Staphylococcus aureus* is the main pyogenic bacterium and the cause of most wound infections. *Staph. epidermidis* and *Staph. saprophyticus* are skin and nasal mucosal organisms with limited pathogenicity. The type species is *Staph. aureus*.

Staphylococcus aureus

Morphology

The usual morphology is Gram-positive cocci which form grape-like clusters.

Cultural characteristics

Growth is abundant on unenriched nutrient agar. Colonies are 1–2 mm in diameter after a 24-hour incubation at 37 °C; they are golden yellow in colour. On horse blood agar, a narrow zone of haemolysis may be present. They are tolerant to high salt concentrations which facilitates their selective culture on salt-containing media. Their ability to produce phosphatase is detected on a solid medium by incorporating phenolphthalein phosphate. The enzyme liberates free phenolphthalein which turns red following exposure of the culture plate to ammonia vapour.

Biochemical reactions

Staphylococci are able to form acid from glucose, both aerobically and anaerobically. In addition to phosphatase, catalase and deoxyribonuclease are also produced. *Staph. aureus* will clump in plasma by reason of the cell wall component known as clumping factor which reacts with fibrinogen. An extracellular coagulase is also produced which causes plasma to coagulate. The presence of the clumping factor and coagulase is used in the rapid identification of *Staph. aureus*.

Toxin production

Staph. aureus is capable of producing a wide range of toxins. General toxins, such as the haemolytic toxins, probably play a role in the pathogenesis of both local and systemic infections. Their general action is to cause damage to cell membranes. The detection of staphylococcal α-haemolysin antibody is used in the diagnosis of deep-seated staphylococcal sepsis. Other general toxins include leucocidins, staphylokinase and hyaluronidase.

Specific toxins are produced by some staphylococcal strains. If strains which produce enterotoxins contaminate food, the toxin will be formed in the food and will survive cooking. Ingestion of the food and, thereby, of the toxin is followed in 1–6 hours by vomiting; this may be severe and be accompanied by muscular cramping and prostration. Staphylococcal food poisoning is a major cause of food-borne illness. The enterotoxins can be detected immunologically.

Staphylococci which produce epidermolytic toxins may cause a severe skin infection – scalded skin syndrome – in which toxins cause splitting of the epidermis with blister formation. The majority of epidermolytic toxin producing strains belong to phage group II with a predominance of type 71.

Antigenic structure

Strains of staphylococci are not antigenically distinct, and antibodies produced to cell wall constituents are not protective. A specific surface antigen, protein A, has been widely studied in consequence of its specific reactivity with immunoglobulins which enables it to be used in many immunological studies.

Bacteriophage typing

Strains of *Staph. aureus* can be typed according to their pattern of susceptibility to a range of bacteriophages. Bacteriophages are viruses which can infect bacterial cells, multiply within them and cause lysis. By employing a range of typing phages, a number of useful epidemiological studies have been undertaken. Also, phage typing is an essential part of the investigation into staphylococcal outbreaks. Certain patterns of lysis occur more often than others which makes possible the division into phage groups I, II, III and IV. Groups I and III have been associated with major outbreaks of hospital-acquired infections. In particular, the strains with the typing pattern 80/81 spread throughout the world, but these have since been replaced by types 84/85 and, more recently, types 94 and 96 have been emerging. Some strains cannot be typed by the standard set of phages and are, therefore, termed 'non-typable'.

Resistance

Staphylococci are well known for their ability to develop resistance to a wide range of antibacterial drugs. Penicillin resistance resulting from the production of a β-lactamase – penicillinase – is common in hospital strains, although the majority of community strains remain sensitive. As new antistaphylococcal drugs were introduced, so resistant strains have developed. Strains resistant to the isoxazolyl penicillins (methicillin, cloxacillin, flucloxacillin, etc.), which are not susceptible to β-lactamase, are now responsible for severe outbreaks of sepsis in some hospitals (Shanson, 1986). These strains may also be resistant to gentamicin, erythromycin, tetracycline and fusidic acid. They are referred to as epidermic methicillin resistant *Staph. aureus* and the outbreaks they cause can be controlled only by strict isolation and control of infection procedures. Life-threatening infections with methicillin resistant *Staph. aureus* may necessitate the use of vancomycin and rifampicin.

Staph. aureus is resistant to drying, especially in the presence of dried protein. Strains may survive in dust for many months, thereby providing an environmental reservoir of infection.

Clinical microbiology

Swabs from infected lesions should be sent to the laboratory in transport medium. Growth will occur within 18 hours on standard culture medium, and suspect colonies are confirmed by using the coagulase test or specific monoclonal agglutination tests. Environmental samples are cultured on a selective medium containing phenolphthalein phosphate. Growth in this case may be slower, although colonies can usually be detected within 24 hours.

Bacteriophage typing is undertaken in specialized laboratories and may take 7–10 days. Individual isolates should not normally be sent for typing, but a collection of strains, for which confirmation or otherwise of an association is required, can be typed.

Haemophilus

Members of this genus are slender Gram-negative bacilli with exacting growth requirements. The first strain to be isolated was termed a 'haemophilic bacillus' and this was thought to be the causative agent of influenza, until the true viral aetiology of the latter was established. The type species *Haemophilus influenzae* may cause primary pyogenic diseases such as meningitis, acute epiglottitis in children and suppurative arthritis. It is often a secondary pathogen in chronic bronchitis and bronchiectasis, and may be present at the site of infection in bronchopneumonia and otitis media. It is frequently present in the upper respiratory tract as part of the normal flora. *H. parainfluenzae* and *H. haemolyticum* have been isolated from patients with acute pharyngitis.

Haemophilus influenzae
Morphology

Fresh clinical isolates generally have a coccobacillary form, although longer rods may occur. They are Gram-negative.

Cultural characteristics

Haemophilic bacilli have characteristic nutritional requirements: almost all require the presence of the 'X factor' (haemin), which is present in blood, with *H. influenzae* also requiring the 'V factor' (NAD). *H. parainfluenzae* requires V but not X factor. Growth will occur on plain agar if the factors are added. In most clinical laboratories, X factor can be provided by heating blood agar to 75 °C for a few minutes in order to break down the red cells, thus releasing their contents ('chocolate' agar). V factor is produced by *Staph. aureus*. If stab cultures are made in the chocolate agar after *Haemophilus* has been spread on the agar surface, *H. influenzae* will grow as satellite colonies around the *Staph. aureus*.

Biochemical reactions

The genus can be divided biochemically but this method has little application in routine clinical laboratories.

Antigenic structure

H. influenzae has a wide antigenic heterogenicity. Strains can be divided into Pittman types, according to the antigenicity of a polysaccharide capsule, by using anticapsular sera. Pittman type b is associated with the severe forms of haemophilus infection. Antibodies provide protective immunity; in the USA, a haemophilus polysaccharide vaccine is recommended for young children.

Resistance

The majority of strains are sensitive to chloramphenicol, co-trimoxazole, erythromycin and the new cephalosporins. Sensitivity to ampicillin depends on whether the strain is capable of producing a β-lactamase. Eight per cent of clinical isolates in the UK are β-lactamase producers. In severe life-threatening infections, chloramphenicol is the drug of choice.

Clinical microbiology

Specimens should be sent to the laboratory in transport media. Growth will occur in 18–24 hours on chocolate agar; and if a source of V factor has been provided, a presumptive identification can be made. Definitive speciation, if required, necessitates subculturing and testing for nutritional requirements.

Bordetella

Although *Bordetella pertussis* does not cause disease in the ear, nose or throat, it can be isolated from the nasopharynx of patients with whooping cough.

The organisms are rod-shaped, coccoid or oval, and Gram-negative. They do not grow on basic media as they require blood or vegetable and tissue extracts. Primary isolation is usually undertaken on Bordet and Gengou medium which contains blood, glycerin, potato extract and charcoal. The plates are incubated in 5–10% carbon dioxide for 3–5 days. Typical colonies are silvery-grey, and confirmation is by agglutination with specific antiserum.

The detection of *B. pertussis* in the nasopharynx is undertaken by means of swabbing the area with a pernasal swab, the latter of which should then be transported to the laboratory in specific transport medium. Culture is on Bordet and Gengou medium.

Enterobacteria

This group includes a wide range of bacteria. These bacteria are not primary pathogens in the ear, nose or throat but may replace part of the normal flora in patients receiving antibacterial chemotherapy, thereby becoming a possible cause of secondary infection in conditions such as chronic sinusitis, and chronic otitis media and externa. The commoner enterobacteria in these situations are *Escherichia coli*, *Klebsiella aerogenes* and *Proteus* species. They are usually associated with urinary tract infection.

They are all Gram-negative bacilli and will grow readily on basic media. Most of the genera are motile. The genera are differentiated according to their biochemical reactions, further subdivision is by both biochemical and serological methods.

Escherichia coli

Morphology

This is a Gram-negative, non-sporing bacillus. Eighty per cent of strains are motile with peritrichate flagella.

Cultural characteristics

Growth occurs readily on basic medium over a wide range of temperatures. After a 24-hour incubation on blood agar at 37°C, colonies are smooth, glistening and about 1–2 mm in diameter. Some discoloration and haemolysis of the medium occurs near the colonies. If lactose and a pH indicator are incorporated in a suitable medium, such as MacConkey agar or cystine lactose electrolyte deficient agar, fermentation and acid production will occur with a change in the colour of the pH indicator.

Biochemical reactions

The full differentiation of *E. coli* necessitates the use of a wide range of biochemical tests, for the reasons that no one test on its own is 100% accurate and that there are many patterns attributable to this species. The majority of strains, however, while being able to ferment lactose, are not able to utilize citrate as the sole carbon source, but produce indole from peptone water and do not produce urease.

Antigenic structure

Three main antigen groups O, H and K are recognized. They enable the species to be subdivided for epidemiological studies.

Toxin production

Some strains produce a range of enterotoxins and are probably the principal cause of travellers' diarrhoea. The lipopolysaccharides in the cell walls are endotoxins.

Resistance

The environmental survival period in dry areas is short but if protected by organic material or moisture, these bacteria may remain viable for lengthy periods. They are sensitive to the main Gram-negative antibiotics although drug resistance does occur, mainly in hospital-acquired strains where the resistance is maintained by keeping an antibiotic selective pressure. Resistance to one or more antimicrobial drugs may be transferred between both strains and species on extrachromosomal genetic material (plasmids).

Clinical microbiology

Provided that the specimen or swab is kept moist, transport to the laboratory is not a problem although the use of transport medium is advised. Characteristic colonies on MacConkey agar or cystine lactose electrolyte deficient agar are recognizable within 24 hours. Biochemical reactions take place after a further 24–48 hours, depending on the purity of the original culture.

Klebsiella aerogenes

K. aerogenes differs from *E. coli* in that it is non-motile, it is able to use citrate as the sole carbon source and it does not produce indole from peptone water. Many strains are capsulated and produce mucoid colonies. The capsular antigens enable them to be typed.

The wide-ranging resistance of this bacillus to antibacterial drugs is of clinical importance, as multiple resistant strains have been involved in a number of outbreaks of infection in intensive therapy units.

Proteus species

The commonest member of this species is *Proteus mirabilis*. This organism has the ability to swarm over non-selective agar instead of forming discrete colonies. It does not ferment lactose and is a potent urease producer.

Pseudomonas

The pseudomonads most familiar to clinicians are those that produce blue or green pigments, are associated with foul smelling pus and are resistant to most antimicrobial agents. Clinically significant infections involving pseudomonads usually occur in patients who have had multiple courses of antibacterial drugs, and these organisms are often associated with a foreign body or an anatomical abnormality. They are ready inhabitants of moist environmental niches. Open bottles of water and solutions including many disinfectants are readily contaminated by pseudomonads and *Ps. aeruginosa*.

Morphology

This is a Gram-negative bacillus, and it is motile.

Cultural characteristics

Growth occurs readily in air on ordinary culture medium. The organisms do not grow in the absence of oxygen. Typical colonies have a matt surface with an irregular edge. In reflected light, the surface often has a metallic sheen. Some strains produce 'coliform' colonies and other profuse amounts of a mucoid substance. The latter type is typical from patients with fibrocystic disease. Most strains produce the pigment pyocyanin on medium which contains magnesium.

Biochemical reactions

The main clinically useful reactions are the inability to ferment lactose, and the positive oxidase reaction. Metabolism of glucose is by oxidation rather than by fermentation.

Toxin production

The ability of many strains to produce soluble bacteriocins which are active against other strains has a practical use inasmuch as the patterns of inhibition can be used for epidemiological typing.

Antigenic structure

The species possess both O and H antigens, although the former are easiest to determine. O antibodies may offer some protection against infection, providing a basis for vaccine development. The lipopolysaccharide in the cell wall has properties similar to the endotoxins of enterobacteria.

Resistance

Ps. aeruginosa is resistant to most antibiotics including ampicillin, sulphonamides, trimethoprim, tetracycline, the majority of cephalosporins, and kanamycin. Most strains are sensitive to gentamicin, tobramycin, carbenicillin, ticarcillin, azlocillin, piperacillin and some specific cephalosporins. However, resistance to colistin is rare.

Most strains are able to grow in aqueous solutions of many disinfectants. Agar which contains cetrimide is used as a selective medium for the isolation of the species.

Clincial microbiology

The organism survives well on moist specimens or swabs. It grows readily on ordinary media and its presence can be detected within 24 hours.

Neisseria

Neisseria gonorrhoeae can cause throat infections, usually following oral sexual practices with men who have genital gonorrhoea. *N. meningitidis* does not cause infection of the throat but may be carried in this area. These genera are Gram-negative diplococci and require media supplemented with blood or animal protein additives. *N. gonorrhoeae* and *meningitidis* are distinguished biochemically. Characteristically, *N. gonorrhoeae* will ferment glucose but not maltose, whereas *N. meningitidis* will ferment both sugars. *N. gonorrhoeae* can also be detected by immunofluorescent techniques. Meningococci can be grouped serologically, with most strains in Britain belonging to group B.

Anaerobic bacteria

There are a large number of different genera and species of anaerobic bacteria. Although not a major cause of infection in the ear, nose and throat, they may be associated with chronic sinusitis and otitis media. *Borrelia vincenti* and anaerobic Gram-negative fusiform bacilli together cause painful ulcers in the throat and an ulcerative gingivitis.

The anaerobic bacteria predominantly associated with human infections are the *Bacteroides* species, anaerobic streptococci, *Actinomyces* and *Clostridium* species.

If an anaerobic infection is suspected, it is essential that any specimens are not exposed to air. Swabs must be transported in transport medium containing a reducing agent. Most strains grow well on media enriched with blood, but it may take 48 hours for colonies to develop. *Actinomyces* spp. take up to 7 days to produce colonies.

All anaerobic bacteria are sensitive to metronidazole. However, their sensitivity to other antimicrobials varies – most clostridia are sensitive to penicillin, wheras anaerobic streptococci and

Bacteroides species may be resistant to multiple drugs.

Mycobacteria

Mycobacteria behave differently from other clinically important bacteria, both in the diseases they cause and in their properties *in vitro*. Infections usually have an extended time course and delayed hypersensitivity reactions are important. *Mycobacterium tuberculosis*, the commonest species infecting man, exists in the human and bovine types. The bovine type also infects cattle, although in many countries it is now successfully controlled. Atypical mycobacteria of clinical importance include *M. avium (intracellulare)*, *M. xenopi*, *M. kansasii* and *M. leprae*. *M. leprae* differs from other mycobacteria in not growing on artificial media. They can, however, be recognized in nasal scrapings from patients with leprosy by their acid fast straining reaction.

Mycobacterium tuberculosis

Morphology

Mycobacteria are bacilli which, on account of the large amount of lipid which they contain, do not take up Gram stains. They will stain with hot carbol fuchsin and resist decoloration with sulphuric acid (Ziehl–Nielsen staining method). They will also take up auramine, when they fluoresce under ultraviolet light.

Cultural charcteristics

M. tuberculosis is normally grown on Löwenstein–Jensen medium which is basically inspissated egg. The growth of bovine strains is encouraged by replacing the glycerol with pyruvate. Colonies usually appear within 1–4 weeks.

Biochemical reactions

Different strains can be distinguished by both growth requirements and biochemical reactions. These tests are normally undertaken in reference laboratories.

Resistance

Mycobacteria survive for long periods in the environment if protected from sunlight. They are more resistant than other bacteria and care must be taken to use recommended concentrations for a sufficient time.

Antituberculous drugs include streptomycin, rifampicin, ethambutol, isoniazid and para-aminosalicylic acid.

Clinical microbiology

Special transport medium is not needed for sending specimens to the laboratory. They are first treated with acid or alkali to destroy other bacteria, and then inoculated on to Löwenstein–Jensen slopes or into Kinchner liquid medium. Colonies may take up to 4 weeks to develop. Confirmation and sensitivity testing may take a further 2 weeks. Ziehl–Neelsen or auramine staining of a film from the specimen may give an early indication of tuberculous infection.

Fungi and yeasts

Fungi and yeasts differ from bacteria in many ways. They all possess chitin in their cell wall; they may have complex structures for multiplication; they may have sexual reproductive cycles; and they may exist in various forms – for example, as yeast cells and hyphal elements. They are resistant to antibacterial drugs and are common secondary invaders in patients who receive multiple antibacterial drugs. Resistance to infection is closely related to the level of cellular immunity.

In Europe, most fungal infections are secondary to an underlying factor. *Candida albicans, Cryptococcus neoformans* and the *Aspergillus* species are the predominant pathogens. Primary fungal infections are associated with geographically defined areas – coccidioidomycosis in the San Joaquin Valley of California and Mexico, blastomycosis in the mid-western and southern parts of the USA, paracoccidioidomycosis in northern South America and histoplasmosis in tropical areas.

Yeasts

C. albicans and *Cr. neoformans* are the two principal yeast pathogens. Candida infections of the ear, nose and throat are associated with distrubances either in the normal flora as a result of antibacterial therapy, or in the local immunity in consequence of corticosteroids, cytotoxic drugs, or radiotherapy to the head and neck. The commonest cryptococcal infection in man is meningitis in an immunocompromised host.

Candida albicans

Morphology

Two distinct morphological phases can be observed. Both are Gram-positive, one as distinct yeast cells, the other as a mycelium of branching hyphae. Chlamydospores are formed in hyphae cultured microaerophilically.

Culture characteristics

Creamy colonies are produced within 24 hours at 37°C on basic culture material containing blood, serum or glucose. A light suspension of *C. albicans* cells in serum will produce germ tubes within 2–3 hours at 37°C.

Biochemical reactions

The ability of yeasts to ferment carbohydrates and to assimilate carbon and nitrogen compounds is used to differentiate between species.

Resistance

Antibacterial drugs have no effect on *C. albicans*. All strains are sensitive to amphotericin B and the imidazoles. Eighty-five per cent of strains isolated in the UK are sensitive to flucytosine; however, because resistance develops rapidly, this drug should always be used in combination with amphotericin B.

Clinical microbiology

C. albicans will survive in clinical specimens without a special transport medium. Yeast cells may be seen in a direct film of the specimen. Culture of typical colonies takes 24–48 hours.

Aspergillus

Aspergillus species are common in the environment. In Europe, *Aspergillus fumigatus* is a frequent pathogen in patients with damaged lungs. Disease may be attributable to direct invasion or hypersensitivity to the spores. *Aspergillus niger* can cause an otitis externa, the black sporing heads being visible through an otoscope. *Aspergillus flavus* is a cause of sinus infection in dry and arid areas such as may occur in the Sudan.

Aspergillus fumigatus
Morphology

The predominant element is the mycelium consisting of a mass of intertwined fungal hyphae. They stain black with a silver stain. Reproductive elements, the conidiophores, are formed and they in turn produce spores. The spores are responsible for the spread of infection between hosts.

Cultural characteristics

Growth will occur on basic culture medium. Colonies appear within 24 hours and if incubation continues they will cover the entire culture medium within a few days. The colonies are greenish in colour and have a powdery surface of spores.

Resistance

The spores are very resistant to drying and survive for long periods in the environment. Amphotericin B is the only effective antifungal drug in the treatment of deep-seated infections.

Clinical microbiology

Culture of this fungus takes 24–48 hours. No special transport medium is necessary if other organisms are not to be sought.

In deep-seated infections, antibodies can be detected in the serum.

Aspergillus niger and flavus

As for *A. fumigatus* except that the colonies are black and yellow respectively.

Viruses

Viruses differ from bacteria, yeasts and fungi in that they are unable to multiply outside living cells. They attach themselves to and then penetrate cells, whereupon they use the intracellular biochemical pathways to reproduce themselves; finally, the new viral particles escape to infect other cells. Viruses are susceptible to host defence mechanisms only in the extracellular phase. The production of specific antibodies is an important factor in the control and prevention of viral infections. Viruses, such as influenza A, which change their antigenic structure are able to infect a host on more than one occasion, whereas those with a fixed structure, such as measles, cause only a single infection.

Some viruses, after entering cells, do not divide and destroy the cell immediately but have a latent phase lasting months or years. An example is the herpes viruses, which may survive for many years in nerve cells before reappearing to cause a recurrent disease.

Antiviral chemotherapy is limited, as the drug must act inside host cells against viral replication without damaging uninfected host cells.

Viruses are probably the commonest cause of upper respiratory tract infection yet the majority cannot be identified in routine microbiology laboratories. As infections, such as the common cold, which result from rhinoviruses are short-lived and usually cause only a mild inconvenience, failure to isolate the virus is of little importance.

The major viral pathogens in the ear, nose and throat are influenza A, rhinovirus, adenovirus, herpes simplex, varicella-zoster and mumps. Hepatitis B and the human immunodeficiency virus (HIV) are important as they may be present in saliva and thus be a source of infection to medical and associated personnel.

Influenza

The influenza A virus has been the cause of major epidemics and pandemics over the centuries. The pandemic of 1918 was well-documented although the causative agent was not recognized. The virus was first isolated from man in 1932 and since then has been studied intensively. Its ability to undergo both major and minor antigenic changes has resulted in the various outbreaks of influenza. Major antigenic shifts led to the Asian influenza of 1957 and the Hong Kong influenza of 1968. The changing antigens have hampered the development of effective vaccines.

Influenza B is associated with smaller outbreaks of influenza; and although small antigenic changes occur, large shifts have not been observed.

Influenza C is a minor cause of respiratory illness.

The influenza viruses belong to the orthomyxoviridae and are similar in structure and properties. They have an RNA genome.

Morphology

Electron microscopy reveals approximately spherical particles with, in fresh clinical isolates, some filamentous forms. The surface is covered with two morphologically different types of spikes – the haemagglutinin and the neuraminidase.

Antigenic structure

The haemagglutinin is the major envelope glycoprotein. During antigenic changes, the peptide composition also changes. There are four major types, namely H0, H1, H2 and H3. The haemagglutinins are responsible for virus attachment to cell surfaces. The neuraminidase is the other main surface antigen and, again, may undergo changes. Two major types, N1 and N2, are recognized in human strains.

Antibodies are produced against both the haemagglutinin and neuraminidase. The major antigen designation of epidemic strains since 1918 are: H1N1 in 1918, H2N2 in 1957, H3N2 in 1968, and H1N1 again in 1977. In between these periods, antigenic drifts occurred which resulted in smaller influenza outbreaks.

Influenza vaccines contain a mixture of recent influenza A and B antigens. Antigenic drift and, possibly, shift means that an outbreak of influenza may be a consequence of a different antigenic strain.

The viral core is also antigenic, serving mainly to distinguish between influenza A, B and C.

Antiviral chemotherapy

Amantadine given before an infection can prevent an attack of influenza A. This is useful in the outbreak situation.

Clinical microbiology

The pernasal aspiration of pharyngeal material, including epithelial cells, enables a rapid diagnosis of influenza to be made. A smear of the aspirate is stained with a fluorescein-labelled antibody, either in a direct or in an indirect technique. Cells infected, which contain the appropriate antigen, will fluoresce under ultraviolet light. If virus isolation is required, a throat swab should be sent to the laboratory in virus transport medium. The virus is cultured in fertile hens' eggs or in susceptible tissue cultures. The measurement of antibody levels in sera collected during the acute and convalescent stage of the illness enables a retrospective diagnosis to be made.

Adenovirus

Adenovirus was first isolated in 1953 from human adenoids. Thirty-five serotypes have been described. Types 1–7 are associated with respiratory disease and types 8 and 19 with epidemic keratoconjunctivitis.

The virus consists of a protein capsid surrounding a dense core containing DNA. The shape of the capsid is an icosahedron with 20 triangular faces. The virus is capable of agglutinating mammalian erythrocytes. It is not susceptible to antiviral agents.

The diagnosis of adenovirus infection is by virus isolation, detection of viral antigen or by serological tests. Throat swabs or pharyngeal secretions should be placed in virus transport medium immediately after collection. A sample of the transport medium is inoculated onto a monolayer of HeLa, H Ep-2 or BK cells.

Adenovirus cytopathic effects take 1–4 weeks to develop. Identification and typing is undertaken by haemagglutination-inhibition or neutralization with specific antisera. A faster diagnosis may be made by fluorescent antibody staining of mucosal cells.

Antibodies are measured by complement fixation.

Rhinovirus

Although it was demonstrated in 1914 that the common cold could be transmitted by bacterial free filtrates, the rhinovirus was not isolated until 1953. A large number of antigenically distinct types has been recognized, and within a type antigenic changes occur.

Rhinoviruses contain RNA. They can be cultured in cell culture, although it is necessary to use the organ culture of trachea or nasal epithelium to isolate some types. Identification is difficult because of the large numbers of serotypes and the absence of a specific group antigen. Neither the isolation of the virus nor the detection of antibodies is routinely undertaken in most clinical microbiology laboratories.

The large number of types has prevented the development of an effective vaccine and explains why repeated common cold infections are common.

Herpes viruses

There are five herpes viruses which may cause infection in man: herpes simplex virus type 1, herpes simplex virus type 2, varicella-zoster virus, Epstein–Barr virus and cytomegalovirus. They are DNA viruses and all have the ability to remain undetected in cells, thereby causing a latent infection. In appropriate situations, all these viruses, with the exception of the varicella-zoster virus, are capable of transforming host cells, a fact which has led to their becoming suspect oncogenic viruses.

The morphology of all the herpes viruses is similar, consisting of a dense nucleocapsid surrounded by an envelope. The distinctive appearance is of practical value in making a diagnosis of herpes virus infection by electron microscopy.

The intracellular multiplication of herpes simplex and varicella-zoster viruses can be inhibited by acyclovir triphosphate, by competing with deoxyguanosine triphosphate and inhibiting viral DNA polymerase. Acyclovir is available for topical, oral or parenteral use. It is of value only when the virus is multiplying within cells and will not, therefore, affect the virus in the latent stage.

Herpes simplex virus type 1 and type 2

Classically, the type 1 virus was associated with oral infection and type 2 with genital infection. There is now a mixture of both types causing either oral or genital infection. In either site, the virus is able to survive for long periods (latency) between recurrent infections. The site of persistence is the ganglia of the sensory nerves serving the area. Resection of the trigeminal ganglia of herpetic carriers for treatment of associated neuralgia stops the recurrent herpes on the operated side. Co-culture of the ganglia with sensitive cells enables the virus to be isolated. Predisposing factors of recurrent infection are often associated with physical or emotional trauma. The exact mechanisms by which the virus becomes active remain a matter of speculation.

The vesicles of acute infection are full of virus particles and constitute an infection hazard.

The diagnosis of herpes simplex infection can be confirmed by the detection of viral antigen in cells scraped from the floor of lesions, by electron microscopy of vesicle fluid or by culturing the virus in sensitive cells. Serological studies are of little value as antibodies are widespread in the population.

Varicella-zoster virus

The primary infection resulting from this virus is chicken pox. This is followed by a latent period with the 'virus' in posterior ganglia. Recrudescence is as herpes zoster. The vesicles of herpes zoster contain the virus, and exposure of non-immune persons may be followed by chicken pox.

Epstein–Barr virus

This virus was discovered from Burkitt's lymphoma tissue. Antibody studies have shown that the virus has a world-wide distribution and is also the causative agent of infectious mononucleosis. This virus is associated with nasopharyngeal carcinoma, the Epstein–Barr virus DNA having been found in virtually every biopsy. However, a definitive aetiological relationship has not been established.

Mumps

The mumps virus contains RNA. It will grow readily in cell culture and is detected by the fusion of cells (syncytia), inclusion bodies and haemadsorption of erythrocytes. The virus has two complement-fixing antigens corresponding to the viral nucleocapsid (S antigen) and the envelope (V antigen). After an infection, the S antibodies develop first but remain active for a shorter time than V antibodies.

The mumps virus causes swelling of the parotid and submaxillary salivary glands. It may also infect the meninges, the ovaries, the testes and other organs.

In patients with mumps, the virus can be isolated from the saliva, throat washings, and from swabs from the parotid ducts.

Hepatitis B

The importance of this virus to otolaryngologists lies not in the infection which it produces in patients, but in the fact that the virus is present in both the blood and saliva. As such, it constitutes an infection hazard to both medical and attendant personnel.

The virus is detected by testing blood for viral antigen and antibody. Three antigens are recognized, namely hepatitis B surface antigen (HB_sAg), hepatitis B core antigen (HB_cAg) and hepatitis B 'e' antigen (HB_eAg). Infectivity is associated with the presence of HB_eAg, although in the absence of anti-HB_e antibody, fluid containing HB_sAg is regarded as potentially dangerous. The commonest antigen detected in serum is the surface antigen, and it is estimated that, in the UK, one in every 1000 persons is a healthy carrier. Antibody to the core antigen represents a recent infection.

A hepatitis B vaccine is available which provides protective immunity. Specific immunoglobulin infected after exposure will also protect against infection.

Human immunodeficiency virus (HIV)

The recognition in 1981 of a new disease, the acquired immune deficiency syndrome (AIDS), was followed in 1982 by the finding of retrovirus in the lymphocytes of patients with AIDS (Barre-Sinoussi *et al.*, 1983; Gallo *et al.*, 1984). The virus was termed the human T-cell lymphotropic III virus by American workers, and the lymphadenopathy associated virus by the French. The evidence is that the two viruses are one and the same. The recognized name is now the human immunodeficiency virus (HIV). The natural history of infection with this virus is not fully known but a high proportion, if not all, of infected persons eventually develop AIDS or a related syndrome such as persistent generalized lymphadenopathy. The immune deficiency results in the acquisition of infection by opportunistic pathogens, with *Pneumocystis carinii* pneumonia predominating. There is also a high incidence of Kaposi's sarcoma. The most commonly known route of spread is transmission through unprotected sexual intercourse. In Europe and North America, the highest incidence is amongst homosexual men, whereas in Central Africa, there is an almost equal distribution between the sexes. It is also spread by the injection of infected blood or blood products.

Antibodies to the HIV virus can be detected in the serum of infected persons approximately 3 months after initial infection, but the fact that they do not neutralize the infectivity means that antibody positive persons are an infection risk.

The risk of transmission through transfused blood has been virtually eliminated by testing all blood donors for HIV antibody. Blood products such as factor VIII also undergo treatment which would inactivate the virus.

Precautions to be taken in the management of patients who are antibody positive are continually being revised in the light of new knowledge (Department of Health and Social Security, 1985, 1986).

Antimicrobial chemotherapy

The wide range of antimicrobial agents, both available and in various stages of development, is a measure of the ability of many microorganisms to develop drug resistance. In the early days of antimicrobials, it was anticipated that infection would soon be a problem of the past; a hope that, as yet, is far from realization. Antimicrobial agents, while life-saving and thus essential in the modern practice of medicine, are in themselves the cause of many iatrogenic infections. The growth of sensitive bacteria will be arrested but resistant strains or mutants may multiply and become hazardous to the patient. The importance of the normal flora in the ear, nose and throat has been discussed. However, it is often not appreciated that antimicrobials used for any infection in the body will also affect the normal flora. There is no safe antimicrobial which will kill all organisms; therefore, there is always a resistant organism waiting to colonize or to superinfect areas.

It must always be remembered when using antimicrobials that it is the patient who is being treated and not the microorganisms.

Antimicrobials to treat infections

Antimicrobials may be the sole treatment for an infection or they may be an adjunct to, for example, the draining of an abscess. The antimicrobial chosen must be active against the infecting organism and, in order to be effective, must reach the site of infection in a sufficient concentration and for a sufficient length of time.

Whenever possible, the infecting organism should be isolated and its sensitivity pattern determined before treatment is initiated. In situations where immediate treatment is necessary, the most likely infecting organism should be assessed and the antimicrobial chosen depending on the local pattern of sensitivities for that organism. Many laboratories provide 'Best Guess Lists' of antimicrobials based on local knowledge.

The route of administration and dosage will depend on the severity and site of the infection, and also on the age, size and, for some drugs, the renal function of the patient.

The length of treatment should be as short as possible but long enough to ensure resolution of the infection. As a 'rule of thumb', antimicrobials should be given for a further 48 hours after the acute symptoms have subsided. For most infections this will mean a 5–7 day course of treatment. Deep-seated infections, such as an osteomyelitis, will require a considerably longer period of treatment.

Repeated courses of antimicrobials should be used only with careful microbiological monitoring in order to detect, at an early stage, the overgrowth of normal flora by multiple resistant organisms.

Antimicrobials to prevent infections

The use of prophylactic antimicrobials has been, and continues to be, the source of much controversy. The aim is to control potentially pathogenic organisms in an area, or to eradicate them from it, before a surgical procedure commences, in order to reduce the possibility of postoperative infection. There is always the danger, however, that the accompanying disturbances in the normal flora will enable organisms resistant to the prophylactic antimicrobial to emerge. Organisms may gain access to a wound directly at the time of operation, or postoperatively during the few hours before surface healing has occurred. Infections at more distant sites, such as on heart valves, are blood borne. The potential infecting organisms are usually part of the normal flora in the operative area. The function of the prophylactic antimicrobial is not to eradicate the organisms from the normal flora but to provide an antimicrobial barrier during the period the host is susceptible to infection. This means, in practice, that prophylactic chemotherapy should begin just before the operation and should continue for a maximum of 24 hours. Resistant strains of bacteria appear rapidly in the normal flora and the continued use of antimicrobials may be positively harmful to the patient.

The choice of antimicrobial agent for prophylaxis will depend on the potential pathogens and whether the patient has recently been exposed to antimicrobials. In uncomplicated surgery of the head and neck, amoxycillin or a first generation cephalosporin will provide suitable cover. In patients with chronic sinusitis or otitis externa, who have received multiple courses of antimicrobials, it may be necessary to use an aminoglycoside or new cephalosporin to combat pseudomonads or multiple resistant enterobacteria.

If active infection is found at the time of operation, the use of a prophylactic antimicrobial may be continued but as a course of treatment.

Using the microbiology laboratory

Infection is a clinical diagnosis, and the role of the microbiology laboratory is to determine the cause of the infection and to provide the information necessary for its control within both the patient and the community. As the facilities in individual laboratories differ, clinicians should always liaise closely with microbiologists, and vice versa, on the use of the laboratory. There are, however, some general aspects applicable to all laboratories.

The specimen

The raw material for laboratory work is the specimen from the patient. It must be relevant to the suspect infection and have been collected according to the correct procedure at the right stage of the illness. Even the best laboratory examination cannot overcome an inadequate specimen. The specimen must be transported to the laboratory in the appropriate transport medium to ensure survival of the pathogens.

Blood for antibody studies

Ten millilitres of blood should be collected during both the acute and convalescent phases of the illness. It should be placed in a plain bottle.

Blood for antimicrobial levels

Approximately 5–10 ml blood should be collected into a plain bottle. The timing of collection will depend on the route of administration of the drug and should be discussed with the laboratory staff.

Blood cultures

Patients with severe infections – especially if there is evidence of septicaemia – should have their blood cultured. Care must be taken to clean the venepuncture site carefully and to avoid contamination of the needle. The volume of blood and the type of medium used vary between laboratories.

Ear swabs

Ordinary swabs are frequently too large to pass into the external auditory meatus, particularly in children, and pernasal swabs should be used.

Nose swabs

The swab should, if possible, be moistened with peptone water or saline, and should be rotated firmly in the anterior nares. Dry swabs can be used if evidence of staphylococcal infection or carriage is required. The swabs should be sent to the laboratory in a suitable transport medium. In many laboratories, swabs are supplied together with the transport medium, the latter of which is usually black in colour on account of the presence of charcoal.

Pernasal swabs

These swabs on fine supple wire are suitable for sampling the posterior nasal area. The patient should sit with the neck extended slightly, while the swab is passed along the floor of the nose. The patient will experience some eye watering and slight discomfort.

Postnasal aspirates

A fine catheter should be passed gently along the floor of the nose and suction applied, thereby collecting the aspirate in a trap. Epithelial cells as well as secretions are required. The trap should be sent directly to the laboratory.

Pus

When pus is present, a small amount should be collected by aspiration into a syringe. A swab dipped into the pus is a poor alternative. As anaerobic bacteria may be present, air should be expelled from the syringe and the nozzle sealed with a cap.

Sinus washings

A sterile bottle should, if possible, be completely filled in order to exclude air.

Throat swabs

The swab must be firmly rolled over the mucosa at the back of the throat, with the tongue depressed. If viral culture is required, it should be placed in virus transport medium.

Ulcers

Ulcers should be firmly swabbed for bacterial and viral isolation. Scraping for immunofluorescent staining should be taken firmly from the ulcer base and smeared directly on to an appropriate slide.

Vesicle fluid

Vesicle fluid for virus isolation is most easily collected using a very small hypodermic needle and a 1-ml syringe. The fluid should be carefully aspirated and then expelled into virus transport medium; or, alternatively, the syringe and needle may be sent directly to the laboratory.

The request form

The request form provides the information which enables the specimen to be correctly examined and the results to be interpreted. This information is extremely important and should be as comprehensive as possible; if only a broad diagnosis, such as '? virus disease', accompanies the blood being submitted for antibody studies, this is both insufficient and meaningless information. It would not be practicable or desirable for the laboratory to examine all such blood samples for every possible viral antibody. If the nature of the illness is stated, the serum can initially be screened for the most likely antibodies.

A throat swab from a suspected diphtheritic patient should have the diagnosis clearly mentioned as many laboratories do not routinely culture specifically for *Co. diphtheriae*. Indeed, in such circumstances the laboratory staff should be notified of the suspected diagnosis by telephone.

The timing of the illness should always be stated, as should any antimicrobial chemotherapy that the patient is receiving.

Safety

All specimens constitute a safety hazard. Their safe transport to the laboratory is the responsibility of the person collecting the specimen. As a general principle, the specimen container should be enclosed in a second container or polythene bag. The request form should not be inside the second container or bag as leakage of the specimen would contaminate the form.

Leaking specimens are generally disposed of by autoclaving. High risk specimens, such as those from known or suspect patients with tuberculosis, hepatitis B virus or human immunodeficiency virus, should, in addition, be specially labelled with the warning 'Infection Risk'.

References

BALDWIN, J. N., RHEINS, M. S., SYLVESTER, R. F. and SCHAFFER, T. E. (1957) Staphylococcal infections in new born infants. Part 3. Colonisation of new-born infants by *Staphylococcus pyogenes*. *American Journal of Diseases of Children*, **94**, 107–116

BARRE-SINOUSSI, F., CHERMANN, J. C., REY, F. NUGEYRE, M. T., CHAMARET, S., GRUEST, J. *et al.* (1983) Isolation of a T-lymphotropic retrovirus from a patient at risk for acquired immune deficiency syndrome (AIDS). *Science*, **220**, 868–871

BOX, Q. T., CLEVELAND, R. T. and WILLARD, C. Y. (1961) Bacterial flora of the upper respiratory tract. *American Journal of Diseases of Children*, **102**, 293–301

EVANS, H. E., AKPATA, S. O. and BAKI, A. (1970) Factors influencing the establishment of the neonatal bacterial flora. 1. The role of host factors. *Archives of Environmental Health*, **21**, 514–519

DEPARTMENT OF HEALTH AND SOCIAL SECURITY (1985) Information for doctors concerning the introduction of the HTLVIII antibody test. *Acquired Immune Deficiency Syndrome Booklet 2*, London: HMSO

DEPARTMENT OF HEALTH AND SOCIAL SECURITY (1986) Guidance for surgeons, anaesthetists, dentists and their teams in dealing with patients infected with HTLV III. *Acquired Immune Deficiency Syndrome Booklet 3*, London: HMSO

FALCONE, G. and CAMPA, M. (1981) Bacterial interference with the immune response. In *Microbial Perturbation of Host Defences*, edited by F. O'Grady and H. Smith, pp. 185–210. London: Academic Press

GALLO, R. C., SALAHUDDIN, S. Z. POPOVIC, M. SHEARER, G. M., KAPLAN, M., HAYNES, B. F. *et al.* (1984) Frequent detection and isolation of cytopathic retroviruses (HTLV III) from patients with AIDS and at risk for AIDS. *Science*, **224**, 500–503

HECZO, P. B., HOFFLER, V., KASPROWICZ, A. and PULVERER, G. (1981) Quantitative studies of the flora of the nasal vestibule in relation to nasal carriage of *Staphylococcus aureus*. *Journal of Medical Microbiology*, **14**, 233–242

HOLMES, M. C. and WILLIAMS, R. E. O. (1954) The distribution of carriers of *Streptococcus pyogenes* among 2413 healthy children. *Journal of Hygiene (Cambridge)*, **52**, 165–179

LAURELL, G., TUNEVALL, G. and WALLMARK, G. (1958) Pathogenic bacteria in the pharynx and naso-pharynx of hospitalised children and their relation to clinical infection. *Acta Paediatrica*, **47**, 34–45

LOVE, G. L., GEZON, H. M., THOMPSON, D. J., ROGERS, K. D. and HATCH, T. F. (1963) Relation of intensity of staphylococcal infections in newborn infants to contamination of nurses' hands and surrounding environments. *Pediatrics (Springfield)*, **32**, 956–965

MARTIN, R. R. and WHITE, A. (1968) The reacquisition of staphylococci by treated carriers: a demonstration of bacterial interference. *Journal of Laboratory and Clinical Medicine*, **71**, 791–797

MYERS, D. M. (1959) An antibiotic effect of viridans streptococci from the nose, throat and sputum and its inhibitory effect on *Staphylococcus aureus*. *American Journal of Clinical Pathology*, **31**, 332–336

NOBLE, W. C. and SOMERVILLE, D. A. (1974) *Microbiology of Human Skin*. London: Saunders

PARKER, M. T. and KENNEDY, J. (1949) The source of infection in pemphigus neonatorum. *Journal of Hygiene (Cambridge)*, **47**, 213–219

PERRY, E. T. and NICHOLS, A. C. (1956) Studies on the growth of bacteria in the human ear canal. *Journal of Investigative Dermatology*, **27**, 165–170

QUINN, R. W., DENNY, F. W. and RILEY, H. D. (1957) Natural occurrence of hemolytic streptococci in normal school children. *American Journal of Public Health*, **47**, 995–1008

ROSS, P. W. (1971) Beta-haemolytic streptococci in the throat: carrier rates in schoolchildren. *Health Bulletin, (Edinburgh)*, **29**, 108–112

ROUNTREE, P. M. and BARBOUR, R. G. H. (1950) *Staphylococcus pyogenes* in new-born babies in a maternity hospital. *Medical Journal of Australia*, **1**, 525–528

RYAN, W. J. (1972) Throat infection and rash associated with an unusual corynebacterium. *Lancet*, **2**, 1345–1347

SARKANY, I. and GAYLARDE, C. C. (1968) Bacterial colonisation of the skin in the newborn. *Journal of Pathology and Bacteriology*, **95**, 115–122

SHANSON, D. C. (1986) Staphylococcal infections in hospital. *British Journal of Hospital Medicine*, **35**, 312–320

SHINEFIELD, H. R., RIBBLE, J. C., BORIS, M. and EICHENWALD, H. F. (1963) Bacterial interference: its effect on nursery-acquired infection with *Staphylococcus aureus*. 1. Preliminary observations on artificial colonisation of newborns. *American Journal of Diseases of Children*, **105**, 646–654 (and 5 papers on succeeding pages)

SPRUNT, K. and REDMAN, W. (1968) Evidence suggesting importance of role of antibacterial inhibition in maintaining balance of normal flora. *Annals of Internal Medicine*, **68**, 579–590

TURK, D. C. (1984) The pathogenicity of *Haemophilus influenzae*. *Journal of Medical Microbiology*, **18**, 1–16

WICKMAN, K. (1970) Studies of bacterial interference in experimentally produced burns in guinea pigs. *Acta Pathologica Scandinavica, B*, **78**, 15–28

WILLIAMS, R. E. O. (1963) Healthy carriage of *Staphylococcus aureus*: its prevalence and importance. *Bacteriological Reviews*, **27**, 56–71

20

Principles of radiotherapy in head and neck cancer

W. F. White

Radium was discovered in 1898 by Marie and Pierre Curie. Within a few years of its discovery, radium was being used in the treatment of cancer, initially by surface application and subsequently by insertion of sealed containers into tumours. In addition, radon gas sealed in a gold capillary tube was implanted into accessible tumours with, what were at the time, amazing results. Even before the Curies' discovery, Wilhelm Röntgen had begun his investigation into the luminescene produced by cathode rays, and in 1895 had discovered a phenomenon which, in view of its uncertain nature, he called X radiation.

During the next 30 years, considerable advances were made in understanding both the production of X-rays and the importance of radioactive substances in the treatment of malignant tumours. Associated with the increasing knowledge of the nature and production of electricity was the development of methods of generating high voltages. This knowledge was used to create a high potential difference (voltage) across an evacuated tube in which electrodes were sealed, permitting the production of X-rays of varying energy. The availability of larger amounts of radium led to the first teletherapy units. In such units, the increased distance of the isotope from the tumour produced a higher absorbed dose at a depth within the patient. The early teletherapy radium units were known as radium bombs.

Subsequent progress was slow until World War II (1939–45), when considerable resources were put into research. This investment led directly to the development of the early machines which still exist today, for example linear accelerators, and other means of producing high energy radiation and particles. Simultaneously, the increase in availability of numerous new radioactive isotopes,

as a byproduct of atomic weapons' manufacture, led to new techniques being developed in both the diagnosis and treatment of cancer. In the last 40 years, there have been a great many advances in all treatment modalities. The main reason for this has been the maintenance of centres of excellence, from which have emanated the results of a wealth of research and development, coupled with the provision of advanced equipment to regional cancer treatment centres and the specialization of medical staff in all forms of cancer therapy. In the field of head and neck malignancy, the scope of treatment methods and the varied expertise available, have meant that treatment by an individual in isolation is no longer the norm. Sometimes, the management of a patient is conducted by a team comprising only an otorhinolaryngologist and a radiotherapist also trained in the use of cytotoxic drugs; more often a medical oncologist, a maxillofacial surgeon and a speech therapist complete the range of expertise available in the joint clinic. The concept of the joint clinic has led to an improvement in the treatment of each individual patient. This is reflected by the longer survival period of patients together with a better quality of life.

The best means of establishing such a joint clinic is to come to an agreement with the specialists involved in the many hospitals served by one cancer treatment centre, as to who will provide which particular expertise and hence become part of the cancer treatment team. This will allow others, for example in the field of otolaryngology, to specialize in otological problems and to establish the same sort of collaboration with other colleagues. Only in this way is it possible for the degree of excellence which should be available to be achieved and for each member of the team to come to know the potential of the other members' special skills.

Radiotherapy – a scientific or clinical speciality?

All radiotherapists would admit that a sound knowledge of the basics of the physics of radiation is essential. Similarly, a surgeon would agree that a detailed knowledge of the different surgical instruments available to him was equally important.

The essential requirements of a radiotherapist and oncologist are a good general training in medicine and, above all, to be a good clinician. Radiotherapy is without doubt a clinical speciality where a scientific knowledge of physics and, probably more important, the biology of tumours and their behaviour, is essential.

The nature of radiation

Electromagnetic radiation

All electromagnetic radiations have the same characteristics and differ only in energy. X-rays and gamma rays of the same energy have precisely the same properties and vary only in the manner by which they are produced. X-rays are produced by the bombardment of a target by electrons, while gamma rays are produced by the nucleus of radioactive atoms. There are many other well-known forms of electromagnetic radiation which have the same properties but behave differently because of their wavelength. Working up the spectrum of electromagnetic radiation, the longest wavelengths are long wave radio, then short wave radio, infrared, visible light, ultraviolet and so up to X-rays and gamma rays, the spectrum spreading from 10^4 Hz to 10^{20} Hz (1 Hz = 1 cycle per second).

Electromagnetic radiation may be thought of as packets of energy which are called photons.

Elementary particles

Radiation emitted from radioactive sources may consist of electromagnetic irradiation (gamma rays) or particles, or of both. Atoms are made up of elementary particles, of which only a few are used clinically. The particles which make up the nucleus are protons, which carry a positive electrical charge, and neutrons, which carry no charge. Electrons carry a negative electrical charge equal to the positive charge on the proton, and are found travelling in orbits around the nucleus. A positron is identical to an electron but has a positive rather than a negative charge.

In clinical radiotherapeutic practice, electromagnetic radiation, electrons and neutrons are used.

Clinical radiotherapy

The radiotherapist has a considerable wealth of radiotherapeutic modalities available for use. The most commonly used form of radiation in clinical practice is high energy photons (electromagnetic radiation), usually produced by linear accelerators but also by the gamma radiation produced by the isotope of cobalt (^{60}Co). One of the advantages of the linear accelerator over cobalt is the former's high output, which results in short treatment times. Cobalt sources decay slowly and have to be changed every 3–5 years, their output becoming less every day, unlike the beam from a linear accelerator which has a constant output.

The older X-ray machines of low energy still have a place in radiotherapy and are used for the treatment of more superficial lesions. This equipment produces X-rays of up to 300 000 volts (300 kV).

The first of the high energy X-ray generators was the Van der Graaf machine. This machine was introduced into clinical practice producing X-rays at an energy of 1.2 million volts (MV), and it was the first equipment to produce megavoltage X-rays, that is over 1 million volts. As the penetration of X-rays depends on their energy, this was a considerable step forward. One advantage of the high energy photon beams of radiation mentioned is the high output of radiation. Of greater importance is the manner in which radiation is absorbed by tissue at different energies. The low energies used to produce diagnostic radiographs make use of photons in the 60–150 kV range. The use for diagnostic purposes of X-rays falling in this range, depending on the method of absorption of the X-rays, is related to the atomic number of the material being irradiated. Because of the considerable variation in the atomic number of body structures, for example in the head and neck, there are considerable differences in methods of absorption by the various structures, and a simple radiograph reveals all the important features, such as bone and different soft tissues, as shades of grey. However, if the same energy of radiation were to be used in the treatment of tumours of the head and neck, great care would be needed as there would be a differential absorption of the radiation, resulting in very high absorbed doses in bone compared with the much lower dose in soft tissue. This variation can approach a ratio of 8:1, bone:soft tissue, and may lead to problems such as bone necrosis. The differential absorption is clearly visible on an ordinary radiograph where the soft tissues show up as black and the bones as white. The white areas show least transmission of X-rays on account of the high absorption, and the black areas demonstrate the high transmission and low absorption. The use of megavoltage radiation overcomes this problem, as all tissues will absorb the same amount of radiation. The absorption of electromagnetic radiation is exponential. For unit depth within the patient or in a water phantom, the same percentage of radiation is absorbed. For example, if in the first centimetre of tissue, 50% of the beam is absorbed, then in the second centimetre, 50% of the remaining 50% will be absorbed, leaving 25% of the original applied amount of radiation and so on. With the increase in energy of the beam, the dose absorbed at a depth will become higher and the greater will be the potential for the treatment of deep-seated tumours.

Electrons have an absorption in tissue which is finite and directly related to their energy. As absorption is not exponential and falls off very much more quickly, this type of therapy is of particular advantage in the treatment of superficial lesions or where a block of tissue is to be treated to a finite depth, for example in the neck following block dissection where the underlying pharynx can be spared. As a working rule, the depth to the 80% isodose is approximately one-third of the energy of the beam expressed in million-electron volts (MeV).

The edge of a beam of irradiation is known as the penumbra, and is mainly related to the size of the source of the radiation. This may be a focal spot on a target of a linear accelerator or a piece of radioactive material such as a ^{60}Co source in a teletherapy machine. The penumbra of the beam produced by a linear accelerator is superior to that produced by other forms of equipment as there is a point source of X-rays, and the scatter of the X-rays within the patient is in a forward direction. The advantage of this property is considerable, especially in the head and neck where it is imperative to administer very accurately a dose of radiation to the tumour volume. This is particularly important, for example, when treating structures around the eye.

Another advantage of megavoltage beams is the skin sparing effect. Beams of radiation with an energy of up to 1 MV always produce the maximum dose on the surface. Unless clever use of multiple beams is employed, with orthovoltage irradiation so that the tumour dose is always very much higher than the skin dose, there will certainly be a very brisk reaction with moist desquamation of the skin. This occurrence tended to give the radiotherapist of the past a reputation for burning the skin. Modern megavoltage beams produce the maximum dose at an approximate

depth of, for example, 1.0 cm with 4 MV X-rays, 2.0 cm with 8 MV X-rays and 7.0 cm with 35 MV X-rays. The last example shows the considerable skin sparing which results from an increase in the energy of the beam. Careful choice of energy may be used to advantage. Many radiotherapists do not favour multi-energy, multifunction accelerators, and it is essential to choose equipment which best suits the practice of the department.

In *Figure 20.1*, all of the curves are drawn to the same scale and demonstrate the dose distribution in a water phantom (tissue equivalent) of: (1) 8 MV X-rays at 100 cm source skin distance; (2) cobalt-60 teletherapy beam at 80 cm source skin distance; and (3) a betatron beam at 11 MeV. All field sizes are for a 10 × 10 cm field. These illustrate the points made relating to the nature of the penumbra, the absorption, and the depth of the maximum dose. The electron beam shows the different type of absorption and the rapid fall-off of the beam.

Other examples of external beam therapy are illustrated in *Figures 20.2, 20.3* and *20.4*, which relate to treatment at sites in the head and neck. *Figure 20.2* illustrates a distribution using three fields of radiation, two lateral 30° wedges and an open anterior field. *Figure 20.3* demonstrates a plan produced using two 45° wedges with the beams angled in such a way as to avoid the spinal cord and the opposite eye. All are drawn to the same scale.

Brachytherapy

The single, most important, landmark in brachytherapy was the standardization of the rules of radium implantation by Paterson (1934) and Parker (1934); the principles set out in their work are still used today. Between 1950 and the latter part of the 1960s there was a general decline in interest in brachytherapy, owing to the introduction of new advanced megavoltage equipment for external beam therapy. The renewal of interest has been aided by three main events: first, the availability of afterloading, which permits longer periods of time for the insertion of non-radioactive carriers into and around a tumour, into which a radioactive source is subsequently placed; secondly, the development of newer and safer radionuclides; and, thirdly, the availability of computerized dosimetry.

The principle of afterloading is very simple and consists of the introduction of hollow applicators; these may be either needles or plastic tubes. With the aid of computer planning, an ideal implant may be computed prior to surgery with unlimited time available to insert the non-radioactive applicators. By using this technique there need be no

475

SL7510
Width 100mm   Wedge No 0

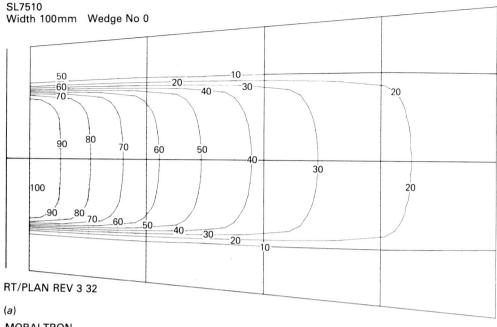

RT/PLAN REV 3 32

(a)

MOBALTRON
Width 100mm   Wedge No 0

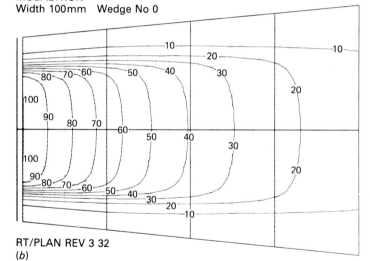

RT/PLAN REV 3 32
(b)

Betatron 11Mev Width 100mm

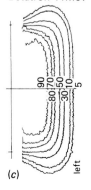

(c)   Figure 20.1

fear on the part of the operator of excessive exposure to radiation. Once the applicators have been inserted, non-active sources may be introduced into the applicators to localize them within the patient; further dosimetric studies are then carried out. When the operator is satisfied with the distribution, the radioactive sources may be loaded. The loading and unloading of radioactive sources is often carried out by hand; however, more sophisticated methods are available, in particular where large amounts of radioactivity are used when the applicators may be loaded mechanically from a safe containing sources of varying intensity. This technique is particularly applicable in gynaecological intracavitary applications. Its use means that not only the operator, but also the nursing staff are protected, as the sources can be removed before nursing procedures are carried out. Once the patient has been left by the nurse, the sources are automatically reintroduced. Two types of afterloading technique have been used: in the past, high dose rate systems were used which

gave the required dose in 20–30 minutes; more recently, the older and more tried, long-exposure techniques have been mimicked using low activity isotopes which are left *in situ* for up to a week.

A number of artificial radionuclides have become available, some of which have physical characteristics which may be preferable to radium or radon. These include caesium-137, iridium-192, iodine-125 and gold-198. The energy of photons emitted from radium and radon can be as high as 2000 kV, whereas that of caesium is 660 kV, that of iridium 350 kV and that of iodine-125 only 28 kV. It is preferable, when the sources of radiation are situated in the tumour, to use low energy photon energies which penetrate short distances into tissue, thus ensuring that relatively little radiation affects the surrounding normal tissue. The patient benefits from a better dose distribution, while nursing and medical personnel are protected, both by the smaller amount of radiation emitted and by the more effective protective shields.

In addition to the advantages of radioactive

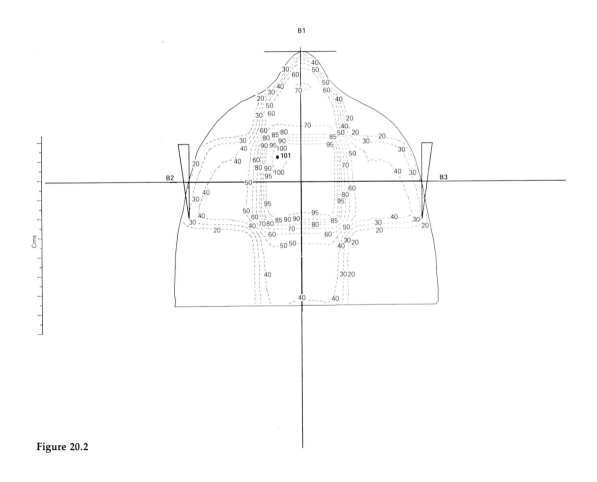

Figure 20.2

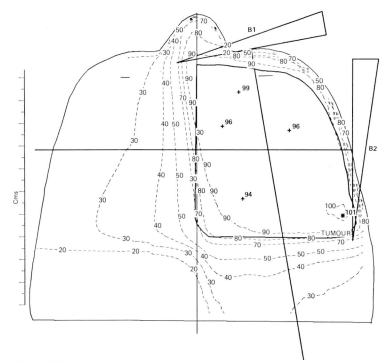

Figure 20.3

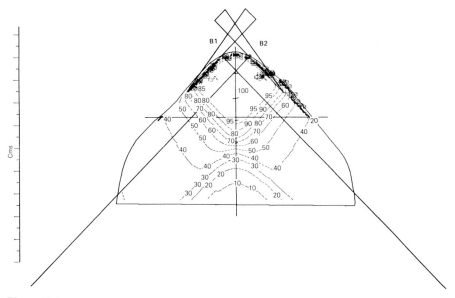

Figure 20.4

sources used for implants, there are three distinct advantages over external beam therapy: the dose distribution is superior, the tumour dose is high while the dose to the surrounding tissues is low, and the dose rate effect is beneficial. The first two advantages can be easily understood whereas the latter may not be so apparent. With an implant, the actual dose rate is considerably lower than with external beam therapy, and the total dose is delivered in a much shorter time; the same total dose may be given in 6 days rather than in 6 weeks. It is recognized that the same dose of radiation delivered in a shorter overall time is more efficient than when given over a longer period (Bedford and Mitchell, 1973). Therefore, it is reasonable to expect a greater destruction of the tumour by delivering the total tumour dose in 1 week rather than in 6 weeks. This would be a disadvantage if normal tissues were subject to the same enhanced radiation damage but with an implant, as was described previously, the dose to the surrounding normal tissue is considerably less and consequently more capable of being tolerated. It has been shown that the oxygen enhancement ratio decreases as the dose rate decreases. Normal tissues are well oxygenated, thus the decrease in dose rate would not make them more susceptible to radiation damage. Malignant tissue, on the other hand, contains a significant number of hypoxic cells which might be more efficiently killed by radiation at the lower dose rate.

Implants of all types are more commonly used in the treatment of small lesions in the oral cavity and pharynx. The method of implantation of radium and caesium varies: the isotope is implanted by being encapsulated in a needle, iridium is implanted in the form of wire, and iodine-125 and gold-198 are implanted as seeds and grains, respectively. The latter remain in place permanently once implanted. Iridium is normally used either as a preshaped 'hairpin' using an introducer, or as a single wire with a looped end for fixation, or in a polyethylene tube by means of the afterloading technique. Seeds or grains require the use of special equipment for insertion.

Radium moulds are now of historical interest only; however, the technique using the less penetrating isotopes is still employed in very selected cases. This technique still applies in the case of carcinoma of the maxillary antrum when there is residual or recurrent disease following surgery. The obturator is marked at the site of persistent disease and a treatment planned with the aid of the planning computer. The radioactive source, or sources, is then placed in the obturator to produce the dose distribution desired. The obturator is worn for the requisite time and a very localized volume in the patient treated.

Where an implant is possible and appropriate, it remains the treatment of choice, surpassing the distribution of external beam therapy and producing better long-term control of tumour.

Factors affecting the efficacy of radiotherapy

The effect of radiotherapy on tumours is dependent on a number of factors, only some of which are at present understood. The immediate effect of radiation on malignant tumours is relatively well understood but of greater significance are the long-term effect and cure rate. The factors affecting the cure of patients with malignant tumours are of considerable importance. Tumours that respond well and disappear with the initial treatment clearly stand a much better chance of being cured than those which appear to be relatively little affected by the initial treatment, but this is by no means the most important factor.

The histology of the tumour may affect its response to radiation therapy and, indeed, its curability. Tumours arising in lymphoid tissue are usually very sensitive to radiation and respond quickly. The chance of curing them is extremely high. Tumours of embryonal origin and those which are anaplastic are also sensitive to irradiation; however, while being initially sensitive and responding well, they may recur at an early stage. Squamous cell tumours and a few adenocarcinomata are sensitive, although they respond slowly after treatment, provided that a sufficiently high dose can be administered and, if possible, in a relatively small volume, for example with an implant. Some slow-growing tumours, however, respond equally slowly and may take many months to disappear completely. This may give cause for anxiety on the part of both patient and clinician in the period immediately after treatment.

Sarcomata arising in soft tissue or in bone are of low sensitivity, with the result that very low cure rates are achieved when treated with radiation. Nevertheless, this form of therapy may be of considerable value when attempting to achieve palliation in patients with widespread or locally advanced disease.

While, in theory, an attempt is being made to destroy all malignant cells in order to achieve a cure, it is unlikely, in practice – even in the case of those tumours in which a cure is achieved – that all cells will have been killed. The tumours most likely to be cured with radiation are obviously the small lesions where high doses can be achieved without the neighbouring structures being affected to an unacceptable degree. Experimental work has shown that in small tumours of as little as 1 cm or less in diameter there may be areas of anoxia. Large tumours definitely contain areas of hypoxia, anoxia and, in some instances, central necrosis, although transplantable and viable cells remain within the necrotic area. Gray *et al.* (1953) demonstrated that hypoxia protects tumour cells from the effects of radiation and is therefore of paramount importance in cases where radiotherapy has failed to achieve a cure. In recognition of the pioneering work of Gray, the new SI unit of absorbed dose of radiation has been named after him; one gray (Gy) is equivalent to 100 of the former unit, the rad.

Attempts have been made to overcome the problems relating to the presence of hypoxic cells within tumours. The first attempt to influence hypoxic cells was made by Churchill-Davidson, Sanger and Thomlinson (1957) with the use of hyperbaric oxygen. The results of the British trials of hyperbaric oxygen used in conjunction with radiotherapy were coordinated by the Medical Research Council and published in 1977 and 1978 (Henk, Kunkler and Smith, 1977; Dische, 1978; Watson *et al.*, 1978). These trials demonstrated a highly significant initial increase in tumour control in patients with carcinoma of both the cervix and uterus, and in those with carcinoma of the larynx. However, disappointing long-term responses were observed at 5 years. The methods used were not without criticism and were difficult to use. It is important to remember that not only are the hypoxic cells supplied with more oxygen but that the tissues with a good blood supply also receive higher concentrations of oxygen under hyperbaric conditions, which may lead to necrosis.

Neutrons or heavily charged particles are densely ionizing and damage cells more effectively than photons. Furthermore, their effect is relatively independent of the presence of oxygen. In tissue culture, Gray showed an enhancement of 2.5–3.0 for X-rays whereas, with neutrons, an enhancement of approximately 1.5–1.8 was seen, indicating an effective increase of 50–80% in dose to hypoxic cells only. It has also been suggested that as cells may be more sensitive to X-rays at different phases of the cell cycle, but that such variations are much smaller with neutrons, there may be fewer surviving cells able to regrow in any such resistant phase if neutron therapy is used. The therapeutic ratio using neutrons is close to one, and necrosis of both normal and tumour tissue is not infrequently observed.

The ideal method of dealing with anoxic or hypoxic cells within a tumour would be that of inducing all the cells, whether normal or hypoxic, to be equally sensitive. Chemical compounds have been developed which have the action of sensitizing hypoxic cells. These compounds reach the hypoxic cells which are inaccessible to oxygen, and they do not sensitize the normal or well-oxygenated cells (Adams, 1972, 1977; Adams *et al.*, 1976; Fowler, Adams and Denekamp, 1976; Fowler and Danekamp, 1979). The concentration required to produce full sensitivity, using the present sensitizers, is unsatisfactory because of the side-effects, in particular neurotoxicity.

Other methods of affecting the sensitivity of tumours to radiotherapy, with no direct relation to the oxygen effect, are under trial. The most interesting of these to date has been the use of hyperthermia. It was initially suggested that whole-body hyperthermia be undertaken, and this was subsequently carried out in patients with disseminated disease who were otherwise fit and, in most cases, young. The combination of hyperthermia and radiation is extremely difficult under such conditions, and the best hope for hyperthermia is unlikely to be the whole-body approach. Whole-body hyperthermia may be of value in association with chemotherapy. Temperatures in the range of 42–45 °C have been achieved for 15 minutes to one hour (Field and Bleehen, 1979). Success using heat alone has been claimed by Hahn *et al.* (1979) in tumours recurring after full doses of radiotherapy. A variety of methods has been employed in clinical practice in order to induce hyperthermia. Whole-body hyperthermia is easily achieved but the methods are cumbersome and the patient often requires a general anaesthetic; no temperature difference is achieved between tumour and normal tissues. Isolated perfusion has been used for many years, often associated with cytotoxic chemotherapy, but this is limited to an easily perfusable site such as a limb. Ultrasonic heating of a limited volume, which may be used with radiation therapy, is more convenient and relatively cheap (Marmor *et al.*, 1979; Marmor and Hahn, 1980). The field of hyperthermia is an interesting and rapidly developing form of potential cancer treatment.

The planning of radiotherapy

As will be apparent from the section dealing with the factors which influence the outcome of radiotherapy, it is essential first to be aware of the nature of the disease and to establish whether other modalities of treatment are to be employed, for example postradiotherapy surgery, or whether surgery and/or chemotherapy have been employed. It is also important to determine from the outset whether the treatment is to be radical or palliative.

The radiotherapist must be aware of the patterns of local and lymphatic spread for each tumour type, thus enabling the design of radiation techniques, which will eradicate the tumour but preserve the normal tissue within the radiation field, to be prepared in advance. Ideally, the field should encompass the primary tumour together with its local spread, and prevent regrowth at the edges of the treatment volume.

The smaller the volume to be treated the better, because if the volume to be treated is small, it is possible to administer a high and hopefully curative dose of radiation. Small volumes may well be treated with interstitial radiotherapy which permits very high doses, but with such a rapid reduction of radiation around the treatment volume that the necessary sparing of the surrounding tissues is achieved.

Clinical examinations, including examination under anaesthetic at the time of biopsy, routine radiology, computerized tomography (CT) and magnetic resonance (MR) give the type of information which is required, particularly in the planning of large volumes. This information must be used in conjunction with knowledge of the behaviour of the type of tumour to be treated.

While the use of high technology is becoming more commonplace, it is important not to place unjustified faith in its use. At present, there is still much to be learnt about the use and abuse of high technology, and there is still no substitute for good clinical judgement and, more importantly, for experience.

When planning treatment in such detail, it is desirable, in the case of tumours of the head and neck, to be able accurately to reproduce treatment plans in the patient at each fraction. A method of comfortably maintaining the position of the patient at each sitting is imperative. It is the normal practice in centres of excellence to produce 'shells' which fit over the patient very accurately. The process of preparation is as follows. After the treatment volume has been decided, the patient is positioned as comfortably as possible in the treatment position on the equivalent of a treatment couch. A substance based on sodium alginate, but also containing diatomaceous earth, lead silicate and calcium sulphate, is mixed with water to a suitable consistency and applied to the face where most detail is required. Over this, moist plaster of Paris bandages are applied to the area of interest on the head and neck; these may be removed after a short time, following the prior application of a releasing agent. Patients usually do not find this a frightening or difficult experience, especially when carried out by an experienced technician. Once the mask has been removed, a releasing agent is placed inside, and the whole filled with plaster of Paris. This should be carried out without undue delay as the alginate will shrink if allowed to dry. After the positive inner plaster has dried, the outer covering is removed and an accurate cast of the patient remains; this is so accurate that even the pores of

the skin are clearly visible. When this cast is completely dry, a shell is produced by vacuum forming with heated cellulose acetate butyrate. This is then used for the planning process and during the subsequent treatment.

In recent years, there has been considerable discussion about the size of each dose and the frequency at which each should be given. Fractionation varies from centre to centre, but the dose and the time period over which it has been given is usually compared to the biological equivalent of 60–65 Gy in 6–6.5 weeks. In some centres, where travelling for the patient is very difficult and hospitalization impossible, single fractions may be given for very small lesions, and treatments once a week for 6 weeks are becoming more common; provided that the site is suitable and the biological protocols are carefully followed, consideration can be given to these forms of fractionation. Hyperfractionation with three fractions each day for approximately 11 days has been administered to advanced cases and, in some of these patients, remarkable results have been obtained.

In the head and neck there are structures which are highly sensitive to radiation and which must always be considered when a decision is being made on a particular treatment plan. These structures are the spinal cord, the lens of the eye, the salivary glands and the lacrimal gland. A dose in excess of 40 Gy in 6 weeks may cause transverse myelitis of the spinal cord. Doses in excess of 6 Gy may cause radiation cataract. Higher and less precise doses give rise to salivary gland dysfunction and very rarely to non-functioning of the lacrimal gland with an ensuing dry eye.

Care of the patient during radiotherapy

Prior to the commencement of radiotherapy, an assessment of the nutritional state of the patient should be made. When afflicted by tumours of the oral cavity or pharynx, patients may well have difficulty and/or pain on swallowing and their nutritional status may well be impaired. The treatment required will depend on the degree of malnutrition and will vary from simple administration of vitamin supplements to feeding with an extremely fine nasogastric tube. As the tube is so well tolerated and easy to use, patients are able to look after themselves at home, thereby avoiding hospitalization. It is usual to feed the patient a proprietary compound which provides sufficient calorie intake as well as the necessary vitamins etc. Some patients may require simple dietary advice, such as the use of puréed food. It may also be of value to administer additional iron if the patient is anaemic as a result of poor food intake in the preceding months.

The treatment of tumours of the mouth exercises the skills of the radiotherapist, because it is important to avoid producing a dry mouth. This can be accomplished by very careful planning in the majority of patients. Unnecessary treatment of the major salivary glands should be avoided where possible, without prejudicing the volume of the mouth or neck which requires treatment. Failure to avoid a dry mouth will usually lead to blackening of the teeth and gross caries, resulting in the necessity for removal. Attempts have been made to save the teeth in the most difficult circumstances by the production of protective splints which are worn until the return of some salivary flow has taken place. Some patients find the splints uncomfortable to wear and a number of departments do not have the facilities for their production.

As a result of endarteritis in the blood vessels in the irradiated area, the blood supply of the mandible and the maxilla may be impaired following radiotherapy, and this is a particular problem in the former. The subsequent removal of teeth may be followed by radiation bone necrosis and this must be avoided by preventative methods. In patients with few and poor quality teeth, removal is best carried out before radiotherapy is commenced. In young patients, where the teeth are of good quality and where care is obviously taken of the dentition, it may be possible to save the teeth. In the event of the teeth's requiring removal following radiotherapy, this is best carried out in a maxillofacial unit, with great care and as gently as possible, creating the least possible trauma, and under antibiotic cover.

During a radical course of radiotherapy, it is inevitable that patients will develop reactions in both the tumour and, more importantly, in normal tissues. Depending on the type of radiation used, there may or may not be a skin reaction. The skin very commonly reacts to electron beam therapy, although this is less likely to occur with megavoltage therapy. It is essential, therefore, before the commencement of treatment to instruct the patient in the care of the skin. Most important is the avoidance of any irritation of the skin. Such irritants may take very many forms including exposure to the sun (another source of electromagnetic irradiation), washing with soap, and dressings which may be required to prevent discharging wounds and sinuses from further irritating the skin. Adhesive plaster of all types must be banned from the treatment area and 'netalast' dressings, a form of stretching, loosely woven material, should be used in preference. The use of a scarf made of silk – a material which is not only soft but also allows free passage of air to the skin, thereby permitting evaporation of any perspiration – should be advised in order both to prevent rough clothes from irritating the area and to protect it from the sun. Male patients should be advised to give up wet shaving during treatment and to shave as gently as possible with an electric razor.

There may be very few indications on the skin of patients during the early part of treatment, but with external beam therapy there will be visible signs on the mucous membrane from a relatively early stage. Initially, some erythema will be visible and this will proceed to a stage where a fibrinous exudate, sometimes called radiation mucositis, becomes apparent. The radiotherapist welcomes this appearance as an indication of a satisfactory reaction to the treatment, but prefers to encounter this on completion of therapy as it is a manifestation that the tissues are approaching the limit of normal tolerance. The patient should, as with the skin, be warned of the kind of trauma which will both advance the onset of mucositis and make the reaction of the tissues worse. The commonest irritants are alcohol, tobacco and strongly spiced foods, which should all be avoided. As the fibrinous exudate increases there is likely to be an increase in pain associated with it, especially on swallowing. The patient will inevitably become more miserable and is likely to become less well nourished, again as a result of treatment. Many types of proprietary medication have been produced to treat the soreness, but simple aspirin mucilage is as effective as most of these. This may be given 20 minutes before meals, and helps by producing not only a local anaesthetic effect but also the systemic effect of analgesia.

Patients who are treated with an implant, usually in the oral cavity, develop the typical radiation mucositis approximately a week or 10 days after the removal of radium or irridium and this may be treated as above. The reaction commonly lasts for 3–4 weeks.

During radiotherapy and especially in debilitated patients who may well have a degree of immune supression, whether local or general, infection is a frequent occurrence. The commonest infection of the oral cavity or pharynx is by *Candida* and is even more predominant when antibiotics are required. Treatment should be immediate and, after swabbing for culture, amphotericin lozenges should be prescribed. As these lozenges dissolve only very slowly, one should be kept in the mouth at all times. Culture may reveal resistant forms of *Candida* and the help of the microbiologist is indispensable in these cases.

While these immediate reactions are visible, it is essential not to lose sight of the long-term reactions. The salivary glands are of importance in this respect. Saliva performs several functions, each of which assists in the prevention of dental caries. It dilutes foods, buffers and dilutes acids produced by fermentation, and constantly washes away food particles and organisms from the mouth. In spite of pre-irradiation precautions, a proportion of irradiated patients will sooner or later develop osteoradionecrosis, a condition which is usually accompanied by pain. Sequestration of dead bone may occur, and this process may take months or indeed years. The availability of megavoltage radiation, with its bone-sparing effect, in no way reduces the need for careful pre-treatment dental evaluation.

The use of electron beam therapy has also led to deafness when treating sites which include the external auditory meatus, as there may be funnelling of the electrons down the canal, which can give rise to late reactions of the temporal bone consisting of atrophy of the membranous labyrinth and osteoradionecrosis.

Adults who as children had retinoblastoma treated with radiotherapy have been known to develop osteosarcoma in the bones of the orbit as much as 20–30 years subsequent to treatment.

Combined radiotherapy and chemotherapy

The treatment of malignant disease of the head and neck is rarely by means of chemotherapy alone. Over recent years, more attention has been paid to the use of combinations of treatment, most commonly surgery and radiotherapy, although the use of chemotherapy in the same way has been gaining support. In those circumstances where surgery is not possible on account of the advanced nature of the disease, the use of chemotherapy either before or after radiotherapy has been adopted as a planned treatment. In addition, a small number of trials have been published, in which chemotherapy has been used at the same time as the administration of radiotherapy. In such circumstances, radiation combined, for example, with bleomycin has given rise to considerable potentiation of the radiotherapy. Perhaps the best known and most used combination of chemotherapy associated with radiotherapy is the regimen suggested by Price and Hill (1978) who have shown that, if it were used before any other form of therapy, their combination induced considerable remission in advanced tumours. This may be extremely beneficial because, as has been explained previously, it is essential to have well-oxygenated tumours to treat with radiotherapy if a cure is to be achieved. There is good evidence to suggest that when the bulk of large tumours has been reduced with chemotherapy, a higher proportion of oxygenated cells remain in the residual tumour. Some of the new cytotoxic drugs, especially some platinum compounds, have shown early promise in the treatment of tumours

of the head and neck. Drugs which for many years have been known to enhance the effect of radiotherapy and which still have a place in this type of treatment are methotrexate and bleomycin. These two drugs have been used by many workers to treat advanced cases, such as inoperable neck nodes. The dose of radiation is frequently reduced by both fraction and total dose as a result of the enhanced reactions encountered. It is very important, however, not to compromise a good therapeutic response by either method, although this might be the unfortunate consequence of reducing the radiation dose to the tumour, or the dose of the cytotoxic drug, to levels where either one might have been better used alone in adequate doses than both used simultaneously. The time–dose relationship with regard to radiotherapy may be further disrupted to disadvantage if it is necessary to rest the patient from therapy as a result of the reactions encountered. In the case of the lymphomata, and especially the non-Hodgkin's lymphomata, the primary tumour and any associated lymph nodes are often treated first with radiation and subsequently with the administration of chemotherapy, usually in the form of combination chemotherapy.

Radiation therapy combined with simultaneous administration of multidrug combination chemotherapy, as reported by O'Connor *et al.* (1982) on behalf of the Radiation Therapy Oncology Group (RTOG) gives hope for future trials of multi-agent radiotherapy treatment regimens.

Attitude to the patient

One of the essential factors in the management of patients with tumours of the head and neck is the attitude of the treating physician to the patient. The majority of patients know they have cancer. Those who do not should, usually, be told of the nature of their disease with sympathy and understanding. Most important is that the patient should be encouraged to look forward to the future with some optimism. The words 'there is nothing we can do to help' should never be used, for, at best, the patient will be cured and, at worst, after good palliation accompanied by a period of good quality life has been achieved, the patient may be helped to die without pain and with dignity. It might well be expected that such an attitude should apply in the case of all patients with malignant disease. However, by virtue of the site of head and neck cancer, in conjunction with the increased use of very extensive and mutilating surgery with the inevitable disfigurement, it is especially important in such cases. Add to this the loss of hair, the nausea and vomiting, and a general discomfort resulting from chemotherapy, and the above attitude becomes imperative. It is hard to explain away some of the necessary therapies which a patient has to undergo without their accepting that a serious problem is being dealt with.

The attitude of all concerned, from the most senior to the most junior member of the therapeutic team, must be one of awareness of what the patient understands about his/her problem and the aims of treatment. The hardest questions are not always asked of the treating doctor. The person confronted with difficult questions is often a student radiographer, a first-year nurse or the new house surgeon or physician. It is important at these times to ascertain the extent of the patient's knowledge by asking what they understand from the information they have been given. The patient's comprehension is often at variance with the meaning which the explanation they were given was intended to convey, and the simple act of talking through what they do understand may provide answers to their questions. If further explanation of a special nature is required then the patient should be referred back to the person who gave the original explanation, but if the remaining question is one concerning the treatment details – for example, of the radiation – then a simple answer may be given.

Under no circumstances should the confidence of the patient be lost by evading or contradicting that which has gone before. This takes time but is of the utmost importance, for patients will almost certainly accept therapy which is unpleasant if they know why they need it and if they have understood that need from the outset. Perhaps the most important words in the clinic are those of encouragement. The patient who has undergone a laryngectomy and who has subsequently made progress with pharyngeal speech should be complimented and urged on to do even better. The establishment of laryngectomy clubs associated with the hospital, but with time spent on social activities, will help the shy or those afraid to use their new found voice. Where appropriate, and where the skills are available, young patients who aspire to take part in activities, should be assisted to achieve their goals. With expert help, some laryngectomy patients are able to swim again. This is merely one example, for there are few limits as to what can be achieved by a fit and well-adjusted patient.

References

ADAMS, G. E. (1972) Chemical radiosensitization of hypoxic cells. *British Medical Bulletin*, **2**, 48–52

ADAMS, G. E. (1977) Hypoxic cell sensitizers for radiotherapy. In *Cancer: A Comprehensive Treatise*, edited by F. F. Becker, Chap. 6, pp. 181–183. New York: Plenum

ADAMS, G. E., DISCHE, S., FOWLER, J. F. and THOMLINSON, R. H. (1976) Hypoxic cell sensitizers in radiotherapy. *The Lancet*, **1**, 186–188

BEDFORD, J. S. and MITCHELL, J. B. (1973) Dose rate effects in synchronous mammalian cells in culture. *Radiation Research*, **54**, 316–327

CHURCHILL-DAVIDSON, I., SANGER, C. and THOMLINSON, R. H. (1957) Oxygenation in radiotherapy. *British Journal of Radiology*, **30**, 406–422

DISCHE, S. (1979) Hyperbaric oxygen and hypoxic cell sensitizers in clinical radiotherapy – present state and prospects. In *High LET Radiations in Clinical Practice*, edited by G. W. Barendsen, J. Broersen and K. Breur, pp. 83–89. Oxford: Pergamon Press

FIELD, S. B. and BLEEHEN, N. M. (1979) Hyperthermia in the treatment of cancer. *Cancer Treatment Reviews*, **6**, 63–94

FOWLER, J. F., ADAMS, G. E., and DENEKAMP, J. (1976) Radiosensitizers of hypoxic cells in solid tumours. *Cancer Treatment Reviews*, **3**, 227–256

FOWLER, J. F. and DANEKAMP, J. (1979) A review of hypoxic cell radiosensitization in experimental tumours. *Journal of Pharmacology and Experimental Therapeutics*, **7**, 413–444

GRAY, L. H., CONGER, A. D., EBERT, M. and HORNSEY, S. (1953) The concentration of oxygen dissolved in tissue at the time of irradiation as a factor in radiotherapy. *British Journal of Radiology*, **26**, 638–648

HAHN, G. M., LI, G., MARMOR, D. and POUND, D. (1979) In *Radiation Research*, edited by S. Okada, M. Imamura, T. Terasima and W. Yamaguchy, pp. 855–859. Tokyo: Japanese association for Radiation Research

HENK, J. M., KUNKLER, P. B. and SMITH, C. W. (1977) Radiotherapy and hyperbaric oxygen in head and neck cancer. Final Report of First Controlled Clinical Trial, *The Lancet*, **2**, 101–103

MARMOR, J. B. and HAHN, G. M. (1980) Combined radiation and hyperthermia in superfical human tumours. *Cancer*, **46**, 1986–1991

MARMOR, J. B., POUNDS, D., POSTIC, T. B. and HAHN, G. M. (1979) Treatment of superficial human neoplasms by local hyperthermia induced by ultrasound. *Cancer*, **43**, 188–197

O'CONNOR, D., CLIFFORD, P., EDWARDS, W. G., DALLEY, V. M., DURDEN-SMITH, J., HOLLIS, B. A. *et al.* (1982) Long term results of VBM and radiotherapy in advanced head and neck cancer. *International Journal of Radiology, Oncology, Biology and Physics*, **8**, 1525–1531

PARKER, H. M. (1934) A dosage system for gamma ray therapy: Part 2. *British Journal of Radiology*, **7**, 612–631

PATERSON, R. (1934) A dosage system for gamma ray therapy: Part 1. *British Journal of Radiology*, **7**, 592–612

PRICE, L. A. and HILL, B. T. (1978) Principles of chemotherapy in head and neck cancer. In *Scott-Brown's Diseases of the Ear, Nose and Throat*, 4th edn, Volume 1, Edited by J. Ballantyne and J. Groves. pp. 665–674. London: Butterworths

WATSON, E. R., HALNAN, K. E., DISCHE, S., SAUNDERS, M. I., CADE, I. S., WIERNIK, G. *et al.* (1978) Hyperbaric oxygen in radiotherapy – a Medical Research Council trial in cancer of the cervix. *British Journal of Radiology*, **51**, 879–887

21

The basic principles of chemotherapy

William J. Primrose

The biology of head and neck cancer

Squamous cell carcinomata, which constitute the majority of upper aerodigestive tract tumours, arise from the cellular unrest of a disturbed epithelium. Light microscopy reveals only one dimension of this complex, chronic process to which descriptive terms such as hyperplasia, dysplasia, metaplasia and anaplasia are applied.

The phenomenon of carcinogenesis involves the interaction of many factors. Ageing, immune competence, hormones, hereditary factors and spontaneous events, which remain essentially beyond our control at present, compound to varying degrees in this process. They are probably inconsequential when compared to the role of environmental factors.

In the area of external stimuli, tobacco and alcohol are the most important factors in the Western world. They act synergistically (Cann, Fried and Rothman, 1985), as both tumour initiators and promotors, on the stem cells of the epithelium. Intermediate cells form, differentiate and die in an uncontrolled fashion, and it is on these cells that tumour promotors exert their effect, causing clones of cells to lose their territorial respect. These are the microinvasive cancers from which large tumours will grow, depending upon blood supply, immunological surveillance and other factors.

The essentials of cytokinetics

Cytokinetics, which is the study of the life cycle of cells, at a cellular level, has developed rapidly since the introduction of radioactively labelled substrates in the late 1940s. It forms the backbone of medical oncology research.

The cell cycle

Fundamental to the understanding of the growth and division of normal as well as of cancerous cells is a dynamic process known as the cell cycle. This is defined as the interval between the midpoint of mitosis of one cell to the midpoint of subsequent mitosis of the daughter cells.

The non-dividing population of cells in any system is said to be in G-0 phase; cells entering the cell cycle go through four phases as follows (*Figure 21.1*):

G-1 phase: the presynthetic/postmitotic phase. The majority of slow growing cell populations spend their time in this phase

S phase: DNA transcription and replication, as well as protein synthesis occur

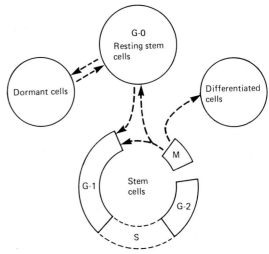

Figure 21.1 The cell cycle

G-2 phase: the postsynthetic/premitotic phase, although RNA and protein synthesis continue

M phase: segregation of genetic material and cell division occur.

Tumour growth

Both normal tissue and tumours grow in volume by:

(1) a net increase in cell numbers (most important)
(2) a net increase in cell size (for example heart muscle hypertrophy)
(3) a net increase in intercellular substance or products (for example colloid goitre).

At any one time, tissue is composed of three distinct populations of cells.

Stem cells. These cells take an active part in the cell cycle and are therefore most sensitive to drugs or radiation. They have the capacity to proliferate, renew themselves, differentiate and be regulated (McCullough and Till, 1971). The last two features may be partly or totally lost in malignant tumours.

Dormant cells. These cells have left the cell cycle temporarily but may re-enter and proliferate when signalled to do so.

Differentiated cells. These cells may have passed through several maturation stages after exiting from the cell cycle, and they usually have a finite function. They do not undergo further mitosis and ultimately die.

The dynamics of any population of tumour cells is governed by the following three indices.

Cell cycle time. This varies as much between different normal tissues as it does between normal and malignant tissue. Normal bone marrow cells may cycle in 18 hours whereas a basal cell carcinoma may cycle in 68 hours.

Growth fraction. This is the percentage of proliferating cells in a tumour, that is those actually traversing the cell cycle at a given point in time. It varies from tumour to tumour and throughout the lifespan of a particular tumour, being greatest in the early stages.

Cell loss. All tumours lose cells by various natural or induced means. Unsuccessful division, death, desquamation, metastasis and migration take their toll on the cell population. Cell loss may range from 30% in a lymphoma to 90% in a poorly differentiated bronchial carcinoma.

Doubling time is an observation which depends on all three of these indices, and hence shows a great variation between tumour classes. A bone sarcoma may take 20 days to double in volume compared to 100 days for a breast carcinoma. If it is assumed that a lung tumour is detected when it reaches $1\,\text{g}$ (approximately 5×10^8 cells), then current mathematical models would suggest that it has been present for up to 7 years. The implications of this concept on the recurrence of tumours after treatment are self-evident.

Chemotherapeutic concepts

Cell kill hypothesis

Basic concepts of drug-induced cell death were elucidated by Skipper, Schabel and Wilcox (1964) from experimental work on L1210 mouse leukaemia. It was recognized that a single inoculated leukaemia cell was capable of multiplying and eventually killing the host. Skipper *et al.* proved that cell destruction by drugs followed first order kinetics, that is a given dose of drug kills a constant fraction of cells, not a constant number, regardless of the number of tumour cells present at the time of treatment. Thus, a drug treatment which reduces a population of 10^6 cells to 10 should reduce a population of 10^5 cells to one cell.

Theoretically, if treatment is started early enough with large enough drug doses, repeated frequently enough, it is possible to reduce a tumour to a small number of cells. Once a 'cure volume' is reached, anatomical and immunological factors may complete the job, as suggested by experiments on tumour transplantation (Fisher and Fisher, 1968). Immunological cell destruction is thought to follow zero order kinetics, that is all foreign cells up to a given number are killed.

Drug scheduling and dosage

Phenomenological models of tumour growth can be devised, with some complicated mathematics, to fit what is observed in reality. Most tumours exhibit exponential growth at some stage in their lifespan, but solid tumours, in particular, show a sigmoid-shaped growth curve called 'Gompertzian growth' (Norton and Simon, 1979) (*Figure 21.2*). This suggests that maximum growth and, by inference, maximum growth fraction occur when the tumour reaches 37% of its expected volume.

Starting the administration of cytotoxic agents when a tumour is reaching its expected maximum volume will have little effect. It is not only the timing of the first treatment which is critical to a successful outcome, but also the timing of successive treatments. If a drug regimen is repeated too soon, the toxic effects on normal tissue will outweigh the benefits of the tumour cell kill, which, as it depends on reasonable numbers of cells re-entering the cell cycle, will be reduced.

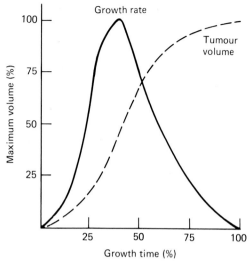

Figure 21.2 Gompertzian growth curve, growth rate superimposed. Growth rate is maximal at 37% of maximum tumour volume, but is very small at the extremes of tumour size

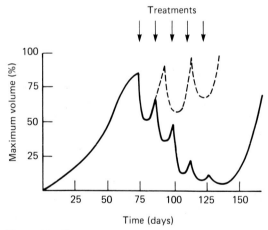

Figure 21.3 Gompertzian growth and theoretical regression induced by an intermittent chemotherapy schedule. The first three cycles have the maximum effect but all the tumour cells are never eradicated. Dotted line indicates progression of disease which occurs if intertreatment level is too long

An optimal intertreatment interval exists (*Figure 21.3*) which maximizes cell kill while allowing bone marrow and other organs to recover. Retreatment delay in the case of a rapidly proliferating tumour may allow progression which may never be brought under control.

The treatment objective of every cytotoxic regimen is to bring about a maximum tumour cell kill with minimum effect on normal stem cells. This narrows the therapeutic index of most drugs so that drug dose and duration of action become

important. Even if the tumour is susceptible to a drug, the drug will not work unless it reaches the tumour site and remains there long enough in tumoricidal concentrations to kill the tumour cells. Hence optimal concentrations (C) and time of action (t) exist for all drugs, but establishing this $C \times t$ ratio is not easy and falls into the complex field of pharmacokinetics. The grey area of risk/benefit is always bordered by black clouds. Too little drug and the tumour progresses; too much and the lethal dose is established. Holding a steady course with the correct dose and scheduling can end all to quickly on the rocks of cumulative organ toxicity.

Selective toxicity

It has for some time been recognized that most cytotoxic agents have a differential action on normal and malignant tissues. The full significance of this was not appreciated until a series of elegant experiments in the 1960s by Bruce, Meeker and Valeriote, who, by studying bone marrow and lymphoma cells in the AKR strain of mouse, were able to develop a quantitative assay of the number of viable clonogenic cells remaining after treatment. Three classes of cytotoxic drug emerged with distinct differential actions.

Class I drugs (Figure 21.4), for example nitrogen mustard. These affect both proliferating and resting cells equally, therefore affecting tumour and normal tissue in an equal dose-related manner. They are said to be 'non-specific'.

Class II drugs (Figure 21.5), for example methotrexate. These kill mainly proliferating cells during a specific part of the latter's cell cycle. These drugs are said to be 'phase specific'.

Class III drugs (Figure 21.6), for example cyclophosphamide. These kill both resting and cycling cells, but the latter are much more sensitive. These drugs are said to be 'cycle specific'.

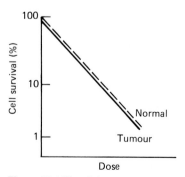

Figure 21.4 Class I drugs

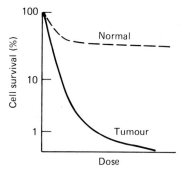

Figure 21.5 Class II drugs

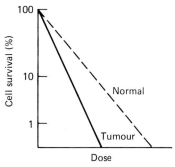

Figure 21.6 Class III drugs

All the major cytotoxic agents have now been studied extensively with regard to their specific sites of action in and out of the cell cycle. Some drugs act at more than one phase (*Figure 21.7*). The knowledge of this and other synergistic effects has become important in designing therapeutic regimens containing more than one drug.

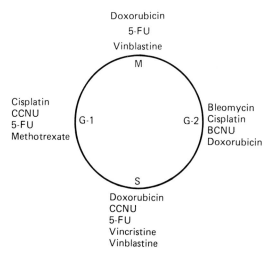

Figure 21.7 Cycle-specific drugs

Rationale for combination drug therapy

The combination of drugs in medicine to treat a single illness has been practised for many centuries. Epilepsy, hypertension and life-threatening infections are a few modern day examples where drug combinations are used. The superiority of combination therapy to single agent therapy was first demonstrated conclusively in the case of childhood acute leukaemia by Frei *et al.* in 1961. This has now been confirmed in certain lymphomata, sarcomata and childhood tumours, to name but a few. The practical benefits of combining drugs may be explained, in part, by the following concepts.

Drug resistance

Drug resistant cell lines develop in most tumours, perhaps in part as a consequence of the mutagenic effects of the drug itself. If a drug which has an associated risk of resistance developing in one in a million cells (10^{-6}) is combined with an unrelated drug with similar risk then the cumulative risk is the product of both, that is 10^{-12}.

Biochemical blockade

Drug combinations can be designed with agents that produce breaks at multiple sites in the tumour cells' essential biosynthetic pathways. 'Sequential blockade' occurs when enzymes are blocked at various steps in the production of an essential metabolite. 'Concurrent blockade' occurs when parallel pathways are affected. 'Complementary blockade' occurs when a drug which blocks the biosynthesis of a macromolecule is combined with a drug which damages the macromolecule directly. Drugs which block DNA repair mechanisms may by synergistic with alkylating agents.

Cell cycle complementation

All tumours are composed of a heterogeneic population of cycling and non-cycling cells, as already described. The combination of alkylating agents and anthracyclines – which are effective against non-cycling cells – with 5-fluorouracil and methotrexate – which are cycle specific – possesses obvious theoretical synergism. Following treatment with non-cycle specific drugs, most tumours show a substantial increase in their growth fraction. This phenomenon is known as 'recruitment' and may also occur in hormone-dependent tumours in response to giving the appropriate hormone. Cycle-specific drugs show more effect after recruitment. 'Synchronization' describes the phenomenon where cells are induced to pass simultaneously through the cell cycle. Cold, shock, thymidine, vincristine and hydroxyurea are capable of producing synchronization *in vitro*. 'Restriction point control' is another theoretical method described for preventing normal cells entering susceptible phases of the cell cycle.

Pharmacological considerations

Some cytotoxic agents may have their effects enhanced when used in combination with other inherently non-toxic agents by a series of unique interactions. Examples of these are:

(1) prolongation of action by probenicid
(2) facilitation of membrane transport by vitamin D
(3) reversal of toxic effects allowing greater cytotoxic dosage, for example folinic acid rescue after methotrexate.

The agents

In the last four decades, perhaps some half-million substances have been screened world-wide for anticancer activity. One hundred or so of them have shown sufficient activity with tolerable toxicity to warrant human trials, and only a handful have found their way into widespread clinical use.

Anticancer drugs can be classified according to their general characteristics (*Table 21.1*), although the specific mode of action of some substances is not fully known.

It must always be borne in mind that cytotoxic agents, by definition, are noxious substances with toxic side-effects; they frequently produce unpleasant adverse reactions which are occasionally lethal. Hypersensitivity, idiosyncratic and unexpected reactions can occur suddenly, thus contraindicating the further use of these drugs. A high risk of abortion and teratogenicity precludes their use in pregnancy.

Drugs and solutions should be carefully prepared and handled by experienced staff, with special regard for labelling and shelf life. Persons gaining experience, or occasional users, should familiarize themselves fully with the appropriate literature and data sheets. Triple checking of dosage and mode of delivery should be carried out, especially by the experienced, as irreversible errors can occur. Intrathecal or intra-arterial injection multiplies the hazards of a miscalculated dose or mistaken drug. Close monitoring of patients in hospital during and after administration is the norm.

The following is a brief pharmacopoeia of the common drugs likely to be encountered in the treatment of head and neck cancer.

Table 21.1 Classification of chemotherapeutic agents

Classification	Drug	Abbreviation
Alkylating agents	Busulphan	BUS
	Chlorambucil	CHL
	Carboplatin	CBDCA
	Cisplatin	DDP
	Cyclophosphamide	CYC
	Mechlorethamine	HN2
	Melphalan	MPL
	Thiotepa	THIO
Antibiotics	Actinomycin D	ACT
	Bleomycin	BLEO
	Daunorubicin	DNR
	Doxorubicin	
	(Adriamycin)	ADR
	Mithramycin	MTH
	Mitomycin C	MTC
Antimetabolites	Cytosine arabinoside	ARA-C
	5-Fluorouracil	5-FU
	Ftorafur	FTOR
	Methotrexate	MTX
	6-Mercaptopurine	6-MP
	Thioguanine	6-TG
Enzymes	L-Asparaginase	L-ASP
Hormones	Adrenocorticoids	PRED
	Androgens	AND
	Oestrogens	ESTR
	Anti-oestrogens	Anti-ESTR
	Progestogens	PROG
Nitrosoureas	Carmustine	BCNU
	Lomustine	CCNU
	Semustine	MCCNU
	Streptozotocin	STZ
Plant alkaloids	Vinblastine	VBL
	Vincristine	VCR
	VM 16	VM 16
	VM 26	VM 26
Random synthetics	Dacarbazine	DTIC
	Dibromomannitol	DBM
	Hexamethylmelamine	HXM
	Hydroxyurea	HYD
	MethylGAG	MGAG
	Mitotane	o,p'DDD
	Procarbizine	PCB

Doxorubicin (Adriamycin)

Doxorubicin is a bright fluorescent red anthracycline antibiotic derived from *Streptomyces peucetius*. It binds between base-pairs of DNA, inhibiting DNA-dependent RNA synthesis, and appears to be most effective during the G-2 phase of mitosis. Intravenous administration results in an initial plasma half-life of 30 minutes, with prolonged hepatic metabolism and excretion in bile and urine.

This drug has one of the widest antitumour spectra known, showing most activity in the acute leukaemias, lymphomata, sarcomata, paediatric malignancies, and breast and lung carcinomata. When it has been used as a single agent in head and neck cancer, response rates of 24% have been described as disappointing (Hong and Bromer, 1983).

The major dose-limiting toxicity is haematological, with nausea, vomiting, diarrhoea, mucositis and alopecia being frequently reported. Of special note is the cardiac toxicity manifested by changes in the electrocardiograph (ECG), and congestive failure resulting from a diffuse cardiomyopathy. The risk of this occurring increases markedly if a total cumulative dose of $550\,mg/m^2$ is exceeded. Synergism with cyclophosphamide may occur. Doxorubicin analogues, for example epirubicin (Epi-adriamycin), are less toxic.

Typical dosages of $60–75\,mg/m^2$ can be given intravenously every 3 weeks. Extravasation at the site of infusion can produce cellulitis and massive tissue necrosis.

Bleomycin sulphate

Bleomycin sulphate is a mixture of glycopeptide antibiotics isolated from strains of *Streptomyces verticullus* by Umezawa (1974). The precise mechanism of acion is unknown, but inhibition of DNA, RNA and protein synthesis occurs. The cycle-specific actions of this drug occur mainly in G-2 and M phases. It concentrates in the skin and lungs but spares haemopoietic tissue. Plasma half-life is approximately 2 hours after intravenous administration, and 60–70% of the administered dose can be recovered in its active form in the urine.

Antitumour activity is seen in most squamous cell carcinomata, lymphomata and testicular tumours. When this drug is used as a single agent in head and neck cancer, 30% of patients show a response which is relatively short lived (Blum, Carter and Agre, 1973). There is a 10% incidence of developing a non-specific pneumonitis, one in 10 of which will progress to a fatal form of pulmonary fibrosis; although age and dose related, its occurrence is unpredictable. Regular chest X-rays and pulmonary function monitoring are necessary. Potentiation of lung damage may occur with oxygen administration, for example during surgery. Rashes, fever, chills and vomiting are frequently reported.

Typical dosages of $10–20\,units/m^2$ are given parenterally, weekly or twice weekly, up to a cumulative maximum of 400 units.

Cisplatin (cis-diammine-dichloroplatinum)

Cisplatin is a heavy metal complex containing a central platinum atom surrounded by two chloride and two ammonia molecules in the *cis* position. It was discovered in 1965 by Rosenberg, Van Camp and Krigas, who noted that platinum compounds produced around an electrode immersed in a culture medium had a bacteriostatic effect. This drug acts as a bifunctional alkylating agent, producing cross-linking of DNA strands, and is apparently cell cycle non-specific. A single intravenous dose concentrates in the liver, kidneys and intestines but spares the central nervous system. It is protein bound in the plasma, demonstrating a biphasic plasma half-life with slow excretion over several days.

Antitumour activity is seen in germinal testicular tumours, ovarian cancer, sarcomata and advanced bladder tumours. When this drug is used as a single agent in squamous cell carcinoma of the head and neck, 30% of patients show a major response (Wittes, 1980).

Renal tubule damage is the major dose-limiting adverse reaction encountered, with urea and creatinine elevations occurring in approximately 30% of patients after a single intravenous dose of $50\,mg/m^2$. Repeated doses are cumulative but intravenous prehydration and mannitol diuresis can reduce nephrotoxicity. Anaphylactic-like reactions, motor toxicity, myelosuppression, severe nausea and vomiting are frequently reported. Electrolyte disturbances and hyperuricaemia occur in relation to renal tubule damage. Neurotoxicity takes the form of peripheral neuropathies and occasional seizures. Sudden death from cerebral herniation has been described and may indicate an occult brain metastasis (Walker, Cairncross and Posner, 1986). Extensive pretreatment work up, including haematological and renal investigations, is necessary. Hearing impairment and platinum compound allergy contraindicate the use of this drug.

Typical dosages of $50–120\,mg/m^2$ are given intravenously over a 2–8 hour period, and adequate hydration and urinary output must be ensured. Subsequent doses should not be given for at least 3 weeks and until the serum creatinine has dropped below $114\,\mu mol/l$.

Cyclophosphamide

Cyclophosphamide is a synthetic white crystalline powder with the molecular formula $C_7H_{15}Cl_2N_2O_2P.H_2O$, and is related to the nitrogen mustards. It is activated by plasma and microsomal enzymes by way of intermediates to intracellular alkylating metabolites. It can be administered orally or parenterally and distributes throughout most body tissues. Serum half-life is 4–6 hours after intravenous administration, and most excretion takes place through the kidneys.

Antitumour activity is seen in a number of malignancies, including lymphomata, multiple myelomata, leukaemias, neuroblastomata, retinoblastomata, and carcinomata of the breast and ovary. As a single agent in squamous cell carcinoma of the head and neck, this drug produces response rates of 36% (Wittes, 1980).

Serious adverse reactions include fatal haemorrhagic cystitis, cardiac toxicity and the development of second malignancies. Alopecia, leucopenia, nausea and vomiting are frequently reported. Potentiation of effects may occur with other cytotoxic agents and with barbiturates. This drug is most frequently used in combination regimens, but a typical intravenous loading dose of 40–50 mg/kg would be given over 2–5 days. An oral maintenance therapy of 1–5 mg/kg has been employed. Total leucocyte counts of less than $3 \times 10^9/l$ may necessitate cessation of treatment.

5-Fluorouracil

5-Fluorouracil is a fluorinated pyrimidine belonging to the antimetabolite group of cytotoxic agents originally discovered by Heidelberger, Chaudhuri and Weston in the 1950s. It is cell-cycle specific with maximum activity in the S-phase. It blocks DNA synthesis by inhibiting thymidylate synthetase, the enzyme responsible for thymidine formation. Intravenous administration leads to a short plasma half-life of 10–20 minutes on account of rapid catabolism in the liver.

Antitumour activity is seen in a variety of carcinomata, including the gastrointestinal tract, breast and bladder. When this drug has been used as a single agent in squamous cell carcinoma of the head and neck, response rates of 15% have been reported, although intra-arterial regional perfusion may improve this. Side-effects include anorexia, nausea, vomiting, mucositis, leucopenia, alopecia and rarely cerebellar ataxia.

Typical dosages of 1000 mg/m^2 can be given daily by intravenous infusion for 4–5 days, repeated at 4-weekly intervals.

Methotrexate

Methotrexate, a sodium salt of 4-amino-10-methylfolic acid, is an antimetabolite acting principally in the S-phase of the cell cycle. It competitively inhibits dihydrofolate reductase, preventing the reduction of dihydrofolate to tetrahydrofolate, a necessary step in the process of DNA synthesis. However, this effect may be reversed by administering tetrahydrofolate (leucovorin) up to 24 hours later.

When this drug is parenterally administered, peak serum levels are seen in 30–60 minutes with a half-life of 2–10 hours, 40% being excreted unchanged in the urine. Daily doses result in sustained serum levels; it essentially does not cross the blood–brain barrier, but may be given intrathecally.

Antitumour activity is seen in trophoblastic tumours, acute leukaemias, lymphomata and a variety of carcinomata. Probably the single most studied cytotoxic agent in squamous cell cancer of the head and neck, it demonstrates response rates approaching 50% when used in high weekly doses with leucovorin rescue in previously untreated patients (Wittes, 1980). The major toxic effects of methotrexate are mylosuppression and gastrointestinal mucositis. Other adverse reactions include abdominal cramps, malaise, rashes, osteoporosis, renal and hepatic toxicity.

Typical dosages of 15 mg/m^2 daily for 3 days, repeated at 3-weekly intervals have prolonged survival in some recurrent cases, with few side-effects. Doses of 500–1000 mg/m^2 given intravenously on a weekly basis combined with leucovorin rescue are possible.

Vinblastine

Vinblastine is a plant alkaloid derived, along with vincristine, from the common garden periwinkle *Vinca rosea*. It inhibits both RNA synthesis and the formation of tubular structures found in the spindle fibres of mitotic metaphase, but the exact mechanisms of tumour cell death are poorly understood. Poor absorption from the gastrointestinal tract dictates intravenous administration, with a plasma half-life of 30 minutes. Liver metabolism and bile excretion occur, and platelets may form a repository for sustained release.

Antitumour activity is broad, with the greatest response seen in the rapidly dividing lymphomata and choriocarcinomata. When this drug is used as a single agent, response rates approaching 30% are seen in squamous cell carcinoma of the head and neck.

Toxic effects include nausea, vomiting, constipation, diarrhoea, granulocytopenia and peripheral neuritis.

Typical dosages range from 4 to 20 mg/m^2 given intravenously on a weekly basis.

Definitions

Medical oncology has developed a jargon unique to the speciality, which lends itself to mesmerism in some, to misunderstanding by many and mistrust by a few, mainly surgeons. The author will attempt to define and expand some of the adjectives and phrases which are essential to the understanding of the subject.

Adjuvant chemotherapy is the use of cytotoxic agents with intent to improve survival before, during or immediately after standard local treatment by surgery, radiotherapy or both.

Induction chemotherapy is the use of cytotoxic agents with intent to improve survival before progressing to standard local treatment as above.

Neoadjuvant chemotherapy is the same as induction chemotherapy, also sometimes described as 'up front' or 'anterior'.

Palliative chemotherapy is the use of cytotoxics, usually single agents, in an attempt to relieve symptoms in an incurable disease process. When administered to some patients with advanced unresectable, recurrent or disseminated disease, it has been known to prolong reasonable quality life in some cases. The question should always be asked, 'Am I prolonging life or prolonging death?'.

Response

Cytotoxic agents should be given to consenting patients only on the basis of a reasonable expectation that a response will be produced in the latter's respective tumours. Although originally intended only as an endpoint in phase II trials, measurement, documentation and correlation of response seem to have assumed a much wider importance to medical oncologists.

Many parameters require consideration. Accurate tumour measurement, by various means, is required at the time of tumour staging. Response is usually measured 2–3 weeks after administration of induction chemotherapy which may consist of one or more cycles. More chemotherapy may be given if the response is favourable. Measurement of response in head and neck tumours is usually clinical and occasionally radiological, and frequently biopsies are taken at the tumour site to assess the 'pathological' response. Response at primary and nodal sites may vary, as may the duration of response if not followed immediately by standard local treatment.

Reassessment by the otolaryngologist who initially staged the patient is advisable. Response is graded according to the following broadly accepted guidelines (Miller *et al.*, 1981).

Complete response (CR) indicates that there is total tumour regression, although a certain amount of tissue distortion or mucosal scarring may be allowed. It should be maintained for at least 4 weeks.

Partial response (PR) indicates that there has been a greater than 50% reduction in the product of the two largest perpendicular diameters of measurable tumour.

No response (NR) indicates no change in the size of the tumour, or a less than 50% reduction of measurable tumour.

Progressive disease (PD) indicates a growth of measurable tumour of 25% or more, or the appearance of new lesions.

'Major' response implies either a complete or partial response.

'Minor' response implies either no response or progressive disease.

Occasionally, responses are quoted after combined modality treatment for example 'a partial response following chemotherapy and radiotherapy'. This can be misleading, and older terms such as 'residual' and 'recurrent' disease are to be preferred.

Survival

Traditionally, the term 'survival' has taken the form of quoting 3- or 5-year survival rates, which, in their crudest form, record only whether the patient is alive or dead. The information can be made a little more sophisticated by recording whether the patient is free of disease or not. Comparison by simple non-parametric tests, for example Fisher's exact or $\aleph^2$, will provide probability values from which significance may be deduced.

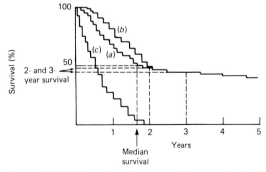

Figure 21.8 (*a*) Typical survival curve following standard treatment for stage III and IV head and neck squamous carcinoma. Most (95%) recurrences occur within 2 years, rendering this a valid approximation for 3- and 5-year survival. (*b*) Standard treatment followed by chemotherapy. (*c*) Control group (no treatment)

The last two decades have witnessed a blossoming of the use of survival curves, sometimes known as actuarial or Kaplan Meier plots, which are now almost mandatory illustrations (*Figure 21.8*). Patients with different lengths of follow-up may be included without fundamentally altering the shape of the curve, and 2- or 3-year survival rates may approximate to what will be observed at 5 years if numbers are large enough. Prognostic inferences may be made from complicated calculations based on the shape of the curves.

Median survival is frequently quoted – this is the time it takes for 50% of the population to die – and may be read off the curve or be calculated. It can vary greatly. In a large series of patients with recurrent intractable squamous cell carcinoma of the head and neck, median survival was reached in only 11 weeks (Stell and McCormick, 1986). Complete responders to chemotherapy, however, may not reach their median survival in 5 years of follow-up. Similarly, patients with malignant salivary gland tumours (Conley and Dingman, 1974) may not reach their median survival in 5 years, but display a completely different survival curve (*Figure 21.9*).

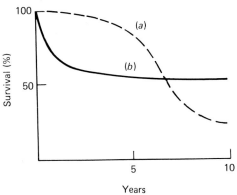

Figure 21.9 (*a*) Slow growing but malignant tumour. (*b*) Treatment initially very toxic but also therapeutic

The timing of entry into a study is an often overlooked but a vitally important consideration. Entry at the commencement of treatment will produce a group of patients who do not complete their ascribed treatment and may not be worthy of comparison. Entry after completing treatment may favourably skew the results by excluding early deaths from disease or treatment. It has been known in some studies, for patients who failed to meet the stringent criteria for treatment on the study arm to be placed into the control arm, thus tipping the balance in favour of the former. If a large number of patients have been lost to follow-up then very close scrutiny is required

before the authors' conclusions can be accepted at face value.

Finally, reports of improved survival with any new treatment regimen over that which was experienced 10 or 20 years ago must be regarded with scepticism, even though numbers are large and statistics convincing. The observed improvement may in fact be attributable to 'stage migration'. This is best illustrated by the 'Will Rogers' phenomenon. This famous American humorist proclaimed that 'when the Oakies moved from Oklahoma to California during the dustbowl crisis, they raised the average IQ of both states'. Feinstein, Sosin and Wells (1985) have produced disturbing evidence which suggests that contemporary improvements of survival rates in patients with lung cancer is a statistical artefact caused by a general drift of patients into higher clinical stages as a result of better diagnostic imaging techniques. Thus patients can move from stage I to stage IV on the basis of a computerized tomographic (CT) scan not available 20 years ago. This has the effect of improving the expected survival of both stage I and stage IV groups.

Clinical trials

Most of the published literature about chemotherapy in head and neck cancer has been based on information obtained from properly conducted clinical trials. Anecdotal reports and retrospective reviews of casually applied but well-intentioned treatment carry little credence. Many agents with proven curability in the case of other tumours are still considered 'investigational' in head and neck cancer. Methotrexate, bleomycin and cisplatin have been extensively investigated at phase I and II levels, but useful phase III trial information is remarkably hard to find.

The backbone of any drug trial is the protocol design: this needs to be 'watertight' with all possible eventualities anticipated before any patients are entered. Objectives need to be clearly defined and finite limits set on numbers and time. Contingency plans of how to deal with 'drop outs' and protocol violations are required.

Eligibility criteria

Eligibility criteria are the set of rigid guidelines which have to be met before any particular patients can be entered into a trial. They are intended to ensure that all the patients in the trial fit into a well-defined population, and to screen against any conditions which may contraindicate chemotherapy. Thus the majority of patients entering phase II and phase III trials are a carefully

Typical 21.2 Typical work up and eligibility criteria required

Full history and physical examination
Routine haematology and biochemistry
    White cell count (WCC)>3 × 10^9/l
    Haemoglobin (Hb)>12 g/100 ml
    Blood urea nitrogen (BUN) < 10 mmol/l
    Creatinine < 114 μmol/l
    Liver function tests normal
Radiology
    Chest X-ray
    Computerized tomographic/magnetic resonance scans
    Ultrasound liver
    Isotope scan liver/spleen/brain
Karnofsky performance status >50%
Pulmonary function tests normal
Cardiac ejection fraction >50%
Audiogram
    Pure-tone audiogram <30 dB; s.d. > 80%
Dental opinion/clearance
Nutritional consultation
Immunobiological staging
    Delayed cutaneous hypersensitivity
    T-lymphocyte levels
    Lymphocyte function *in vitro*
    IgA and IgE determinations

selected group who do not necessarily reflect a typical sample of patients with advanced head and neck carcinoma. A fairly typical work up with criteria is given in *Table 21.2*. Common exclusions from entry into a trial include:

(1) another synchronous primary tumour
(2) another recent primary tumour, for example within 3 years
(3) previous chemotherapy
(4) poor renal and lung function
(5) refusal to consent.

Phase I trials

Phase I trials are intended to be the initial evaluation of a new drug in humans. Ideally, the drug will have been evaluated in rodents, dogs and monkeys, and information gained about its absorption, blood levels, distribution, excretion and toxicity. The objectives of the trial are to

(1) establish antitumour activity
(2) establish toxicity
(3) establish the maximum tolerated dose
(4) gain information about uptake, metabolism excretion and organ distribution.

These trials are often performed on patients with advanced disease refractory to other treatments, so interpretation of the results may be difficult and a false negative result can condemn a truly active drug to the shelf.

Phase II trials

Phase II trials are intended to identify the therapeutic efficacy of a single new drug or new drug combination. Definitive answers about the ultimate value or precise role of each drug or combination are not expected. Ideally, the drugs should be given at levels close to the maximum tolerated dose and the dose schedule varied, if possible.

The objectives of a phase II trial are to assess response and measure duration of response, if possible.

'Broad' trials may include a variety of 'signal' tumours such as lymphomata, leukaemias, and carcinomata of the breast, colon and lung. Head and neck cancer trials are much narrower 'disease-orientated studies' in which patient characteristics, site and stage are variables. Again, safeguards have to be taken to avoid wrong conclusions, with false negative results high on the list.

Phase III trials

Phase III trials are comprehensive studies of an active drug or drug combination, usually involving a large controlled clinical trial. Historical controls are virtually meaningless for this type of study as there is a great danger that two different populations will be compared. Patients should be matched, stratified, and randomized into study and control arms before treatment is begun.

The main objective of a phase III trial is to measure and compare length of survival. Crossovers should be avoided as they defeat the objectives and confuse the issues. Protocol design should include calculations of necessary sample size, details of statistical analysis and instructions of how to deal with excluded or 'non-evaluable' patients. A multicentre trial may be required to obtain a sufficient number of patients within the time period allotted.

The Veterans Administration study no. 268 is a good example of such a multicentre approach. Induction chemotherapy followed by radiotherapy is presently being compared with surgery and radiotherapy for resectable stage III and IV laryngeal cancer. The goal is to detect a projected difference of a 40% 2-year survival in the standard arm with a projected 55% 2-year survival in the experimental arm with a significance level of 0.05 and power of 0.80. It is estimated that 348 patients will be required to prove this hypothesis; therefore, allowing for a 3% loss to follow-up, 360 patients will be entered into the trial. Fourteen hospitals are participating over a 3-year entry period and minimum follow-up is 2 years.

Ethical problems may arise in large trials like this when it becomes obvious that one arm is performing much better than the other, but happily guidelines exist to deal with such a dilemma (Rubinstein and Gail, 1982).

Chemotherapy in practice

The role of chemotherapy in the treatment of head and neck cancer is under critical scrutiny at present, with many otolaryngologists maintaining an open mind on the subject. Palliative chemotherapy is comprehensively covered in Volume 5, Chapter 24. Some aspects of induction chemotherapy, drawn mainly from North American sources, will be discussed in this section.

Strong theoretical and practical arguments have been put forward to support or condemn the use of induction chemotherapy (*Table 21.3*). Some experts hold the view that it is only a matter of time until the 'breakthrough' seen in haematological and some other solid tumours occurs in head and neck cancer. Some signs of this must surely exist in the accumulated knowledge of the last decade.

The significance of a complete response

Achieving a complete response after induction chemotherapy, followed by a standard treatment modality, appears to be associated with a significantly enhanced survival (Ensley *et al.*, 1984; Primrose *et al.*, 1985). Whether this survival benefit can be attributed, wholly or in part, to the chemotherapy, is open to debate. Achieving a lesser response, as in other solid tumours, is much less predictive of ultimate cure. It is possible that complete responders have biologically favourable tumours which will do well with any established treatment modality.

Radiotherapy alone, following a complete response, may be adequate treatment (Primrose *et al.*, 1985), as the total tumour burden is obviously very small after chemotherapy.

Histological specimens of tumour sites, following a complete response, are difficult to interpret. Increased differentiation, manifested by cellular enlargement, glycogen formation, desmosome activity and marked keratinization have been described (Michaels, Grey and Rowson, 1973). Is the persistent tumour, seen histologically (Spaulding *et al.*, 1982; Decker, Drelichman and Jacobs, 1983), still viable? Ironically, this question can be answered by examining closely the inevitable drop-outs from the larger trials, most of which have a few patients who achieve a complete response and then refuse all further treatment. Of the 100 patients reported by the present author, two such patients are identified (complete remission after cisplatin and bleomycin), both of whom eventually died with disease at 5 and 6 years respectively. Four such patients are identified by Weaver *et al.* (1982) (complete remission after cisplatin and 5-fluorouracil). Tumour recurrence was noted in three of these patients at 4, 6 and 7 months after chemotherapy; the fourth patient, with a base of tongue tumour, was noted to be clinically and histologically disease free at 18 months after chemotherapy.

Table 21.3 Theoretical and practical arguments for and against induction chemotherapy

	Advantages	*Disadvantages*
(1)	Effective drug levels obtained because tumour vascularity unaffected by surgery or radiotherapy	Time spent giving chemotherapy delays surgery and radiotherapy which may be of more benefit
(2)	Better drug tolerance allows full effective courses to be given	Toxicity
(3)	Micrometastases eradicated	Immunosuppression promotes survival of micrometastases
(4)	Unresectable tumours rendered resectable	Tumour shrinkage confuses the surgical margin
(5)	Radiotherapy field and dose may be reduced, thus lowering morbidity	Potentiation of side-effects of radiotherapy, for example mucositis, may compromise treatment
(6)	Chemotherapy predicts response to radiotherapy	Complete responders occasionally refuse further treatment until too late
(7)	Radiotherapy alone may be sufficient after a major response	Prolonged hospitalization

The Royal Marsden experience

Chapter 22 is devoted to the experiences of Price and Hill.

The Wayne State University experience

Virtually every self-respecting induction chemotherapy phase II or III trial at present under way in North America includes cisplatin in some combination. The head and neck group at Wayne State University, Detroit (Kish *et al.*, 1984), have been pioneering its use since 1977, and have reported their experience with 188 patients. Seventy-seven patients received two courses of cisplatin, cyclophosphamide and bleomycin. Twenty-six patients received two courses of cisplatin and 5-fluorouracil (days 1–4) and 85 patients received three courses of cisplatin and 5-fluorouracil (days 1–5). All patients received standard treatment of surgery and/or radiotherapy following chemotherapy. The major response rate was 80%, 88% and 93% respectively for the different regimens, but the last regimen produced a complete response rate of 54%. In this last group, 79% of T4N0 patients had a complete response.

Synergism between cisplatin and 5-fluorouracil was reported as far back as 1971 in experimental animal tumours. Many oncologists have adopted the Wayne State regimen of cisplatin $100 \, mg/m^2$ followed by 5-fluorouracil $1000 \, mg/m^2$ per day for 5 days, repeated in three cycles, as the 'state of the art' regimen.

The National Cancer Institute trial (HNCP-128)

The National Cancer Institute trial is, to date, the largest prospective randomized trial of induction chemotherapy for resectable stage III and IV head and neck carcinoma, with 13 participating institutions. A total of 462 patients were randomized to one of three arms:

(1) standard treatment of surgery followed by radiotherapy
(2) induction chemotherapy (cisplatin $100 \, mg/m^2$ and bleomycin) followed by standard treatment
(3) induction chemotherapy and standard therapy followed by maintenance chemotherapy (cisplatin $80 \, mg/m^2$ monthly for 6 months).

Of the 282 patients receiving induction chemotherapy there was a 37% major response rate with minimal toxicity. The study closed in April 1982, with 443 evaluable patients.

No statistical difference in overall (0.56–0.59) or disease-free survival existed at 2 years between the three treatment arms (Jacobs *et al.*, 1984). Of the 148 patients with recurrent disease, 48% had distant metastases. Several prognostic factors influenced survival – for example site, stage and performance status. The writing committee concluded that adjuvant chemotherapy in this trial did not improve survival when compared with standard treatment. This massive trial has been criticized by some, with the benefit of hindsight, because only one cycle of induction chemotherapy was given. The 3-year survival status and detailed study report is still pending.

The Milwaukee experience

Two prospective randomized induction chemotherapy trials have been performed by Toohill and colleagues between 1979 and 1985 (Toohill *et al.*, 1986). In the first study, 43 patients received bleomycin, cyclophosphamide, methotrexate and 5-fluorouracil in two cycles (one cycle if no tumour response was noted), followed by standard treatment. Forty control patients received only standard treatment. Despite a 'major' response rate of 68% in the chemotherapy arm, 2-year survival was better in the control group (43% against 31%).

In the second study, 27 patients received cisplatin and 5-fluorouracil in three cycles prior to standard treatment. Thirty control patients received only standard therapy. Despite an improved 'major' response of 85% in the chemotherapy arm, control patients fared better with survival rates of 69% against 46% at 19 months. The largest statistically significant differences were seen in stage IV patients. The relative risk of having persistent disease was calculated to be 2.9 times greater for patients who received chemotherapy. These trials show convincingly that the inherent delay in giving chemotherapy (66 days average in the first study and 95 days in the second) is responsible for their negative findings.

Control of micrometastases

Widely varying estimates are reported of the incidence of distant metastases from squamous cell carcinoma of the head and neck. Merino, Lindberg and Fletcher (1977) reviewed 5019 cases with a minimum follow-up of 2 years, and found an overall incidence of 11%. Site and stage influenced their occurrence with incidences of 7.5% from the oral cavity compared to 15% from the supraglottic larynx and 23.6% from the hypopharynx. Merino *et al.* estimated that the incidence doubles if the patient has a recurrence above the clavicles and that the lung accounts for more than 50% of the first recognized sites of distant metastasis. Micrometastases present at the time of pretreatment work-up are unlikely to be detected by available diagnostic methods. Surgery and radiotherapy cannot be expected to eradicate such disease, whereas some form of systemic treatment might do so. This question was addressed by Hong *et al.* (1985), who projected their 5-year local recurrence rate to be 39% and their distant failure rate to be 26%. They concluded that their combined modality approach with induction chemotherapy does not seem significantly to reduce the incidence of distant metastases.

Cost

The cost of induction chemotherapy cannot be overlooked in these days of financial audit and restraint. A single dose of cisplatin for an average adult costs the National Health Service £50–£60. The typical 1984 cost of four courses of cisplatin and bleomycin (outpatient treatment) in the USA is estimated at $6452 (Million and Sigal, 1984). Five days hospitalization with leucopenia may cost another $2000.

New dimensions and new directions

The search for effective new drugs and drug combinations continues, with carboplatin (*cis*-diammine-1,1-cyclobutane dicarboxylate platinum II) receiving much attention. This platinum compound is undergoing phase II evaluation in head and neck cancer in the USA, with National Cancer Institute support. Good risk patients appear to tolerate $400\,mg/m^2$ repeated after 4 weeks with less nephrotoxicity, ototoxicity and vomiting than is experienced with high dose cisplatin (Koeller, 1986).

'Protective agents' – substances which affect epithelial growth and maturation – have recently been the subject of renewed interest. Reversal of leucoplakia and erythroplasia has been observed after long-term administration of 13-*cis*-retinoic acid (Hong and Doos, 1985). Whether such substances can prolong survival or prevent second primary tumours in at-risk patients remains to be proven.

Finally, the otolaryngologist is occasionally confronted by an aggressive salivary gland tumour, mucosal melanoma or basal cell carcinoma. A multimodality approach to some of these tumours may show more promise than has been the case with squamous cell carcinoma. The discovery of oestrogen receptors in some salivary gland carcinomata has stimulated interest in the use of tamoxifen. Combination drug therapy in malignant melanoma based on dacarbazine or a platinum compound may yield an effective regimen in the treatment of mucosal melanomata.

References

BLUM, R., CARTER, S. and AGRE, N. (1973) A clinical review of bleomycin – a new antineoplastic agent. *Cancer*, **31**, 903–914

BRUCE, W., MEEKER, B. and VALERIOTE, F. (1966) Comparison of the sensitivity of normal haematopoietic and transplanted lymphoma colony-forming cells to chemotherapeutic agents administered *in vitro*. *Journal of the National Cancer Institute*, **37**, 233–245

CANN, C., FRIED, M. and ROTHMAN, K. (1985) Epdemiology of squamous cancer of the head and neck. *Otolaryngologic Clinics of North America*, **18**, 367–388

CONLEY, J. and DINGMAN, D. (1974) Adenoid cystic carcinoma of the head and neck. *Archives of Otolaryngology*, **100**, 81–90

DECKER, D., DRELICHMAN, A.and JACOBS, J. (1983) Adjuvant chemotherapy with cis-diamminodichloroplatinum II and 12 hour infusion of 5-fluorouracil in stage III and IV squamous carcinoma of the head and neck. *Cancer*, **51**, 1353–1355

ENSLEY, J., KISH, J., JACOBS, A., WEAVER, J., CRISSMAN, J., KINZIE, J. *et al.* (1984) Superior survival in complete responders with chemotherapy alone compared to those requiring chemotherapy and radiation in patients with advanced squamous cell carcinoma of the head and neck. *Proceedings of the American Society of Clinical Oncology*, **3**, 181 (Abstracts)

FEINSTEIN, A., SOSIN, D. and WELLS, C. (1985) The Will Rogers phenomenon. Stage migration and new diagnostic techniques as a source of misleading statistics for survival in cancer. *New England Journal of Medicine*, **312**, 1604–1608

FISHER, B. and FISHER, E. (1968) The proliferation and spread of neoplastic cells. In *21st Annual Symposium on Fundamental Cancer Research*. M.D. Anderson Hospital Tumour Institute, pp. 552–582. Baltimore: Williams and Wilkins

FREI, E., FREIREICH, E., GEHAN, E. and RINKEL, D. (1961) Studies of sequential and combination antimetabolite therapy in acute leukaemia: 6-mercaptopurine and methotrexate. Acute leukaemia group B. *Blood*, **18**, 431–454

HEIDELBERGER, C., CHAUDHURI, N. and WESTON, E. (1958) The metabolism of 5-fluorouracil-2-C in humans. *Proceedings of the American Association of Medicine*, **73**, 897–900

HONG, W. and BROMER, R. (1983) Chemotherapy in head and neck cancer. *New England Journal of Medicine*, **308**, 75–79

HONG, W., BROMER, R., AMATO, D., SHAPSHAY, S., VINCENT, M. and VAUGHAN, C. (1985) Patterns of relapse in locally advanced head and neck cancer patients who achieve complete remission after combined modality therapy. *Cancer*, **56**, 1242–1245

HONG, W. and DOOS, W. (1985) Chemoprevention in head and neck cancer. *Otolaryngologic Clinics of North America*, **18**, 543–549

JACOBS, C., WOLF, G., MAHUCH, R. and VIKRAM, B. (1984) Adjuvant chemotherapy for head and neck squamous carcinomas. *Proceedings of the American Society of Clinical Oncology*, **3**, 182 (Abstract)

KISH, J., ENSLEY, J., WEAVER, A., JACOBS, J., KINZIE, J., CUMMINGS, G. *et al.* (1984) Improvement of complete response rate to induction adjuvant chemotherapy for advanced squamous carcinoma of the head and neck. In *Adjuvant Therapy of Cancer IV*, pp. 107–115. New York: Grune and Stratton

KOELLER, J. (1986) Phase 1 clinical trials using CBDCA. *Cancer*, **57**, 282

McCULLOUGH, E. and TILL, J. (1971) Regulatory mechanisms acting on haematopoietic stem cells. *American Journal of Pathology*, **65**, 601–614

MERINO, O., LINDBERG, R. and FLETCHER, G. (1977) An analysis of distant metastases from squamous cell carcinomas of the upper respiratory and digestive tracts. *Cancer*, **40**, 145–151

MICHAELS, L., GREY, P. and ROWSON, K. (1973) Effects of bleomycin on human and experimental squamous carcinoma. *Journal of Pathology*, **109**, 315–321

MILLER, A. B., HOOGSTRATEN, B., STAQUET, M. and WINKLER, A. (1981) Reporting results of cancer treatment. *Cancer*, **47**, 207–214

MILLION, R. and SIGAL, M. (1984) Cost of management of head and neck cancer. In *Management of Head and Neck Cancer, a Multidisciplinary Approach*, pp. 647–649. Philadelphia: J. B. Lippincott and Co

NORTON, L. and SIMON, R. (1979) New thoughts on the relationship of tumour growth and characteristics to sensitivity to treatment. In *Methods in Cancer Research vol XVII Cancer Drug Development, part B*, edited by V. T. De Vita Jr. and H. Busch, pp. 53–90. New York: Academic Press

PRIMROSE, W., VAUGHAN, C., HONG, W., KARP, D., WILLETT, B. and STRONG, M. (1985) Three year survival rates in advanced head and neck cancer after induction chemotherapy ; significance of initial response. In *New Dimensions in Otorhinolaryngology – Head and Neck Surgery*, edited by E. N. Myers, vol. II, pp. 1077–1078. Amsterdam: Excerpta Medica

ROSENBERG, B., VAN CAMP, L. and KRIGAS, T. (1965) Inhibition of cell division in *Escherichia coli* by electrolysis products from a platinum electrode. *Nature*, **205**, 698–699

RUBINSTEIN, L. and GAIL, M. (1982) Monitoring roles for stopping accrual in comparative survival studies. *Controlled Clinical Trials*, **3**, 325–343

SKIPPER, H., SCHABEL, F. and WILCOX, W. (1964) Experimental evaluation of potential anticancer agents. *Cancer Chemotherapy Reports*, **35**, 1–111

SPAULDING, M., KAHN, A., SANTO, R., KLOTCH, D. and LORE, J. (1982) Adjuvant chemotherapy in advanced head and neck cancer, an update. *American Journal of Surgery*, **144**, 432–436

STELL, P. M. and McCORMICK, M. S. (1986) The design of phase III palliative chemotherapy trials in head and neck cancer. *Clinical Otolaryngology*, **11**, 21–29

TOOHILL, R., HOFFMAN, R., GROSSMAN, T., DUNCANVAGE, J. and MALIN, T. (1986) The effects of delay in standard treatment due to induction chemotherapy in two randomised, prospective trials. *Otolaryngology, Head and Neck Surgery* (in press)

UMEZAWA, H. (1974) Chemistry and mechanism of action of bleomycin. *Federation Proceedings*, **33**, 2296–2302

WALKER, R., CAIRNCROSS, J. and POSNER, J. (1986) Acute neurological deterioration after cisplatin therapy for primary and metastatic brain tumours. *ASCO Abstracts*, **5**, 135

WEAVER, A., FLEMMING, S ., KISH, J., VANDENBURGH, H., JACOBS, J., CRISSMAN, J. *et al.* (1982) Cisplatinum and 5-fluorouracil as induction therapy for advanced head and neck cancer. *American Journal of Surgery*, **144**, 445–448

WITTES, R. (1980) Chemotherapy of head and neck cancer. *Otolaryngologic Clinics of North America*, **13**, 515–520

22

Chemotherapy in head and neck cancer

L. A. Price and Bridget T. Hill

The role of chemotherapy in squamous cell carcinomata of the head and neck has been undergoing intensive re-evaluation during the last decade. The traditional approach to treatment of head and neck cancer (summarized in *Figure 22.1*) involved some form of surgery, preceded or followed by radiotherapy. In the one-third of

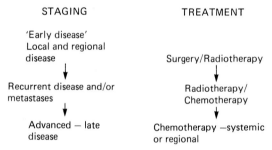

STAGING	TREATMENT
'Early disease' Local and regional disease	Surgery/Radiotherapy
Recurrent disease and/or metastases	Radiotherapy/ Chemotherapy
Advanced — late disease	Chemotherapy —systemic or regional

Figure 22.1 The traditional approach to the management of head and neck tumours. (Adapted from Carter and Soper, 1974)

patients presenting with local disease, the use of such measures resulted in a significant cure rate. However, most patients present with advanced stage III or IV local and regional disease. Although combined surgery and radiotherapy have provided greater local control, the incidence of local failure remains high, at 70%, and distant metastases develop in 20–30% of patients (Probert, Thompson and Bagshaw, 1974; Grunberg, 1985). Therefore, in spite of the best local therapy, most patients with squamous cell carcinoma of the head and neck die from their disease.

Traditionally, only patients with recurrent or disseminated head and neck tumours were considered eligible for chemotherapy. These patients have a poor prognosis, with an average survival period of six months or less. Despite the fact that several antitumour drugs have proved highly effective in shrinking bulky lesions, palliative chemotherapy, using single agents, has had no impact on the survival rate. Indeed, not for several decades has this traditional approach to the management of head and neck tumours resulted in any overall improvement in disease-free survival rates. Identification of a large number of active single agents and their potential in drug combinations has led to consideration of a new role for chemotherapy. This chapter reviews these developments and describes a logical scientific approach towards earlier integration of safe and optimum chemotherapy into a multidisciplinary attack, in an attempt to improve the prognosis for this group of tumours.

Traditional approach to chemotherapy in advanced disease

The evaluation of chemotherapy data pertaining to head and neck cancer is complicated by the heterogeneity of prognostic variables associated with this tumour type (Carter and Livingston, 1982). These include: the site of the primary lesion, the clinical stage, prior therapy, and nutritional and performance status. Most studies report on a relatively small number of patients so that the analysis of response, even according to only one of these parameters, leads to numbers which are too small to be meaningful. The overall impression is that each of these variables may be prognostically significant.

Single agents

The history of chemotherapy for head and neck cancer began with a demonstration that methotrexate was capable of shrinking clinically evident tumour masses. Results from many studies have established an approximate 40% response rate to this agent, although the optimal schedule is still not known. The general recommendation for routine administration with acceptable toxicity is for methotrexate to be used systemically, in moderate dose, on an intermittent basis. This avoids the definite morbidity associated with intra-arterial cannulation. Bertino, Boston and Capizzi (1975), in a detailed analysis by site (*see Table 22.1*), reported the highest response rates to methotrexate in oral cavity and oropharyngeal lesions, and the lowest in nasopharyngeal and hypopharyngeal tumours. The response duration was longest (four months) in tonsillar and oral tongue lesions, and was shortest (two months) in tumours of the palate, oropharynx, floor of mouth and hypopharynx.

Bleomycin is the second most studied single agent in head and neck cancer. In 298 assessable patients, 48 showed a 25% response or greater, 54 showed responses of 50% or greater and 10 had a complete response (Carter, 1977). The highest rates were noted in tumours of the tonsil, nasopharynx and sinuses, while the longest durations of response (four to six months) were seen in tonsillar, palatal and nasopharyngeal lesions (*Table 22.1*). The optimum dose of bleomycin in this compiled study was considered to be 0.25–0.50 units/kg administered weekly or twice weekly by either intravenous or intramuscular routes.

Cisplatin is the newest single agent to demonstrate definite activity in head and neck cancer (Carter and Livingston, 1982; Million, Cassissi and Wittes, 1985). Its major toxicities are nausea and vomiting, dose-related renal damage and ototoxicity. These side-effects can be reduced by appropriate antiemetics, prehydration and diuresis. Cisplatin is effective when administered intravenously over 30–60 minutes or as a 24-hour infusion. A recent randomized study (Veronesi *et al.*, 1985), confirming earlier reports, found no evidence of drug–dose dependency, which would suggest that patients may be spared the toxicity of high dose cisplatin without a consequential undermining of their chances of benefiting from treatment.

Data on the remaining standard antitumour drugs are far less extensive (*see Table 22.2*) with some activity indicated with cyclophosphamide, doxorubicin (Adriamycin), vinblastine, dibromodulcitol (Mitolactol) and the newer agent methylglyoxal bisguanylhydrazone (methyl-GAG). For most drugs tested, only small numbers of patients were evaluated and response rates of less than 20% reported.

It must be emphasized that nearly all these studies were carried out on patients with recurrent and previously treated disease. Although respectable response rates have been achieved in a significant number of patients treated with

Table 22.1 Advanced squamous cell carcinomata of the head and neck: responses to single agent methotrexate or bleomycin as a function of tumour site

Tumour site of origin	Methotrexate			Bleomycin		
	Number of patients evaluated	Response* rate (%)	Median response duration (months)	Number of patients evaluated	Response† rate (%)	Median response duration (months)
Palate	6	67	2.0	34	32	5.6
Oropharynx	5	60	2.0	32	28	1.9
Alveolar ridge	9	56	2.8	–	–	–
Tonsil	10	50	4.5	42	52	4.2
Mouth	–	–	–	12	33	1.8
Tongue	16	50	3.5	73	26	1.8
Floor of mouth	10	50	2.0	–	–	–
Larynx	9	44	2.5	–	–	–
Nasopharynx	4	25	–	15	53	4.0
Hypopharynx	17	18	2.3	–	–	–
Sinuses	–	–	–	22	59	1.9
Gingiva	–	–	–	24	38	1.9
Epiglottis	–	–	–	16	50	2.5

* Definition of response not stated.
† Response defined as 25% or greater reduction in tumour size.
Adapted from Bertino, Boston and Capizzi (1975) and Carter (1977).

Table 22.2 Activity of systemically administered single agents in head and neck cancer

Drug	Antitumour activity*	Number of evaluated patients	Response† (%)
Methotrexate	++	630	47
Bleomycin	++	298	21
Cisplatin	++	255	24
Cyclophosphamide	+	77	36
Doxorubicin	+	112	28
Dibromodulcitol	+	50	22
Vinblastine	+	35	29
Methyl-GAG‡	+	72	21
5-Fluorouracil	+	118	15
Methyl-CCNU‡	+	40	15
Chlorambucil	+	34	15
Hexamethylmelamine	+	75	12
6-Mercaptopurine	+	45	12
Vindesine	−	40	10
Procarbazine	−	31	10
Nitrogen mustard	−	66	8
CCNU‡	−	50	8
VP-16-213‡	−	40	8
PALA‡	−	50	6
DTIC‡	−	24	5
Mitoxantrone	−	35	3
Aclacinomycin A	−	31	3

* ++, adequate evaluation, drug definitely active; +, inadequate evaluation, some evidence of drug activity; −, adequate evaluation, drug inactive.
† Response, 50% or greater shrinkage of all measurable lesions.
‡ Methyl-GAG = methylglyoxal bisguanylhydrazone; CCNU = 1-(2-chloroethyl)-3-cyclohexyl-1-nitrosourea; VP-16-213 = etoposide; PALA = *N*-(phosphonacetyl)-L-aspartate; DTIC = dacarbazine.
After Bonadonna *et al.*, 1975; Wasserman *et al.*, 1975; Aapro and Alberts, 1984; Mattox *et al.*, 1984; Taylor, 1984; Eckenrode, Wheeler and Forastiere, 1985; Grunberg *et al.*, 1985; Million, Cassisi and Wittes, 1985.

methotrexate, bleomycin or cisplatin, the median durations of response have been of the order of three to six months only (*see*, for example, *Table 22.1*). In the few reported randomized studies comparing these three agents, no major differences in response or survival rate have been noted, although methotrexate was much better tolerated than cisplatin, and the lack of myelosuppression associated with bleomycin was considered particularly beneficial. In an attempt to improve the results, combinations of drugs were tested next in advanced disease.

Drug combinations

Many different drug combinations have been tried in advanced head and neck cancer (*see Table 22.3* for some examples), based mainly on the following agents: methotrexate, 5-fluorouracil, cisplatin, bleomycin and vincristine. Reported response rates range from 14% to 73%, thereby providing an indication of increased overall response rates with combination chemotherapy as opposed to single agents. However, durations of response remain short, that is about six months. Furthermore, in the few reported randomized studies comparing single agents with combinations of drugs, no significant differences were reported in response or survival rates, and in certain cases the drug combinations were associated with increased toxicities (*see*, for example, Vogl *et al.*, 1985; Williams *et al.*, 1986).

The conclusion to be drawn from these studies, using the traditional approach in managing

Table 22.3 Combination chemotherapy for advanced disease

Drug combination*	Number of evaluated patients	Response (%)	Duration of response (months)
MTX + 5FU	67	54	3.6–5.5
5FU + MTX	39	62	5.5
CDDP + MTX	39	33	4.4
CDDP + ADR	19	53	2.7
CDDP + BLM	16	13	12
CDDP + BLM	14	21	3
CDDP + VCR + BLM	94	33	4
CDDP + MTX + BLM	25	52	11
BLM + VCR + MTX	20	25	6
CDDP + ADR + CYC	18	44	Not stated
CDDP + VCR + MTX + BLM	63	67	4
CDDP + MTX + BLM + HU	23	48	4
BLM + VCR + MTX + 5FU + CYC + levamisole + PRED	30	73	3–9
ADR + CYC + MMC + VCR + BLM + MTX + 5FU	51	33	5.5

* ADR = doxorubicin (Adriamycin); BLM = bleomycin; CDDP = cisplatin; CYC = cyclophosphamide; 5FU = 5-fluorouracil; HU = hydroxyurea; MMC = mitomycin C; MTX = methotrexate; PRED = prednisone; VCR = vincristine.
Adapted from Taylor (1984).

advanced tumours of the head and neck, is that, in spite of an occasional dramatic response rate being achieved with specific antitumour drugs, there has been considerable morbidity and no significant increase in the survival rate. The next step forward has involved a more logical approach to the use of chemotherapy, based on certain principles derived from experimental and theoretical studies.

A logical scientific approach to optimal adjuvant combination chemotherapy

Although the search for new agents or combinations of agents continues, it is the more logical use of drugs already available which offers the best prospect for increasing survival times, and even cure rates. This approach is based on certain recent advances in tumour biology, results from experimental animal studies and theoretical concepts of drug resistance.

Experimental studies with clinical relevance

Rationale for the combined modality approach

In many experimental animal tumours and certain human tumours, where accurate measurements have been possible, there is a constant relationship between the increase in tumour cell number and time period, and these cells are said to grow exponentially. Exponential growth is especially characteristic of the early period of tumour development, but as the tumour mass increases, the growth rate tends to slow. *Figure 22.2* provides a diagrammatic representation of the correlation

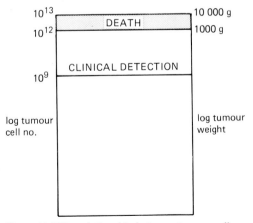

Figure 22.2 The relationship between tumour cell number, tumour weight, clinical detection and the death of the patient. (Reproduced from Hill and Price, 1977, with the kind permission of William Heinemann Medical Books Ltd)

between tumour cell number and tumour weight, the ability to detect the tumour clinically and the death of the patient. Present methods of investigation in man are unable to detect tumours until about 1 g of tumour is present, consisting of approximately 10^9 cells. As the patient is likely to die when the total tumour burden reaches between 10^{12} and 10^{13} cells (that is 1–10 kg tumour weight), it follows that, by the time the tumour can be detected, it is already at least two-thirds of the way through its lifespan. By definition, most tumours are late or advanced at the time of presentation. The same theoretical point applies to the detection of secondary deposits of all tumour cells not removed or destroyed by local therapy. This, therefore, provides an explanation of why even the best techniques of surgery and/or radiotherapy have been unable to cure many advanced head and neck cancers, as undetectable malignant cells will have been left behind. It follows, therefore, that any attempt to increase the cure rate must include a systemic form of treatment, namely antitumour drugs, as part of the initial combined attack on the tumour.

Rationale for optimal adjuvant chemotherapy

Experimental animal studies as early as the mid-1950s provided evidence in favour of combining local therapy with chemotherapy (Shapiro and Fugmann, 1957). Subsequent studies in the 1960s by Skipper, Schabel and Wilcox (1965) emphasized that this combined approach was more effective against smaller tumours than against larger ones (*see Figure 22.3a*), and that superior results were produced with 'full-doses' of drugs (*see Figure 22.3b*). To summarize, these studies showed that chemotherapy was optimal when full-dose intensive drug combinations were used to treat unrecognized regional or metastatic disease before the latter became clinically evident. This use of chemotherapy has been termed 'adjuvant chemotherapy' and, in this chapter, the term is used to describe the administration of antitumour drugs before, during or immediately after local treatment by surgery and/or radiotherapy. These experimental studies also showed that suboptimal adjuvant chemotherapy, like any other kind of inadequate treatment, produced inadequate results.

More recently, Goldie, Coldman and Bruchovsky (1983) have described a mathematical model relating the probability of curing a tumour with drugs to the length of time that the tumour has been present. This concept is illustrated in *Figure 22.4*. Essentially, the model proposes that as tumour cells multiply there is an increased likelihood of cells with drug-resistant phenotypes emerging by chance. The probability of cure is

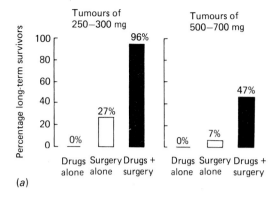

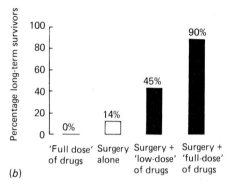

Figure 22.3 Effects of combining chemotherapy and surgery in the treatment of animal tumours: (*a*) advantages of using combined treatments when tumours are small; (*b*) advantages of using full-dose intensive adjuvant chemotherapy. (Reproduced from Hill and Price, 1984, with the kind permission of Pharmacy International, Elsevier Science Publishers)

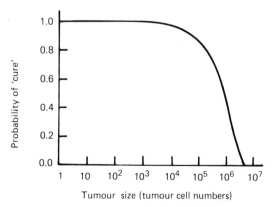

Figure 22.4 The relationship between the probability of 'cure' (zero drug-resistant cells) and the size of the tumour. (Adapted from Goldie, Coldman and Bruchovsky, 1983, with the kind permission of Alan R. Liss, Inc.)

high early in the lifetime of the tumour, but as the tumour increases in size the number of drug-resistant mutants also increases and, consequently, the probability of cure falls sharply, ultimately reaching zero. Combination chemotherapy will have the effect of reducing the mutation rate, thereby making treatment more effective. In summary, this work emphasizes that any delay in starting chemotherapy will greatly reduce the likelihood of 'cure'. Adjuvant combination chemotherapy should be started in conjunction with, or should even precede, the local attack on the primary tumour. Furthermore, Goldie and co-workers (Goldie, Coldman and Gudauskas, 1982; Goldie, Coldman and Bruchovsky, 1983) have shown, in an extension of their model, that prolonged therapy with a single agent (or combination of agents), which allows the unimpeded growth of subpopulations resistant to it, will increase the probability of mutants developing which are resistant to all available therapies. Therefore, when a number of drugs are available which cannot be used simultaneously – perhaps, for example, because of toxic side-effects – then the most effective strategy for delaying or preventing the emergence of drug-resistant tumour cells is to administer two equally effective combinations alternately and not sequentially. This has led to the testing of 'alternating non-cross-resistant drug combinations'.

These observations have major implications for future adjuvant studies, showing how chemotherapy can be used more logically and more acceptably. Verification of these predictions rests on appropriate clinical studies.

Rationale for administering safe, yet effective, combination chemotherapy

One of the main objections to adjuvant chemotherapy has been that the use of antitumour drugs is associated with extremely toxic side-effects. However, there now exists a proven method of giving intensive chemotherapy much more safely than in the past (reviewed in Price, Hill and Ghilchik, 1981; Price and Hill, 1983, 1985). This major contribution to chemotherapy, in terms of safety and minimal toxicity to normal bone marrow stem cells, has come from the clinical application of certain fundamental experimental concepts of cell cycle kinetics. Stem cells, by definition, have the capacity for unlimited proliferation. It is the stem cell population which is responsible for maintaining the integrity and continued survival of any population (reviewed in Hill, 1978). The object of chemotherapy is to inflict the maximum damage to malignant stem cells while doing minimal damage to normal stem cells.

In the 1960s, a technique was developed which enabled a comparison to be made between the differing effects on the survival of the normal bone marrow stem cells and lymphoma stem cells in tumour-bearing mice, of a 24-hour exposure to various chemotherapeutic agents (Bruce, Meeker and Valeriote, 1966). Results showed that drugs could be divided into two categories: those which, after an initial reduction in survival rate, did not cause increasing damage to normal bone marrow stem cells with increasing dosage (class II); and those where the bone marrow stem cell kill was accelerated with increasing dosage (class III). In both cases, there was maximal selective kill of malignant stem cells (*see Figure 22.5*). This selectivity appeared to be based on the fact that, in untreated mice, most of the normal haematopoietic stem cells were resting, while all the detectable lymphoma stem cells appeared to be cycling. Therefore, short courses (that is over 24 hours) of class II and class III drugs would cause a much greater kill of malignant as opposed to normal stem cells. If the time of drug exposure is prolonged, however, this kinetic difference between normal and malignant stem cells is abolished and increasing damage to the normal bone marrow occurs. These initial studies have now been extended to include other agents (reviewed by Hill, 1978) and form the basis for a kinetic classification of antitumour drugs. *Table 22.4* classifies the drugs used in the treatment of head and neck cancer. Bleomycin and hexamethylmelamine have not been included as data suggest that

Table 22.4 Kinetic classification of antitumour drugs used in the treatment of head and neck cancer

Class II drugs	Class III drugs
Hydroxyurea	Doxorubicin
6-Mercaptopurine	Cisplatin
Methotrexate	Cyclophosphamide
Vinblastine	Dibromodulcitol
Vincristine	5-Fluorouracil
	Methyl-CCNU*
	Methyl-GAG*
	Mitomycin C

* Methyl-GAG = methylglyoxal bisguanylhydrazone; CCNU = 1-(2-chloroethyl)-3-cyclohexyl-1-nitrosourea.

they have little effect on normal bone marrow stem cells.

The experimental findings from this model system show that the following principles should be applied in the chemotherapy of head and neck cancer.

(1) Chemotherapy should be given over periods of 24–36 hours in intermittent courses (at approximately 2–3 week intervals) as this approach would markedly reduce toxicity and lead to safer chemotherapy.
(2) A knowledge of the kinetic classification of antitumour agents is essential if chemotherapy is to be safely administered. The toxicity of class II agents to normal stem cells (for example bone marrow) is not dose dependent.

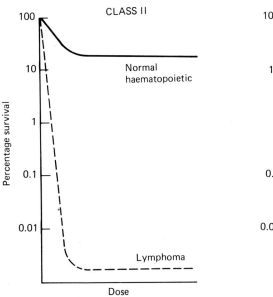

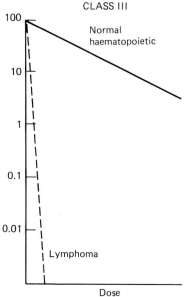

Figure 22.5 The basis of a kinetic classification of antitumour drugs. Dose survival curves for both normal haematopoietic and lymphoma colony-forming units. (After Bruce, Meeker and Valeriote, 1966)

Class II drugs may, therefore, be added to combinations without necessitating a reduction in their dose, provided that the total treatment does not exceed 24–36 hours. Combinations of class III drugs will be additively toxic to normal bone marrow and doses should, therefore, be reduced proportionately.

(3) The practice of giving small daily doses of drugs from either class should be avoided, as under these conditions normal bone marrow stem cells will be drawn into the cycle and killed. This approach would increase the toxicity to normal bone marrow and may reduce the number of malignant cells that are killed because the treatment has to be postponed or interrupted.

Clinical implications of these theoretical concepts

The theoretical points outlined previously show that chemotherapy can be given much more safely than in the past and also that it should be given early in the disease, that is either before, in conjunction with, or as soon as possible after, local treatments. The traditional use of drug therapy in head and neck cancer should be reviewed and replaced by the logical approach shown in *Figure 22.6*. In this way, the safe integration of chemotherapy into a combined attack with surgery and radiotherapy can be achieved in head and neck cancer.

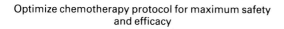

Identify potentially effective drugs from available clinical and/or experimental data

↓

Optimize chemotherapy protocol for maximum safety and efficacy

↓

Integrate optimal chemotherapy protocol with surgery and/or radiotherapy. Use as a primary treatment of 'bad-risk' local and regional disease
Evaluate in large, randomized, prospective controlled clinical trials

Figure 22.6 A suggested approach towards the integration of chemotherapy with surgery and/or radiotherapy in a multidisciplinary attack on head and neck cancers

Clinical results using this scientific approach

The aforementioned principles have direct clinical application, whether head and neck cancer is treated with single agents or with drug combina-

tions. For example, it is possible to give methotrexate in very high doses with increased therapeutic effect provided that certain precautions are rigorously observed. A safe approach is to infuse the drug in 1–2 litres of normal saline over periods of 12–30 hours in doses of 100–20 000 mg, followed by a folinic acid 'rescue' (Goldie, Price and Harrap, 1972). It is essential to maintain a good diuresis during the infusion and to extend the folinic acid rescue appropriately in patients with impaired renal function, as judged by low creatinine clearance (Price and Hill, 1977). Similarly, up to 40 g of hydroxyurea, a class II agent, can be given over 24 hours (Hill and Price, 1982).

The greatest step forward, however, in terms of the response rate, has been the use of the foregoing concepts in designing combination chemotherapy protocols which are not only safer but also more effective than previous multiple drug treatments given over several days. In 1975, the use of a seven-drug kinetically designed combination produced not only an 80% response rate in advanced squamous cell carcinoma (T3 and T4 lesions in the TNM classsification), but also caused no significant myelosuppression (Price *et al.*, 1975). Forty per cent of the patients in this study survived for at least one year, even though they were all considered 'terminal' when treatment was started.

Therefore, contrary to widespread belief, even among 'experts', intensive chemotherapy can be given with safety, provided that the standard medical precautions, listed in *Table 22.5*, are

Table 22.5 Precautions to be observed in all cases receiving chemotherapy

(1) Never give another treatment unless the peripheral blood count has returned to its original level
(2) Patients with impaired renal function receiving methotrexate must have an extended folinic acid 'rescue', that is at least 3 hours longer than normal
(3) Doses of cyclophosphamide, doxorubicin (Adriamycin) and 5-fluorouracil should be halved in patients who have had thoracic, abdominal or pelvic irradiation
(4) Doses of class III agents should be reduced proportionately if more than one of them is included in a combination
(5) Doxorubicin should not be given to patients with a history of cardiac failure. The total dose of doxorubicin must never exceed 550 mg/m². The dose of doxorubicin should be halved in patients who have impaired hepatic function
(6) Patients receiving drugs which are excreted in the urine, for example methotrexate, cisplatin and hydroxyurea, must be adequately hydrated and passing urine while they are having the drug
(7) Bleomycin should not be given to any patients with impaired respiratory function

rigorously observed. Furthermore, the authors' 24-hour approach has enormous advantages for the patient, and these are as follows: patients spend only one night in hospital every three or four weeks; there is no serious myelosuppression, thus obviating the need for intensive supportive therapies, such as platelet transfusions and anti-septicaemia regimens; the patients spend 90% of their time at home and can plan their lives accordingly; and there is no loss of therapeutic effect. Several other groups (Bezwoda, de Moor and Derman, 1979; Shah *et al.*, 1979; Malaker, Robson and Schipper, 1980; Sergeant and Deutsch, 1981) have now confirmed the efficacy and significant lack of toxicity using either the present authors' original seven-drug protocol or a modified version (schedule A chemotherapy).

It is of major significance, however, that this 24-hour method of administering antitumour drugs has definite implications for optimal adjuvant chemotherapy, as summarized in *Table 22.6*. Indeed, the present authors have now carried out a detailed evaluation of a simplification of the 1975 protocol, using a kinetically sequenced

combination of vincristine, bleomycin, methotrexate, 5-fluorouracil and hydrocortisone (schedule A) given over 24 hours with a folinic acid 'rescue' as initial treatment in advanced head and neck cancer (Price and Hill, 1977, 1982; Hill, Price and MacRae, 1986). Two hundred and eight patients have now been entered into this study. Chemotherapy was administered on days 1 and 14 before 'curative' local therapy. Toxicity was minimal and patient compliance was 100%. Chemotherapy response was assessed in 200 patients on day 28: 132 (66%) had an objective response and 68 (34%) were judged as non-responders. The complete remisison rate following local therapy was significantly greater in chemotherapy responders (78%) than in non-responders (49%), $P < 0.001$. The overall seven-year survival time of this entire patient group was 33%, with median survival figures of 32 months for all patients, 37 months for all chemotherapy responders, and 69 months for all patients achieving a final complete remission. Analysis by tumour site shows that patients with oral cavity or nasopharyngeal tumours responded well to initial chemotherapy ($P < 0.05$ and $P < 0.01$) compared with those with tumours at all other sites (*see Table 22.7*). This high response rate was not, however, necessarily associated with increased survival, for although the median survival time in patients with nasopharyngeal tumours was 64 months, in the case of oral cavity lesions, the median survival time of chemotherapy responders was only 22 months. Furthermore, the longest median survival time was observed in patients with laryngeal tumours, in spite of these patients having had one of the lower response rates to initial chemotherapy. Therefore, in this series, survival figures are markedly influenced by the tumour site, and the response to initial chemotherapy is not *automatically* a favourable prognostic sign.

Table 22.6 Advantages of the 24-hour approach to adjuvant chemotherapy

(1) Full-dose intensive combination chemotherapy can be administered early and safely
(2) Intervals between the courses of chemotherapy can be the minimum consistent with clinical tolerance for the first few cycles, since there is no severe myelosuppression
(3) These chemotherapy protocols can be integrated successfully and safely with surgery or radiotherapy
(4) The 24-hour approach can be used in designing alternating non-cross-resistant combination chemotherapy protocols

Table 22.7 Analysis of response rate to initial schedule A chemotherapy by tumour site and medial survival figures

Tumour site	Response rate to initial schedule A chemotherapy*	Median survival duration (months)		
		All patients	Chemotherapy responders	Patients in final complete remission
Nasopharynx	19/20 (95)	51	64	64
Oropharynx	20/36 (56)	34	41	>84
Oral cavity	36/45 (80)	21	22	30
Hypopharynx	10/21 (48)	11	12	48
Larynx				
Supraglottic	17/31			
Glottic	22/34 } (61)	69	71	>84
Subglottic	2/0			

* Values in parentheses are the percentage.

The authors' results would appear to indicate that initial schedule A chemotherapy may be of significant benefit in prolonging good quality life for patients with tumours at certain specific sites, for example in the larynx and nasopharynx, but not at others. Different chemotherapy protocols may be required for tumours at other sites. On the basis of these data, it is suggested that squamous cell carcinomata of the head and neck should no longer be grouped as if they were a single disease entity, but that randomized, prospective, controlled clinical trials should be carried out using initial chemotherapy protocols to see which particular sites would benefit in terms of increased good quality survival.

Combined modality approaches

Head and neck cancer is a disease in which many various combinations of drugs with surgery and/or radiation outlined in *Figure 22.7* have been considered. The increasing evidence that chemotherapy given after surgery and radiotherapy is poorly tolerated, and is associated particularly with severe local toxicity, has meant that the two most favoured approaches have involved the use of initial induction chemotherapy before local treatment, or the synchronous use of chemotherapy and definitive irradiation, with salvage surgery as appropriate. The alternative strategy, that of using chemotherapy after complete response has been achieved by means of primary local therapy, has not been widely tested, mainly because of associated side-effects. Indeed, Ervin, Clark and Weichselbaum (1985) reported that 50% of patients refused 'adjuvant' chemotherapy under these circumstances on account of the toxicity and disability induced by surgery and/or irradiation. It is significant also that in a large randomized trial, with one arm consisting of one initial course of cisplatin plus bleomycin, followed by eight cycles of cisplatin after local control, exceedingly poor compliance was reported (Jacobs *et al.*, 1984).

Initial induction chemotherapy

There are a number of theoretical advantages to using induction chemotherapy, some of which have already been discussed, and they are summarized in *Table 22.8*. Initial induction chemotherapy has now been widely tested in previously untreated patients with locally advanced stage III and IV head and neck tumours, with reported response rates ranging from 60% to 90%. These results are clearly superior to those achieved in patients who have undergone prior surgery and/or radiotherapy. Several studies have confirmed that, after such induction chemotherapy, it is feasible to proceed to either surgery or radiotherapy, or to both, without any obvious increase in morbidity. The higher complete remission rate noted among responders to chemotherapy in many of these

Table 22.8 Theoretical advantages of using induction chemotherapy

(1) The intact vascular supply to the tumour present before radiation or surgery might allow better vascular access of the drugs to the tumour
(2) The generally better nutritional status and performance status of patients earlier in the course of their disease might permit effective chemotherapy to be given
(3) Chemotherapy response of the previously untreated tumour can be determined and this might serve as a chemosensitive assay *in vivo* which could direct later therapy
(4) Treatment of the tumour with chemotherapy early in the course of the disease might allow eradication of micrometastases prior to the development of drug-resistant clones
(5) Reduction in size of the tumour might allow surgery or radiotherapy that would not previously have been possible
(6) Preoperative shrinkage of the tumour might help the surgeon and/or radiotherapist to reduce the extent of locoregional therapy, thereby decreasing local morbidity and mutilation

Adapted in part from Hong and Bromer (1983) and Grunberg (1985).

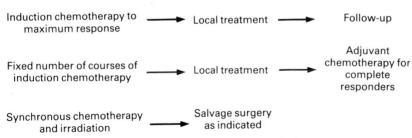

Figure 22.7 The multidisciplinary approach to advanced squamous cell carcinoma of the head and neck. (Adapted from Ervin, Clark and Weichselbaum, 1985)

studies argues in favour of this approach, resulting in increased local control with subsequent surgery or radiotherapy. However, at present, induction chemotherapy should still be considered as additional treatment to *standard* surgery and radiation. Local treatments should not be changed because of tumour reduction following induction chemotherapy. Furthermore, firm evidence that these high initial response rates translate eventually into increased overall survival rates is still not available. It is unfortunate that the great majority of reported induction chemotherapy trials are, in fact, only pilot studies with a small number of patients and a relatively short follow-up. As shown in *Table 22.9*, the authors' results obtained by using schedule A chemotherapy in the largest

reported series with the longest follow-up, compare very favourably with data from other studies. However, these pilot studies, while providing interesting leads, do not justify the use of initial drug treatment as part of everyday practice but rather point to the requirement for large-scale randomized trials.

The necessity for large numbers of patients to be incorporated into such studies is frequently stated and can also be appreciated by considering the many variables which need to be evaluated (*see Table 22.10*). Unfortunately, there have been relatively few reports of the successful setting up of multicentre studies.

The most commonly used preoperative chemotherapy protocols have included cisplatin (*see Table*

Table 22.9 Induction chemotherapy trials for advanced squamous cell carcinomata of the head and neck: response rates and survival data

*Drugs used and reference**	*Number of cycles*	*Number of patients*	*Response to chemotherapy (%)* CR	PR+CR	*Percentage NED after all therapy†*	*Survival data*
CDDP + 5FU						
Kish *et al.*, 1984	2	26	19	88	ns	Median survival = 13 months
Kish *et al.*, 1984	3	85	54	93	ns	Median survival = 18+ months
Amrein and Weitzman, 1985	1–4	31	23	84	ns	At 2 years – 59% alive
CDDP + BLM + VLB						
Perry *et al.*, 1984	3	63	22	65	84	Median survival CR to chemo = 52 months PR to chemo = 12 months At 5 years – 17% NED
BLM + CDDP						
Hong *et al.*, 1984, 1985	1–2	101	14	64	75	Median survival Final CRs = 46 months CR to chemo = 58 months PR to chemo = 26 months
CDDP + BLM + MTX						
Sridhar *et al.*, 1985	1	14	7	93	ns	Median survival = 48 weeks At 2 years – 30% alive
Weichselbaum *et al.*, 1985	2	109	26	78	51	Median survival = 24 months
CDDP + VLB + 5FU						
Spaulding *et al.*, 1986	2	25	4	76	ns	At 24 months follow-up – 36% NED
CDDP + VCR + 5FU						
Spaulding *et al.*, 1986	2	46	23	65	ns	At 41 months follow-up – 41% NED
VCR + BLM + MTX + 5FU						
Hill *et al.*, 1984; Hill, Price and Macrae (1986)	2	208	7	66	69	Median survival Final CRs = 69 months PR to chemo = 37 months At 5 years – 38% NED

* For abbreviations *see* footnote to *Table 22.3*.   CP = complete remission.
† NED = no evidence of disease.   PR = partial remission.
ns = not stated.

22.9). Response rates as high as 80–90% have been reported, in spite of the fact that most of these studies have involved fewer than 100 patients.

Table 22.10 Variables in induction chemotherapy trials

Tumour characteristics
  Site
  Stage
  Differentiation
Patient characteristics
  Age
  Sex
  Nutritional status
  Performance
Drug treatment
  Drugs selected
  Number of induction cycles
  Route of administration
  Dose intensity
Local treatment
  Surgery only
  Radiotherapy only
  Surgery → radiotherapy
  Radiotherapy → surgery
  Criteria for operability
  Surgical technique
  Radiation dose and schedule
Chemotherapy *after* local treatment(s)
  Included or excluded
  Drug(s) selected
  Pre- or postradiotherapy

Adapted from Carter (1985).

Considerable interest has recently been created by the very high complete response rate (approximately 54%) achieved with three courses of initial chemotherapy consisting of cisplatin plus a 5-fluorouracil infusion (Kish *et al.*, 1984). Median survival had not been achieved in this group of patients at 18 months, but the results of long-term follow-up are awaited. It remains to be established whether higher complete response rates achieved by chemotherapy alone produce improved survival figures. The authors' observation that a high response to initial schedule A chemotherapy does not necessarily translate into an increased survival rate, for example in oral cavity lesions, emphasizes the heterogeneity of this group of tumours (Hill, Price and MacRae, 1986). The value of chemotherapy programmes in head and neck cancer should, therefore, be based on significant prolongation of good quality life and not just on achievement of high initial response rates.

Monitoring of good quality survival raises the question of toxicities associated with the administration of initial induction chemotherapy. Many authors consider that the toxicity associated with their protocols is acceptable. However, a survey of some recent presentations (*see Table 22.11*) shows that significant toxicity is frequently associated with cisplatin-containing protocols. Therefore, in evaluating initial chemotherapy programmes, there is a need to justify, in randomized studies, the now almost automatic inclusions of cisplatin, by demonstrating improved survival figures.

Table 22.11 Summary of toxicities from some recent studies using cisplatin-containing drug combinations

Drugs used and reference	Number of patients	Days on treatment per course	Nausea and vomiting (%)	Significant myelotoxicity (%)	Renal toxicity (%)
CDDP + BLM					
*Pennachio *et al.*, 1982	41	9	100	5	20
*Israel *et al.*, 1983	57	5	100	4	0
CDDP + VCR + BLM					
*Spaulding *et al.*, 1982	48	7	100	2	19
Rooney *et al.*, 1985	77	5	71	27	10
CDDP + BLM + MMC					
*Israel *et al.*, 1983	53	5	100	6	0
CDDP + 5FU					
Amrein and Weitzman, 1985	31	5	41	24	28
Kies *et al.*, 1985	40	5	35	13	5
Rooney *et al.*, 1985	26	4	70	27	27
Rooney *et al.*, 1985	61	5	57	41	43
CDDP + BLM + VCR					
Sridhar *et al.*, 1985	14	12	100	14	14
Weichselbaum *et al.*, 1985	114	22	46	20	21
VCR + BLM + MTX + 5FU					
Hill *et al.*, 1984	208	2	9	2	0

* Reference cited in Hill *et al.* (1984).
For abbreviations of drugs *see* footnote to *Table 22.3*.

Objective evidence of the effects of this combined modality approach on overall survival awaits definitive results from large, randomized, prospective, controlled clinical studies. Although preliminary results from a few of these randomized studies are not very encouraging, they do show that single-agent methotrexate or a single course of an initial cisplatin and bleomycin combination are inadequate (Jacobs *et al.*, 1984; Taylor *et al.*, 1985). Therfore, the impact of *optimal* initial chemotherapy in these tumours remains to be established.

Synchronous chemotherapy and radiation therapy

An extensive literature on the combination of irradiation with chemotherapy, dating back many years, is available. In the past, the most commonly used drugs were methotrexate, 5-fluorouracil and hydroxyurea and, in a review of these studies, Goldsmith and Carter (1975) reported somewhat contradictory, but essentially negative, results. These studies were designed to test the hypothesis that such antitumour drugs were acting as

Table 22.12 Synchronous chemotherapy and radiotherapy for advanced squamous cell carcinoma of the head and neck

Drugs	Radiotherapy schedule	Number of patients	Complete response rate (%)	Comment	Reference
VCR + BLM + MTX	60–66 Gy total (2 Gy × 5/week)	198	83	Overall survival rate at 60 months of 41% 5-year DFS of 52% Increased DFS versus historical control 7.5% toxic deaths	O'Connor *et al.*, 1982
	60 Gy total (2 Gy × 5/week)	33	34	Overall survival rate at 30 months of 31% 3% toxic deaths Moderate haemotological and gastrointestinal toxicity	Rosso *et al.*, 1984
MTX + BLM + CDDP	20 Gy/10 fractions	20	74	Overall survival rate at 40 months of 45% Median survival of 17 months 17% toxic deaths	Pearlman *et al.*, 1985
CDDP + 5FU	30 Gy/15 fractions	20	90	Median DFS exceeds 9 months (range 4–22) Significant toxicity	Adelstein *et al.*, 1985*
	10 Gy/week × 4–7	33	59	2-year DFS of 56% Significant toxicity – 4 deaths	Murphy *et al.*, 1985*
CDDP	65 Gy total (10 Gy/week)	22	45	Median survival of 18 months Increased DFS versus historical control	Miller *et al.*, 1985*
	45–50 Gy total (9–10 Gy/week)	34	53	Median survival of 13 months Significant toxicity – no deaths	Bloom *et al.*, 1985*
5-FU 120-h infusion	50 Gy total (10 Gy/week)	18	75	2-year DFS of 50% Mucositis only significant toxicity	Byfield *et al.*, 1984*
MMC + 5FU	50 Gy total (2 Gy/treatment)	42	64	Toxic complications in only 5% No survival data yet	Kaplan *et al.*, 1985

For abbreviations of drugs *see* footnote to *Table 22.3*.
* Reference cited in Ervin, Clark and Weichselbaum, 1985.
DFS = disease-free survival.

radiation sensitizers which would improve both the extent and duration of local control. However, patients demonstrated a poor tolerance of these therapies on account of moderate to severe local toxicities that frequently necessitated the interruption of planned radiation treatment. More recently, the concurrent use of drugs, such as bleomycin, 5-fluorouracil and cisplatin, with irradiation has received renewed attention. Evidence from studies *in vitro* has also indicated that these drugs can potentiate the killing effects of ionizing radiation. Recent studies of synchronous irradiation and chemotherapy are summarized in *Table 22.12*. By altering the irradiation schedules to include occasional breaks in treatment, and by using chemotherapy on as many radiation treatment days as possible, it would appear that the local toxicities (mucositis, skin reaction, radionecrosis) can be more readily controlled (Ervin, Clark and Weichselbaum, 1985). Therefore, encouraging data from some of these small pilot studies have provided the impetus for larger prospective studies. The Northern California Oncology Group is currently performing a prospective study comparing 7000 cGy alone to 7000 cGy plus bleomycin in patients with stage III and stage IV disease who are deemed to be inoperable (Carter, 1985). The code has not been broken, but one arm seems to be superior. In addition, the Eastern Cooperative Oncology Group has begun a randomized trial of radiation alone against cisplatin with radiation (Taylor, 1984).

It would appear that chemotherapy combined synchronously with radiation, in schedules that allow for intermittent repair of sublethal injury to normal tissues, represents another avenue in the treatment of head and neck tumours which needs to be more thoroughly explored.

Current trends and prospects

The 1980s should be the decade in which head and neck cancer is added to the list of curable tumours. This is most likely to be achieved when there is full cooperation between surgeons, radiotherapists and medical oncologists.

There is ample evidence that head and neck tumours respond to currently available antitumour drugs and that the highest response rates are obtained using chemotherapy 'up-front'. The need remains to find effective salvage regimens for recurrent disease. However, the main focus of attention must be on obtaining improved good quality survival figures in previously untreated patients. As these studies must involve large numbers of patients, it is essential that multicentre trials are organized and encouraged. It could then be established whether:

(1) it is necessary to include cisplatin, with its associated toxic side-effects, in initial combination chemotherapy or whether comparable results can be achieved using combinations of other drugs
(2) certain chemotherapy protocols are particularly beneficial for tumours at specific sites within the head and neck region
(3) increased complete response rates to initial chemotherapy improve survival
(4) the use of initial chemotherapy and radiotherapy or synchronous drugs and radiation can replace surgical intervention and minimize mutilation for tumours at certain sites
(5) the identification of a safe and effective chemotherapy protocol and its use after initial chemotherapy and the completion of local therapy will improve overall survival figures.

In this way, the initial benefits of chemotherapy in head and neck cancer can be fully realized and lead to the successful achievement of an increased cure rate in the near future.

References

AAPRO, M. S. and ALBERTS, D. S. (1984) Phase II trial of mitoxantrone in head and neck cancer. *Investigational New Drugs*, **2**, 329–330

AMREIN, P. C. and WEITZMAN, S. A. (1985) Treatment of squamous-cell carcinoma of the head and neck with cisplatin and 5-fluorouracil. *Journal of Clinical Oncology*, **3**, 1632–1639

BERTINO, J. R., BOSTON, B. and CAPIZZI, R. L. (1975) The role of chemotherapy in the management of cancer of the head and neck: a review. *Cancer*, **36**, 752–757

BEZWODA, W. R., DE MOOR, N. G. and DERMAN, D. P. (1979) Treatment of advanced head and neck cancer by means of radiation therapy plus chemotherapy – a randomised trial. *Medical and Paediatric Oncology*, **6**, 353–358

BONADONNA, G., BERETTA, G., TANCIN, G., BRAMBILLA, C., BAJETTA, E., De PALO, G. M. *et al.* (1975) Adriamycin (NSC-123-127) studies at the Istituto Nazionale Tumori, Milan. *Cancer Chemotherapy Reports*, Part 3, **6**, 231–245

BRUCE, W. R., MEEKER, B. E. and VALERIOTE, F. A. (1966) Comparison of the sensitivity of normal hematopoietic and transplanted lymphoma colony-forming cells to chemotherapeutic agents administered *in vivo*. *Journal of the National Cancer Institute*, **37**, 233–245

CARTER, S. K. (1977) The chemotherapy of head and neck cancer. *Seminars in Oncology*, **4**, 413–424

CARTER, S. K. (1985) Combined modality chemotherapy in head and neck cancer. In *Head and Neck Cancer*. Proceedings of the International Conference, Baltimore, Maryland, July, 1984. Edited by P. B. Chretien, M. E. Johns, D. P. Shedd, E. W. Strong and P. H. Ward, Vol. 1, pp. 60–68. Philadelphia: B. C. Decker

CARTER, S. K. and LIVINGSTON, R. B. (1982) The chemotherapy of head and neck cancer. In *Principles of Cancer Treatment*, edited by S. K. Carter, E. Glatstein and R. B. Livingston, pp. 644–651. New York: McGraw-Hill

CARTER, S. K. and SOPER, W. T. (1974) Integration of chemotherapy into combined modality treatment of solid tumours. *Cancer Treatment Reviews*, **1**, 1–13

ECKENRODE, J. L., WHEELER, R. H. and FORASTIERE, A. A. (1985) A phase II trial of aclacinomycin-A in advanced squamous cell carcinoma of the head and neck. *Investigational New Drugs*, **3**, 389–392

ERVIN, T. J., CLARK, J. R. and WEICHSELBAUM, R. R. (1985) Multidisciplinary treatment of advanced squamous carcinoma of the head and neck. *Seminars in Oncology*, **12** (Suppl. 6), 71–78

GOLDIE, J. H., COLDMAN, A. J. and BRUCHOVSKY, N. (1983) A quantitative model for drug resistance in cancer chemotherapy. In *Rational Basis for Chemotherapy*, edited by B. A. Chabner, pp. 23–39. New York: Alan R. Liss

GOLDIE, J. H., COLDMAN, A. J. and GUDAUSKAS, G. A. (1982) A rationale for the use of alternating non-cross resistant chemotherapy. *Cancer Treatment Reports*, **66**, 439–449

GOLDIE, J. H., PRICE, L. A. and HARRAP, K. R. (1972) Methotrexate toxicity: correlation with duration of administration, plasma levels, dose and excretion pattern. *European Journal of Cancer*, **8**, 409–414

GOLDSMITH, M. A. and CARTER, S. K. (1975) The integration of chemotherapy into a combined modality approach to cancer chemotherapy. V. Squamous cell cancer of the head and neck. *Cancer Treatment Reviews*, **2**, 137–158

GRUNBERG, S. M. (1985) Future directions in the chemotherapy of head and neck cancer. *American Journal of Clinical Oncology*, **8**, 51–54

GRUNBERG, S. M., FELMAN, I. E., GALA, K. V., JOHNSON, K. B. and OWENS, J. C. (1985) Phase II study of etoposide (VP-16) in the treatment of advanced head and neck cancer. *American Journal of Clinical Oncology*, **8**, 393–395

HILL, B. T. (1978) Cancer chemotherapy: the relevance of certain concepts of cell cycle kinetics. *Biochimica Biophysica Acta: Cancer Reviews*, **516**, 389–417

HILL, B. T. and PRICE, L. A. (1977) Concepts and prospects in adjuvant chemotherapy. In *Secondary Spread in Breast Cancer*, edited by B. A. Stoll, pp. 193–212. London: William Heinemann Medical

HILL, B. T. and PRICE, L. A. (1982) An experimental biological basis for increasing the therapeutic index of clinical cancer therapy. *Annals of the New York Academy of Sciences*, **397**, 72–87

HILL, B. T. and PRICE, L. A. (1984) The potential role of chemotherapy in improving survival in some common cancers. *Pharmacy International*, **5**, 268–272

HILL, B. T., PRICE, L. A., BUSBY, E., MacRAE, K. and SHAW, H. J. (1984) Positive impact of initial 24-hour combination chemotherapy without cis-platinum on 6-year survival figures in advanced squamous cell carcinomas of the head and neck. In *Adjuvant Therapy of Cancer IV*, edited by S. E. Jones and S. E. Salmon, pp. 97–106. Orlando: Grune & Stratton

HILL, B. T., PRICE, L. A. and MacRAE, K. (1986) Importance of primary site in assessing chemotherapy response and seven-year survival data in advanced squamous carcinomas of the head and neck treated with initial combination chemotherapy with cisplatin. *Journal of Clinical Oncology*, **4**, 1340–1347

HONG, W. K. and BROMER, R. (1983) Chemotherapy in head and neck cancer. *New England Journal of Medicine*, **308**, 75–79

HONG, W. K., BROMER, R. H., AMATO, D. A., SHAPSHAY, S., VINCENT, M., VAUGHAN, C. et al. (1985) Patterns of relapse in locally advanced head and neck cancer patients who achieved complete remission after combined modality therapy. *Cancer*, **56**, 1242–1245

HONG, W. K., POPKIN, J., STRONG, M. S., BROMER, R., VAUGHAN, C., SHAPSHAY, S. et al. (1984) Adjuvant chemotherapy as initial treatment of advanced head and neck cancer: survival data at three years. In *Adjuvant Therapy of Cancer IV*, edited by S. E. Jones and S. E. Salmon, pp. 127–133. Orlando: Grune & Stratton

JACOBS, C., WOLF, G. T., MAKUCH, R. W. and VIKRAN, B. (1984) Adjuvant chemotherapy for head and neck squamous carcinomas. *Proceedings of the American Society of Clinical Oncology*, **3**, 182

KAPLAN, M. J., HAHN, S. S., JOHNS, M. E., STEWART, F. M., CONSTABLE, W. C. and CANTRELL, R. W. (1985) Mitomycin and fluorouracil with concomitant radiotherapy in head and neck cancer. *Archives of Otolaryngology*, **111**, 220–222

KIES, M. S., GORDON, L. I., HUACK, W. W., KRESPI, Y., OSSOFF, R. H., PECARO, B. C. et al. (1985) Analysis of complete responders after initial treatment with chemotherapy in head and neck cancer. *Otolaryngology, Head and Neck Surgery*, **93**, 199–205

KISH, J. A., ENSLEY, J. F., WEAVER, A., JACOBS, J. R., KINZIE, J., CUMMINGS, G. et al. (1984) Improvement of complete response rate to induction adjuvant chemotherapy for advanced squamous carcinoma of the head and neck. In *Adjuvant Therapy of Cancer IV*, edited by S. E. Jones and S. E. Salmon, pp. 107–115. Orlando: Grune & Stratton

MALAKER, K., ROBSON, F. and SCHIPPER, H. (1980) Combined modalities in the management of advanced head and neck cancers. *Journal of Otolaryngology*, **9**, 24–30

MATTOX, D. E., CLARK, G. M. BALCERZAK, S. P., O'BRYAN, R. M., OISHI, N. and STUCKEY, W. J. (1984) Southwest oncology study of mitoxantrone for treatment of patients with advanced squamous cell carcinoma of the head and neck. *Investigational New Drugs*, **2**, 405–407

MILLION, R. R., CASSISI, N. J. and WITTES, R. E. (1985) Cancer of the head and neck. In *Cancer Principles and Practice of Oncology*, edited by V. T. DeVita, S. Hellman and S. A. Rosenburg, pp. 407–506. Philadelphia: S. B. Lippincott

O'CONNOR, D., CLIFFORD, P., EDWARDS, W. G., DALLEY, V. M., DURDEN-SMITH, J., HOLLIS, B. A. et al. (1982) Long-term results of VBM and radiotherapy in advanced head and neck cancer. *International Journal of Radiation Oncology, Biology and Physics*, **8**, 1525–1531

PEARLMAN, N. W., JOHNSON, F. B., BRAUN, R. J., KENNAUGH, R. C., SPOFFORD, B. F., BORLASE, B. C. et al. (1985) A prospective study of preoperative chemotherapy and split-course irradiation for locally advanced or recurrent oral/pharyngeal squamous carcinoma. *American Journal of Clinical Oncology*, **8**, 490–496

PERRY, D. J., DAVIS, R. K., ZAJTCHUK, J. R. and BAUMANN, J. C. (1984) Vinblastine, bleomycin and cisplatin in the treatment of squamous carcinoma of the head and neck. In *Adjuvant Therapy of Cancer IV*, edited by S. E. Jones and S. E. Salmon, pp. 135–143. Orlando: Grune & Stratton

PRICE, L. A. and HILL, B. T. (1977) A kinetically-based logical approach to the chemotherapy of head and neck cancer. *Clinical Otolaryngology*, **2**, 339–345

PRICE, L. A. and HILL, B. T. (1982) Safe and effective

induction chemotherapy without cisplatin for squamous cell carcinoma of the head and neck: impact on complete response rate and survival at five years following local therapy. *Medical and Pediatric Oncology,* **10,** 535–548

PRICE, L. A. and HILL, B. T. (1983) An experimentally based safe method of administering intensive cancer chemotherapy. *South African Medical Journal,* **64,** 987–993

PRICE, L. A. and HILL, B. T. (1985) Safer cancer chemotherapy using a kinetically based experimental approach. *Mount Sinai Journal of Medicine,* **52,** 452–459

PRICE, L. A., HILL, B. T. and GHILCHIK, M. (1981) *Safer Cancer Chemotherapy,* pp. 1–124. London: Baillière Tindall

PRICE, L. A., HILL, B. T., CALVERT, A. H., SHAW, H. J. and HUGHES, K. B. (1975) Kinetically-based multiple drug treatment for advanced head and neck cancer. *British Medical Journal,* **3,** 10–11

PROBERT, J. C., THOMPSON, R. W. and BAGSHAW, M. A. (1974) Patterns of spread of distant metastases in head and neck cancer. *Cancer,* **33,** 127–133

ROONEY, M., KISH, J., JACOBS, J., KINZIE, J., WEAVER, A., CRISSMAN, J. *et al.* (1985) Improved complete response rate and survival in advanced head and neck cancer after three-course induction therapy with 120-hour 5-FU infusion and cisplatin. *Cancer,* **55,** 1123–1128

ROSSO, R., MERLANO, M., SERTOLI, M. R., CAMPORA, E., SCARPATI, D., BORASI, F. *et al.* (1984) Multidrug chemotherapy (vincristine, bleomycin and methotrexate) with radiotherapy in stage III–IV squamous cell carcinoma of the head and neck. *Cancer Treatment Reports,* **68,** 1019–1021

SERGEANT, R. and DEUTSCH, G. (1981) A preliminary report of the combination of initial chemotherapy and radiotherapy in the treatment of advanced head and neck cancer. *Journal of Laryngology and Otology,* **95,** 64–74

SHAH, J. R., SHAH, P. C., VOHRA, R. M., GIHOSH, B. K., HAZENFIELD, H. N. and PATEL, A. R. (1979) Multiagent chemotherapy in head and neck cancer. In *Proceedings of the Eleventh International Congress of Chemotherapy,* edited by J. D. Nelson and C. Grassi, Volume II, pp. 1652–1654. Washington DC: American Society of Microbiology

SHAPIRO, D. M. and FUGMANN, R. A. (1957) A role for chemotherapy as adjunct to surgery. *Cancer Research,* **17,** 1098–1101

SKIPPER, H. E., SCHABEL, F. M. and WILCOX, W. S. (1965) Experimental evaluation of potential anticancer agents. XIV. Further study of certain basic concepts underlying chemotherapy of leukemia. *Cancer Chemotherapy Reports,* **45,** 5–28

SPAULDING, M., ZIEGLER, P., SUNDQUIST, N., KLOTCH, D., LEE, K., KHAN, A. *et al.* (1986) Induction therapy in head and neck cancer – a comparison of two regimens. *Cancer,* **57,** 1110–1114

SRIDHAR, K. S., OHNUMA, T., BILLER, H., HOLLAND, J. F., AMBINDER, E. P. and BARBA, J. (1985) Combination chemotherapy with high-dose methotrexate, bleomycin and cisplatin in management of head and neck squamous cell carcinoma. *American Journal of Clinical Oncology,* **8,** 55–60

TAYLOR, S. G. (1984) Head and neck cancer. In *Cancer Chemotherapy Annual 6,* edited by H. M. Pinedo and B. A. Chabner, pp. 285–298. Amsterdam: Elsevier

TAYLOR, S. G., APPLEBAUM, E., SHOWEL, J. L., NORUSIS, M., HOLINGER, L. D., HUTCHINSON, J. C. *et al.* (1985) A randomized trial of adjuvant chemotherapy in head and neck cancer. *Journal of Clinical Oncology,* **3,** 672–679

VERONESI, A., ZAGONEL, V., TIRELLI, U., GALLIGIONI, E., TUMULO, S., BARZAN, L. *et al.* (1985) High-dose versus low-dose cisplatin in advanced head and neck squamous carcinoma: a randomized study. *Journal of Clinical Oncology,* **3,** 1105–1108

VOGL, S. E., SCHOENFELD, D. A., KAPLAN, B. H., LERNER, H. J., ENGSTROM, P. F. and HORTON, J. (1985) A randomized prospective comparison of methotrexate with a combination of methotrexate, bleomycin and cisplatin in head and neck cancer. *Cancer,* **56,** 432–442

WASSERMAN, T. H., COMIS, R. L., GOLDSMITH, M., HANDELMAN, H., PENTA, J. S., SLAVIK, M. *et al.* (1975) Tabular analysis of the chemotherapy of solid tumours. *Cancer Chemotherapy Reports,* **6,** 399–419

WEICHSELBAUM, R. R., CLARK, J. R., MILLER, D., POSNER, M. R. and ERVIN, T. J. (1985) Combined modality treatment of head and neck cancer with cisplatin, bleomycin, methotrexate-leucovorin chemotherapy. *Cancer,* **55,** 2149–2155

WILLIAMS, S. D., VELEZ-GARCIA, E., ESSESSEE, I., RATKIN, G., BIRCH, R. and EINHORN, L. H. (1986) Chemotherapy for head and neck cancer – comparison of cisplatin plus vincristine plus bleomycin versus methotrexate. *Cancer,* **57,** 18–23

23

The principles of laser surgery

J. A. S. Carruth

It has been said that when the time in which we live is finally named, it will be known as the 'laser age' rather than the atomic or space age. However, we are still only at the dawning of this age. The first laser was not produced until 1960, but since that time a large number of laser systems have been developed with a vast range of scientific, industrial and military uses. Astronomers have measured, to within centimetres, the distance to the moon; huge numbers of telephone calls can be transmitted by way of flexible glass fibres; and physicists have probed plasmas hotter than the sun. In addition, the role of lasers in the 'star wars' programme is currently being researched with amazing defence possibilities and an equally amazing and horrifying potential for offence.

These diverse uses of the laser (light amplification by stimulated emission of radiation) are nevertheless all dependent on the basic characteristics of the laser beam: an intense beam of pure, monochromatic light which does not diverge and in which all the light waves are of the same length, travel in the same direction and are in phase, rising and falling together. The beam can be focused to a fine point producing very high energy levels.

The development of lasers

The essential physics of stimulated emission, which produces coherent laser light, was developed by Albert Einstein in 1917. Planck had proposed the 'quantum theory' embracing the principle that systems had to be restricted in the energy which they could attain, that is their energy was quantized. As a development of this theory, Einstein proposed the idea of stimulated emission which was new to science. Until that time, only two interactions had been known to exist between matter and light, namely absorption and spontaneous emission. An atom is normally in the low energy ground state, but it may be excited by the absorption of a photon (a quantum of light) if that photon has the correct frequency and concomitant energy to bridge exactly the gap between the two energy levels. Conversely, if an atom has been excited, for example by collision with an electron, it can return to the low energy ground state with the spontaneous emission of a photon.

Einstein proposed that if an atom in the excited state were struck by a photon with the same energy as that which would normally be emitted spontaneously, it would be stimulated to emit an identical photon travelling in the same direction as the original stimulating photon. From this concept, it was possible to imagine that in a population of excited atoms a series of collisions would result in the release, by stimulated emission, of an increasing number of identical photons.

The first device to exploit this phenomenon was the maser (microwave amplification by stimulated emission of radiation) produced in 1955 by Townes and his students at Columbia University. Three years later, Schawlow and Townes (1958) proposed that the principle of the maser could be extended to the infrared and visible areas of the spectrum. In 1960, T. H. Maiman, working at the Hughes Research Laboratory, produced the first laser using a synthetic ruby as the lasing medium, which emitted deep-red light at a wavelength of 694 nm, but at short pulses of less than a millisecond.

At about the same time, the xenon photo-coagulator was introduced into ophthalmology by Meyer-Schwickerath (1956), and early experimental work suggested that the laser was superior to this instrument for the purpose of retinal photocoagulation. However, it soon became apparent that for much clinical work, the pulsed ruby laser was too harsh and uncontrollable, and it was eventually shown (Minton *et al.*, 1965; Ketcham, Hoye and Riggle, 1967) that in the destruction of tumours with the pulsed laser, viable malignant cells were contained in the debris produced explosively by the laser impact, and with the additional significant risk of forcing malignant cells into adjacent, normal tissues.

The helium neon laser was the first continuous wave machine to be developed producing low power red light, and it is still in use both as an aiming beam and in alignment, but is too low powered for therapeutic use, although its role in biostimulation is being investigated.

In 1965, Patel produced the continuous wave carbon dioxide laser which has become the laser most commonly used as a high precision, blood-less, light scalpel and which has unique value in gynaecology and in otolaryngology. Early animal experiments with laboratory bench machines were carried out, and in some studies it was necessary to use moving tables on which to move the anaesthetized animals beneath the fixed, focused laser beam. However, these experiments demonstrated the potential of this laser as a surgical tool and the first clinical CO_2 laser system was developed by the American Optical Corporation in 1969.

At the same time as the CO_2 laser was being investigated, the argon laser was being developed, and this continuous wave device is now widely used for retinal photocoagulation based on the orginal work of Zweng (1971). The pulsed neodymium glass laser was also investigated and rejected by surgeons in the mid-1960s, but in the early 1970s, the continuous wave neodymium-YAG (yttrium aluminium garnet) laser was developed which produces near infrared coherent light. This is used for thermal tissue destruction and blood vessel coagulation. The pulsed Nd-YAG laser has recently been introduced which delivers nanosecond (10^{-9}) pulses of energy into the eye. These produce precisely localized lesions in which the temperature is higher than that of the sun, and shock waves from these are used to destroy opaque structures within the eye, such as the posterior lens capsule after the removal of a cataract. Pulsed lasers are also being investigated for the destruction of renal stones and gallstones by photomechanical effects.

These three lasers – carbon dioxide, argon and Nd-YAG – are the three most commonly used in clinical practice, with the krypton laser being widely used for retinal photocoagulation.

The dye laser is under investigation for use in two main areas: first, the photoactivation of intratumour haematoporphyrin derivative for the treatment of malignant disease by photodynamic therapy and, second, in both pulsed and continuous waveforms, for the selective destruction of blood vessels within the skin in the treatment of the port wine stain and other cutaneous vascular malformations. Pulsed metal vapour lasers are now being evaluated in these areas: copper vapour on the skin and gold vapour in photodynamic therapy.

Within the last few years, the excimer lasers have been developed and these appear to have enormous potential for producing remarkably precise incisions. The name is derived from 'excited dimer' and the lasing medium is made up of molecules comprising two atoms of the same species (XeF or ArF) which are bound in the excited state but repel on decaying to the ground state.

The laser

Production of coherent laser light

The lasing medium is contained within the laser tube which has a fully reflective mirror at one end and a partially reflective mirror at the other, which allows access to the laser beam (*Figure 23.1*).

The lasing medium is pumped or excited electrically, or by a high energy light source, to create a population inversion of atoms in the high laser energy state compared to the low energy laser state, which, in a collection of excited atoms, normally has an excess in the lower state.

The energy of an atom is raised to the high energy laser level and, with the spontaneous emission of a photon, it decays to the low energy laser level and then back to the ground state. For the population inversion to be achieved, the high laser level must have a long lifetime compared to the low level, allowing the high laser level to build up (*Figure 23.2*).

As proposed by Einstein, stimulated emission then occurs as atoms spontaneously emit photons which, on collision with other excited atoms, stimulate these to emit identical photons travelling in the same direction as the original stimulating photons (*Figure 23.3*). The release of these photons is in all directions, but from time to time a photon will be released exactly in the axis of the laser tube and will then be reflected back into the lasing medium from the mirrors, with further collisions causing the release of increasing numbers of identical photons, all travelling in the axis of the

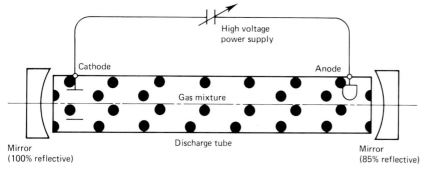

Figure 23.1 Gas laser configuration

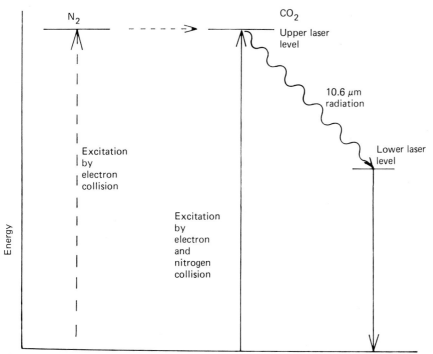

Figure 23.2 Laser energy diagram

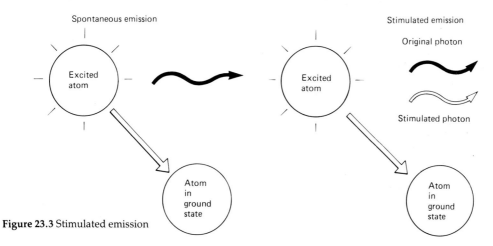

Figure 23.3 Stimulated emission

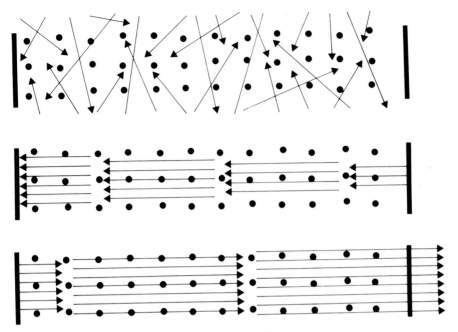

Figure 23.4 Production of the laser beam: the cascade effect

tube. There is a rapid build-up of light energy in the laser tube – the cascade effect (*Figure 23.4*) – and the beam is then emitted through the partially reflective mirror.

Beam characteristics

The laser beam is an intense, collimated (parallel) beam of pure, monochromatic, single wavelength light in which all the light waves are the same length and travel in phase in the same direction. This beam can be focused by a lens or concave mirror into a small spot producing extremely high energy densities.

Beam transmission

The coherent light from visible and low infrared lasers can be transmitted by fine flexible fibres to appropriate delivery devices. However, as yet, no flexible fibre has been found which will transmit efficiently the far infrared CO_2 laser energy, although a number of fibres are currently under investigation and it appears certain that an efficient fine fibre will soon be available. The CO_2 laser tube of some early models was mounted directly on to the operating microscope and the beam was aimed at the target by a concave mirror on the laser/microscope assembly, controlled by a micromanipulator. This made the system both unstable and cumbersome and, in more modern machines, the laser tube is mounted on the console or on the microscope stand and the beam is transmitted to the microscope attachment, hand piece or bronchoscope by way of a self-supporting articulated arm which is hollow, with mirrors at the articulations. The length of the arm and the number of articulations and, therefore, range of movements, vary from machine to machine (*Figure 23.5*).

The argon laser is used with a slit lamp or operating microscope and both incorporate a shutter, which closes when the laser is fired, to protect the eyes of the operator. It may also be used with a hand piece in dermatology or by means of a delivery fibre for endoscopic work. The Nd-YAG laser may also be used with a microscope or slit lamp, with the operator's eyes protected by filters. Filters or goggles will also be used for protection when an endoscopic delivery fibre is used. The design of the tip of the endoscopic fibre appears to be critical. The laser fibre is surrounded by a metal-tipped Teflon sheath, down which compressed air is blown to keep the fibre tip free from debris and secretions. If these touch the tip they will absorb energy causing thermal damage to the fibre which may have to be removed for cleaning and even for recutting during a long treatment session. In addition, the metal tip may become so hot that it causes the Teflon sheath to swell, making it impossible to remove the fibre from the biopsy channel of the endoscope.

shorter working distances may be used and Anderson (1981) described the use of a laser focused at 400 mm, with a microscope lens of 250 mm focal length, to give a wide defocused beam of 2 mm in diameter for work on the cervix.

The laser/microscope attachment incorporates a micromanipulator which moves the final focusing mirror enabling the aiming and working beams to be positioned with great accuracy.

With the bronchoscope, the working beam may be 'fixed' into the centre of the distal opening of the bronchoscope with no aiming beam, or static aiming with thumbscrews may be available. Others have full aiming facilities with a small micromanipulator on the bronchoscope coupler.

Laser beam parameters

Beam power

The power levels vary from laser to laser with milliwatt powers for mid-laser therapy to 100 watts in high-powered CO_2 or Nd-YAG surgical lasers.

Power density

For all medical and surgical laser applications, it is essential to know not only the power but also the power density or irradiance measured as power per unit area.

The laser energy will have a greater effect if it is delivered within a small spot rather than if it is spread over a large area. The power density, recorded in watts or milliwatts per square centimetre, is measured by dividing the power by the area of the imprint.

Energy distribution within the beam

In spite of the parallel laser beam, there may be profound differences in the energy distribution within the beam resulting from differences within the optical cavity, such as the radii of the mirrors and their spacing.

There are, therefore, a number of different transverse electromagnetic modes (TEM). The commonest is the fundamental or TEM_{00} mode in which the distribution is circular but the power level does not have a sharp cut-off, and the spot size is measured between points at which the power has fallen to 14% of the central level. This means that in this mode there will be effects on the tissue outside the boundaries of the quoted spot size. With TEM_{01} the power distribution is doughnut shaped, and with other modes the energy may be distributed in a number of points with the TEM number indicating the number of nodes or points of zero energy.

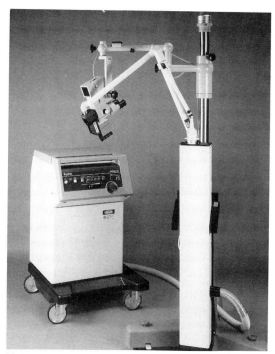

Figure 23.5 Carbon dioxide surgical laser mounted on operating microscope

The CO_2 laser is used with the microscope when the operator's eyes are protected by the optics of the microscope, or with the hand piece when the laser is used as a light scalpel. There are a number of different types of hand piece and it must be said that some are far too bulky and clumsy for precise work, particularly in the oral cavity. A rigid bronchoscope may be coupled to the articulated arm, and there are considerable differences in the design of the couplers with particular reference to the beam aiming facilities.

Beam aiming

Before the 'working' laser beam is activated, it must be aimed accurately at the target. With lasers operating in the visible wavelengths, an attenuated beam is used to define the beam path and target area; but with the invisible near and far infrared lasers, a coaxial low-powered visible helium neon laser is used for aiming. With the CO_2 laser, a concave mirror may be used to focus the beam, but some use a zinc selenide lens as this is a substance which will transmit both the infrared and red wavelengths.

When used with the operating microscope for laryngology, the focal point of the beam is adjusted to the focal length of the lens, which for most microlaryngeal surgery is 400 mm. However,

Total energy delivered

This is measured in joules (watts/seconds) per unit area and is measured by the power, exposure time and spot size.

Laser/tissue interaction

The qualitative nature of the laser/tissue interaction is wavelength dependent, as this determines the pattern of absorption of the laser beam by the tissues and its effects on them. The quantitative extent of the interaction will depend on the intensity of the irradiation, the total energy delivered and the rate of delivery of the energy.

Biostimulation

In a paper summarizing the work of Mester and his colleagues in Hungary in the 1960s, published after his death by his sons (Mester, Mester and Mester, 1985), it has been stated that very low levels of laser energy are biostimulative and at higher levels become inhibitory, ultimately having a thermal effect on tissues.

Mid-laser therapy has developed on the basis of this work and is used for improving wound healing and for pain relief in sports injuries and in 'rheumatological' conditions. Much of the early work was uncontrolled and anecdotal and could not be repeated in other centres. It is indeed difficult to define a mid-laser, as in this field the essentially low-powered, red helium neon and infrared gallium arsenide lasers and therapeutic CO_2, argon and Nd-YAG lasers at very low subtherapeutic power levels have been used. However, some controlled studies have recently been reported which do show some value in these lasers for the purpose of pain relief and in the promotion of wound healing. Dyson and Young (1986) have shown that both wound contracture and cellularity are affected by mid-laser treatment. Further results from carefully constructed studies must be awaited with interest.

Thermal effects

When tissues absorb laser energy, the temperature rises. No changes in tissue structure are evident between 37 and 60 °C, but above that temperature tissues begin to coagulate. The protein in the collagen fibres denatures owing to a randomization of the protein chains, and this results in contraction. This contraction of collagen in both the blood vessel wall and in perivascular tissues accounts for the haemostatic properties of laser energy.

When the temperature of soft tissues is raised to 100 °C, intracellular water is boiled and this conversion into steam with a thousand-fold expansion results in almost instantaneous vaporization. Once the water has been removed from tissues in this way, residual cellular debris is burnt at a temperature of 400–500 °C, but as there is poor thermal contact between this debris and residual tissues, this burning should not cause any significant damage to normal tissues adjacent to the laser wound.

Non-thermal effects

The non-thermal effects may be photomechanical or photochemical. An example of the mechanical effects is the use of the pulsed Nd-YAG laser for destruction of opaque bodies within the eye. Nanosecond (10^{-9}) pulses create minute balls of plasma in which the temperature is higher than that of the sun, and shock waves from these are used to destroy the lesions. This laser, using longer pulses, is being investigated for the photomechanical destruction of renal stones and gallstones.

A direct interaction between laser photons and molecules is responsible for photochemical effects in, for example, the photoactivation of haematoporphyrin derivative within a malignant tumour for photodynamic therapy, and in the ultraviolet laser tissue interaction with excimer lasers in the reshaping of the cornea or in the removal of atheroma from arteries.

Surgical lasers

The name of each laser is taken from the lasing medium, which also determines the wavelength of coherent light produced by that laser. The wavelength determines the absorption of the laser beam by body tissues and this defines the clinical role of the laser. As each laser produces essentially one wavelength of coherent light, it has one main clincial role, and to change role, one must change laser. There is, however, considerable overlap in the roles of the three lasers most commonly used in clinical practice, as can be seen in *Table 23.1*.

Table 23.1 The most commonly used roles for lasers

Laser	Tisue destruction	Vessel coagulation
Carbon dioxide	+ +	±
Argon	±	+ +
Neodymium-YAG	+	+

The CO_2 laser is used as a high precision, bloodless, light scalpel with an ability to seal blood vessels of up to 0.5 mm in diameter. The role of the argon laser is in blood vessel coagulation and, at higher power levels, slow and relatively imprecise thermal tissue destruction can be performed. The Nd-YAG laser is used for slow, imprecise, but adequate tissue destruction, with better haemostasis than is possible with the CO_2 laser.

The carbon dioxide laser

The carbon dioxide (CO_2) laser produces continuous wave, far infrared, coherent light at a wavelength of 10 600 nm which is absorbed by water and, therefore, by body soft tissues which contain 70–90% water. Intracellular water absorbs the energy and is boiled, causing a thousand-fold increase in volume and sudden, almost instantaneous, cell vaporization, which releases the cell contents into the beam where they are carbonized and fall as carbon soot around the laser wound.

It has been shown in several studies that there are no viable cells or cell components in the debris released by cell vaporization. Mihashi *et al.* (1976) studied the debris following vaporization of the tongues of dogs and found that, although some epithelial cells were recognizable, they had lost their 'functional vitality'. Oosterhuis *et al.* (1982) vaporized Cloudman mouse melanomata and found no viable tumour cells on culture *in vitro* or on intramuscular or intraperitoneal implantation *in vivo*, whereas controls of cells mixed with debris and smoke remained viable.

There is no shock impact when the beam strikes the tissues and, therefore, no tendency to force cells into adjacent normal tissues.

Cell vaporization takes place at the relatively low temperature of 100 °C (the boiling point of water) and, as tissues conduct heat poorly, there is a very thin layer of damaged cells adjacent to the laser wound which may be as little as 50 μm wide. It has been shown by Kiefhaber, Nath and Moritz (1977) that the CO_2 laser energy is 90% absorbed in a depth of 100 μm. This laser, therefore, removes a layer of cells by vaporization, exposing subjacent layers which are then vaporized, so deepening the wound as with a scalpel.

Two methods are available for the removal of tumours with this laser. First, after a representative biopsy has been taken, the laser is used to vaporize the whole lesion and adjacent normal tissues until a tumour-free defect to appropriate margins has been achieved. This technique destroys the greater part of the lesion, thus making it unavailable for microscopic assessment. The second, and better, method is to use the laser beam where possible as a scalpel to excise the lesion with appropriate margins. The anterior border is first cut to an appropriate depth, and then the lesion is undercut. The specimen must be kept under tension to prevent heat contracture, and with this technique the final defect is no larger, and is more precisely cut, and the whole specimen is available for histological study.

As a result of this method of tissue removal, the features of CO_2 laser surgery, in appropriate fields are:

(1) immediate tissue destruction
(2) bloodless dissection
(3) minimal instrumentation
(4) precise dissection
(5) minimal damage to adjacent normal tissues.

Immediate tissue destruction

Tissue destruction by instantaneous vaporization is an obvious advantage over cryotherapy, in which a period of many days is needed to allow the tissue destroyed by freezing to separate. This period is accompanied by pain, oedema and slough which are minimal or absent after CO_2 laser surgery.

Bloodless dissection

The focused CO_2 laser beam will seal blood vessels of up to 0.5 mm in diameter, and if a defocused beam with lower power density is used, larger vessels may be controlled. As with the monopolar diathermy, if high cutting power is used, coagulation is less efficient, and for all work a 'compromise' power will be used which provides both rapid cutting and good haemostasis. Surgery within the larynx is essentially bloodless, but if extended endoscopic resections are performed, some vessels will be encountered which will require diathermy coagulation. In surgery to the mouth and tongue, some diathermy will be required with ligatures for control of the major vessels.

The beam also seals lymphatics and it has been suggested that this may reduce the spread of malignant cells by this route. Oosterhuis (1978) studied the lymphatic spread of labelled Cloudman S91 melanoma cells after scalpel and laser incisions, and found significantly higher spread after a scalpel incision, with the spread after laser incision no higher than in the controls in which no incision had been made.

The beam also seals nerve endings. Holzer and Ascher (1979) studied severed peripheral nerves and showed that the ends were smooth with a sealing of the endoneurium and that there was no incidence of neuroma formation.

Minimal instrumentation

When a CO_2 laser is used with the operating microscope, no instruments are needed to deliver the beam to the tissues, but a sucker is needed at the point of surgery to remove the steam produced by tissue vaporization, both for visual access and to prevent damage to adjacent normal tissues by the scalding steam. This relative lack of instrumentation is vitally important when access is limited, as in paediatric laryngology.

The CO_2 laser beam cannot, at present, be transmitted by way of a fine flexible fibre and the target area must be accessible to a rigid, straight endoscope. However, stainless steel mirrors equipped with suction are available to reflect the beam to treat lesions in inaccessible areas, such as the undersurface of the vocal cords, laryngeal surface of the epiglottis or nasopharynx.

Precise dissection

In otolaryngology, almost all the work is done under the operating microscope, although some resections in the anterior part of the mouth may be carried out with the hand piece. The microscope provides a well-illuminated, magnified operative field in which the bright-red helium neon aiming beam spot is positioned with great accuracy using the micromanipulator on the laser/microscope attachment (*Figure 23.6*).

The amount of tissue destruction produced by each activation of the laser with the foot switch can be 'preset' by selecting an appropriate power of the beam and its exposure time on the tissues. The power is continuously adjustable to a maximum of about 40 watts in most clinical machines and a mechanical shutter controls the exposure, permitting exposure times of 0.1, 0.2, 0.5 and 1 second, and 'continuous' when the exposure time will be controlled by the foot switch.

A large number of techniques have been described for removal of tissue in various sites. For much of the early work on the larynx, low power levels of 5–10 watts or even lower were used. For removal of mouth or tongue lesions, 20–25 watts with continuous exposure was often used as this permitted rapid cutting with good blood vessel coagulation. However, many modern machines offer 'super pulsing' of the beam with a high peak power and exposure times measured in milliseconds. Both the theoretical evidence provided by McKenzie (1983) and early clinical evidence indicate that the use of a super pulsed beam with a 'short, sharp' dissection technique may reduce damage to adjacent normal tissues and reduce charring in the wound.

In addition, no instruments or blood are present in the wound and, as the beam does not significantly denature the tissue adjacent to the wound, the progress of dissection can be followed with great accuracy under the microscope.

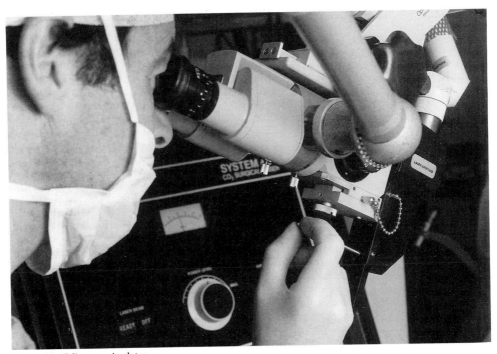

Figure 23.6 Micromanipulator

Minimal damage to adjacent normal tissues

The absorption of the far infrared CO_2 laser beam by intracellular water causes an instantaneous explosive destruction of cells by vaporization, but at the relatively low temperature of 100 °C. As tissues conduct heat poorly, there is an extremely thin layer of damaged cells, only a few micrometres in width, between the laser wound and adjacent normal tissues. As a result, there is minimal postoperative oedema.

Healing of skin incisions cut by CO_2 laser would appear to be slower, with a reduced tensile strength after seven days, compared with an incision cut by scalpel, although the final strength is the same (Cochrane *et al.*, 1980).

In the healing of CO_2 laser wounds of the larynx, reported by Tranter, Frame and Brown (1985), little inflammatory response and few myofibroblasts with little collagen formation in the wounds were found, which meant that minimal scarring or deformation of tissues would result. Similar findings were reported in the case of wounds of the oral mucosa by Fisher *et al.* (1983).

These findings suggest that there are no particular advantages to cutting skin incisions with the CO_2 laser, except in patients with a haemorrhagic tendency where better haemostasis will be achieved, but that it is essentially a mucosal tool of value in gynaecology and otolaryngology, and also in neurosurgery for the performance of precise, atraumatic 'no touch' surgery.

Carbon dioxide surgical lasers

A number of CO_2 surgical lasers are now available, and the majority deliver up to 40 watts of power at the tissues by way of an articulated arm system. The power level is relatively meaningless unless the area of the laser imprint is also known, enabling the power density to be calculated in W/cm^2.

With the hand piece, very small spot sizes of a fraction of a millimetre can be produced; but at a focal length of 400 mm, which is commonly used with the operating microscope, spot sizes of between 0.9 and 1.7 mm diameter are commonly found, although in some machines the spot diameter can be changed over a wide range of sizes and with this are associated changes in power density.

All machines are supplied with a hand piece for use as a light scalpel, although in otolaryngology these are of limited value as they tend to be somewhat bulky. Many machines supply a coupler for use with a rigid bronchoscope, and a number of trials are in progress to compare the role of the CO_2 laser with that of the Nd-YAG laser in endobronchial tumour destruction.

In the selection of a clinical machine, a number of features must be considered including: power and spot sizes available; length, number of articulations and range of movement of the articulated arm; ease of use of micromanipulator; availability of hand piece and bronchoscope with distal suction and good beam aiming facilities; reliability and quality of service; and, inevitably, price.

The argon laser

The argon laser produces continuous wave coherent light at a number of wavelengths, but most of the energy is at 488 and 514 nm which can be transmitted by way of a flexible fibre.

Coherent light at these wavelengths will pass through water and clear colourless structures without absorption and without causing thermal damage. The light is selectively absorbed by tissues which have its complementary colour red.

In skin, the beam is scattered but absorption by chromophores, such as blood, is significant; it has an absorption depth of about 230 μm whereas in blood it is 170 μm. The selective absorption pattern of argon laser energy means that it is predominantly used for the photocoagulation of both normal and abnormal blood vessels. Jain (1983) compared the use of the laser for blood vessel coagulation in neurosurgery with the bipolar coagulator. He commented that the laser could perform photocoagulation by delivering a precisely calculated dose of energy to create discrete lesions with no spread of energy to adjacent tissues and without contact with the vessel. He commented further that the coagulator had to touch the vessel, with a risk of dislodgement of the clot when the instrument was removed; the amount of energy delivered was imprecise, and there was electrical current leakage and diffuse vessel wall damage. However, he pointed out that the coagulator is simple and cheap whereas the laser is complex and expensive.

In the field of photocoagulation, the argon laser was first used on the retina where, attached to a slit lamp, avascular areas of retina in diabetic retinopathy were photocoagulated to reduce the stimulus to new vessel formation. This treatment can be carried out through, and without damaging, the clear anterior parts of the eye, and it is still widely used in this field, alongside the krypton laser. It is also used in dermatology to treat the hitherto untreatable port wine stain by photocoagulation of the abnormal capillaries in the outer dermis through, and without damaging, the clear overlying normal epidermis. Another unique advantage in this field is the potential to coagulate small vessels lying on vital structures such as the vasa nervorum as suggested by Di Bartolomeo (1981).

The absorption pattern of this laser means that slow and relatively imprecise thermal tissue destruction can be carried out. Some early work on the photodestruction of bronchial tumours was performed with this laser by Hetzel *et al.* (1983). However, for tumour destruction it has largely been replaced by the Nd-YAG laser, although it is still used on occasion to 'gut' tumours which are small, adjacent to vital structures and inaccessible to the CO_2 laser.

Early machines required a continuous flow of water for cooling the laser tube and this, plus the requirement for three-phase electricity, made it necessary to plumb and wire in the machine giving a fixed and relatively immobile installation. Recently, air-cooled machines have been introduced which are readily movable, and even portable, and which are, therefore, much more suitable for multidisciplinary use, appearing not to overheat if used continuously. A majority of machines produce about 5 watts of power but 20-watt lasers are available; these more powerful machines will be necessary only for the control of haemorrhage from upper gastrointestinal ulcers and for some tumour work.

Transmission of the beam is by way of a single flexible fibre of approximately 100 µm in diameter embedded in a protective sheath; at the distal end, the diverging beam is refocused by a lens. When used with a slit lamp or microscope, spot sizes of 50–100 µm are available and aiming is provided by an attenuated beam controlled by a micromanipulator. With the hand piece used in dermatology, a spot size of about 1 mm diameter is used. With the CO_2 laser, the optics of the microscope would absorb the laser energy in case of reflection of the beam and, as such, the operator is not at risk of eye damage. However, the operator could be at great risk of suffering retinal damage with lasers of visible wavelength, and both slit lamp and microscope incorporate a shutter which closes when the main beam is activated; this mechanism is fail safe in that the beam cannot be activated unless the shutter is closed.

The Nd-YAG laser

The Nd-YAG laser is the only one of the three most commonly used lasers in clinical practice which does not have a gas as its lasing medium. It has a crystal rod, 100 mm long and about 6 mm wide, of yttrium aluminium garnet with dopant neodymium ions embedded in the lattice. The exciting energy is provided by a powerful light source which is usually a krypton arc lamp focused on the crystal rod. This is the most powerful surgical laser currently in use, as more neodymium ions can be contained in a given volume compared to a gas, and power levels of up to 100 watts are available.

The near infrared coherent light at a wavelength of 1060 nm can be transmitted by way of a flexible fibre and it is aimed by a visible low-powered helium neon laser. The beam at this wavelength is deeply absorbed in the tissues without colour or tissue specificity. Early work suggested that the absorption length of this wavelength could be as long as 90 mm and there was concern that damage could be caused to subjacent tissues even beyond the organ being treated. However, more recent work by Kiefhaber, Nath and Moritz (1977) showed that the beam is absorbed in tissue within a few millimetres. The beam is scattered and diffused by tissue inhomogeneities and so great is the scattering/absorption ratio that a near infrared photon may be scattered many times before it is absorbed.

This pattern of absorption means that the beam affects a far larger volume than the CO_2 laser and that at a given power level the temperature rise is far less (*Figure 23.7*). The Nd-YAG laser is used at high power levels to perform relatively slow, but adequate, tissue destruction with better control of bleeding than is possible with the CO_2 laser. Kelly *et al.* (1983) have stated that the Nd-YAG laser can control vessels of up to 1.5 mm in diameter compared to 1.0 mm with the argon laser, and it has been estimated that vessels of up to 0.5 mm in diameter can be controlled with the focused CO_2 beam.

In the thermal destruction of tissue with the Nd-YAG laser, it would appear that there are three distinct layers of damage. First, a layer which has been vaporized; second, one which has been coagulated and will subsequently slough; and third, one in which death of cells occurs, these then being replaced by fibrous tissue without loss of physical integrity. This means that, in the treatment of a tumour involving the whole wall of the oesophagus or trachea, there is only a small risk of perforation.

Tissue removal with this laser lacks the precision which is obtainable with the CO_2 laser, but recently the Nd-YAG laser has been coupled to a synthetic sapphire 'blade' and this is used as a laser scalpel. The performance of a wide range of general surgical procedures using this system has been described indicating good healing and low patient morbidity. Results from controlled clinical trials with this laser scalpel must be awaited with interest.

The laser tissue interactions produced by the pulsed Nd-YAG laser which are used to destroy opaque lesions in the eye, and renal stones and gallstones have already been described.

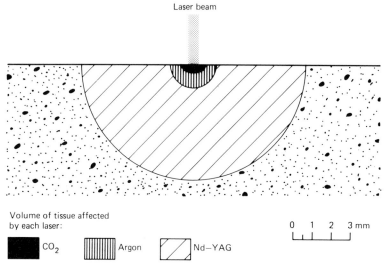

Laser beam

Volume of tissue affected
by each laser:

CO_2 Argon   Nd–YAG

0 1 2 3 mm

Figure 23.7 Depth of tissue affected by different lasers

The dye laser

The dye laser is under investigation in two main clinical areas: for the photoactivation of intra-tumour haematoporphyrin derivative for the treatment of malignant tumours by photodynamic therapy, and for the selective destruction of blood vessels within the skin, for which both continuous wave and pulsed lasers are being evaluated. Early work was carried out with laboratory bench machines which required the constant attention of a laser physicist. Recently, however, more stable and, clinical 'hands off' machines have been introduced.

The dye laser uses an organic rhodamine dye as the lasing medium and this is continuously circulated to avoid heating. The dye laser is excited either by a flash lamp or by an argon or copper vapour laser. As each dye molecule is composed of many atoms, it gives rise to a spectrum of laser lines and each dye can be made to lase over a range of about 50 nm. By changing the dye, coherent light in almost all parts of the visible spectrum can be obtained. The required laser line is selected from the available spectrum by the insertion of a birefingent filter which allows only one wavelength of light to pass through it depending on its angle in the beam.

The ability to tune a dye laser is an important feature, of potential value for the photoactivation of other tumour sensitizers which will be developed in the future and which may be photo-activated at different wavelengths. However, a disadvantage is that the power available is, at best, only 25% of that of the exciting laser.

The light from the dye laser can be transmitted by way of flexible fibres, and a number of delivery fibre tips for surface irradiation of tumours are available, together with a cylinder for implantation into tumour tissue and for the treatment of a circumferential lesion, and also a diffusing bulb tip for the irradiation of the whole of the inside of a hollow viscus such as the bladder.

Metal vapour lasers

A wavelength of approximately 630 nm is required for the photoactivation of an intratumour haematoporphyrin derivative, and an alternative light source for this is the gold vapour laser. This machine can produce much higher power levels and is more stable and easier to use than many dye laser systems. It is, therefore, more suited to clinical practice as shown by Carruth and McKenzie (1986).

This laser produces red light at a fixed wavelength of 628 nm which is pulsed at a rate of 10 kHz, meaning that for practical purposes it is a continuous wave beam. However, it has been suggested by Hisazumi *et al.* (1985) that the pulsed beam penetrates the tissues better than the continuous wave dye laser beam, but this work has not been confirmed elsewhere and McKenzie's investigations (1986, personal communication) do not support these findings.

It might be thought that when other tumour photosensitizers are developed, which are excited at different wavelengths, this gold vapour laser would become obsolete. However, it appears certain that for the next five years at least, haematoporphyrin derivative, or one of its components, will be the only sensitizer in clinical use. Furthermore, when other sensitizers are developed, it is reasonably easy to change the metal in the laser from gold to copper, and the copper vapour laser could be used to drive a tunable dye laser.

Safety

The lasers used in medicine and surgery are, obviously, much less powerful than many of those used in science and industry, but all the therapeutic lasers are in the highest power class (class 4) and 'their use requires extreme caution'.

A wide range of national and international safety codes, pertaining to the safe use of lasers, are in existence. In the UK, the relevant codes are the British Standards Code BS 4803, *Radiation Safety of Laser Products and Systems 1983*, and BS 5724, for electrical safety of laser equipment. In addition, the document *Guidance on the Safe Use of Lasers in Medical Practice* has recently been published by the Department of Health and Social Security (DHSS).

Safety administration

The local health authority has overall responsibility for the implementation of health and safety advice, and it is stated by the codes of safe practice that a laser safety officer should be appointed who will advise on all aspects of this problem and produce a code of safe practice for each laser in each clinical situation.

The laser safety officer is usually a medical physicist with a wide experience of lasers, and may be responsible for several hospitals within a district or region. Therefore, a local laser protection supervisor will be appointed who may be a doctor or a member of the operating theatre staff, and he/she will be responsible for the implementation of the safety codes when lasers are being used clinically.

It is suggested that a list of 'nominated users' should be drawn up and access to the machine by the key control should be limited to doctors on this list. It is essential to ensure that lasers do not fall into the wrong hands, and the problem of identifying those who have had appropriate training in medical laser techniques and safety remains unsolved. The British Medical Laser Association, founded in 1982, has introduced the idea of accreditation for suitably trained doctors and a mechanism has been set up whereby the

curriculum vitae of those wishing to be accredited is studied by the appropriate specialist representative on the committee of the Association and by one or two others appointed by the appropriate national specialist body. However, the concept of accreditation has not been widely accepted and remains a topic of regular and often heated debate.

It would be both impossible and inappropriate to discuss all aspects of laser safety, but some of the more important points must be mentioned.

The machine

The machine must comply with the British Standards codes for electrical and laser safety and a number of specific features have been recommended in the DHSS guide.

Key control

All class 3A, 3B and 4 lasers must incorporate a master key control.

Emission warning

A visible or audible warning should be provided when the laser is switched on and operating.

Remote interlock

This should be available to lock the operating theatre doors electrically when the laser is operating.

Aiming beam

An aiming beam must be fitted and it must not be possible to operate the laser if this beam fails.

Emergency shut-off switch

An instant switch must be fitted.

Beam transmission system

The fibre or articulated arm should be securely fitted and a tool required for detachment.

Warning labels

Appropriate labels must be fitted.

Environmental

The room in which the laser is operated must be designated a 'laser controlled area' and access to this area must be strictly limited to those essential to the procedure, and to specified visitors.

Warning signs must be displayed outside and, ideally, these should be illuminated when the laser is switched on. Remote door interlocks which are activated when the laser is working should be used, particularly if there is a significant risk of accidental entry to the controlled area.

The eye hazard

The part of the eye which could be damaged by laser radiation depends on the wavelength of the coherent light. Far infrared light produced by the CO_2 laser would be absorbed by the cornea and a retinal injury could not occur until the beam had penetrated the whole globe. However, the near infrared laser light produced by the Nd-YAG laser and visible wavelengths would be focused on the retina with an increase of power per unit area of 10^5 times the energy incident on the cornea.

The maximum permissible exposure has been calculated and, for wavelengths transmitted on to the retina, this is a factor of 10 below the level of exposure for which there is a 50% chance of detecting a retinal injury. Maximum permissible exposure tables are available in the British Standards Code, and the DHSS Code states that these levels should be used as a guide on the control of exposure and should not be regarded as precisely defined lines between safe and dangerous levels.

Eye protection

Adequate eye protection must be provided for the patient and for all the staff in the laser controlled area if the maximum permissible exposure level for the particular laser can be exceeded (*Figure 23.8*). It is obviously extremely unlikely that a member of staff could be exposed to the direct beam, but it is possible that the laser beam could be reflected back into the operating theatre from an instrument or retractor. The design of and specifications for the 'laser proof' eye wear which should be provided are clearly defined in the safety codes. The eye wear must be marked to indicate the wavelengths against which protection is provided and the absorbance of the filter at these wavelengths. The glasses must attenuate the laser beam to below the maximum permissible exposure, even if direct exposure occurs, and must not shatter or puncture if exposed directly to the maximum power of the laser.

Different eye wear will be required for use with each laser, and glasses which conform to these specifications are available and must be provided. The eyes of the patient will be protected by glasses or by appropriate, carefully fixed pads which, in the case of the CO_2 laser, must be soaked in water

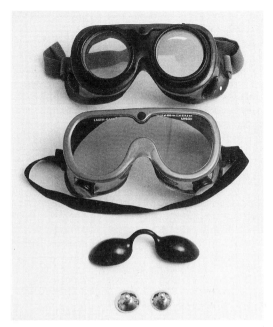

Figure 23.8 Eye protection from the top – CO_2 laser goggles, argon laser goggles and eye shields and contact lenses for use with the argon laser

– as described by Colman and Conway (1985) – to absorb the energy should the beam miss the target (*Figure 23.9*). Argon laser goggles or eye shields are available; and if work is to be performed close to the patient's eyes, stainless steel contact lenses are available and must be used.

When using the operating microscope, the surgeon will have the optics to protect his eyes

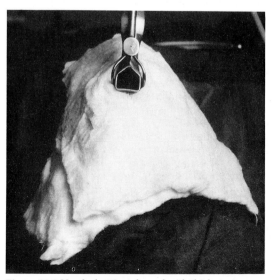

Figure 23.9 Head of patient draped with thick, wet swabs for CO_2 laser surgery to the larynx

against CO_2 laser radiation when the microscope or slit lamp is used with the argon laser, shutters which operate when the laser is activated are used for protection. With the Nd-YAG laser, filters on the endoscope will be used to protect the eyes of the surgeon and goggles or pads are provided for the patient. However, for all other usage, particularly with hand pieces, the surgeon must wear appropriate laser-proof glasses.

Skin injury

Unless accidental exposure to the direct beam occurs, skin injury from a reflected beam would be insignificant, and protective clothing is not thought to be necessary for operating theatre personnel.

Anaesthetic safety

A hazard unique to otolaryngology is the danger of anaesthetic tube combustion when the CO_2 laser is used, particularly in laryngology. A number of endotracheal fires have been recorded with some fatalities.

If an endotracheal tube, made of combustible material, is struck by the CO_2 laser beam, it will ignite. Research has shown that a continuous beam, at normally used power levels, will cause a rise in temperature of the tube of approximately 5000 °C per second (A. C. Wainwright and J. A. S. Carruth, unpublished results).

A number of 'laser-resistant' tubes have been developed and several will not ignite if surrounded by a gas mixture with low oxygen and nitrous oxide content, or if used with a flow of carbon dioxide or nitrogen around the upper part of the tube above the cuff. However, all the tubes tested to date will ignite if surrounded by oxygen, and the use of nitrous oxide does not ameliorate the situation as this gas supports combustion as well as oxygen.

A very large number of materials have been tested which could be used to produce a smooth, flexible anaesthetic tube and these have been plated with a number of metals using a variety of techniques. It has been found that all these materials, when surrounded by oxygen or nitrous oxide, will ignite and burn if struck by the laser. After metal plating the tube appeared to be entirely smooth with a complete coating of metal, but microscopy showed that 'peaks and troughs' on the surface of the tube allowed islands of plastic to appear in the metal coat and these could be ignited. When a thick metal plate was applied the tube became rigid and when flexed the coating cracked.

However, in spite of the lack of a totally laser-proof disposable, soft, flexible anaesthetic tube, a number of 'laser-safe' anaesthetic techniques have been developed, either without an endotracheal tube or using a protected plastic or metal tube. It is essential for the laryngologist to work as a team with an anaesthetist who is fully conversant with this hazard and the techniques to overcome it.

Anaesthetic techniques for microlaryngeal laser surgery

(See Figure 23.10)

Jet ventilation with no endotracheal tube

The Venturi ventilation principle, first suggested by Bernoulli, has been known since the eighteenth century. With this technique, the patient is anaesthetized routinely and a fine endotracheal tube is inserted. When the patient has been positioned on the operating table, a laryngoscope is inserted and appropriately fixed. The tube is then removed, a 'jet ventilator attachment' is fastened to the laryngoscope and the paralysed patient is oxygenated by intermittent jet ventilation of oxygen.

There are a number of disadvantages to this technique which, nevertheless, is totally laser safe as there is no combustible material in the airway. First, some patients are not suitable for the technique, particularly those who are grossly obese or who have severe chronic obstructive airways disease. Secondly, the cords abduct and vibrate on each injection of gas, and surgery has to take place between injections. However, when working with the same anaesthetist, the surgeon soon learns the rhythm of injection and surgery can be carried out easily when this technique is employed. Thirdly, the subglottis cannot be protected with a wet swab, although there have been no reports of problems from injuries to this area from the defocused laser beam. Fourthly, it has been suggested that jet ventilation may blow viable particles of papillomata into the lower airways with a risk of seeding the disease. However, this risk, which could also be present with malignant disease, would appear to be theoretical only and there is no clinical evidence to support it.

Other jet ventilation techniques employ metallic catheters inserted into the trachea, but it is considered by some that the risk of causing a pneumothorax with these catheters, particularly in children, is significant.

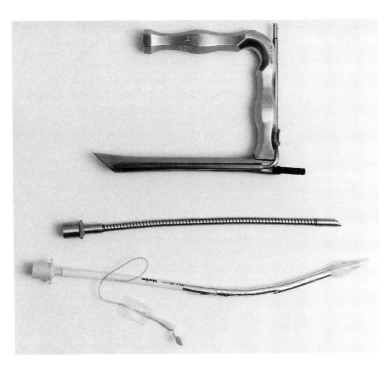

Figure 23.10 Anaesthetic equipment: top – jet injector attached to laryngoscope, metal tube, portex tube wrapped with aluminium foil

Nasopharyngeal airway with spontaneous respiration

With this technique, described by Vivori (1980), a nasopharyngeal airway is inserted and kept well out of the operative field. Steward and Fearon (1981) suggested that the technique should be supplemented by topical analgesia to lighten the depth of anaesthesia. It is essential to ensure that there is a constant flow of gas down the airway as, without it, there could be a chance, in the expiratory phase, of incandescent carbon particles being blown into the catheter with a risk of fire.

The technique appears to be particularly appropriate for children with recurrent respiratory papillomatosis.

Protected endotracheal tube

If an endotracheal tube is in place, it is easier to control and maintain adequate ventilation in difficult patients and it is also possible to protect subglottic structures with wet swabs. The tube may be protected by a wrapping of metal foil, which must be relatively thick as it will absorb some of the laser energy if hit and must, to some extent, act as a 'heat sink'. Narrow 0.5–1 inch (1.3–2.6 cm) adhesive aluminium tape is wound up the tube from the proximal edge of the cuff to a point where the tube is well outside the operative field. The wrapping must start distally to avoid spaces appearing in the wrapping when the tube is flexed, as these might allow passage of the laser beam to strike the tube and cause ignition. The cuff cannot be wrapped and must be protected with a wet swab in the subglottis.

However, this wrapping makes the tube rough and rigid and can cause soft tissue damage to the larynx and pharynx; the tube must never be passed through the nose. It has been suggested that tubes can be protected with wet gauze, but this is generally difficult to apply and to keep in place and it must be kept very wet.

When work is to be carried out in the mouth or pharynx, the upper end of the tube is wrapped and the distal end protected with an appropriate wet throat pack.

Metal tube

Norton and de Vos (1978) developed a flexible metal tube which is totally laser proof, but it has some disadvantages. It is somewhat rough and a little traumatic for the patient and to seal the airway a cuff must be attached for each procedure which, even though it is filled with saline, must be protected. The inside diameter of these tubes is small in relation to the outside diameter when compared with similar sized plastic tubes, and many use these metal tubes with some form of jet ventilation. A malleable copper catheter has also been described by Herbert, Berlin and Eberle (1985) and by Benke *et al.* (1985).

Other techniques

A number of other techniques are being evaluated including high frequency positive pressure ventilation by way of a metal cannula and the use of a metal cricothyrotomy cannula has also been suggested.

Conclusions

With further research, it seems likely that a soft, flexible, disposable, endotracheal tube will be developed which will not ignite in any gas mixture and will, therefore, be totally laser- and foolproof.

Clinical use of lasers in otolaryngology

In all medical and surgical laser usage, it is not sufficient to show that a laser can be used to perform a specific task; it must also be shown why a laser, rather than conventional instruments, should be used. A laser should be used only when it can be clearly demonstrated that it can perform a specific medical or surgical task better than established, conventional techniques, and the words of one of the fathers of laser surgery, Dr Leon Goldman, must never be forgotten – 'If you don't need a laser, don't use one'.

In all clinical situations, it must be demonstrated that a safe machine is being used in a totally safe manner by fully trained medical personnel in appropriate clinical conditions.

The carbon dioxide laser

Instrumentation and technique

For work in the larynx, a rigid laryngoscope with an appropriate support system will be used.

With standard microsurgical instruments, work at the somewhat awkward standard distance of

400 mm can pose some problems for the surgeon, particularly during a prolonged procedure, and some employ an arm rest to avoid fatigue and to prevent shaking of the instrument. However, many laser micromanipulators incorporate a hand rest enabling the aiming beam to be positioned within the operative field with 'shake-free' accuracy.

It has already been stressed that, where possible, lesions should not be vaporized totally after biopsy, but should be excised using the laser as a scalpel, thus enabling the whole lesion to be studied under the microscope. This is of great importance for leucoplakic lesions of the oral cavity and larynx which may show a different histological pattern in various areas, making a single biopsy unrepresentative.

To enable the surgeon to excise laryngeal lesions, special instruments are required. The lesion must be retracted medially with microlaryngeal forceps to enable the pedicle to be divided with the laser; the beam must be aimed with the micromanipulator and suction must be provided at the point of surgery to allow visual access, and to prevent the steam from damaging the normal laryngeal structures with the production of oedema. The only instrument which could be used by an assistant is the suction tube, and this is not practical as there would a significant risk of hitting the assistant's hand with the direct beam. A number of instruments have been designed for laser laryngeal microsurgery including those described by the author (Carruth, 1985b) (*Figure 23.11*).

Microlaryngeal suction forceps are available with a fine suction catheter built into an angled cupped forceps as is a malleable adjustable suction tube which can easily be clamped into any size or type of laryngoscope to provide adequate distal suction without encroaching significantly into the lumen of the laryngoscope. Rhys-Evans has designed a double-suction tissue holding device

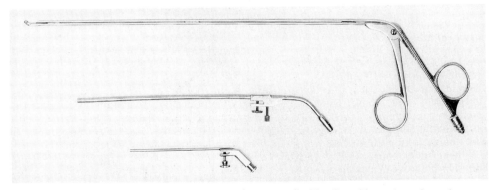

Figure 23.11 Microlaryngeal instruments: suction forceps, malleable adjustable suction tube and attachment for jet ventilation

which enables the tissues to be held and retracted with the distal suction hole, with steam aspirated through a more proximal opening.

A number of other retractors and metal 'paddles' are available with built-in suction, both to retract tissues in the exposure of lesions and to prevent damage, by the beam or by steam, to other areas of the larynx. Despite some early evidence to the contrary, it has been shown that it is not possible to remove mucosa from the anterior ends of both vocal cords without a significant risk of webbing.

For work in the mouth, a number of standard mouth gags can be used and the lesion will be kept under tension by sutures. Further retraction and suction will be provided by an assistant who is able to observe the dissection directly and, with the use of a long metallic suction tube, there will be no significant risk of injury.

Microlaryngeal surgery

All the features of tissue removal with the CO_2 laser make it an ideal tool for these procedures, which can be performed precisely, with no bleeding and with minimal damage to normal laryngeal structures, resulting in minimal postoperative oedema and contracture of the surgical defect (*Figure 23.12*).

Benign lesions

Traumatic vocal cord nodules

It would be preferable to excise all lesions from the larynx for histological examination, but 'classical' vocal cord nodules lying at the junction of anterior and middle thirds of the cords are almost invariably smaller than the laser 'spot size' at the microscope's working distance of 400 mm.

Suspicious or atypical nodules should be removed for histology and cupped forceps will be needed for this procedure. However, if there is no doubt about the diagnosis, the lesions may be destroyed using the CO_2 laser. A suitably protected anaesthetic tube is inserted and the cuff and subglottis are protected with wet swabs. The CO_2 laser beam is then aimed at the wet swab, turned on and moved towards the lesion, allowing the edge of the beam to shave the nodule off the vocal cord edge without damaging the underlying fibrous cord. Postoperative speech therapy will then be given, as appropriate.

Polyps

Localized polyps can be drawn medially with microlaryngeal suction forceps and excised by division of the pedicle. If more sessile lesions cannot be excised, then they can be readily vaporized after representative biopsies have been taken.

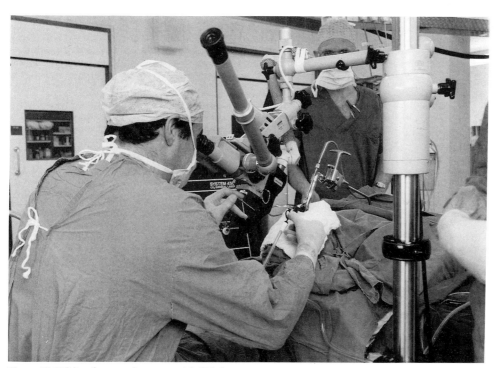

Figure 23.12 Microlaryngeal surgery with CO_2 laser

Vocal cord oedema

It has been shown by Moesgard-Nielsen, Højslet and Karlmose (1986) that if, after surgical vocal cord stripping, the patient continues to smoke there will be a high chance of recurrence. In their series of 120 cases treated by a standard microsurgical technique, only six stopped smoking with a recurrence rate of 58%, although 81% had persistent voice problems.

The vocal cord mucosa and oedematous tissue may be vaporized and, under the microscope, this can be done without causing damage to the fibrous cord. However, a number of more detailed, sophisticated techniques have been described in the literature, including the submucosal enucleation of polypoid cords performed by Yates and Dedo (1984). They made an incision in the mucosa of the superior part of the vocal cord following the arcuate line. The mucosal edge was then retracted medially and the submucosal oedematous tissue vaporized until the fibres of the thyroarytenoid muscle could be seen. The mucosa was then turned back and laid on the denuded cord. This technique is essentially similar to that described by Kolle, Iverson and Paulsen (1985) who, where possible, removed the oedematous tissue by suction and then fixed the mucosa to the surface of the vocal cord with intermittent pulses of laser energy.

In the Yates and Dedo short series of 11 patients, nine had good or excellent results and, in the Paulsen series, the results were better than in previously reported series in which routine microsurgical techniques had been used.

Laryngeal stenosis

It was hoped that the minimal tissue reaction adjacent to the CO_2 laser wound might make it possible endoscopically to 'core out' both congenital and acquired stenoses in which the cartilaginous support of the airway was maintained, without recurrence or with a much reduced rate of recurrence compared to conventional endoscopic techniques. A study of the literature shows that this hope has, in part, been realized and, if laser vaporization of the stenosis is combined with the endoscopic insertion of a 'stent', a majority of patients can be 'cured', if a cure is defined as an adequate voice and airway with no tracheostomy.

Vocal cord webs

Vocal cord webs may be congenital or post-traumatic following external trauma or the endoscopic stripping of the mucosa from the anterior ends of both vocal cords.

Using the CO_2 laser, it is extremely easy to divide the web. However, if such a division is carried out, many webs will recur, as this procedure, in itself, denudes the anterior ends of both cords of mucosa. Nevertheless, the recurrent web is almost always smaller than the original and, in many cases, one or two laser procedures will reduce the web to insignificant proportions.

Several techniques have been described to overcome the problem of recurrence. The first technique is to open only the anterior end of the web, leaving a bridge at the posterior edge of the web which is divided when the anterior opening has epithelialized. The second technique is to remove the fibrin endoscopically from the healing cords at regular intervals to prevent reformation of the adhesions, and the third technique, is to provide cover for one cord, using either an absorbable gelatin sponge or a plastic splint. The fourth and most commonly used technique is to insert an endoscopic 'keel' into the anterior commissure, but debate continues on the length of time that the keel should be left in place.

Division of the web alone will be more successful in thin diaphragmatic webs, and a keel or another technique will almost always be needed to prevent recurrence after laser division of thick, post-traumatic webs.

Subglottic stenosis in children

This condition may be congenital or acquired from prolonged endotracheal intubation. Traditionally, it was managed by performing a tracheostomy with a fenestrated tube which incorporated a speaking valve. This allowed the child to breathe out through the larynx, enabling normal laryngeal growth to occur and the child to speak. However, in a series of 25 children reported by Fearon and Cotton (1974), six (24%) died of causes related to their tracheostomy. In contrast, in a similar series of 85 children who required a tracheostomy, described by Hollinger et al. (1976), 10 children died, but only five from causes related to the tracheostomy.

Evans and Todd first reported their technique of laryngotracheoplasty in 1974, and since then a number of surgical procedures have been developed to correct the stenosis, but all are associated with a significant morbidity.

In a series of 13 patients reported by Kaufman, Thompson and Kohut (1981), 11 were children under the age of three years. These patients with subglottic stenosis, predominantly from prolonged intubation, were managed by injection of steroids into the lesion before laser vaporization. Stents were used in three patients, but did not appear to be of benefit in this series. Kaufman et al. suggested that circumferential removal of the subglottic mucosa should not be performed as it would encourage scar formation and would interrupt the mucociliary cleansing system of the tracheobronchial tree. They considered that dilatation and both antibiotics and steroids given systemically or by injection into the lesion, had a part to play in the management of these cases. At presentation, eight patients had a tracheostomy; of these, three could be decannulated and two had normal airways, but were not decannulated for various reasons. However, two other patients needed tracheostomies during the course of treatment, but a satisfactory airway was achieved in 10 of the 11 children treated.

Holinger, in a preliminary report in 1982, described the use of the laser in the mangement of six children with severe subglottic stenosis who would have needed a tracheostomy but could be managed without one. The children needed from one to 11 endoscopic resections (average 6.5), but a successful outcome was achieved in all cases. He concluded that an infant with subglottic stenosis who, while needing a tracheostomy, was able to breathe spontaneously and undergo a general anaesthetic, was a suitable candidate for management with the laser. However, in the paper, mention was made of a further five children with the same problem who, for logistic or timing reasons, could not be treated with the laser, and of one child who needed an urgent tracheostomy for very severe obstruction. A further requirement for this management technique is that the child should be in, or should be safely transportable to, a centre in which there is a paediatric laryngologist with experience in the use of the laser.

Post-traumatic stenosis

This may be caused by external trauma, prolonged endotracheal intubation, by an imperfectly performed tracheostomy or it may follow laryngeal surgery. Each case is unique and it is difficult, therefore, to compare series and results.

Management has always posed serious problems; many endoscopic procedures are followed by a disappointingly high rate of recurrence and open surgical procedures are associated with a significant morbidity.

A number of experimental animal studies on the role of the CO_2 laser, in the management of post-traumatic laryngeal stenosis, were performed by McGee, Nagle and Toohill (1981), Healey (1982) and Toohill, Campbell and Duncavage (1984). These studies suggested that in cases of severe stenotic lesions, partial or complete resection of the obstruction alone would both be followed by recurrence, but the use of a stent with antibiotics would improve the results.

In 1980, Lyons *et al.* reported the use of the CO_2

laser in the management of six patients, five of whom had had previous treatment. After a relatively short period of follow-up, the tracheostomies in four could be 'plugged' and two patients had been decannulated. For the treatment of supraglottic and isolated glottic stenosis, Lyons *et al.* excised the false and true cords on both sides and one arytenoid, and for other causes excised the stenosis on one side and combined this with an injection of steroids. They concluded that the technique appeared promising but further follow-up was needed.

Shugar, Som and Biller (1982) described the management of 16 patients with the laser. Seven had redundant supraglottic soft tissues following hemilaryngectomy; after this was removed, six could be decannulated and in one a tracheostomy was avoided. However only two of the other cases could be decannulated; one had a web which was excised and a keel inserted for two weeks, and another suffered postradiotherapy scarring which recurred nine months after decannulation following laser excision of the stenosis. A further resection in the same case had been successful in maintaining the airway but for only three months.

In a comprehensive paper, Simpson *et al.* (1982) described the management of 60 patients with a wide range of stenotic lesions of the larynx and upper trachea. In 39 of them, soft Silastic stents were used. Success was defined as an adequate voice and airway without a tracheostomy, and this was achieved in 41 patients. However, it is somewhat difficult to compare exactly results for laser surgery alone with results for laser surgery followed by stenting. Simpson *et al.* concluded that features indicating a poor prognosis were circumferential scarring, stenosis longer than 1 cm, posterior inlet scarring with arytenoid fixation and bacterial infection of the tracheostomy.

Duncavage, Ossoff and Toohill (1985), in an elegant review paper, reported a successful outcome in 11 out of 20 patients treated with the CO_2 laser. Seventeen were managed by laser excision of the stenosis alone and, in the remainder, 'supplemental treatment' was given with dilatation, intralesion steroids, grafts and, in three patients, the use of a stent. They concluded that success could be anticipated with small thin scars and redundant soft tissues and they shared the views expressed by Simpson *et al.* (1982) on poor prognostic features. They felt that the use of submucosal 'micro-trapdoor flaps', stents and steroids should improve results.

The micro-trapdoor flap was described by Dedo and Sooy (1984) for the management of stenosis in the posterior glottis, subglottis and trachea. They made an incision on the superior surface of the scar and the submucosal tissue was then removed with the laser. Incisions with a knife or micro-scissor were then made on either side of the trapdoor, enabling it to be laid on the raw area. Suturing was not necessary as the mucosa readily adhered to the denuded area. They achieved success in eight of nine patients.

It would appear appropriate and ethical to attempt to treat stenotic leisons of the larynx and upper trachea with the CO_2 laser, ideally carrying out a submucosal dissection of the stenotic area rather than a simple vaporization. A careful follow-up will show whether improvement is being achieved and, if so, surgery with the laser should continue until decannulation is possible. However, if there is no significant improvement, a stent should be employed after the stenosis has been resected and, in this way, it should be possible to manage many patients endoscopically and avoid the morbidity of an open procedure.

There is recent anecdotal evidence that the use of a super pulsed laser for the treatment of laryngeal and upper tracheal stenosis may produce results which are superior to those achieved with the standard continuous wave models. It has been suggested that the super pulsed beam may cause even less damage to adjacent, normal tissues, and this may be significant in reducing the rate of recurrence. Further work with these machines must be awaited with interest.

Bilateral vocal cord paralysis

In the past, this condition was managed by endoscopic arytenoidectomy, with standard microlaryngeal instruments, or by an external approach, such as Woodman's operation.

A number of techniques have been described to perform endoscopic cordectomy with the CO_2 laser with, in some, either partial or complete removal of the arytenoid in the treatment of this condition.

In all reported series, excellent results have been obtained and it would seem that the CO_2 laser is now the preferred treatment modality for this problem.

The technique was first introduced by Strong *et al.* in 1976 (1976a), and Croft presented a series of cases (1984) in which a wide resection of the true cord was performed with good results in a short series. Shaheen (1984) described his own procedure for the removal of the posterior third of one cord, with 'enhanced effects' if the arytenoid were also removed.

Ossoff *et al.* (1984) updated their 1983 paper and reported success in 10 of 11 patients treated by laser arytenoidectomy, in which the cartilage was exposed and vaporized with the laser. They concluded that the use of the laser offered refinements over the operation performed by conventional instruments. Prasad (1985) also reported a successful outcome in a short series of 10 patients who had been subjected to CO_2 laser vaporization of part of the cord and of the vocal process of the arytenoid.

It has been stated that the use of the CO_2 laser to vaporize the 'non-water-containing' arytenoid cartilage is time-consuming and creates very high temperatures. Further series will show whether it is significantly better to excise rather than to vaporize this cartilage.

Recurrent respiratory papillomatosis

This condition, thought to be caused by the human papilloma virus, often begins between the ages of 2 and 5 years and was once known as 'juvenile laryngeal papillomatosis' in the expectation that a remission would occur at about the time of puberty. However, in many patients the disease may continue into, or even begin in, adult life and the newer name of 'recurrent respiratory papillomatosis' has been suggested.

In the past, the disease has been treated by a number of surgical techniques to remove the papillomata in order to preserve the airway and by a number of 'medical' techniques in an attempt to prevent or reduce the rate of recurrence.

Routine surgical excision of papillomata is accompanied by significant nuisance bleeding, and diathermy techniques cause significant thermal damage to normal tissues with postoperative oedema and the risk of late scarring with contraction. Treatments given to prevent a recurrence have ranged from antibiotics to antimetabolites, and from ultrasound to radiotherapy, but no technique has given consistently good results and some were either harmful or had an unacceptable morbidity. It was hoped that vaccines would be of value but only one series, reported by Professor C. Freche (personal communication), regularly gave good results, but his vaccine required 2 grams of papilloma tissue and a high pressure press, and his results have not been repeated elsewhere.

Several papers have suggested the use of interferon (Haglund *et al.*, 1981; Goepfert *et al.*, 1982; McCabe and Clark, 1983; Saito *et al.*, 1985). All series showed a significant regression of the papillomata while the adminstration of interferon continued, but there was a rapid recurrence of the disease in most patients when the drug was withdrawn. This drug has to be given by intramuscular injection and toxic side-effects were reported. However, treatment appeared to be well tolerated by most patients and had to be discontinued in very few. All state that the drug is of obvious value in this condition, but that they found it hard to define the optimum treatment programme. In the author's series of six patients treated with inosine pranobex (Immunovir), five showed significant improvement, and one child, aged two years, who had needed the removal of papillomata every three weeks to maintain his airway, has had no evidence of disease for almost two years while on treatment. The drug has low toxicity and can be given by mouth.

Further studies will determine whether these drugs may be used to reduce the recurrence rate in patients with this condition and, if so, how this may be done; however, until further evidence is available, children will be managed by surgical removal of the papillomata. As children often require dozens of operations, the CO_2 laser should be used as it reduces the morbidity of each procedure.

With the CO_2 laser, complete removal of all visible disease can be performed without nuisance bleeding and with minimal damage to underlying, normal laryngeal tissues; there should, therefore, be no postoperative oedema and less contracture of the mucosal defects.

McCabe has pointed out that the laser can, if used inexpertly or excessively, cause significant damage with webbing and scarring, particularly to the posterior and anterior commissures, and he has suggested that a debulking rather than a total extirpation of disease should be carried out.

With the use of the laser, it should be possible to avoid a tracheostomy which, in itself, has a significant morbidity in small children, and which has been followed in some cases by the development of papillomata in the trachea and in the tracheostome. In 109 patients treated by laser and by the application of podophylum, Dedo and Jackler (1982) reduced the need for a tracheostomy from an average figure reported in the literature of 25% to 1.8% and the mortality from 7% to 0.

Two methods of managing the patients have been described, and some maintain that by debulking the papillomata at regular intervals, a prolonged remission can be obtained. Strong (personal communication) maintains, however, that in his large series he has not been able to achieve this and advocates an 'on-demand' technique. This technique requires intelligent, alert parents and an ever-ready surgical team, but, in practice, 'out of hours' procedures are extremely rare and the child has the least number of operative procedures.

The CO_2 laser is, undoubtedly, the instrument of choice for the surgical removal of papillomata, but it must be used with care to take advantage of its minimal damage to normal tissues and to avoid excessively deep damage with webbing and scarring. It is to be hoped that one of the new 'antiviral' agents will reduce the need for any form of surgical intervention in this distressing condition.

Intubation granuloma

Vocal cord granulomata may follow intubation, and surgical removal is often followed by recurrence. The CO_2 laser is an ideal tool for their removal as the lesion can be excised to the point of exposing the arytenoid cartilage. However, as shown by Benjamin and Croxson (1985), its use does not seem to produce improved recurrence rates.

Malignant granuloma

The larynx may be involved in one of these unpleasant conditions with complete obstruction and the need for a tracheostomy. Obstructing tissue may be removed with the laser to provide both an airway and a voice, but the ease of surgery and the rate of recurrence will depend on the activity of the disease. If the disease is active and not under control, surgery will be accompanied by significant bleeding and recurrence will be rapid; on the other hand, if the disease is inactive, surgery will be bloodless and recurrence will be slow or may not take place.

Leucoplakia

Histology of a leucoplakic patch may vary from a simple hyperkeratosis to an invasive carcinoma and different patterns may be seen in different parts of an individual lesion. It is essential, therefore, to excise these lesions with the laser, thus enabling the whole specimen to be examined histologically, as a single biopsy taken before the lesion is vaporized may be unrepresentative.

Further management will depend on the histology, but almost all patients will be advised, where relevant, to cut down or, ideally, to stop smoking. If the lesion is found to be a carcinoma *in situ*, which has been excised with adequate margins, then the patient should be regularly and carefully followed up. The management of early invasive lesions is discussed in the next section, but, at present, if an invasive carcinoma is found, the patient should be considered for a course of radiotherapy.

Malignant disease of the larynx

It is difficult to write authoritatively about the management of carcinoma of the larynx as treatment varies between clinics and countries. However, in a majority of centres in the UK, T1 N0 carcinoma of the vocal cord would be treated by radiotherapy, with the expectation of a 'cure rate' of 80–90% and without any significant incidence of complications or of radionecrosis. The course of radiotherapy has a significant morbidity with, where relevant, the risk of radiation-induced malignant change after several decades. However, after a well given, successful course of radiation, the voice should essentially return to normal.

In 1975, Strong introduced the idea of treating early vocal cord carcinoma by laser excision and the experience of the Boston group was updated by Blakeslee *et al.* in 1984.

In Strong's first series of 11 patients, three had failed radiotherapy, all had free margins at excision, and no patient had a recurrence. In one patient, a tumour was removed from the other cord one year later. Strong commented that if margins were found to be involved by tumour, other treatment by radiotherapy or surgery would be necessary, and that the voice was 'as good as the remainder of the larynx would allow'.

In 1984, in the updated paper by Blakeslee *et al.*, and in the paper by Ossoff, Sisson and Shapshay (1985), a total of 113 non-irradiated patients were treated in essentially the same way: the lesion was excised with appropriate margins and biopsies taken from the edge of the defect, which were then studied by frozen section. The removal of tumour was continued until either the margins of the defect were shown to be tumour free or the thyroid cartilage was reached when it was considered that further resection was inappropriate and radiotherapy should be given.

Blakeslee *et al.* defined the criteria for a successful treatment by excision biopsy as follows. The lesion must be completely exposed at laryngoscopy, it must not extend to the vocal process of the arytenoid or anterior commissure, and it should be confined to the mucous membrane. No residual tumour should be evident at high magnification and frozen section from the defect should be tumour free, as must be the margins of the specimen when examined by multiple routine sections. If these criteria were met, then excision was considered to be curative; but if the excision extended to the thyroid cartilage, or if the specimen margins showed involvement by tumour, then further therapy with radiotherapy or surgery was considered to be essential. The results from the two series are shown in *Table 23.2*.

In Blakeslee's paper, reference is made to 15 patients who had failed radiotherapy, only six of whom were disease free after a period of three years. These findings were confirmed in the series of Annayas *et al.* (1984), who obtained good results in non-irradiated patients and poor results when laser salvage surgery was attempted for radiation failures.

With regard to the effect on the voice of laser excision, Blakeslee *et al.* reported the voice to be serviceable following the removal of small lesions, and breathy and rough when larger tumours had been resected. Ossoff *et al.* (1985) found the voice

Table 23.2 Carcinoma of the larynx

Treatment	No.	Free at 3 years	%
Excision biopsy			
Blakeslee	50	46	92
Ossoff	17	17	100
Excision + radiotherapy			
Blakeslee	34	29	85
Ossoff	6	6	100
Excision + surgery			
Blakeslee	4	4	100
Ossoff	2	1	50
Total	113	103	91

after laser excision to be good to excellent; and in a study of patients after unilateral laser cordectomy, Vercerina and Krajina (1983) stated that the vocal function was good.

The advantages of excision biopsy were summarized by Blakeslee *et al.* as: the ability to establish the diagnosis and stage, and to provide an adequate treatment for 'mini' and 'micro'-tumours and squamous carcinoma if the margins were found to be clear. The technique is very appropriate for radiotherapy-resistant tumours and for exploring recurrent lesions after unsuccessful radiotherapy. This treatment technique offers several advantages. If the excision is found to be complete, the patient will have been spared the short- and long-term problems of a course of radiation and will have had treatment carried out under one anaesthetic. The treatment can be repeated as often as necessary, but the voice will not be as good as after a well given, successful course of radiotherapy. In the long term, it appears that 'cure rates' will be as good as those obtained by radiation.

Some cases have been reported by Motta (1985) in which more extensive tumours were resected endoscopically until the sphincter function of the larynx has been threatened in some cases. The period of follow-up is too short to draw significant conclusions, but early results are encouraging.

In the management of advanced tumours, the laser offers three potential advantages, but trials have not yet shown whether these will prove to be significant. The tumour can be debulked at the time of biopsy, enabling more accurate staging and reporting of results. It also presents the radiotherapist with a reduced tumour bulk to treat, which may possibly improve results. In the past, if a patient has presented with laryngeal obstruction from a tumour, only two treatment techniques have been available: urgent laryngectomy after frozen section confirmation of the diagnosis, or, alternatively, a tracheostomy, but with this there is a risk of tumour seeding around the stoma. Using the CO_2 laser, it is possible to vaporize sufficient tumour to restore the airway allowing further treatment to be planned at leisure.

Tongue and oral cavity

From the early work of Strong *et al.* (1979b, c), it has been evident that the CO_2 laser can be used to remove lesions from the tongue and oral cavity with advantages over conventional instruments. Much of the work has been carried out under the operating microscope which provides a well-illuminated, magnified view of the operative field. However, the system is a little 'rigid' and it is important to check regularly the lines of resection. The hand piece can also be used for work in the anterior part of the mouth but many hand pieces are rather bulky for intraoral work. As in all other areas, lesions should be excised where possible rather than vaporized.

In the removal of lesions from the mucosa of the oral cavity, underlying soft tissues on the floor of the mouth, fauces and cheek may be removed *en bloc* with the lesion, and as the healing of laser wounds is associated with a low number of myofibroblasts and little collagen in the defect, it appears that there is significantly less contracture of laser cut wounds, and large defects may be left open and ungrafted.

If the lesion involves bone, it may be exposed during the dissection if radiotherapy has not been given, and bone may be removed slowly and at a high temperature. However, if radiotherapy has been given there is a significant risk of osteoradionecrosis if bone is exposed or damaged.

Benign, premalignant and malignant lesions may be removed without significant bleeding and with low postoperative morbidity. Rhys-Evans *et al.* (1984) reported the management of 51 lesions, 44 of which were leucoplakia in 34 patients, and their series confirms the advantages of the CO_2 laser in this field.

Lesions of the tongue can also be removed transorally and the limitations of transoral surgery apply, namely that the lines of resection must be visible at the outset or become visible during the course of the dissection. The lines of resection are first marked out and then cut using the laser at about 25 watts, which gives both good cutting and coagulation of vessels. Bleeding should be minimal and haemostasis can be achieved with a few points of diathermy and ligatures on the lingual artery.

Standard 'cancer margins' must be observed for malignant lesions as the CO_2 laser does not, in itself, cure cancer and the ability of the surgeon to control malignant disease will depend on the removal of a specimen with histologically free margins. However, it has been suggested that the limited tissue manipulation and sealing of lymphatics may lead to improved 'cure rates', but confirmation of this from controlled trials is needed.

It has been shown that muscle in the mouth epithelializes rapidly and defects may be left ungrafted and unsutured. This enables residual tongue muscle to hypertrophy and, untethered by sutures, the tongue regains maximal residual function.

Healing appears to be relatively rapid, although it has been shown that laser defects heal rather more slowly than scalpel cut wounds. There is minimal postoperative oedema and postoperative pain is also slight. Patients can resume their normal diet in the evening on the day of surgery and nasogastric feeding is rarely, if ever, needed.

In the author's series (Carruth, 1985a) of 100 major tongue procedures performed by laser, 45% needed no analgesics, 32% mild oral analgesics and 85% could be discharged on the first or second postoperative day.

The management of carcinoma of the tongue has not changed significantly, except that slightly larger lesions may be removed by laser for cure by excision biopsy and, occasionally, larger lesions will be excised in the elderly, infirm patient in whom a laser excision has a lower morbidity than a course of radiation. Primary excision may also be performed in young patients where radiotherapy is relatively contraindicated. In all other cases, the laser will be used to resect residual or recurrent tumour after radiation failure.

In the author's series, in which the majority of patients have been follwed up for two to three years, 100% of T1N0 tumours treated by excision biopsy are disease free, and for larger T2 and T3 tumours a 'cure rate' of more than 60% has been achieved, which compares favourably with historical controls.

Pharyngeal pouch

The pharyngeal pouch or hypopharyngeal diverticulum may be treated either by external excision, followed by cricopharyngeus myotomy, or by an endoscopic technique based on the procedure described by Dohlman (1949).

In a recent update of their earlier paper by van Overbeek, Hoeksema and Edens (1984), the endoscopic treatment of 377 patients is described, in which 308 were treated by electrocoagulation and excision and 69 were treated by laser excision of the 'party wall' between pouch and oesophagus. With the laser technique under microscopic control and with the use of a specially developed endoscope, the bridge is excised with accuracy and with minimal bleeding.

It might be thought that the lack of tissue reaction adjacent to the laser wound would not encourage adhesions between pouch and oesophagus and might, therefore, lead to leakage and the development of mediastinitis. Although three cases of mediastinitis were reported in 69 laser cases, compared to five in 308 cases treated by the standard technique, van Overbeek considered that this was acceptable and that the final results were better without any of the circumferential scarring which was found on occasions with the electrocoagulation and excision technique.

Endobronchial surgery

Both the CO_2 and Nd-YAG lasers are in use for the removal of lesions from the tracheobronchial tree, and in some of the early work described by Hetzel *et al.* (1983), the argon laser was used although, for fibreoptic work, this has now been almost totally replaced by the Nd-YAG laser.

The use of the CO_2 laser in this field was first described by Strong *et al.* (1974), and since that time bronchoscopic adaptors have been developed for use with almost all CO_2 surgical lasers (*Figure 23.13*). There are considerable design differences in the adaptors, as described previously, and in particular the aiming facilities vary from a fixed

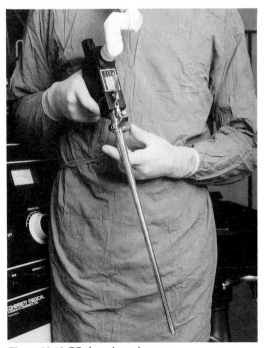

Figure 23.13 CO_2 laser bronchoscope

beam through a static readjustment with thumb-screws, to continuous aiming with a micromanipulator. Almost all bronchoscopes provide adequate distal suction.

Nd-YAG laser energy can be transmitted by a flexible fibre and it can, therefore, be used with a fibreoptic bronchoscope. In theory, it could be used to remove more peripherally placed lesions which are inaccessible to the rigid instrument that has to be used with the CO_2 laser. However, in practice, palliation can be achieved regularly only by the removal of tumour from the trachea or main bronchi, and this may be done through either bronchoscope. Much of the work with the Nd-YAG laser is done using a rigid bronchoscope to enable fragments of necrotic tumour to be removed with forceps and to provide better suction.

A relatively small number of cases using the CO_2 laser have been reported in the literature, and McElvein and Zorn (1983) described the management of 43 patients with malignant disease of the trachea and bronchi, treated for palliation which was achieved immediately in 39.

Several series of cases of carcinoma of the bronchus treated for palliation with the Nd-YAG laser have been reported by Toty *et al.* (1981), Dumon *et al.* (1982), Hetzel *et al.* (1983) and McDougal and Cortese (1983). The series all include between 22 and 50 patients, and in at least 50% of these considerable palliation could be achieved, but not in cases where there was total obstruction of a bronchus with collapse of the lung. In these, although re-expansion could, on occasions, be achieved, the risk of pneumonia appeared to be extremely high.

Benign tumours may be removed and the recurrence rate will depend on the histology and natural history in each case. Stenoses may also be 'cored out' and the chance of cure depends on the integrity of the cartilaginous support of the airway, the thickness of the stenosis, the amount of the circumference of the airway which it occupies, and carinal involvement, as reported by Ossoff *et al.* (1985) who successfully treated eight of 14 patients.

The CO_2 laser produces better and more precise tissue destruction and the Nd-YAG laser better haemostasis, although severe problems with bleeding have not been regularly reported with the use of the CO_2 laser.

The oesophagus

A number of series have been reported by Fleischer and Kessler (1983), Mellow, Pinkus and Frank (1983). Krasner and Beard (1984), and Swain *et al.* (1984) to show that obstructing tumours of the oesophagus may be treated for palliation by removal of the tumour by means of the Nd-YAG laser. Many treatment sessions may be needed initially to relieve the dysphagia, but prolonged palliation may be achieved by repeating the procedure as often as is necessary. As mentioned previously, this laser produces three layers of thermal tissue damage: the first, a vaporized layer; the second, a coagulated layer, which will subsequently slough; and a third layer in which cell death occurs and which is replaced by fibrous tissue but without loss of physical integrity. This means that the risk of perforation, even if the tumour involves the whole thickness of the oesophageal wall, is slight.

It is not possible to palliate untreatable tumours of the postcricoid region by the passage of an indwelling tube and, in such cases, where cure is not possible, the laser may be of great value in providing palliation.

Otology

The role of lasers in otology is currently being evaluated, and although the argon laser offers some potential advantages, these await confirmation by controlled trials. The value of lasers in this field is not widely accepted.

Some work has been carried out with the CO_2 laser to perform myringotomies and to vaporize the stapes footplate in experimental animals. However, many believe that this laser is not suitable for otological work.

The argon laser has been used to perform atraumatic 'no touch' stapedectomies in the hope that the lack of manipulation might lead to less inner ear damage. Critics suggest that when the argon laser beam has penetrated the footplate of the stapes, it could pass through the perilymph and be absorbed by a vascular structure on the saccule. However, as yet, neither the advantages nor the potential hazard have been shown clearly in the reported clinical work.

The argon laser is coupled to the operating microscope which incorporates a safety shutter which closes when the laser is fired. An attenuated beam is used for aiming, guided by a micromanipulator, and spot sizes of 50–100 μm are used.

Perkins (1980) reported a series of argon laser stapedectomies and suggested that the atraumatic technique might result in better preservation of high tone hearing and less vestibular disturbance. In his technique, the laser was used for haemostasis during the tympanotomy and for dividing the stapedius and the posterior crus of the stapes, and partially dividing the anterior crus. A rosette of perforations was then made in the footplate,

enabling a small piece to be removed to accept a prosthesis.

McGee (1983) compared 100 small fenestra stapedectomies with 100 performed with the argon laser and found that the postoperative course in the laser cases was smoother, but he could not find any significant difference in audiometric results.

The argon laser has also been used for the removal of granulation tissue, for the removal of dense fibrous tissue from the mastoid in revision procedures, and to spot weld a graft of fascia on to the drum remnant in myringoplasty.

Otoneurosurgery

Glasscock, Jackson and Whitaker (1981) reported the use of the argon laser in the removal of 25 acoustic neuromata in a series of 48 tumours. They exposed the lesion and then, by applying a power of 3–3.5 watts, used the laser first to 'gut' the tumour and then to remove the capsule. At these power levels, tumour removal was slow, but they found the laser to be of value in the management of small inaccessible lesions which were difficult to remove with forceps.

Gardner, Robertson and Clark (1983) used the CO_2 laser in 15 cerebellopontine angle tumours in a series of 105, and found it to be of value for the rapid atraumatic removal of tumour tissue. However, Powers *et al.* (1984) initially used the CO_2 laser and then changed to an argon laser, which they found to be more suitable for the removal of acoustic neuromata.

Nasal surgery

The CO_2 laser can be used to perform precise 'dermabrasion' for the treatment of rhinophyma, whereas the argon laser is of great value in the management of cutaneous vascular abnormalities of the skin of the nose. In addition, the argon laser can be used to coagulate the telangiectatic spots of Osler's disease, but, as with all other techniques, there is a tendency for the lesions to recur elsewhere.

With regard to the nasal cavity, Simpson *et al.* (1982) reported on the use of the CO_2 laser for the removal of a wide range of lesions including papillomata, nasal polyps, adhesions and granulomata. The series also included one malignant case treated for palliation through a lateral rhinotomy. The use of both the CO_2 and argon lasers for the performance of turbinate reduction has also been reported.

If adequate access is possible then the CO_2 laser can be used to remove lesions from the nose, but its advantages in this field are limited.

However, Healey *et al.* (1978) reported that the CO_2 laser can be used transnasally to resect the obstructing partition in choanal atresia; and Williams (1983) has suggested that in the performance of a vidian neurectomy for intractable rhinorrhea, the CO_2 laser may be used to destroy the contents of the vidian canal after a standard bony approach, and has stated that the operation could be performed as a day case procedure with improved patient comfort.

The CO_2 laser can undoubtedly be used to ablate untreatable fungating tumours for palliation, as reported by Rontal and Rontal (1983).

Photodynamic therapy

This technique represents a new and exciting approach to the management of many forms of localized, malignant disease.

Research is concentrated, at present, on the indentification of an ideal tumour sensitizer which should be selectively taken up or retained by malignant tissues, giving a high tumour/normal tissue ratio. Such a sensitizer should be non-toxic in clinically useful doses; it should have a high level of photochemical activity; and it should be activated by a wavelength of light which provides adequate tissue penetration.

To date, the only tumour sensitizer which has been developed to a point at which clinical trials are appropriate, is the haematoporphyrin derivative which is activated by red light at a wavelength of 630 nm produced by either a tunable dye or gold vapour laser.

The tumour sensitizer

Although many substances have been investigated, most of the work has been on the porphyrins and on haematoporphyrin derivative in particular, which was first used by Lipson, Baldes and Olsen (1964) for the identification of malignant tumours. Recently, Dougherty, Potter and Weishaupt (1983) have reported the identification of the active component from the mixture of porphyrins as dihaematoporphyrin ether, but others consider that further work on the identification of the active component is appropriate.

Much of the research into the development of a new sensitizer is concentrated on the phthalocyanines and these appear very promising. Uroporphyrin I was also hailed as the ideal sensitizer by El Far and Pimstone (1983), but their results have not yet been confirmed.

It seems certain that other better sensitizers than haemtoporhyrin derivative will be developed, but it will be several years before another is ready for clinical trials.

Light sources

The laser is somewhat peripheral to the technique of photodynamic therapy and many early studies were carried out with a wide range of both filtered and unfiltered light sources. However, it became apparent that lasers provided the ideal source of pure light, and, of sufficient power, which could be transmitted via a flexible fibre.

The first laser to be used was the tunable dye laser, described previously, which has the advantage that the wavelength can be changed to activate other sensitizers which may be developed in the future, but has the disadvantage that the power output is limited to, at best, 25% of the power of the driving argon laser. The gold vapour laser produces pulsed, red light at a fixed wavelength of 628 nm and high power levels are available. It has been suggested that the pulsed light might penetrate more deeply into tissues than the continuous wave light produced by the dye laser, but subsequent work has not confirmed these findings. As this laser has a fixed wavelength, it cannot be tuned to activate other sensitizers. However, it is relatively easy to change the metal in the tube to copper and the copper vapour laser could be used to drive a tunable dye laser.

Haematoporphyrin derivative is activated best by ultraviolet light but this does not adequately penetrate tissues. Therefore, the 'compromise' wavelength of 630 nm is used which activates haematoporphyrin derivative and, with surface irradiation, penetrates most tissues to a depth of up to 1 cm.

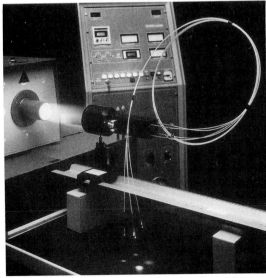

Figure 23.14 Gold vapour laser with multifibre delivery system

A number of delivery fibres are now available with a straight cut or microlens tip for surface irradiation, a diffusing cylinder to treat circumferential lesions or for implantation into tumours, and a diffusing bulb to irradiate the whole of the inner wall of a hollow viscus.

Mode of action

Much of the credit for the development of this technique must be given to Dr Tom Dougherty and his colleagues at Roswell Park Memorial Institute, Buffalo, USA. It has been shown that after an intravenous injection, haematoporphyrin derivative is widely distributed in body tissues and is then selectively retained by malignant tumours. The mechanism for this retention remains uncertain, but it is thought to be related to the abnormal tumour circulation.

It has been shown by Weishaupt, Gomer and Dougherty (1976) that when haematoporphyrin derivative is exposed to red light, singlet oxygen is produced by energy transfer from the excited porphyrin molecule. This highly reactive, transient state of the oxygen molecule is cytotoxic by oxidation of sensitive bonds.

There appears to be photodynamic activity within the vascular stroma, as shown by Henderson and Dougherty (1983), and also at cellular level, as shown by Moan *et al.* (1982).

Diagnosis

When a tumour which contains haematoporphyrin derivative is exposed to ultraviolet light, it will fluoresce. Some exciting work has been reported on the diagnosis of early lung tumours by a fluorescent bronchoscopic technique, which uses a krypton laser as the source of ultraviolet light, and an image intensifier used with a fibreoptic bronchoscope to identify the areas of fluorescence. Some of these tumours have been treated when surgery was refused or deemed inappropriate and there have been some exciting early results. The technique is also used to diagnose malignant areas in multifocal disease of the bladder.

Treatment technique

In all the clinical studies, essentially the same technique has been used. On day one, the patient is given haematoporphyrin derivative or dihaematoporphyrin ether by intravenous injection, in a dose of 3 mg/kg body weight for haematoporphyrin derivative (dihaematoporphyrin ether, 1.5–2 mg/kg). No significant side-effects have been reported from the injection, but all patients develop severe skin photosensitization which lasts for three to four weeks.

After 72 hours, the tumour is photoirradiated using a laser and delivery fibre. Subcutaneous disease is treated to a dose of 25 joules/cm^2 which will destroy the tumour but preserve the overlying skin; whereas ulcerated lesions are treated to a total dose of 100–200 joules/cm^2 which will cause maximal tumour necrosis to a depth of 1 cm with surface irradiation.

The treatment can be repeated as often as necessary, both to remove further layers of thick tumour or to treat other new lesions.

The time taken will depend on the power output of the laser and the area to be treated, but for large tumours with a low power laser the time may be measured in hours.

Clinical trials

It has been estimated that more than 5000 patients have now been treated by this technique, and much of the work has been carried out on primary and secondary skin tumours. Dougherty has estimated that local control can be achieved in 60–80% of patients with multinodular metastatic disease of the chest wall from breast carcinoma. Basal cell carcinoma which has failed other modalities, and in particular multiple lesions, can readily be treated, with excellent results. Several head and neck series have now been reported. These tumours appear ideal for this form of therapy as they are relatively small, remain localized, are accessible, and surgery is always mutilating, either to the cosmetic appearance of the patient or to his ability to talk and swallow.

The largest number of patients has been treated by Wile *et al.* (1982, 1984) who treated 114 tumour sites in 39 patients. In 28 sites, complete tumour response was obtained and 'several' remained tumour free for more than one year. A partial response was obtained in 42 patients but the others were either not measurable or showed no response. They found that patients with persistent or recurrent disease in the primary site benefited substantially from treatment and that tumours of the tongue appeared to be particularly sensitive to this form of therapy.

Other series, reported by Carruth and McKenzie (1985), Keller, Doiron and Fisher (1985) and Schuller, McCaughan and Rock (1985), have shown that in the advanced tumours which are ethically permitted to be treated in pilot studies, it is possible to produce tumour necrosis, with the result that palliation can be achieved in many cases and local control in some.

Basal cell carcinomata have appeared to respond well, and this treatment is particularly appropriate for multiple lesions which are extremely difficult to treat by other modalities. When, on occasions, small recurrent tumours have been treated where no other modality is available, for example in the nasopharynx, local control has been achieved, but the period of follow-up remains short.

Head and neck tumours appear to be most suitable for treatment by photodynamic therapy and it appears likely that this modality will soon be introduced into controlled trials of combined therapy.

References

ANDERSON, M. C. (1981) Treatment of cervical intraepithelial neoplasia with the carbon dioxide laser: report of 543 patients. *Obstetrics and Gynecology*, **55**, 541

ANNYAS, A. A., VAN OVERBEEK, J. J. D., ESCAJADILLO, J. R. and HOEKSMA, P. E. (1984) CO_2 laser in malignant disease of the larynx. *The Laryngoscope*, **94**, 836

BENJAMIN, B. and CROXSON, G. (1985) Vocal cord granulomas. *Annals of Otology, Rhinology and Laryngology*, **94**, 538

BENKE, A., GLANINGER, J., FISCHER, P. L. and PRAMESBERGER, G. (1985) A new anaesthetic technique for laser surgery of the larynx. *Proceedings of the Sixth Conference of the International Society for Laser Surgery*, Jerusalem, 27

BLAKESLEE, D., VAUGHAN, C. W., SHAPSHAY, S. M., SIMPSON, G. T. and STRONG, M. S. (1984) Excisional biopsy in the selective management of T_1 glottic cancer: 3-year follow-up study. *The Laryngoscope*, **94**, 488

CARRUTH, J. A. S. (1985a) Tongue resection with the CO_2 laser: 100 cases. *Journal of Laryngology and Otology*, **99**, 887

CARRUTH, J. A. S. (1985b) Laryngeal microsurgery: instrumentation and technique. *Journal of Laryngology and Otology*, **99**, 573

CARRUTH, J. A. S. and McKENZIE, A. L. (1985) Preliminary report of a pilot study of photoradiation therapy for the treatment of superficial malignancies of the skin, head and neck. *European Journal of Surgical Oncology*, **11**, 47

CARRUTH, J. A. S. and McKENZIE, A. L. (1986) New concepts in cancer therapy: photoradiation therapy. In *Head and Neck Oncology*, edited by H. J. Bloom, pp. 315–318. New York: Raven Press

CARRUTH, J. A. S., MORGAN, M. J., NIELSEN, M. S., PHILLIPPS, J. J. and WAINWRIGHT, A. C. (1986) The treatment of laryngeal stenosis using the CO_2 laser. *Clinical Otolaryngology*, **11**, 145–148

COCHRANE, J. P. S., BEACON, J. P., CREASEY, G. H., and RUSSELL, R. C. G. (1980) Wound healing after laser surgery: an experimental study. *British Journal of Surgery*, **67**, 740

COLMAN, M. F. and CONWAY, M. (1985) Prevention of facial burns during laser laryngoscopy. *The Laryngoscope*, **95**, 349

CROFT, C. B. (1984) The use of the carbon dioxide laser in the treatment of bilateral abducta paralysis of the vocal cords. *Proceedings of the Third Annual Conference of the British Medical Laser Association*

DEDO, H. H. and JACKLER, K. (1982) Laryngeal papilloma: Results of treatment with the CO_2 laser and podophyllum. *Annals of Otology, Rhinolology and Laryngology*, **91**, 425–430

DEDO, H. H. and SOOY, C. D. (1984) Endoscopic laser repair of posterior glottic, subglottic and tracheal stenosis by division and micro trapdoor flap. *The Laryngoscope*, **94**, 445

DI BARTOLOMEO, J. R. (1981) The argon and CO_2 lasers in otolaryngology: which one, when and why? *The Laryngoscope*, Suppl. 26, 1–16

DI BARTOLOMEO, J. R. and ELLIS, M. (1980) The argon laser in otology. *The Laryngoscope*, **90**, 1786–1796

DOHLMAN, G. (1949) Endoscopic operations for hypopharyngeal diverticula. *Proceedings of the 4th International Congress of Otolaryngology*

DOUGHERTY, T. J., POTTER, W. R. and WEISHAUPT, K. R. (1983) The structure of the active component of hematoporphyrin derivative. In *Porphyrins in Tumour Phototherapy*, edited by A. Andreoni and R. Cubeddu, pp. 23–35. New York: Plenum

DUMON, J. F., REBOUD, E., GARBE, L., AUCOMTE, F. and MERIC, B. (1982) Treaatment of tracheobronchial lesions by laser photoresection. *Chest*, **81**, 278–284

DUNCAVAGE, J. A., OSSOFF, R. H. and TOOHILL, R. J. (1985) Carbon dioxide laser management of laryngeal stenosis. *Annals of Otology, Rhinology and Laryngology*, **94**, 565

DYSON, M. and YOUNG, S. (1986) Effect of laser therapy on wound contraction and cellularity in mice. *Lasers in Medical Science*, **1**, 125

EL FAR, M. A. and PIMSTONE, N. R. (1983) Superiority of Uroporphyrin I over other porphyrins in selective tumour localization. *Proceedings of the Clayton Foundation Symposium on Porphyrin Localization and Treatment of Tumours*. Santa Barbara, California

EVANS, J. N. G. and TODD, G. B. (1974) Laryngotracheoplasty. *Journal of Laryngology and Otology*, **88**, 589

FREARON, B. and COTTON, R. J. (1974) Surgical correction of subglottic stenosis of the larynx in infants and children: progress report. *Annals of Otology, Rhinology and Laryngology*, **83**, 428

FISHER, S. E., FRAME, J. W., BROWNE, R. M. and TRANTER, R. M. D. (1983) A comparative histological study of wound healing following CO_2 laser and conventional surgical excision of canine buccal mucosa. *Archives of Aural Biology*, **28**, 287

FLEISCHER D. and KESSLER, F. (1983) Endoscopic Nd-YAG laser therapy for carcinoma of the oesophagus: a new form of palliative treatment. *Gastroenterology*, **85**, 600

GARDNER, G., ROBERTSON, J. H. and CLARK, W. C. (1983) 105 patients operated upon for cerebello-pontine angle tumours – experience using combined approach and CO_2 laser. *The Laryngoscope*, **93**, 1049

GLASSCOCK, M. E., JACKSON, C. E. and WHITAKER, S. R. (1981) Argon laser in acoustic tumour surgery. *The Laryngoscope*, **91**, 1405

GOEPFERT, H., SESSIONS, R. B., GUTTERMAN, J. U., CANGIR, A., DICHTEL, W. J. and SULEK, E. (1982) Leukocyte interferon in patients with juvenile laryngeal papillomatosis. *Annals of Otology, Rhinology and Laryngology*, **91**, 431

HAGLUND, S., LUNDQUIST, P. G., CANTELL, K. and STRANDER, H. (1981) Interferon therapy in juvenile laryngeal papillomatosis. *Archives of Otolaryngology*, **107**, 327

HEALEY, G. B. (1982) Experimental models for the endoscopic correction of subglottic stenosis with clinical applications. *The Laryngoscope, 92,* 1103

HEALEY, G. B., McGILL, T., STRONG, M. S., JAKO, G. J. and VAUGHAN, C. W. (1978) Management of choanal atresia with the carbon dioxide laser. *Annals of Otology, Rhinology and Laryngology, 87,* 2–5

HENDERSON, B. W. and DOUGHERTY, T. J. (1983) Studies on the mechanism of tumour destruction by photoradiation therapy (PRT). *Proceedings of the Clayton Foundation Symposium on Porphyrin Localization and Treatment of Tumours.* Santa Barbara, California

HERBERT, J. J., BERLIN, I. and EBERLE, R. (1985) Jet ventilation via a copper endotracheal tube for CO_2 laser surgery of the auropharynx. *The Laryngoscope, 95,* 1276

HETZEL, A. R., MILLARD, F. J. C., AYESH, R., BRIDGES, C., NANSON, A. and SWAIN, C. B. (1983) Laser treatment of carcinoma of the bronchus. *British Medical Journal, 286,* 12–16

HISAZUMI, H., NAITO, K., MISAKKI, T., KOSHIDA, K. and YAMAMOTO, H. (1985) An experimental study of photodynamic therapy using a pulsed gold vapour laser. In *Photodynamic Therapy of Tumours and Other Diseases,* edited by G. Jori and C. Perria, pp. 251–254. Padova: Edizioni Libreria Progetto

HOLINGER, L. D. (1982) Treatment of severe subglottic stenosis without tracheostomy: preliminary report. *Annals of Otology, Rhinology and Laryngology, 91,* 407–412

HOLLINGER, P. H., KUTNICK, S. L., SCHILD, J. and HOLINGER, L. D. (1976) Subglottic stenosis in infants and children. *Annals of Otology, Rhinology and Laryngology, 85,* 591

HOLZER, P. and ASCHER, P. W. (1979) Laser surgery of peripheral nerves. In *Laser Surgery,* edited by I. Kaplan and P. W. Ascher, Vol. 3, part 2, p. 149. Jerusalem: Academic

JAIN, K. K. (1983) Lasers in neurosurgery: A review. *Lasers in Medicine and Surgery, 2,* 217–230

KAUFMAN, J. A., THOMPSON, J. N. and KOHUT, R. I. (1981) Endoscopic measurement of subglottic stenosis with the CO_2 surgical laser. *Otolaryngology Head and Neck Surgery, 89,* 215

KIEFHABER, P., NATH, G. and MORITZ, K. (1977) Endoscopical control of massive gastrointestinal hemorrhage by irradiation with a high power Nd-YAG laser. *Progress in Surgery, 15,* 140–155

KELLER, G. S., DOIRON, D. R. and FISHER, G. U. (1985) Photodynamic therapy in otolaryngology – head and neck surgery. *Archives of Otolaryngology, 111,* 758

KELLY, D. F., BOWN, S. G., CALDER, B. M., PEARSON, H., WEAVER, B. M. Q., SWAIN, C. P. *et al.* (1983) Histological changes following Nd-YAG laser photocoagulation of canine gastric mucosa. *Gut, 24,* 914–920

KETCHAM, A. S., HOYE, R. C. and RIGGLE, G. C. (1967) A surgeon's appraisal of the laser. *Surgical Clinics of North America, 47,* 1249–1263

KOLLE, I., IVERSON, P. and PAULSEN, J. (1985) CO_2 laser stripping in polypoid degeneration of the vocal cords. *Proceedings of the Sixth Congress of the International Society for Laser Surgery and Medicine,* p. 32. Jerusalem

KRASNER, N. and BEARD, J. (1984) Laser irradiation of tumours of the oesophagus and cardia. *British Medical Journal, 288,* 829

LIPSON, R. L., BALDES, E. J. and OLSEN, A. M. (1964) A further evaluation of the use of hematoporphyrin derivative as a new aid for the endoscopic detection of malignant disease. *Diseases of the Chest, 46,* 676

LYONS, G. D., OWENS, R., LOUSTEAU, R. J. and TRAIL, M. L. (1980) Carbon dioxide laser treatment of laryngeal stenosis. *Archives of Otolaryngology, 106,* 255

McCABE, B. F. and CLARK, K. F. (1983) Interferon and laryngeal papillomatosis. The Iowa experience. *Annals of Otology, Rhinology and Laryngology, 92,* 1

McDOUGAL, J. C. and CORTESE, D. A. (1983) Neodymium YAG laser therapy of malignant airway obstruction. *Mayo Clinic Proceedings, 58,* 35

McELVEIN, R. B. and ZORN, G. (1983) The treatment of malignant disease in trachea and main stem bronchi by carbon dioxide laser. *Journal of Thoracic and Cardiovascular Surgery, 86,* 858

McGEE, T. M. (1983) Argon laser in surgery for chronic ear disease and otosclerosis. *The Laryngoscope, 93,* 1177

McGEE, K. C., NAGLE, J. W. and TOOHILL, R. J. (1981) CO_2 laser repair of subglottic and upper tracheal stenosis. *Otolaryngology Head and Neck Surgery, 89,* 92

McKENZIE, A. L. (1983) How far does thermal damage extend beneath the surface of CO_2 laser incisions. *Physics in Medicine and Biology, 28,* 905–912

MAIMAN, T. H. (1960) Stimulated optical radiation in ruby. *Nature, 187,* 493–494

MELLOW, M., PINKUS, H. and FRANK, J. (1983) Endoscopic therapy for oesophageal carcinoma with Nd-YAG laser prospective evaluation of efficacy, complications and survival. *Gastrointestinal Endoscopy, 29,* 161

MESTER, E., MESTER, A. and MESTER, A. (1985) The biomedical effects of laser application. *Lasers in Surgery and Medicine, 5,* 31

MEYER-SCHWICKERATH, G. (1956) Erfaroungen mit der Licht Koagulation der Netzhaut und der Iris. *Documenta Ophthalmologica, 10,* 91–131

MIHASHI, S., JAKO, G. J., INCZE, J., STRONG, M. S. and VAUGHAN, C. W. (1976) Laser surgery in otolaryngology: interaction of CO_2 laser and soft tissue. *Annals of the New York Academy of Science, 267,* 263–295

MINTON, J. P., CARLTON, D. M., DEARMAN, J. R., McKNIGHT, W. B. and KETCHAM, A. S. (1965) An evaluation of the physical response of malignant tumour implants to pulsed laser radiation. *Surgery in Gynaecology and Obstetrics, 121,* 538–544

MOAN, J., JOHANNESSEN, J. V., CHRISTENSEN, T., ESPERIK, T. and McGHIE, J. B. (1982) Porphyrin-sensitized photoinactivation of human cells in vitro. *American Journal of Pathology, 109,* 184

MOESGARD-NEILSEN, V., HØJSLET, P. E. and KARLMOSE, M. (1986) Surgical treatment of Reinke's oedema (long term results). *Journal of Laryngology and Otology, 100,* 187

MOTTA, G. (1985) Endoscopic resection of malignant tumours of the larynx. *International Laser Conference, Bolognia*

NORTON, M. L. and De VOS, P. (1978) A new endotracheal tube for laser surgery of the larynx. *Annals of Otology, Rhinology and Laryngology, 87,* 554–558

OOSTERHUIS, J. W. (1978) Lymphocytic migration after laser surgery. *The Lancet, i,* 446

OOSTERHUIS, J. W., VERSCHUEREN, R. C. J., EIBERGEN, R. and OLDHOFF, J. (1982) The viability of cells in the waste products of CO_2 laser evaporation of the Cloudman mouse melanoma. *Cancer, 49,* 61

OSSOFF, R. H., SISSON, G. A., DUCAVAGE, J. A., MOSELLE, H. I., ANDREWS, P. E. and McMILLAN, W. G. (1984) Endoscopic laser arytenoidectomy for treatment of bilateral vocal cord paralysis. *The Laryngoscope*, **94**, 1293

OSSOFF, R. H., SISSON, G. A. and SHAPSHAY, S. M. (1985) Endoscopic management of selected early vocal cord carcinoma. *Annals of Otology, Rhinology and Laryngology*, **94**, 560

OSSOFF, R. H., TUCKER, G. F., DUNCAVAGE, J. A. and TOOHILL, R. J. (1985) Efficacy of bronchoscopic carbon dioxide laser surgery for benign strictures of the trachea. *The Laryngoscope*, **95**, 1220

PERKINS, C. R. (1980) Laser stapedectomy for otosclerosis. *The Laryngoscope*, **90**, 228–241

POWERS, S. K., EDWARDS, M. S. B., BOGGAN, J. E., PITTS, L. H., GUTIN, T. H. and HOSOIBUCHI, Y. (1984) Use of the argon surgical laser in neurosurgery. *Journal of Neurosurgery*, **60**, 523

PRASAD, U. (1985) CO_2 surgical laser in the management of bilateral vocal cord paralysis. *Journal of Laryngology and Otology*, **99**, 891

RHYS-EVANS, P. H., FRAME, J. W., DASGUPTA, A. R. and DALTON, G. A. (1984) Use of the carbon dioxide laser in the management of pre-malignant lesions of the oral mucosa. *Journal of Laryngology and Otology*, **98**, 1251

RONTAL, M. and RONTAL, E. (1983) Treatment of recurrent carcinoma at the base of the skull with carbon dioxide laser. *The Laryngoscope*, **93**, 1261

SAITO, R., DATE, R., UNO, K., UEDA, S., QUIJANO, M. and OGURA, Y. (1985) Treatment of juvenile laryngeal papilloma with a combination of laser surgery and Interferon. *Auris-Nasus-Larynx (Tokyo)*, **12**, 117

SCHAWLOW, A. L. and TOWNES, C. H. (1958) Infrared and optical masers. *Physics Review*, **112**, 1940–1949

SHAHEEN, O. H. (1984) The carbon dioxide laser in the treatment of bilateral vocal cord paralysis. In *Problems in Head and Neck Surgery*, p.9. London: Baillière Tindall

SHUGAR, J. M. A., SOM, P. M. and BILLER H. F. (1982) An evaluation of the carbon dioxide laser in the treatment of traumatic laryngeal stenosis. *The Laryngoscope*, **92**, 23

SCHULLER, D. E., McCAUGHAN, J. S. and ROCK, R. P. (1985) Photodynamic therapy in head and neck cancer. *Archives of Otolaryngology*, **111**, 351

SIMPSON, G. T., SHAPSHAY, S. M., VAUGHAN, C. W. and STRONG, M. S. (1982) Rhinologic surgery with the carbon dioxide laser. *The Laryngoscope*, **92**, 412–415

SIMPSON, G. T., STRONG, M. S., HEALEY, G. D., SHAPSHAY, S. M. and VAUGHAN, C. W. (1982) Predictive factors of success or failure in the endoscopic managment of laryngeal and tracheal stenosis. *Annals of Otology, Rhinology and Laryngology*, **91**, 384–388

STEWARD, D. J. and FEARON, B. (1981) Anaesthesia for laryngoscopy. *British Journal of Anaesthetics*, **53**, 320

STRONG, M. S. (1975) Laser excision of carcinoma of the larynx. *The Laryngoscope*, **85**, 1286

STRONG, M. S., HEALEY, G. B., VAUGHAN, C. W., FRIED, M. P. and SHAPSHAY, S. (1979a) Endoscopic management of laryngeal stenosis. *Otolaryngology Clinics of North America*, **12**, 797

STRONG, M. S., JAKO, G. J., VAUGHAN, C. W., HEALEY, G. B. and POLANYI, T. (1976a) The use of the CO_2 laser in otolaryngology. A progress report. *Transactions of the American Academy of Ophthalmology and Otolaryngology*, **82**, 595–602

STRONG, M. S., VAUGHAN, C. W., HEALEY, G. B., GOOPERBAND, S. R. and CLEMENTE, M. A. (1976b) Recurrent respiratory papillomatosis. *Annals of Otology, Rhinology and Laryngology*, **85**, 508

STRONG, M. S., VAUGHAN, C. W., HEALEY, G. B., SHAPSHAY, S. M. and JAKO, G. J. (1979c) Transoral management of localised carcinoma of the oral cavity using CO_2 laser. *The Laryngoscope*, **89**, 897–905

STRONG, M. S., VAUGHAN, C. W., JAKO, G. J. and POLANYI, T. (1979d) Transoral resection of cancer of the oral cavity: The role of the CO_2 laser. *Otolaryngology Clinics of North America*, **12**, 207–218

STRONG, M. S., VAUGHAN, C. W., POLANYI, T. and WALLACE, R. (1974) Bronchoscopic carbon dioxide laser surgery. *Annals of Otology, Rhinology and Laryngology*, **83**, 769

SWAIN, C. P., BOWN, S. G., EDWARDS, D. A. W., KIRKHAM, J. S., SALTION, P. R. and CLARK, C. J. (1984) Laser recanalisation of obstructing foregut cancer. *British Journal of Surgery*, **71**, 121

TOOHILL, R. J., CAMPBELL, B. H. and DUNCAVAGE, J. A. (1984) CO_2 laser management of laryngeal stenosis. *Conference Presentation 1984*

TOTY, L., PERSONNE, C., COLCHEN, A. and VOURCH, G. (1981) Bronchoscopic management of tracheal lesions using the neodymium yttrium aluminium garnet laser. *Thorax*, **36**, 175–178

TRANTER, R. M. D., FRAME, J. W. and BROWNE, R. M. (1985) The healing of CO_2 laser wounds of the larynx. *Journal of Laryngology and Otology*, **99**, 895

VAN OVERBEEK, J. J. M., HOEKSEMA, P. E. and EDENS, E. T. (1984) Microendoscopic surgery of the hypopharyngeal diverticulum using electrocoagulation or carbon dioxide laser. *Annals of Otology, Rhinology and Laryngology*, **93**, 34–36

VECERINA, S. and KRAJINA, Z. (1983) Phonatory function following unilateral laser cordectomy. *Journal of Laryngology and Otology*, **97**, 1139

VIVORI, E. (1980) Anaesthesia for laryngoscopy. *British Journal of Anaesthetics*, **52**, 638

WEISHAUPT, K. R., GOMER, C. J. and DOUGHERTY, T. J. (1976) Identification of singlet oxygen as the cytotoxic agent in photo-inactivation of a murine tumour. *Cancer Research*, **36**, 2326

WILE, A. G., DAHLMAN, A., BURNS, R. G. and BERNS, M. W. (1982) Laser photoradiation therapy of cancer following hematoporphyrin sensitization. *Lasers in Surgery and Medicine*, **2**, 163

WILE, A. G., COFFEY, J., NAHOBEDION, M. Y., BAGHDESSARIAN, R., MASON, G. R. and BERNS, M. W. (1984) Laser photoradiation therapy of cancer: An update of the experience at the University of California, Irvine. *Lasers in Surgery and Medicine*, **4**, 5

WILLIAMS, J. D. (1983) Laser vidian neurectomy. *Annals of Otology, Rhinology and Laryngology*, **92**, 281

YATES, A. and DEDO, H. H. (1984) CO_2 laser enucleation of polypoid vocal cords. *The Laryngoscope*, **94**, 731

ZWENG, H. C. (1971) Lasers in ophthalmology. In *Laser Applications in Medicine and Biology*, edited by M. L. Wolbarsht, Vol. I, p. 239. New York: Plenum

24

Physiological aspects of wound healing

Principles of head and neck plastic operations and repair

William Panje

The physioclinical aspects of wound healing

Wound healing is the process by which the body seals off an injury from the external environment and restores the site to structural integrity. Although successful healing depends on the complex and simultaneous coordination of various cells and tissues, the process can be broken down into the stages of inflammation, epithelialization, mesenchymal healing, contraction, and scar formation. Some scientists refer to the various stages of wound healing as the cellular–humoral phase, the phase of glycosaminoglycan accumulation, the phase of collagen deposition and polymerization followed by remodelling of the scar.

Inflammation

Inflammation is the body's means of protecting itself against alien substances, and of disposing of dead and dying tissues, in preparation for repair of the wound. Celsus in the first century AD described the initial process of wound healing, 'Notae vero inflammationia stunt quator:rubor et tumor cum calore et dolore.' (Take heed, however, of inflammation's four indicators: redness and swelling with heat and pain.) Centuries later the response was identified with the local release of humoral substances that mediate redness, swelling, heat, and pain. A noxious agent or stimulus rather than just cell death (necrosis) appears to be the prerequisite for producing inflammation and scarring. Wound healing always follows the same sequence of processes, irrespective of the type of noxious agent which induced the tissue damage

(that is, surgery, trauma, burns, frostbite, infections), the site of the injury, or the sex or age of the patient. The only difference which may be evident is the duration or magnitude of the inflammatory response and subsequent cicatrix formation.

Immediately upon injury there is constriction of the small vessels in the area. Vascular occlusion may occur at the actual point of injury, to reduce haemorrhaging. After 5–10 minutes, vasoconstriction gives way to vasodilation. At the same time as these vascular changes are taking place, intracellular materials are being released into the extracellular compartment of injured tissue. These materials then migrate through the wound, with some of them, such as histamine and serotonin, causing increased permeability of the microcirculation. Proteolytic enzymes also help to increase permeability of the microcirculation. This increased permeability causes, in turn, an increase of proteins and cells in the area of the wound. Certain enzymes destroy noradrenaline, thereby helping to increase vasodilation.

Kallikreins – derived from the Greek word for pancreas, *kallikreas* – are enzyme(s) which convert a precursor protein into biologically active polypeptides, the kinins. One such kinin, bradykinin, is a potent local tissue hormone which mediates the four cardinal signs of inflammation described by Celsus.

During inflammation, prostaglandin levels increase. Certain prostaglandins aid vasodilation, permeability, and lymph flow. Other types of prostaglandin, including leukotrienes and lymphokines, are believed to mediate the final stages of the acute inflammatory response, thus playing a role in the initial stages of wound repair.

The cellular phase of inflammation is initially identified by the presence of blood platelets, red blood cells, polymorphonuclear leucocytes and macrophages. Other cells that subsequently participate in the inducement of inflammation are mast cells, lymphocytes and eosinophils.

Wound hypoxia and tissue bleeding usually occur in the initial stages of wound healing. Low wound oxygenation stimulates the macrophage to produce a growth factor that promotes fibroblast proliferation. Blood clot fibrin serves as a substrate for the attachment and ingrowth of cells, mainly fibroblasts.

Epithelialization

The epithelium, which covers all of the body's surfaces, acts as a barrier between the body and the environment. It keeps harmful agents from entering the body, and prevents the loss from within of essential materials, such as water. The surface layer, in particular, undergoes a good deal of wear and must constantly be replaced by the process of cell regeneration. Accordingly, the epithelium responds to a wound by intensifying the normal process of cell replacement.

The primary epithelial regeneration activity takes place in the basal cell layer of the epidermis. The epithelium is a cellular tissue composed of stratified squamous epithelial cells resting on a basal cell layer on dermal connective tissue. Injury causes the basal cells to come loose from their normally firm attachment to the dermal papillary layer, and they migrate upwards to the defective area, travelling as a sheet rather than as individual cells (Ross and Odland, 1967). Once they reach the site of injury, the cells proliferate by mitosis; cells already at the site increase their rate of mitosis. Epithelial cells migrate centripetally to cover open wounds when there are no epidermal formative cells left in the wounded area – for example following an avulsion injury or after the removal of a skin cancer. Precursor cells that give rise to skin can originate from epidermal appendages that include sweat glands, hair follicles and sebaceous glands. These structures represent an important source of the regenerating layer of epidermis when the overlying epidermis is removed, as in providing donor sites for split thickness skin grafts.

Mesenchymal healing

Repair of the connective tissue begins immediately upon injury. In the initial or cellular–humoral phase, the ground substance undergoes changes to prepare the wound for the production of collagen. The damaged tissues are replaced by collagen in order to strengthen the wound. The collagen is produced by fibroblasts that migrate to the wound area approximately 3 days after injury. This later stage of wound healing coincides with the collagen deposition and polymerization phase.

In the early stages of healing, the production of collagen exceeds the production of collagenase (which causes the breakdown of collagen). This overproduction of collagen causes the scar to be temporarily hypertrophied and to feel hard and stiff from the second week after injury until 3 or 4 months afterwards. Later, collagen breakdown may overtake collagen production, until a balance is finally reached; the healed wound will now feel soft and pliable. Widening and depression of scars are evidence of this phenomenon. The process of softening may take several months, and usually becomes clinically evident at 4–6 months. Insufficient collagen can cause scars to weaken; too much collagen can result in the formation of keloids or hypertrophic scars.

Contraction

The terms 'contraction' and 'contracture' should not be confused. Contraction is the natural process by which a wound closes, through the centripetal movement of the surrounding skin (Hunter, 1794; Carrel and Hartmann, 1916; Zahir, 1964). Contracture is the condition or the result of excessive collagen production, usually produced in response to motion; it can also be caused by contraction, or by tissue damage such as muscle fibrosis.

Wound contraction can be either desirable or detrimental, depending on the location and condition of the wound. In an area of great skin mobility, contraction can result in a wound closure with minimal scarring. When the skin is attached to underlying structures, contraction can lead to the distortion of surrounding tissues – for example the pulling down of an eyelid, which is called 'ectropion' (*Figure 24.1*). If wound contraction proceeds about a joint, permanent flexion may occur, a condition called 'flexion contracture'. In head and neck operations involving the jaw muscles, such flexion can lead to scar contraction, which can result in limited mouth opening, a condition called 'trismus'.

During contraction, the entire dermis moves over the bed of granulation tissue (*Figure 24.2*). The movement involves existing tissue at the wound edge and not newly formed tissue. Therefore, the tissue around the wound is stretched and thinned. In compensation, new epithelial cells are formed under these areas of tension, and new connective tissue is formed in the underlying dermis.

Although the skin covering a contracted wound

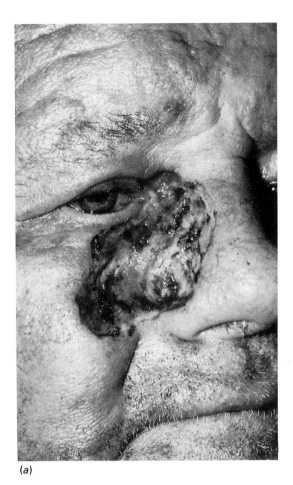

(a)

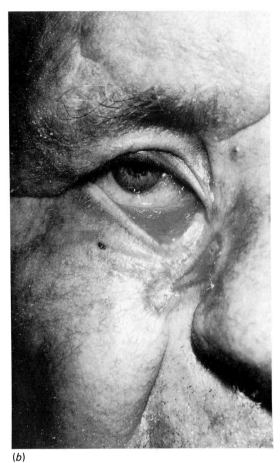

(b)

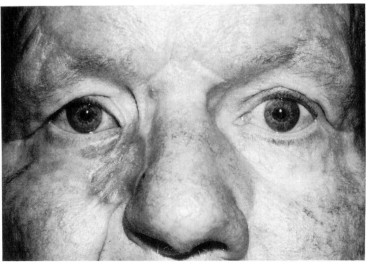

(c)

Figure 24.1 (*a*) Patient has had a skin cancer (basal cell carcinoma) removed from the side of his nose and cheek. The wound was allowed to heal by secondary intention. (*b*) Appearance of wound 4 weeks later. Note how the natural forces of wound contraction have produced a severe distortion of the eyelid (ectropion). (*c*) To repair the ectropion, scar was removed and a full thickness skin graft was applied to the area. Appearance one month following skin grafting

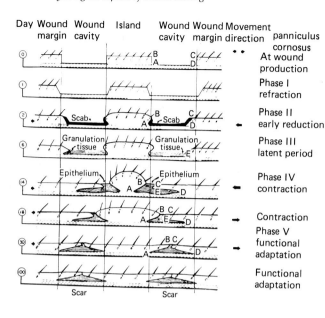

Figure 24.2 Schematic representation of closure of a full-thickness excisional wound, leaving a central island of tissue. Note that the period of most active tissue contraction occurs around day 14 following wound production. (After Luccioli, G. M., Kahn, D. S., and Robertson, H. R., 1964, *Annals of Surgery*, **160**, 1030)

may appear normal, it is nevertheless inferior to uninjured skin. Many components of the dermis are unable to regenerate; only epithelium and collagen fill in for the stretching and thinning of the skin. In addition, a scar of the connective tissue the size of the original wound exists underneath the skin.

Wound size does not affect the rate of contraction. The wound closes most rapidly after a lag phase of 5–7 days following tissue loss. However, wound geometry does affect the rate and amount of closure. Generally, circular wounds close more slowly than rectangular wounds; circular wounds also contract incompletely, if at all, because the force of contraction causes compression of the wound edges.

Remodelling of scar

During remodelling of a scar, new collagen fibres are laid down, while others are destroyed. Those that remain are usually orientated along the tension lines of the scar. For the wound to remain closed, the new collagen must be securely attached to the old collagen in the surrounding tissue. It is believed that the old and new collagen fibres become interwoven, with the new collagen fibres convolutedly cross-linked to the old (Peacock, 1984a). Remodelling of a scar is the final and long-lasting phase of fibroproductive inflammation.

As the scar ages (3–12 months), it loses water and mucopolysaccharides. This results in tighter packing of the collagen fibres and fibre bundles, which in turn aids the molecular cross-linking. As

cross-linking occurs, the collagen becomes more insoluble and more resistant to collagenase. Clinically, the incision becomes lighter in colour and scar widening ceases.

Wound healing: response to injury

Wounds heal through the processes of cell migration, cell division and the synthesis of various proteins. The result is a fibrous product, that, even when it appears close to normal, is far inferior to undamaged tissue. Rather than simply allow the body to take its own course in wound healing, the surgeon must consider all available options for the manipulation of such aspects of healing as timing, placement and closure. It is important to understand the response to injury of each of the body's components.

Skin and mucosa

The skin is a complex organ and, like other such organs, is incapable of complete regeneration. It responds to injury by contraction, epithelialization and the synthesis of fibrous tissue. Contraction plays a much greater role in wounds where there is loss of full thickness dermis than in those in which the dermis remains (*Figure 24.3*). Skin thickness varies between 0.025 and 0.233 cm depending on body location. Eyelid skin and postauricular skin are approximately 0.036 cm thick, while leg and back skin thicknesses vary from 0.147 cm to 0.233 cm respectively. Hence the removal of 0.036 cm thickness of skin from the

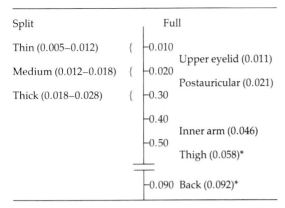

Split	Full

Thin (0.005–0.012) { ⊢0.010
                        Upper eyelid (0.011)
Medium (0.012–0.018) { ⊢0.020
                        Postauricular (0.021)
Thick (0.018–0.028) { ⊢0.30

⊢0.40
                        Inner arm (0.046)
⊢0.50
                        Thigh (0.058)*

⊢0.090 Back (0.092)*

* Thigh and back skin are too thick to act as full thickness skin grafts.

Figure 24.3 Comparison of split-thickness and full-thickness skin graft size and location

thigh leaves the dermis and adnexal structures fairly intact. Donor site contraction and scarring are usually minimal. Re-epithelialization occurs from the dermis, principally from hair follicles, sebaceous glands or sweat glands (Bell, 1973) (*Figure 24.4*). Thus another skin graft can be taken from the original donor site after 6–8 weeks of healing. If the dermis is violated, a host of variables are introduced which influence wound healing. Contraction, increased collagen production and disorganization of tissue forces can produce unsightly scarring.

After epidermal disruption, when there is not enough tissue to allow for immediate approximation of epidermis to epidermis, a graft of epidermis can be used to bridge the defect, thereby reducing

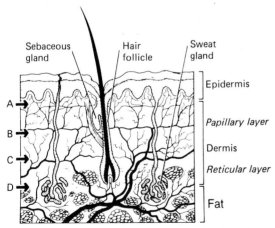

Figure 24.4 Illustration of a cross-section of a piece of skin. An incision at A produces an epidermal graft. Incisions at B or C produce a split-thickness skin graft. A full-thickness skin graft is obtained by making an incision at level D

contraction and subsequent scarring. Full thickness skin grafts which include dermis are more effective in initiating primary intention wound healing than grafts of epidermis only (Bell, 1973). Immediately following skin disruption, reapproximation of the epidermis by suturing or taping allows for reduced scar formation. This process is referred to as primary intention healing. If the epidermis cannot be immediately reapproximated, because of insufficient tissue or fear of infection, the wound can be allowed to heal by secondary intention (*Figure 24.5*) – that is, the wound closes itself naturally, influenced by such factors as location, amount of tissue loss, wound geometry, general health of patient, age and motion. Healing by secondary intention usually produces more scarring, and takes a longer period of time. The advantage of secondary healing is that the potential for infection is reduced. In fact, most head and neck surgical wounds were allowed to heal by secondary intention when antibiotics were not available.

Bone

Bone is one of the few organs of the human body capable of regeneration. Bone has exceptional reparative properties in that it can heal without scarring and can alter in response to functional demand (Pritchard, 1969).

Bone healing occurs in two phases. The first is a cellular phase which lasts 2–4 weeks, followed by the remodelling phase which may continue for a full lifespan (Ray and Sabet, 1963; Urist, 1964).

The cellular phase is stimulated by the hypoxic tissue environment around the necrotic ends of fractured bone and torn soft tissues. Specialized cells derived from the bone marrow and also the cortex produce tropocollagen which is mineralized into callus. Periosteum produces osteoprogenitor cells that form an external callus. Osteoclasts, of histiocytic blood origin, appear at the junction of living and dead bone and begin to resorb the non-viable bone. Capillary ingrowth soon occurs, which reverses the hypoxia and stimulates osteoblastic production of new bone.

New bone production is induced by a glycoprotein substance called bone morphogenic protein. In cancellous bone, the process of bone opposition or replacement takes place on the trabecular surface by means of a process called creeping substitution. In the cortical bone, by contrast, osteoclasts first have to burrow into the dead bone to produce an opening for vascular ingrowth and osteoblast production. The osteoblastic penetration of cortical bone may allow for primary bone union.

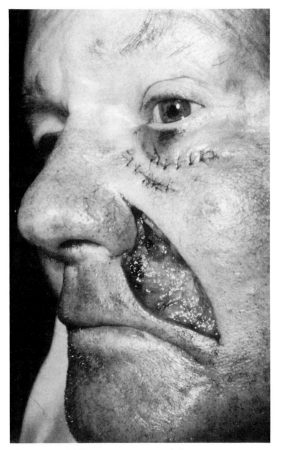

Figure 24.5 (*a*) Patient appearance following removal of a large skin cancer involving the lip and cheek

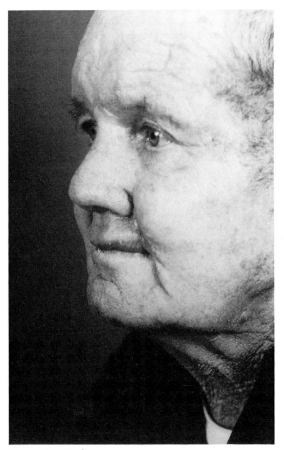

Figure 24.5 (*b*) Four weeks later the wound has completely healed by secondary intention without the use of grafts or flaps

Two types of bone exist in the facial skeleton (Rowe and Killey, 1968). Endochondral or long bone and intramembranous or flat bone are differentiated both by their anatomy and by the way in which they ossify. Bone that has epiphyses and cartilage, and forms new bone by cartilage formation, cartilage calcification, cartilage resorption and then by bone formation, is called endochondral bone. New bone formed at the epiphyseal plate during growth is called endochondral ossification. Flat bones which make up 95% of the facial skeleton and skull do not have epiphyses and are formed by direct ossification, also termed intramembranous ossification.

The blood supply of a bone determines how it will heal and also differentiates the two types of bone (Trueta and Little, 1962; Ray, 1972). Endochondral bone has three principal vascular supplies, namely nutrient, epiphyseal and periosteal. Flat bones have only a periosteal blood supply. Removal of periosteum from long bones minimally affects bone growth and repair, whereas the same

procedure carried out on flat bones significantly alters the process of bone healing.

Another differing property of endochondral and intramembranous bone is the lack of callus formation associated with the healing of the latter. Callus, initially fibrous tissue, quickly calcifies providing an internal and external biological splint for the healing of long bone fragments. From a technological point of view, it is extremely fortunate that intramembranous bone does not heal by callus formation in that facial plastic operations, such as rhinoplasty and mandibular recessions, as well as facial fractures, would produce hideous bulging deformities if callus participated in the healing process of facial bones.

Nerve

When the axon of a nerve is severed, the cell body swells for 4–20 days, until regeneration has been achieved (Cajal, 1928; Grabb, 1977). The closer the site of injury is to the cell body, the greater the amount of swelling. The ends of the severed nerve also swell; this swelling subsides about one week after injury.

The distal portion of the axon undergoes a process called wallerian degeneration. Unmyelinated fibres degenerate more rapidly than myelinated fibres. About 48 hours after injury, the myelin sheaths will begin to degenerate. Other parts of the nerve, such as the blood vessels and endoneurium, survive in the expectation that the axon will be repaired. Within 2–3 weeks, the debris of the disintegrated axons and sheaths is removed, and the vacant sheath of Schwann awaits the regenerated axon.

Although the proximal portion of the nerve also degenerates, this degeneration, unlike wallerian degeneration, extends only a few millimetres beyond the site of severance.

Within 2–21 days after injury, sprouting or budding begins on the intact segment of the axon. Six to seven days after injury, myelin sheaths begin to appear on regenerating myelinated axons. Depending on the size of the cylinders, myelin will continue to regenerate for up to one year. Recovery of motor and/or sensory functions takes from several months to as long as 5 years.

Immediate repair of a cut nerve gives the best chance for recovery. Likewise, waiting 21 days after nerve transection for optimum axon sprouting also gives a good chance for a satisfactory repair of the nerve. The assessment of cranial nerve function soon after head or facial injury is important in order to determine whether or not surgical exploration is necessary. If, following injury, the tested facial or mouth part does not move on command or stimulation, the nerve has probably been transected. On the basis of what has been learned from experimental and clinical nerve injuries, the surgeon would either repair the nerve immediately or wait 21 days. The latter situation would be preferred in situations where the patient had received multiple trauma, and there was a possibility of morbidity or mortality if a long and tedious nerve repair were undertaken.

Functional integrity of a cranial nerve can be evaluated through electrophysiological means. Sufficient direct electrical stimulation of a cranial motor nerve will cause that particular muscle group innervated by the nerve tested to contract. The muscle will contract upon electrical nerve stimulation for up to 72 hours following injury whether or not the nerve has been transected. Stimulating the nerve proximal to the transection will obviously not produce muscle contraction regardless of the intensity of the electrical stimulation. The residual capability of a nerve to function for up to 72 hours after severance aids the surgeon to find the distal part of a nerve for subsequent

repair. A surgeon confronted with the problem of whether to repair a nerve immediately or whether to wait 21 days before doing so must give consideration to this basic knowledge.

Severity of injury (*Figure 24.6*)

Nerve injuries can be classified into the following five categories:

(1) *First-degree injury.* Although conduction in the axon has been interrupted, the nerve remains intact. Sensory and motor function may be absent for a period of time ranging from a few days to several months. Some authors refer to this condition as neuropraxia. Expected recovery of nerve function is complete. Bell's palsy or idiopathic facial nerve paralysis is an example of this phenomenon.

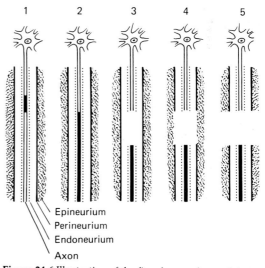

Figure 24.6 Illustration of the five classes of nerve injury

(2) *Second-degree injury.* Minimal crushing of the nerve causes wallerian degeneration of the distal portion of the axon. The endoneural tubes remain intact. Complete functioning is recovered over a period of months. This condition is frequently seen after facial trauma and temporal bone fracture. If facial movements are observed immediately following the injury with subsequent loss of function this would suggest a second-degree injury. Watchful waiting will allow time for the nerve to regenerate.

(3) *Third-degree injury.* Continuity of the nerve fibres is interrupted, but the perineurium and funicular arrangements are preserved. This condition is sometimes described as neurotmesis. Degeneration of the proximal portion of

the axon is more severe, and regeneration is delayed. Because endoneural tubes have been disrupted, budding axons frequently grow into other tubes. Recovery of sensory and motor functions is incomplete. For example, in such an injury to the facial nerve the face would, after regeneration, move in unison upon blinking the eyelids or smiling, with loss of selective facial movement. This is often referred to as synkinesis.

(4) *Fourth-degree injury.* The nerve trunk in the damaged segment becomes a disorderly strand of connective tissue, Schwann cells and re-generating axons called a neuroma. Excision of the neuronal segment with repair of the nerve is necessary. Recovery of sensory and motor functions is incomplete.

(5) *Fifth-degree injury.* The peripheral nerve is completely severed. Axotmesis is another term to describe this condition. There is no return of function unless the cut nerve is repaired. Even so, function will be reduced. In this case, the face would have no function from the time of the accident, and would never regain function unless a repair were carried out.

As the injured axon regenerates down its empty sheath, it eventually reaches either a muscle and a motor end-plate, or an area such as the skin, where the sensory nerve endings will perceive sensation. Because regenerating motor axons do not know which empty sheaths will proceed to muscle, approximately 50% of them will grow down pathways intended for sensory nerves. This can be a limiting factor in recovery of motor and sensory functions.

Muscle

Muscles of the trunk and limbs are primarily striated (Peacock, 1984b). A unique property of facial and laryngeal musculature is that it is of branchomeric origin, unlike other striated muscles which are somatic in origin. Branchomeric muscles can potentially be reinnervated for many years after neural damage; this is unlike somatic musculature which regains function poorly even if reinnervation is established immediately following injury. Nerve repair, nerve grafts, and neuro-muscular implants have all produced significant restoration of facial and laryngeal function follow-ing paralysis.

Direct muscle injury usually produces some form of ischaemia which, if severe enough, will result in fibrosis. Muscle shortening is the usual end result of fibrosis. Therefore, injury to muscle about the jaw can produce significant limited mouth opening.

One of the most important steps in either primary or secondary muscle repair is to excise carefully all of the old scar tissue or damaged muscle. The biological key to the healing of muscles is the knowledge that muscle cells do regenerate. Muscle does not grow by mitosis and development of new cells, but old myofibrils have the capability of regenerating if they are not strangled by extensive fibrous tissue. Moreover, healing between muscle ends by fibrous protein synthesis is not as desirable as the regeneration of myofibrils. Careful excision of old scar in secon-dary repair and precise debridement of damaged muscle, so that fibrous tissue replacement will not occur, offer the best chance of maximal muscle regeneration and minimal fibrous protein syn-thesis following an acute injury.

An interesting feature of skeletal or striated muscle is that of the atrophy associated with denervation. Branchomeric musculature, on the other hand, undergoes very slow degeneration and atrophy. In fact, facial muscles have been found to exist even 20 years after denervation. Conversely, somatic muscle would atrophy and become fibrotic within months after denervation. An example of skeletal muscle atrophy is often seen after transplantation of musculocutaneous flaps for reconstruction of head and neck cancer defects.

Fascia

Fascia is significant in an injury primarily when the undamaged fascia fails to provide sufficient tensile strength and structural support. Although fascia heals well, by means of protein synthesis and collagen remodelling, it is able to regenerate to only a limited degree. Structural stability usually has to be achieved through transplantation of fascia from other sources.

Fascia is frequently used to close soft tissue defects requiring support and/or closure. Dural defects, following removal of temporal bone and ethmoid sinus cancers, are often repaired with grafts of fascia. The otologist uses fascia to repair tympanic membrane perforations. Strips of fascia are also used to suspend the lower lip in order to correct drooling following major resections of the jaw and oral cavity tissues.

Tendon

A tendon consists basically of collagen and a few fibroblasts or tenocytes. The tendon's function is to transmit the force generated by the muscle to the skeleton. Therefore, the objective of repairing a tendon is to restore maximum strength without restricting motion.

It is necessary to regard tendon repair as 'one wound–one scar' (Peacock, 1984c). The cavity containing a disrupted tendon also contains injured fat, blood vessels, dermis, and perhaps bone or cartilage. These layers are ultimately connected by a single medium as healing proceeds. Basically, there is a single wound and a single scar.

Cartilage

Cartilage is an elastic skeletal tissue, which, when injured, is replaced not by cartilage but by undifferentiated fibrous tissue (Fry, 1977). An example of this phenomenon is the 'cauliflower' ear so frequently found in wrestlers who do not bother to wear ear protectors and thus suffer ear trauma. Although the three traditional classifications of cartilage are elastic cartilage (pinna, alar cartilage or the nose), hyaline – or chondroid – cartilage (thyroid ala, cricoid cartilage), and fibrocartilage (found in the intervertebral disc, and in the intra-articular discs of the knee joint and temporomandibular joint), it is important to view each specific cartilage as a specific structure adapted to a specific function.

In elastic cartilage, the perichondrium – the fibrous capsule surrounding the cartilage – is closely bound to the cartilage itself and not easily separated from it. In hyaline cartilage, there is a more distinct division between the perichondrium and the cartilage, and the latter can be separated more easily.

Any segment of cartilage contains a complex balanced system of forces (Fry, 1966). For example, if one surface is interrupted, the more intact surface – released from the opposing tensile surface – will shorten. Because a material is weaker in tension than in compression, the convex side of any curve will be damaged more than the concave side. When cartilage is thus deformed, as in an untreated nasal injury, the collagen will remould over a period of 6–12 months, and the new shape will be considered neutral, that is with the forces of tension and compression in balance. By making incisions on one side of fibroelastic cartilage, such as the nasal septum, the shape will change according to where the incisions are placed. A deviated septum can sometimes be straightened without removal of any cartilaginous tissue.

Fat

Fat provides for insulation, protection, energy storage, and bulk. In the face and neck region, fat is mainly located over the cheeks and under the chin.

Fat is made up of rather large cells containing various lipids in combination with proteins and cholesterol. Fat injury usually produces inflammation with subsequent fibrosis and shrinkage. Liposuction is a technique to remove fat which is frequently used in facial plastic surgery. Essentially, the fat cells are broken and removed by passing a metal sucking rod through the adipose tissues. The damaged fat cells produce inflammation with subsequent scarring and atrophy (Watson, 1959).

Factors that affect wound healing

Extrinsic

In treating a wound, it is important to consider all the effects and possible side-effects of any drugs administered to the patient (Boucek, 1984). For example, anti-inflammatory drugs that cause vasoconstriction can interfere with blood flow to the wound. Cytotoxic drugs, which are used to treat cancer patients, interfere with cell proliferation, an important element of wound healing.

Several vitamins may affect wound healing. For example, adequate levels of vitamin C are important, as there is a constant turnover of ascorbic acid in scar tissue. Vitamin A can reverse the inhibition of wound healing, sometimes caused by diabetes, the use of glucocorticoids or high doses of vitamin E. Vitamin E can retard collagen production; this very fact might account for the improvement in scar appearance when vitamin E is topically applied to recently closed incisions. Sufficient levels of vitamin K are necessary for proper blood coagulation. As vitamin K is normally synthesized by intestinal bacteria, certain conditions of the gastrointestinal tract (sprue, antibiotics) may prevent adequate production of vitamin K.

Zinc and copper have been found to influence wound healing through their participation in the synthesis of certain enzymes necessary for epithelial and/or fibroblast proliferation. The two minerals are actually antagonistic to each other. High levels of zinc make copper unavailable for enzyme synthesis. If tissue zinc levels are low – for example in fad diets, poor nutrition, alcoholism, or following irradiation, during chemotherapy, or in cancer – administration of zinc can assist in restoring normal healing. Conversely, excess zinc can be detrimental by inhibiting macrophage migration and phagocytosis and also by interfering with enzyme synthesis of collagen. Zinc administration to patients with normal zinc levels has no accelerating effect on wound healing.

Adequate nutrition is important during healing. Particular attention should be paid to the protein intake (>1 g protein/kg body weight per day).

Inadequate protein can increase susceptibility to infection. A high protein diet will increase the rate of tensile strength gain during the fibroblastic period.

Mechanical

Skin tension is an important fact in the way in which a wound heals. In general, it is preferable to place any incision along the lines of relaxed skin tension, as a scar that forms across a tension line is more likely to stretch or bunch up into a hypertrophic scar. Relaxed skin tension lines, sometimes referred to as Langer's lines, are found to lie parallel to facial and neck wrinkles.

Genetic

Black and oriental people are more susceptible than white people to the formation of hypertrophic scars and keloids. Heredity does seem to play a role in identifying patients that may be susceptible to bad scarring. Young individuals are much more severely affected by scarring than are adults. The face is particularly vulnerable to hypertrophic scars (*Figure 24.7*).

Physical

Thickness, tension and extensibility of the skin all change with age (Gibson, Stark and Evans, 1969). The epidermis and dermis thicken during childhood and adolescence, remain constant throughout adulthood, and then grow thinner during old age. Tension and elasticity decrease noticeably from around the age of 40 onwards.

Skin wounds can be caused by both long-wave or thermal radiation (sun exposure, sun drying or mechanical irritation) and by short-wave or X-radiation. Injuries produced by short-wave radiation are much more likely to result in carcinoma than are those produced by long-wave radiation. In addition, the lapse of time between injury and development of invasive cancer appears to be directly proportional to the wavelength of the radiation (*Figure 24.8*).

Blood supply

Good wound healing depends on the oxygen and nutrients supplied by the microcirculation (Irvin, 1981). Therefore, anaemia, haemorrhage, arteriosclerosis and shock can all inhibit healing. In cases of severe trauma, microvascular constriction or sludging can also limit the supply of oxygen and nutrients.

Irradiation, which is frequently used to treat head and neck cancer, causes irreparable damage to the skin's microvasculature (Archer *et al.*, 1970). As a consequence of reduced blood supply,

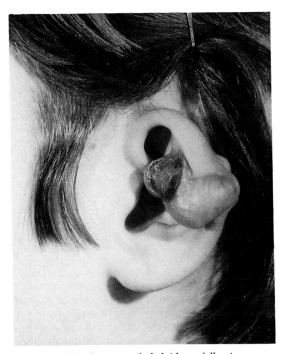

Figure 24.7 Development of a keloid scar following surgical repair of an ear injury

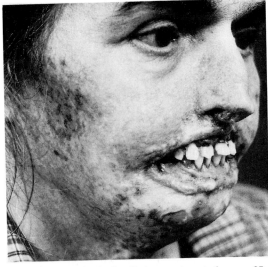

Figure 24.8 Patient had radiation treatments for acne 25 years previous to this photograph. Her lips are now infiltrated with invasive cancer. Note the extensive facial scarring resulting from the previous radiation

resulting from irradiation, wounds heal poorly and are much more susceptible to infection than are non-irradiated tissue beds. A reduction in blood supply to the skin may have some influence on the bacterial population, in that there is a notable shift to Gram-negative organisms, responsible for wound infections, following irradiation. It has been conclusively demonstrated that prophylactic antibiotics are indicated when major head and neck cancer operations which enter the upper aerodigestive tract are being carried out (Panje and McCabe, 1979). If the patient has previously undergone irradiation, an antibiotic that kills Gram-negative organisms – such as gentamicin – should be included to provide adequate prophylaxis against subsequent wound infection.

Blood supply plays a very important role in wound healing on the face and neck. Wounds about the face and neck tend to heal more readily than wounds below the clavicle. In fact, the surgeon is encouraged to remove sutures on day 5 rather than day 10 when dealing with face and neck skin wound closures. Leaving sutures in the face and neck for longer than 5 days usually predisposes the area to inflammation and subsequent scarring.

Lacerations

Initial decisions regarding the treatment of a skin wound depend on the ability to discern whether the wound is contaminated or infected. A contaminated wound (bacteria, foreign body, animal bite) can usually be made surgically clean by debridement so that it can be closed primarily. An infected wound (abscess, human bite) cannot be made clean quickly, and therefore cannot be closed mechanically. Particularly in the case of the head and neck – principally because of their profuse blood supply – there is no hard and fast rule as to how long after injury a wound can be safely closed mechanically. Wounds have been closed as long as one day following injury without undue risk of infection. The most common contraindication to wound closure is the presence of inflammation, puncture wounds, or of high risk wounds such as human bites.

Principles of head and neck plastic operations and repair

Principles of head and neck plastic operations and repair are based upon basic understanding of wound healing as it applies to tissues above the clavicles. The uniqueness of the head and neck in respect of their function and appearance are all integral to proper repair of tissue dysfunction. Tissue blood supply, the defect and its location are of paramount importance when considering the technical aspects of head and neck plastic operations. Just as important as the technical factors to a satisfactory plastic operation is the necessary understanding of the patient's psychological and sociological needs. Of paramount importance is that the patient should be justly satisfied, followed closely by the surgeon's own sense of satisfaction. The surgeon's 'golden' rule must be the answer to the question 'Would I do (recommend) this operation to members of my family?'

In order to perform head and neck plastic and repair operations, the surgeon must understand basic clinical tenets that individually are intriguing, but together consummate the necessary 'art' work for the repair of head and neck defects. The following are succinct descriptions of the basic clinical tenets necessary for performing plastic and reconstructive surgical repair of the head and neck.

Primary intention closure

Suturing a wound closed with some form of material is the basic method for a surgeon mechanically to produce primary intention wound healing (*Figure 24.9*). The way in which the wound is closed greatly affects its final appearance and function. The tissues must be handled gently to reduce the possibility of further injury and ischaemia. Reduced tissue blood supply or ischaemia contributes to infection and excessive scar formation. Fine non-absorbable monofilament suture (for example 6-0 or 7-0 nylon) is best for closing facial lacerations and incisions. Absorbable sutures (catgut, polyglycolic acid) are best used for closing mucosal wounds and where the suture is buried into the tissues beneath the mucosa or skin.

The avoidance of haematoma and dead space formation is tantamount to satisfactory wound healing. A haematoma provides a medium for bacterial growth and consequential wound infection or abscess formation. Infected wounds will usually heal poorly, with attendant excessive scar formation. Wound drainage with rubber drains is helpful in avoiding haematoma formation. Wound haemostasis is important before closure. Dead space is an opening or cavity which contains air located within the tissue. Dead space is usually produced from tissue loss and/or poor wound closure. Although drains placed in the wound help to eradicate dead space and/or haematoma, by producing a negative pressure, reliance should not be placed on them alone for dealing with this problem. Proper wound closure – that may include transplantation of tissue into the wound to

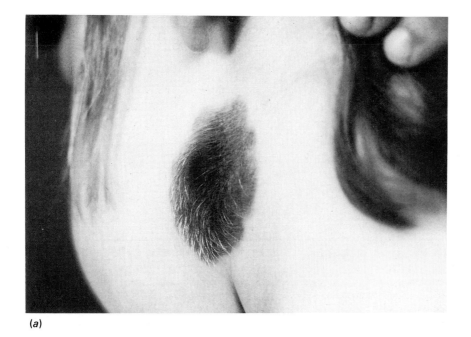

(a)

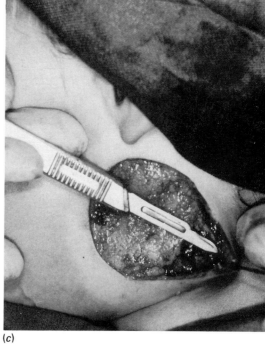

(b)   (c)

Figure 24.9 (*a*) Congenital pigmented hairy cell nevus involving the neck of an 8-year-old girl. (*b*) Appearance of wound following removal of nevus. Note how the wound has become larger because of elastic tissue forces *in situ*. (*c*) Edges of wound are undermined to reduce tissue retraction forces

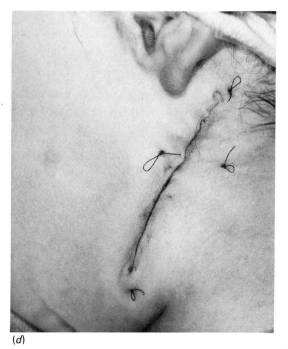

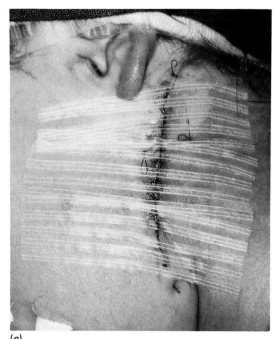

(*d*)   (*e*)

Figure 24.9 (*d*) Wound is closed by primary intention. A subcuticular running suture(s) was utilized for the closure. (*e*) In order to reduce incision motion and reduce tension small strips of tape are applied perpendicular to the incision

fill the dead space, or placement of absorbable sutures in the wound to approximate the deep tissues – will greatly reduce the problems of dead space or haematoma formation.

Face, scalp and neck wounds heal more rapidly than skin wounds located below the clavicle. Again, this phenomenon is related to the excellent blood supply afforded the face and neck. Sutures used to close wounds above the clavicles should be removed by the fifth or sixth day to avoid infection and scarring. Sutures left in for 10 or more days will cause excessive scarring where the suture pierces the skin. The 'zipper' scar is characteristic of this healing problem (*Figure 24.10*).

Tension across a closed wound can produce infection and hypertrophic scars. To reduce tension, the surgeon will frequently employ pieces

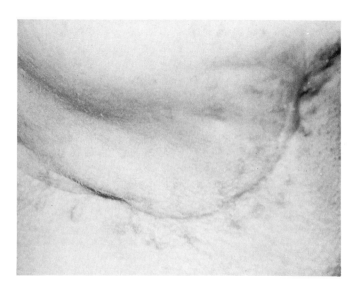

Figure 24.10 Appearance of a healed neck incision in which thick sutures were left *in situ* for 2 weeks before removal. Note 'zipper' appearance of scar

of tape applied across the wound after sutures have been removed. The tape, often referred to as 'steri-strips', will distribute the tension over a larger surface area and also reduce motion at the wound site. Steri-strips are usually left on for an additional 2–3 weeks following suture removal to facilitate the establishment of wound closure strength and to reduce scarring.

Sutures

Sutures can be classified as absorbable and non-absorbable, and as monofilament and multi-filament (*Table 24.1*). Generally, absorbable sutures (catgut, cotton) lose strength much more rapidly (10–20 days) than non-absorbable sutures (nylon, silk). Absorbable sutures are usually used beneath the skin and in the mouth and throat; non-absorbable sutures are commonly used on the skin surface. Sometimes, non-absorbable sutures are placed below the skin to give added strength to a wound closure over a longer period of time. However, the use of non-absorbable suture-like silk within the wound's environment can potentially give rise to serious wound infection. More recently, fabricated absorbable sutures (polygly-colic acid (Vicryl), polyglactin 910 (Dexon) and polydioxanone (PDS)) have been introduced. These sutures have unique properties, when compared with the more common absorbable sutures, in that they are much stronger, are less inflammatory, and yet are resorbed. Multifilament (silk) sutures are usually easier to handle than monofilament (nylon) sutures. Although multifila-ment sutures are more pliable and easier to tie, they do have the serious drawback of being more prone to producing wound infection, even if used only on the skin's surface; 'wicking' of skin surface bacteria along the multiple little strands into the wound is felt to be the cause. This is the reason why a patient is often admonished not to allow a wound to be exposed to water until the sutures have been removed. The basic principle in choosing a suture is to choose one of a material of sufficient strength to last until the wound has healed. For example, a wound that is expected to take a long time to heal will require a suture which maintains its strength for an equally long time (maybe weeks) and which causes minimum inflammation.

Handling of tissue

Fundamental to satisfactory wound repair is that healing should be rapid with minimal scar formation. Atraumatic tissue handling is impor-tant to good wound healing, as tissue damage will produce necrosis, infection and subsequent scar-ring. Handling tissues with fine instruments, such as small hooks or grasping forceps, produces the least amount of tissue injury. Excessive clamping and retraction of tissue usually produces non-favourable wound healing. Lesser tissue injury is produced with thin sutures and needles. The length of an incision has no bearing on how the wound will heal.

Table 24.1 Absorbable and non-absorbable sutures

Type	Strength (b)	Half-life	Reactivity	Throws required	Comment
Absorbable					
gut	±3.3	5–20 days	++++	3–4	Low knot security until moist; non-uniform, can fray
collagen	±3.3	5–20 days	++++	3–4	Low knot security until moist
Dexon	6	10 days	++	3–4	Half-life pH dependent
Vicryl	6	10 days	++	4–5	Half-life pH dependent
Polydiaxone (PDS)	±4	4.5 weeks	+	4–5	New, promising monofilament
Non-absorbable					
silk	3	0.5–1 year	+++	3–4	Inconsistent strength
cotton	≤3	>1 year	+++	2–3	Drags, cuts tissue
Dacron	4	*	+++	2–3	Rough surface causes capillary action
coated Dacron	4	*	+++	4–5	Coatings may fragment
nylon monofilament	3.6	0.5–1 year	+	5	Can fracture
nylon braided	4	≤1 year	++	3–4	Dead spaces
polypropylene	3.5	*	+	5+	Can fracture
stainless steel	9.5	*	+	2–3	Poor handling

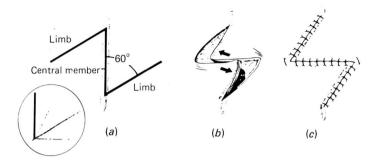

(a) (b) (c)

Figure 24.11 Z-plasty: note how central member of Z lies along scar. This area will be elongated by transposing the two triangular flaps

Z-plasty

The Z-plasty (McGregor, 1980), a widely used technique in plastic and reconstructive surgery, is a form of double transposition flap, the purpose of which is to gain length in one direction at the expense of width in the other (*Figure 24.11*). The basic Z-plasty consists of two triangular flaps of skin and subcutaneous tissue formed by three connecting incisions of equal length and at a 30–60° angle to one another. Essentially, the two flaps are moved until they have exchanged places. Greater elongation is achieved by the use of wider flaps with concomitant larger angles to the vertical axis (*Figure 24.12*). The Z-plasty retards contracture, as the stress that is transmitted to surrounding tissues in a straight scar is cancelled out by the two opposing triangular flaps. The Z-plasty can

increase the length of skin (direction of final central member) and change the direction of a scar so that it will lie in the same direction as relaxed skin tension lines.

In any Z-plasty, the limbs should be along either the lines of minimal tension – that is, the relaxed skin tension lines – or the pre-existing skin wrinkle lines. If necessary, the angles formed between the wrinkle line and the triangular flaps may be a good deal less than 60°. Depending on the specific conditions – for example the skin on one side may be looser and require less elongation – the triangular angles of each flap may be of unequal size (for example a 30° and a 60° flap). The Z-plasty has been used for releasing cervical contracture scars following neck surgery, and for facial scars, burns and skin grafted sites (*Figure 24.13*).

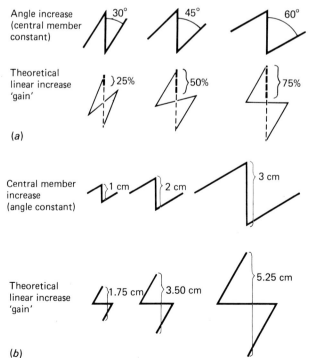

Figure 24.12 (*a*) Increasing the angle between the central member and arms of the Z will result in a theoretical linear increase of the central arm.
(*b*) Similarly keeping the angle constant, but increasing the central member length, will also produce lengthening in the direction of the original central member

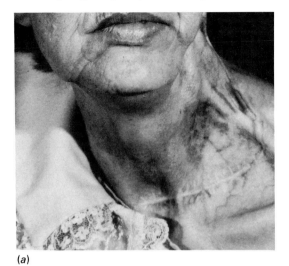

(a)

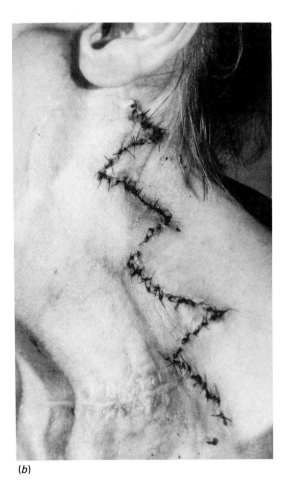

(b)

Figure 24.13 (*a*) Cervical contracture scar following radical neck dissection. (*b*) Contracture released with multiple Z-plasty

W-plasty

The W-plasty is a technique using multiple triangular incisions along either side of an unsightly scar. The W-plasty resembles the blade of a hand-saw. Although the triangles opposite each other are of equal size, those towards the ends of the scar become smaller, and the length of the limbs tapers to avoid puckering at the ends of the incision.

Both the Z-plasty and W-plasty break up the linear scar into smaller components, and move the scar into a better relation to the lines of relaxed skin tension. The visual appearance of a scar is an important factor in the way in which it is perceived; an irregular line is less perceptible than a straight line.

Rotation flaps

The rotation flap is among the flaps most commonly used to close skin tissue defects in head and neck plastic and reconstructive surgery (*Figure 24.14*). This flap usually has the appearance of a semicircle. It is cut adjacent to the defective area and then rotated around a pivot point until it covers the defect. Because a diagonal line of tension is created from the base of the flap to its leading point, the larger the flap, the more the tension is diffused across the flap. As the flap rotates, it becomes shorter. Therefore, extra tissue must be taken to achieve the desired coverage. Of prime importance in achieving sufficient rotation of a flap is its 'back cut'. An incision placed at less than 90° to the arc of the flap's rotation provides the main impetus to flap rotation.

Advancement flaps

An advancement flap is stretched or slid along a single axis or plane to cover an adjacent defective area. Advancement flaps can be used progressively; at each stage, as the skin loses its tension, the flap can be further stretched, or advanced.

Advanced flaps are most successful with infants, whose skin is highly elastic and well vascularized. In essence, stretch or tension does not usually interfere with the flap's blood supply. By contrast, it should be remembered that in the case of the advancement flap, tension usually does retard flap blood supply.

Rotation advancement flaps

Typical examples of rotation advancement flaps would include the Millard repair of cleft lip

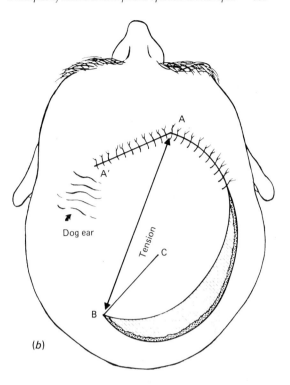

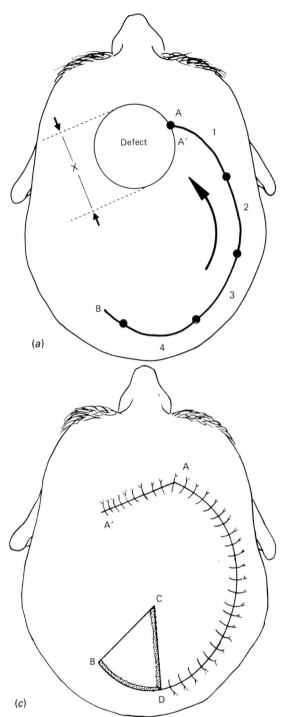

Figure 24.14 (*a*) Example of a rotation flap to close a scalp defect. Note that the diameter (*x*) of the defect determines the length of the incision of the flap (A → B). (*b*) When the flap has been rotated to close the defect, a 'dog ear' or a skin bulge is produced. A raw crescent area is also produced. (*c*) A back cut is performed to close the crescent area

deformities and that used by the author to repair scalp defects. The flap conforms to a semicircular appearance but, to cover a tissue defect, it must be advanced over the tissue deficiency in order to complete the closure.

Transposition and interpolation flaps

A transposition flap is a rectangular section of skin and subcutaneous tissue that is turned on its pivot point to an adjacent defect. An interpolation flap is like a transposition flap except the recipient site is nearby, thus the flap must pass over or under intervening tissue. Transposition and interpolation flaps usually have a narrower base than rotation or advancement flaps. As a general clinical rule, the length of a transposition flap should be no more than three times its width. Clinical examples of a transposition flap would include the cervical apical flap or the deltopectoral flap to close an adjacent neck defect. The midline forehead flap frequently used in nasal reconstruction, the deltopectoral flap used in head and neck ablative cancer reconstructive surgery, and the lip switch flap used to repair lip defects are all examples of interpolation flaps (*Figure 24.15*).

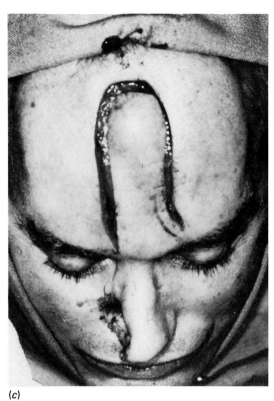

(a)

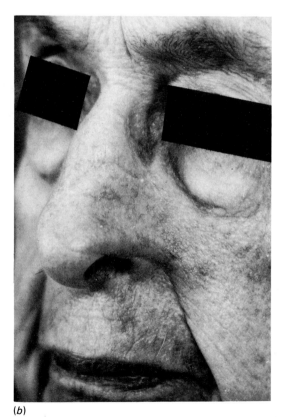

(b)

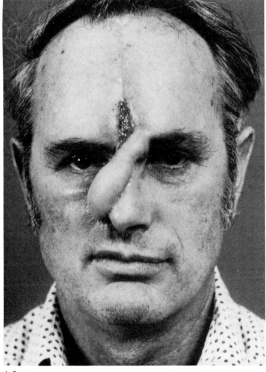

(c)

Figure 24.15 Examples of transposition flaps to close nasal defects produced by cancer ablation. (*a, b*) A nasolabial flap is used to close a lateral nasal defect. (*c, d, e*) A midline forehead flap to close a through-and-through nasal defect

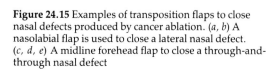

(d)

Secondary intention closure

Secondary intention closure, or delayed healing, is often used after breakdown of a primary wound closure, wound infections, cleft palate defects, cryotherapy, cauterization, and CO_2 laser therapy when there is a possibility of finding cancer. Frequently, large wounds are allowed to develop abundant 'proud' flesh to fill in depressions before closure – for example donor defect forehead flap, following the excision of skin cancers (Panje, Bumsted and Ceilley, 1980). In many cases, the combined use of delayed healing to reduce the wound's size, and subsequent simple reconstructive methods can be used to achieve an acceptable cosmetic and functional result (Goldwyn and Rueckert, 1977). The successful head and neck plastic and reconstructive surgeon always strives to use the more basic and simple rules of tissue closure.

Wound contraction, wherein the margin of the wound closes in on itself, becomes active during delayed healing at 4–5 days after injury. Approximately 24 days after injury, contraction slows markedly. The application of skin grafts or flaps, especially full thickness grafts, as soon as possible after injury is an effective means of reducing contraction.

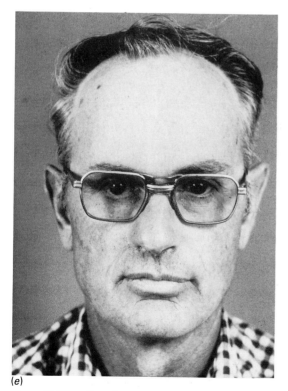

(e)

Figure 24.15 continued

Up to 80% of a wound's closure can be achieved by contraction of adjacent tissue into the defect (Higton and James, 1964). The presence of lax skin around the soft tissue defect appears to allow dramatic wound closures without producing significant facial distortions. If tissue adjacent to a wound is firmly attached to underlying bone, as on the scalp, there appears to be minimal contraction of the surrounding skin. Instead, granulation tissue builds up until epithelialization or skin coverage occurs (James and Newcombe, 1961). Excessive granulation may develop in the area of tight skin to such a degree that the depressed wound will be significantly filled in. It must be remembered that the more the granulation tissue accumulates, the more connective tissue will make up the closure.

If the wound extends from a densely adherent cutaneous area to a loose area, the most significant part of contraction will occur from the latter. With wounds around the eyes, lips and nose, the surgeon should strive to replace lost tissue in order to prevent distortion of these structures. If the greater part of the wound remains over bone, minimal facial distortion will occur.

Wound contraction is influenced by motion of structures adjacent to the wound area. In general, greater contraction takes place in areas of greater motion. Surface tension lines and geometry of the wound will also influence contraction. Therefore, shaping and location of the wound can be useful in avoiding distortions.

Delayed healing must be used judiciously, as it can cause the development of much more scar tissue than is the case with primary intention healing. A thicker scar will produce more tension, which may distort the facial features. Indiscriminate use of delayed healing can cause ectropion, stenotic nares, lip retraction, microstomia, velopharyngeal incompetence, stridor, aspiration, drooling and other problems.

Transplantation and replantation

The term 'transplantation' refers to the transfer of tissue or an organ from one part of the body to another, or from one body to another. A graft is basically similar to a transplant. Replantation refers to the surgical replacement of tissue to its original site. An autograft is a piece of tissue that is transferred from one area to another on the same person. An allograft (homograft) refers to a graft transplanted between individuals belonging to the same species. An isograft usually refers to an allograft between extremely inbred, or genetically pure, strains of animals. Syngenesiotransplantation is the transplantation of tissue between individuals who are closely related genetically. A xenograft (heterograft) is the graft of tissue between individuals of different species. Alloplasts are biologically inert foreign materials used for implantation into tissue for augmentation or reconstruction.

Skin grafts

A skin graft consists of both the epidermis and dermis. If the entire thickness of dermis is used, the tissue is called a full thickness skin graft; if only a portion of the dermis is included with the epidermis, it is called a split thickness skin graft. A split thickness skin graft would vary in thickness between 0.0025 and 0.0046 cm. Obtaining a 0.0051 cm thickness skin graft from the postauricular area would include all of the dermis and epidermis, thereby exposing subcutaneous fat. A flap would include skin, subcutaneous fat, fascia and, in some cases, muscle. In general, the successful transplantation or replantation of tissue without a blood supply *in situ* is limited. Thus a split thickness skin graft is more likely to be viable after transplantation than a full thickness graft. Similarly, a full thickness graft will be significantly more successful than a flap transferred without any blood supply. A successful skin graft depends on initial diffusion of oxygen into the graft, then rapid revascularization and disposal of metabolic waste products (Smahel and Ganzoni, 1970; Smahel, 1971). Researchers are not certain whether revascularization occurs through a connection between existing capillaries in the graft and vessels in the recipient area, or whether an entirely new vascular network develops.

Full thickness grafts

Because full thickness grafts revascularize more slowly than split thickness grafts, the former require optimal wound care. The grafted site must be immobilized and kept free of haematoma formation. The advantages of the full thickness graft are that it is less likely to contract or pigment, and it often produces a superior skin coverage.

Common donor sites for full thickness grafts are the retroauricular area, the supraclavicular area, the upper eyelid and the inside of the upper arm. Although the abdomen and thigh are also good donor sites, the colour match is usually not as good. In addition, the skin of the abdomen and thigh is so thick that split thickness grafts from these areas are usually preferred.

Split thickness grafts

Split thickness grafts are used when the recipient area is either too large or of too poor vascularity to take a full thickness skin graft. The abdomen, hip and thigh are usually considered the best donor sites for split thickness grafts, as they can be covered by clothing to conceal the scarring and they constitute relatively large flat areas for easier procurement of the graft. When a good colour match is desired, the face, neck or upper back is a better donor site. Usually any skin graft site is particularly painful to the patient unless covered by some type of plastic membrane-like material. Because hair follicles and sebaceous glands remain after removal of a split thickness skin graft, the donor site will recover itself with new skin from these sites. In fact, another split thickness skin graft can be taken from these sites once healing has taken place.

Mesh skin grafts

A mesh skin graft is a thin split thickness graft in which multiple slits have been made by means of multiple rotating blades. The graft, which can be stretched in two directions, can be used to cover an area many times its original size. Mesh skin grafts are used to cover extensive burns and other traumatic wounds to facilitate drainage and provide more coverage of an area with a certain amount of skin. If the skin graft is not meshed, it can be incised with a knife in a number of different areas to provide for some expansion and, most importantly, for drainage.

Flaps

A flap is a composite of various tissues transplanted from one location to another to replace or cover similar tissue losses. The flap must have a vascular supply for survival.

Two systems of flap classification have been developed on the basis of the anatomical vascularity of the flap. One system (McGregor and Morgan, 1973) divides flaps into the random pattern flap, which lacks a recognized arteriovenous system, and the axial pattern flap, which exhibits at least one axial arteriovenous system. In the latter case, easily identifiable blood vessels entering the flap would be evident.

Another system (Daniel and Williams, 1973) classifies flaps as cutaneous, arterial and island (*Figure 24.16*). Most cutaneous flaps, like the random pattern flap, lack a specific vascular system. Arterial flaps have a skin bridge and at least one direct cutaneous artery and vein located along the longitudinal axis of the flap. Island flaps have a pedicle containing the nutrient artery and vein, but do not contain any skin. Arterial and island flaps, because of their superior blood supply, are much more hardy flaps than

(a) Cutaneous flap

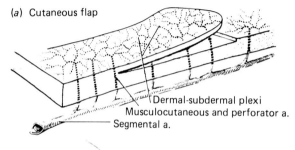

Dermal-subdermal plexi
Musculocutaneous and perforator a.
Segmental a.

(b) Peninsula arterial flap

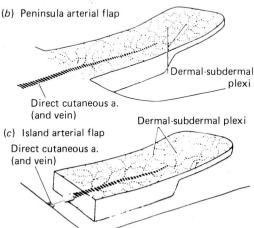

Dermal-subdermal plexi

Direct cutaneous a.
(and vein)

Dermal-subdermal plexi

(c) Island arterial flap

Direct cutaneous a.
(and vein)

Figure 24.16 Examples of cutaneous and arterial flaps.
(After Daniel and Williams)

cutaneous (random pattern) flaps. In order to improve a cutaneous flap's blood supply, the surgeon will sometimes employ a surgical method, called flap delay, to augment its vascularity. This is done by removing some of the flap's blood supply, waiting 2 weeks and then transplanting the flap into its new position. Delay makes a flap more reliable and enables a larger flap to be used.

Skin flaps

A skin or cutaneous flap consists of skin, subcutaneous tissue and small blood vessels. A skin flap can be used as a local, regional or distant flap. The skin flap can be either a random pattern or an arterialized flap, again depending upon its vascular supply.

A local flap usually means the transposing of skin subcutaneously from an adjacent area into the defect site. Commonly used local flaps on the face include the transposition, interpolation or rotation advancement flap.

A regional flap is considered a tissue transplanted from a site away from the defect to be reconstructed, but yet in close enough proximity

to allow closure of the area. Examples of a regional flap include the deltopectoral (Bakamjian), forehead (McGregor), midline forehead, scalp, nape of neck (Zovickian), retroauricular, cervical and so on.

A local or regional flap is usually elevated from its place of origin on to a skin bridge or bridges. Where the flap remains attached to the body is called the pedicle. A flap may be either unipedicle, bipedicle or multipedicle. A unipedicle flap is when the flap remains attached to the body at one site. A bipedicle flap is attached at two different loci and resembles a bucket handle. The more pedicles a flap has, the greater the potential blood supply and, concomitantly, the greater the likelihood of its surviving. On the other hand, the more pedicles a flap has, the less its manoeuvrability when it is being moved to its new location. Making the pedicle wider or increasing the number of pedicles at one end of a flap does not necessarily increase its length of survival (Milton, 1970). Length of survival usually relates to the long axis of the flap drawn perpendicular to its base or pedicle. To increase the likelihood of flap survival or to increase the flap's length of survival, pedicles must be added to the middle or other end of the flap. Similarly, the inclusion of an identifiable artery in the flap will greatly increase its viability and length of survival.

There have been no statistically significant medical ways of improving the chances of length of flap survival. Vasoactive drugs, regardless of how much they vasodilate, cannot improve the tissue's chances of living as the main determinant of its viability is the surgical construction of the flap. Once the flap has been constructed, technical factors influence flap survival more than any others. The presence of either flap tension, stretching, kinking, twisting, compression or constriction can severely compromise a flap's chance of survival. In head and neck flap cases, proper patient positioning can alleviate tension, stretching, kinking, or twisting of the flap. Tracheostomy tapes used to secure a tracheostomy tube in place can compress or constrict the flap's pedicle and simultaneously reduce blood supply to the distal end of the flap. Diseases, such as diabetes, arteriosclerosis, polycythaemia vera, hyperlipidaemia, vasculitides, multiple myeloma and leukaemia, can all increase the chance of flap death or necrosis. The vasculitides decrease the amount of microcirculation to the skin by decreasing the number and diameter of the blood vessels. Conditions that increase blood viscosity reduce the amount of blood flow to the skin. Elementary thinking would indicate that the occurrence of such flap problems would be inevitable as the basic laws of fluid mechanics are adversely affected by the foregoing conditions (Panje, 1984).

Poiseuille developed a mathematical equation to explain the flow (F) of the fluid through a rigid cylinder. His equation constitutes a useful approximation of blood flow in a skin flap's vascular system

$$F = \frac{\pi\, r^4\, (P1 - P2)}{8\eta l}$$

where $\pi = 3.14159$, r = the radius of the cylinder, η = the fluid viscosity, l = the cylinder length, and $P1–P2$ = the hydrostatic pressure difference between the two ends of the cylinder. From this equation it is apparent that haemodynamic resistance (R) is given by

$$R = \frac{8\eta l}{\pi r^4}$$

By substituting R into the original equation, the formula then states that

$$F = P/R$$

Poiseuille's equation states that blood flow can be essentially affected by the size of the blood vessel(s), the pressure difference between the entrance and exit sites, the length of the blood vessel, and the viscosity of the blood. Although the Poiseuille equation was not derived from the study of human tissue blood flow, it does provide a convenient, albeit severely simplified, means of understanding flap physiology.

Myocutaneous (musculocutaneous) flaps

The greater part of the human integument is supplied by small blood vessels called musculocutaneous perforators. These vessels arise from segmental arteries deep to the musculature, traverse the muscle bed, and turn into a candelabra pattern of very small blood vessels that pierce the subcutaneous fat and dermis to communicate with the dermal–subdermal plexus of the skin. The myocutaneous flap consists of a patch of skin and muscle with an identifiable vascular pedicle (*Figure 24.17*). Some of the most commonly used myocutaneous flaps for head and neck reconstructive surgery are the pectoralis major, trapezius, latissimus dorsi and sternocleidomastoid myocutaneous flaps.

The myocutaneous flap has revolutionized head and neck reconstructive surgery. It has allowed the head and neck surgeon immediately to repair major head and neck tissue losses, with a greater than 90% chance of success (Panje, 1987). The technique is highly reproducible. The myocutaneous flap is today used more than any other type of flap in head and neck cancer reconstructive surgery. This flap is so hardy that the surgeon can

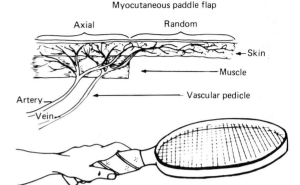

Figure 24.17 Illustration of a myocutaneous flap. In this case the skin being extended beyond the muscle represents the 'paddle' part of the flap

confidently repair contaminated and previously irradiated mouth and throat wounds. Irradiation, although quite effective in eradicating a number of head and neck cancers, does produce severe microvascular damage and scarring. Infection as well as bone and cartilage necrosis are potential complications of operating on a previously irradiated head and neck tumour patient. The myocutaneous flap, by reason of its abundant blood supply, seems to reduce the incidence of wound infection and impede the development or continuation of osteoradionecrosis/chondoradionecrosis.

Before the advent of the myocutaneous and free flaps, previously irradiated head and neck wounds were often treated as though it were inevitable that they would all become infected and break open. Therefore, controlled openings (fistulae) were made between the mouth or throat and the neck skin to reduce the chance of saliva and bacteria penetrating beneath the closed neck and upper aerodigestive tract. Such controlled salivary fistulae markedly reduced complications and the risk of infection, but resulted in prolonged hospitalization and the need for subsequent operations.

The primary problems with myocutaneous flaps are donor site morbidity, including deformed appearance and functional muscle loss, and bulkiness of the flap. Use of the pectoralis major myocutaneous flap probably involves the most significant potential for donor site scarring and deformity, depending on the amount of tissue removed. The trapezius mycocutaneous flap can produce the most disabling deformity by paralysing the trapezius muscle and thus severely weakening the shoulder (Panje and Cutting, 1980). For this reason, most head and neck surgeons will not use the trapezius muscle flap unless the accessory nerve (XI) has previously been sacrificed (that is, through radical neck dissection).

The latissimus dorsi myocutaneous flap is taken from the back, and is either passed up through the axilla and neck or is transplanted as a free flap with microvascular anastomosis (*Figure 24.18*). This flap has been used primarily for the reconstruction of massive face, mouth and throat defects. It suffers from the disadvantage of being the myocutaneous flap with the greatest potential for complications (Maves, Panje and Shagets, 1984).

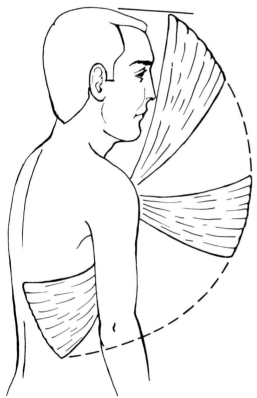

Figure 24.18 Illustration of arc of rotation of the latissimus muscle to reach the head and neck

At the present time, the most frequently used myocutaneous flap for head and neck reconstructive surgery is the pectoralis major (Ariyan, 1979; Back *et al.*, 1979; Biller *et al.*, 1981). Because this flap is taken from the chest, it can be used without any repositioning of the patient. The pectoralis major myocutaneous flap has been used to repair a host of defects that include: temporal bone, scalp, mid-face, palate, oropharynx, oral cavity, jaw, through and through defects, pharynx, cervical oesophagus, and neck.

Free flaps

Beginning in the early 1960s, surgeons have transplanted tissue by microvascular anastomosis to reconstruct head and neck defects (Nakayama *et al.*, 1964). Free flaps are arterialized islands of tissue that have been severed from their original location and transplanted to a different place on the body. The small blood vessels in the flap are connected to similar size blood vessels at the recipient site. Blood vessels usually range in size from 1 to 3 mm in diameter. These microscopic blood vessels are connected either by very fine sutures (the size of a strand of hair) or by small metal rings. Free flaps of skin, scalp, toes, bone, stomach and intestine have been utilized to replace head and neck tissues lost as a result of cancer surgery, trauma and congenital deformities. Major advantages of the free flap technique over other flap procedures include: one stage operation, reduced stays in hospital, and minimal donor site deformity.

Free flaps have been taken from more or less any place on or inside the body where there is tissue connected to an artery and a vein with a diameter greater than 1 mm (Serafin and Buncke, 1985). The free flap can consist merely of skin and subcutaneous fat based on a vascular supply. The more commonly used examples include the groin skin flap based on the superficial iliac artery and its vein, the forearm skin flap based on the radial artery and cephalic vein, and the top of the foot skin based on the dorsalis pedis artery and accompanying veins. A free flap can be a myocutaneous flap severed from its blood supply and transplanted to a new area of the body. Some of the most commonly used free myocutaneous flaps include the latissimus dorsi based on the long thoracic artery and accompanying veins, and the rectus abdominus based on the inferior epigastric artery and vein.

Free flaps can be made up of a muscle and its vascular supply. Muscles such as the latissimus dorsi, the gracilis and extensor hallucis longus, and the pectoralis minor have all, at some time, been transplanted to the face for restoration of facial animation. The latissimus muscle has also been utilized as a free flap to rebuild the tongue.

Bone has been used as a free flap primarily to reconstruct the jaw after ablative cancer surgery (Ostrup and Fredrickson, 1975). Bone used for the transplantation is usually based either on a blood vessel that is the nutrient artery or its collateral supply, or on a blood vessel that is connected to an accessory nutrient artery (Panje, 1981). Basing the endochondral bone on its periosteum alone has not proven to be reliable for long-term (years) jaw reconstruction. Examples of bone free flaps include the iliac crest based on either the superficial or the deep circumflex iliac artery – with the latter being preferred – the fibula, the scapula, the radius, or even the second phalanx of the foot.

Viscus

Stomach, intestine and colon have all been used as free flaps to replace upper aerodigestive tract defects, usually following cancer or trauma (lye ingestion). The advantage of using these tissues for the repair of mucosal defects in the head and neck is that like tissue is being replaced by like tissue. In other words, mucosa is replacing mucosa. Frequently, head and neck defects are repaired by some form of skin graft. Skin is capable of repairing the mucosal defect but it does not restore graft moisture in the way that viscous replacements do. Another disadvantage of skin replacement of the upper aerodigestive tract is the possibility of hair growth within the mouth or throat, which is an undesirable situation.

Grafts

Grafting is defined as the implantation of skin or other tissue from a different site or source to replace damaged structures. A graft could thus also be a flap. In general, however, a graft does not immediately have a blood supply. In some cases the graft will never have a blood supply. Grafts are very useful to the head and neck reconstructive surgeon. Grafts are usually readily obtainable, with minimal morbidity to the patient, and can be rapidly employed for repair of a defect.

Cartilage

Cartilage has traditionally been classified into hyaline, elastic, and fibrocartilage, based principally on the kind of fibre make-up of the tissue. Hyaline cartilage, for example, includes the costochondral cartilages, the nasal septum, the alar cartilages, and those of the trachea and larger bronchi. Human cartilage is usually regarded as a unique structure whose physical and mechanical properties are adapted for a specific function. Transplanting rib cartilage to the ear does not cause the cartilage to change into the cartilage associated with that particular location. Each type of cartilage is adapted to a specific function. Cartilage used as an autograft includes the costochondral portion of the rib, the nasal septum and the ear cartilages.

The balance of stresses in intact cartilage may be released when cartilage is excised for a graft. The portion chosen for a graft should as closely as possible resemble the desired size and shape of the defect. As it takes time for the maximum amount of deformation to occur, a piece of cartilage that is carved and immediately grafted will have warped by the time the dressings are removed. For best results, at least 30 minutes should be allowed to elapse before the cartilage graft is inserted, unless there is a specific wish to exploit the anticipated warp to achieve a particular effect.

Cartilage can be grafted with or without its perichondrium. When transplanted with the perichondrium, the mechanics of nutrition remain unchanged for the cartilage itself. When cartilage is transplanted without the perichondrium, the grafted piece must re-establish its means of nutrition. Revascularization of the perichondrium, or of the naked cartilage, is developed through the apposition of the graft and the tissues at the new site. As with any graft, the greatest risk of rejection results from haematoma formation.

Some immature cartilage grafts exhibit growth after transplantation, while others do not. The reason for the inability to grow may be insufficient nutrition, haematoma, or the incomplete apposition of surrounding tissues.

Surgeons have experimented with the use of preserved cartilage because dead cartilage does not warp, and thus will not change shape after implantation. However, one disadvantage is that, because the matrix cannot be sustained in the absence of live chondrocytes, such grafts are sometimes absorbed. Irradiation of the cartilage before implantation appears to reduce the rate of absorption. Absorption may be an immunological process.

Tendon, collagen grafts

The subject of tendon grafts is as controversial as that of fat grafts. Opinion is divided as to whether the tendon autograft survives completely, or whether it becomes reorganized. In order to survive, a tendon autograft must receive a blood supply from the recipient bed. This revascularization can be achieved through direct anastomosis of the bed vessels with those of the graft (primary revascularization), or through the establishment of a new vascular network by the ingrowth of capillaries (secondary revascularization). Although either primary or secondary revascularization can occur, it is believed that tendon graft survival is usually achieved by secondary revascularization (Peacock, 1959).

After a tendon graft, the healing process takes place in three phases. During the first phase – the phase of cellular reaction – the wound fills with blood clot, and granulation tissue is formed, whereupon fibroblast development and then collagen synthesis begin. During the second phase

– the phase of fibrous protein synthesis – fibroblast production reaches a peak at about 14 days, and then declines, as does the level of collagen synthesis. The collagen fibres change their orientation from a transverse to longitudinal axis, strengthening the union between the tendon and graft ends. During the third phase – the phase of secondary remodelling of the scar tissue – the union gains enough strength to allow slight mobility. By 8 weeks, the adhesions between the graft and the peritendinous tissue should have loosened. However, it takes 6–9 months for the intertendinous collagen fibres to arrange themselves in their characteristic bundles.

Age is a significant factor in the success of tendon grafts. The grafts are most successful in persons below the age of 40 years. However, they are somewhat less successful in children below the age of 6 years. Tendon grafts have been used in the head and neck to reconstruct larynges following cancer operations.

Fascia grafts

Facial plastic and reconstructive surgeons frequently use fascia transplant to repair facial paralysis by attaching slings or strips of fascia to an active muscle for static support. The fascia for most transplants is taken from the fascia lata of the thigh or temporalis muscle.

Fat grafts

The behaviour of transplanted fat cells remains in dispute. There are two basic theories, namely the host cell replacement theory and the cell survival theory. Proponents of the host cell replacement theory believe that none of the fat in a graft actually survives, but that host histiocytes take the lipid released from the dead fat cells and become new adipose cells. Proponents of the cell survival theory believe that the transplanted cells themselves survive.

Fat is most successfully grafted in conjunction with the dermis, as this allows revascularization of the fat through the dermal vessels, thereby helping to limit absorption of the grafted fat (*Figure 24.19*). Dermis–fat grafts are considered by some to be the best substitute for soft tissue deficiencies of the cheeks. Fat grafts have been used to augment significant facial depressions (radical parotidectomy, congenital deficiencies) (Leaf and Zarem, 1972). The main advantage of reconstituting blood supply (microvascular anastomosis) to a fat graft is its reliability in maintaining tissue thickness. Maintenance of vascular integrity apparently retards or prevents resorption and substitution.

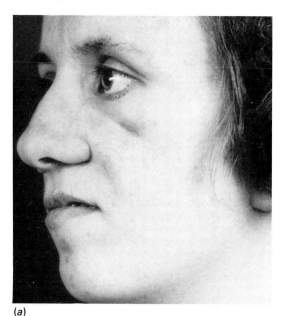

(a)

(b)

Figure 24.19 (a) Patient appearance following removal of large tumour involving the maxilla. (b) Same patient's appearance one year following fat graft transplantation from groin to the cheek

A fat transplant should never be carried out in the presence of infection. If the transplant becomes infected, the fat will liquefy and the dermis will then be extruded as a necrotic mass with fat attached. However, if this does occur, the wound will heal and another graft can be carried out. Fat grafts have been utilized with considerable success to fill body defects such as the frontal sinus, the mastoid cavity and in the repair of cerebrospinal fluid leaks.

The fat graft should be larger than the desired end result, as it will reduce to approximately 20–30% of its former size over a period of several months.

Bone grafts

Bone transplants are used to induce healing in fractures, to bridge gaps caused by compound wounds or after removal of bone tumours, and to restore missing bones, such as after a mandibulectomy (Peacock, 1984d).

Bone grafts heal through a process called creeping substitution. Most of the transplanted cells do not survive, but are replaced by mesenchymal cells from the host bed. The new cells provide support as they slowly remodel the matrix to help reduce stress in the area. These cells are also believed to promote bone formation in the connecting areas between the graft and the other segments. Four to six weeks of healing are usually required before sufficient bone substitution and revascularization have occurred to allow for removal of bone stabilization. In the case of the mandible, a biphasic appliance consisting of a rigid bar attached to the jaw by bone screws provides for stabilization and fixation until bone graft healing has occurred.

The necessary ingredients for successful bone grafting in mandibular reconstruction include: adequate soft tissue replacement, strict immobilization of the bone graft and remaining jaw, antibiotics, avoidance of oral cavity contamination of the graft site, and revascularization of the graft area or graft if the bone deficiency being repaired is in an irradiated area.

The technique of transplanting revascularized bone has for some time been used to restore mandibular deficiencies. Ostrup and Fredrickson (1975) supplied some of the first experimental evidence to support this innovative method of restoring jaw losses. The author has found the technique reliable but trying to both the surgeon and the patient. This type of grafting may require 14–20 hours of operating time before completion.

Iliac bone

The ilium is one of the best sources of bone graft. Its accessibility makes removal simple and the secondary defect easy to cover. The bone consists almost entirely of cortical bone, with a good supply of cancellous bone. However, morbidity after removal, in the form of bleeding, pain, ileus, and muscle spasm, is considerable relative to the amount of bone taken. The ilium is also a good source of bone graft in children, particularly because it remains a separate bone until later in life. The hip also provides a convenient source of marrow when a freeze-dried mandible or some type of alloplastic basket is utilized to reconstruct the jaw. The marrow is packed into the jaw replacement section to provide a matrix and osteocytes for new bone formation.

Rib bone

Rib bone is useful for grafts because of its capacity for repeated self-regeneration. In the early part of the century, however, grafts were performed using whole ribs, which allowed vascular penetration only through the ends of the graft. This made it difficult for the grafts to survive. The introduction of the use of split rib grafts greatly improved the results of transplantation.

Clavicle

The clavicle has been used to repair mandibular losses. The clavicle is endochondral bone and therefore requires a periosteal and intramedullary blood supply if it is to remain completely intact upon transplantation. Maintaining the vascular supply to the clavicle necessitates the preservation of the sternocleidomastoid muscle attachments. In practice, however, this method of mandibular reconstruction would have only limited application as in a number of cancer cases the sternocleidomastoid muscle would be removed for oncological reasons.

Scapula

The scapula is a membranous bone and consequently needs its periosteal blood supply only for the purpose of surviving as a complete bone. Membranous bone can be transplanted without a vascular supply and be expected to live, provided that the graft is placed into a well-vascularized bed. The spine and the lateral border of the scapula have been successfully used for the reconstruction of particularly difficult jaw deficiencies after cancer ablation. Proximity and sufficient bone for partial mandibular reconstruction provide the main impetus for using the scapula for jaw reconstruction. The scapula can also be utilized as a free (microvascularized) bone graft.

Calvarium

The calvarium is a membranous bone. The calvarium has been used for reconstruction of various head and neck defects. Recently, the calvarium has been used to reconstruct the mandible.

Composite grafts

Composite grafts of skin and cartilage from the auricle or nasal ala have all been used to repair nasal deficiencies. Composite grafts of skin and fat, and of skin, fat, and cartilage have also been used. Composite grafts have been used to correct cleft lip and partial losses of the nasal columella.

Alloplastic grafts

Although autografts have traditionally been considered to be the most desirable in replacement of body losses, there are cases where an inorganic implant better meets the needs of the situation. Some determining factors might be insufficient donor tissue, replacement of the autograft by scar tissue, absorption and shrinkage of the autograft, uncertainty of future treatment that might interfere with autograft success, that is, irradiation, and infection.

In general, the body responds to the presence of an insoluble foreign substance by extruding it, if possible, or by closing it off. Some specialized materials, such as titanium, hydroxyapatite, bioglass, ceramic and carbon, appear to be readily integrated into bone tissue. It has demonstrated conclusively that titanium becomes so well incorporated into various facial bones that new teeth, ears, hearing aids, jaws and noses can easily be fabricated and attached to the face and neck. Other materials may produce different reactions in the body according to the form of the implant. Teflon, for example, usually causes only a mild reaction when used in the form of a fibre, cloth or paste, yet in powder form it can cause extensive granulation. Even with those materials that cause minimal reaction, such as silicones and polypropylene, the body responds by walling off the foreign substance with a layer of mononuclear cells and a thin collagenous sheet. Teflon paste has been used successfully for a number of years to restore vocal cord function following a laryngeal paralysis. Teflon paste has also been injected into the nasopharynx for the purpose of overcoming the hypernasal speech associated with cleft palates or neurological conditions.

It is important to try to prevent haematoma formation around an implant, as this can result in extensive fibrosis. Silicone implants, in particular, have been associated with the development of a hard fibrous capsule. Sometimes a degree of fibrosis is desired as an aid to fixation. Plastics are generally more popular than metals for use in implants, as their malleability makes them easier to handle. The exceptions are the hard plastics such as polypropylene and polyethylene. Polypropylene mesh has found an important role in facial and nasal augmentation (Stucker, 1982). The mesh is a porous malleable material that makes this allograft more acceptable as a graft material.

Silicone

Silicones are especially popular for implants because of their availability in a wide variety of forms, that is as sponges, gels, meshes, foams, liquids, and rubbers. The body's response to the implantation of silicone is usually mild inflammation and the formation of a thin collagen pseudosheath. The tissue around the implant reacts by forming a granulation layer that eventually converts to fibrous tissue.

Dacron and Teflon induce a bodily reaction similar to that induced by silicone.

References

ARCHER, R. R., GREENWELL, E. J., WARE, T. and WEEKS, P. M. (1970) Irradiation effect on wound healing in rats. *Radiation Research*, **41**, 104–112

ARIYAN, S. (1979) The pectoralis major myocutaneous flap. *Plastic and Reconstructive Surgery*, **63**, 73

BAEK, S. M., BILLER, H. F. and KRESPI, Y. P. (1979) The pectoralis major myocutaneous flap for reconstruction of the head and neck. *Head and Neck Surgery*, **1**, 293

BELL, R. C. (1973) *The Use of Skin Grafts*. London: Oxford University Press

BILLER, H. F., BAEK, S. M., LAWSON, W. and KRESPI, Y. P. (1981) Pectoralis major myocutaneous island flap in head and neck surgery. *Archives of Otolaryngology*, **107**, 23

BOUCEK, R. J. (1984) Factors affecting wound healing. *Otolaryngologic Clinics of North America*, **17**, 243–261

CAJAL, S. R. (1928) *Degeneration and Regeneration of the Nervous System*. London: Oxford University Press

CARREL, A. and HARTMANN, A. (1916) Cicatrization of wounds: I. the relation between the size of a wound and the rate of its cicatrization. *Journal of Experimental Medicine*, **24**, 429

DANIEL, R. K. and WILLIAMS, H. B. (1973) The free transfer of skin flaps by microvascular anastomoses. *Plastic and Reconstructive Surgery*, **52**, 16

FRY, H. J. H. (1966) Interlocked stresses in human nasal septal cartilage. *British Journal of Plastic Surgery*, **19**, 276

FRY, H. J. H. (1977) The healing of cartilage. In *Biological Aspects of Reconstructive Surgery*, edited by D. Kernahan and L. Vistnes, ch. 19, pp. 351–365. Boston: Little, Brown & Co

GIBSON, T., STARK, H. and EVANS, J. H. (1969) Directional variation in extensibility of human skin *in vivo*. *Journal of Biomechanics*, **2**, 201

GOLDWYN, R. M. and RUECKERT, F. (1977) The value of healing by secondary intention for sizeable defects of the face. *Archives of Surgery*, **112**, 285–292

GRABB, W. C. (1977) The healing of nerve. In *Biological Aspects of Reconstructive Surgery*, edited by D. Kernahan and L. Vistnes, p. 391. Boston: Little, Brown & Co

HIGTON, D. I. R. and JAMES, D. W. (1964) The force of contraction of full-thickness wounds of rabbit skin. *British Journal of Surgery*, **51**, 462

HUNTER, J. (1794) *A Treatise on the Blood, Inflammation, and Gun-Shot Wounds*. London: George Nicol

IRVIN, T. T. (1981) *Wound Healing. Principles and Practices*. London: Chapman and Hall

JAMES, D. W. and NEWCOMBE, J. F. (1961) Granulation tissue resorption during free and limited contraction of skin wounds. *Journal of Anatomy*, **95**, 247

LEAF, N. and ZAREM, H. A. (1972) Correction of contour defects of the face with dermal and dermal–fat grafts. *Archives of Surgery*, **105**, 715–719

McGREGOR, I. A. (1980) *Fundamental Techniques of Plastic Surgery*. Edinburgh: Churchill Livingstone

McGREGOR, I. A. and MORGAN, R. G. (1973) Axial and random pattern flaps. *British Journal of Plastic Surgery*, **26**, 202

MAVES, M. D., PANJE, W. R. and SHAGETS, F. W. (1984) Extended latissimus dorsi myocutaneous flap reconstruction of major head and neck defects. *Otolaryngology, Head and Neck Surgery*, **92**, 551

MILTON, S. H. (1970) Pedicled skin flaps – the fallacy of the length–width ratios. *British Journal of Surgery*, **57**, 502

NAKAYAMA, K., YAMAMOTO, K. and TAMIYA, T. (1964) Experience with free autografts of the bowel with a new anastomosis apparatus. *Surgery*, **55**, 796

OSTRUP, L. T. and FREDRICKSON, J. M. (1975) Reconstruction of mandibular defects after irradiation using a free living bone graft transferred by microvascular anastomosis. *Plastic and Reconstructive Surgery*, **55**, 563

PANJE, W. R. (1981) Free compound groin flap reconstruction of anterior mandibular defects. *Archives of Otolaryngology*, **107**, 17

PANJE, W. R. (1984) Musculocutaneous and free flaps: physiology and practical considerations. *Otolaryngologic Clinics of North America*, **17**, 401–412

PANJE, W. R. (1987) Immediate reconstruction of the oral cavity. In *Comprehensive Management of Head and Neck Tumors*, edited by S. E. Thawley and W. R. Panje, pp. 563–595. London: W. B. Saunders

PANJE, W. R. and CUTTING, C. (1980) Trapezius osteomyocutaneous island flap for reconstruction of the anterior floor of the mouth and mandible. *Head and Neck Surgery*, **3**, 66

PANJE, W. R. and McCABE, B. F. (1979) A review: antibiotics in head and neck surgery. *Journal of Surgical Practice*, **28**, 56–60

PANJE, W. R., BUMSTED, R. M. and CEILLEY, R. I. (1980) Secondary intention healing as an adjunct to the reconstruction of mid-facial defects. *Laryngology*, **90**, 1148–1154

PEACOCK, E. E. JR (1959) A study of circulation in normal tendons and healing grafts. *Annals of Surgery*, **149**, 415

PEACOCK, E. E. JR (1984a) Structure, synthesis and interaction of fibrous protein and matrix. In *Wound Repair*, ch. 4, pp. 56–101. Philadelphia: W. B. Saunders

PEACOCK, E. E. JR (1984b) Fascia and muscle. In *Wound Repair*, ch. 9, pp. 332–362. Philadelphia: W. B. Saunders

PEACOCK, E. E. JR (1984c) Repair of tendons and restoration of gliding function. In *Wound Repair*, p. 264. Philadelphia: W. B. Saunders

PEACOCK, E. E. JR (1984d) Healing and repair of bone. In *Wound Repair*, pp. 395–416. Philadelphia: W. B. Saunders

PRITCHARD, J. J. (1969) Bone. In *Tissue Repair*, edited by R. McMinn, pp. 492–568. New York: Academic Press

RAY, R. D. (1972) Vascularization of bone grafts and implants. *Clinical Orthopedics*, **87**, 45

RAY, R. D. and SABET, T. Y. (1963) Bone grafts: cellular survival versus induction. *Journal of Bone and Joint Surgery*, **45A**, 337

ROSS, R. and ODLAND, G. (1967) The fine structure of human skin wounds. *Quarterly Journal of Surgical Science*, **3**, 2

ROWE, N. L. and KILLEY, H. (1968) *Fractures of the Facial Skeleton*, 2nd edn. Baltimore: Williams and Wilkins

SERAFIN, D. and BUNCKE, H. J. JR (1985) Editors. *Microsurgical Composite Tissue Transplantation*, 2nd edn. St Louis: C. V. Mosby

SMAHEL, J. (1971) Biology of the stage of plasmatic imbibition. *British Journal of Plastic Surgery*, **24**, 140

SMAHEL, J. and GANZONI, N. (1970) Contribution to the origin of the vasculature in free skin autografts. *British Journal of Plastic Surgery*, **23**, 322

STUCKER, F. J. (1982) The autoallograft – an alternative in facial implantation. *Otolaryngologic Clinics of North America*, **15**, 161

TRUETA, J. and LITTLE, L. (1962) The vascular contribution to osteogenesis: II: studies with electron microscope. *Journal of Bone and Joint Surgery*, **42B**, 367

URIST, M. R. (1964) Recent advances in physiology of calcification. *Journal of Bone and Joint Surgery*, **46A**, 889

WATSON, J. (1959) Some observations on free fat grafts with reference to their use in mammoplasty. *British Journal of Plastic Surgery*, **12**, 263

ZAHIR, M. (1964) Contraction of wounds. *British Journal of Surgery*, **51**, 456

25

Intensive care and resucitation in otolaryngology

Julian M. Leigh

The intensive care unit in a district general hospital offers a service to a wide variety of patients. The types of management available for patients may, broadly speaking, be subdivided into specific therapy, expectant monitoring and routine system maintenance.

Examples of therapy would be management of diabetic ketoacidosis with insulin, fluid replacement and alkali; the treatment of severe chest infection by antibiotics and physiotherapy; or the treatment of renal failure by dialysis.

The classic service under the heading of expectant monitoring is carried out for patients with myocardial infarction who are in danger of suffering from acute dysrhythmias or cardiogenic shock. This category would also include patients with upper airway problems which are within the province of otolaryngological surgery.

Finally, under routine maintenance would come care of nutrition, fluid and electrolyte balance in any patient unable to control these, even though the primary problem under treatment may be principally in another physiological system.

Relationships between intensive care and otolaryngology

A service to otolaryngological patients is provided by the intensive care unit in the case of children with upper airway obstruction. This is seen not only in acute epiglottitis but also in the inspissated secretion syndrome, which may occur with severe pneumonias and dehydration in small children. Adult admissions to the intensive care unit tend to be for upper airway obstruction caused usually by pharyngeal or laryngeal carcinoma. These patients are sometimes admitted for management before

surgery, but are mostly admitted postoperatively to provide the intensive nursing observation and management of the airway which are necessary in the first 24 hours.

Although admission may be less important after laryngectomy, it is still regarded as a reasonable policy for such patients to receive 24 hours of management in the intensive care unit, not only for the airway but also because lengthy surgery may have caused problems with fluid balance and body temperature maintenance.

The other important relationship with the otolaryngology department arises from what might be called the 'tracheostomy service' for patients requiring that manoeuvre for long-term intermittent positive pressure ventilation (IPPV), such as patients with head injuries, and multiple trauma cases with chest complications. It is also important that the otolaryngology department should be involved in the formulation of intensive care unit policies for the 'routine' management of tracheostomies. This includes not only the policy on surgical technique but also policies on what types of tube should be used, dressings, humidification and suction, and so on. The details of the policies are not as important as their being agreed and standardized.

The intensive care service

In intensive care units, general management procedures of problems in the different body systems are not necessarily influenced by the specific cause of admission. General policies and management techniques of major body systems will now be discussed under separate headings.

Respiratory system

The corner-stone of intensive care is respiratory management, particularly intermittent positive pressure ventilation. Many surgical patients in the past have died from insidious respiratory failure in the postoperative period. Age, previous respiratory disease, prolonged surgery and, particularly, postoperative pain and endotoxaemia with humoral pneumonitis, all contribute to inadequate alveolar ventilation, sputum retention and respiratory death.

Many patients, particularly the elderly, undergoing oesophageal and arterial surgery and/or other emergency major intra-abdominal procedures, are currently ventilated postoperatively in the intensive care unit. Fluid and electrolyte balance is adjusted and continuous analgesia is provided either by intravenous narcotic administration or with epidural opiates. Weaning from intermittent positive pressure ventilation takes place after about 24 hours and feeding regimens are introduced. The result of this type of management is a profound reduction in morbidity and mortality.

Physiotherapy and fibreoptic bronchoscopy are important when sputum retention is a problem, as is full hydration of the patient. The newly available technique of inserting an indwelling 'mini-trach' laryngotomy suction tube is a useful adjunct to clinical practice.

When upper airway obstruction is a problem, time can be bought by medical means by using oxyhelium therapy. This mixture of 21% oxygen with 79% helium has one-third of the density of air and, as turbulent flow at such sites is predominantly influenced by gas density, the flow of respired gases past an obstruction can take place with one-third of the pressure drop.

Table 25.1 summarizes respiratory function, failure, diagnostic points, causes and treatment. In practice, any or all types of respiratory failure may coexist in a given patient. The situation must be unravelled by using clinical criteria as well as blood gas analysis.

Cardiovascular system

An understanding of the cardiovascular system is fundamental to the practice of clinical medicine (*Table 25.2*).

The object of the cardiovascular system is that the tissues should be perfused for the exchange of nutrients. The requirements are: first, that the heart should function as a demand pump, responsive to the magnitude of the venous return; and, second, that there should be an adequate distributive system to individual organ capillary beds. The heart pump requires the following: that its power output is kept within its own capability to supply itself with nutrients via the coronary

Table 25.1 Schema of respiratory system

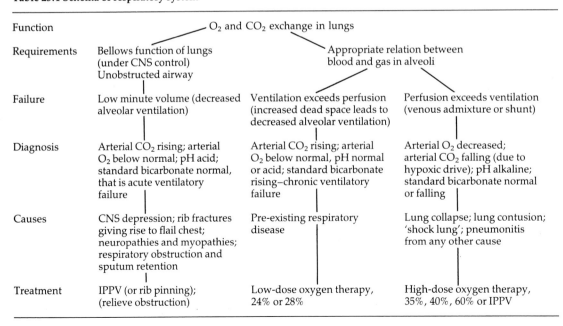

Function	O_2 and CO_2 exchange in lungs		
Requirements	Bellows function of lungs (under CNS control) Unobstructed airway	Appropriate relation between blood and gas in alveoli	
Failure	Low minute volume (decreased alveolar ventilation)	Ventilation exceeds perfusion (increased dead space leads to decreased alveolar ventilation)	Perfusion exceeds ventilation (venous admixture or shunt)
Diagnosis	Arterial CO_2 rising; arterial O_2 below normal; pH acid; standard bicarbonate normal, that is acute ventilatory failure	Arterial CO_2 rising; arterial O_2 below normal, pH normal or acid; standard bicarbonate rising–chronic ventilatory failure	Arterial O_2 decreased; arterial CO_2 falling (due to hypoxic drive); pH alkaline; standard bicarbonate normal or falling
Causes	CNS depression; rib fractures giving rise to flail chest; neuropathies and myopathies; respiratory obstruction and sputum retention	Pre-existing respiratory disease	Lung collapse; lung contusion; 'shock lung'; pneumonitis from any other cause
Treatment	IPPV (or rib pinning); (relieve obstruction)	Low-dose oxygen therapy, 24% or 28%	High-dose oxygen therapy, 35%, 40%, 60% or IPPV

IPPV: intermittent positive pressure ventilation

Table 25.2 Schema of cardiovascular system

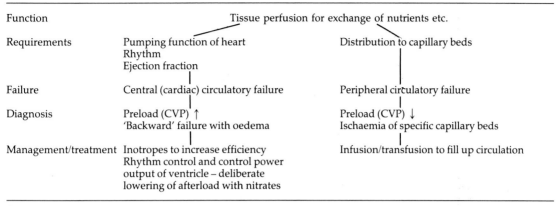

Function	Tissue perfusion for exchange of nutrients etc.	
Requirements	Pumping function of heart Rhythm Ejection fraction	Distribution to capillary beds
Failure	Central (cardiac) circulatory failure	Peripheral circulatory failure
Diagnosis	Preload (CVP) ↑ 'Backward' failure with oedema	Preload (CVP) ↓ Ischaemia of specific capillary beds
Management/treatment	Inotropes to increase efficiency Rhythm control and control power output of ventricle – deliberate lowering of afterload with nitrates	Infusion/transfusion to fill up circulation

CVP: central venous pressure

circulation, that it has a near normal rhythm; and that the ejection fraction of the ventricle is also near normal.

Failure in the system produces conditions known as central circulatory (cardiac) failure and peripheral circulatory failure. In the former, the central venous pressure (the preload) is high, indicating pump failure, and is attended by backward oedema. In the latter, the preload is low and ischaemia of specific capillary beds may be manifest, for example skin vasoconstriction.

The management of pump failure may require inotropic support to increase the efficiency of the myocardium and to control rhythm and, finally, measures to reduce the power output of the heart by means of vasodilators such as nitrates. Treatment of peripheral circulatory failure usually requires infusion or transfusion of the appropriate fluids.

Renal management

The function of the renal system (*Table 25.3*) may be summarized as the excretion of non-volatile waste products, and of surplus water and electrolytes in order to maintain the milieu interieur.

The way in which this is achieved is that the million nephrons in the kidneys filter the plasma volume over 50 times per day, whereupon the 40 miles of tubules elaborate this filtrate according to the requirements of acid–base balance, water and electrolyte surpluses or deficiencies and nitrogen excretion.

The system requires local autoregulation of blood flow at glomerular level, and active and passive processes within the tubules under the control peripherally of hormonal and humoral mechanisms initiated in the kidney by the renin–angiotensin system and, *centrally*, in the

Table 25.3 Schema of renal function

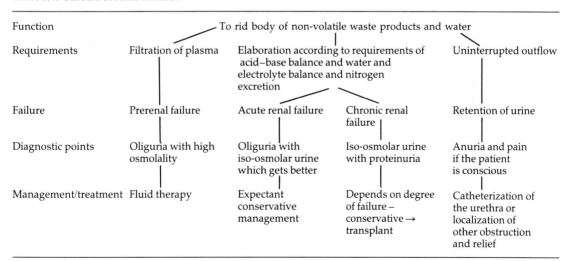

Function	To rid body of non-volatile waste products and water			
Requirements	Filtration of plasma	Elaboration according to requirements of acid–base balance and water and electrolyte balance and nitrogen excretion		Uninterrupted outflow
Failure	Prerenal failure	Acute renal failure	Chronic renal failure	Retention of urine
Diagnostic points	Oliguria with high osmolality	Oliguria with iso-osmolar urine which gets better	Iso-osmolar urine with proteinuria	Anuria and pain if the patient is conscious
Management/treatment	Fluid therapy	Expectant conservative management	Depends on degree of failure – conservative → transplant	Catheterization of the urethra or localization of other obstruction and relief

hypothalamus and pituitary. An additional requirement is that the elaborated urine can be voided to the exterior by an uninterrupted genitourinary tract.

From the clinical point of view, failure of urine elaboration may be prerenal, renal or postrenal. Prerenal failure occurs when the filtration pressure is low in consequence of, for example, hypotension and hypovolaemia. Postrenal failure occurs with genitourinary tract obstruction. Renal (nephron) failure may be either acute or chronic; the former commonly occurs in surgical patients as a consequence of severe hypotension and endotoxaemia, while the latter has a variety of causes including pyelonephritis and atherosclerosis.

Clinically, a distinction usually has to be made between prerenal and acute renal failure in the context of surgery. Both are characterized by oliguria, but in prerenal failure the osmolarity of urine is high, so the clearance of osmolar particles is not reduced, whereas in acute nephron failure the urine is isotonic. Retention of water, sodium, potassium, urea, creatinine and hydrogen ions will follow to a greater or lesser extent. In practice, two *clinical* forms of oliguric renal failure with nitrogen retention are seen postoperatively; one of these is relatively benign and potassium and hydrogen ion excretion are unaffected, while in the second type significant potassium retention and acid–base disturbance occurs.

The former condition requires fluid intake of a volume equal to the urine output plus insensible loss, by using high concentration carbohydrate solutions. In the latter condition, this management must be accompanied by bicarbonate (alkali) therapy to combat metabolic acidosis, and glucose/insulin infusions plus potassium exchange resin in an attempt to lower potassium levels. If these measures are not effective, then either peritoneal dialysis, haemodialysis or ultrafiltration must take place.

Symptoms appear when the glomerular filtration rate (measured by creatinine clearance) falls from 120 to less than 30 ml/minute. If the glomerular filtration rate is less than 3 ml/minute, then dialysis and/or transplantation is required.

Management of nutrition

As malnutrition is not uncommon in certain types of otolaryngological patient, this topic will be dealt with in some detail.

Types of patient requiring nutritional support

Patients requiring nutritional support are those suffering from the following conditions:

(1) interference with gastrointestinal function: poor dentition; dysphagia; obstruction; prolonged paralytic ileus from any cause, for example peritonitis, pancreatitis, major surgery; gut fistulae; malabsorption and short bowel syndrome
(2) renal failure
(3) severe burns, trauma and sepsis and other hypermetabolic states
(4) cachexia caused by severe cardiac or respiratory disease
(5) severe psychological disturbances, for example anorexia nervosa.

Types of malnutrition

Basically there are two types of protein/energy malnutrition: first, the chronic fasting-adapted starvation known as marasmus; second, the fasting-unadapted starvation of critical illness accompanied by the stress response, which may be made worse by surgical intervention. If protein and energy requirements are chronically unsatisfied because of a lack of exogenous replacement, catabolism of somatic protein and fat stores follows, leading to a kwashiorkor-like state.

A mixed condition occurs when, for example, a patient with dysphagia resulting from pharyngeal carcinoma and marasmus undergoes surgery without prior protein/energy replacement.

Fasting-adapted starvation

In chronic starvation, there is a progressive fall in both energy requirements and nitrogen loss. Once the carbohydrate stores have been utilized, it is the fat metabolism which supplies energy requirements, while glucose deficits are made up from the carbon skeletons of deaminated amino acids. Early on, the ratio of fat utilization to protein is about 2.5:1, while at full adaptation this ratio increases to 7.5:1, which means that, to some extent, body protein is spared in relation to fat. This adaptive process breaks down if the stress response is initiated. Breakdown of endogenous protein is a significant source of energy under these circumstances, and the metabolic expenditure closely parallels nitrogen losses. These losses can be reversed by feeding traumatized patients with high calorie/protein diets. A full explanation of the role of protein and fat in starvation may be understood with reference to the schema of intermediary metabolism shown in *Figure 25.1*.

Carbohydrate metabolism

Carbohydrate is the usual source of energy. Glucose is metabolized via glucose 6-phosphate to

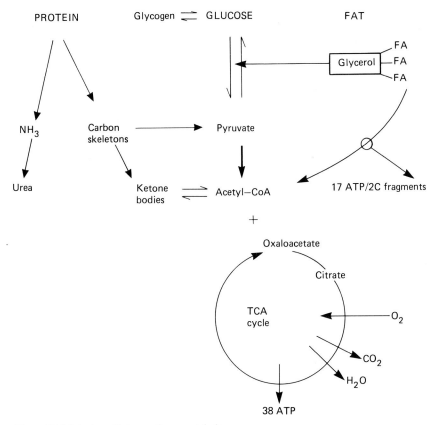

Figure 25.1 Schema of intermediary metabolism

pyruvate and thence to acetyl coenzyme A which is incorporated into the citric acid cycle by combining with oxaloacetate to form citrate. This pathway, in which glucose finally becomes carbon dioxide and water, liberates 38 molecules of energy-rich ATP. Carbohydrate yields 40 cal/g.

When metabolism of glucose is not required, excesses are stored as glycogen. Glycogen stores occur in the liver (up to 8%) and in muscle (up to 2%). As there is much more muscle than liver, the former constitutes the major store of glycogen, although it can be utilized only by muscle.

The steps on the main glycolytic pathway are all reversible *apart* from the last one, where pyruvate is metabolized to acetyl-CoA.

Fat metabolism

The metabolism of fat yields 9 cal/g. The main fats of interest in animal metabolism are glycerides. These consist of glycerol combined with up to three substituted chains of fatty acids. Metabolism yields glycerol which, by way of α-glycerophosphate, is incorporated in the glycolytic sequence, as shown in *Figure 25.1*. The fatty acids

are metabolized to acetyl coenzyme A by being split off two-carbon atoms at a time, each yielding 17 energy-rich ATP molecules. When, for example, palmitic acid is totally broken down, the side chains yield 130 molecules of ATP, which explains why fat has such a high energy yield.

As acetyl coenzyme A cannot be resynthesized to pyruvate, fat metabolism does not yield glucose intermediates (other than glycerol in small quantities) for energy transport; nor does it supply energy for tissues which can use only glucose – predominantly the brain. Thus fat metabolism is incapable of maintaining the blood glucose level.

Protein metabolism

Protein metabolism, by contrast, can maintain the blood glucose level. Amino acids are deaminated, thereby yielding ammonia (which is converted in the ornithine cycle to form urea). The carbon skeletons which remain are either glucogenic, forming pyruvate which can be converted to glucose or, in lesser quantities, ketogenic, forming the ketone bodies (acetoacetic acid, β-hydroxybutyrate and acetone).

When there is very decreased glycolysis, as in carbohydrate starvation, the citric acid cycle slows down because oxaloacetate, which combines with acetyl coenzyme A, is not regenerated in sufficient quantities. Although there is an alternative direct path for the production of oxaloacetate by carboxylation of pyruvate, the lack of consumption of acetyl-CoA, from fatty acid degradation and from the ketogenic carbon skeletons of protein, results in the accumulation of ketone bodies; of these, β-hydroxybutyrate can quite easily be measured in the blood.

The problem for the body in starvation/catabolism is that the carbohydrate stores – as circulating glucose or glycogen – are depleted well within 24 hours. Metabolism must, therefore, switch to the high energy yielding fat, and glucogenesis has to occur from amino acid metabolism.

The role of insulin and glucagon

Insulin regulates glucose metabolism and also controls the anabolism of both lipids and amino acids, whereas glucagon, broadly speaking, exerts the opposite effect. Insulin has a dual mechanism for lowering of the blood glucose level. First, it increases glucose uptake in the peripheral tissues, particularly striated muscle and adipose tissue; and, second, it decreases the hepatic glucose output. Therefore, when insulin is present, glucose enters cells readily from the extracellular fluid and becomes available for intracellular metabolism or fatty acid or amino acid synthesis.

The biological half-life of insulin in the blood is of the order of 2–5 minutes. However, its biological action may persist for longer and reactive hypoglycaemia can occasionally develop when glucose infusions are stopped.

In the liver, insulin decreases gluconeogenesis and glycogenolysis and encourages glycogen synthesis. Therefore, when insulin is deficient, gluconeogenesis and glycogenolysis increase with an output of glucose from the liver into the extracellular fluid. The blood glucose level further builds up, as the glucose is inhibited from entering the tissues in the absence of insulin, and glycosuria may ensue. As the glucose cannot be metabolized, ketosis follows fatty acid breakdown and thus is seen both in starvation and, more severely, in diabetics.

Insulin promotes triglyceride synthesis in the adipose tissue cells. As lipase activity is normally inhibited by the presence of insulin, the consequence of insulin deficiency is the occurrence of unopposed lipolysis. For these reasons, insulin should be added to total parenteral nutrition regimens to inhibit catabolism.

The metabolic response to trauma

The metabolic response to trauma consists of disordered carbohydrate metabolism with ketosis, negative nitrogen balance, increased oxygen consumption and salt and water retention. Various triggering mechanisms are responsible and include soft tissue trauma, haemorrhage, other types of fluid losses, severe illness, burns, sepsis, and both pain and psychological stress.

Mediation seems to be integrated in the hypothalamus with hormonal changes from the anterior and posterior pituitary, the adrenal cortex and medulla, the pancreas, thyroid and kidney. Humoral mechanisms, involving kallikreinin and prostaglandins, are also instrumental in the initiation of the response. The metabolic phenomena can be blocked during surgery, either in part or wholly, by combinations of epidural or spinal analgesia, barbiturates, morphine, neuroleptanalgesia and adrenergic blocking agents.

Metabolic changes in stress

The interaction of catecholamines, growth hormone, cortisol and glucagon together with diminished insulin secretion and increased resistance to its activity, cause hyperglycaemia and inhibit both the intracellular transfer and metabolism of glucose, as indicated earlier.

Mineralocorticoid secretion and altered renal perfusion suggest that the primary disturbance at cell membrane level consists of inhibition of the sodium pump. This would explain the intracellular sodium retention with extracellular hyponatraemia, the simultaneous opposite effects on potassium, and the consequent shifts in water. The potassium losses are also exacerbated by the increase in nitrogen excretion.

Evidence for a single 'biochemical lesion' in this area of intermediary metabolism has been demonstrated by its successful inhibition by means of glucose, potassium, and insulin regimens.

Feeding the otolaryngological patient

The vast majority of otolaryngological patients do not require extra feeding as they are neither starved beforehand nor do they get sufficient stress response. However, those patients with upper digestive tract carcinoma and/or dysphagia often present with fasting-adapted starvation. Most of these patients do not have an ileus and can be fed before surgery either by sip feeding or by continuous or bolus administration by way of a tube which bypasses the lesion.

Tube feeding may be through a nasal or orogastric narrow bore tube, if either of these can be tolerated, or by way of a jejunostomy. A homogenized diet, which can contain useful roughage and microorganisms as well as the essential food elements cannot pass through very narrow bore tubes. If a small bore tube is passed, then only a liquid diet can be given. Under these circumstances, it is usual for a proprietary synthetic elemental diet to be used. These preparations contain all food principals, including trace elements and vitamins, usually in such a concentration that they supply 1 cal/ml. These solutions are thus hyperosmolar and may cause purgation; to avoid this problem, it is advisable initially to dilute the solutions to half strength. Proprietary elemental diets are obtainable in lactose- and gluten-free forms, such as Ensure, or a milk-based diet such as Clinifeed. Supplementation by other proprietary preparations, such as Complan (carbohydrate and protein) or Hycal (carbohydrate only), is possible. Milk, eggs and natural orange juice are also frequently employed as supplements to the diet.

Table 25.4 Intravenous nutrition via a central venous catheter

Requirements for normal nutrition:

Calories	30–40 cal/kg per day $\simeq$ 2000/day
Nitrogen	0.15–0.20 g N_2/kg per day $\simeq$ 10–14 g N_2/day $\simeq$ 60–90 g protein
Water	40 ml/kg per day $\simeq$ 2.5–3 l/day

These figures are raised by up to 50% in fever and severe trauma
Insensible water loss is 10 ml/kg per day $\simeq$ 700 ml/day which increases by 10%/°C of pyrexia
Normal kidney function will sort out a moderate excess of fluid intake
Additional requirements supplied by:

Parentrovite I and II daily	i.v.
Konakion (vit K) 10 mg daily	i.m.
Folic acid 15 mg twice weekly	i.v.
Neo-Cytamen (vit B_{12}) 500 µg monthly	i.m.

After one month, consider vitamin and trace element preparations Vitlipid and Addamel (10 ml vials added to Intralipid and Vamin glucose twice weekly). Start sooner if the patient is nutritionally deprived beforehand

A regimen for intravenous feeding might reasonably be A + B with one from C, D or E, depending on requirements. Common sense should prevail

A	*20% Intralipid 500 ml Vamin glucose	} given together over 6–8 h		Supplying 2650 cal with 9.4 g N_2 $\simeq$ 60 g protein in 2 litres – Na 50, *K* 20, Ca 2.5, Mg 1.5, Cl 55 mmol, essential fatty acids and phosphates
	50% glucose 500 ml and 20 units soluble insulin Vamin glucose 500 ml	} given together over 6–8 h		
B	Hartmann's solution 1000 ml	in 6–8 h		Na 131, K 5, Ca 2, Cl 111, HCO_3 29 mmol. KC1 supplement should be added according to daily requirements
C	Synthamin-17 500 ml	in 6–8 h		Supplying 8.25 g N_2 $\simeq$ 54 g protein, Na 36.5, *K* 30, Mg 2.5, acetate 75, Cl 35, phosphate 15
D	Glucose 20% 500 ml or Glucose 50% 500 ml	in 3–4 h	400 kcal 1000 kcal }	Soluble insulin should be added to prevent hyperglycaemia
E	Plasma protein fraction Freeze-dried plasma Whole blood (Weigh bag to determine amount and bear in mind that SAGM blood† is now the commonest product supplied)	400 ml 500 ml 200–500 ml } in 3–4 h		Given only if required Fresh frozen plasma may be needed for extra clotting factors.

*NB The equivalent number of calories (1000) can be supplied in 500 ml of 50% glucose at approximately one-seventh of the cost

†SAGM blood: saline–adenine–glucose–mannitol blood

Insulin at one unit per hour given subcutaneously should be given for its anabolic effect. Glucose levels should be monitored with BM-sticks and a colorimeter; this is especially important if the energy administration regimen is interrupted for other fluids

Total parenteral nutrition

It may be easier in some of these patients to begin nutrition with an intravenous regimen, and if ileus follows surgery then it becomes mandatory. Some authorities recommend the provision of all nutrition, water and electrolyte requirements in a 3-litre bag for 24-hour administration. This may be possible once a stable situation has been achieved, but acutely ill patients require more frequent evaluation and alteration of their regimens.

The requirements for the common electrolyte substances may be determined on a daily basis by plasma estimation and, where necessary, urinary excretion measurements. The requirement for potassium is likely to be higher than normal as its excretion is accelerated if there is excessive nitrogen excretion. Other than this, the necessary supplies of these substances are covered in the total parenteral nutrition regimen, given in *Table 25.4*.

It remains axiomatic from the biochemical information given earlier that a positive nitrogen balance is not possible if insufficient non-protein calories are given. The ratio of non-protein calories to nitrogen should be of the order of 200 cal/g.

Obtaining circulatory access

The choice lies between peripheral and central venous administration. If, for any reason, venous access is impossible then nutrition can be administered intra-abdominally after the insertion of a peritoneal dialysis catheter, and the amino acid, fat or carbohydrate solutions will subsequently be absorbed through the peritoneum.

As ill patients may require other non-nutritional fluids, the carbohydrate and amino acid solutions tend to be hypertonic in order that the maximum amount of nutrient may be administered with the minimum amount of fluid. The advantage of central venous cannulation is that these hypertonic fluids are rapidly diluted in the large blood vessels, and thus a central line is the commonest method of administering total parenteral nutrition.

A radiopaque catheter is inserted so that its tip lies in the superior vena cava or right atrium. Transcutaneous access is achieved by way of the basilic vein in the antecubital fossa or by way of either the internal jugular vein or the subclavian vein.

Central venous catheterization may be unnecessary in patients who are on enteral feeding but who are as yet unable to tolerate total enteral nutrition. These individuals can have their diet supplemented by peripheral venous feeding using combinations of fat with either amino acid or glucose solutions, so that the mixture delivered into the vein is essentially isotonic.

Assessing nutrient requirements

Caring for the metabolically compromised patient requires: first, the treatment of the stress component, such as pain, haemorrhage, tissue necrosis and sepsis, as mitigation in this way will diminish the hormonal and humoral triggering of the catabolic stress response; second, assessments to be made of the dietary components which need to be administered, including electrolytes, trace elements and vitamins.

Assessment techniques

The proteins can be separated into visceral and somatic compartments. The visceral compartment consists of all the secretory proteins which play an important role in the survival of the organism. Included here are serum albumin, transferrin and cell-mediated immunocompetence proteins.

The search for protein nutrition markers among these secretory proteins has been protracted. The ideal marker would be affected promptly by any alteration in nutritional status; it would be unaffected by catabolism and non-nutritional therapies; and it would have a low extracellular fluid concentration and a short half-life. Albumin does not fulfill these requirements and measurements of transferrin have not proved useful. More recently, retinol binding protein and thyroxine binding pre-albumin have been assessed in this respect, but have also not proved useful.

The somatic protein compartment is muscle – the so-called 'lean body mass'. Estimation of 24-hour urea nitrogen excretion reflects the status of the metabolism of the lean body mass, that is an increased nitrogen excretion indicates that protein catabolism is occurring.

The 24-hour creatinine excretion is proportional to somatic muscle mass in normal individuals. However, an increased excretion may occur when there is heightened protein catabolism in the presence of a depleted lean body mass and its measurement is inconclusive.

Even the standard anthropomorphic techniques of nutritional assessment used for the non-critically ill are less reliable. Arm circumference, triceps skin fold and body weight may all be affected by fluid shifts as a result of 'third spacing' in the extracellular compartment of oedema fluid.

In the final analysis, reliance has to be placed on clinical judgement of the status of the lean tissue mass, and on common sense. The crude, but nevertheless useful, tool of 24-hour urine urea nitrogen determination and comparison with the 24-hour intake of nitrogen, is probably the only practical method of deciding whether lean tissue anabolism or catabolism is taking place.

Complications associated with total parenteral nutrition

The insertion of central lines is beset with a number of problems. Perforation of the pleura and pneumothorax has been described both with the internal jugular and subclavian approach. Additionally, air embolism can theoretically occur during insertion of the cannula. This may be avoided by ensuring that the patient is in a head-down tilt during the procedure.

Thrombosis and phlebitis are risks more commonly associated with peripheral infusion, and they may be avoided by using solutions which are not hypertonic in combination with regular changing of the cannulation site. Long lines from the antecubital fossa produce the biggest risk of venous thrombosis.

Infection

Infection may arise for a number of reasons attributable to faulty aseptic technique:

(1) during insertion
(2) during subsequent dressings of the insertion site
(3) when changing bottles, bags or lines
(4) contamination of the infusate during manufacture or when additives are given.

More recently, subcutaneous tunnelling of the central catheter has been advocated. However, unless strict aseptic technique is adhered to during this procedure, this method will not reduce the risk of infection. The use of this technique also assumes that central line infections occur by contamination of the wound and spread down the outside of the catheter. In reality, it is almost certain that catheters are infected more often by blood-borne organisms.

Ideally, there should be a specific line for intravenous feeding only. However, in the critically ill patient this may not be possible. Therefore, regular handwashing and strict adherence to written policies/procedures is of vital importance. The practice in the author's unit is to use 70 cm lines for subclavian central venous insertion. The advantage is that the excess line outside the patient allows the points of contact with taps, etc., to be distal to the wound, which is dressed in the prescribed manner every 48 hours.

Monitoring of white cell count daily and of temperature, pulse and respiration 4-hourly may give a clue to infection of the central venous line.

Other complications

Other complications relate to circulatory overload with fluid and to glycaemic instability. Hyper-osmolar (hyperglycaemic) non-ketotic syndrome and coma may ensue, as may excessive fluid losses with glycosuria. Regular blood glucose measurements at the bedside, with a chemical 'stick test' read colorimetrically, and urine analysis avoid this complication, provided that the insulin administration is adjusted accordingly. Insulin may be given mixed with the substrates in the infusion solutions, in which case allowances have to be made for binding of the insulin to the containers; or, alternatively, in concentrated form by way of a syringe pump through a separate line. The disadvantage of the latter occurs when nutrients are discontinued, and care must be taken to avoid disastrous hypoglycaemia.

Evaluation of feeding regimens

As has been indicated earlier, evaluation of feeding regimens may prove extremely difficult in practice. Measurement of β-hydroxybutyrate in plasma is now fairly easy and levels in excess of 0.3 mmol/l indicate that non-carbohydrate metabolism (catabolism) is occurring. Under these circumstances, the blood sugar level is of no help in assessing nutritional status but is monitored to help promote glycaemic stability. β-Hydroxybutyrate measurements can be combined with 24-hour nitrogen balance to assess the status of the lean body mass.

Weaning once total parenteral nutrition is discontinued

A patient recovering from serious illness, who has been receiving long-term total parenteral nutrition, will require a gentle introduction to oral or nasogastric feeds. The onset of gut sounds and diminution of nasogastric aspiration to a minimum indicate that water may be introduced initially. If this is absorbed then nutrient substances can be introduced. As the gut which is recovering from ileus is very often lactose intolerant, it is usually wise to introduce a lactose-free synthetic elemental diet, such as Ensure, before proceeding by means of milk to a homogenized diet, whereupon the nasogastric tube can be removed.

The gastrointestinal hormones will have been in abeyance during total parenteral nutrition, and the hepatic enzymes will have adapted to the total parenteral nutritional regimen, arriving in the systemic circulation, rather than with partially processed nutrients which arrive by way of the portal vein. Consequently, as re-adaptation will be necessary, all feeding should be introduced slowly and intravenous feeding should be concomitantly reduced.

Haematological considerations

Anaemia

Anaemia has many causes but in the final analysis can be the result of either abnormal red cell production or excessive loss of blood. It may be congenital or acquired, and primary or secondary.

From a clinical point of view, the important consideration is when and by what method correction should be carried out. Clearly, if a patient is bleeding and anaemic, correction needs to be carried out by transfusion. However, for more chronic forms, medical measures will suffice. The signs of absent compensation would be breathlessness and tiredness, together with palpitations, dyspnoea on exertion, and possibly effort angina with an ejection systolic murmur.

Oxygen transport

Haemoglobin is *not* the most important factor in oxygen transport. A full understanding of oxygen transport is important for the clinician because its consideration has to be balanced against the quality of blood available for transfusion in the surgical situation.

The oxygen transported to the tissues in unit time is a function of the haemoglobin concentration, oxygen saturation of the haemoglobin in arterial blood, and the cardiac output.

O_2 availability = $K(Hb \times SaO_2 \times Qt)$, where

Hb = haemoglobin level in g/100 ml whole blood
SaO_2 = percentage oxygen saturation of the haemoglobin in arterial blood
Qt = cardiac output in ml/minute
K = constant, derived from the oxygen capacity of haemoglobin and appropriate decimal corrections, with a resulting value of 0.000139.

Considering some normal values:

$$O_2 \text{ availability} = K(14.5 \times 100 \times 5000)$$
$$\approx 1000 \text{ ml/minute}$$

As basal oxygen consumption is of the order of 250 ml/minute there is still a considerable reserve under normal conditions.

The relative contributions of the foregoing factors can be placed in perspective as follows:

(1) each litre change in cardiac output, when the haemoglobin level is normal and there is full saturation, accounts for a change of 200 ml/minute in oxygen availability
(2) each gram change in haemoglobin, when the cardiac output is 5 l/minute and there is full saturation, accounts for a change of 69 ml/minute in oxygen availability

(3) each 1% change in saturation, when the cardiac output is 5 l/minute and the haemoglobin level is normal, accounts for 10 ml/minute in oxygen availability.

The impact of anaemia on a patient, especially for routine surgery, must be weighed against the disadvantages of delaying surgery until medical correction can be achieved. In the emergency situation, the disadvantage of anaemia has to be offset against the disadvantages of whole blood available for transfusion.

The quality of blood for transfusion

It is an unfortunate fact that blood is usually only made available for transfusion late in its shelf life of 3 weeks, by which time it contains clots and microaggregates of dead white cells and effete red cells. Depending on the anticoagulant used – the blood may be acid in the case of acid–citrate–dextrose blood and have a high serum potassium – it may be infected, incompatible and so on. In addition, with the modern presentation as saline–adenine–glucose–mannitol blood, the plasma – which is perhaps the most important component of blood – will have been depleted. It is not too cynical to state that if blood were classified as a medicine, it would probably not pass the stringent regulations of the various safety organizations around the world. As an acute replacement for lost blood volume, plasma protein fraction (human albumin) is much safer.

If, in spite of these considerations, a blood transfusion is still deemed necessary, it is mandatory in present times that the blood be filtered with a device capable of removing particulate matter down to 20 µm because, *if it is not filtered beforehand, the lungs will do so subsequently.* Debris from transfused blood in the lungs causes a humoral response and pneumonitis, resulting in shunting or venous admixture, and this is an avoidable additional risk factor.

Sickle-cell trait and disease

Normal adult haemoglobin is given the designation HbA. In the heterozygous condition of sickle-cell trait, there is a mixture of HbA with HbS, whereas in the homozygous condition of sickle-cell disease, the haemoglobin is all HbS, and the sufferer has the designation HbSS. Equally serious are the combination of the sickle-cell gene with HbC, giving the sickle-cell C disease (HbSC), or the combination with thalassaemia, giving sickle-cell thalassaemia (HbS-thal).

Sickling of the red cells occurs with apparent crystallization of the abnormal haemoglobin at low oxygen tension and pH. There is aggregation of abnormal cells, which causes microinfarctions in the tissues, and the disease manifestations depend on the distribution of the infarcts.

Sufferers from this disease tend to be coloured patients of African or West Indian origin or from the Mediterranean region.

Homozygous patients will usually give a history of sickling crises with haemolytic anaemia, but the heterozygous patients may be found by screening with a bedside test such as the 'Sickledex'. If this test is positive and the patient has no concurrent anaemia, it is unlikely that the patient will have a significant clinical problem as the positive test suggests the heterozygous condition. However, if there is time, the patient should be genotyped and a blood film examined. The care required by these patients is no more meticulous than that offered to any other. Therefore, even in countries with large populations of the type just described, management of the condition is passive rather than active. Even the use of tourniquets in orthopaedic procedures is not proscribed in these countries, although their use would not appear to be justifiable.

Bleeding disorders

Clinical medicine in the UK is no longer carried out without access to consultant haematologists. However, it is clearly the duty of the ordinary clinician to be able to differentiate between large diagnostic groups, for example, to determine whether a bleeding tendency is lifelong or whether there is a family history of such a condition.

Purpura and excessive bleeding from superficial cuts and mucosal haemorrhages suggest a platelet disorder, whereas the occurrence of deep bruising, bleeding into joints and haematuria, or delayed wound healing after previous surgery, would be indicative of coagulation factor deficiencies. In the laboratory, the bleeding time and platelet count can detect quantitative and qualitative platelet deficiencies, while a prothrombin time is sensitive to defects of the coagulation factors II, V, VII and X and is also prolonged in liver failure, vitamin K deficiency and during the use of anticoagulants. The activated partial thromboplastin time indicates a deficiency of factors V, VIII, IX and X and is used to detect haemophilia (factor VIII deficiency) and Christmas disease (factor IX deficiency).

In the condition of disseminated intravascular coagulation, there is an increased level of fibrin degradation products, and both fibrinogen and platelet levels are lowered. At the present time, disseminated intravascular coagulation is treated with antibiotics for the triggering sepsis and by the transfusion of fresh frozen plasma and platelets, rather than by trying to inhibit the process of accelerated intravascular coagulation with heparin. None of these conditions should be treated without reference to, and without the close cooperation of, the haematologist.

Prophylaxis of deep vein thrombosis

Intra- and postoperative prophylaxis of deep vein thrombosis is carried out not only in the wards after surgery but also in the intensive care unit. It might be considered an area for controversial discussion as many disciplines are involved. Moreover, there is a shifting ground of fashion in the management of these problems.

The position used to be less problematical in the case of women taking the contraceptive pill as it had been considered beneficial for the woman simply to stop therapy. However, in the light of experience this assumption has been questioned and many have now ceased this practice. Nevertheless, a history of obesity and previous deep vein thrombosis would indicate active prophylaxis. On the other hand, a decision is more difficult when, for example, a patient has varicose veins unrelated to the current surgical/medical problem, and treatment must depend on the reasoned opinion of the individual clinician. The author has found the advice of Browse (1977), in his excellent article: 'What Should I Do about Deep Vein Thrombosis and Pulmonary Embolism', to be of great use in this respect. Crandon *et al.* (1980) have also made an attempt to identify high-risk patients for selective prophylactic anticoagulant therapy. The present author's current practice, once a patient is in the intensive care unit, is to use subcutaneous heparin therapy (5000 units, 8-hourly) and anti-embolism stockings on the basis that both these measures have been shown to be effective in the prophylaxis of deep vein thrombosis. Heparin is the anticoagulant of choice as it can be easily reversed with protamine.

Haemolytic transfusion reactions

Haemolytic transfusion reactions are usually the result of ABO incompatibility. More rarely, IgM antibodies acting against other blood group antigens may be the cause. Invariably, the fault lies with the transfusor rather than with the cross-matching process. In the conscious patient there is pain along the vein, flushing, palpitations and headaches, with a feeling of chest constriction and pain in the lumbar region. The full picture is rather anaphylactoid in nature, with tachycardia, hypotension, urticaria, peripheral circulatory collapse, rigors and pyrexia. If the patient is anaesthestized or sedated during this period in the intensive care unit, then much of this picture may be abolished. Tachycardia, hypotension and rigors with increased blood loss from drains or into dressings may be suggestive. The diagnosis can be confirmed by inspection of a blood film, a positive direct antiglobulin test and free haemoglobin-aemia.

The treatment depends on the severity of the reaction. First, the blood transfusion is stopped, whereupon adrenaline, antihistamines and steroids are administered. Sodium bicarbonate is given if there is a metabolic acidosis; volume expanders are given if there is hypotension; a dopamine infusion is set up to promote renal blood flow; disseminated intravascular coagulation is looked for and is treated if it occurs. The patient may develop renal failure and this condition must be appropriately handled.

Management of the collapsed otolaryngological patient

Otolaryngological surgery is carried out on age groups at both ends of the spectrum. The commonest problem with the younger age groups is postoperative bleeding which is manifestly obvious to all concerned and does not pose a problem in differential diagnosis. However, in the case of adults, particularly the elderly, a collapse with hypotension, pallor and a change in pulse rate (tachycardia or bradycardia) can occur without postoperative haemorrhage, and a differential diagnosis needs therefore to be made.

In general surgery, a common cause of postoperative collapse is endotoxic shock and/or septicaemia as a consequence of complications in which parts of the gut have been breached. This situation would be rare in otolaryngological practice except when combined laryngopharyngeal and oesophageal surgery has been carried out with mobilization of stomach or large bowel up through the chest. Consequently, endotoxic shock is an infrequent cause of collapse in an otolaryngological patient, but it should nevertheless be borne in mind, as the condition can follow instrumentation of the urethra if the patient requires catheterization following postoperative retention of urine. Additionally, any patient, irrespective of surgical procedure, can acquire an ileus as part of the humoral response to trauma and may, as a consequence, absorb bacterial endotoxin from the gut.

Other possible causes of collapse commonly originate in the cardiovascular system, and coronary thrombosis and/or arrhythmias would be the commonest of these. Pulmonary embolism can also occur, and other less likely causes would be gallbladder colic, peptic perforation, acute pancreatitis or dissection of an aortic aneurysm.

Faced with a hypotensive shut-down and an oliguric patient, how should the clinician arrive rapidly at the diagnosis? It is imperative that there be a high index of suspicion that the cause of collapse is a surgical one before a medical cause of collapse is espoused.

Previous history

The type of surgery performed and the possibility of bleeding, together with significant events in the previous history, such as ischaemic heart disease, form the background on which to build the pathway to diagnosis.

The timing of the collapse in relation to the surgical intervention is important. Collapse from endotoxic shock can follow within a very short time of, for example, instrumentation of the urethra, but it can also occur at any time during the postoperative period. A rigor may be a presenting feature in septicaemic shock and would indicate the diagnosis from the outset. Primary surgical haemorrhage usually manifests itself well within the first 12 hours. Fortunately, in otolaryngological practice, haemorrhage is usually apparent from the beginning as a drainage loss. However, in the rare event of haemorrhage to the exterior not being immediately apparent, the most obvious manifestation, distinguishing it from other causes of collapse/shock, is the waxen appearance of the lips and mucous membranes of the gums. In both myocardial infarction and pulmonary embolism the features tend to be blue/grey. However, the pulmonary embolism case is typically marked by agitation, while the patient with severe myocardial infarction and shock has a resigned attitude.

Current history

One of the most helpful indices, on taking a history from the patient, is the character and distribution of any pain. The pain of myocardial infarction is characteristically central, and crushing or vice-like, and may radiate to either arm or jaw. In pulmonary embolism there may be no pain at all or, if it does occur, it will be lateralized and pleuritic in nature. In the case of sepsis or haemorrhage, chest pain is invariably absent.

The pulse rate is rapid in haemorrhagic shock, usually rapid in septicaemic shock and may be slow, rapid or unchanged in both myocardial infarction and pulmonary embolism.

The temperature may be raised in septicaemic shock but this is often not the case. A small rise in temperature does occur in myocardial infarction.

The jugular venous pressure is unequivocally lowered in haemorrhagic shock and may be raised in the other three conditions. Characteristically, however, the patient with pulmonary embolism can lie flat, whereas in severe myocardial infarction the patient cannot. In both the latter conditions, the patients may have a cough: in myocardial infarction the patient may cough up frothy pink sputum, while in pulmonary embolism the sputum will be normal in consistency but blood stained. Auscultation in cardiogenic shock may reveal crepitations at the lung bases and a third heart sound or a gallop. Initially, in pulmonary embolism, there will be no chest signs, although bronchial breathing may develop later if there is a pulmonary infection. However, a right sternal edge fourth heart sound may be heard.

Haemorrhagic shock itself is not usually associated with sputum production. A patient with septicaemic shock, however, may have infected-looking sputum if the septicaemia originates from the lungs.

A chest X-ray which shows bats-wing pulmonary oedema would be an indication of left ventricular failure associated with cardiogenic shock. A picture of widespread patchy infiltration may be consistent with the 'shock lung' syndrome associated with septicaemic shock or, if there is a consolidated patch with an air bronchogram, this may be consistent with a focus of lung sepsis associated with septicaemia. The chest X-ray in haemorrhagic shock will probably be normal, and in pulmonary embolism may be unaffected unless a pulmonary infarction occurs later on. Postoperative collapse may result from aspiration of acid gastric contents, although this is rare. In the event of its occurring, the patient will be cyanosed and may have bronchospasm and a tachycardia, and the chest X-ray will show fluffy blotched areas of consolidation.

An erect abdominal or lateral decubitus X-ray may show free gas if septicaemia is associated with gut perforation, or it may show pelvic collections of gas if gas-producing anaerobic abscesses are present. Gut fluid levels with ileus may be present in all the named conditions.

The electrocardiogram (ECG) is an important means of investigation to assist in these cases. However, it is important to recognize that generalized ischaemic ECG changes can occur when the hypotension is not in fact caused by myocardial infarction but is merely a result of myocardial hypoxaemia.

In myocardial infarction, ST segment changes occur initially with elevation in the leads which overlie the damaged areas of myocardium. If there is full thickness myocardial infarction, then Q waves develop in the relevant leads. It is usually assumed that a pathological Q wave must be more than 0.4 second in duration and more than 25% of the succeeding R wave. It is important to realize that Q waves do not appear until muscle necrosis occurs and thus may be delayed for some hours.

If the infarction is anterior, then the most affected leads are I, AVL and the chest leads; in anteroseptal infarction, the early chest leads show the maximal changes; if the infarction is antero-lateral, then V4 to V6 demonstrate the main effects; and, on some occasions, extensive infarction may be manifest in all the anterior chest leads. In inferior infarction, the main changes are in leads II, III and AVL.

In pulmonary embolism, the ECG changes are characteristic. There is right axis deviation and, with the onset of right ventricular strain, the development of an S wave in lead I, a Q with an inverted T wave in lead III, and T wave inversion in V1 to V3. There is a pronounced atrial wave (P pulmonale) and right bundle-branch block. In acid aspiration syndrome, the picture is not dissimilar from pulmonary embolism with marked right ventricular strain and P pulmonale; and more widespread ST changes may be associated with severe hypoxaemia.

Enzyme changes

A rise in the serum creatinine phosphokinase (CPK) begins to occur 6 hours after myocardial infarction and reaches a peak in about 24 hours, whereas in pulmonary embolism a small rise occurs. Another isoenzyme, CPK-MB, which is said to be specific for the myocardium, may prove invaluable in the future but is still not as totally specific as was hoped. Aspartate aminotransferase (SGOT) rises after 12–24 hours, while lactic dehydrogenase (LDH) rises after 72 hours. The white cell count is of little use in differential diagnosis. In septicaemic shock, it may not be significantly raised above that found in other postoperative patients.

Direct central venous pressure measurements

A central venous pressure line will be a further aid in diagnosis. The catheter is inserted via the subclavian vein, usually approached infraclavicularly, and connected to a saline manometer zeroed at the level of the right atrium. This will certainly enable the accurate detection of the low central venous pressure of haemorrhagic shock and thereafter enable monitoring of the response to transfusion. The central venous pressure is often lowered in septicaemic shock as well. By contrast, it will be raised in pulmonary embolism and is usually raised in cardiogenic shock.

First line treatment

If the patient appears to have a myocardial infarction, he will be taken over by the appropriate team. However, initial management should consist of pain relief with diamorphine which is a vasodilator in addition to being a narcotic analgesic. In pulmonary embolism, full heparization should be commenced immediately.

In haemorrhagic shock, initial resuscitation should be by colloidal infusions, such as Haemaccel or Hespan, while awaiting cross-matched blood and, at the same time, organizing surgical intervention.

If endotoxic shock is a possible diagnosis, management is aimed at initial definitive diagnosis, very early medical treatment and delayed surgical intervention, if indicated.

Initially, two samples of blood should be drawn under sterile conditions and should be inoculated into culture medium before being sent for incubation, whereupon the administering of antibiotics must be commenced immediately, with metronidazole 1 g intravenously, gentamicin 120 mg and ampicillin 1 g. This regimen will cover Gram-negative rods, staphylococci and haemolytic streptococci. Fluid therapy with Haemaccel or HPPF should be started in order to raise central venous pressure and improve renal perfusion. Steroids in the form of methylprednisolone 30 mg/kg should be given initially and every 6 hours thereafter, for 24–48 hours, to combat the effect of endotoxin which will persist in the circulation even following the destruction of the offending bacteria.

The bladder should be catheterized and, if there is oliguria, then dopamine should be administered in 'nephrogenic' doses, that is 3–5 µg/kg per h. Any necessary surgery to rectify soiling from gut spillage or to secure leaks as appropriate, must then be contemplated. All these patients are prone to develop acute renal failure unless renal perfusion is ensured. While diuretics are appropriate in severe myocardial infarction, the use of dopamine, as described, as a prophylactic measure, even in the absence of oliguria, is advisable.

Other causes

The pain of a perforated peptic ulcer has a characteristic distribution in the upper central hypochondrium, together with gas under the diaphragm on X-ray. However, it is unusual for these patients to be grossly shocked.

Pain and, indeed, septicaemia may follow gallbladder colic and cholecystitis. The incidence of gallbladder symptoms should be sought from the patient, and stones may be present on the abdominal X-ray. Pain radiating through to the back would assist in establishing the gallbladder as a source of problem if other characteristic features of the main diagnoses are not present. Similar pain could also be caused by acute dissection of the thoracic aorta. Theoretically, pericarditis might be a cause of the pain but, in this case, the patient should also exhibit a pericardial rub on auscultation and possibly the signs of cardiac tamponade. Acute pancreatitis can be excluded by the finding of normal serum amylase levels.

General supportive measures

In the circumstances under discussion, oxygen therapy will benefit all groups. If the patient is in severe pain then it is cruel to withold analgesics, even if final diagnosis might not yet have been made. Short-acting drugs, such as diamorphine or fentanyl, can be used at this stage, and should be given in small doses *intravenously*. Patients in extremis from the causes discussed pass rapidly into a situation of respiratory failure and should be intubated and undergo intermittent positive pressure ventilation. All of these patients should be transferred to the intensive care unit.

Haemorrhage and disseminated intravascular coagulation

If it is considered that haemorrhage is in fact associated with disseminated intravascular coagulation, the occurrence of this syndrome should be confirmed in the laboratory, and management should be as indicated earlier.

Extreme emergency situations

When the situation is rapidly deteriorating and the differential diagnosis between cardiac infarction, pulmonary embolism and septicaemic shock is unclear, then the regimen outlined previously for the immediate treatment of septicaemic shock *must* be initiated. Such a step will not further harm the patient with an infarct or embolism, but will produce dramatic improvement in the septicaemic patient. The longer the delay the worse the outlook in the case of the latter condition, with the onset of multiorgan microcirculatory failure and its consequences – shock lung syndrome, acute respiratory distress syndrome, acute renal failure, and so on. Many clinicians and their patients have, in the past, been thankful that this approach has been adopted.

Reference

CRANDON, A. J., PEEL, K. P., ANDERSON, J. A., THOMPSON, V. and McNICOL, G. P. (1980) Postoperative deep vein thrombosis; identifying high-risk patients. *British Medical Journal*, **281**, 343–344

26

Anaesthesia for otolaryngology

Henry J. L. Craig

The wider range and the increase in technical skills developed in otolaryngology over the last 20 years have greatly increased the demands made on the skill and knowledge of the anaesthetist. Anaesthetic problems and the very real influence of anaesthetic techniques on the ultimate outcome of the surgery, quite apart from morbidity and mortality resulting from ordinary anaesthetic complications, are now well recognized. There is no branch of surgery in which good communication and cooperation between surgeon and anaesthetist are more important than in otolaryngology. Central to all anaesthesia in otolaryngology is the control of the airway, and problems are particularly likely in operations around the nose, pharynx and larynx as a consequence of the anaesthetist having to share the airway with the surgeon. In a few cases the airway may be compromised by disease even before operation, and in such patients the problems will necessarily be compounded. In this chapter, both local and general anaesthetic techniques in the adult are discussed, while anaesthesia for infants and young children is dealt with in the relevant chapter in Volume 6. The aim of this chapter is not to try to teach the surgeon general anaesthetic techniques but to help him to understand some of the anaesthetist's problems in this field.

Preoperative preparation and preanaesthetic medication

As in all surgery, it is important to evaluate the physical condition of each patient and to achieve the healthiest possible state before surgery, this being an important determinant of peri- and postoperative morbidity and mortality (Goldman

et al., 1977). Patients for minor surgery who are judged fit at an earlier outpatient general medical examination can be admitted as day cases on the morning of operation or kept in overnight after operation. In all other cases, except where associated medical problems require earlier admission, patients should be admitted to hospital on the day before surgery.

Preoperative assessment

A careful assessment of general medical history, with particular attention to cough, sputum production, breathlessness or pain in the chest, is essential. A physical examination must pay particular attention to the cardiovascular and respiratory systems.

Cardiovascular disease

Pre-existing cardiovascular disease is seldom a contraindication to general anaesthesia and surgery, provided that the patient is treated to attain optimum fitness before operation. Avoidance of anxiety is particularly important and good general anaesthesia, after adequate premedication, may well be preferable to surgery under local anaesthesia. Adequate control of hypertension will ensure better stability of the blood pressure during anaesthesia (Prys-Roberts, Meloche and Foex, 1971), and therapy should be continued up to the time of the operation. Cardiac failure should be adequately treated with digoxin and diuretics.

Patients with stable angina which is controlled by drugs are able to tolerate both surgery and anaesthesia well, as myocardial work is decreased under general anaesthesia. However, patients with unstable, poorly controlled angina, and those who experience pain at rest, are in a high-risk category for any operative procedure. In the latter case, otolaryngology should, if possible, be postponed until the condition of such patients has been improved by drugs or by coronary artery surgery. Patients with angina should have their usual coronary artery dilator drug included in the premedication. Elective surgery should be postponed for 6 months after myocardial infarction.

A severe degree of heart block requires careful preoperative assessment by both anaesthetist and cardiologist, and the insertion of a pacemaker may be indicated before operation.

Respiratory disease

Upper respiratory tract infection is a contraindication to elective surgery, as it is a cause of excessive secretions together with hyperaemia and irritability of the respiratory tract with a predisposition to laryngospasm and increased surgical bleeding. In the presence of an active chest infection, anaesthesia should also be avoided and appropriate antibiotics administered. Patients with a chronic productive cough should have physiotherapy, and bronchodilators may be required to improve the respiratory function; in these patients, premedication with promethazine will help to reduce the respiratory secretions and bronchospasm. However, some chronic infections, such as nasal discharge secondary to obstruction of the nasal passages, may never clear up without surgery. It is essential that all factors are taken into consideration before a decision on the postponement of an operation is made.

Asthmatic patients tolerate general anaesthesia well, as most inhalational agents are bronchodilators. The patient should use his usual bronchodilatory medication up to the time of operation, and premedication should avoid bronchoconstrictors such as morphine; phenothiazines or benzodiazepines are suitable, and an aminophylline suppository may also be helpful. Postponement of surgery will be indicated in cases where the patient suffers acute attacks of bronchospasm immediately before the operation or during the induction of anaesthesia.

Diabetes

Diabetics should be properly controlled before surgery, and this is generally possible except in emergencies. A suitable regimen is to omit the oral hypoglycaemic agent or insulin on the morning of the operation; then to perform a blood glucose estimation and to administer a 5% dextrose infusion with an appropriate amount of soluble insulin added to the solution. This intravenous fluid is run at about 1.5 ml/kg per hour with additional fluid, if required, being given as physiological saline. Many patients are able to return to oral feeding on the day of the operation, thus eliminating the need to add potassium to the infusion fluid. It is usually not necessary to switch patients from oral hypoglycaemic agents to soluble insulin before the day of the operation. Indeed, it may not be necessary for patients for minor surgery to undergo any change in their treatment regimens. The blood glucose level should be checked immediately after an operation or intraoperatively during long procedures, and maintained at around 10 mmol/l. The subject of perioperative management of diabetes is fully discussed by Walts *et al.* (1981) and Bowen *et al.* (1982).

Concurrent drug therapy

Concurrent drug therapy should be noted and given proper consideration, particularly for those on beta-adrenergic blocking drugs, monoamine oxidase inhibitors, corticosteroids, contraceptive drugs or tricyclic antidepressants.

Beta-adrenergic blocking drugs

The administering of beta-adrenergic blocking drugs, which are widely used in the treatment of hypertension and angina, should be continued up to the time of the operation. It may be advisable to substitute short-acting agents for long-acting members of the same group but, on the whole, problems are not usual when combined with modern anaesthetic agents. If necessary, adverse effects of beta blockade can be controlled by drugs producing inotropic and chronotropic stimulation by way of alternative pathways.

Monoamine oxidase inhibitors

The use of pressor amines will be contraindicated in the presence of antidepressant monamine oxidase inhibitors as the combination will produce a dangerous hypertension. This antidepressant therapy would also preclude the use of nasal decongestants such as ephedrine and phenylephrine. Narcotics, particularly pethidine, can produce dangerous side-effects such as excessive respiratory depression, hypo- or hypertension, sweating, nausea and collapse. In addition, any drug metabolized by the liver will be potentiated. If possible, general anaesthesia should be avoided for 3 weeks after stopping these drugs.

Corticosteroids

Patients on prolonged steroid therapy may need steroid cover during operation and in the immediate postoperative period. Patients undergoing minor surgery should either not be given any steroid cover, or be given a single dose of hydrocortisone hemisuccinate along with their premedication or at the time of induction of general anaesthesia.

Contraceptive pill

Patients on contraceptive pills should probably stop taking these tablets for at least one complete month before surgery; but for emergency operations, prophylaxis with subcutaneous heparin (Minihep) or dextran infusion should be considered to reduce the risk of postoperative venous thrombosis.

Pregnancy

Pregnancy in the first or last trimester is usually considered a contraindication to elective surgery. There may be a small increase in the risk of miscarrying in the early stages of pregnancy and, if a miscarriage should occur, the operation will certainly be blamed. In the final weeks of pregnancy, increased intra-abdominal pressure may lead to respiratory embarrassment, and the risk of gastric regurgitation will be increased, with very serious consequences should aspiration into the respiratory tract occur. In the middle trimester, there is no containdication to general anaesthesia.

Preoperative investigations

Routine investigations include haematological and electrolyte screening and, at the same time, blood can be taken for grouping and cross-matching if significant operative blood loss is anticipated.

When anaemia is detected, the cause should be sought and treated. Patients originating from Africa, the Middle-East, the eastern Mediterranean, India and the West Indies should be screened for sickle-cell disease. Patients with the homozygous form (90% of haemoglobin in the abnormal sickle HbS form) run a very high risk of haemolysis and multiple infarctions under general anaesthesia, as the abnormal HbS forms crystals when oxygen tension is reduced. A haematological opinion should be sought before surgery, and the latter should be performed under local anaesthesia, if possible. Patients with the heterozygous form, the so-called sickle-cell trait (not more than half the haemoglobin in HbS), are able to withstand both the operation and the anaesthesia well, provided that they are in optimum condition before surgery and that dehydration and hypoxia (both global and regional) are avoided.

If the patient gives a history of abnormal bleeding and disease is suspected, and if platelet count or bleeding, clotting or prothrombin times reveal any abnormality, then consultation with a haematologist may be necessary.

Diuretics taken over long periods may produce electrolyte disturbances, particularly hypokalaemia; and a serum potassium level of less than 3 mmol/1 should be treated before surgery.

Serial blood glucose estimations are required in diabetic patients.

Urine examination is carried out routinely and, if there is any doubt about renal function, particularly in patients requiring hypotensive anaesthesia, plasma creatinine levels should be checked.

Elderly patients, and all subjects with a history suggestive of cardiovascular disease, should have an ECG and chest X-ray to check for myocardial ischaemia, incipient failure and cardiac enlargement. In other cases, a chest X-ray is of questionable value and greater emphasis should be laid on a physical examination of the respiratory system. Other special investigations, such as thyroid and respiratory function tests, should be carried out as indicated.

Preoperative medication

Sedative drugs

A careful and reassuring explanation, with respect to the operation itself, the method of inducing anaesthesia and the immediate postoperative period, is more likely than any sedative drug to dispel the apprehensions of the patient. This information should be given well in advance of surgery and can be repeated with advantage on the night before the operation.

In the case of the very anxious patient, reassurance alone may not be sufficient and sedation may be required from the time of admission to hospital – diazepam 2–5 mg thrice daily being suitable. A good night's sleep before surgery should be the aim, and many patients require a sedative such as nitrazepam 5–10 mg. Patients who are accustomed to taking night sedation should be given their usual drug in a slightly increased dose. The elderly are not usually apprehensive, and a preoperative explanation, together with reassurance, is frequently all that is required.

Various premedicants can be given 1–2 hours before surgery, depending on the patient's condition and the anaesthetist's individual preference. Preoperative pain is unusual in elective otolaryngology and there is no rational requirement for the traditional opiates such as morphine or papaveretum; an oral anxiolytic drug is usually adequate and diazepam 0.2 mg/kg has become popular in recent years.

Anticholinergic drugs

The use of anticholinergic drugs, such as atropine, has been questioned (Mirakhur *et al.*, 1978). These drugs produce subjective discomfort with a dry mouth and throat and loss of visual accommodation. Atropine is usually omitted before the induction of controlled hypotensive anaesthesia because of the potential problem of tachycardia. If necessary, such drugs can be given during operation; however, if a dry mouth and throat are required during surgery, preoperative i.m. atropine is more effective than intraoperative i.v. administration. When atropine is omitted, bradycardia is more likely to occur during laryngoscopy, particularly with the use of the suspension laryngoscope, and during application of topical anaesthesia to the larynx; so careful monitoring and readily available intravenous atropine are necessary. Glycopyrrolate (5–10 µg/kg i.m. or i.v.) is an alternative to atropine, providing both a better drying effect and more cardiostability (Mirakhur and Dundee, 1983).

Prophylactic antibiotics

Bacteraemia is common during any oral operation, including endoscopies (Bayliss *et al.*, 1983). Patients with congenital heart disease or valve lesions, who run the risk of bacteraemia during surgery, require antibiotic cover before and during operation. Amoxycillin 20 mg/kg to a maximum of 1 g i.m. at the time of premedication or, more logically, i.v. during induction, followed by a single oral or i.m. dose of amoxycillin 10 mg/kg (to a maximum of 500 mg) 6 hours later, is recommended. Patients with prosthetic valves or those who have had endocarditis are at special risk, and they should be given gentamicin in addition to amoxycillin. Patients who are already taking penicillin, or who are allergic to penicillin, can be given oral erythromycin (20 mg/kg) 1 hour before operation and half that dose 6 hours later (Simmons *et al.*, 1982).

Prophylactic anticoagulants

The risk of venous thrombosis is less following operations on the head and neck than it is compared with some other sites. Nevertheless, patients having prolonged surgery with extensive dissection, or who are otherwise especially at risk, should be considered for prophylactic subcutaneous heparin: 5000 units being given before operation and 5000 units at 12-hourly intervals thereafter, until the patient is fully ambulant. Unfortunately, this treatment will increase bleeding during operation and also increase the risk of postoperative haemorrhage.

Local anaesthesia

With modern anaesthesia and the general availability of trained anaesthetists, the demand for local anaesthesia has declined; however, there are still circumstances and operative procedures where the latter will be indicated. Local anaesthesia plays an important part in minor outpatient and day case surgery, and also in more major operations when specialist anaesthetic services are not available. Some of these procedures are used primarily to produce vasoconstriction, rather than analgesia, and are then frequently combined with general anaesthesia.

Patients who have a dread of general anaesthesia should, when practicable, be offered local anaesthetic blocks as an alternative; but if there is a patient who is temperamentally unsuited for any type of surgery under local anaesthesia, this should be recognized. Knowledge of regional blocks is necessary when permanent nerve destruction for the relief of intractable pain is required, this being accomplished either by injecting alcohol or phenol, or by using percutaneous radiofrequency thermocoagulation techniques.

Pharmacology of local anaesthetic agents

Local effects

Clinically useful local anaesthetic agents are either aminoesters or aminoamides which, when applied in sufficient concentration to the site of action, prevent the conduction of electrical impulses by the membranes of nerve and muscle. Local anaesthetics may provide analgesia by topical application to mucosal surface or by being injected around peripheral nerve endings or in the vicinity of nerve trunks. The ideal agent should have adequate potency, short latency, good penetration and diffusion, low toxicity and controllable duration of action with complete reversibility; it should also be water-soluble and stable in solution to permit heat sterilization; in addition, it should be non-irritant, non-antigenic and not interfere with wound healing. Excellent local anaesthetics are available, but the search for the ideal drug is still continuing.

In a myelinated nerve, the site of action of these drugs is at the nodes of Ranvier where the myelin sheath is thin or absent; two or three adjacent nodes must be exposed to the agent (6–10 mm of nerve) as the electrical impulse is capable of jumping one or two nodes. The conduction of nerve impulses is interrupted because the generation of an action potential has been prevented by the obstruction of the inward flow of sodium ions through the nerve membrane. A certain minimum concentration of local anaesthetic agent is necessary in order to block impulse conduction in a nerve fibre within a reasonable time, and the greater the diameter of the fibre, the greater is the concentration required. The duration of action depends on the firmness of the bond between the analgesic agent and the nerve membrane, and on the rate of drug removal, which occurs as a result of dilution by tissue fluid, diffusion away from the nerve, bloodstream uptake and metabolic inactivation.

Local anaesthetic drugs in solution exist in two forms, namely the uncharged base and the charged cation, with the degree of ionization depending on the pH of the solution and the buffering effect of the tissue fluid at the injection site. It is only the lipid-soluble free base that can penetrate the fat barrier of the nerve sheath. The greater the acidity of the tissue fluid, the higher is the ratio of ionized particles to the free base. When a local anaesthetic solution is injected into inflamed tissues, which have poor buffering properties and a low pH (pus has an acid pH), it tends to be ineffective.

All local anaesthetics, with the exception of lignocaine and cocaine, cause peripheral vasodilatation by their direct action on arterioles; in contrast, lignocaine has little effect, whereas cocaine causes vasoconstriction.

General systemic effects

In addition to local effects, local anaesthetic agents have important actions on other systems in the body. These actions become manifest when toxic plasma levels are reached as a result of too rapid absorption for destruction and excretion to maintain a safe equilibrium. Systemic effects are sometimes used therapeutically, for example the effect of intravenous lignocaine can be used to control ventricular extrasystoles, but they are usually regarded as side- or toxic effects depending on the severity of the patient's response which is determined both by the nature of the drug and the plasma concentration. Factors controlling plasma concentration are those of the dose and concentration of the drug used, the vascularity of the injection site (or mucosal surface) and the rate of the drug's removal from the plasma. The most important toxic manifestations are in the central nervous and cardiovascular systems.

Central nervous system

Local anaesthetic agents pass readily from the bloodstream to the brain but, at recommended clinical doses, serum levels remain well below toxic concentrations unless inadvertent intravascular injection occurs. Toxic plasma levels initially depress cortical inhibitory pathways, thus allowing unopposed excitatory activity which causes restlessness, visual and auditory disturbances (tinnitus), garrulousness, slurred speech, shivering and muscular tremors leading to convulsions; a state of generalized central nervous system depression will follow. However, in the case of some drugs, such as lignocaine, the excitatory phase may not be manifest, with toxicity becoming apparent initially as depression.

Cardiovascular system

The cardiovascular effects of local anaesthetics can occur either indirectly by the inhibition of autonomic pathways – for example during epidural anaesthesia – or directly by depression of the myocardium and its conducting system, and relaxation of the vascular smooth muscle. These direct actions result in the slowing of the heart, a reduction in cardiac output and a fall in blood pressure.

Respiratory system

Central stimulation causes an increase in the rate and depth of respiration but, as the medulla becomes depressed, breathing in turn becomes rapid and shallow. Respiration ceases during convulsions and, unless resuscitative measures are taken, severe hypoxia will result.

Prevention and treatment of toxic effects

In both head and neck surgery, the toxic effects of local anaesthetics are unlikely to be a consequence of absolute overdosage, as large amounts are seldom injected. High plasma concentrations can result from direct intravascular injection (particularly intra-arterial), or from excessive amounts being placed on mucous membranes which will facilitate quick absorption. Toxic features resulting from intravascular injection occur rapidly, usually within 10–20 seconds. Clinical features are caused mainly by central nervous system reactions to the drug. Cardiovascular changes are usually the result of hypoxia caused by respiratory depression. If signs of toxicity occur, the infiltration of local anaesthetic solution must cease, 100% oxygen should be administered by way of a face mask, and a good venous line secured. Frequently, such measures will be sufficient, but if muscle twitching continues, 5–10 mg diazepam should be given intravenously. An anaesthetist must be summoned so that the patient can be paralysed with a muscle relaxant, the trachea intubated and respiration controlled should convulsions occur. Cardiovascular depression, as indicated by hypotension and poor peripheral circulation, is treated by correction of hypoxia, moderate head-down tilt and infusion of crystalloid fluids together with inotropic agents, if necessary.

Hypersensitivity reactions to local anaesthetic agents

Hypersensitivity reactions are rare, and toxic reactions to small doses are usually the result of intravascular injection. True hypersenstivity reactions result in cardiovascular collapse, bronchospasm and cutaneous oedema. The treatment consists of rapid intravenous infusion of crystalloid solutions together with bronchodilators, such as aminophylline or adrenaline, and artificial ventilation with 100% oxygen. Again, hypoxia is the greatest danger and primary treatment must be directed towards achieving adequate oxygenation.

Local anaesthetic agents

The flexibility of local anaesthetic techniques is in large part due to the wide variety of agents now available, and it is possible to select a drug that will fulfil most of the requirements of any particular type of block.

Properties of special concern are those of effectiveness, speed and duration of action, spreading power, toxicity and surface activity. The surgeon should limit his repertoire of local anaesthetic drugs in order to familiarize himself thoroughly with the use of each one of them. Therefore, in the following sections on specific anaesthetic drugs, only the few most commonly used agents will be discussed.

Cocaine

Cocaine is an ester of benzoic acid that is hydrolysed by plasma cholinesterase. It is heat labile and is broken down by autoclaving. Cocaine is employed solely for topical application because it is too toxic for parenteral use. It is an excellent surface analgesic with a marked vasoconstrictor effect which is due to its ability to block the re-uptake of catecholamines released by adrenergic nerve endings; catecholamines thus accumulate at the active receptor sites. The effect of any additional sympathetic stimulation or catecholamines (either exogenous or endogenous) is potentiated and excessive sympathetic activity is responsible for many of the signs of cocaine toxicity.

Cocaine stimulates the central nervous system from above downwards causing euphoria and a reduction in the sense of fatigue; because this is an addictive effect, the drug is in the controlled category. Medullary stimulation causes an increase in both blood pressure and respiratory rate which can lead to depression, with coma or convulsions and respiratory failure. Cocaine sensitizes the myocardium to adrenaline, and toxic plasma levels can cause ventricular fibrillation. The addition of adrenaline to cocaine is both unnecessary and dangerous as the risk of cardiac arrhythmias is thereby increased.

Cocaine is absorbed from mucosal surfaces, and stronger solutions may be absorbed more slowly than weaker solutions because of more intense vasoconstriction. Nevertheless, the weaker solutions may well be safer. Cocaine is used as a 4–20% solution or as a 20% paste, the maximum dose being about 3 mg/kg with an absolute maximum of 200 mg in the fit adult. The duration of its action is about 60 minutes. On account of cocaine's toxicity, its use is best confined to the nose, where only small quantities are required. For the purpose of inducing anaesthesia of other mucosal surfaces, such as the larynx and trachea, lignocaine is much safer than cocaine.

Lignocaine hydrochloride

Lignocaine (Xylocaine, lidocaine USP) is an amino-acyl amide, a derivative of acetanilide, which is heat stable and can be autoclaved. It is metabolized in the liver, the metabolites being excreted in the urine. Lignocaine is a very effective local anaesthetic with a rapid onset of action and good diffusing properties. It does not cause vasoconstriction but, unlike most local anaesthetics, neither does it cause much dilatation. On injection, it has a duration of action of about 1 hour which can be prolonged to 2–3 hours by the addition of vasoconstrictor agents. When injected intravenously, lignocaine has antiarrhythmic properties on the heart. The absorption of large doses of lignocaine may produce drowsiness and amnesia as a result of depression of the the central nervous system.

Lignocaine is absorbed effectively from mucous membranes and is a useful surface anaesthetic in concentrations of 2–4%. The 2% preparation is available in viscous form for oral analgesia. The more effective 4% solution can be used in hand-operated sprays or in the form of nasal packs and applicators. There is also a pressurized 10% aerosol spray which gives 10 mg lignocaine per dose. Ointments and gels in 2–5% concentrations can be used for lubricating tubes and instruments. For topical use the maximum safe dose is about 3 mg/kg with an upper limit of 200 mg in the fit adult. The onset of action is rapid but of short duration (approximately 20 minutes).

Infiltration anaesthesia can be accomplished with 0.5% lignocaine, with or without the addition of adrenaline (1:200 000), but nerve blocks require 1–1.5%. The maximum dose depends on the concentration of solution used and on whether or not adrenaline is added. The maximum dose of plain 0.5% lignocaine is 3 mg/kg (not exceeding 200 mg total) and 7 mg/kg when adrenaline is added (total maximum 500 mg). These doses should be reduced in the following cases: when stronger solutions are used; when patients are elderly or are not physically fit; and when the injection is into very vascular regions.

Prilocaine hydrochloride

Prilocaine (Citanest) is an effective local anaesthetic; it is chemically related to lignocaine, but is less toxic and longer acting. Prilocaine is as effective as lignocaine for surface analgesia and its systemic effects are similar. Dose for dose, prilocaine is less potent than lignocaine, but with large doses (over 500 mg) cyanosis may occur as a result of the formation of methaemoglobin which is harmless, unless accompanied by severe anaemia or circulatory impairment, and usually disappears within 24 hours. If necessary, the condition can be treated with intravenous methylene blue 1 mg/kg. The maximum safe dose without a vasoconstrictor is 6 mg/kg (0.5% solution), and with a vasoconstrictor it is 8 mg/kg, these doses being reduced in elderly and frail patients. Concentrations used are similar to those for lignocaine. The addition of adrenaline improves the duration and quality of the action of prilocaine but less impressively than with lignocaine. Prilocaine is the agent of choice when adrenaline is contraindicated.

Bupivacaine hydrochloride

Bupivacaine (Marcain) is a potent, effective and long-lasting local anaesthetic agent, with the addition of adrenaline marginally increasing the length of action. Bupivacaine remains active for about 4 hours (6 hours with the addition of adrenaline), but residual anaesthesia may be present for up to 36 hours. This is particularly useful in cases where postoperative analgesia is required or where the duration of surgery is uncertain. It is not an effective surface analgesic. Bupivacaine is about four times as potent as lignocaine although this is offset by its greater toxicity. It is used in concentrations of 0.25–0.5% for peripheral nerve blocks, with or without adrenaline, the maximum safe dose being 2 mg/kg. In otolaryngology, the main use for bupivacaine lies in regional nerve blocks where a prolonged action is required.

Other local anaesthetic agents

There are many other local anaesthetic agents, some of which are just as effective as those mentioned; but others, such as procaine which is less effective than lignocaine, and amethocaine which is much more toxic, have been superseded by these newer agents.

Vasoconstrictors

The addition of a vasoconstrictor to a local anaesthetic solution has the effect of delaying the rate of absorption, prolonging the anaesthetic's action and reducing the maximum plasma level attained for any given dose, thereby decreasing the danger of toxic reactions. Vasoconstrictors will reduce tissue bleeding, which is particularly important when working in very vascular areas.

Adrenaline

Adrenaline (epinephrine) is the vasoconstrictor most commonly used in association with local anaesthetic agents, and it is present in many commercial preparations of lignocaine, prilocaine and bupivacaine. These preparations are convenient but their concentration of adrenaline is often too high: 1 in 80 000 being common, whereas 1 in 200 000 is all that is required. In addition, these preparations tend to have a low pH (on account of the antioxidant added to prevent oxidation of the adrenaline), which results in a decrease in the free base and in a reduced penetration of nerve axons. It is often more satisfactory, therefore, to add adrenaline just before using the local anaesthetic. The dose of adrenaline by injection should not exceed 0.01 mg/kg, with a total maximum of 0.5 mg (0.5 ml of 1:1000 solution) in the fit adult. Overdosage, usually the result of intravascular injection, may cause anxiety, vertigo, pallor and palpitations. Systolic blood pressure rises while the diastolic pressure falls and cardiac output increases. However, severe tachyarrhythmias (which can terminate in ventricular fibrillation) and the consequent fall in cardiac output may lead to a fall in blood pressure and peripheral circulatory failure.

When combined with a local anaesthetic solution, or saline, infiltration of adrenaline causes ischaemia of the skin and related tissues, which both reduces bleeding and aids surgical vision, but adrenaline usually dilates blood vessels which supply muscle. Adrenaline must not be infiltrated into tissues supplied by end arteries lest arterial insufficiency and tissue necrosis result. The use of adrenaline is contraindicated in patients who are receiving drugs which sensitize the myocardium to catecholamines. These include the general anaesthetic agents halothane, methoxyflurane and trichloroethylene. Tricyclic antidepressants (but not monoamine oxidase inhibitors) inhibit the destruction of catecholamines and can potentiate the systemic effects of adrenaline (Boakes *et al.*, 1973). Advanced ischaemic heart disease, marked hypertension and thyrotoxicosis also contra-indicate the use of adrenaline.

Felypressin

Felypressin (Octapressin) is a synthetic vasocon-strictor with a low systemic toxicity which has little effect on blood pressure and does not increase myocardial irritability. The main disadvantage of felypressin is that it may take 15 minutes for the maximum vasoconstrictor effect to occur. Felypressin is a possible alternative to adrenaline when that drug is contraindicated. It is more effective than adrenaline in prolonging the action of prilocaine (Goldman and Evers, 1969), and is commercially available with 3% prilocaine in a 2 ml dental cartridge (felypressin 0.03 unit/ml).

Phenylephrine hydrochloride

Phenylephrine (Neosynephrine, Neophryn) is a synthetic vasoconstrictor but compared to adrena-line its action is weak; it is used in a concentration of 1:20 000. Phenylephrine does not produce tachycardia but does sensitize the myocardium to catecholamines, and probably has the same contraindications as adrenaline.

Local anaesthetic techniques

Nose and paranasal sinuses

Topical anaesthesia, using 4–10% cocaine or 4% lignocaine with adrenaline, is widely used for minor surgery on the nose, such as the removal of polyps, local electrocautery and antral puncture. The nasal cavities are first sprayed with the anaesthetic solution, the patient having been warned not to swallow any excess solution – this is particularly important when cocaine is being used, for fear of gastric absorption. After a few minutes, with good illumination and using a speculum and forceps, each side of the nose is packed with half-inch (12.7 mm) wide ribbon gauze soaked in the anaesthetic solution. The packs are removed after about 10 minutes and a wool applicator, soaked in the anaesthetic solution, is inserted at an angle of 20° to the floor of the nose until bone is felt at a depth of 6–7 cm, the end now lying adjacent to the sphenopalatine foramen (*Figure 26.1a*). A second applicator is inserted along the anterior border of the nasal cavity until the

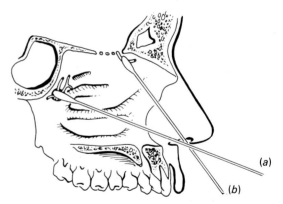

Figure 26.1 Applicators placed in nasal cavity in such a way that tip of (*a*) is adjacent to the sphenopalatine foramen and (*b*) near the cribriform plate. (From Macintosh and Ostlere, 1955, by courtesy of the author and publisher)

anterior end of the cribriform plate is reached at a depth of about 5 cm (*Figure 26.1b*). Before surgery on the nose under general anaesthesia, a similar technique is used to provide vasoconstriction, with the applicators being omitted.

For extensive surgery on the nose, a more thorough technique of inducing anaesthesia of the nasal mucosa may be required, using a modifica-tion of Moffet's technique (Curtiss, 1952). The nasal cavity is sprayed as before and the patient is then put into a supine position, with a pillow under the shoulders to extend the head until it is upside-down (*Figure 26.2*). The patient is told to

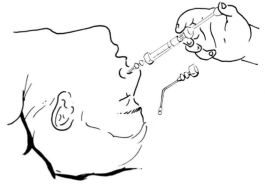

Figure 26.2 Position of head before instillation of cocaine into nasal cavity. (From Macintosh and Ostlere, 1955, by courtesy of the author and publisher)

breathe through the mouth and 2 ml of 5% cocaine solution are injected into each side of the nasal cavity, as near to the roof of the nose as possible, using a special angulated cannula (*Figure 26.3*). The patient remains in this position for 10 minutes and then, after pinching the nose to prevent any

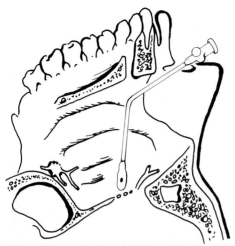

Figure 26.3 Angulated cannula in position for injection of cocaine into nose. (From Macintosh and Ostlere, 1955, by courtesy of the author and publisher)

solution being sniffed back and swallowed, is helped to roll into a prone position, with the head being kept down throughout. The remaining fluid drains out of the anterior nares, and if any runs down the back of the patient's throat, he should be instructed to spit it out and not to swallow it. A similar technique can be used to produce vasoconstriction of the nasal mucosa for surgery under general anaesthesia. The procedure can be carried out after induction of anaesthesia, with the patient placed in the tonsillectomy position, any excess solution being removed by suction. The anaesthetic solution may extend through the sphenopalatine foramen to the maxillary nerve, and then analgesia will be sufficient for operations on the antrum; otherwise a separate maxillary nerve block is necessary for surgery in this region. If there is any possibility of the ethmoidal air cells being entered the anterior ethmoidal nerve must also be blocked. Infiltration of the columella of the nose with lignocaine through a fine needle will provide analgesia of that area not supplied by the anterior ethmoidal nerve and also help to separate mucous membrane from the septal cartilage, aiding operations on the nasal septum.

For external ethmoidectomy, a block of the anterior ethmoidal and infratrochlear nerves and infiltration along the line of incision is required; and a maxillary block is a wise precaution against the possible danger of surgery extending into its territory.

Maxillary nerve block

The maxillary division of the trigeminal nerve is blocked as it crosses the upper part of the pterygomaxillary fissure. An 8 cm needle, with a

marker 5 cm from the tip, is inserted 1 cm below the inferior margin of the zygoma and overlying the anterior border of the masseter muscle, where a vertical line from the lateral orbital margin crosses a horizontal line through the middle of the upper lip (*Figure 26.4*). The needle is directed

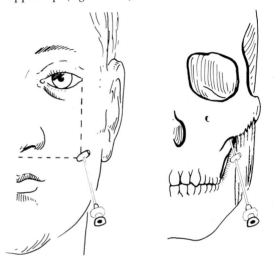

Figure 26.4 Maxillary nerve block. From Macintosh and Ostlere, 1955, by courtesy of the author and publisher)

backwards at an angle of 30° from the horizontal and upwards and inwards, in such a direction that when viewed from the front, the shaft of the needle lies in a line which passes through the pupil (*Figure 26.5*). The marker indicates the

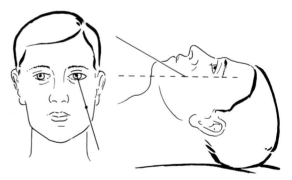

Figure 26.5 Maxillary nerve block. (From Macintosh and Ostlere, 1955, by courtesy of the author and publisher)

maximum depth of insertion and the needle point will then lie in the pterygomaxillary fissure. The needle may be arrested at a depth of 4 cm by the upper part of the lateral pterygoid plate, but even here an injection is effective. After an aspiration test, 4 ml of local anaesthetic solution are injected and then a further 4 ml as the needle is slowly withdrawn over a distance of 1 cm.

Anterior ethmoidal nerve block

The anterior ethmoidal and infratrochlear nerves can be blocked together at their origin from the nasociliary nerve in the upper half of the medial wall of the orbit, 2.5 cm from the orbital margin. A 5 cm needle, with a marker 2.5 cm from the tip, is inserted 1 cm above the inner canthus and directed horizontally backwards (*Figure 26.6*). The needle

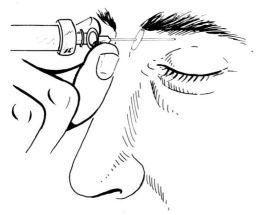

Figure 26.6 Anterior ethmoidal nerve block

passes between the medial rectus and the inner wall of the orbit, well away from the eyeball. At a depth of 2.5 cm, the tip lies close to the anterior ethmoidal nerve where it enters its foramen (*Figure 26.7*). One millilitre of local anaesthetic

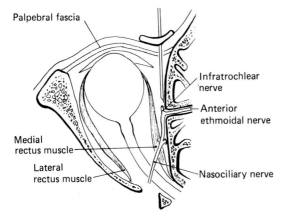

Palpebral fascia

Infratrochlear nerve

Anterior ethmoidal nerve

Medial rectus muscle

Lateral rectus muscle

Nasociliary nerve

Figure 26.7 Course of needle for anterior ethmoidal nerve block

solution is injected and then a further 1 ml as the needle is slowly withdrawn. If bone is encountered at a depth of less than 2.5 cm, the needle should be withdrawn almost to the skin before it is redirected.

Pharynx, larynx and trachea

Topical anaesthesia can be used for direct laryngoscopy, and it is also of great value in the case of tracheal intubation in the awake patient with a compromised airway, in whom general anaesthesia may precipitate complete respiratory obstruction. A similar technique can be used for fibreoptic or rigid bronchoscopy, but for the latter general anaesthesia is to be preferred. Local infiltration anaesthesia may also be used for tracheostomy.

Topical anaesthesia of the oropharynx is obtained by giving the patient 5–10 ml of 2% Xylocaine Viscous, and instructing him to spread it around his mouth and retain it on the back of his tongue. After a few minutes, any remaining fluid should be spat out. With the patient sitting up, any remaining pharyngeal reflexes can be obtunded by spraying the soft palate and oropharynx with 4% lignocaine. With the tongue held forwards, a swab, soaked in 4% lignocaine and held by Krause's laryngeal forceps, is inserted in turn into each piriform fossa by sliding it over the back of the tongue and keeping close to the lateral pharyngeal wall. Once in the fossa, the swab is held there for about 1 minute, to block the internal laryngeal nerve which at this point lies just deep to the mucosa. This will produce anaesthesia in the region extending as far as, and including, the upper surface of the vocal cords. Anaesthesia of the trachea can be obtained by spraying lignocaine through the cords under direct vision, or by injecting 1–2 ml of 4% lignocaine through the cricothyroid membrane in the midline. With the latter technique, aspiration of air confirms the correct position of the needle, which must be withdrawn rapidly after injection before the patient coughs. The total dose of lignocaine should not exceed 3 mg/kg. Rigid bronchoscopy under topical anaesthesia is an unpleasant experience for the patient, and a fairly heavy premedication should be used which is consistent with the patient's ability to cooperate during the examination and to cough on command at the end. The combination of a narcotic and a sedative such as diazepam or midazolam is suitable.

In the case of fibreoptic bronchoscopy, sedative premedication will probably not be required (Pearce, 1980). Here, the instrument is passed through the nose, thereby necessitating surface anaesthesia of the nose, pharynx, larynx and trachea. A 4% lignocaine aerosol from a hand nebulizer is used to anaesthetize the nose, and this usually penetrates to the pharynx and sometimes to the larynx. When the nose has become numb, the bronchoscope is introduced and advanced far enough into the pharynx to obtain a view of the vocal cords which are then sprayed through the bronchoscope. After 1 or 2 minutes, the instrument is passed through the cords and into the trachea. If there is any coughing, small doses of 2% lignocaine should be injected through the instrument as it is being advanced (Clarke and Knight, 1977).

Alternatively, excellent topical anaesthesia of the tracheobronchial tree can be obtained by using an aerosol in association with a ventilator. Most patients will accept positive pressure ventilation from a face mask for the few minutes that are required to nebulize 5 ml of 4% lignocaine, using a Bird Mk7 ventilator (Newton and Edwards, 1979).

Local anaesthesia for tracheostomy

The simple infiltration of the skin and subcutaneous tissues in the region of the intended incision is usually quite adequate. Alternatively, complete anaesthesia of the lower half of the neck can be obtained by blocking the clavicular branches of the superior cervical plexus. This is done on each side by injecting about 5 ml of local anaesthetic solution just beneath the midpoint of the posterior border of the sternomastoid muscle. Deeper layers of the wound are managed by simple infiltration. The injection of 2–3 ml of 4% lignocaine transtracheally into the lumen will reduce coughing and straining when the trachea is opened.

Ear

Local anaesthesia has been used for almost all types of ear surgery and it is effective for simple brief procedures such as removal of lesions of the pinna. For long operations, local anaesthesia can be trying for both patient and surgeon; the delicate nature of the operation and the use of the operating microscope mean that the patient must lie absolutely still, the slightest movement being greatly magnified. The advantages claimed are that an awake patient will be in a position to evaluate a hearing change and that a dry operative field can be maintained, but it has never been a popular technique in Britain for major ear surgery. If the operation involves working anywhere near the labyrinth, then dizziness, nausea and even vomiting can make the procedure impossible.

Local anaesthetic solutions will not normally penetrate the drum but can be forced through it by means of an electric current, iontophoresis. This is a method whereby a direct current is passed through an anaesthetic solution which has been instilled into the external auditory meatus. The positive electrode, a stainless steel needle, is put into the meatus and the negative terminal is placed over the mastoid, forcing the positively

charged ions of local anaesthetic into the tympanic membrane, thereby inducing anaesthesia of the drum.

For permeatal operations, analgesia can be obtained by injecting 0.5 ml of 1% lignocaine with adrenaline posteriorly, just lateral to the junction of the bony and cartilaginous parts of the meatus, while 0.25 ml of the anaesthetic are injected superiorly, inferiorly and anteriorly at the same depth. Analgesia is enhanced by two further injections, of 0.2 ml each, being given superiorly and inferiorly at points 5 mm lateral to the margin of the tympanic membrane. This technique provides analgesia to the meatus adjacent to the drum, but more extensive blocks are required if other parts of the meatus, the auricle or skin over the mastoid are involved in the incision.

The auriculotemporal nerve can be blocked by injecting 1.5–2.0 ml lignocaine just anterior to the meatus. The operator's index finger is placed in the auditory canal and advanced until arrested by its bony part; the needle point is then advanced until it is adjacent to the tip of the finger (*Figure 26.8*). The great auricular and auricular nerves can

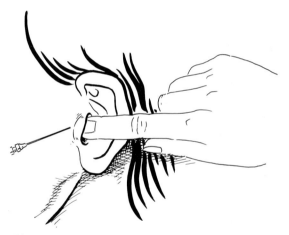

Figure 26.8 Nerve block of auriculotemporal nerve. (From Morrison, Mirakhur and Craig, 1985, by courtesy of the publisher)

be anaesthetized behind the pinna, using a common skin puncture. A weal is raised in front of the lower anterior border of the mastoid process, a 7 cm needle is inserted and directed upwards, and 2–3 ml of anaesthetic are placed between the mastoid process and the meatus. The needle is then withdrawn and redirected upwards and backwards to pass posteriorly to the ear canal until its tip is cranial to that structure; 2–4 ml of solution are injected as the needle is being withdrawn (*Figure 26.9*).

If anaesthesia is required within the tympanic cavity, 4–6 drops of sterile 4% lignocaine may be

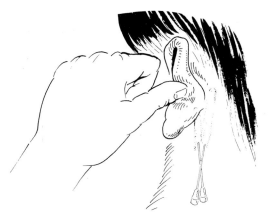

Figure 26.9 Nerve block of great auricular and auricular nerves. (From Morrison, Mirakhur and Craig, 1985, by courtesy of the publisher)

instilled; but it may be necessary to repeat this process because the irregular shape of the tympanic cavity can result in the uneven distribution of the anaesthetic. Local anaesthetic solutions injected in this way can cause dizziness and nausea lasting up to 8 hours; this is thought to result from diffusion of the anaesthetic through the round window membrane (Simmons, Glattke and Downie, 1973).

General anaesthesia

Drugs used in general anaesthesia

It is not possible to describe the pharmacology of all the drugs used in general anaesthesia, but some of the principal agents will be mentioned. General anaesthetic agents can be divided into inhalational and intravenous categories, although some of the latter can be given by other routes. Inhalational agents can be subdivided into gases and volatile liquids.

Nitrous oxide

At the present time, nitrous oxide is the only widely used anaesthetic gas. It is non-flammable, colourless, slightly heavier than air and has a sweetish odour. It is a weak anaesthetic and, if hypoxia is to be avoided, it is very difficult to produce general anaesthesia by using this agent alone. Subanaesthetic doses (50%) are used for analgesia, but for general anaesthesia, 60–70% nitrous oxide in oxygen is supplemented with other agents. Nitrous oxide depresses the central nervous system, causes a slight depression of myocardial contactility together with some alpha- and beta-adrenergic stimulation and, after prolonged use, causes depression of the bone marrow function.

Nitrous oxide is 34 times more soluble than nitrogen in the blood (Thomsen, Terkildsen and Arnfred, 1965) and because of this disparity, it will diffuse into any air-containing cavity more rapidly than nitrogen will exit. In the normal middle ear, an increase in pressure (limited by the passive opening of the eustachian tube) and a slight increase in volume, resulting from the outward bulging of the tympanic membrane, occur during inhalation of the gas. The rate of rise of pressure with the inhalation of 70% nitrous oxide is about 0.1–0.2 kPa/min (10–20 mmH$_2$O/min), reaching a maximum of 3.9 kPa (400 mmH$_2$O) in 30 minutes (Davis, Moore and Lahiri, 1979). The rate of rise of pressure will be increased if respiration is assisted, using a bag and mask, because gas can be forced into the ear cavity from the nasopharynx (Casey and Drake-Lee, 1982). The rate of diffusion is even more rapid into ear clefts with a markedly subatmospheric pressure (Drake-Lee, Casey and Ogg, 1983). When nitrous oxide is discontinued, a negative middle ear pressure may develop on account of the gas diffusing out more rapidly than nitrogen can enter to replace it (O'Neill, 1980). Nitrous oxide can have no effect on a middle ear cavity which is completely filled with fluid, as there will be no air-containing space with which the gas can equilibrate (Gates and Cooper, 1980). This situation is probably unusual because some air remains, at least in the mastoid air cells, in most fluid-filled ear clefts.

These pressure changes can be either beneficial or harmful. An atelectatic tympanic membrane may be forced into a normal position and contour (Graham and Knight, 1981) and serous fluid may be displaced (Marshall and Cable, 1982). Tympanic membrane rupture has been reported after nitrous oxide inhalation (Man, Segal and Ezra, 1980), particularly in patients with pre-existing ear pathology. A conductive hearing loss, lasting 1 or 2 days (Waun, Swietzer and Hamilton, 1967), and the displacement of ossicular reconstruction and tympanic membrane grafts have also been reported (Patterson and Bartlett, 1976). During middle ear surgery, it may be advisable to discontinue nitrous oxide for a few minutes before the ear is closed with a tympanic graft, in order to avoid both the ballooning of the graft while it is being fixed in position and the retraction of the graft after the operation.

Halothane, enflurane and isoflurane

Halothane, enflurane and isoflurane are the three volatile anaesthetic agents most widely used today. They are all non-flammable. Halothane is twice as potent as enflurane, with isoflurane occupying an intermediate position. These agents are administered from calibrated, temperature compensating vaporizers, each liquid having its own specific vaporizer. Halothane is used in a concentration of 0.5–2% for maintenance of anaesthesia, and higher concentrations can be used for induction. All three have a depressant action on respiratory and cardiovascular systems which is proportional to the depth of anaesthesia. The hypotension that results from halothane is due to myocardial depression and a reduction in cardiac output, while with isoflurane, the fall in blood pressure can be attributed to reduction in peripheral vascular resistance. Halothane sensitizes the myocardium to catecholamines, and arrhythmias are not infrequent, especially if marked hypercarbia is allowed. For this reason, the use of halothane is contraindicated if it is planned to use adrenaline infiltration during surgery. Enflurane or isoflurane are compatible with adrenaline, with isoflurane being noted particularly for the maintenance of a stable cardiac rhythm during anaesthesia.

There is evidence that halothane may cause gross disturbance of liver functions, with severe and often fatal jaundice; this is more likely to occur if repeated administrations are given within 6 months. The complication is fortunately very rare, but, when repeated anaesthesia is necessary within this period, consideration should be given to the use of an alternative agent.

Intravenous anaesthetic agents

The induction of anaesthesia in the adult today is almost always by the intravenous route, one notable exception being in the patient with a compromised airway. Sodium thiopentone is still the most commonly used drug and it produces a smooth quiet induction in one arm–brain circulation time. Much emphasis has been placed on the respiratory and cardiovascular depressant effects of thiopentone, but in the healthy patient these are, in practice, minimal. If it is used with care, and given slowly and in reduced dosage to the ill patient, thiopentone is a very satisfactory agent in skilled hands. Like all intravenous anaesthetic agents, it should never be given by those unskilled in airway maintenance, tracheal intubation and artificial respiration. Recovery from thiopentone results from the redistribution of the drug in the body and not from rapid detoxication, as a large amount of unmetabolized drug remains for at least 12 hours after its administration. Thiopentone is not ideal for day case anaesthesia. Methohexitone, while not giving as smooth an induction as thiopentone, is more rapidly metabolized and will produce less of a hangover effect; thus it is a more suitable intravenous barbiturate for outpatient anaesthesia.

Many other drugs have been developed for intravenous anaesthesia but most have been discarded, either because they had no obvious advantages over thiopentone, or produced hypersensitivity reactions in too high a proportion of patients, or had other toxic effects. Of these drugs, two remain at present (1985): etomidate, which is rapidly metabolized but produces a high incidence of involuntary movement during induction, and propofol (diisopropyl phenol), also rapidly metabolized, which is still undergoing clinical trials and shows considerable promise.

Muscle relaxant drugs

Since the introduction of tubocurarine into anaesthetic practice, a large number of myoneural blocking agents have been developed over the last four decades, all capable of producing profound relaxation of striated muscle during light general anaesthesia. Tubocurarine is still in use and is popular in the technique of controlled hypotensive anaesthesia as it produces a fall in blood pressure by histamine release and ganglionic blockade, as well as a non-depolarizing myoneural blockade. Suxamethonium, the only depolarizing relaxant in common use, is valuable when a short period of relaxation is required, for example, to facilitate laryngoscopy and tracheal intubation. Pancuronium is widely used in general anaesthetic practice, its main disadvantage being the propensity to cause tachycardia. The newer relaxants, atracurium and vecuronium, which do not have any significant effect on the cardiovascular system and are easy to reverse, even after prolonged administration, are gaining wide acceptance.

Narcotic drugs in general anaesthesia

Opiates are frequently given either intramuscularly before operation or, more logically, intravenously during surgery, to augment the effects of general anaesthetic agents and to provide a carry-over effect of analgesia into the postoperative period. Morphine (0.15–0.2 mg/kg) or papaveretum (0.2–0.25 mg/kg), with a duration of action of about 4 hours, is often used. The longer-acting levorphanol (25 µg/kg), with an action lasting 6–8 hours, may be more appropriate if the main aim is that of postoperative pain relief. The short-acting narcotic drugs, such as fentanyl (with a duration of action of about 20 minutes with a single 1–2 µg/kg dose) or ultrashort-acting alfentanil (with action lasting about 4–5 minutes after 5–7 µg/kg) may also be used intraoperatively to prevent reaction to painful stimuli. Narcotic drugs cause dose-related respiratory depression, most marked after intravenous administration, which can be reversed by intravenous naloxone

(0.4 mg). Repeated or very large doses of fentanyl can, after excretion in the bile, be reabsorbed from the gut and cause unexpected delayed respiratory depression about 6–8 hours after administration. Nausea and vomiting frequently ensue from the use of narcotics, and will require treatment with antiemetics.

Antiemetic drugs

If antiemetic drugs are not used, about one-third of all patients undergoing anaesthesia and surgery will suffer nausea and vomiting afterwards, and in certain types of surgery (for example operations on the middle ear), the proportion is very much higher. The cause may be peripheral or central in origin, the latter arising either from the stimulation of the chemoreceptor trigger zone or by the activation of labyrinthine reflexes. Antiemetic drugs act either in the periphery or on the vomiting centre or both. The most useful drugs belong to the antihistamine or phenothiazine groups. Perphenazine is one of the most effective of these drugs, particularly in doses of about 5 mg, but the drug is liable to produce distressing extrapyramidal side-effects in a proportion of patients if it is repeated too frequently. It is much less likely to produce side-effects if the dosage is halved, but it thereby becomes less effective than cyclizine. Cyclizine, an effective antiemetic with few side-effects, can be given parentally as the lactate (50 mg every 6–8 hours) or by mouth as 50 mg hydrochloride tablets. In severe cases of vomiting, such as that associated with labyrinthine disturbances, there is often an associated agitation, so the addition of a benzodiazepine (e.g. diazepam) can be helpful in settling the patient.

When opiates are used in premedication, the addition of an antiemetic will decrease the probability of nausea. This is particularly useful if atropine, which has an antiemetic action, has been omitted.

Techniques of general anaesthesia in otolaryngology

The majority of adult patients will have induction of anaesthesia with an intravenous barbiturate (for example thiopentone 4–6 mg/kg) followed by a muscle relaxant and, when the muscles of the jaw and larynx are relaxed, a direct laryngoscopy can be performed followed by tracheal intubation, with the tube being passed through either the mouth or the nose. Anaesthesia is maintained either by artificially ventilating the paralysed patient through the tracheal tube with nitrous oxide, oxygen and an inhalational anaesthetic agent or, if a short-acting relaxant (suxamethon-

ium) is used, by allowing spontaneous breathing of the anaesthetic mixture. If artificial ventilation is being used, a cuff will be necessary on the tracheal tube to provide an airtight seal. Oral tracheal intubation is preferable to the nasal route as the former avoids damage to delicate nasal mucosa and allows the passage of a larger tube with less resistance to respiration. However, intubation does not guarantee a free airway, for tubes can become kinked (less likely with modern kink-resistant tubes), obstructed with secretions or the tip can be occluded by resting on the carina or against the wall of the trachea. If the tube is too long it will pass into a bronchus, usually the right, resulting in ventilation of one lung only with consequent cyanosis. If the tube is too short it may become dislodged, which is particularly likely if the patient's head is flexed or rotated. A tracheal tube does not ensure protection of the air passages from soiling by blood or secretions. A carefully placed throat pack and an inflated cuff on the tube, to make an airtight fit with the tracheal wall, are necessary; a cuffed tube without a pack will not always prevent blood seeping past into the trachea.

If anaesthetic hoses between the tracheal tube and the anaesthetic machine become disconnected during spontaneous respiration, the patient will become too lightly anaesthetized; but with a paralysed, ventilated patient, respiration will cease and life-threatening hypoxia result. These disconnections can occur very easily, often as the result of the patient's head being moved by the surgeon, and pass unnoticed when the head is covered with sterile towels; therefore, the surgeon should give a warning, and the anaesthetist should check the circuit, each time the position of the head is altered. The use of a disconnection alarm, fitted to the anaesthetic circuit, is a wise precaution.

The aim is to establish and maintain a perfect airway and, while minor degrees of obstruction may not be life-threatening, the resultant venous congestion will increase bleeding. Light anaesthesia which results in coughing and straining on the tracheal tube, particularly likely if the tube is moved as occurs when the position of the patient's head is altered, will have the same result.

Anaesthesia for tonsillectomy

The fact that adenoidal tissue is normally absent in the adult means that a nasotracheal tube is suitable for this type of operation, but a kink-resistant reinforced oral tube, together with a gag with a split tongue plate, can also be used. Spontaneous breathing is usually allowed and the standard tonsil position is used with the nasopharynx dependent to protect the airway from blood;

therefore, a cuffed tube is not necessary. Stiff plastic nasal tubes should be softened in warm water before use to reduce trauma to the nasal mucosa; many anaesthetists still prefer the older softer red rubber tubes. There is no place nowadays to attempt a tonsillectomy under general anaesthesia using an insufflation technique without a tracheal tube.

Post-tonsillectomy bleeding

Reoperation to control secondary or reactionary bleeding after tonsillectomy presents a considerable hazard for the patient and poses formidable problems for the anaesthetist. Bleeding in the early postoperative period may be largely masked until blood loss is of significant proportions; this is because the patient, drowsy or even asleep, may swallow blood as quickly as it is lost from the circulation, and the first external sign of bleeding may be vomiting of blood. It is essential at this stage that a reliable intravenous line be established and blood sent for grouping and cross-matching, if this has not already been done. It is ill-advised to give sedative drugs in the hope that bleeding will stop, as these will tend to mask further bleeding and also increase the risk of aspiration of blood into the respiratory tract. It is important not to anaesthetize the patient until resuscitative measures are well in hand and cross-matched blood is available, with adequate volumes of crystalloid solution being given while awaiting the blood. While it must be assumed that the patient's stomach is full of blood, most of these patients will be too distressed to tolerate the passage of a gastric tube, and the attempt may further aggravate the bleeding.

Problems during induction of anaesthesia include the probability of blood in the stomach, with the risk of vomiting or regurgitation, and the danger of aspiration. An additional hazard is the presence of varying amounts of blood clot and active bleeding in the pharynx which can obscure the larynx, or even cause respiratory obstruction. The anaesthetist must decide whether there will be any difficulty in intubating the trachea, and careful inspection of the pharynx in the awake patient is necessary. If no difficulty is anticipated, a rapid sequence intravenous induction is generally acceptable; that is preoxygenation, an intravenous induction agent and suxamethonium, cricoid pressure (to prevent passive regurgitation of stomach contents) and intubation using a cuffed oral tube, avoiding, if possible, positive presure ventilation of the patient before intubation. In the presence of active bleeding or numerous large blood clots, it is advisable to maintain spontaneous respiration until there is absolutely no doubt that intubation can be achieved. The

technique then is to induce anaesthesia with oxygen and halothane with the patient in the head-down left lateral position, with cricoid pressure being applied by an assistant from the time of loss of consciousness. When the patient is deeply anaesthetized, direct laryngoscopy and intubation, again with a cuffed oral tube, is carried out. Adequate suction must be available at all times and an adequate selection of working laryngoscopes and a variety of tracheal tubes must always be to hand. Most of the disasters from pharyngeal bleeding occur as the result of loss of control of the airway.

Anaesthesia for the patient with an obstructed airway

Respiratory obstruction, of varying aetiology and severity, may occur in any part of the respiratory tract; trismus may or may not be present.

In patients with severe obstruction, who are in obvious distress and using the accessory muscles of respiration, the only safe method of inducing general anaesthesia is by first establishing the airway in the conscious patient. If the obstruction is in the region of the glottis, it may be possible to perform a direct laryngoscopy under local anaesthesia and intubate the trachea, thereafter rapidly inducing intravenous general anaesthesia. However, if the obstruction is higher or trismus is present, then the only safe choice may be a tracheostomy performed under local anaesthesia. The cardinal rule is that general anaesthesia should not be induced until the airway is secured.

With lesser degrees of obstruction, induction of anaesthesia may be attempted by using an inhalational technique and maintaining spontaneous respiration until direct laryngoscopy shows that intubation is possible, but the surgeon must be available for emergency tracheostomy or cricothyrotomy, should this be necessary. Intravenous induction of anaesthesia is dangerous as respiration can cease and the anaesthetist may not be able to ventilate the patient or visualize the larynx.

In some cases, it may be feasible to use a fibreoptic bronchoscope. First, a suitably sized nasotracheal tube is threaded over the instrument and then, under local anaesthesia, the tube and endoscope are passed together through the nose, the larynx visualized, and, once the tip of the instrument is through the glottis, the tube is pushed down into the trachea. Because of swelling and anatomical distortion, the procedure can be very difficult and should be attempted only by those skilled in the use of this instrument.

Blind nasal intubation should not be attempted when the airway is compromised as, on account of the distorted anatomy, it is unlikely to succeed and it may precipitate complete obstruction. This manoeuvre is of value in the unobstructed patient in whom laryngoscopy is impossible; for example, a patient with a wired fractured mandible.

In all cases where a partially obstructed airway is present, medication with opiates is dangerous because depression of the respiratory centre may lead to a complete cessation of breathing. In lesser degrees of respiratory embarrassment, a benzo-diazepine (for example diazepam) may be helpful.

Anaesthesia for nasal surgery

The principles of anaesthesia during surgery on the nose are those of faultless maintenance of anaesthesia and protection of the airway, with recognition of the probability of blood and debris draining into the pharynx during operation, of the possibility of systemic effects from the use of vasoconstrictor drugs, and of the likelihood of preoperative and postoperative nasal obstruction. A cuffed oral tube together with a pharyngeal pack should be used to prevent soiling of the respiratory tract. Throat packs should be moistened with water, not with paraffin or other insoluble lubricants which may cause lipid pneumonia if they enter the lungs. Spontaneous ventilation is satisfactory for most nasal operations. If cocaine or catecholamines are used topically, it is safer to avoid the use of halothane; enflurane or isoflurane are suitable alternatives as they are much less likely to be associated with arrhythmias. Controlled ventilation using muscle relaxants, nitrous oxide and oxygen, with narcotic or inhalational supplementation, is particularly suitable in very prolonged procedures or where a rapid recovery of consciousness is desired. It is also a valuable technique in patients with a respiratory disease with an irritable respiratory tract, in whom deep anaesthesia would otherwise be necessary to prevent coughing or straining on the tracheal tube.

The patient should be put in a slightly head-up position to help reduce bleeding and improve surgical access. At the end of the operation, care must be taken to remove the pharyngeal pack, clear the pharynx of blood by suction, turn the patient into the semi-prone position and insert a pharyngeal airway before removal of the tracheal tube. If a nasal pack is to be left in place, the security of this must be checked to ensure that there is no likelihood of it becoming displaced and thus liable to being inhaled. A good airway, adequate anaesthesia, correct position of the patient and efficient use of topical vasoconstrictors are usually adequate to reduce bleeding to a minimum, but with the occasional difficult rhino-plasty or extensive cancer surgery, the use of controlled hypotension may be considered.

Anaesthesia for endoscopy

Laryngoscopy and microlaryngoscopy

During laryngoscopy, the surgeon requires a clear view, immobile cords and adequate space for inspection and instrumentation; while good anaesthetic practice demands overall safety, adequate respiratory exchange, protection of the lower airways and reliable and speedy recovery of reflexes at the end of the procedure. Very many different anaesthetic techniques have been described to try to meet these requirements. Light premedication, such as oral diazepam, is preferred in order to facilitate quick postoperative recovery. It is important to avoid narcotics if airway patency is suspect, and the precautions already described for induction in this situation must be taken. Most cases for laryngoscopy have a clear airway, and the main argument about anaesthetic technique is whether or not a tracheal tube should be used and, if not, how adequate ventilation should be maintained.

Using a tracheal tube

The use of a small nasal or oral cuffed tracheal tube secures the airway, provides protection from soiling and allows adequate ventilation. The 31 cm long, 5 mm tracheal tube, described by Coplans (1976), with a high volume (10 ml) low pressure cuff is suitable. Airway resistance is high in tubes of this size, so controlled ventilation using muscle relaxants is essential. The main disadvantage is that of interference with good surgical access, particularly for lesions on the posterior aspect of the vocal cords. In addition, tubes can become occluded as the result of surgical manipulation and they are a fire hazard if laser surgery is used.

Using a catheter

Instead of a 5–6 mm tracheal tube, a small catheter (14 FG or smaller) can be positioned with the tip midway between the cords and the carina. After an intravenous induction, anaesthesia is deepened using an inhalational agent and the larynx and trachea are thoroughly sprayed with 4% ligno-caine before introduction of the catheter. Oxygen and anaesthetic agents are insufflated through the catheter, with the patient being allowed to breathe spontaneously (Hadaway, Page and Shortbridge, 1982). Although this method is claimed to give better surgical access, the disadvantages are the lack of protection of the lower airway, some slight movement of the cords with each respiration and the surgeon being subjected to exhaled anaesthetic gases.

Using jet ventilation

Variants of the Sanders (1967) technique of jet ventilation for bronchoscopy have been adopted for microlaryngoscopy, the great advantage being the unobstructed view of the larynx. The method uses the Venturi principle of entrainment of air by means of a tube within a tube, the larger tube being the trachea or the laryngoscope. The gas (oxygen) in the inner tube is under pressure and thus it expands at the point of exit, producing a suction effect which entrains the surrounding gas (air) in the larger tube, the result being a magnified gaseous thrust (*Figure 26.10*). Basic equipment consists of a bayonet-fitting nipple plugged into

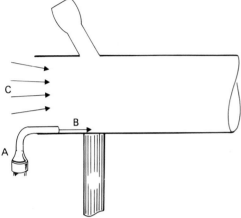

Figure 26.10 Diagram to show entrainment effect of Venturi jet. Gas under high pressure in tube A expands at B producing a suction effect at C. (From Morrison, Mirakhur and Craig, 1985, by courtesy of the publisher)

the high pressure oxygen outlet, connected by high pressure tubing to a manual valve, which permits control of both the frequency and length of inspiration (*Figure 26.11*). From the valve, plastic tubing connects the system to a jet ventilating needle or catheter. Different points of delivery of the jet have been used and all have relative advantages and disadvantages.

If the tip of the jet is kept within the laryngoscope, then, in order to maintain effective ventilation, the tip of the laryngoscope must be kept close to the cords and the lumen of the instrument kept in line with the axis of the trachea. The cords must be fully relaxed and the lesion must not cause mechanical obstruction to air flow. Large tumours can have a ball valve effect and thus render ventilation ineffective. In these circumstances, it is best to use a tracheal tube in the first instance in order that the bulk of the tumour can be surgically reduced before jet ventilation is started. The advantage of having the jet in this position is that it avoids the need for a tube of any kind having to pass through the glottis.

The tip of the jet can protrude beyond the laryngoscope (*Figure 26.12*) and pass a short way through the glottis (Ruder *et al.*, 1981). Again, there must be no obstruction to air flow through the larynx, otherwise dangerously high intracheal pressure may be generated with resultant baro-trauma. The size of the ventilating needle will vary according to the weight and age of the patient, a 14-gauge needle being suitable for most adults. A plastic nasal catheter can be used instead of a needle, the tip being placed 3–5 cm above the carina (Tobias, Nasser and Richards, 1977).

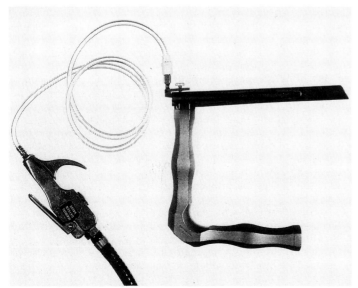

Figure 26.11 Equipment for jet ventilation. (From Morrison, Mirakhur and Craig, 1985, by courtesy of the publisher)

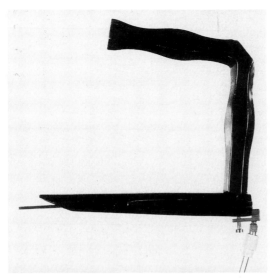

Figure 26.12 Laryngoscope with tip of jet cannula extending beyond the break. (From Morrison, Mirakhur and Craig, 1985, by courtesy of the publisher)

A more recent method of jet ventilation during laryngoscopy involves the use of the modern high frequency ventilator (Eriksson and Sjöstrand, 1977; Smith, 1982). Ventilation at about 100 breaths per minute, with small tidal volumes, can provide good gas exchange with low airway pressures. The gas can be delivered by a nasal or oral catheter with the tip well below the level of the cords (Babinski, Smith and Klain, 1980). A fairly stiff catheter, 3.5–4.0 mm in diameter, is necessary for this procedure because fine flexible catheters vibrate quite violently with the rapidly alternating pressures and this can damage laryngeal or tracheal mucosa. The ventilator driving pressure can be varied, but although lower pressures decrease the vibratory cord movement, they tend at the same time to produce less effective ventilation. The advantages over conventional jet ventilation include a decreased risk of mucosal trauma and the resultant risk of surgical emphysema, and more effective ventilation in patients with respiratory disease.

Jet ventilation techniques are not without risk and fatalities have been reported (Vivori, 1980). The risk of barotrauma is increased if the jet exit is inside the trachea. Factors such as any obstruction to expiration, small mucosal tears or the use of too high gas pressures further increase the risk of surgical emphysema or pneumothorax. The risk is decreased if the jet is kept within the laryngoscope, precautions are taken to ensure that the airway is clear and ventilation is not started until the laryngoscope is in place and the relaxed unobstructed cords can be seen. Chest movements

must be observed at all times and it is wise to commence with a low ventilating pressure (100–130 kPa in the adult). If a plastic catheter is used, it should be of reasonable stiffness to avoid a whiplash injury to the trachea (Ruder *et al.*, 1981) and it is important that the tip is in the correct position at all times. If the catheter becomes displaced out of the trachea, large volumes of gas can be jetted into the gastrointestinal tract. When using a catheter with side holes, it is possible for gas to be forced down the oesophagus while the catheter tip lies below the glottis and ventilation appears to be normal (Chang *et al.*, 1978). If the catheter tip goes beyond the carina, one-lung anaesthesia will result and dangerously high intrabronchial pressures may be generated.

When the jet needle is placed within the laryngoscope, gas can be forced down the oesophagus if the axis of the instrument is not kept in line with the trachea. In addition to the dangers of gross abdominal distension, even small amounts of gas forced into the stomach will greatly increase the risk of regurgitation of gastric contents. If it is suspected that gas has entered the stomach, it is a wise precaution to pass a gastric tube and to keep it in place until the patient is awake.

Jet ventilation systems may not be able to ensure adequate ventilation in patients with a very low lung compliance. In obese patients and those with obstructive airways disease it may be safer to use a small cuffed tracheal tube and manual ventilation.

Laser surgery of the larynx

Laser surgery poses special problems for the anaesthetist. If rubber or plastic tubes are used they must be protected from the laser beam because, if hit directly or contacted by a beam reflected off a shiny metal surface, they are liable to be ignited. Flammable anaesthetic agents must not be given and it is wise to avoid high concentrations of oxygen. Nitrous oxide, which supports combustion at high temperatures, should not be used. Similarly, lubricants should be restricted to aqueous solutions because ointments and other greases may be flammable. Combustible tracheal tubes must be protected by being wrapped in aluminium foil tape as far down as the cuff (*Figure 26.13*), or by being covered with muslin which has been previously soaked in saline. Cuffs can be protected by saline-soaked cotton swabs, but great care must be taken to ensure that they are all removed at the end of the procedure. If the patient has a tracheostomy with a plastic tube, the latter can be protected in a similar manner. It is difficult to maintain adequate protection of tracheal tubes at all times; gaps can appear between the layers of tape, and if the tape is

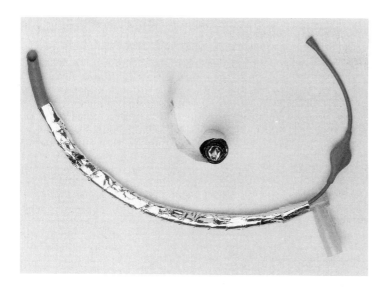

Figure 26.13 Tracheal tube protected by metal foil tape. (From Morrison, Mirakhur and Craig, 1985, by courtesy of the publisher)

broken the sharp edges can injure mucosa (Patil, Stenlurg and Zauder, 1979). Flexible all-metal tubes can be used but they are liable to be traumatic and it is not possible to provide a cuff. Tracheal tubes made of silicone elastomer, and coated with a layer of silicone containing reflective aluminium oxide, are claimed to be non-flammable. The aforementioned problems can also be avoided by using jet ventilation through a metal needle jet.

Cardiovascular risks during laryngoscopy

Manipulation in and around the larynx may cause a rise in blood pressure, tachycardia, dysrhythmias, mycocardial ischaemia and even cardiac arrest. The risks are particularly great if coronary artery disease is present and in patients with uncontrolled hypertension. The risks can be minimized by preoperative treatment of hypertension, adequate anaesthesia and ventilation, and by careful monitoring. Beta-adrenergic blocking drugs before or during induction may be helpful, as may small intravenous doses of lignocaine. Tachycardia and the hypertensive response to laryngoscopy can be moderated by careful application of topical anaesthesia to mouth, pharynx and larynx after the patient is asleep. The procedure must be carried out slowly, one stage at a time, to avoid triggering the reflex; and although this may be tedious, it may be of great value to the high risk patient. Levels of anaesthesia which are too light, hypercarbia or hypoxia are all liable to increase the incidence of dysrhythmias. The most dangerous combination is tachycardia and hypertension, with the former decreasing the time available for coronary perfusion of the deeper layers of the

myocardium, and the latter increasing the workload of the heart. Strong *et al.* (1974) reported a 1.5% incidence of myocardial infarction or myocardial ischaemia following microlaryngoscopy, but the incidence rose to 4% in those with a previous history of cardiac disease. As many of these infarctions are symptomatically silent, a routine postoperative ECG is recommended for those patients thought to be at risk.

ECG monitoring and frequent blood pressure measurements are essential during laryngoscopy. If hypertension or dysrhythmias should develop during the operation, it may be necessary to release the suspension laryngoscope for a few minutes, deepen anaesthesia and sometimes to give beta-adrenergic blocking drugs.

Bronchoscopy

General anaesthetic techniques for bronchoscopy are as numerous and as varied as those for laryngoscopy. The procedure may be diagnostic or therapeutic using a rigid or fibreoptic bronchoscope. As in laryngoscopy, the aim is to provide a quiet patient with fully obtunded gag and cough reflexes, who will quickly recover both consciousness and protective reflexes once the examination is completed. The choice of general anaesthetic technique is dependent, to some extent, on the purpose of the examination, how long it is likely to take and the condition of the patient. Retention of spontaneous respiration is preferred in those cases where there is a foreign body, where there are copious bronchial secretions or where a bronchopleural cyst or fistula is present. In all techniques, sufficient general anaesthesia, topical anaesthesia and intravenous narcotics should be provided to prevent the occurrence of hypertension and dysrhythmias associated with stimulation of the tracheobronchial tree.

For rigid bronchoscopy, anaesthesia can be induced in any suitable way and continued with the patient breathing a mixture of oxygen and inhalational anaesthetic agent. When the anaesthetic is deep enough, the glottis and upper trachea are sprayed with a local anaesthetic solution and a ventilation pattern bronchoscope is inserted. Spontaneous ventilation may continue with the anaesthetic mixture being delivered through the side port of the bronchoscope, and with the eyepiece-obturator in position as often as possible. It is quite possible to assist or even control ventilation in these circumstances. An alternative is to use the short-acting muscle relaxant, suxamethonium, in intermittent doses and to control ventilation throughout.

Another option is to use the jet injector technique already described for laryngoscopy. The high pressure jet of oxygen is applied at the operator's end of an open bronchoscope and room air is entrained during flow through the jet so that the lungs are inflated with a mixture of oxygen and air (Sanders, 1967; Komesaroff and McKie, 1972). The advantage of this method is that adequate ventilation can be maintained while the surgeon is able to work unimpeded by eyepieces. The disadvantages are that blood and particulate matter may be blown down the tracheobronchial tree, and anaesthesia cannot easily be maintained with inhalational agents. The use of the injector requires an anaesthetized and paralysed patient.

High frequency jet ventilation techniques have also been used employing rates of up to 300 breaths per minute (Smith, 1982; Vourc'h *et al.*, 1983). Movements in the bronchial tree are reduced to a minimum with these techniques – a particular advantage during laser surgery – and an additional benefit is the minimal spread of blood and debris.

The use of general anaesthesia is not common for fibreoptic bronchoscopy but may be performed by passing the fibreoptic bronchoscope through a tracheal tube, with ventilation of the patient continuing using the space between the tracheal tube and the bronchoscope (employing a 'chimney' or side-arm connector for the breathing circuit). In some patients with tracheostomies it may be possible to pass the fibrescope through the nose or mouth and along the trachea behind the tracheostomy tube, thus allowing ventilation to be continued more easily than when the instrument has to be passed through the tracheal tube.

Bronchoscopy is well tolerated by patients who have no obvious loss of cardiac or pulmonary reserves. However, in the case of those patients with grossly impaired cardiac or ventilatory function, it is not a procedure to be undertaken lightly as complications can occur as a consequence of the inevitable increase in hypoxaemia. While trauma to the teeth and oropharyngeal tissue during the passage of the endoscope may result from inappropriate manipulation of the instrument, trauma to the tracheobronchial tree is more likely to be attributable to coughing or movement of the patient. Bleeding, even to a minor degree following a biopsy, may pose a threat to life by obstructing the airway; therefore, tracheobronchial suction through the bronchoscope must be continued until bleeding has stopped or become insignificant. Pneumothorax is rare, usually only occurring when excessive airway pressure has been allowed to develop as a result of a ventilatory obstruction or the use of injector ventilation with an inadequate expiratory airway. Any cardiovascular disturbances which may arise are similar to those seen during laryngoscopy and, as such, they respond to the same treatment.

Pharyngoscopy and oesophagoscopy

General anaesthesia for these procedures does not present any problems because tracheal intubation provides safety for the patient and good access for the surgeon. Good muscle relaxation is necessary for passage of the oesophagoscope and will also prevent sudden movement which could result in laceration or perforation of the oesophagus while the endoscope is in place. Cardiac dysrhythmias do sometimes occur as the instrument passes behind the pericardium, but they are rarely troublesome.

Tracheostomy

The key to a satisfactory tracheostomy is the prior securing of the airway by tracheal intubation or bronchoscopy, thus allowing the surgeon to perform an unhurried operation in an uncongested field. If the patient has significant airway obstruction, the technique for induction of anaesthesia already described for the patient with an obstructed airway must be used. While anaesthesia and intubation are always desirable for the optimum operating conditions, general anaesthesia may, in a few cases, be too dangerous and a tracheostomy should be performed under local anaesthesia. The anaesthetist must never be persuaded to embark on a general anaesthetic against his better judgement, as he is the only person who can fully appreciate both the difficulties that may be encountered and the extent of his own experience and capability in overcoming them.

Major head and neck surgery

Laryngectomy

Careful preoperative preparation is necessary in laryngectomy patients as many suffer from chronic obstructive airways disease and require intensive preoperative physiotherapy. An assessment of laryngeal airway patency is essential. Most patients will have had a laryngoscopy and biopsy carried out a few days before, so an accurate assessment of the airway will already have been made by both anaesthetist and surgeon. If a different anaesthetist is to be involved with the laryngectomy, then consultation with the surgeon and anaesthetist who were present at the biopsy is advisable. Some patients may develop oedema after the trauma of biopsy, so a good airway at the time of the biopsy is not an absolute guarantee that all will be well a few days later. When there is doubt, the procedure described for induction of anaesthesia in the patient with a partially obstructed airway is followed. Occasionally, preliminary tracheostomy under local anaesthesia may be the safest course.

Care must be taken during intubation to avoid trauma to the neoplastic area, and bleeding; therefore, a smaller tube than usual may be necessary. A cuffed oral armoured tube is less likely to be occluded during surgical manipulation than an unarmoured type. Once the airway is established, there will be few problems in most cases. If spontaneous ventilation is allowed, then anaesthesia should be based on an inhalational agent. It is usually more satisfactory to employ muscle relaxants and controlled ventilation throughout what is often a long operation in a poor risk patient. Before the trachea is divided, the patient is ventilated with 100% oxygen; after the division, the tracheal tube is removed and a sterile cuffed tracheostomy tube inserted into the tracheostome by the surgeon. The change-over should be performed as quickly and smoothly as possible. The surgeon who does not appreciate the need for speed in this manoeuvre may cause the anaesthetist considerable anxiety, as may the sudden discovery of a missing or inappropriate connection or piece of tubing. At this stage, care must be taken that blood does not enter the trachea. If spontaneous ventilation is allowed, anaesthesia must be deepened before the change-over period to prevent the patient from coughing, but as the patient is breathing spontaneously there will not be quite the same urgency. Bleeding can be quite brisk at times, particularly if a block dissection of neck glands is necessary, and controlled hypotension may have to be considered.

Pharyngolaryngectomy

A radical one-stage operation using a stomach transplant together with total oesophagectomy is a procedure that is used for the surgical treatment of some types of hypopharyngeal cancer. Anaemia, malnutrition and electrolyte imbalance may be present at the preoperative stage. Nutrition of those patients who have difficulty in swallowing liquids can be improved by nasogastric feeding, with parenteral nutrition rarely being required. There is a high incidence of postoperative chest infection after this particular operation, and the importance of preoperative physiotherapy and attainment of maximum respiratory function before surgery must be emphasized.

Access to the patient may be difficult during the operation because of the number of operators and their assistants who are present; therefore the anaesthetist may be more dependent than usual on monitoring devices, and must insist on having access to one arm on an armboard.

Controlled ventilation is used throughout the operation and deliberate lowering of the arterial blood pressure may be helpful at certain stages. Graft circulation can be compromised by hypotension, so blood pressure must be restored to normal levels before the stomach is brought up into the neck. However, the use of controlled hypotension is not without risk in these debilitated patients, and many anaesthetists feel it to be both unnecessary and dangerous (Condon, 1971; Plant, 1982). Blood loss is substantial, particularly during mobilization of the thoracic oesophagus by blind digital dissection, and this may be largely concealed in the thorax. Dysrhythmias and dramatic falls in blood pressure, resulting from interference with venous return, are not infrequent at this stage.

When the trachea becomes unsupported after mobilization of the oesophagus, the fragility of the posterior wall of the trachea can cause rupture in the membranous part at the site of the tracheostomy tube cuff, thus making inflation of the lungs difficult or impossible (Bains and Spiro, 1979). Manual ventilation with 100% oxygen until the stomach is drawn up into the neck to tamponade the leak may cope with the situation (Plant, 1982), but a short cuffed tracheal or endobronchial tube may be necessary and should be available. The pleura on one or both sides is frequently torn during blind dissection of the oesophagus, so the routine placement of bilateral chest drains is advisable.

Tracheal reconstruction

Operations involving the resection or repair of the trachea are a challenge to the anaesthetist. The problems of providing adequate oxygenation and facilitating carbon dioxide removal with an open trachea, combined with the need to provide good operating conditions, are formidable. Periods of hypoventilation may be unavoidable and careful monitoring is required in order to detect quickly the onset of serious hypoxaemia. Airway management usually necessitates a multi-stage approach, and each step must be fully planned before operation, with the nature, site and extent of the obstructed segment and the proposed method of surgical repair all being taken into account.

The anaesthetic technique depends on the degree of narrowing of the trachea and the level of the lesion. Controlled ventilation using an uncuffed small bore orotracheal tube inserted into the distal segment is a suitable technique, provided that the narrowing is not too severe (Heifetz, 1974; Borgan and Privitera, 1976). If the trachea is deviated, the bevel of the tube should be cut in such a way that the opening does not lie against the tracheal wall. With a very tight stenosis, it may be unwise to force through even a small diameter tube, for fear of subsequent bleeding and oedema, and in this case an ordinary tracheal tube is positioned just proximal to the stenosis.

The presence of the tracheal tube interferes with the surgical access during the anastomosis. This can be overcome by withdrawing the tracheal tube into the proximal segment and passing a catheter down the orotracheal tube into the distal segment of the trachea after its division, with ventilation being maintained by means of an injector or high frequency ventilation (Lee and English, 1974; Ellis, Hinds and Gadd, 1976; Rogers *et al.*, 1985). If the stenosis is very low, two tubes may be passed, one down each bronchus. The catheter(s) must be secured by a stitch to the tracheal or bronchial walls. As soon as the anastomosis is completed, the catheter(s) should be withdrawn and ventilation continued through the tracheal tube. Alternatively, a cuffed tube may be inserted into the distal cut end of the trachea or into a main bronchus (Kamvyssi-Dea *et al.*, 1975), which is then removed before completion of the anastomosis, at which time an orotracheal tube is passed down through the cut ends. A technique using spontaneous ventilation may occasionally be employed in high tracheal stenosis, but the danger of opening the pleurae during the operation must be borne in mind.

Anaesthesia during the period of the tracheal anastomosis is usually maintained with intravenous drugs (Vyas, Lyons and Dundee, 1983), except where a tracheal tube has been passed into the distal segment when inhalational agents can be used. When spontaneous ventilation is used, the wound is flooded with oxygen by way of a tracheal tube placed in the proximal segment during the anastomosis.

Monitoring during major head and neck surgery

Monitoring should include continuous ECG display and blood pressure measurement, preferably using a direct method with radial artery cannulation which also allows access for blood gas analysis both during and after the operation. Central venous pressure measurement can be useful to help estimate fluid replacement; however, neck catheters are impracticable, while central venous catheters placed by way of an arm vein are reasonably satisfactory but their position must be checked by radiography.

Air embolism, although rare, is a potential complication. Air may sometimes be seen entering one of the neck veins, but the condition is best detected by using an end-tidal carbon dioxide monitor which will indicate a sudden fall in the gas tension should this mishap occur. A precordial Doppler flow transducer can also be used for the diagnosis, whereas hypotension, tachycardia and ECG changes (dysrhythmias and evidence of right heart strain) are late signs. Treatment consists of any measure which will increase venous pressure, such as continuous positive pressure ventilation and compression of jugular veins. The patient is ventilated with 100% oxygen and, as soon as is practicable, is placed in the left lateral head-down position. It may be possible to aspirate air through the central venous catheter. In extreme cases, external cardiac massage and transthoracic aspiration of air from the right ventricle with needle and syringe may be necessary. General supportive measures include the use of inotropic agents and correction of metabolic acidosis.

Long procedures can result in marked falls in body temperature and this should be monitored by means of a rectal or oesophageal temperature probe; falls in temperature are minimized by using a heating blanket. The use of a peripheral nerve stimulator will provide a useful guide to the state of neuromuscular blockade and the timing of further doses of muscle relaxants.

Patients should be transferred to an intensive care unit after most types of major head and neck surgery.

Controlled hypotension

Ever since surgery began, bleeding has been a problem both to the surgeon, when blood obscures the operative field and makes precise technique difficult, and to the anaesthetist, when the volume of blood lost is large. The difficulties for the surgeon are greater when the operation involves very small structures, often in confined cavities such as the middle ear. In these situations, even small amounts of blood make successful reconstructive surgery very difficult or sometimes impossible, and it is generally agreed that a reduction in blood pressure is useful, indeed often essential, in this type of surgery. Indications for controlled hypotension in other types of head and neck surgery are less clear-cut.

The aim of the anaesthetist is to provide conditions which give the surgeon the best operating field possible, while at the same time not endangering in any way the life or well-being of the patient. The exact relationship between the level of blood pressure and the degree of reduction of bleeding has not been firmly established, and there is no evidence that profound hypotension, with systolic pressures as low as 30 mmHg, or even less (Kerr, 1977), is any more effective than a more moderate lowering of arterial pressure (Donald, 1982).

There are other factors in addition to arterial pressure which are important in wound bleeding. Venous pressure, which plays an important part in venous oozing, can be reduced at the operation site by careful posturing of the patient, securing a free airway and by ensuring a complete absence of any coughing or straining on the tracheal tube. Local vasoconstriction can be produced by means of a vasoconstrictor. Infection will result in vasodilatation and increased bleeding.

Arterial blood pressure is directly proportional to cardiac output and peripheral resistance, and is maintained in normal circumstances by the autonomic nervous sytsem and by hormonal control. These mechanisms tend to resist attempts to lower the arterial pressure with the result that resistance to drugs and techniques aimed at producing hypotension is frequently experienced, particularly in the young, robust patient.

The safety of any state of lowered blood pressure will be determined by the ability of the reduced perfusion pressure to maintain an adequate blood flow to vital organs, particularly to the brain and the heart. Both these organs are able to maintain their perfusion over a wide range of presure change by local autoregulation, provided that their vasculature is normal. Serious reductions in blood flow in the healthy brain or heart are unlikely to occur provided that the arterial pressure is not reduced too rapidly (so that autoregulatory mechanisms have time to come into play) nor to too low a level (not less than 60 mmHg except in exceptional circumstances). When the patient is tilted feet downwards, to reduce venous pressure at head level, adequate allowance must be made for the difference in arterial pressure between the point of measurement and the brain, allowing a 2 mmHg fall in pressure for every 2.5 cm difference in vertical height.

A fall in arterial oxygen tension occurs when arterial blood pressure is reduced in anaesthetized patients (Wildsmith, Drummond and MacRae, 1975). This is a consequence of ventilation/perfusion inequalities in the lung caused by a reduction in cardiac output, a fall in pulmonary pressure and a depression of the normal hypoxic vasoconstrictor mechanism which diverts blood flow from parts of the lung with a low alveolar oxygen tension.

Preoperative assessment is very important before controlled hypotension to exclude the possibility of cardiovascular, cerebrovascular and pulmonary disease. Anaemia is a contraindication. Hypertensive patients should be regarded as having a diseased cardiovascular system and many anaesthetists would therefore be reluctant to induce hypotension in such patients. Diabetic patients likewise are prone to atheroma, and those with severe long-standing disease are not suitable for hypotensive techniques. Similarly, a history of angina or coronary artery occlusion or cerebral vascular accident would be a contraindication.

If lung disease is present, pulmonary function tests may be helpful in assessing its severity, as may a blood gas analysis; however, caution is required if arterial pressure is to be lowered, and arterial carbon dioxide and oxygen tensions should be monitored during surgery.

Pregnancy or the use of contraceptive medication are also contraindications.

Age is not of itself a contraindication and older patients, if they are normotensive and fit, will tolerate a moderate reduction in pressure. Elderly patients are very sensitive to hypotensive techniques and care must be taken to avoid excessive reductions in blood pressure.

Blood pressure should not be reduced when a hypotensive technique is thought to carry a significantly increased risk, as will be indicated by the general condition of the patient, the past history or abnormal findings in ECG, chest X-ray, pulmonary function tests or routine blood analysis. If factors which increase wound bleeding are avoided, reasonably satisfactory results can often be obtained without recourse to a reduction of arterial pressure. Local injections of vasoconstrictor solutions may also help in these situations.

Techniques of controlled hypotension

Blood pressure is reduced by lowering peripheral vascular resistance or decreasing cardiac output, or by a combination of both. Tilting the patient head-up will hydrostatically decrease arterial

Table 26.1 Drugs commonly used to produce controlled hypotension

Drug	Method and rate of administration	Dose
Trimetaphan camsylate	Infusion 3–4 mg/minute	Maximum dose 1 g
Sodium nitroprusside	Infusion 50–500 µg/minute Maximum 10 µg/kg per minute	Maximum dose 1.5 mg/kg*
Nitroglycerin	Infusion 150–500 µg/minute	
Labetalol	Test dose followed by single bolus	0.1 mg/kg 0.15–0.4 mg/kg

* Rarely necessary to exceed 0.5 mg/kg

pressure at the operation site, as well as decreasing cardiac output by pooling blood in the lower parts of the body, thereby reducing venous return to the heart. Inhalational anaesthetic agents decrease blood pressure either by myocardial depression, as in the case of halothane, or by peripheral vasodilatation as occurs with isoflurane. Some muscle relaxants increase cardiac output by increasing the heart rate (e.g. gallamine), and so are unsuitable for hypotensive anaesthesia, while others have no effect on the heart rate or peripheral resistance (e.g. vecuronium and atracurium) and are, therefore, quite suitable for this technique. Tubocurarine, with its hypotensive action, is also popular.

Drugs which are used specifically to lower blood pressure are many and varied; the four most commonly used are listed in *Table 26.1*. With the exception of labetalol, the drugs are administered by continuous infusion and the blood pressure reduction is controlled by the rate of infusion.

Trimetaphan camsylate

Trimetaphan camsylate has a direct dilatory effect on vascular smooth muscle and causes histamine release, but its hypotensive effect is mainly due to ganglionic blockade (Adams and Hewitt, 1982). Blood pressure falls within 4 minutes of beginning the infusion and the full effect is produced within 10 minutes. Likewise, blood pressure usually returns to prehypotensive levels within a few minutes of stopping the infusion, but recovery may be delayed following prolonged administration or the giving of large doses (Adams, 1975). The hypotensive action is markedly potentiated by halothane and other inhalational agents. Tachycardia is often a problem, particularly in the young adult, causing a rise in cardiac output, increased wound bleeding and difficulty in lowering arterial blood pressure; it can usually be controlled by beta-adrenergic blocking drugs.

Sodium nitroprusside

Sodium nitroprusside acts directly on vascular smooth muscle causing relaxation in both resistance and capacitance vessels. The onset of action is very rapid and the duration of its effect transient, the rapidity of response making it necessary to control accurately the rate of administration, preferably with an infusion pump. When the infusion is stopped, arterial pressure will rise spontaneously and rapidly, provided that the blood lost has been replaced; vasopressors are not required (Cole, 1978). Tachycardia can be troublesome but it can be minimized by adequate analgesia, and by the use of inhalational agents and beta-adrenergic blockers.

Large doses of nitroprusside can lead to toxic effects resulting from the release of cyanide during metabolic breakdown (Vesey and Cole, 1975), so the total dose should not exceed 1.5 mg/kg and the rate of administration should be limited to 10 µg/kg per minute. In practice, there is rarely a need for 0.5 mg/kg to be exceeded, provided that use is made of inhalational agents to potentiate the hypotensive effects. Patients suffering from metabolic disorders may be unduly susceptible to the toxic effects of nitroprusside. The use of the drug is contraindicated in cases of Leber's optic atrophy (a rare inherited disease), and tobacco amblyopia and in the presence of neuropathies secondary to vitamin B_{12} deficiency, in all of which cyanide metabolism is abnormal. It is also to be avoided in patients with hepatic or renal failure.

Nitroglycerin

Nitroglycerin (glyceryl trinitrate) produces dilatation of the peripheral veins, with a lesser vasodilatory effect on the resistance vessels. It has a slower, less effective and less certain action than nitroprusside in producing hypotension, and the return of pressure to normal levels is also slower.

This can be an advantage in that it makes abrupt swings in blood pressure easier to avoid (Fahmy, 1978); however, the difficulty in obtaining adequate hypotension in some patients is a disadvantage (Chesnut *et al.*, 1978).

Labetalol

Labetalol is an amide with both alpha- and beta-adrenergic blocking properties, decreasing blood pressure by a reduction in peripheral vascular resistance and by a decrease in cardiac output (Richards, 1976). The drug shows a remarkable synergism with the volatile anaesthetic agents in producing a hypotensive effect, and arterial pressure can be quickly and easily controlled by adjustment of the inspired concentration of the volatile agent. Blood pressure can be raised after operation by withdrawing the volatile agent and, if necessary, giving atropine intravenously to increase the heart rate.

Monitoring during hypotensive anaesthesia

Careful monitoring of the patient is essential during controlled hypotension and, although particular attention must be paid to the level of arterial pressure, other vital observations must not be ignored.

Blood pressure

The choice of the method of measuring blood pressure depends on the drugs used for producing hypotension, the degree of reduction in pressure desired and the nature of the operation. If a rapidly acting and powerful agent such as nitroprusside is to be used then direct invasive monitoring with a cannula in the radial artery, providing a beat-by-beat observation of the pressure, is essential (Cole, 1978). When slower acting, less powerful agents are used to produce moderate falls in pressure, and when little blood loss is likely, a non-invasive method of pressure measurement is adequate. At low pressures, palpation of peripheral pulses is difficult, and a Doppler sensor placed over the radial or brachial artery and a reliable sphygmomanometer, or an automatic monitor working on the oscillotonometry principle (e.g. Dinamap, Critikon), should be used. A simple mechanical oscillotonometer (von Recklinghausen) is also quite accurate in the presence of vasodilatation, provided that the anaesthetist is familiar with its use.

ECG

A continuous display of the ECG is necessary during controlled hypotension, for observing cardiac rhythm and for detecting the occurrence of myocardial ischaemia. A preoperative ECG should always be available for comparison.

Carbon dioxide tension

A large decrease in arterial carbon dioxide tension, resulting from overventilation during controlled breathing, may be dangerous during controlled hypotension as the resultant cerebral vasoconstriction will further decrease cerebral blood flow. Monitoring of the end-tidal carbon dioxide tension will act as an effective guide to the arterial gas tension, and it will provide a warning should excessive ventilation lead to the washing out of carbon dioxide.

Blood loss

Adequate replacement of blood loss is essential because the normal circulatory defence mechanisms which compensate for a reduction in blood volume will have been abolished by the hypotensive technique. Direct measurement of blood loss by weighing swabs and, whenever possible, by estimating the haemoglobin content of the fluid in the suction bottles, is necessary during those operations where significant haemorrhage occurs. Central venous pressure measurement can be helpful in monitoring fluid replacement, but central venous pressure can be decreased by some of the agents used to produce arterial hypotension.

Temperature

Temperature should be monitored during long procedures; a mid-oesophageal or rectal temperature probe is satisfactory.

EEG

Monitoring of the cerebral function would seem to be an ideal means of obtaining a warning when an excessive decrease in arterial pressure is compromising cerebral perfusion. The conventional EEG has marked limitations because of the complexity of the equipment and the difficulty in interpreting the record, but the cerebral function monitor is a portable and much simpler machine providing a continuous integrated record of overall cerebral electrical activity. Unfortunately, factors other than arterial pressure can have marked effects on the level of cerebral electrical activity, including those of depth of anaesthesia, blood carbon dioxide tensions and hypothermia. However, during stable conditions a decrease in the level of the cerebral function monitor trace could indicate a decrease in cerebral perfusion with cortical depression and act as a warning to increase arterial pressure.

References

ADAMS, A. P. (1975) Techniques of vascular control for deliberate hypotension during anaesthesia. *British Journal of Anaesthesia*, **47**, 777–792

ADAMS, A. P. and HEWITT, P. B. (1982) Clinical pharmacology of hypotensive agents. *International Anesthesiology Clinics*, **20**, 95–109

BABINSKI, M., SMITH, R. B. and KLAIN, M. (1980) High frequency jet ventilation for laryngoscopy. *Anesthesiology*, **52**, 178–180

BAINS, M. S. and SPIRO, R. H. (1979) Pharyngolaryngectomy, total extrathoracic esophagectomy and gastric transposition. *Surgery, Gynecology and Obstetrics*, **149**, 693–696

BAYLISS, R., CLARKE, C., OAKLEY, C. M., SOMERVILLE, W., WHITFIELD, A. G. W. and YOUNG, S. E. J. (1983) The microbiology and pathogenesis of infective endocarditis. *British Heart Journal*, **50**, 513–519

BOAKES, A. J., LAURENCE, D. R., TEOH, P. C., BARAR, F. S. K. and BENEDIKTER, L. T. (1973) Interactions between sympathomimetic amines and antidepressant agents in man. *British Medical Journal*, **1**, 311–315

BORGAN, C. P. and PRIVITERA, P. A. (1976) Resection of stenotic trachea: a case presentation. *Anesthesia and Analgesia*, **55**, 191–194

BOWEN, D. J., NANCEKIEVILL, M. L., PROCTOR, E. A. and NORMAN, J. (1982) Perioperative management of insulin dependent diabetic patients. Use of continuous intravenous infusion of insulin-glucose-potassium solution. *Anaesthesia*, **37**, 852–855

CASEY, W. F. and DRAKE-LEE, A. B. (1982) Nitrous oxide and middle ear pressure. *Anaesthesia*, **37**, 896–900

CHANG, J. L., MEEVWIS, H., BLEYAERT, A., BABINSKI, M. and PETRUSCAK, J. (1978) Severe abdominal distension following jet ventilation during general anesthesia. *Anesthesiology*, **49**, 216

CHESNUT, J. S., ALBIN, M. S., GONZALEZ-ABOLA, E., NEWFIELD, P. and MAROON, J. C. (1978) Clinical evaluation of intravenous nitroglycerin for neurosurgery. *Journal of Neurosurgery*, **48**, 704–711

CLARKE, S. W. and KNIGHT, R. K. (1977) Fibreoptic bronchoscopy. *The Practitioner*, **218**, 119–122

COLE, P. (1978) The safe use of sodium nitroprusside. *Anaesthesia*, **33**, 473–477

CONDON, H. A. (1971) Anaesthesia for pharyngo-laryngo-oesophagectomy with pharyngo-gastrostomy. *British Journal of Anaesthesia*, **43**, 1061–1065

COPLANS, M. P. (1976) A cuffed naso-tracheal tube for microlaryngeal surgery. *Anaesthesia*, **31**, 430–431

CURTISS, E. S. (1952) Postural nerve block for intra-nasal operations. *The Lancet*, **1**, 989–991

DAVIS, I., MOORE, J. R. M. and LAHIRI, S. K. (1979) Nitrous oxide and the middle ear. *Anaesthesia*, **34**, 147–151

DONALD, J. R. (1982) Induced hypotension and blood loss during surgery. *Journal of the Royal Society of Medicine*, **75**, 149–151

DRAKE-LEE, A. B., CASEY, W. F. and OGG, T. W. (1983) Anaesthesia for myringotomy. *Anaesthesia*, **38**, 314–318

ELLIS, R. H., HINDS, C. J. and GADD, L. T. (1976) Management of anaesthesia during tracheal resection. *Anaesthesia*, **31**, 1076–1080

ERIKSSON, I. and SJÖSTRAND, U. (1977) A clinical evaluation of high-frequency positive-pressure ventilation (HFPPV) in laryngoscopy under general anaesthesia. *Acta Anaesthesiologica Scandinavica*, **64**, 101–110

FAHMY, N. R. (1978) Nitroglycerine as a hypotensive drug during general anaesthesia. *Anesthesiology*, **49**, 17–20

GATES, G. A. and COOPER, J. C. (1980) Effect of anesthetic gases on middle ear pressure in the presence of effusion. *Annals of Otology, Rhinology and Laryngology*, **89** (Suppl.), 62–64

GOLDMAN, L., CALDERA, D. L., NUSSBAUM, S. R., SOUTHWICK, F. S., KROGSTAD, D., MURRAY, B. *et al.* (1977) Multifactorial index of cardiac risk in non-cardiac surgical procedures. *New England Journal of Medicine*, **297**, 845–850

GOLDMAN, V. and EVERS, H. (1969) Prilocaine-felipressin: a new combination for dental analgesia. *Dental Practitioner*, **19**, 225–231

GRAHAM, M. D. and KNIGHT, P. R. (1981) Atelectatic tympanic membrane reversal by nitrous oxide supplemented general anaesthesia and polyethylene ventilator tube insertion. *The Laryngoscope*, **91**, 1469–1471

HADAWAY, E. G., PAGE, J. and SHORTBRIDGE, R. T. (1982) Anaesthesia for microsurgery of the larynx. *Annals of the Royal College of Surgeons of England*, **64**, 279–280

HEIFETZ, M. (1974) Management of anaesthesia during tracheal resection. *Anaesthesia*, **29**, 760–761

KAMVYSSI-DEA, S., KRITIKOU, P., EXARHOS, N. and SKALKEAS, G. (1975) Anaesthetic management of reconstruction of the lower portion of the trachea. *British Journal of Anaesthesia*, **47**, 82–84

KERR, A. R. (1977) Anaesthesia with profound hypotension for middle ear surgery. *British Journal of Anaesthesia*, **49**, 447–452

KOMESAROFF, D. and McKIE, B. (1972) The bronchoflator: a new technique for bronchoscopy under general anaesthesia. *British Journal of Anaesthesia*, **44**, 1057–1068

LEE, P. and ENGLISH, I. C. W. (1974) Management of anaesthesia during tracheal resection. *Anaesthesia*, **29**, 305–306

MACINTOSH, Sir R. and OSTLERE, M. (1955) *Local Analgesia: Head and Neck*. Edinburgh: E & S Livingstone

MAN, A., SEGAL, S. and EZRA, S. (1980) Ear injury caused by elevated intratympanic pressure during general anaesthesia. *Acta Anaesthesiologica Scandinavica*, **24**, 224–226

MARSHALL, F. P. F. and CABLE, H. R. (1982) The effect of nitrous oxide on middle-ear effusions. *Journal of Laryngology and Otology*, **96**, 893–897

MIRAKHUR, R. K., CLARKE, R. S. J., ELLIOTT, J. and DUNDEE, J. W. (1978) Atropine and glycopyrronium premedication: a comparison of the effects on cardiac rate and rhythm during induction of anaesthesia. *Anaesthesia*, **33**, 906–912

MIRAKHUR, R. K. and DUNDEE, J. W. (1983) Glycopyrrolate: pharmacology and clinical use. *Anaesthesia*, **38**, 1195–1204

MORRISON, J. D., MIRAKHUR, R. K. and CRAIG, H. J. L. (1985) *Anaesthesia for Eye, Ear, Nose and Throat Surgery*, 2nd edn. Edinburgh: Churchill Livingstone

NEWTON, D. A. G. and EDWARDS, G. F. (1979) Route of induction and method of anaesthesia for fibreoptic bronchoscopy. *Chest*, **75**, 650

O'NEILL, G. (1980) Middle ear pressure measurements during nitrous oxide anaesthesia. *Clinical Otolaryngology*, **5**, 355

PATIL, V., STENLURG, L. C. and ZAUDER, H. L. (1979) A modified endotracheal tube for laser microsurgery. *Anesthesiology*, **51**, 571

PATTERSON, M. E. and BARTLETT, P. C. (1976) Hearing impairment caused by intratympanic pressure changes during general anesthesia. *The Laryngoscope*, **86**, 399–404

PEARCE, S. J. (1980) Fibreoptic bronchoscopy: is sedation necessary? *British Medical Journal*, **281**, 779–780

PLANT, M. (1982) Anaesthesia for pharyngo-laryngectomy with extrathoracic oesophagectomy and gastric transposition. *Anaesthesia*, **37**, 1211–1213

PRYS-ROBERTS, C., MELOCHE R. and FOEX, P. (1971). Studies of anaesthesia in relation to hypertension: 1. Cardiovascular responses of treated and untreated patients. *British Journal of Anaesthesia*, **43**, 122–137

RICHARDS, D. A. (1976) Pharmacological effects of labetalol in man. *British Journal of Clinical Pharmacology*, **3**, 721S–723S

ROGERS, R. C., GIBBONS, J., COSGROVE, J. and COPPEL, D. L. (1985) High frequency jet ventilation for surgery. *Anaesthesia*, **40**, 32–36

RUDER, C. B., RAPHAEL, N. L., ABRAMSON, A. L. and OLIVERIO, R. M. Jr (1981) Anesthesia for carbon dioxide laser microsurgery of the larynx. *Otolaryngology and Head and Neck Surgery*, **89**, 732–737

SANDERS, R. D. (1967) Two ventilating attachments for bronchoscopes. *Delaware Medical Journal*, **39**, 170–176

SIMMONS, F. B., GLATTKE, T. J. and DOWNIE, D. B. (1973) Lidocaine in the middle ear: a unique cause of vertigo. *Archives of Otolaryngology*, **98**, 42–43

SIMMONS, N. A., CAWSON, R. A., CLARKE, C., EYKYN, S. J., McGOWAN, D. A., OAKLEY, C. M. *et al.* (1982) The antibiotic prophylaxis of infective endocarditis. Report of the working party of the British Society for Antimicrobial Chemotherapy. *The Lancet*, **2**, 1323–1326

SMITH, R. B. (1982) Ventilation at high respiratory frequencies. *Anaesthesia*, **37**, 1011–1018

STRONG, M. S., VAUGHAN, C. W., MAHLER, D. L., JAFFE, D. R. and SULLIVAN, R. G. (1974) Cardiac complications of microsurgery of the larynx. *The Laryngoscope*, **84**, 908–920

THOMSEN, K. A., TERKILDSEN, K. and ARNFRED, I. (1965) Middle ear pressure variations during anesthesia. *Archives of Otolaryngology*, **82**, 609–611

TOBIAS, M. A., NASSER, W. Y. and RICHARDS, D. C. (1977) Nasotracheal jet ventilation for microlaryngeal procedures. *Anaesthesia*, **32**, 359–362

VESEY, C. J. and COLE, P. V. (1975) Nitroprusside and cyanide. *British Journal of Anaesthesia*, **47**, 1115

VIVORI, E. (1980) Anaesthesia for laryngoscopy. *British Journal of Anaesthesia*, **52**, 638

VOURC'H, G., FISCHLER, M., MICHON, F., MELCHOIR, J. C. and SEIGNEUR, F. (1983) High frequency jet ventilation *v.* manual jet ventilation during bronchoscopy in patients with tracheo-bronchial stenosis. *British Journal of Anaesthesia*, **55**, 969–972

VYAS, A. B., LYONS, S. M. and DUNDEE, J. W. (1983) Continuous intravenous anaesthesia with Althesin for resection of tracheal stenosis. *Anaesthesia*, **38**, 132–135

WALTS, L. F., MILLER, J., DAVIDSON, M. B. and BROWN, J. (1981) Perioperative management of diabetes mellitus. *Anesthesiology*, **55**, 104–109

WAUN, J. E., SWIETZER, R. S. and HAMILTON, W. K. (1967) Effect of nitrous oxide on middle ear mechanics and hearing acuity. *Anesthesiology*, **28**, 846–850

WILDSMITH, J. A. W., DRUMMOND, G. B. and MacRAE, W. R. (1975) Blood gas changes during induced hypotension with sodium nitroprusside. *British Journal of Anaesthesia*, **47**, 1205–1211

27

Biomaterials

J. J. Grote

Biomaterials are synthetic or treated materials employed to replace or augment tissues and organs. The potential usefulness of alloplastic materials in the fabrication of prostheses has been known for a long time; however, the adaptation of materials technology for the purposes of surgical implant manufacture did not take place until about 25 years ago (Calman, 1963).

Biomaterials science is the study of living and non-living materials. Biomaterials themselves have always been of interest to the otologist concerned with reconstructive middle ear surgery (Grote, 1984a). In the past, the results obtained from using alloplastic implant materials in the middle ear have been disappointing because of the problems associated with extrusion (Guilford, 1964; Portmann, 1967). Nevertheless, it is worth noting that the most successful middle ear reconstruction in otosclerosis patients has been that performed with alloplastic implants (Shea, 1969). The recent advances in biomaterials science and the concomitant increase in knowledge have effected a revival in the development of middle ear prostheses. Furthermore, in maxillofacial surgery, implants are being used for the reconstruction of bony defects. In cases of head and neck surgery and in rhinology, the use of biomaterials has so far been reported only in experimental studies.

Scientific methods and surgical criteria must be applied if good results with alloplastic materials are to be achieved; the interrelationship between these criteria, however, necessitates their combined application. The dissimilarity between the surgical aims and the demands to be made on the implants used in orthopaedics and those used in otology will obviously be reflected in the different implant materials employed by surgeons in these respective fields. The same is true in the case of middle ear reconstruction, where the requirements for the reconstruction of the canal wall are different from those for an ossicular chain reconstruction.

The selection of alloplastics for reconstructive surgery is based on aspects derived from a variety of physical, chemical, biomechanical and surgical concepts (Homsy, 1970). With the ever increasing number of implants on the market, it is essential that the otolaryngologist has a fundamental knowledge of biomaterials science to complement his surgical aims.

Biocompatibility

The reaction of the body to the implant has to be studied in terms of both local and general reactions – the cytotoxicity of the implant material; however, the influence of the body on the prosthesis is also of importance. These reactions can eventually lead to degradation and loss of function. This phenomenon is called the biofunctionality of the implant.

Biocompatibility is the first prerequisite for a useful implant material and this must be tested extensively *in vitro*, in animal experiments, and in clinical studies with long postoperative follow-up periods. The interaction between the implant and the body must ultimately lead to a good and permanent integration. Such a successful integration is dependent on the surface activity of the implant material, and on the breakdown and likely remodelling of the implant by the body.

Surface activity

An implant material can be regarded as bioinert if the body does not react at all to the implant material; as biotolerant if the body regards the implant material as a foreign body but, after incorporation, ceases to react to the implant; and as bioactive if the body has an active surface compatibility with the implant material, which leads to a firm integration between the body and the foreign material.

An implant material will always be placed in a wound, and thus normal wound reactions will inevitably take place (Silver, 1980). A foreign body will be encapsulated by a fibrous capsule with a varying number of reactive cells, particularly foreign body giant cells. In the case of bioinert material, where no reaction of the surface to the body occurs, the encapsulation will be in the form of only a small fibrous capsule, without further reaction taking place. A biotolerant material will have a good fibrous capsule around the implant material, an indication of cellular activity; giant cells, in particular, can be present even after longer postoperative periods, but the integration will be stable. A bioactive material will achieve a real bond with the surface of the surrounding tissue, because of active ion exchange, leading to a firm bond between the implant material and the body.

Structure

In the past, implant materials had a solid structure. However, during the last decade, several investigators have developed porous materials which enable the host tissue to grow into the porous part of the implant, resulting in a good integration with the body (Friedenberg, 1963; Klawitter and Hulbert, 1971; Homsey and Anderson, 1976; Spector, Fleming and Kreutner, 1976). It was found that macropores of 100 µm were ideal for the ingrowth of fibrous tissue, especially of bone tissue, if adjacent to the implant material. Micropores of several micrometres seemed to be essential, particularly if the implant materials had to be resorbed and remodelled in living tissue. In contrast, the micropores can be a problem in those materials which are not meant for degradation.

It is important to understand, however, that all materials will be affected by the body and will be resorbed to some degree, depending on the surface activity. If there is a large surface area, the response of the body tissue to the implant material will be greater, with the production of large numbers of macrophages and giant cells (Brown, Neel and Kern, 1979; Kerr, 1981). The corrosion of implants can lead to the release of potentially harmful substances into the body; for example metals such as nickel, cobalt, chromium and aluminium which can be released from metal implants, may cause allergic responses, for which nickel, in particular, is notorious (Barranco and Solomon, 1972; Benson, Goodwin and Brostoff, 1975). Polymers can undergo degradation as a result of water or lipid absorption, by leaching of low-molecular-weight molecules, or by chain scission through oxidation or hydrolysis. It is probable that some additives, which are necessary for the stability of the polymer, will be released from the implant material, and some of these can be very toxic (*US Pharmacopeia* 1975, XIX). Even ceramics, such as alumina, which are very inert, can release substances into the body, and a characteristic of alumina is that it can be stored in the brain. Small particles from the implant can stimulate a non-specific fibrocytic response, which leads to the destruction of surrounding tissue.

A most important criterion is the potential carcinogenic property of some substances which may be released – in particular from certain polymers. It has been demonstrated in animal experiments that large smooth surfaces may enhance the development of sarcomata, but the same is not reported from clinical studies (Oppenheimer *et al.*, 1964).

A foreign body placed in a wound can attract bacteria which colonize the surface of the implant in a protected environment that is ideal for the proliferation of such organisms, thereby rendering conventional antibiotic treatment ineffectual (Gristina *et al.*, 1976). Therefore, the behaviour of the implant material should also be studied in an infected surrounding.

An aspect of the structure of the material which must be considered is the density, including the porosity which will indicate the macropores and micropores, as this will have an influence on both the integration capacity and the wound reaction and remodelling capacity. In the case of ceramics, the crystallographic structure must also be indicated.

Generic names

Many implants are marketed with trade names, which give no information on the capacity of the material; therefore, the generic name of the material used must be indicated.

In addition to the generic names of the materials, the additives which might be part of the implant material must also be listed. The generic names can give the information on biocompatibility.

Specific materials

In reconstructive surgery, three classes of biomaterials are used: metals, polymers and ceramics. The different classes of biomaterials have both advantages and disadvantages with regard to biocompatibility, integration capacity and surgical application.

Metals

Metals are used less frequently in otolaryngology than in other disciplines. Over 100 years ago, it was noticed that metal, in the form of bullets, gave rise to inflammation, but occasionally the metal would be walled off in a pocket of scar tissue, thus creating few problems. However, metal implants were a considerable infection risk and caused a great deal of wound reaction; the exceptions were gold and silver devices, although their applicability had been restricted by the softness of these two metals. Metallurgic developments gave rise to a large variety of alloy steels (the patent for stainless steel was recorded in 1913), but none of the steels had sufficient resistance to corrosion.

Cobalt–chromium alloys – first invented by Haines – were developed before 1930, and in the late 1930s a cobalt–chromium alloy (Vitalium) began to be used, particularly in arthroplasty. After the Second World War, when knowledge about corrosion resistance had increased, metal implants achieved a wide application, especially in the field of orthopaedics. There are three classes of alloys: the cobalt–chromium group, the stainless steel group and the titanium group. The cobalt–chromium alloy group is especially popular, and is covered by several trade names, Vitalium being used most frequently. All cobalt–chromium alloys are corrosion resistant to tissues (Cohen, 1983). These types of prosthesis are generally not used in the middle ear but can be used in maxillofacial surgery.

According to the patent description of 1930, the definition of stainless steel is a steel that has a chromium content of between 11 and 30%, with the higher amount of chromium giving the steel a relative resistance to many corrosive fluids. The most corrosion resistant are those such as 316 low carbon steel and these are the most widely used. Stainless steel prostheses, especially in the form of wire prostheses, are well known in middle ear surgery and have proven to be reliable, particularly when integrated into a mobile middle ear chain (Schuknecht, 1958). Stainless steel plates for the purpose of reconstruction are also used in maxillofacial surgery.

The development of a metal alloy based on titanium began during the Second World War when it was used in the airplane industry. These metals are mostly used in orthopaedic devices. There is a reasonable level of corrosion resistance, but experience has shown that tissue surrounding the implant can be dark, indicating an initial loss of titanium to the tissues. Titanium wires are also used in middle ear surgery.

In some metals, corrosion products can be observed in the cells around the implant. As with all implant materials, one important consideration is that concerning the possibility of inducing malignancy. In orthopaedics, in particular, there are large numbers of individuals who have had metal implants for long periods of time, and there is no evidence to support an aetiological connection between the use of these metals and any type of neoplasm. A second very important aspect is that of hypersensitivity reactions to implants. Dermatologists are well aware of the sensitivity of some patients to certain metals, particularly nickel. However, whether that sensitivity also applies in the case of implants under the skin is not known. The conclusion must be that metal implants should not be widely used in otolaryngology, apart from their application in maxillofacial surgery and, in some cases, in middle ear surgery, especially for reconstruction of the middle ear chain. Integrated into a mobile middle ear chain remnant, these implants are reliable; placed against a mobile tympanic membrane, they are extruded (Plester, 1968).

Polymers

Large quantities of plastics were being manufactured as early as the 1930s and 1940s. The application of these industrial polymers to surgical procedures was dictated by both the availability of the product and the intuition of the clinician. The first use of a biomaterial in reconstructive middle ear surgery was by Wullstein in 1952. He implanted a columella of Palavit in the middle ear for the reconstruction of the middle ear chain. Initial hearing results were good, but the implant was extruded. At that time, commercial plastics such as polyethylene, Teflon, and Silastic were used. Only a few polymers had been designed and tested specifically for surgical application. Later, many polymers were used for different types of columella reconstruction. At the end of the 1960s, the use of plastic implant materials was abandoned, particularly in reconstructive middle ear surgery, because of the high extrusion rate (Sheehy, 1965). Apart from the body's reaction to the different polymers, many materials, which were originally intended for industrial use, frequently demonstrated the presence of low-molecular-weight impurities and pharmacologically active trace components in the polymer system.

Many classes of polymers are unsuitable for reconstructive surgery. In otolaryngology, the principal generic classes of interest are low density polyethylene (LDPE or LDP), high density polyethylene (HDPE or HDP), polytetrafluoroethylene (PTFE, also called Teflon) and polydimethyl-xylothene (Silastic).

Some polymers may also consist of more than one chemical entity. To test the different polymers for their potential application in the field of reconstructive surgery, classic procedures are a necessity, depending on either intradermal reaction tests or systemic toxicity tests, the latter of which uses extracts of the materials. These tests are not very sensitive methods for testing biocompatibility; therefore, testing procedures in tissue culture and in cell growth inhibition are more appropriate alternatives (Autian, 1977). Long-term animal and clinical studies are essential. Following the implantation of polymer implants, chemical reactions, as well as wound reaction, will take place, leading to the formation of a fibrous capsule. The thickness of this capsule is an indication of the level of tolerance of the material. In the cellular reaction around the implant, the foreign body reaction with giant cells and macrophages is of primary importance. It has been shown that giant cell reaction around polymers will continue for a long time. This foreign body reaction will also take place in the case of more tolerant materials, especially at sites where there is mechanical irritation (Kuijpers, 1984).

At the beginning of the 1970s, a new concept for implant materials was invented, namely the concept of the porous implant materials. Friedenberg, in 1963, was the first to report on the possibility of adapting an open pore sponge material which, in his case, was made of polytetrafluoroethylene, especially for surgical reconstructive use. This initial work generated a great deal of further research into porous implant materials, especially where ingrowth was apparent when the material was in contact with the bony skeleton. Two porous alloplasts, Proplast and Plastipore, have been promoted in otolaryngology (Janeke and Shea, 1975; Shea, 1976). Proplast is a composite of polytetrafluoroethylene and carbon, and Plastipore is a trade name for a porous polyethylene polymer. These materials show ingrowth of fibrous tissue and capillaries during the first month and, if exposed to bone, bony ingrowth as well. During the implantation periods, the giant cells predominate in the transitional areas between implant and soft tissue. After longer survival periods, hyalinization of the fibrous tissue in the pores has been demonstrated in some studies (Kuijpers, 1984). The resorption of these materials by macrophages has also been demonstrated (Kerr, 1981). It has to be expected that a variety of other polymers will be developed in porous and solid form, and the same test results can be expected. Of the porous materials, total ossicular replacement prostheses (TORPS) and partial ossicular replacement prosthesis (PORPS), which are used as columellae between the footplate and the tympanic membrane, or between the stapes superstructure and the tympanic membrane, have been used in middle ear reconstructive surgery. In the absence of cartilage between the tympanic membrane and the prosthesis, an increase in extrusion rate has been reported (Smyth *et al.*, 1978). Whether this can be blamed only on the materials or whether surgical procedures with regard to the columella technique are also culpable, has not yet been established.

Porous materials have also been used in maxillofacial surgery. Apart from these materials, Silastic has also been used in otolaryngology, especially as plastic sheeting in the middle ear (Sheehy, 1973). Teflon is used in different situations in the middle ear as well as in head and neck surgery for stenting of the larynx and trachea. It must be stated that a precise knowledge of the chemistry and physics of the surface of different polymer implants does not yet exist. The chemical and physical reactions that take place in those areas where the implant is in contact with surrounding tissue, as well as with blood, must be understood. Better physical criteria have to be established in order to facilitate an optimum selection of polymer materials for implantation.

Ceramics

Biologically, ceramics can be classified as bioinert materials (most oxide ceramics or a different modification of carbon) and reactive materials (glass ceramics and calcium phosphate ceramics). Some of these ceramics are used in otolaryngology.

Bioinert ceramics

The Al_2O_3 ceramic is a bioinert ceramic which is used in otolaryngology. It is a polycrystalline material consisting of corundum crystals. The advantage of this material is that it can be used under full load application. Although this is not of importance in the middle ear, it may be of significance in maxillofacial surgery. It has already been demonstrated in animal experiments that the implant is covered with a delicate membrane within 3 weeks; there is also a normal subepithelial cell layer with active fibroblast–collagen fibres and blood vessels. Because it is a bioinert ceramic, integration will be less than with other implant materials, although there will be the fibrous capsule. Prostheses of corundum crystals are very hard and not easy to shape; however, as has been proven in long-term clinical studies with columella prostheses, these bioinert materials behave well in the middle ear (Jahnke, Plester and Heimke, 1979). Other applications in maxillofacial surgery are being developed.

Bioactive ceramics

Glass ceramics

Glass ceramics were developed in order to achieve a direct chemical bond between the implant and the living tissues. They are available in different compositions of surface active glasses (Ceravital, Bioglass, and Macor). Each glass ceramic has its own distinct composition, and the different reactivity can be explained in terms of this individual composition. The basic reactivity depends on the ion exchange at the surface of the implant material. The surface of glass ceramics is lysed after implantation, and is coated with an amorphous gel layer, which probably contains SiO_2, CaO and P_2O_5 and is about 0.1 μm thick. Into this gel layer, the osteoblasts lay down and embed collagenous fibres. Calcium phosphate precipitates as apatite on the surface. This fixes the collagenous fibres on the surface of the implant, thereby preventing its further corrosion. All glass ceramics will be degradable to a certain extent (Hench and Paschall, 1973).

Glass ceramics are used in otolaryngology mainly for reconstruction of the middle ear chain, in the form of columella prostheses (Reck, 1984). Glass material can be difficult to shape during surgery.

Calcium phosphate ceramics

Because their composition resembles that of bone tissue, calcium phosphate ceramics have been studied for many years. These materials are used to fill defects in the bone, Dreesman (1984) being the first to publish the clinical results. The problem is that the biomaterial usually disappears faster than new bone can fill the empty spaces. Different calcium phosphates of the bone matrix have been studied and used, for example B-whitlockite ($Ca_3(PO_4)_2$) and hydroxyapatite ($Ca_{10}(PO_4)_6(OH)_2$) in otolaryngology. Hydroxyapatite is present in the bony tissue and B-whitlockite is present in the body in only a soluble form and can, by means of sintering techniques, be reproduced in ceramic. A selection has to be made according to the reactivity of the body, but there is general agreement that calcium phosphate ceramics are very compatible with the body, especially with bony tissues (de Groot, 1981).

B-whitlockite

Tricalcium phosphates, as a bioactive implant material, behave in the same manner as all calcium phosphates in viable tissues. However, the control on degradation and remodelling is less than with hydroxyapatite, particularly when some impurities are present in the ceramic, the remodelling cannot be controlled and trace elements of the implant may be found in the macrophages around the implant. The degradation process takes place in two stages. As a result of the physicochemical dissolution of the necks between sintered powder particles, individual particles are released, which are subsequently digested and presumably dissolved by cells. If degradation occurs rapidly, the cells cannot dissolve all particles intracellularly before these reach the lymph nodes. This will result in a temporary presence of tricalcium phosphate crystals in the lymph nodes.

Tricalcium phosphates (B-whitlockite) have been used for the obliteration of mastoid cavities (Zöllner *et al.*, 1983; Wullstein, Schindler and Döll, 1984).

Hydroxyapatite

Hydroxyapatite has been studied extensively both *in vitro* and *in vivo*, and in long-term clinical studies (van Blitterswijk *et al.*, 1986a,b; Grote, 1984b, 1986). It has proven to be a bioactive material which achieves a real integration with bone tissue, without any encapsulation. There is controlled remodelling if a porous material is used. These calcium phosphate ceramics can be made in porous as well as in dense forms, depending on the surgical requirements. The continuation of remodelling of the porous forms is also compatible in infected surroundings. The interaction with epithelium and connective tissue has been shown to be excellent, with a direct bond and then integration between the material and the tissue in continuity with the surrounding materials. The attachment of epithelium to dense apatite surfaces has been shown to take place by means of hemidesmosomes, while connective tissue fibres do not encapsulate the implant but run perpendicular to the ceramic surface.

Biologically, B-whitlockite or tricalcium phosphate ceramics behave in the same manner as hydroxyapatite, the one difference being that the B-whitlockite ceramic may be more biodegradable than the hydroxyapatite. This means that an implant in bony tissue will be degraded in an uncertain way. Calcium phosphate materials are resorbed and remodelled in the same way as a living bone tissue matrix; thus they are released and resorbed by macrophages. The resorption and remodelling is not only dependent on the macropores, but also on the micropores, and this in turn is dependent on the crystallography and stoichiometry of the calcium phosphate materials and on the sintering procedures. The disadvantage of calcium phosphate ceramics is their brittleness. As it has insufficient tensile strength, this type of ceramic is not useful as a replacement in large bony defects; only smaller defects in the bone and maxillofacial surgery can be repaired. The use of this ceramic in long-term clinical studies in middle ear surgery has validated its biocompatibility and usefulness. An extensive application in the fields of nasal and maxillofacial surgery has now begun.

Conclusions

Many criteria must be met before an implant can be used effectively. Apart from the biomaterial criteria, a combined application of these with good surgical criteria is a prerequisite for a lasting result. The site where the implant is to be used will determine the selection of the material. The ideal implant material will closely resemble the tissue it is designed to replace in such factors as the size, shape and consistency of the defect. It will be structured in such a way that neither infection nor healing response will alter its characteristics. As the implant becomes established it will assume the characteristics of the tissue which it replaces or augments, thereby ensuring its permanent toleration by the body.

Autologous and homologous materials are often considered to be ideal for the reconstruction of defects in the body. However, after preservation techniques have been carried out, the remodelling of the body with these materials will take place in the same way as with alloplastic implant materials. Advances in biomaterials science will increase the fundamental knowledge of the surface activity of these alloplastic implant materials and of their interaction with the body. The more the material resembles the human body, the better will be its compatibility with the body. The surgical criteria employed in implantation techniques have to be developed and refined for the different surgical areas. It is obvious that the increase in knowledge will lead to the development of innovative implant materials, devices and artificial organs in the near future. The prefabrication of these reliable materials will more than compete with all the problems associated with the transplantation of autologous materials and with the preservation and shaping of homologous materials. A critical evaluation of the materials concerned and some fundamental knowledge of biomaterials science are necessary for the successful use of alloplastic implant materials in the field of reconstructive surgery.

References

AUTIAN, J. (1977) Toxicological testing of biomaterials. *Artificial Organs*, **1**, 59

BARRANCO, V. P. and SOLOMON, H. (1972) Eczematous dermatitis from nickel (letter). *Journal of American Medical Association*, **220**, 1244

BENSON, M. K. D., GOODWIN, P. G. and BROSTOFF, J. (1975) Metal sensitivity in patients with joint replacement arthroplasties. *British Medical Journal*, **4**, 374–375

BROWN, B. L., NEEL III, H. B. and KERN, E. B. (1979) Implants of Supramid, Proplast and Plastipore and Silastic. *Archives of Otolaryngology*, **105**, 605–609

CALMAN, J. (1963) The use of inert plastic material in reconstructive surgery. *British Journal of Plastic Surgery*, **16**, 1

COHEN, J. (1983) Metal implants: historical background and biological response to implantation. In *Biomaterials in Reconstructive Surgery*, edited by L. Rubin, Chapter 6, 46–61. St Louis: C. V. Mosby Company

DE GROOT, K. (1981) Degradable ceramics. In *Biocompatibility of Clinical Implants Materials*, vol I, edited by D. F. Williams, pp. 199–224. Boca Raton, Fla: CRC Press

DREESMAN, H. (1984) Über Knochenplombierung. *Beitraege Klinik Chirurgica* 9200

FRIEDENBERG, T. B. (1963) Bone growth into Teflon sponge. *Surgery, Gynecology and Obstetrics*, **116**, 588

GRISTINA, A. G., ROVERE, G. D., SJOHI, H. and NICASTRO, J. F. (1976) An *in vitro* study of bacterial response to inert and reactive metals and to methyl methacrylate. *Journal of Biomedical Materials Research*, **10**, 273–281

GROTE, J. J. (1984a) *Biomaterials in Otology*. Boston: Martinus Nijhoff Publishers

GROTE, J. J. (1984b) Tympanoplasty with calcium phosphate. *Archives of Otolaryngology*, **110**, 197

GROTE, J. J. (1986) Reconstruction of the middle ear with hydroxyapatite implants. *Annals of Otology, Rhinology and Laryngology*, **95**, (suppl. 123), 1–12

GUILFORD, F. R. (1964) Tympanoplasty: use of prosthesis in conduction mechanism. *Archives of Otolaryngology*, **80**, 80–86

HENCH, L. L. and PASCHALL, H. A. (1973) Direct bond of bioactive glass ceramic materticls to bone and muscle. *Journal of Biomedical Materials Research*, Symp. 4, 25–42

HOMSY, C. A. (1970) Biocompatibility in selection of materials for implantation. *Journal of Biomedical Materials Research*, **4**, 341–356

HOMSY, C. A. and ANDERSON, M. S. (1976) Functional stabilization of soft tissue and bone prostheses with a porous low modulus system. In *Biocompatibility of Implant Materials*, edited by D. F. Williams, p. 85. Tunbridge Wells: Sector Publications Ltd

JAHNKE, K., PLESTER, D. and HEIMKE, G. (1979) Aluminiumoxide Keramik, ein bioinertes Material für die Mittelohrchirurgie. *Archives of Oto-Rhino-Laryngology*, **223**, 373–376

JANEKE, J. B. and SHEA, J. J. (1975) Self-stabilizing total ossicular replacement prostheses in tympanoplasty. *The Laryngoscope*, **85**, 1550–1556

KERR, A. G. (1981) Proplast and Plastipore. *Clinical Otolaryngology*, **6**, 187–191

KLAWITTER, J. J. and HULBERT, S. F. (1971) Application of porous ceramics for the attachment of load bearing internal orthopedic application. *Journal of Biomedical Materials Research*, Symp. 2, 161–229

KUIJPERS, W. (1984) Behaviour of bioimplants in the

middle ear, an experimental study. In *Biomaterials in Otology*, edited by J. J. Grote, 18–27. Boston: Martinus Nijhoff Publishers

OPPENHEIMER, B. S., WILLHITE, M., STOUT, A. P., DANISHEF-SKY, I. and FISHMAN, M. M. (1964) A comparative study of the effects of imbedding cellophane and polystyrene films in rats. *Cancer Research*, **24**, 379

PLESTER, D. (1968) Die Anwendung prothetischen Materialion im Mittelohr. *Laryngologie, Rhinologie und Otologie*, **102**, 105–109

PORTMANN, M. (1967) Management of ossicular chain defects. *Journal of Laryngology and Otology*, **81**, 1309–1323

RECK, R. (1984) Bioactive glass-ceramics in ear surgery. Animal studies and clinical results. *The Laryngoscope*, **94**, (suppl. 33), 1–54

SCHUKNECHT, H. F. (1958) Stapedectomy and graft prostheses operation. *Acta Oto-Laryngologica*, **49**, 71–80

SHEA, J. J. (1969) A technique for stapes surgery in obliterative otosclerosis. *Otolaryngologic Clinics of North America*, **1**, 199–215

SHEA, J. J. (1976) Plastipore total ossicular replacement prosthesis. *The Laryngoscope*, **86**, 239–240

SHEEHY, J. L. (1965) Ossicular problems in tympanoplasty. *Archives of Otolaryngology*, **81**, 115–122

SHEEHY, J. L. (1973) Plastic sheeting in tympanoplasty. *The Laryngoscope*, **83**, 1144

SILVER, I. A. (1980) The physiology of wound healing. In *Wound Healing and Wound Infection*, edited by T. K. Hunt. New York: Appleton-Century Crofts

SMYTH, G. D., HASSARD, T. H., KERR, A. G. and HOULIHAN, F. P. (1978) Ossicular replacement prostheses. *Archives of Otolaryngology*, **104**, 345–351

SPECTOR, M., FLEMING, W. R. and KREUTNER, A. (1976) Bone ingrowth into porous high density polyethylene. *Journal of Biomedical Materials Research*, **7**, 595

US PHARMACOPEIA XIX (1975) Biological tests: plastic containers. Easton, Pa: Mack Publishing Co

VAN BLITTERSWIJK, C. A., GROTE, J. J., KUIJPERS, W., DAEMS, W. TH. and DE GROOT, K. (1986a) Macropore tissue ingrowth: a quantitative and qualitative study on hydroxyapatite ceramic. *Biomaterials*, **7**, 137–144

VAN BLITTERSWIJK, C. A., KUIJPERS, W., DAEMS, W. TH. and GROTE, J. J. (1986b) Epithelial reactions to hydroxyapatite. *Acta Oto-Laryngologica*, **101**, 231–241

WULLSTEIN, H. L. (1952) Operationen am Mittelohr mit Hilfe des freien spaltlappen Transplantates. *Archives of Otolaryngology*, **161**, 422–435

WULLSTEIN, S. R., SCHINDLER, K. and DÖLL, W. (1984) Further observations on application of Plasticin in ear surgery. In *Biomaterials in Otology*, edited by J. J. Grote. Boston: Martinus Nijhoff Publishers

ZÖLLNER, CH., STRUTZ, J., BECK, CHL., BÜSING, C. M., JAHNKE, K. and HEIMKE, G. (1983) Verödung des Wartenforsatzes mit poröser Trikalciumphosphat Keramik. *Laryngologie, Rhinologie und Otologie*, **62**, 106–111

Volume index

Cumulative index

This index is intended as a general guide only of the main heading entries covered in the six volumes of *Scott-Brown's Otolaryngology*, and is not comprehensive. For more detailed treatment of a subject refer to the individual volume indexes.

Entries are indexed by volume and page number, volume numbers are indicated by **bold** type.